WE 190 WIE £64

LIBRA

Orthopedic Surgery: Principles of Diagnosis and Treatment

EDITORS

BRENT B. WIESEL, MD

Chief, Shoulder Service
Department of Orthopaedic Surgery
Georgetown University Hospital/MedStar Health
Washington, District of Colombia

WUDBHAV N. SANKAR, MD

Assistant Professor of Orthopaedic Surgery
Division of Orthopaedic Surgery
The Children's Hospital of Philadelphia
Philadelphia, Pennsylvania

JOHN N. DELAHAY, MD

Professor of Orthopaedic Surgery
Department of Orthopaedic Surgery
Georgetown University Hospital/MedStar Health
Washington, District of Colombia

SAM W. WIESEL, MD

Chair and Professor of Orthopaedic Surgery
Department of Orthopaedic Surgery
Georgetown University Hospital/MedStar Health
Washington, District of Colombia

Wolters Kluwer Health | Lippincott Williams & Wilkins

Philadelphia • Baltimore • New York • London
Buenos Aires • Hong Kong • Sydney • Tokyo

Executive Editor: Robert Hurley
Developmental Editor: Sarah M. Granlund
Vendor Manager: Bridgett Dougherty
Product Manager: Dave Murphy
Senior Manufacturing Manager: Ben Rivera
Design Manager: Stephen Druding
Marketing Manager: Lisa Lawrence
Compositor: Aptara, Inc.

© 2011 by LIPPINCOTT WILLIAMS & WILKINS, a WOLTERS KLUWER business
Two Commerce Square
2001 Market Street
Philadelphia, Pa. 19103 USA
LWW.com

All rights reserved. This book is protected by copyright. No part of this book may be reproduced in any form by any means, including photocopying, or utilized by any information storage and retrieval system without written permission from the copyright owner, except for brief quotations embodied in critical articles and reviews. Materials appearing in this book prepared by individuals as part of their official duties as U.S. government employees are not covered by the above-mentioned copyright.

Printed in China

Library of Congress Cataloging-in-Publication Data

Orthopaedic surgery : principles of diagnosis and treatment / editors, Brent B. Wiesel . . . [et al.].
p. ; cm.
Includes bibliographical references and index.
ISBN 978-0-7817-9751-1 (hardback : alk. paper) 1. Orthopedic surgery. I. Wiesel, Brent B.
[DNLM: 1. Orthopedic Procedures. 2. Musculoskeletal Diseases–diagnosis. 3. Musculoskeletal Diseases–therapy. WE 190]
RD731.O7745 2010
617.4′7–dc22 2010037456

Care has been taken to confirm the accuracy of the information presented and to describe generally accepted practices. However, the authors, editors, and publisher are not responsible for errors or omissions or for any consequences from application of the information in this book and make no warranty, expressed or implied, with respect to the currency, completeness, or accuracy of the contents of the publication. Application of the information in a particular situation remains the professional responsibility of the practitioner.

The authors, editors, and publisher have exerted every effort to ensure that drug selection and dosage set forth in this text are in accordance with current recommendations and practice at the time of publication. However, in view of ongoing research, changes in government regulations, and the constant flow of information relating to drug therapy and drug reactions, the reader is urged to check the package insert for each drug for any change in indications and dosage and for added warnings and precautions. This is particularly important when the recommended agent is a new or infrequently employed drug.

Some drugs and medical devices presented in the publication have Food and Drug Administration (FDA) clearance for limited use in restricted research settings. It is the responsibility of the health care provider to ascertain the FDA status of each drug or device planned for use in their clinical practice.

To purchase additional copies of this book, call our customer service department at (800) 638-3030 or fax orders to (301) 223-2320. International customers should call (301) 223-2300.

Visit Lippincott Williams & Wilkins on the Internet: at LWW.com. Lippincott Williams & Wilkins customer service representatives are available from 8:30 am to 6 pm, EST.

10 9 8 7 6 5 4 3 2 1

CCS1110

I dedicate this book to my wife, Katie, whose love, support, and patience over the past 10 years have made this possible. Also to my mentors in shoulder surgery: Charlie Getz, Mark Lazarus, Matt Ramsey, and Gerald Williams—it took 6 years and two institutions but you all can train anybody.

-BBW

I dedicate this book to my wife, Ariana, who constantly inspires me to be the best that I can be. She is and always will be my closest friend. Also to the best role model any young surgeon could ask for, Vernon Tolo. The strength of his Cobb is exceeded only by the size of his heart. Thanks for everything.

-WNS

I dedicate this effort to Maggie, Jack, Jimmy, Katie, Luke, Julia, Ryan, Brigid, and Ben and to their grandmother, Cathy, who keeps me sane when I am with them all.

-JND

I dedicate this book to my grandchildren: Anneliese Holland Wiesel, Sam Augustus Wiesel, and Maxwell Vickery Wiesel—they are giving their parents "hell" and I am enjoying every minute of it. They represent the future.

-SWW

Contents

Contributors

JACOB N. ABLIN, MD Internal Medicine, Sackler School of Medicine, Tel Aviv University; Director Fibromyalgia Clinic, Department of Rheumatology, Sourasky Medical Center, Tel Aviv, Israel

KEITH D. BALDWIN, MD, MSPT, MPH Resident, Department of Orthopaedic Surgery, Hospital of the University of Pennsylvania, Philadelphia, Pennsylvania

PEDRO K. BEREDJIKLIAN, MD Chief, Division of Hand Surgery, The Rothman Institute; Associate Professor of Orthopaedic Surgery, Thomas Jefferson University School of Medicine, Philadelphia, Pennsylvania

DANIEL J. CLAUW, MD Professor of Anesthesiology, Medicine (Rheumatology) and Psychiatry, University of Michigan, Ann Arbor, Michigan

JOHN N. DELAHAY, MD Professor of Orthopaedic Surgery, Department of Orthopaedic Surgery, Georgetown University Hospital, Washington, District of Colombia

JOHN L. ESTERHAI, MD Professor, Department of Orthopaedic Surgery, Hospital of the University of Pennsylvania, University of Pennsylvania School of Medicine, Philadelphia, Pennsylvania

BRIAN G. EVANS, MD Professor and Vice Chairman of Operations and Finance, Department of Orthopaedic Surgery, Georgetown University Hospital, Washington, District of Colombia

JOHN M. FLYNN, MD Associate Chief of Orthopaedic Surgery, Children's Hospital of Philadelphia, Philadelphia, Pennsylvania

FREDDIE FU, MD Professor and Chair of the Department of Orthopaedic Surgery, University of Pittsburgh, Pittsburgh, Pennsylvania

BRIAN P. GLADNICK, MD Resident, Department of Orthopaedic Surgery, Hospital for Special Surgery, New York, New York

F. WINSTON GWATHMEY JR., MD Resident, Department of Orthopaedics, University of Virginia, Charlottesville, Virginia

JOSEPH M. HART, PhD, ATC Assistant Professor of Orthopaedic Surgery, Department of Orthopaedics, University of Virginia, Charlottesville, Virginia

R. BRUCE HEPPENSTALL, MD Attending Orthopaedic Surgeon, Professor of Orthopaedic Surgery, Vice Chairman of the Department of Orthopaedic Surgery, Hospital of the University of Pennsylvania, Philadelphia, Pennsylvania

HARISH HOSALKAR, MD Attending Orthopedic Surgeon, Co-Director of International Center for Pediatric and Adolescent Hip Disorders, Director, Hip Research Program, Rady Children's Hospital, UCSD, San Diego, California

G. RUSSELL HUFFMAN, MD, MPH Assistant Professor, Shoulder and Elbow Division, Department of Orthopaedic Surgery, Hospital of the University of Pennsylvania, Philadelphia, Pennsylvania

JOHN A. JOHANSEN, MD Chief Resident, Georgetown University Hospital, Department of Orthopaedic Surgery, Washington, District of Colombia

ATUL F. KAMATH, MD Clinical Instructor, Department of Orthopaedic Surgery, Hospital of the University of Pennsylvania, Philadelphia, Pennsylvania

ROBERT M. KAY, MD Associate Professor, Department of Orthopaedic Surgery, Keck-University of Southern California School of Medicine; Vice Chief, Department of Pediatric Orthopaedics, Children's Hospital Los Angeles, Los Angeles, California

JOHN KLIMKIEWICZ, MD Chief, Division of Sports Medicine, Department of Orthopaedic Surgery, Georgetown University Hospital, Washington, District of Colombia

ANDREW F. KUNTZ, MD Resident, Department of Orthopaedic Surgery, Hospital of the University of Pennsylvania, Philadelphia, Pennsylvania

MICHAEL K. KUO, MD Assistant Professor, Department of Rehabilitation Medicine, Georgetown University Hospital, Washington, District of Colombia

RICHARD D. LACKMAN, MD Professor and Chief, Orthopaedic Oncology, Department of Orthopaedic Surgery, University of Pennsylvania, Philadelphia, Pennsylvania

JOSEPH M. LANE, MD Professor of Orthopaedic Surgery, Weill Cornell Medical College; Chief, Metabolic Bone Disease Service, Department of Orthopaedics, Hospital for Special Surgery, New York, New York

WILLIAM LAUERMAN, MD Professor, Department of Orthopaedic Surgery, Georgetown University Hospital, Washington, District of Colombia

BRIAN MAGOVERN, MD Clinical Instructor, Harbor-UCLA Medical Center; Private Practice, Orthopaedic Institute, Torrance, California

BENJAMIN D. MARTIN, MD Chief Resident, Department of Orthopaedic Surgery, Georgetown University Hospital, Washington, District of Colombia

JONAS L. MATZON, MD Chief Resident, Department of Orthopaedic Surgery, University of Pennsylvania, Philadelphia, Pennsylvania

BENJAMIN A. MCARTHUR, MD Resident, Department of Orthopaedics, Hospital for Special Surgery, New York, New York

MOIRA M. MCCARTHY, MD Resident, Deparment of Orthopaedics, Hospital for Special Surgery, New York, New York

FRANCIS X. MCGUIGAN, MD Professor, Department of Orthopaedic Surgery, Georgetown University Medical School, Washington, District of Colombia

SAMIR MEHTA, MD Assistant Professor, University of Pennsylvania School of Medicine; Chief, Orthopaedic Trauma & Fracture Service, Hospital of the University of Pennsylvania, Philadelphia, Pennsylvania

J. STUART MELVIN, MD Resident, Department of Orthopaedic Surgery, University of Pennsylvania, Hospital of the University of Pennsylvania, Philadelphia, Pennsylvania

MARK D. MILLER, MD S. Ward Casscells Professor of Orthopaedic Surgery, Head, Division of Sports Medicine, University of Virginia Department of Orthopaedic Surgery; Charlottesville, Virginia: Team Physician, James Madison University

KAREN MYUNG, MD, PhD Assistant Professor of Orthopaedic Surgery, Children's Hospital Los Angeles, Assistant Professor of Orthopaedic Surgery, Department of Orthopaedic Surgery, University of Southern California Keck School of Medicine, Los Angeles, California

CHARLES L. NELSON, MD Attending Orthopaedic Surgeon; Associate Professor, Hospital of the University of Pennsylvania, Philadelphia, Pennsylvania

NICK PAPPAS, MD Resident, Department of Orthopaedic Surgery, University of Pennsylvania, Philadelphia, Pennsylvania

WILLIAM F. POSTMA, MD Resident, Department of Orthopaedic Surgery, Georgetown University Hospital, Washington, District of Colombia

MATTHEW L. RAMSEY, MD Shoulder and Elbow Service, The Rothman Institute; Associate Professor of Orthopaedic Surgery, Jefferson Medical College, Thomas Jefferson University, Philadelphia, Pennsylvania

TODD RIMINGTON, MD Resident, Department of Orthopaedic Surgery, Georgetown University, Washington, District of Colombia

WUDBHAV N. SANKAR, MD Assistant Professor of Orthopaedic Surgery, Children's Hospital of Philadelphia, Philadelphia, Pennsylvania

STEVEN SCHERPING, MD Department of Orthopaedic Surgery, Georgetown University Hospital, Washington, District of Colombia

BENJAMIN SHAFFER, MD Washington Orthopaedics and Sports Medicine, Washington, District of Colombia

NEIL P. SHETH, MD Resident, Department of Orthopaedic Surgery, University of Pennsylvania, Hospital of the University of Pennsylvania, Philadelphia, Pennsylvania

DAVID L. SKAGGS, MD Professor of Orthopaedic Surgery, University of Southern California School of Medicine; Chief of Orthopaedic Surgery and Endpwed Chair of Pediatric Spinal Disorders, Children's Hospital Los Angeles, Los Angeles, California

AASIS UNNANUNTANA, MD Fellow, Department of Orthopaedic Surgery, Weill Cornell Medical College; Fellow, Department of Orthopaedic Surgery, Hospital for Special Surgery, New York, New York

TURNER VOSSELLER, MD Fellow, Foot and Ankle Surgery, Hospital for Special Surgery, New York, New York

SAM W. WIESEL, MD Professor of Orthopaedic Surgery, Chair Deptartment of Orthopaedic Surgery, Georgetown University Hospital, Washington, District of Colombia

BRENT B. WIESEL, MD Chief, Shoulder Service, Department of Orthopaedic Surgery, Georgetown University Hospital/ MedStar Health, Washington, District of Colombia

GERALD R. WILLIAMS JR., MD Professor, Department of Orthopaedic Surgery, Jefferson Medical College; Chief, Shoulder and Elbow Service, The Rothman Institute at Jefferson, Thomas Jefferson University Hospitals, Philadelphia, Pennsylvania

JOHN A. ZAVALA, MD Chief Resident, Department of Orthopaedic Surgery, Georgetown University Hospital, Washington, District of Colombia

Preface

The goal of this book is to create a comprehensive, readable resource for orthopedic residents during the early years of their training. We envision *Principles* as a book that interns can read from cover to cover during the course of their PGY1 year to gain a broad base of knowledge before they start their orthopedic rotations. The individual subspecialty chapters will again be helpful during their PGY2 and PGY3 years as a concise review of an entire subspecialty that they can read prior to starting a new rotation.

The book is divided into two sections. The general principles portion presents orthopedic basic science in sufficient detail to prepare the reader for the in-training and board examinations. It contains chapters on the basics of the various modalities commonly used for patient evaluation in orthopedics and the evaluation and treatment of musculoskeletal infection, metabolic bone disease, and musculoskeletal oncology. In addition, an overview of rheumatologic diseases affecting the musculoskeletal system and the principles guiding the treatment of orthopedic trauma and sports medicine patients are included.

In the subspecialty section, each chapter addresses the functional anatomy, patient evaluation (history, physical examination, and imaging), traumatic injuries, and atraumatic conditions for a specific region of the body. For each diagnosis, the typical presentation, options for nonoperative and operative management, and expected outcomes are discussed.

Creating a text of this size always requires the assistance of a several creative and capable people. We would first like to thank Bob Hurley, Dave Murphy, and Eileen Wolfberg at Lippincott Williams & Wilkins whose help and support have been invaluable in transforming this project from a one-page proposal into a nearly 1,000-page book.

We have also had the privilege of working with a number of orthopedic and nonorthopedic colleagues throughout the country. For each chapter, we have sought to include at least one junior and one senior author. The junior authors have either recently completed or are in the final years of their training and are included to make sure the information is presented at a level that will be understandable by junior residents. The senior authors, many of whom are leaders in their fields, are included to assure that the information is accurate and up to date. We are very appreciative of all of their contributions and hope the book provides each reader with a strong foundation in the fundamentals of orthopedics.

Brent B. Wiesel, MD
Wudbhav N. Sankar, MD
John N. Delahay, MD
Sam W. Wiesel, MD

Basic Science

1

Section 1 Development of the Musculoskeletal System and the Growth Plate

John A. Zavala John N. Delahay

INTRODUCTION

A thorough understanding of genetics, embryology, and postnatal development of the musculoskeletal system is needed to engage in a discussion of musculoskeletal anomalies. Approximately 5% of babies are born with some type of congenital defect. Many defects require a period of growth and development before they become apparent. An appreciation of normal development of the musculoskeletal system is integral to a more complete understanding of these congenital defects of the musculoskeletal system.

One of the most well-studied areas of musculoskeletal development is the physis or growth plate. A thorough understanding of this structure is essential for the treatment of many pediatric orthopaedic diseases and fractures. Furthermore, many of the biologic processes that naturally create bone in the growing skeleton are currently being explored for manipulation in an attempt to improve bone healing in problematic adult fractures.

GENETICS

Although there have been more than 3000 genetic disorders identified, very few genes are responsible for musculoskeletal diseases. Most genetic diseases fall into one of three categories. The first group consists of isolated gene defects that are governed by the principles of Mendelian inheritance. Chromosomal abnormalities, such as deletions and translocation, are included in the second group. Lastly, a heterogeneous group of polygenic defects are the result of an interplay between genetic and environmental factors.

Genetic defects can present at any age from infancy to adulthood. The prevalence of genetic defects will also vary widely. It is important to perform a careful family history and family pedigree in the complete evaluation of a child with a genetic abnormality. Genetic counseling, the determination of inheritance patterns, and an assessment of the likelihood that siblings will be affected all depend on this information.

The common patterns of Mendelian inheritance are specifically predicated upon the presence or absence of an abnormal gene on a chromosome. Patterns may be dominant, requiring only a single allele to express the trait, or recessive, requiring the expression of both alleles. The four patterns that are typically seen are autosomal dominant, autosomal recessive, X-linked dominant, and X-linked recessive.

Autosomal dominant inherited conditions typically produce nonfatal structural abnormalities. Heterozygotes will express the condition. Expression of a genetic trait suggests a wide variation in the severity of the manifestation. There is no male/female preference, and half of the offspring will be affected (Fig. 1.1).

Generally, autosomal recessive conditions tend to be enzymatic defects (inborn errors of metabolism). Both alleles must be abnormal for the condition to be expressed; therefore, only homozygotes can express the condition. It is possible for parents to be unaffected but carriers of the gene. Twenty-five percent of offspring are affected, and there is no male/female predominance (Fig. 1.2).

X-linked conditions are described as being either dominant or recessive. In X-linked dominant conditions, the heterozygote manifests the condition, but it is the affected mother who transmits the X-linked gene to 50% of her daughters and 50% of her sons. An affected father will transmit the gene to 100% of his daughters and none of his sons. Male children typically have more severe involvement than do females. In X-linked recessive conditions, the

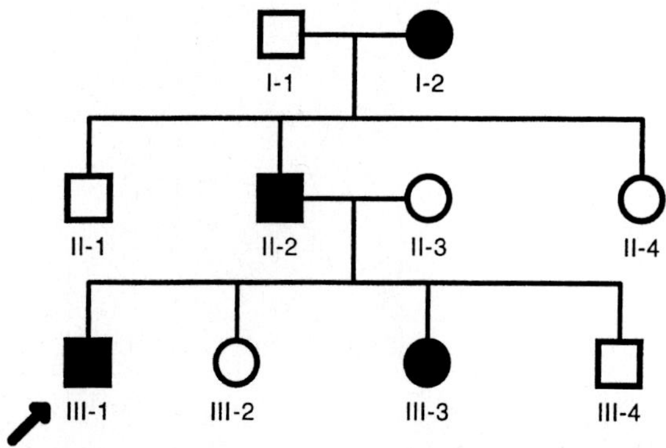

Figure 1.1 Autosomal dominant pedigree. Men are indicated by squares and women by circles. Filled symbols indicate clinically affected individuals. (*Reprinted with permission from* Morrissy RT, Weinstein SL. *Lovell and Winter's Pediatric Orthopaedics*. Philadelphia, PA: Lippincott Williams & Wilkins, 2006.)

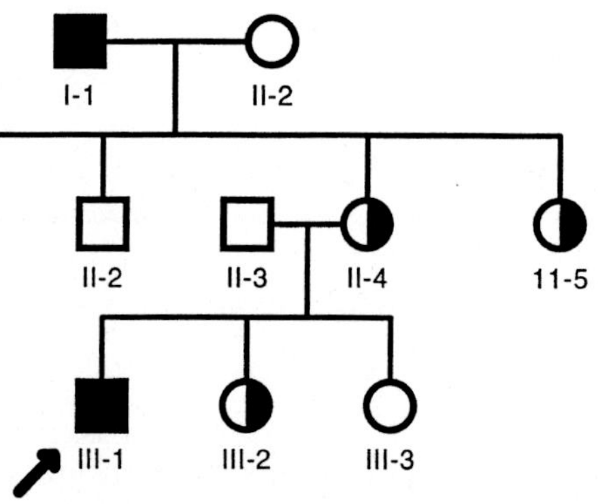

Figure 1.3 X-linked recessive pedigree. Affected hemizygous men are indicated by *filled squares*. Asymptomatic female carriers are indicated by *half-filled circles*. (*Reprinted with permission from* Morrissy RT, Weinstein SL. *Lovell and Winter's Pediatric Orthopaedics*. Philadelphia, PA: Lippincott Williams & Wilkins, 2006.)

female homozygote will be a carrier for the disease (Fig. 1.3). Because males have only one X chromosome they will be affected by the conditions. Affected fathers will transmit the gene to all their daughters, who will be carriers. Carrier females will transmit the gene to 50% of their daughters, who will be carriers, and all of their sons. Important diseases to remember in this category are hemophilia and Duchenne's muscular dystrophy.

Polygenic inheritance occurs in the setting of multiple genes that interact with environmental factors to produce a given trait. The Gaussian curve (Fig. 1.4) is used to depict what has been referred to as "the threshold of risk" in a given population. If there is a first-degree relative who has a given trait, such as scoliosis, there is clearly an increased risk for other relatives to manifest the trait. This can be represented by a shift of the curve or a lowering of the threshold. The threshold of risk is affected by race, sex, and to some degree by geography.

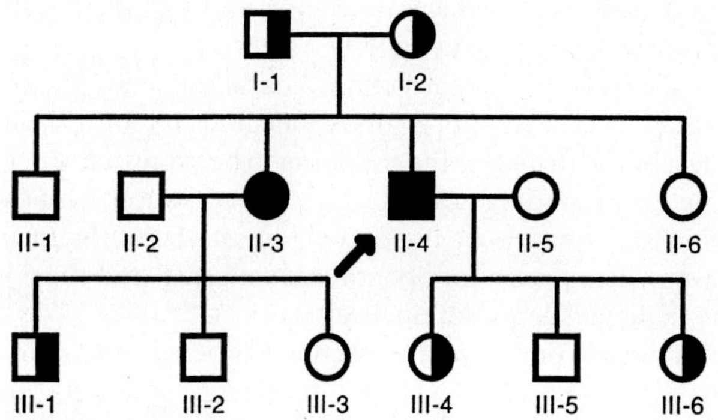

Figure 1.2 Autosomal recessive pedigree. Homozygous affected individuals are indicated by *filled* symbols. Asymptomatic carriers, who are heterozygotes, are indicated by *half-filled* symbols. (*Reprinted with permission from* Morrissy RT, Weinstein SL. *Lovell and Winter's Pediatric Orthopaedics*. Philadelphia, PA: Lippincott Williams & Wilkins, 2006.)

The third category of genetic disease results from rearrangements within a given chromosome. These abnormalities can include extra chromosomes, referred to as "trisomy, or partial or complete loss of a chromosome." In addition, mosaics and translocations can be grouped under this heading. Many of these chromosomal abnormalities result in spontaneous abortions. It has been estimated that approximately 1% of live-born children have some type of chromosomal aberration. Trisomy 21 (Down syndrome) is the most common disease in this category with an incidence of 1 per 700 live births.

ORTHOPAEDIC EMBRYOLOGY

Intramembranous and Enchondral Ossification

All bones of the musculoskeletal system begin as mesenchymal condensations from a primary germ layer with multiple mechanical and chemotactic factors actively influencing the cellular differentiation. These condensations of cells typically form bone in one of two ways. Intramembranous bone formation occurs with the condensation of

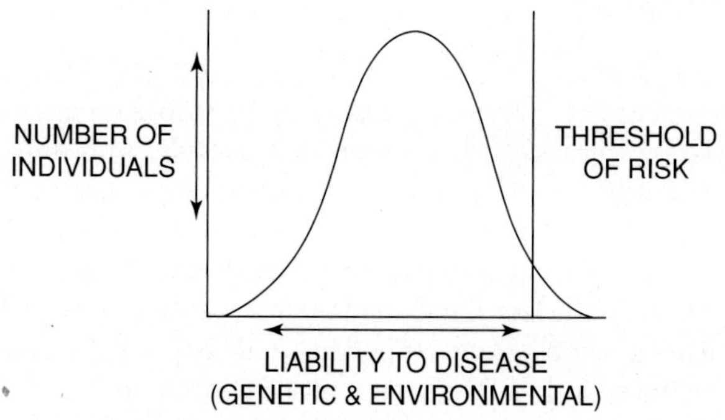

Figure 1.4 Gaussian curve: depiction of polygenic inheritance.

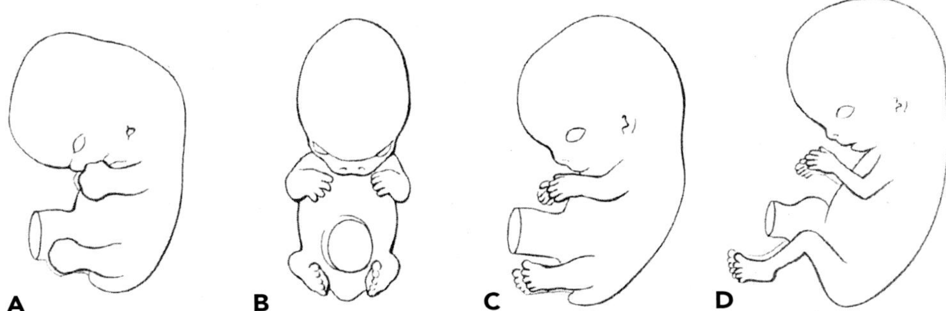

Figure 1.5 Normal limb rotation. **A:** At 48 days, the hand and foot plates face each other. **B:** At 51 days, elbows are bent laterally. **C:** At 54 days, the soles of the feet face each other. **D:** The lateral rotation of the arms and medial rotation of the legs result in caudally facing elbows and cranially facing knees. (*Reprinted with permission from* Morrissy RT, Weinstein SL. *Lovell and Winter's Pediatric Orthopaedics*. Philadelphia, PA: Lippincott Williams & Wilkins, 2006.)

mesenchymal cells. They produce a mucoprotein matrix in which collagen becomes embedded. Subsequent mineralization converts the anlage to bone without an intermediate cartilage step. The second way is the more classic enchondral ossification where bone replaces a cartilage model.

Intramembranous bone formation is well demonstrated by the example of the calvarium of the skull. This process involves the direct elaboration by osteoblasts of bone matrix without a cartilage template. Initially a small group of cells aggregate, divide, and form random cords of cells. These cells are high in alkaline phosphatase, and as one would expect, rapid calcification occurs and subsequent ossification forms primary trabecular bone. Intramembranous formation is also responsible for the appositional growth of long bones.

The long bones of the skeleton form by the process of enchondral ossification. The major components originate from the mesodermal layer of the trilaminar embryo. One can trace the development of the major long bones through the enchondral process. The primitive limb bud appears around the fifth week of embryonic life (Fig. 1.5). It is about that time that a tubular condensation of mesenchyme develops centrally in the limb bud. During the sixth week, the mesenchyme differentiates into cartilage through the process of chondrification. Both interstitial and appositional growth occurs. In the seventh week, the cartilage model is penetrated by a vascular spindle, and subsequently, a sleeve of primitive bone is seen surrounding it. Progressively, necrosis of the central cartilage occurs. Once this vascular spindle is established, the central portion of the model is populated by osteoblasts. As matrix is secreted, immature bone is formed. Once the central portion of the model is ossified, it is referred to as the "primary ossification center." Further ossification of this primary ossification center can occur both enchondrally and intramembranously. Keep in mind that bone formed under the primitive periosteum does so intramembranously, whereas the bone formed at the ends is made enchondrally.

From the second through the sixth embryonic months, progressive changes occur in the tubular bones. First, the central (medullary) canal cavitates, leaving a hollow tube of bone with a large mass of cartilage persisting at each end. Within these masses of cartilage, the secondary ossification center, or epiphysis, will form. A cartilage plate persists between the developing metaphysis and epiphysis. This structure, the physis, is responsible for longitudinal growth of the long bone. On the other hand, the periosteum is primarily responsible for latitudinal growth, thereby increasing girth.

Neuromuscular Development

In the second week of life, the embryo itself is bilaminar, that is, ectoderm and endoderm. At the caudal end of the bilaminar embryo is an area referred to as the "primitive streak," a cluster of cells that invaginates between the two layers of the bilaminar embryo. The third layer subsequently formed is referred to as the "mesoderm." This mesoderm is critical to the development of the bulk of the muscular and skeletal systems. It should be remembered that the neural structures of the central nervous system are ultimately developed from cells originating from the ectoderm.

Around the third week, ectodermal induction results in the formation of a neural plate. The edges of this plate curl dorsally to form a neural tube (Fig. 1.6). Beginning in the center and continuing to each end this neural tube will begin to close (Fig. 1.7). Obviously, failure to close cranially results in anencephaly, and failure to close caudally results in spina bifida. A population of ectodermal cells parallel to the closed neural tube, referred to as "neural crest cells," are the precursors of the dorsal root ganglia and much of the peripheral nervous system. Most of the neural tube development is guided by notochordal induction. The notochord, which has been previously derived from the primitive knob, a cellular aggregate of the bilaminar embryo,

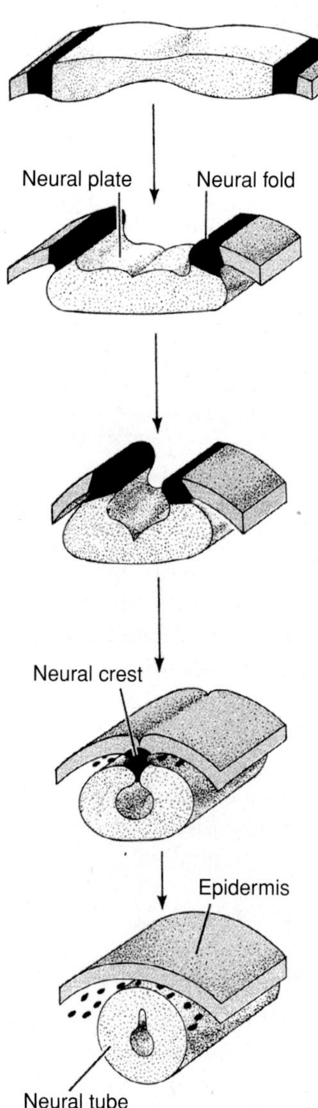

Figure 1.6 Diagrammatic representation of neural tube formation. The ectoderm folds in at the most dorsal point, forming a neural tube that is connected by neural crest cells, and an outer epidermis. (*Reprinted with permission from* Gilbert SF. *Developmental Biology*. 3rd ed. Sunderland, MA: Sinauer Associates, 1991.)

has been cited to be the pacemaker of the neural tube. The mesodermal plate parallels the notochord in its development, thus elongating at the anterior end first, with more caudal elements being added later.

Mesodermal Differentiation

Two large masses of mesoderm are seen on each side of the neural tube and are thus referred to as "paraxial mesoderm." Three distinct areas in this paraxial mesoderm have been identified: (1) medial mesoderm ultimately will form axial musculature, (2) the intermediate portion of the paraxial mesoderm in large part develops into the genitourinary (GU) system, and (3) the lateral mesoderm will give rise to the musculature of the thoracic and abdominal cavities, as well as the rib cage (Fig. 1.8). The intimate proximity of the medial and intermediate mesoderm clearly demonstrates why GU system anomalies are the most common associated defects in congenital musculoskeletal disease. Next in frequency are cardiac anomalies, owning to the fact that the heart is also of mesodermal origin.

At about 4 weeks of embryologic life, the paraxial mesoderm will segment into blocks of cells referred to as "somites." The somites will number between 42 and 44. Once the somites have segmented, beginning cranially and progressing caudally over a 10-day period, they will further differentiate into three cell masses—a dermatome, a myotome, and a sclerotome, forming skin, muscle, and skeleton respectively (Figs. 1.9 and 1.10). The limb buds will develop from progressive differentiation of these somites. As mentioned earlier, the limb buds are identifiable around the fifth week of embryonic life.

Development of Joints

Condensations occur in the limb bud where mesenchyme aggregates. Ultimately, these tubular condensations are separated by a discrete area referred to as the "interzone." This interzone marks the primitive joint and typically has three layers of cells—two parallel chondrogenic layers and a third intermediate layer. The intermediate zone of cells will ultimately form the synovium and the intra-articular structures. Cavitation of this primitive joint usually awaits contouring of the joint surfaces. It has been suggested that cavitation is primarily an enzymatic process and is independent of fetal movement. The joint spaces are typically well established by the 10th week of embryonic life. Classically, the embryo becomes a fetus by the 12th week. At that point all the embryonic organ systems and their respective organs have formed. The remaining 6 months of fetal development is simply further growth and maturation of these previously formed embryologic structures.

THE GROWTH PLATE

As previously stated, the bones of the fetus are developing through the two mechanisms of intramembranous and enchondral bone formation. Following birth, these processes continue at an accelerated pace. The periosteal surfaces of all long bones, as well as large portions of the flat bones, continue to grow as a result of intramembranous bone formation. Bone is directly formed in a collagenized matrix by the activity of osteoblasts without the benefit of a cartilage model.

The most critical mechanism in postnatal bone maturation is the activity of the physis or growth plate. Significant knowledge currently exists as to the anatomy and

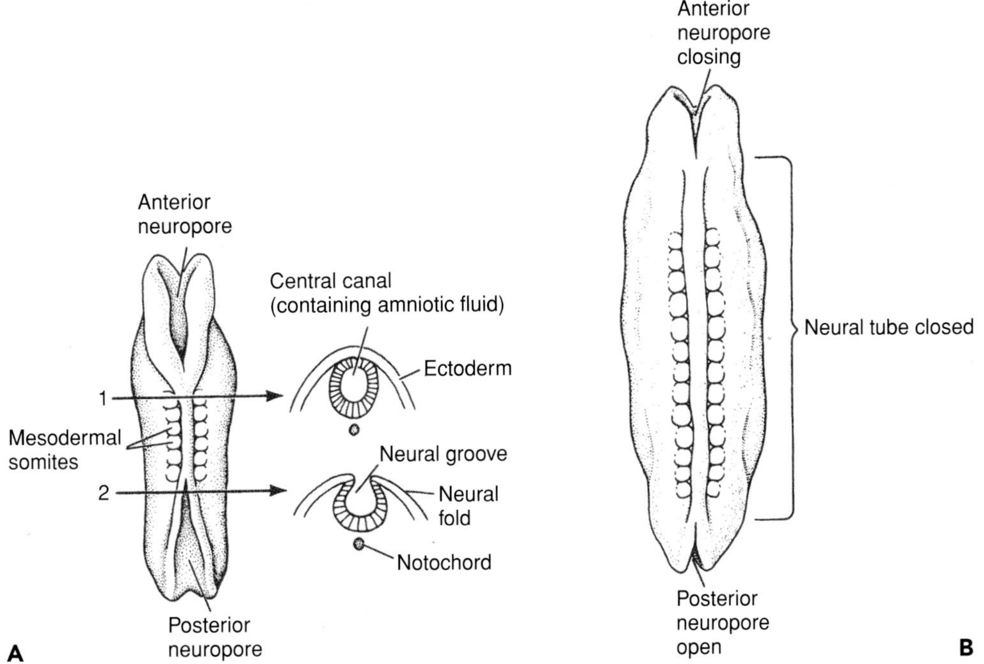

Figure 1.7 **A:** At the initial stages, both anterior and posterior neuropores are open. **B:** Closing of the neural tube progresses both cranially and caudally. (*Reprinted with permission from* Gilbert SF. *Developmental Biology*. 3rd ed. Sunderland, MA: Sinauer Associates, 1991.)

physiology of the normal growth plate, as well as its biochemistry and its mechanical properties. This growth plate is a unique anatomic structure. It is the essential mechanism by which mammals are able to enlarge their endoskeleton. Whereas lesser animals must molt an exoskeleton in an effort to grow, the physis allows for longitudinal growth of the higher organism. It is clear, however, from the beginning that this unique anatomic structure has its own obsolescence built in. Not only does it stop producing bone, but it is in large measure consumed by its own product. During the time it exists, the physis, for all its unique and critical importance, creates a mechanical flaw in the bone. The growth plate is a critical entity in postnatal bone development and maturation.

The Physis (Fig. 1.11)

The characteristic cytoarchitectural pattern of the growth plate is typically present by the fourth month of fetal life. For most long bones, the discoid configuration is typical. This is, of course, characterized by a planar area of rapidly differentiating cartilage, which blends into, but is nonetheless structurally distinct from, hyaline cartilage covering the chondroepiphysis. This discoid physis is located between the metaphysis and the epiphysis of a long bone.

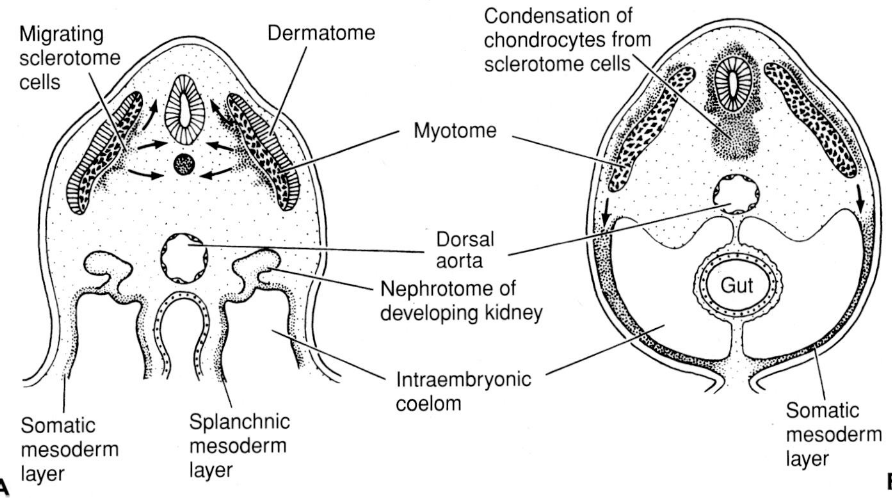

Figure 1.8 Mesoderm formation in human embryo. Transverse section through the trunk of an early 4-week embryo **(A)** and a late 4-week embryo **(B)**. Sclerotome cells migrate from the somite, and these cells ultimately become chondrocytes. The remaining dermatome cells will form the dermis. The myotome cells will give rise to the striated muscles of the back and limbs. (*Reprinted with permission from* Gilbert SF. *Developmental Biology*. 3rd ed. Sunderland, MA: Sinauer Associates, 1991.)

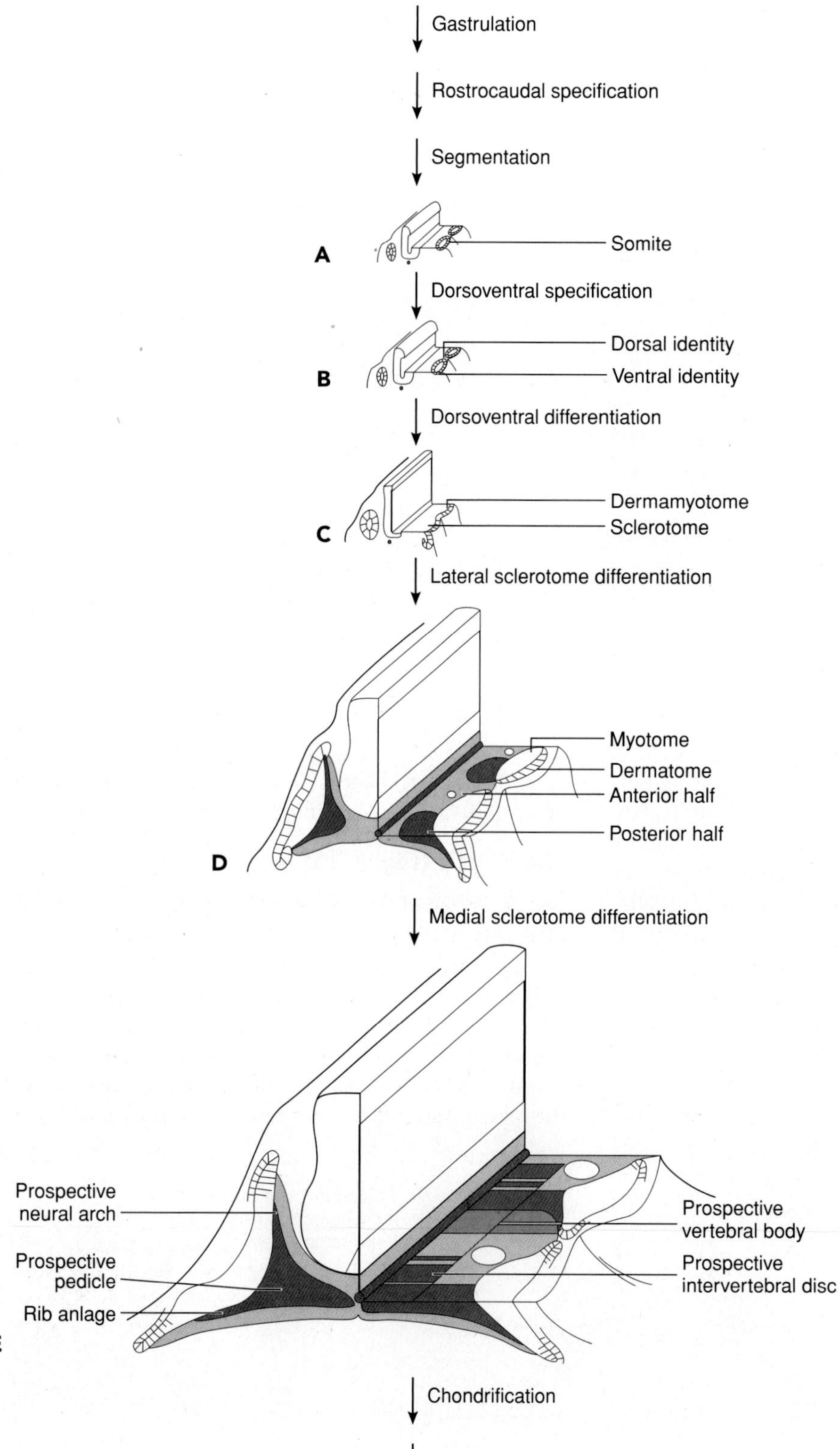

Figure 1.9 The progressive differentiation of the vertebral column. (*Reprinted with permission from* Thorogood P. *Embryos, Genes and Birth Defects*. New York, NY: John Wiley & Sons, 1997:282.)

The epiphysis is a secondary ossification center and typically ossifies from a central area, which then grows centrifugally (Fig. 1.12). The epiphysis is normally subjected to compressive forces. Conversely, an *apophysis* is also a secondary ossification center, but one that ordinarily forms a point for muscle attachment and therefore is subjected to tensile forces. Both of these secondary ossification centers typically sit astride a discoid physis.

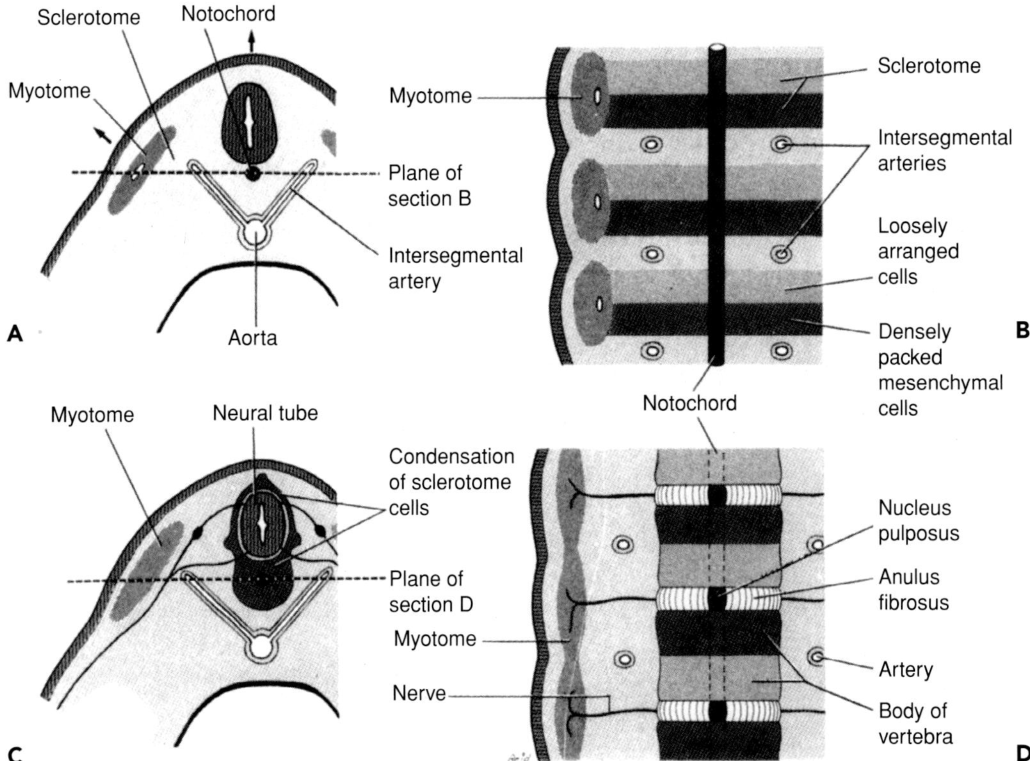

Figure 1.10 **A:** Transverse section through a 4-week-old embryo. The top arrow shows the direction of growth of the neural tube and the side arrow shows the dorsolateral growth of the somite remnant. **B:** Coronal section of the same-stage embryo showing the condensation of sclerotomal cells around the notochord with loosely packed cells cranially and densely packed cells caudally. **C:** A transverse section through a 5-week-old embryo depicting the condensation of sclerotome cells around the notochord and neural tube. **D:** Coronal section illustrating the formation of the vertebral body cranial and caudal halves of adjacent sclerotomes resulting in the segmental arteries crossing the bodies of the vertebrae and the spinal nerves lying between the vertebrae. (*Reprinted with permission from* Moore KI, Persaus TVN. *Before We Are Born. Essentials of Embryology and Birth Defects.* 4th ed. Philadelphia, PA: WB Saunders, 1993:257.)

The growth plate histologically can be shown to have four distinctly separate zones: (1) resting, (2) proliferating, (3) hypertrophic (degeneration), and (4) provisional calcification. Each zone has its own unique anatomy as well as its own function. Type II collagen has been demonstrated to be the predominant collagen in the growth plate.

The Resting (Reserve) Zone

This histologic region is immediately subjacent to the bony epiphysis. The cells are roundish and occur in either singlets or doublets. There is a high ratio of extracellular matrix to cell volume. Studies demonstrate a rather abundant endoplasmic reticulum, suggesting active synthetic activity. Blood vessels pass through this zone without significant perfusion resulting in a decreased oxygen tension. The location and histology of this region suggest that it has the capacity to produce cartilaginous matrix.

The Proliferating Zone

The cells in this region are typically flattened and arranged in longitudinal columns parallel to the long axis of the bone. Again, a significant amount of endoplasmic reticulum has been demonstrated in this region. The top cell in each of the columns is thought to be the germinal cell for the longitudinal growth of the column below. There is a high level of proteoglycan in this zone. Matrix vesicles are also present in high numbers, suggesting their role in matrix mineralization. Oxygen tension levels are highest in this zone due to the rich vascular supply seen here. Considering the anatomy and biochemistry of this region, the major functions of the proliferating zone are cell proliferation and matrix production, both of which are required for linear growth.

The Hypertrophic (Degeneration) Zone

The cells identified in this region are approximately five times the size of those in the zones above. Intracellular matrix gradually decreases in content as one goes deeper into this zone. The longitudinal septa of intracellular matrix persist into the deepest regions of the hypertrophic zone. However, thin transverse septa become progressively more sparse, the deeper one goes into the plate. Similarly,

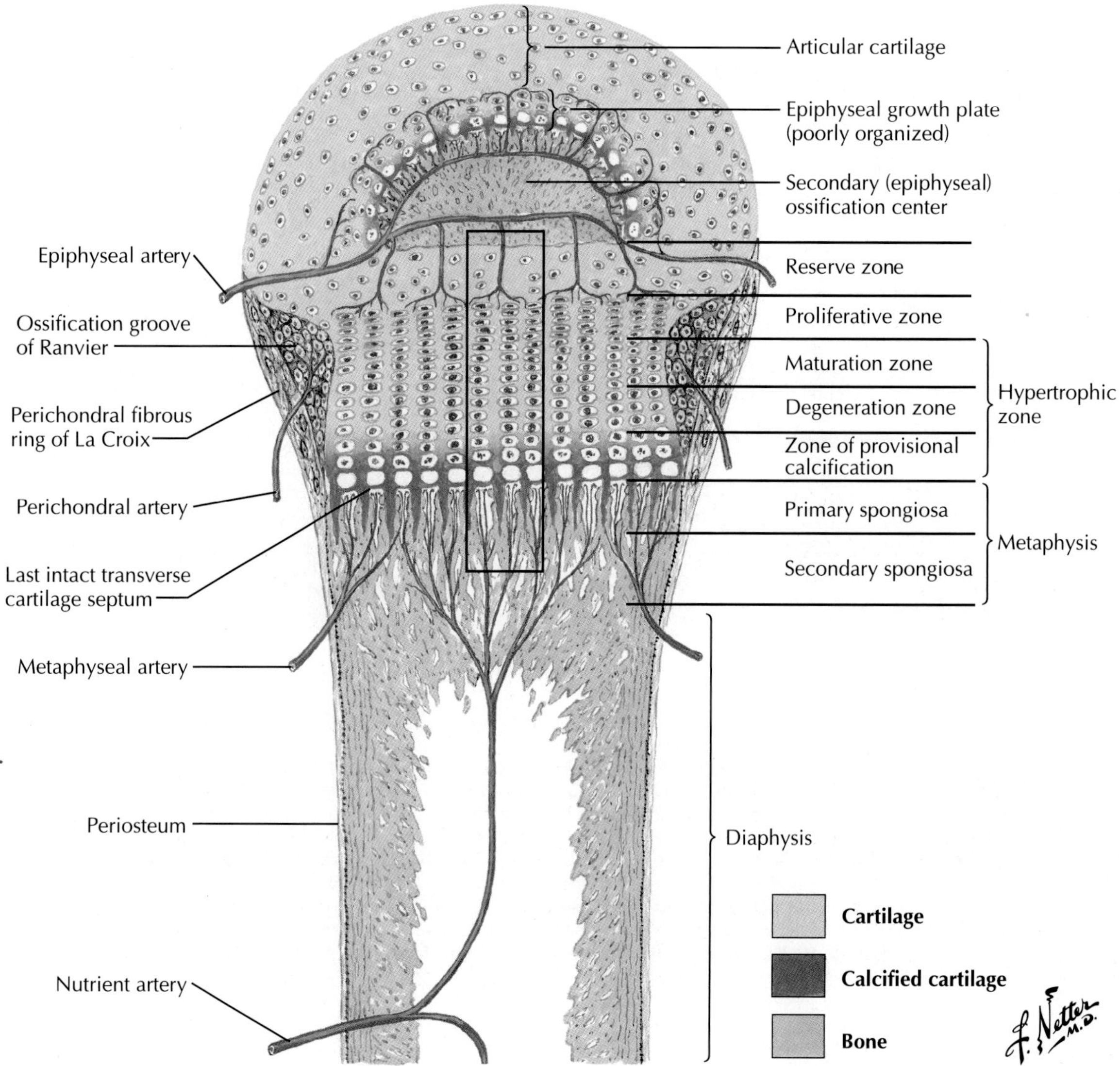

Figure 1.11 Structure and blood supply of the growth plate. *([2011]. Used with permission of Elsevier. All rights reserved.)*

glycogen, which is identified in the upper regions of the hypertrophic zone, is gradually lost in the lower half. The concentration of lysosomal enzymes is extremely high, and the concentration of proteoglycans and hydroxyproline is markedly low. Electron microscopy reveals the presence of an endoplasmic reticulum in the cells with increased vacuolation, cytoplasmic swelling, and increased numbers of mitochondria and lysosomes throughout this region. In addition, the previously noted matrix vesicles appear to be not only more prevalent but also more active in this region. It appears clear that the ultimate fate of the vessels in this region is necrosis. Similarly, the relatively low levels of oxygen tension indicate poor vascularity. All of these features—lysosomal enzymes, vacuolation, marginal blood supply—support the idea that the role of the hypertrophic zone is to prepare the matrix for calcification.

The Zone of Provisional Calcification

The lowest region of the growth plate is the area where calcification of the cartilaginous matrix occurs. It is here that the matrix vesicle concentration is highest, and it is here that these vesicles are most active. The mechanisms for the delivery and liberation of the calcium are still under active investigation. It is felt that the relative anoxia of this region plays a role in calcium release from the mitochondria. Clearly, the function of this region is calcification. Typically, the mineral is deposited only in the longitudinal bars of matrix and not in the transverse septa.

The Metaphysis

Any discussion of the growth plate would not be complete without a word about the subjacent metaphysis.

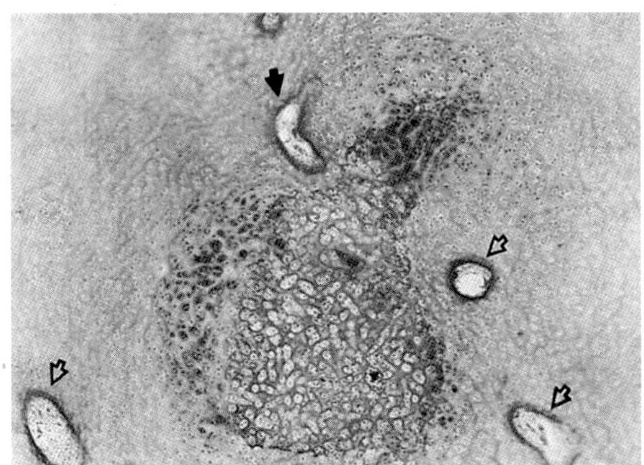

Figure 1.12 Early formation of the secondary ossification center within the epiphyseal cartilage. The solid arrow indicates a well-vascularized cartilage canal with a branch into the hypertrophic cells, triggering the ossification process. (*Reproduced with permission from* Beaty JH, Kasser JR. *Rockwood and Wilkins' Fractures in Children.* 6th ed. Philadelphia, PA: Lippincott Williams & Wilkins, 2006.)

Metaphyseal bone begins just distal to the last intact transverse septum. This specific region where the calcified cartilage becomes vascularized is referred to as "primary spongiosa bone" (Fig. 1.11). Osteoblasts can be identified lining up on the longitudinal bars of calcified cartilage. Assuming this cartilage to be calcified, the process of ossification can begin spontaneously. In certain metabolic disease states, specifically rickets, in which calcification has not occurred, ossification cannot proceed normally. As one goes deeper in the metaphysis, the calcified cartilage cores of the trabeculae will be seen to disappear. At the point at which no calcified cartilage is present, the trabeculae are referred to as "secondary spongiosa bone." The functions of the metaphysis are vascular invasion, bone formation, and bone remodeling. In regard to bone remodeling, resorption occurs on the internal surface of the cortical bone resulting in "cut back" or funnelization of the end of the long bone. This mechanism is exactly the opposite of what one will see at the level of the diaphysis.

Finally, two peripheral structures surrounding the growth plate are noteworthy. The first structure is the *ossification groove of Ranvier,* which is a wedge-shaped ring of cells surrounding the margins of the plate at the level of the resting zone. This structure is felt to provide support and allow for latitudinal growth of the physis. The second peripheral structure is the *perichondrial ring of La Croix*. This is a fibrous sleeve that merges with the periosteum and provides additional mechanical support.

Blood Supply of the Growth Plate

Essentially, the vasculature of the plate can be subdivided into three major groups: epiphyseal vessels, metaphyseal vessels, and a small group of perichondral vessels (Fig. 1.11). The epiphyseal vessel enters the epiphysis and terminally arborize in the upper portions of the proliferating zone. The entry point of this vessel depends on the amount of articular cartilage covering the bony epiphysis. Ordinarily, the vessel enters the bony epiphysis between the articular margin and the growth plate. In the case of the proximal femur, the vessel must travel beneath cartilage to the plate. During its very tortuous course, it is extremely vulnerable to shear injury. The metaphyseal vessels terminate in many straight branches, which penetrate the lowest regions of the growth plate. It is their presence that in some measure participates in the calcification of the matrix. The perichondral vessels supply the peripheral cells and do not enter the depths of the epiphysis. As previously noted, the proliferating zone is the only area receiving a blood supply. The remainder of the plate is largely avascular. Nutrition and oxygen for cell metabolism are obtained by diffusion.

Patterns of Growth

Characteristically, long bone growth is generally considered to be a longitudinal phenomenon. The anatomy of the previously described physis clearly emphasizes its linear orientation and its predisposition to grow in this fashion. However, some latitudinal growth is essential for normal plate development. This growth is accomplished both by interstitial growth within the plate and appositional growth at the periphery in the region of the groove of Ranvier. Latitudinal expansion of the physis will obviously be precluded in areas that are juxtaposed to the subchondral plate once the subchondral plate has developed.

There are a number of regional variations in plate growth. Most of the time these variations result from mechanical limitation to interstitial expansion. As mentioned earlier, the subchondral plate is one of the major mechanical factors limiting plate growth. Differential growth of the various ossification centers is also typical. The distal humerus is a good example of such differential growth. The trochlea and capitellum are initially equal in size. The ossification center of the capitellum tends to develop earlier and more rapidly, and in doing so, it restricts its own interstitial expansion. The trochlea does not appear until later and therefore can ultimately achieve a larger size because it has a longer period of interstitial growth. Ultimately, when both of these centers fuse, latitudinal growth of the distal humerus becomes a peripheral function at the level of the epicondyles.

Control of the Growth Plate

As one would expect, a number of factors affect normal plate growth and development. Both local and systemic factors have been clearly identified as manipulating the plate and the way in which growth is accomplished.

The Heulter-Volkmann law is an important local factor. Increasing compression forces across the physis will slow longitudinal growth. Conversely, increasing tension on the physis will result in increased longitudinal growth (Delpach law). This principle helps to explain the progression on angular deformities of the lower extremities. The integrity of the periosteum acts as another mechanical restraint on the plate. Because it attaches directly to the perichondral ring of Lacroix, it will control the amount of latitudinal and longitudinal growth seen.

Obviously, the vascular supply to the plate is critical for growth integrity. Any disruption or damage to this supply of the plate will clearly impede its ability to function and grow normally.

A number of systemic factors have also been implicated in normal plate function. Genetic as well as nutritional factors certainly play a role in physeal manipulation. However, most indications are that hormonal control is the primary regulator of plate function.

Growth hormone is a peptide hormone produced by the pituitary gland that stimulates physis activity by affecting cellular proliferation via its mediators, somatomedins and sulfation factor. Excessive levels of this hormone will cause an anticipated growth plate widening and ultimately gigantism. Should the plate be closed at the time of excessive growth stimulation, acromegaly results. This condition is typified by increased appositional bone growth. On the other hand, deficiency of this hormone typically slows the plate growth. However, because the plate tends to remain open longer, the ultimate height is variable. This finding suggests that growth hormone has no effect on plate closure, but rather a regulatory effect on the rate of proliferation and osteogenesis.

Thyroid hormone has a primarily trophic effect on cartilage growth and is essential to the normal health and growth of cartilage. Recently, a synergistic effect with insulin-like growth factor has been suggested. Excess levels of thyroid hormone have wide-ranging systemic effects but relatively few musculoskeletal manifestations. Low levels of thyroid hormone, however, result in growth retardation, erosion of the chondroepiphysis, and degradation of mucopolysaccharides.

Glucocorticoids are steroid hormones produced by the adrenal cortex and similarly seem to exert a trophic effect on cartilage. A physiologic level is required for normal physeal function. In the face of excessive levels, derived either endogenously or exogenously, there is a stunting effect on the chondrocytes with decrease in mitotic and synthetic activity. Inadequate levels of adrenal steroids can also result in stunting, but to a lesser degree.

Sex hormones, androgens and estrogens both, are steroid hormones. The androgens are felt to exert their effect in the hypertrophic zone. Testosterone seems to stimulate rapid cell division, calcification, and premature physeal closure. Conversely, deficiency states of androgenic hormones are characterized by a marked delay in physeal closure, resulting in the typical eunuchoid body habitus. Estrogen, on the other hand, apparently has a more complex effect on the plate. Some suppressive activity on plate function has been demonstrated with excessive levels of estrogen activity.

Plate Closure

Physiologic closure of the growth plate is a complex phenomenon. Clearly, there are hormonal as well as local factors that manipulate this process. Once physeal growth has stopped, initial closure of the plate begins. The portion of the plate that closes first and the pattern of closure vary from bone to bone. Ultimately the growth plate, as we know it, disappears, and the metaphysis fuses to the secondary ossification center.

Females close their physes earlier than males, probably due to estrogens, which accelerate cartilage replacement and osseous maturation. In any event, the process begins with the formation of an ossified bridge between the epiphysis and the metaphysis. It ends with a complete disappearance of the cartilaginous physis. As mentioned previously, the location of the initial bridge in the transverse plane of the plate varies from bone to bone.

Biomechanics of the Growth Plate

The cartilaginous physis is clearly a mechanical defect at the end of a long bone. It is vulnerable not only to a number of chemical and toxic effects but to mechanical disruption as well. As with all biologic tissues, injury to the plate can occur when the load exceeds the ultimate tensile strength. At that point, failure will occur. The result will be a function of the strength of the plate, as well as the magnitude of the load applied.

The cross-sectional anatomy of a physis varies from bone to bone. Some plates are relatively planar with few metaphyseal interdigitations. Others are contoured to a significant degree, making failure patterns more complex. These interdigitations, referred to as "mammillary processes," confer a certain resistance to shear forces. Unfortunately, the greater constraint conferred by these processes, the greater the risk of premature physeal closure should the plate fail in shear resulting in mamillary process fracture. Such is the case of the distal femoral physis; fractures disrupt the mammillary processes, frequently resulting in premature physeal closure. As a generalization, it is fair to say that the plate is most vulnerable when it is actively growing. Therefore, in the prepubertal and pubertal individuals, one would anticipate the plate to be most susceptible to excessive mechanical load. Plate failure and its long-term complications can be relatively wide ranging and is further explored in the chapter on pediatric trauma.

RECOMMENDED READINGS

Ballock RT, O'Keefe RJ. Current concepts review: the biology of the growth plate. *JBJS Am* 2003;85-A:715–726.

Day TF, Yang Y. Wnt and hedgehog signaling pathways in bone development. *JBJS Am* 2008;90:19–24.

Dietz FR, Mathews KD. Current concepts review: update of the genetic bases of disorders with orthopaedic manifestations. *JBJS Am* 1996;78-A:1583–1598.

Section 2 Basic Science of Cartilage and Bone

John A. Zavala John N. Delahay

INTRODUCTION

Cartilage and bone are the basic building blocks of the musculoskeletal system. This chapter describes the cellular composition, microscopic structure, and basic physiology of these important tissues.

CARTILAGE

Cartilage is a specialized, fibrous connective tissue. Its function varies on the basis of its histologic type. There are essentially three histologic types of cartilage. In addition, the growth apparatus of the skeleton includes physeal and epiphyseal cartilage, which are variants of these basic subtypes. Table 1.1 shows the composition of the various types of cartilage.

Types of Cartilage

Hyaline cartilage: This tissue covers the ends of long bones, forming their articular surfaces. Hyaline cartilage is important for its ability to resist compressive forces and provide a relatively frictionless surface for smooth joint motion.

Fibrocartilage: The matrix of fibrocartilage is high in collagen fibers. These fibers tend to be visible by light microscopy. The menisci, the annulus fibrosus, and the symphysis pubis are largely fibrocartilage. Biomechanically, fibrocartilage is designed to resist tensile load.

Elastic cartilage: Elastic cartilage is composed primarily of elastic fibers. It is found in the external ear, the epiglottis, and the tip of the nose. Elastic cartilage has a moderate ability to resist tensile load, but it also allows for some controlled deformation.

Articular Cartilage

From an orthopaedic standpoint, the most important histologic type of cartilage is hyaline cartilage. It is a very tough, resilient, firm material that allows for almost frictionless motion of the joints. The average thickness of the articular surface is between 2 and 4 mm, with some surfaces being as thick as 7 mm. Normal adult human articular cartilage is typically described as being divided into four histologic zones (Fig. 1.13).

Histologic Zones

Tangential (Gliding) Zone

The tangential zone is the most superficial zone of flattened cells. Collagen fibers are arranged parallel to the joint surface and help limit shear forces.

Transitional (Intermediate) Zone

The cells in this zone are round or ovoid and are randomly distributed throughout the matrix in this region. These cells manifest small membrane processes, which are noted to extend into the matrix. There is a higher level of metabolic activity in this zone.

Radial Zone

The cells in this zone are arranged perpendicular to the articular surface. Membrane processes are similarly noted in this region and interconnect the cells. In addition, glycogen-containing storage granules can be found in these cells. This zone contains the highest content of proteoglycans and the lowest content of water.

Calcified Zone

Small irregular cells with pyknotic nuclei are found in lacunae surrounded by huge amounts of hydroxyapatite crystal.

Tidemark

This is a wavy basophilic line that appears when the growth plate closes. This line is seen to be interposed between the radial zone and the calcified zone. No blood vessels can be seen to cross this line in normal articular cartilage.

Lamina Splendens

This surface layer consists of tightly packed collagen bundles tangential to the surface and slightly subjacent to it. It is felt that this material causes surface undulations seen in articular cartilage and represents part of the complex lubricating system.

Morphology and Physiology

The cells that are integral to the articular surface are called "chondrocytes." They account for only 0.1% of the volume of the tissue. The shape of chondrocytes varies depending on the zone in which they are found. Typically, the nucleus is located in the lacunae of articular cartilage and is eccentric and basophilically stained. Numerous organelles such as a Golgi complex, endoplasmic reticulum, mitochondria, and vacuoles have all been identified in these cells. Articular tissue is isolated in that it does not have a neural, lymphatic, or vascular supply.

TABLE 1.1
APPROXIMATE COMPOSITION OF THE VARIOUS TYPES OF CARTILAGE

			Solids (%)		
Cartilage	**Water (%)**	**Collagen (%)**	**GAG**	**Elastin**	**Other***
Articular	72	66	18	—	16
Epiphyseal	81	37	15	—	48
Fibrocartilage	74	78	2	0.6	19
Elastic	71	53	12	19	16

*Includes monocollagen proteins, calcium phosphorous, other ions, and macromolecules such as DNA and RNA.
Reprinted with permission from Wiesel SW, Delahay JN. *Principles of Orthopaedic Medicine and Surgery.* Philadelphia, PA: Saunders; 2001.

The chemistry of articular cartilage is essentially the chemistry of its matrix (Table 1.2). As noted, the chondrocytes are distributed in the cartilage matrix. This matrix primarily is composed of water, accounting for 65% to 80% of the wet weight of cartilage. Approximately 10% to 20% of the wet weight of cartilage matrix is collagen and approximately 5% to 7% is a unique proteoglycan commonly referred to as "aggrecan." In addition, electrolytes are present in this fluid.

Collagen constitutes 10% to 20% of the matrix when wet and approximately 50% to 60% when dry. Type II collagen account for 90% to 95% of collagen seen in articular cartilage. In the superficial layer, collagen fibers are arranged parallel to the joint surface, whereas in other layers, they are uniformly distributed. The collagen meshwork gives cartilage its tensile strength and form and maintains the location of the chondrocytes. Each tropocollagen molecule is composed of three alpha-1 chains.

The third matrix constituent is a complex proteoglycan macromolecule, referred to as "aggrecan" (Fig. 1.14). This molecule consists of a large protein core to which are attached upwards of 100 chondroitin sulfate molecules and 40 to 50 keratan sulfate chains. These substances are polysaccharide molecules and are unique to articular cartilage. The polysaccharide molecules, specifically the chondroitin and keratin sulfate, are attached roughly perpendicular to the protein core, which, in turn, is attached to a central filamentous core of hyaluronic acid via a link protein. The distribution of the aggrecan molecules is not homogeneous. The highest concentrations of these molecules can be found in the perilacunar areas, whereas their concentrations seem to be less in the superficial zones. Similarly, based on the age, the location, and the disease state, there is a variation in the amount of chondroitin-4-sulfate, chondroitin-6-sulfate, and keratan sulfate. The importance, however, of these macromolecules remains unquestioned.

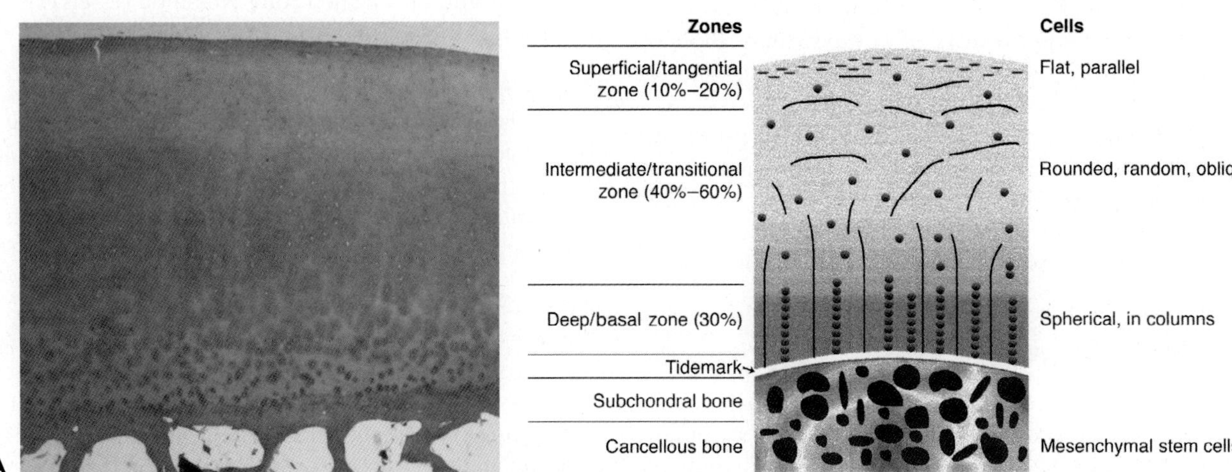

Figure 1.13 Cartilage morphology: **(A)** superficial layer collagen stains red with eosin; intermediate layer proteoglycan stains bluish with hematoxylin. The basal layer with increasing collagen, binding the cartilage to the bone and stains predominantly red with eosin. The subchondral bone below, primarily collagen and mineral, stains densely red. **(B)** Diagram on right outlines the corresponding zones and cellular morphology. (*Reprinted with permission from* Damron T. *Orthopaedic Surgery Essentials. Oncology and Basic Science*. Philadelphia, PA: Lippincott Williams & Wilkins, 2008.)

TABLE 1.2
ADULT ARTICULAR CARTILAGE COMPOSITION

Component	Cartilage Content (%)
Cells	95
Matrix	5
Water	70
Mineral	—
Organic	30
Collagen	60
Proteoglycan	25
Protein	15

Reprinted with permission from Damron TA, Morris CD, Tornetta P, Einhorn TA. *Oncology and Basic Science*. Philadelphia, PA: Lippincott Williams & Wilkins; 2007.

They create huge electronegative fields around them. These large electrostatic domains bestow upon articular cartilage its biomechanical resiliency and resistance to deformity. The ability to hydrate the matrix largely depends on the concentrations of these large macromolecules.

Because cartilage is an avascular material, its nutrition depends on diffusion. Adult articular cartilage essentially must depend on diffusion from synovial fluid through the surface layers to provide cartilage nutrition. Obviously, the rates of diffusion are a function of the size of the molecule and the concentration gradient. Permeability is slower in the deeper layers because of the greater fixed charge. As this fixed charge decreases, as in the case of osteoarthritis and other disease states, permeability rates tend to increase.

As one would expect, given its relative avascularity, the metabolism of articular cartilage is primarily anaerobic. Although there are a few aerobic pathways, they are far less developed and of relative little importance. Articular cartilage, which was once thought to be metabolically inert, has clearly been shown to be quite the opposite. The chondrocytes are capable of synthesizing protein, specifically collagen, using standard pathways of DNA/RNA transcription. In addition, they can synthesize the glycosaminoglycan (aggrecan) component of the matrix. Most studies have indicated that synthetic rates are linear with time. Although quite rapid in the immature, in the adult the rates are relatively constant, despite aging.

Turnover does exist in the articular surface and the matrix. While mitotic activity is seen in the immature animal, this generally ceases once maturation is achieved. While there is generally no mitotic activity seen in normal adult articular cartilage, under certain circumstances chondrocytes can become active as chondroblasts.

The continued ability of cartilage to withstand shear, compression, and tensile forces depends on the composition of the extracellular matrix. Maintenance of this matrix requires chondrocyte-mediated synthesis, assembly, and degradation of proteoglycans, collagens, and other matrix molecules. Cartilage enzymes are felt to be at the heart of this remodeling system. Proteolytic enzymes (proteinases) that are synthesized by the chondrocytes appear to be key in the degradation of articular cartilage. Two major groups of proteinases are currently receiving attention: metalloproteinases, such as collagenase and gelatinase, and the cathepsins. Collagenase is key to the breakdown of the

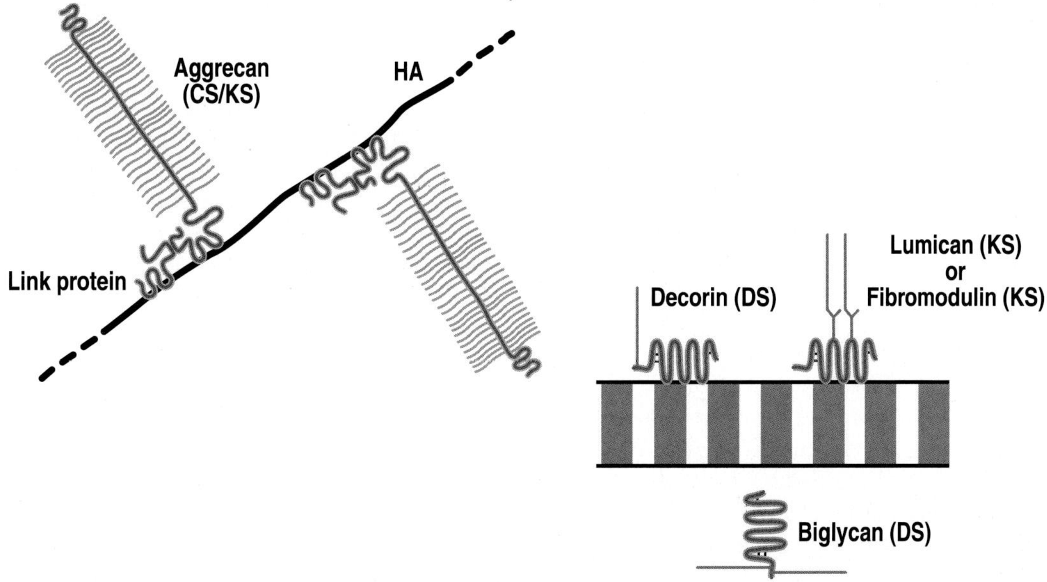

Figure 1.14 Cartilage proteoglycans. Aggrecan is the major aggregating proteoglycan (25% of dry weight): it is associated with compression and linked to hyaluronic acid (HA). The other proteoglycans are nonaggregating and associate with and stabilize fibrils. (*Reprinted with permission from* Damron T. *Orthopaedic Surgery Essentials. Oncology and Basic Science*. Philadelphia, PA: Lippincott Williams & Wilkins, 2008.)

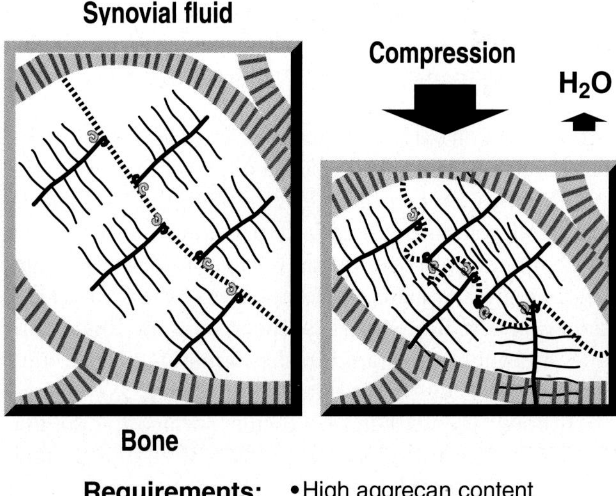

Figure 1.15 Resistance to compression: on the left, articular cartilage is in equilibrium, with the swelling pressure of the proteoglycan balanced by the tensile force in the collagen fibril. With compression, water is squeezed out of the cartilage and a new equilibrium is reached, with an increased swelling pressure of the proteoglycan balancing the applied compression. When the compression is removed, water is drawn in and the former steady state is achieved. (*Reprinted with permission from* Damron T. *Orthopaedic Surgery Essentials. Oncology and Basic Science.* Philadelphia, PA: Lippincott Williams & Wilkins, 2008.)

protein collagen. Cathepsins are critical for the degradation of aggrecan.

Cartilage as a tissue serves a favorable biomechanical role. It is an amazingly indentable tissue. This property is a function of its hyperhydrated state, which allows it to return to its original shape when indented (Fig. 1.15). The ability of cartilage to deform over time, or "creep," is a function of the thickness of the articular surface. Cartilage is also able to provide the diarthrodial joint with a certain level of shock absorption. This ability can occur passively, as a result of cartilage's deformation on impact, and actively, as a function of joint motion and muscle lengthening. Joint congruence, especially with loading, depends on the cartilage thickness and its pliability. There is an inverse relationship between cartilage thickness and joint congruence. Specifically, the thicker the articular surface, such as the patellofemoral joint, the less congruent the joint will be. As the articular surface becomes damaged from various pathologic states, the ability of this cartilage to function normally in its biomechanical modes is markedly altered. This change simply compounds the rate of joint breakdown in a number of different pathologic situations.

Pathologic Changes

Aging

The chondrocytes in the aging articular surface tend to increase in size, increase their content of lytic enzymes, and no longer reproduce. There is an overall decrease in the glycosaminoglycans and a relative increase in the protein content of the articular surface. As the aggrecan component of articular cartilage matrix decreases, the overall water content decreases. With loss of water and proteoglycan, the cartilage becomes stiffer and less pliable.

Trauma to the Articular Surface

Mechanical injury, such as superficial and deep laceration, is not uncommon. The healing of these chondral defects, however, varies depending on whether or not the subchondral plate is violated. Superficial laceration that does not cross the tidemark will cause chondrocyte proliferation but little healing due to avascularity. With a deep laceration, one will ordinarily see a vascular response and resultant adherent fibrous plaque forms. This becomes populated with proliferating fibroblasts, and over a period of 2 to 6 months, healing with fibrocartilage occurs. This fibrocartilage provides articular surface continuity but is biomechanically less efficient than the normal hyaline surface. Unfortunately, many of these new fibrocartilage plaques are quite vulnerable.

Chemical damage to the articular surface is generally the result of deposition of metabolic end products and can be seen in gout, pseudogout, ochronosis, and hemachromatosis. The deposition of these end products in the articular cartilage layer alters the normal cartilage matrix, typically resulting in increased stiffness. As a result, shear and impact load injury may occur, damaging the articular surface.

Osteoarthritis

Both biomechanical and biochemical mechanisms are seen in the degradation of cartilage leading to osteoarthritis. Three overlapping stages can be seen: cartilage matrix damage, chondrocyte response to tissue damage, and the decline of the chondrocyte synthetic response and progressive loss of tissue.

With the disruption of the matrix, there is a concomitant increase in the water content. There is a decrease in proteoglycan aggregation and aggrecan concentration. Decreases in length of glycosaminoglycan chains are also seen. The collagen content tends to remain relatively constant. There are generally some distribution changes of collagen between the various layers. Chondrocytes detect tissue damage and release mediators that result in both anabolic and catabolic alterations in cartilage metabolism. Early, there is an increased rate of DNA synthesis and cell replication. There is an increased rate of protein and glycosaminoglycan synthesis. Ultimately, the entire reparative effort fails, and at this point, water content, glycosaminoglycan content, and, to a lesser degree, collagen content gradually decrease. As these changes occur, the mechanical properties of the articular surface suffer and mechanical failure of the cartilage is imminent (Fig. 1.16).

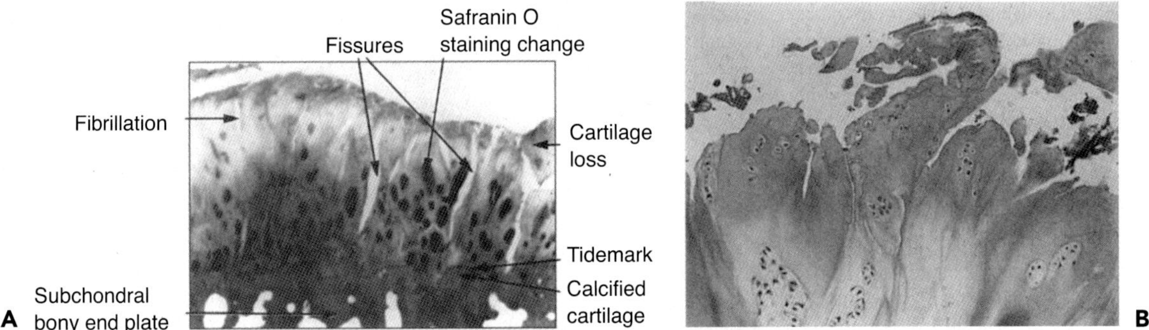

Figure 1.16 **(A)**: Low-power magnification of a section of a glenohumeral head of osteoarthritic cartilage removed at surgery. **(B)** A high-power magnification of surface fibrillation showing the vertical cleft formation and widespread large, necrotic regions of the tissue devoid of cells. (*Reprinted with permission from* Buckwalter JA, Einhorn TA, Simon SR. *Orthopaedic Basic Science: Biology and Biomechanics of the Musculoskeletal System.* 2nd ed. Rosemont, IL: American Academy of Orthopaedic Surgeons, 2000.)

BONE

Bone is a connective tissue that serves major roles as a structural support for the musculoskeletal system and as a dynamic reservoir for calcium. This latter function is essential in the maintenance of normal skeletal homeostasis as well as calcium and phosphate metabolism. Bone is in a constant state of flux between continual bone formation and bone resorption; the processes are normally finely balanced. The balance between resorption and formation is controlled by a number of local and systemic factors. The alteration in any of these systems will clearly affect the way in which the normal bone turnover is regulated.

Bone Morphology and Physiology

Bone is a connective tissue, as is cartilage, ligament, and tendon. It is unique, however, in that its extracellular matrix becomes impregnated with a mineral. On a macroscopic level, bone is typically described as being cortical or cancellous. Cortical (compact) bone is the bone typically found in the diaphysis of long bones as well as in subchondral plates, the outer and inner table of the skull, and the outer and inner table of the pelvis. Cancellous (trabecular) bone is more typically seen in areas such as the metaphysis of a long bone and the diploic space of the skull. Cancellous bone is extremely responsive to mechanically applied stress and is primarily affected by Wolfe's law. Simply stated, this law emphasizes the observed fact that bone will be formed in areas where it is needed and will be resorbed in areas where it is not needed.

Microscopically, there are two levels of organization. Normal bone is lamellar and can be either cortical or cancellous. Lamellar bone has a highly ordered arrangement of collagen and cells. The differentiation is determined on the basis of the distribution of the collagen fibers in the matrix as well as the orientation of the cells. Immature bone is referred to as "woven bone" in which the collagen fibers are randomly and loosely arranged. The cells are large and irregular and are located in very rudimentary lacunae. While commonly seen in the fetus and prepubertal child, after growth completion, woven or immature bone is not seen except in the presence of pathologic states. In these situations, the presence of woven bone indicates high rates of bone turnover.

In the adult skeleton, all the bone present is lamellar bone. In cancellous bone, the lamellar bone is configured in a very loose honeycomb with few blood vessels entering the bone surface of the trabeculae. Cortical bone (haversian bone), on the other hand, is a very highly ordered, geometrically arranged structure. The basic unit of cortical bone is the osteon or Haversian system that is built around a central capillary canal. This canal is surrounded by layers of mineralized bone matrix. The matrix collagen in each successive layer has a different orientation (Fig. 1.17), giving the bone "ply strength." The osteocytes are located in lacunae, and the cellular processes radiate from the lacunae in small channels called "canaliculi" (Fig. 1.18).

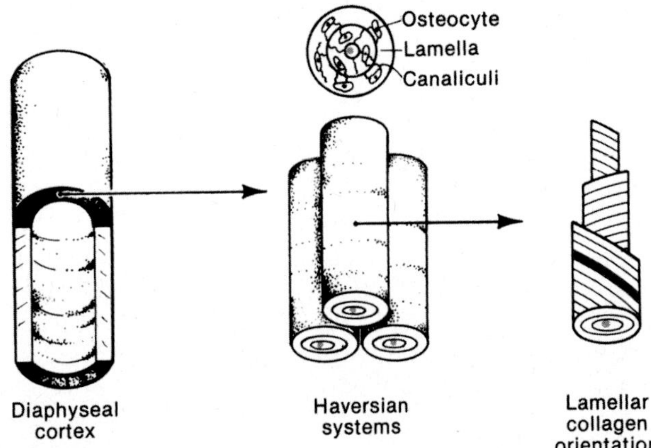

Figure 1.17 Diaphyseal cortex of a long bone. (*Reprinted with permission from* Gamble JG. *The Muscoloskeletal System: Physiologic Basics.* New York, NY: Raven Press, 1988.)

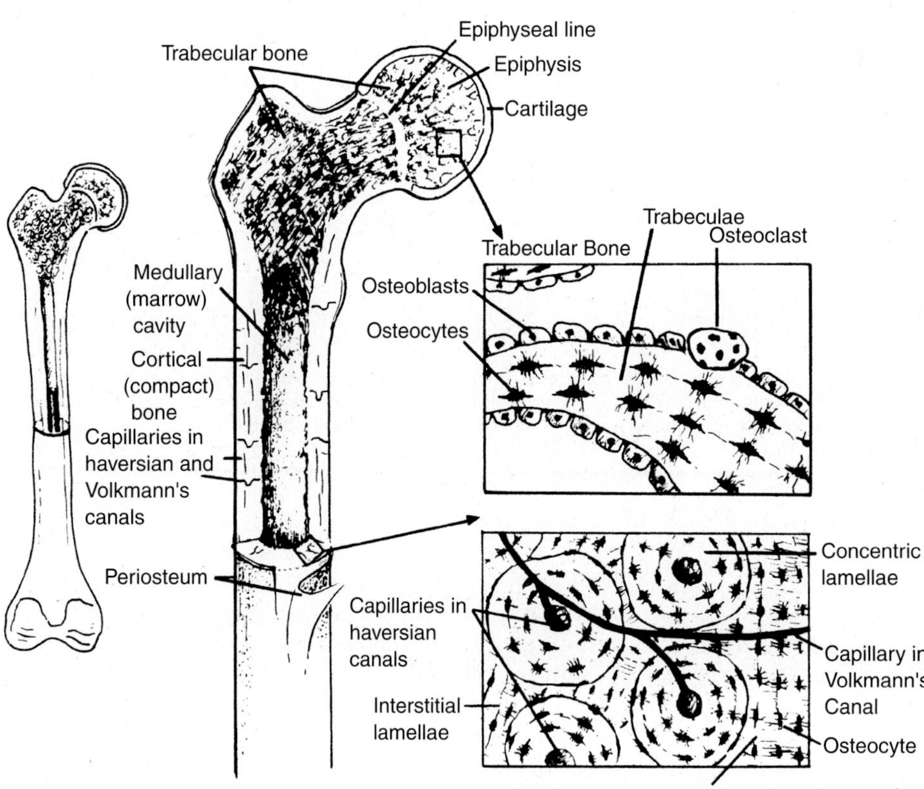

Figure 1.18 Schematic diagram of cortical and trabecular bone showing the different microstructures. (*Reprinted with permission from* Hayes WC. Biomechanics of cortical and trabecular bone: implications for assessment of fracture risk. In: Mow VC, Hayes WC, eds. *Basic Orthopaedic Biomechanics.* New York, NY: Raven Press, 1991.)

In any given section of haversian bone, there are multiple osteonal systems. Between osteonal systems, there is additional lamellar bone filing the void. These lamellae are referred to as "interstitial lamellae." In addition, surrounding the whole cortex itself is a layer of lamellar bone, referred to as the "outer circumferential lamellae."

Bone Circulation

Bone has a vascular flow accounting for 8% of the cardiac output in the normal resting state. Most of the cells in adult bone are within 0.1 mm of a small blood vessel. On a macroscopic level, the blood vessel enters the bone typically through the nutrient foramen (Fig. 1.19). Once interiorized, the blood vessels arborize extensively through the medullary canal and periphery to the periosteum. In addition, blood vessels supplying the periosteum arborize over the surface of the bone. The nutrient artery system is a high-pressure system, whereas the periosteal system is a low-pressure system with resultant centrifugal flow. This reverses in the setting of disruption of the endosteal system. Periosteal blood supply is adequate to feed the outer third of the cortex, whereas the interosseous or medullary supply carries the inner two-thirds of the cortex.

Bone Cells

Bone cells have the usual cellular structure and cellular organelles. In bone, there are several different cell lines. One rudimentary population of progenitor cells is capable of differentiating into an osteoblastic line, and the other is capable of differentiating into an osteoclastic line. The basic bone-forming cell or osteoblast (Fig. 1.20) measures approximately 20 to 30 μm in diameter. The cell has a single nucleus and basophilic cytoplasm and is usually polyhedral in shape. Typically, these cells are found in layers lined up on the surface of bony trabeculae. They contain more endoplasmic reticulum, Golgi apparatus, and mitochondria given their function of matrix production. Initially, the organic matrix (osteoid) they lay down is unmineralized. Matrix is made at the rate of 1 μm/day and takes about 15 days to ossify. Therefore, the normal width of osteoid on the surface of any given trabecula remaining unmineralized is approximately 15 μm. As the osteoid is formed by the osteoblast, the cells become incorporated into the matrix at regular intervals. The area of incorporation is referred to as a "lacuna," and the osteoblast having buried itself in a lacuna becomes known as an "osteocyte."

The osteocytes vary in shape and size on the basis of their age. These cells have a high nucleus-to-cytoplasm ratio with numerous cellular processes extending into the canalicular system. These cellular processes are critical for mineral exchange and the maintenance of calcium homeostasis. The canalicular system ultimately links the cellular processes of the osteocyte with the vascular channel in the central canal of the osteonal system. In addition to their role in the maintenance of skeletal homeostasis and calcium metabolism, the osteocytes have been shown

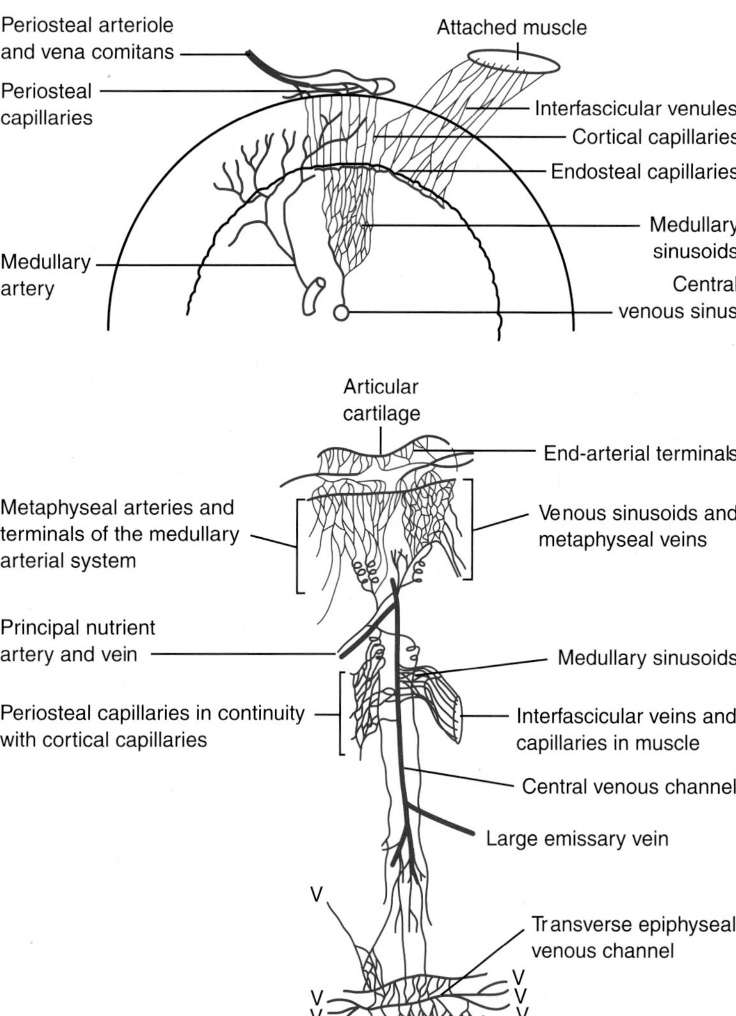

Figure 1.19 Blood supply of a long bone. Three basic blood supplies are shown: (1) nutrient; (2) metaphyseal, which anastomoses with epiphyseal after epiphyseal closure; and (3) periosteal. The numerous metaphyseal arteries arise from periarticular networks and anastomose with terminal branches of ascending and descending medullary arteries. Periosteal capillaries emerge from the cortex (efferent blood flow). (4) A periosteal arteriole feeds capillaries that provide afferent blood flow to a limited outer layer of cortex. (*Adapted from* Rhinelander FW. Circulation of bone. In: Bourne GH, ed. *The Biochemistry and Physiology of Bone*. 2nd ed. New York, NY: Academic Press, 1972.)

to be capable of a limited amount of bone resorption. This phenomenon is referred to as "osteocytic osteolysis." However, this limited amount of resorption is felt to be important in the physiologic maintenance of skeletal mass.

The osteoclast is a large, multinucleated cell containing numerous mitochondria and very dense granules. Of significance is the presence of an unusual ruffled border of the active surface of these cells. This ruffled border appears to be the "active end" of the osteoclast where there are numerous channels and vesicles present (Fig. 1.21). The major function of the osteoclast is to resorb bone. They synthesize tartrate-resistant acid phosphatase. Based on its size, the osteoclast is far more efficient than the osteoblast. It is capable of undoing the work of 20 osteoblasts. The nuclear ratio (osteoclast-to-osteoblast ratio) is 6:1.

The osteoblast and osteoclast work in tandem. There is always a population of both cell lines active in the skeleton. Measurable levels of bone resorption and formation are ongoing. When bone resorption ceases and bone formation begins, this event is marked by the formation of a "cement" or reversal line. This histologic mark emphasizes the continuously reciprocating bone-forming and bone-resorbing activity essential for normal skeletal homeostasis. The average cement line is approximately 1 μm in width. It is easily stained with the usual techniques because of its biochemical differences with the surrounding matrix.

Bone Matrix and Formation

Bone is a unique material in that it is biphasic. It is a composite structure, combining a blend of mineral in matrix. The mineral phase, accounting for 70% of bone by weight, is primarily calcium hydroxyapatite. The organic phase, or matrix, constitutes approximately 30% of bone by weight. This organic matrix is composed primarily of collagen, accounting for 95% of its weight. Therefore, like cartilage, collagen is an important component of the tissue matrix. In addition to collagen, small amounts of mucoprotein, phospholipid, and sialoproteins are present. Along with these chemical components, 2% by weight is water and the cells account for an additional 2% (Table 1.3).

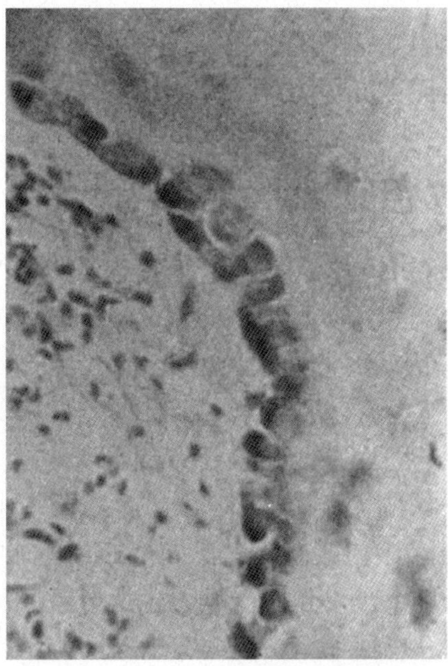
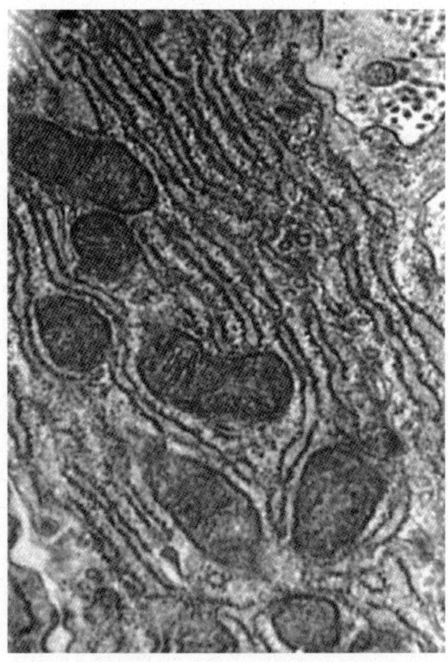

Figure 1.20 Light **(A)** and electron **(B)** photomicrographs of osteoblasts. (*Reprinted with permission from* Buckwalter JA, Einhorn TA, Simon SR. *Orthopaedic Basic Science: Biology and Biomechanics of the Musculoskeletal System.* 2nd ed. Rosemont, IL: American Academy of Orthopaedic Surgeons, 2000.)

Bone collagen, which is predominantly type I, behaves differently from collagen in soft tissue. It is only sparingly soluble. It has a lower shrinkage temperature, and it does not denature. The tropocollagen molecules overlap each other by 25% of length or quarter staggers. In addition, there are small pores, or "hole zones," which exist between the sides of adjacent parallel molecules. The net effect of the quarter stagger and "hole zones" is to make it more accessible for the deposition of mineral. These properties are the result of the unique cross-linking.

There are numerous types of collagen, all of which preserve its characteristic triple helical structure. Those most important to the musculoskeletal system are type I collagen, which is seen in bone, skin, tendon, and blood vessel wall, and type II collagen, which is seen in articular cartilage and the nucleus pulposus. Investigations into collagen polymorphism and the molecular bases are actively ongoing. Numerous collagen dysplastic diseases, as well as their genetic defects, continue to be elucidated (Table 1.4).

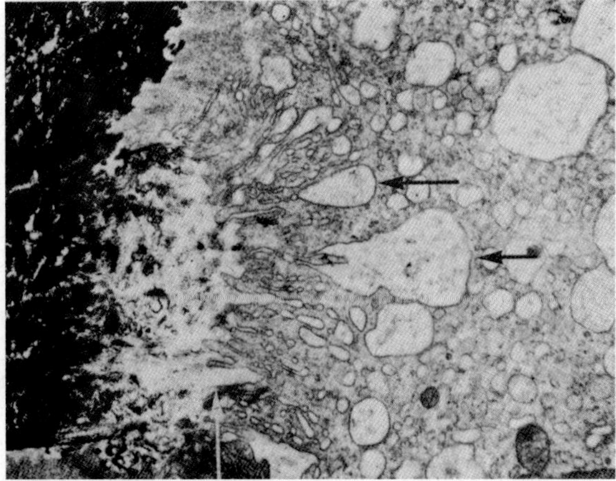

Figure 1.21 Electron micrograph of a section of a bone surface undergoing resorption. Calcified bone appears black on the left. The main part of the picture is occupied by the cytoplasm of the osteoclast: it consists of complex folds and projections that abut on the bone at the left. (*Reprinted with permission* from Hayes WC. Biomechanics of cortical and trabecular bone: implications for assessment of fracture risk. In: Mow VC, Hayes WC, eds. *Basic Orthopaedic Biomechanics.* New York, NY: Raven Press, 1991.)

TABLE 1.3
THE GENERAL COMPOSITION OF BONE

Component	Percentage
Solids	92%
Water	8%
Solid composition	
Mineral phase	65%
Organic phase	35%
Mineral phase composition	
Calcium	60%
Phosphorous, Mg, Na, other ions	40%
Organic phase composition	
Collagen	95%
Cells	3%
Lipids, glycosaminoglycans, noncollagen proteins, etc.	2%

Reprinted with permission from Wiesel SW, Delahay JN. *Principles of Orthopaedic Medicine and Surgery.* Philadelphia, PA: Saunders; 2001.

TABLE 1.4
MOLECULAR DEFECTS IN THE HERITABLE DISEASES OF COLLAGEN

Syndrome	Defect
Ehlers–Danlos syndrome	
Types I–III	Fibrillogenesis defects
Type IV	Decreased type III collagen
Type VI	Lysyl hydroxylase
Type VII	Persistence of N-propeptide
Type IX	Defective cross-linking
Marfan syndrome	Abnormal pro-α 2(I) affecting the structure of type I collagen
Osteogenesis imperfecta	
Type I	Probable deletion of d(1) gene
Type II	Defective secretion of α-chains
Type III	Decreased pro-α 2(I) chains
Menkes syndrome	Cu metabolism abnormality causing defective cross-linking

Reprinted with permission from Wiesel SW, Delahay JN. *Principles of Orthopaedic Medicine and Surgery*. Philadelphia, PA: Saunders; 2001.

Mineral Phase of Bone

Approximately two-thirds of bone matrix by weight and approximately one-half by volume are mineral. The most common form is calcium hydroxyapatite crystal. These crystals are 580 Å and are described as tubular hexagons. Although hydroxyapatite is the most common form of the mineral present, there is also a small amount of amorphous calcium phosphate. Debate still exists as to whether this form of mineral is merely a finely divided apatite crystal.

As noted earlier, the unique feature of the bone mineral is its ordered association with bone collagen. The mineral is arranged along the long axis of the collagen fibril with an interval of 600 to 700 Å. This periodicity is identical to the normal periodicity of the unmineralized collagen fibril. Studies have clearly indicated that the mineral is found in the "hole zones" of the quarter stagger arrangement of the collagen molecules. Approximately 50% of the total mineral in bone is contained in these "hole zones." Similarly, noncovalent "interactions" have been identified between the collagen and the apatite. This "bonding" bestows on this two-phase material properties that are greater than the sum of the parts. The remaining bone mineral is postulated to be contained in the central core of the collagen fibril.

Mineralization

The process of mineralization occurs in two distinct phases: initiation followed by proliferation or accretion. The process of *initiation* requires a combination of events. Specifically, increase in the local concentration of precipitating ions, followed by exposure of those ions to mineral nucleators, begins the propagation process. Inhibitors and regulators modulate the formation of apatite. The process of initiation requires more energy than does the addition of mineral to already existing crystals. Because sufficient energy is not always readily available, some have proposed that the initial mineral deposited is a metastable precursor of apatite, and as more energy becomes available, this unstable precursor is converted to the more stable forms of apatite crystal.

Within the extracellular environment are small structures referred to as "matrix vesicles." These structures have been credited with the ability to facilitate calcification by concentrating calcium ions, by providing a microenvironment free of inhibitors, and by providing the needed enzymes for matrix modification.

Once the initial process of deposition occurs, the second phase of *proliferation* or *accretion* can begin. At this time, additional mineral is added to that which is already present. As previously discussed, this mineral is inserted into the "hole zones" of the collagen fibers. Obviously, the further deposition of mineral will serve to improve the rigidity of the overall matrix.

Recently, the importance of calcium-binding proteins within the bone matrix has been emphasized. These noncollagenous proteins are felt to be critical in the facilitation of mineralization within the collagen. Specifically, phosphoproteins, osteonectin, and some of the GLA proteins have been cited. Osteocalcin, one of the recently isolated GLA proteins, is said to account for 10% to 20% of all the noncollagenous proteins in bone. The role of these GLA proteins is still being actively investigated.

Bone Resorption

The process of bone formation clearly appears to be more complex than that of bone resorption. This process involves the hydrolysis of collagen and the dissolution of bone mineral. It is well documented that the osteoclast must simultaneously do both. There is no mechanism in place for the simple dissolution of bone mineral, leaving unmineralized osteoid. As described earlier, the osteoclast is the critical cell for the resorption of bone. The brush border of this multinuclear cell is always in contact with the bone that is actively being resorbed. Electron micrographs of these cells demonstrate an increased number of mitochondria adjacent to the brush border, suggesting their function in the transcellular transport of calcium ion. In addition, numerous lysosomes are identified in this area, which seems appropriate, considering the fact that these organelles contain numerous hydrolytic enzymes.

The process is thought to be initiated by the lysosomal degradation of bone collagen. Once the initial degradation begins, fragments of the disrupted collagen are taken up by the cell and are further hydrolyzed. Collagenase cleaves tropocollagen into two major fragments. Parathyroid hormone seems to directly increase the local concentration of collagenase enzyme. Considering the role of parathyroid hormone in calcium release, this effect seems appropriate. Coincident with the degradation of the collagen is the solubilization of the hydroxyapatite crystal.

Bone Remodeling

The removal of bone and its subsequent redeposition are an ongoing process. The process is somewhat age dependent. Approximately 80% of total skeletal mass is cortical bone, and approximately 20% of skeletal mass is cancellous bone. In the young skeleton, turnover rates can be as high as 50% per year in certain diaphyseal bones. With aging, this number decreases to 2% to 3% per year. The process of resorption begins with a wave of osteoclastic activity in the form of "cutting cones." These osteoclastic cutting heads remove old bone, and in their wake, new osteoblastic activity can be seen. The process of bone remodeling and the rates of this process are under the control of numerous local and systemic factors.

RECOMMENDED READINGS

Buckwalter JA, Glimcher MJ, Cooper RR, Recker R. Instructional course lecture: bone biology. Part I: structure, blood supply, cells, matrix, and mineralization. *J Bone Joint Surg Am.* 1995;77:1256–1275.

Buckwalter JA, Glimcher MJ, Cooper RR, Recker R. Instructional course lecture: bone biology. Part II: form, modeling, remodeling, and regulation of cell function. *J Bone Joint Surg Am.* 1995;77:1276–1289.

O'Driscoll SW. Current concept review: the healing and regeneration of articular cartilage. *J Bone Joint Surg Am.* 1998;80-A(12):1796–1812.

Section 3 Biomechanics and Biomaterials

John A. Zavala John N. Delahay

INTRODUCTION

The study of mechanics is critical to understanding of the principles of orthopaedic surgery, in terms of both the normal functioning of the musculoskeletal system and the aberrant behavior due to alterations of the mechanical environment. The study of biomaterials is also an integral part of the field inasmuch as many implants are used in the management of musculoskeletal afflictions. An understanding of these implants and the properties of the material from which they are made is critical to an appreciation of their use. The purpose of this chapter is to assist the reader in understanding the basic principles of biomechanics and biomaterials.

BIOMECHANICS

Forces

A *force* is simply defined as a push or pull and technically is one of three types.

1. Tensile force, which tends to pull objects apart
2. Compressive force, which tends to push objects together
3. Shearing force, which tends to make one part of an object slide over an immediately adjacent part.

Forces can act separately or in combination with one another. It is important to understand that forces are essentially vector quantities. That is, they have a magnitude, a line of application, a direction or sense, and a point of application. If any one of these four characteristics is changed, the entire vector itself is altered.

When multiple forces act on a structure, it is possible to resolve these forces into a single vector. Most loading situations feel the effect of forces. Therefore, the techniques of vector analysis permit the summation of these forces and a graphic demonstration of their combination. Joints are no exception. Multiple muscle forces tend to pull structures with varying magnitudes, points of attachment, and directions. These forces require resolution in order to be able to evaluate the loading environment. By resolving these multiple forces into a single vector, their net effect can be anticipated (Fig. 1.22).

Forces that act at different points on a body tend to result in moments. Moments cause bending or rotation of the body in question. A moment can be expressed as the product of the force and the perpendicular distance from the line of action of the force to the axis of rotation. It is important to keep in mind that the distance (d) in the standard formula for moment ($M = F \times d$) is the perpendicular distance from the line of application to the axis of rotation. In the seesaw example, each child creates a bending moment on the board. This moment tends to bend the board at the fulcrum. In Figure 1.23, these two moments are represented by Ba and Cb. For the system to be in equilibrium, these moments must be equal.

There are numerous examples in the musculoskeletal system of the effects of a moment. The classic example frequently used is that of the bending moment felt by a dynamic hip compression screw used to fix an intertrochanteric fracture. A moment is created by the vertical

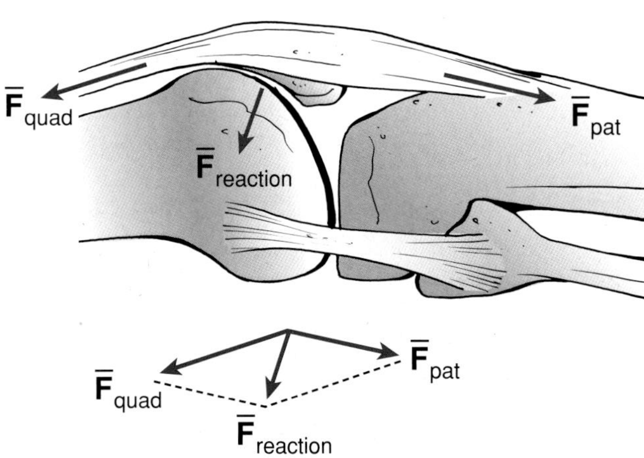

Figure 1.22 Example of calculation of forces in the knee joint. The patellofemoral joint reaction force, $F_{reaction}$, is the vector parallelogram sum of the quadriceps force, F_{quad}, and the patellar tendon force, F_{pat}. (*Reprinted with permission from* Damron TA, Morris CD, Tornetta P, et al. *Oncology and Basic Science*. Philadelphia, PA: Lippincott Williams & Wilkins, 2007.)

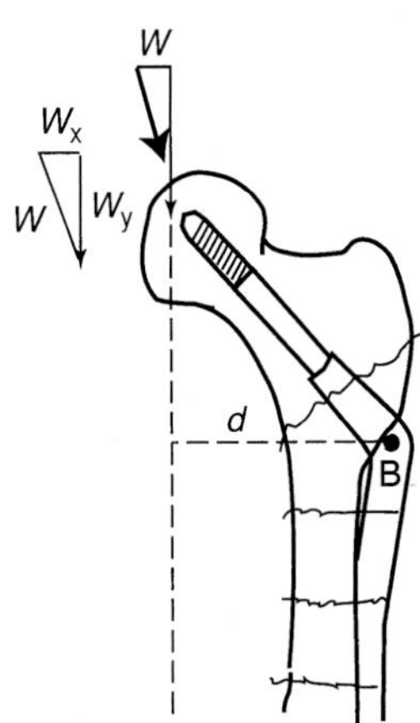

Figure 1.24 Bending moment (M) on a compression hip screw is calculated as follows: $M = Wy \times d$ Where d = distance from line of application to axis of rotation (B) and Wy = component of force W (body weight) acting along the y axis. (*Reprinted with permission from* Wiesel SW, Delahay JN. *Principles of Orthopaedic Medicine and Surgery*. Philadelphia, PA: Saunders, 2001.)

force (Wy) acting at distance (d), which is tending to bend the plate. With a higher angle plate, d will decrease; hence, the bending moment will decrease (Fig. 1.24).

The term *torque* is occasionally used to indicate a moment that produces rotational motion about an axis. Essentially, a moment and a torque can be considered to be the same. Despite the fact that the formulas for these forces are different, they produce similar results—bending or rotation about an axis. A special example of torsional moments is the force couple. This force system is created by two equal, parallel forces that are not collinear. Their resultant effect is additive and is represented by $F \times d$.

For an object to be in equilibrium, all of the forces must equal zero *and* all of the moments must equal zero. The concept of equilibrium is important, if one is to use mathematical models to determine the loading of various joints and the effect of load on various implants.

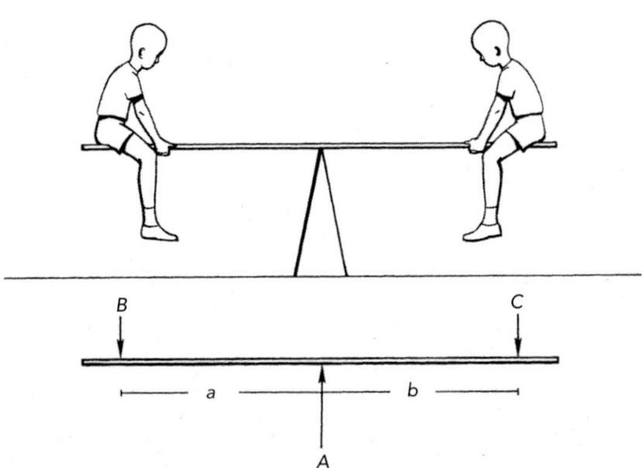

Figure 1.23 Forces on opposite sides of the axis. In equilibrium, $B + C$ (downward forces) $= A$ (upward force). (*Reprinted with permission from* Le Veau B. *Williams and Lissner: Biomechanics of Human Motion*. Philadelphia, PA: Saunders, 1977.)

The formula for force is $F = m \times a$ (mass $\times$ acceleration), which allows one to define force in terms of any unit desired. The standard force unit is the Newton, which is defined as the force needed to accelerate 1 kg of mass 1 m/s^2. Inertia is the resisting force that tends to keep the 1 kg of mass in its existing state of motion. The term *weight* represents a special form of force, specifically that which results from gravity. The force with which a given mass is attracted toward the center of a gravitational body is represented by its weight. Unfortunately, the term kilogram is widely used to indicate weight and mass. Therefore, the use of that term creates confusion as to the force. The term Newton is the preferred term to indicate force.

Elasticity, Stress, and Strain

The orthopaedic surgeon deals with many solid structures, some biologic, such as bone and cartilage, and others nonbiologic, such as metals and plastics. In the pure science of mechanics, one assumes that the objects or bodies analyzed are rigid. In biologic systems, this is not a valid assumption. It is important to be able to consider the change in shape or volume of an object as external forces are applied. The elasticity of matter is demonstrated simply by a diving board that bends under load and returns to its original shape when the load is removed. For many materials, this ability to return to its original configuration is nearly perfect; these materials are said to be elastic (Fig. 1.25). The behavior of elastic materials is governed by Hooke's law, which states that the deformation of an elastic body is directly proportional to the magnitude of the applied force provided that the elastic limit is not exceeded.

The analysis of the behavior of a material hinges on the principles of stress and strain. *Stress* is defined as a force per unit area of material and is a measurement of the intensity

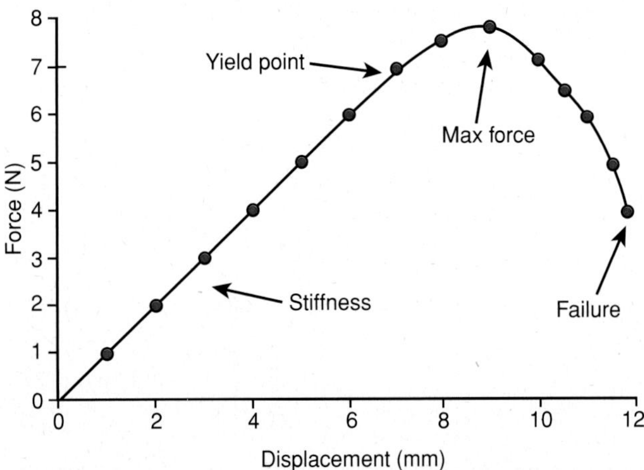

Figure 1.25 Example of a force-displacement loading curve for a linear, elastic structure. (*Reprinted with permission from* Damron TA, Morris CD, Tornetta P, et al. *Oncology and Basic Science.* Philadelphia, PA: Lippincott Williams & Wilkins, 2007.)

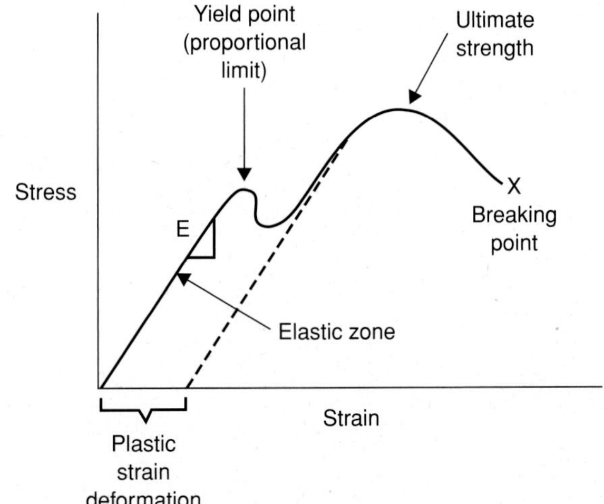

Figure 1.26 The stress–strain curve. (*Reprinted with permission from* Miller MD. *Review of Orthopaedics,* 2nd ed. Philadelphia, WB Saunders, 2008.)

of the force. Stress essentially represents the intermolecular resistance within an object to the action of an outside force that has been applied. Stress cannot be measured directly; however, its magnitude can be calculated by various formulas. The use of these formulas to determine a material's stress-related properties is predicated upon the fact that the material is isotropic. This description implies a homogeneity of the material such that the physical properties are the same regardless of the direction of testing. Conversely, in an anisotropic material, the physical properties vary with the direction of testing.

There are two basic types of stress. *Normal stress* is perpendicular to the plane of any cross section of material. Therefore, compressive forces and tensile forces will generate a normal stress in the structure. *Shear stress* is defined as the intensity of force parallel to the surface on which it acts.

When forces create stress within a structure, they typically produce strain. *Strain* is defined as the deformation within a structure. Before a structure or a material breaks, it usually stretches or bends. This stretching or bending prior to failure is called "strain," and it is defined as the change in unit length or angular deformation of a material subjected to load. Similar to stress, there are two types of strain: *normal strain,* which is caused by either stretching, which results from tensile force, or shortening, which results from compressive force, and *shear strain,* which is defined as the angular deformation suffered by an object subjected to a shearing force.

At this point it is necessary to clarify the terms force, deformation, stress, and strain. Force and deformation are said to be structural properties. Thus, when a force is applied to a given structure, some degree of deformation is produced. Stress and strain, on the other hand, are said to be material properties; that is, they are the same for a given material no matter what structure is made from that material. Essentially, stress is force normalized per unit area.

Stress–Strain Curve

When an elastic material is subjected to an increasing tensile stress that carries the material beyond the elastic limit, a stress–strain curve can be plotted (Fig. 1.26). In considering this curve, the line between zero and the yield point is straight, showing that stress is proportional to strain for small strains in accordance with Hooke's law. A specimen will exhibit linear elastic behavior up to a certain limit, which is referred to as the "yield point." Beyond the yield point stress is no longer proportional to strain, and the deforming object is no longer capable of regaining its original length when the disturbing force is removed. If the force is removed beyond the yield point, the strain retraces the broken line back to the baseline and the object is left with permanent deformation. The important features of this curve are as follows:

Yield point is the stress at which marked increase in deformation occurs without an increase in load.

Ultimate tensile strength (UTS) is the highest point on the curve. This is the maximum apparent stress that the material can withstand. UTS is frequently referred to as the strength of the material.

Elastic region is the portion of the curve from zero to the yield point. This portion of the curve is typically linear. It is within this portion that stress is proportional to strain and Hooke's law is valid.

Plastic region is the portion beyond the yield point where the deforming strain is not proportional to the applied stress.

Modulus of Elasticity is represented by the slope of the line in the elastic portion. The modulus is also a material property. The higher the number, the greater the hardness of the material. Essentially, this modulus indicates the pounds per square inch (psi) of stress that must develop to gain a certain amount of strain.

These curves can be used to compare the behavior of various materials. Specifically, in orthopaedics, one can compare the material properties of the commonly used metals; cobalt-chrome alloy, titanium alloys, and stainless steel as they relate to cortical and cancellous bone.

Loading

Forces can load an object in a number of ways. The object frequently used to model loading mechanisms is a solid bar of material or a beam. This bar of material can be used to compare the changes that are seen as various loads are applied and as the direction of these loads is altered. *Tensile koading* results from a force applied along the long axis of the bar, stretching the bar and causing any given cross-sectional area to decrease in size. *Compressive loading* conversely will tend to shorten the bar and will tend to increase any given cross-sectional area. The specific dimensions of the change can be determined using Poisson's ratio.

Bending is actually a form of composite loading. Using the model of a cantilever beam in which the material is fixed at one end and loaded at the other, isolated loading patterns can be appreciated as the beam is bent. On the convex side of bending, tensile stresses are generated and tensile strain is observed. On the opposite, or concave, side of the bend, compressive strain is noted, resulting from compressive stresses generated. Located in the center of the beam is a neutral plane, where the stresses are zero. The principles are applicable to the failure of long bones. When subjected to bending loads, the bones behave much like a cantilever beam, that is, tensile stress on the convex side and compressive stress on the concave side.

The way in which the material is distributed over the cross section in any beam of material will alter the loading pattern. An important property, the area moment of inertia, defines this material distribution to bending of a structure under static loading.

Torsional loading results when a torque is applied to a cylinder of material. In doing so, stresses are created within this cylinder. The *polar moment of inertia* is that property of the cross-sectional area of a cylindrical structure that is a measure of the distribution of the material about an axis perpendicular to the cross section (Fig. 1.27). For example, the distribution of the material at greater distances from this central axis tends to improve the torsional rigidity of the cylinder in question. The polar moment of inertia can dramatically affect torsional loading and, as such, plays an important role in the fracture patterns seen in long bones. For example, the polar moment in the proximal tibia is greater than in the distal tibia. Therefore, torsional failure is predictably more likely to occur distally, and clinically, that is the case.

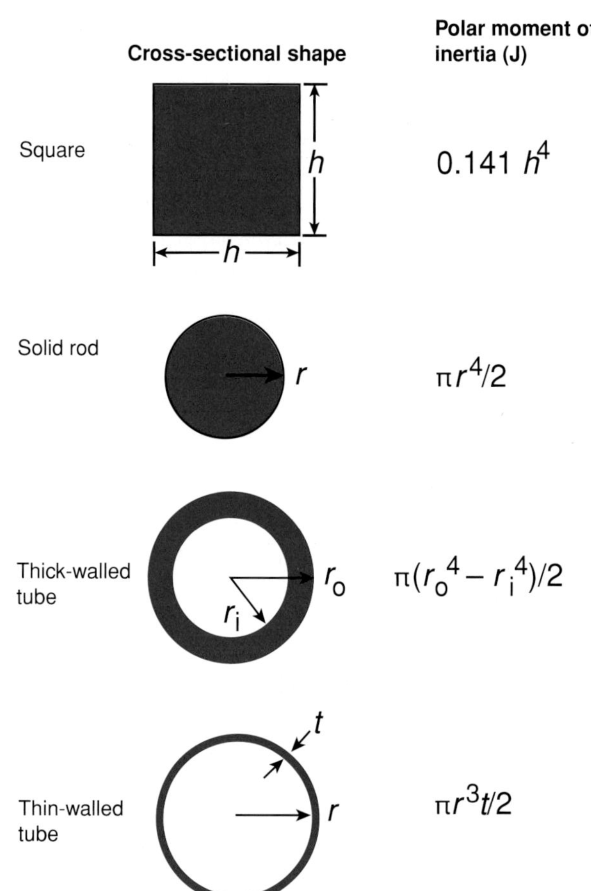

Figure 1.27 Cross-sectional views and the corresponding moments of inertia. (*Reprinted with permission from* Damron TA, Morris CD, Tornetta P, et al. *Oncology and Basic Science*. Philadelphia, PA: Lippincott Williams & Wilkins, 2007.)

Combined loading occurs in most structures, biologic and nonbiologic. Most fractures are the result of a combination of mechanisms: compression, tension, shear, bending, and torsion.

Stress Concentration Effects

Stress of a smooth bar of an isotropic material is rather easy to calculate. However, if the material is anisotropic or if there is a missing section, the calculation becomes far more complex. The principle of stress concentrators (stress raisers) has broad clinical significance. Animal studies have demonstrated that the presence of a screw or drill hole can decrease the ability of that bone to store energy by 70% when stressed torsionally. Additionally, following removal of a screw from a long bone, 8 to 10 weeks are required for the stress concentration effect to be negated. An open section defect is created when a large segment of bone is removed from the circumference of a long tubular bone. The cortical discontinuity functions as a large stress raiser. In the human tibia, an open defect can reduce load to failure and ability to store energy by up to 90%.

Viscoelasticity

Many nonbiologic materials behave in a purely elastic manner. That is, the stress and strain are linearly proportional and constant. Most of the metals and ceramics that are used in orthopaedics behave in a classically elastic fashion. Polymers, on the other hand, behave differently. Polymers show a degree of rate dependence. That is, the stress developed depends not only on the strain but also on the time taken to reach that strain. This behavior of rate dependence is referred to as "viscoelasticity."

For a viscoelastic material, the stress developed depends on the strain and the time, that is, the stress–strain curve can be altered by changing the strain rate. The model frequently used to demonstrate biologic viscoelastic behavior is the earlobe (Fig. 1.28).

Using this curve as a reference one can identify three phenomena that are typical of a viscoelastic material.

Damping

This phenomenon is explained by the syringe in which the resistance or force required to move the plunger into the syringe increases as the rate of movement of the plunger increases. This property of a material, offering greater resistance as the speed is increased, is called "damping."

Creep

Following the sudden application of a given load, there is an initial deformation, followed by a subsequent additional deformation, which occurs as a function of time under the same initial load. For example, we lose some height during the course of the day. This loss of height is due to creep of the intervertebral disks. Slowly over time, they thin down; the net effect when summated is loss of height.

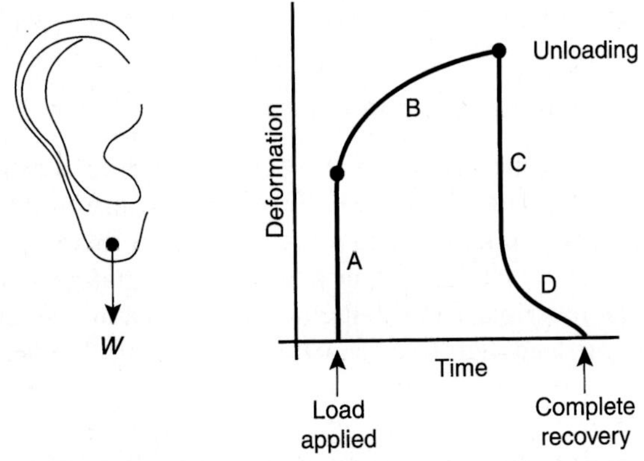

Figure 1.28 Principles of Viscoelastic behavior. As load is applied to a viscoelastic material, immediate deformation **(A)** occurs. With the load held constant, slow progressive additional deformation (creep) continues to occur with time **(B)**. When unloading occurs, there is immediate recoil **(C)**, followed by a prolonged period of stress relaxation **(D)**. (*Reprinted with permission from* Wiesel SW, Delahay JN. *Principles of Orthopaedic Medicine and Surgery.* Philadelphia, PA: Saunders, 2001.)

Relaxation

Relaxation describes a decrease in stress within a deformed structure over time, when the deformation is held constant. When a Harrington rod is used on the concave side of a scoliotic curve to straighten the spine, there is an immediate tightening of the ligamentous structures on the concavity of the curve. The stresses within those ligamentous structures lessen with time.

Mechanical Properties of Tissues

Bone

Cancellous bone is an organized, load-bearing material. By its very nature, cancellous bone is anisotropic; therefore, its behavior varies in the direction of loading. It tends to be stiffer in tension than in compression. It also fails at lower strain in the direction parallel to the axis of the spicule.

The major difference between cortical and cancellous bone is the degree of porosity. Because of its greater porosity, cancellous bone behaves very poorly during compression. Despite its ability to absorb energy upon impact, the application of significant loads will cause failure at strain rates of 0.5. At that point, crushing of the trabeculae has already begun to occur. As is the case in a vertebral body compression fracture, once a certain amount of compression and failure has occurred, the overall construct does become somewhat stiffer. This ability to become stronger with the application of compressive load is in contrast to the application of tensile load. Once yielding of cancellous bone occurs in tension, rapid fracture is likely to follow. The ability to absorb energy in tensile loading is markedly less than in compressive loading.

Cortical bone is a unique tissue. In light of its organized, mineralized structure, it is clearly designed to carry load. The classic lamellae are 3 to 4 μm thick. The haversian systems are suited and designed to withstand bending about their long axis. Cortical bone, although viscoelastic by nature, is characterized by its elastic properties, especially at low strain rates. The ability of bone to deform plastically is a function of its hydration. In the fully hydrated state, cortical bone exhibits elastic behavior up to 0.3% strain. When it is dry, bone exhibits a higher modulus in both tension and compression, but it is more brittle. Therefore, in its normal hydrated state, bone has a far greater ability to absorb strain energy. The fact that bone is viscoelastic only enhances its behavior in the mechanical environment within which it must function. This ability to behave differently at different strain rates protects the structure from failure within a wide range. The mechanical properties of bone are intimately related with its chemistry.

Articular Cartilage

The biomechanical behavior of articular cartilage can best be understood by appreciating the fact that it is a biphasic tissue. Cartilage is a fluid-filled porous medium. The chemical constituents of the organic matrix and the interstitial water interact with each other to create a unique tissue capable of impact load absorption and near frictionless interfaces. Articular cartilage is viscoelastic and therefore is capable of creep. The ability of cartilage to creep is important in the normal lubricating mechanics of diarthrodial joints. As the cartilage is loaded, fluid is expressed, creating what has been referred to as "an elastohydrodynamic mechanism of joint lubrication."

Collagenous Tissues

Ligament and tendon are essentially passive structures and inherently are not responsible for active motion. They are composed of three fiber types: collagen, elastic fibers, and reticular fibers. Both ligament and tendon function primarily in tension. Their mechanical properties are a function of the orientation of the fibers, the material properties of the fibers, and the relative proportion of collagen to elastin.

Structurally, the direction of the fibers varies between the tendon and the ligament. In tendon, the collagen bundles are parallel, as one would expect, making them the ideal tissue to withstand high tensile load. Ligament must function throughout the full range of a given joint. Therefore, the fiber orientation must be far more diverse. Typically, nonparallel arrays of collagen fibers are seen. While ligaments, like tendons, are primarily composed of collagen fibers, they contain a much larger portion of elastic fibers. The properties of the two fibers are somewhat different. Collagen is a ductile material, showing a stress–strain curve similar to that of bone. The elastic fibers show significant deformation or strain with relatively minimally applied load, but once failure occurs, it occurs quickly.

The size and shape of a ligament are critical issues in its behavior. As one would expect, the larger the cross-sectional area, the stronger the ligament. The speed of loading, as is the case with other viscoelastic biologic tissues, also plays a role in ligament failure. The anterior cruciate ligament (ACL) has been shown to function much like bone in that, as the loading rate increases, the ligament is able to store more energy prior to failure. Unfortunately, when the ligament does fail at these high rates, it tends to be within the substance of the ligament with disastrous consequences. At lower loading rates, the bony insertion of the ligament is more vulnerable and therefore the tibial spine avulsion is more likely. This data suggest that with an increase in loading rate, the strength of the bone increases more than the strength of the ligament. Hence, the ligament failure occurs at higher loading rates.

BIOMATERIALS AND IMPLANTS

In this section, the principles of biomaterials will be reviewed as they relate specifically to orthopaedic implants. Obviously, any foreign implant needs to survive in the environment in which it is placed. Biocompatibility is one of the major concerns in implant development. As implant use has become more widespread, the problems related to the strength of the implant have been carefully studied. At the present time, it is probably fair to say that most implants currently available are able to adequately withstand the loads placed upon them.

TABLE 1.5
GENERAL ADVANTAGES AND DISADVANTAGES OF STAINLESS STEEL

Advantages
- Cheap raw elements
- Good biocompatibility

Disadvantages
- Some grades not suitable for long-term implantation due to fatigue failure
- Galvanic corrosion to CoCr and titanium
- Nickel sensitivity
- Poor wear properties

Reprinted with permission from Damron TA, Morris CD, Tornetta P, et al. *Oncology and Basic Science*. Philadelphia, PA: Lippincott Williams & Wilkins, 2007.

Metals

In orthopaedic surgery, essentially, three metallic alloys are employed for implant fabrication: (a) stainless steel, (b) chrome-cobalt, and (c) titanium. Stainless steel is a mixture of primarily iron and nickel. It has the lowest yield strength of the three alloys. However, its benefit is a long plastic region of the stress–strain curve, making it the most ductile of the three materials. Therefore, it is able to absorb large amounts of strain energy prior to failure (Table 1.5). Most fracture fixation implants are fabricated from stainless steel.

Chrome–cobalt alloy has the highest UTS, and it is therefore the strongest. It also has the highest modulus of elasticity, making it the stiffest of the three materials (Table 1.6).

Titanium-based alloys include aluminum and vanadium to harden the material. These alloys have excellent corrosion resistance and good fatigue properties (Table 1.7). However, wear has been a significant problem. Their modulus is the lowest of the three alloys. Therefore, many suggest that these are the best for implant applications, because their modulus is closest to that of bone. However, it is important to realize that modulus values of none of the three are even close to the modulus value of bone. In addition, their UTS is below that of chrome-cobalt, despite the fact that their yield strength is somewhat higher. Additionally, their ability to deform plastically is limited.

The choice of a metal for a given application has historically been somewhat idiosyncratic. Depending on the application, the cost, the surgeons' prejudice, and other factors, different metals have been chosen over the years.

TABLE 1.6
GENERAL ADVANTAGES AND DISADVANTAGES OF COBALT-BASED ALLOYS

Advantages
- Good biocompatibility
- Fatigue resistant
- Wear resistant
- Low galvanic corrosion to titanium

Disadvantages
- Galvanic corrosion to stainless steel
- Concerns regarding nickel content
- Cobalt and chromium ion release
- High elastic modulus
- Expensive
- Difficult to process

Reprinted with permission from Damron TA, Morris CD, Tornetta P, et al. *Oncology and Basic Science*. Philadelphia, PA: Lippincott Williams & Wilkins, 2007.

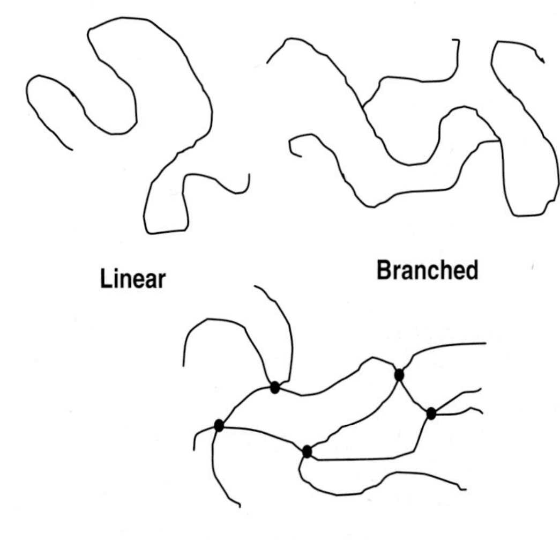

Figure 1.29 Polymer chain arrangements. (*Reprinted with permission from* Damron TA, Morris CD, Tornetta P, et al. *Oncology and Basic Science*. Philadelphia, PA: Lippincott Williams & Wilkins, 2007.)

Polymers

Ultra High Molecular Weight Polyethylene

At the present time, the polymer of choice in the fabrication of implant components is ultra high molecular weight polyethylene (UHMWPE), which is essentially a long-chain threadlike molecule of very high molecular weight chains of varying lenghts (Fig. 1.29). These chains are mesomorphic, in that they have regular atomic arrangements in some directions, but not in others. As one would expect, the polymers get stronger as the chain length increases. Strength can be improved by increasing the cross-linking. Polyethylene itself is a whole class of compounds, which differ by molecular weight, branching, density, and capacity for crystallization. In general, the higher the molecular weight, the higher the crystallinity, and the harder the product. The mechanical properties depend on the molecular weight, the density, and the crystallinity. UHMWPE is a thermoplastic resin. This means that the polymer softens with increasing temperature, making molding and manufacture feasible and allowing a superior finish to be achieved. This process is reversible with reheating of the material. This property explains the reason that implant components cannot be heat sterilized. They will distort and their properties will be altered.

TABLE 1.7
GENERAL ADVANTAGES AND DISADVANTAGES OF TITANIUM-BASED ALLOYS

Advantages
- Excellent biocompatibility
- Relatively low elastic modulus
- Spot welding to itself in taper junctions
- Low galvanic corrosion to Co–Cr–Mo alloy

Disadvantages
- Poor wear properties
- Notch sensitive
- Concern with vanadium and aluminum content in specific alloys

Reprinted with permission from Damron TA, Morris CD, Tornetta P, et al. *Oncology and Basic Science*. Philadelphia, PA: Lippincott Williams & Wilkins, 2007.

Polymethyl Methacrylate

Polymethyl methacrylate (PMM) has frequently been referred to as "cement" and is frequently used to secure orthopaedic implants. It is essentially a luting agent, which creates a mechanical interlocking bond between adjacent surfaces. A "glue" or adhesive, on the other hand, creates a chemical bond between the surfaces. PMM is supplied in the form of a white powder, which consists of small balls of PMM polymer, and a vial of monomer that contains a stabilizer to prevent polymerization until after mixing. When the monomer is mixed with the polymer, benzoyl peroxide catalyzes the process of polymerization. This particular polymeric material is a thermosetting resin. The polymerization occurs in the presence of heat. However, once the material has set, no amount of heating can reverse its configuration. The single most important factor in the setting time of PMM is the ambient temperature of the room. The cooler the room, the longer the setting time. In addition, the type of mixing, the rate of mixing, and the patient's body temperature all will alter the rate of setting.

Implant Failure

A number of mechanisms can cause the failure of a given implant. Metal, plastics, and cement are all vulnerable to

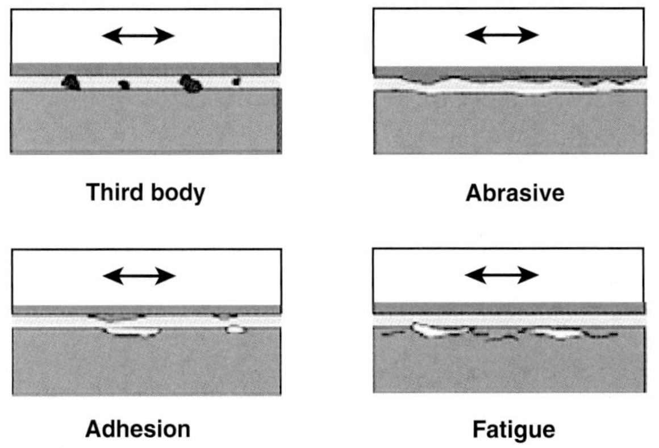

Figure 1.30 Examples of material wear. (*Reprinted with permission from* Damron TA, Morris CD, Tornetta P, et al. *Oncology and Basic Science*. Philadelphia, PA: Lippincott Williams & Wilkins, 2007.)

various types of failure. Mechanical as well as chemical breakdown of the implant can occur.

Fatigue

Most implants are made to tolerate the loads encountered below their yield point. Some implants will fail under extreme cyclic loading conditions due to the process of fatigue. Fatigue is the result of repetitive or fluctuating application of load. Each measured load application is below the yield point, but when applied cyclically, fatigue failure with crack propagation can occur. The endurance limit is that critical load below which no amount of cyclic loading will produce failure. Implants should be designed to function below the endurance limit. As loads exceed the endurance limit or are applied cyclically, fatigue of the implant may occur. Ductility does not in and of itself preclude fatigue, because only a moderate amount of plastic deformation of an implant can be tolerated before failure is seen. Imperfections in design or fabrication such as cracks, notches, impurities, and sharp angles predispose the implants to fatigue failure.

Wear

Wear is the mechanical removal of material from the surfaces in relative motion to each other (Fig. 1.30). For example, the sliding of one object over another produces wear. It is key to remember that wear is a mechanical process. When two surfaces are loaded together in intimate contact, the surface roughness or asperities create points of frictional contact. It has been demonstrated that fragments from one surface may adhere to the opposite surface. Typically, this adherence results from intermolecular actions. As the surfaces continue to rub against one another, further disruption of surface smoothness can occur. This process is referred to as "adhesive wear."

Abrasive wear occurs when a hard rough surface slides on a softer material. The harder material tends to cut grooves in the softer material. The presence of particulate debris between the surfaces that may have arisen from the process of adhesive wear accentuates the process of abrasive wear. When fragments are present between the bearing surfaces, the process is referred to as "third-body wear." As the distance over which the bearing surfaces slide will increase over time, there tends to be a volumetric increase in the number of wear particles.

Corrosion

Corrosion is the electrochemical breakdown of a metallic surface. The ionic transfer, from one metal to a more base level, produces the surface breakdown of a metallic implant. Stainless steel is the best example of the corrosion problem. If the surface coating of a metallic implant were to be disrupted, the underlying base metal is exposed to the surrounding milieu. Depending on the base metal, corrosion may then proceed. In the case of stainless steel, exposure of the base metal (iron) usually stimulates an obvious corrosive response. If extensive, blackening of the adjacent soft tissues can be seen. The surface protective layer of an implant is referred to as the "passivation layer." The coating is designed to protect the implant from a corrosion attack and is applied at the time of manufacture.

RECOMMENDED READINGS

Jazrawi LM, Kummer FJ, DiCesare PE. Alternative bearing surfaces for total joint arthroplasty. *J Am Acad Orthop Surg* 1998;6(4):198–203.

Lucas GL, Cooke FW, Friis EA. *A Primer of Biomechanics*. New York, NY: Springer, 1998.

Schmalzried TP, Callahan JJ. Current concepts review: wear in total hip and knee replacements. *JBJS Am* 1999;81:115–136.

2

Epidemiology and Biostatistics in Orthopaedic Surgery

Keith D. Baldwin ***G. Russell Huffman***

INTRODUCTION

Epidemiology, biostatistics, and evidence-based medicine are the tools by which new knowledge is attained and incorporated into the practice of orthopaedic surgery. The methodology that these fields utilize is applied in everyday practice. It is therefore critically important that the orthopaedic surgeon be familiar with the tools and methods of biostatistics in order to critically evaluate available evidence surrounding the diagnosis and treatment of orthopaedic populations and musculoskeletal disease.

Epidemiology is the study of the distribution and risk factors for disease. ***Biostatistics*** is the application of statistical or mathematical methods to the collection, organization, and interpretation of clinically relevant biological, medical, or functional data. ***Evidence-Based Medicine*** is the practice of applying the results of scientific studies to the practice of medicine in general, and orthopaedic surgery in specific. ***Inference*** is the derivation of logical conclusions from existing knowledge regarding a specific condition. Biostatistical procedures allow inferences to be made with a quantifiable certainty. Inferences are made regarding probable causes and associations with disease, success of treatments, and factors that may influence a specific condition. This provides the framework of epidemiological study.

DATA

Data are a collection of facts from which conclusions may be drawn or derived. Data are used during patient interviews in order to make treatment decisions. Data can be used to decide what car to buy or, alternatively, which specific treatment option is most appropriate. In the realm of biomedical study, data can be classified into three types: continuous, ordinal, or categorical. The type of data that exists in a data set will in large part determine which statisitical tests are appropriate for data analysis.

VARIABLES

Information acquired for a given characteristic of a unit of interest (most often a patient in clinical studies) can be referred to as a "variable." For example, in a study of patients with proximal humerus fractures, one may be interested in knowing the age of the patient, the gender of the patient, how many "parts" the fracture was, whether or not the patient was a smoker, what the occupation of the patient was, and whether or not the patient was treated operatively. Each defined parameter is gathered and then recorded in a database for subsequent analysis. For the above example, suppose the variable of interest is time until union. Various statistical tests may be used to assess for an association between the variable of interest and the other variables in the study, such as age of the patient or number of "parts" in the fracture.

Independent variables are variables that determine (or are thought to determine) the value of the dependent variable according to their value. In an experimental design, the independent variable of interest is under the control of the researcher (operative versus nonoperative treatment of proximal humerus fractures). ***Dependent variables*** are variables of interest that are thought to be affected in some way by the independent variable(s) (e.g., time to union in the above example). ***Confounders*** are variables that may be related in some way to both dependent and independent variables and, therefore, may affect the size of the relationship between the dependent and independent variable(s) (e.g., four-part proximal humerus fractures may be more likely to get surgery, but also may be more likely to have delayed or nonunion). In addition, other factors such as smoking and increasing age may put patients at a higher risk for both the dependent variable (nonunion) and the independent variable (a fracture requiring surgery).

TYPES OF DATA

Data are organized by whether they are strictly numeric (continuous), ordered (ordinal), or categorical (qualitative). ***Continuous variables*** are numeric values where the data can theoretically take any value within a range of values. Numbers such as range of motion, newtons of force, and temperature can be considered continuous. For comparing two different treatments or populations with continuous variables, the Student's t test can be used for statistical analysis. For three or more groups with continuous variables, the analysis of variance (ANOVA) test can be used, and for comparing one group to itself at a later date, the paired t test can be used. ***Ordinal variables*** are data that are represented in an ordered (valued) fashion, but in which there is no specific scale by which the values differ. These data are represented by integers (i.e., 1, 2, 3, ...). A prime example of ordinal data in orthopaedic surgery is the pain scale. Typically, nonparametric tests are appropriate for statistical analysis of this type of data, as they are often not normally distributed. The Mann–Whitney U test is appropriate for two independent groups, the Kruskal–Wallis test is appropriate for more than two groups, and the Wilcoxin Signed-Rank test is often appropriate for paired or test–retest data. ***Categorical (Nominal) variables*** are qualitative categories in which there is no specific value assigned to the data, but the data differ in some qualitative way. For example, suppose one wanted to compare injury rates in the NBA, one may break the players down by position. Each position has no inherent value, but they differ from each other in some qualitative way. A special type of categorical data is the ***binary variable***, a variable in which a patient either has or doesn't have a certain characteristic, for example, that patient is either alive or dead, got treatment A or did not, and played or did not play. Fisher's exact test may be used to compare two categorical groups, Pearson's chi-square test may be used to compare two or more groups, and McNemar's test can be used for paired variables.

DATA DISTRIBUTION

Continuous data may be parametric or nonparametric. ***Nonparametric*** data are data in which the distribution of the population values is not similar to any specific standard distribution. ***Parametric***, or distributional, data can often be described by one mathematical equation. These equations assume that the population from which the sample came is distributed similar to a standard distribution. The most common distribution that data follows is a Gaussian, or "normal," distribution. This distribution is bell shaped and is illustrated by Figure 2.1.

The y axis ($f(x)$) represents the probability (or percentage frequency) of observing a certain value. The x axis represents the range of potential values. The area under the curve is equal to 1 and is the cumulative probability of observing any value under the curve. The mean value is assumed to be the apex of the curve. In a normal distribution, 95% of values fall within ±2 standard deviations (SD) of the population mean; this represents the ***95% confidence interval***. Furthermore, 69% of values fall within ±1 SD, and 99% of values fall within ±3 SD. In a normal distribution, mean, median, and mode are all equivalent. In general, the ***mean*** is the sum of all observations divided by the number of observations (the average). The ***median*** value is the 50th percentile value, or the value under which half of the observations occur. For nonparametric data, median values are more robust because they are not influenced by outliers (the skewness of the data) to as great a degree. The ***mode*** is the most frequently observed value. Chi-square distribution and the binomial (logit function) distribution are other standard distributions used to make inferences about data. ***Skewness*** represents more data being clustered in low values of x or high values of x, in other words, an asymmetry in the data (Fig. 2.2). ***Kurtosis*** is when the data are more or less peaked than normal (more or less close to the mean). Statistical tests for skewness and kurtosis are available in most commercially available statistical packages to determine whether or not parametric testing is appropriate.

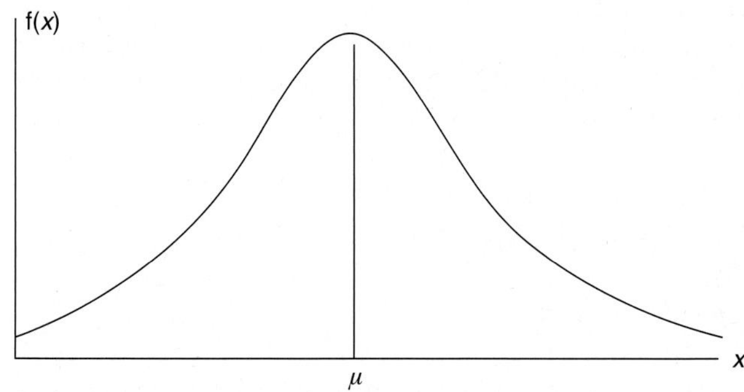

Figure 2.1 The normal distribution.

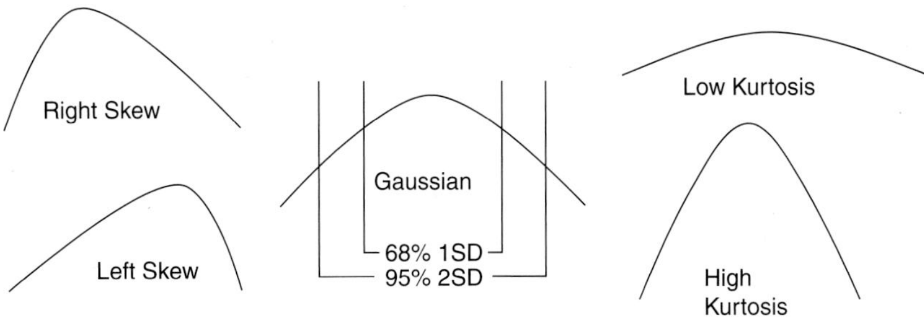

Figure 2.2 Skewness and kurtosis.

INFERENCE

The main purpose of biomedical research is to help us gain knowledge about the truth or reality of a clinical problem. This is the purpose of inference, a systematic usage of data to derive a broader conclusion. By using statistical methods, we can draw conclusions about populations on the basis of a sample drawn from that population. Our ability to do this can be compromised by error. ***Systematic error*** is error that can be characterized by bias, confounding, or chance. ***Random error*** is error built into measurement tools due to imperfection of the tool being used. Systematic error can be minimized by rigorous study design and attention to detail. Random error often cannot be controlled for unless a better test with more precise measurements is available. Alternatively, random error (or chance) may be diminished by increasing the size of the sample studied so that it more closely resembles the entire population about which an inference is made. Our confidence in inference derived from statistical tests is measured by a studies' power and by the ability to reject the null hypothesis.

ERRORS IN INFERENCE

Bias is a nonrandom systematic error in the design or execution of a study that may result in mistaken inference about association of causation between the independent and dependent variables. There are a few common types of bias about which every researcher should be aware. ***Selection bias*** involves situations in which two groups differ in some significant way other than the independent variable of interest. For example, suppose a study was conducted in which union rates were observed for two different treatments of tibial fractures. Now suppose one group had more women and the other had more men, there is selection bias between treatments that leads to a potential for ***confounding*** of the effect of treatment method on union rate by sex of the patient; this bias may be minimized by randomization or matching controls. ***Recall bias*** is common in retrospective studies, and it can occur when a patient is asked to remember qualities about his or her condition at some point in the past. The patient may not remember his or her story perfectly. This bias may be minimized by controls, so that at least bias is consistent, or by performing prospective studies in which all pertinent data are recorded as these occur. ***Measurement bias*** can be noted if an investigator asks questions, or records data, in such a way that more accurate data are collected in one treatment group (i.e., surgical) than in another group (i.e., nonsurgical). This bias can be minimized by blinding researchers to the treatment type or by having independent reviewers. ***Sampling bias*** occurs when patients in the sample are significantly different, in some crucial ways, from the population in which the researcher is interested in making inferences. This may lead to a decrease in ***external validity*** or generalizability of results to populations outside the study sample. ***Publication bias*** is noted when published studies tend to have a greater effect size than all completed studies. Another type of publication bias is publication of only positive or significant results. This can be assessed for during meta-analysis using funnel plots (Fig. 2.3). ***Missing data***, or ***nonresponse bias***, can lead to its own special types of challenges. Most commercially available software packages deal with missing data by ***listwise deletion***. That is to say, if a patient is missing any parameter, then that patient is eliminated for the purposes of analysis. If the data are missing completely at random, this method of dealing with missing data is probably the most robust and does not introduce additional bias into the study, but it does decrease power by making the sample size smaller. Essentially, you are left with a subsample of the original sample. When the data are not missing completely at random, it is often necessary to employ a statistician to perform special tests on the data to determine the most appropriate way to deal with the missing data.

Confounders are variables that have an association with both the independent and dependent variables of a study. Variables such as age, gender, socioeconomic status, medical comorbidities, and injury severity are common examples of confounders. Suppose an investigator wants to determine whether a cemented or cementless implant has greater longevity. The researcher would need to factor in by statistical adjustment, matching, or randomization age and activity level; otherwise, the effect may be confounded by these factors (Table 2.1). When the study is retrospective, there should be a demographic table that clearly evaluates potential confounders, and if there is a difference, consideration should be made to statistically adjust for confounding

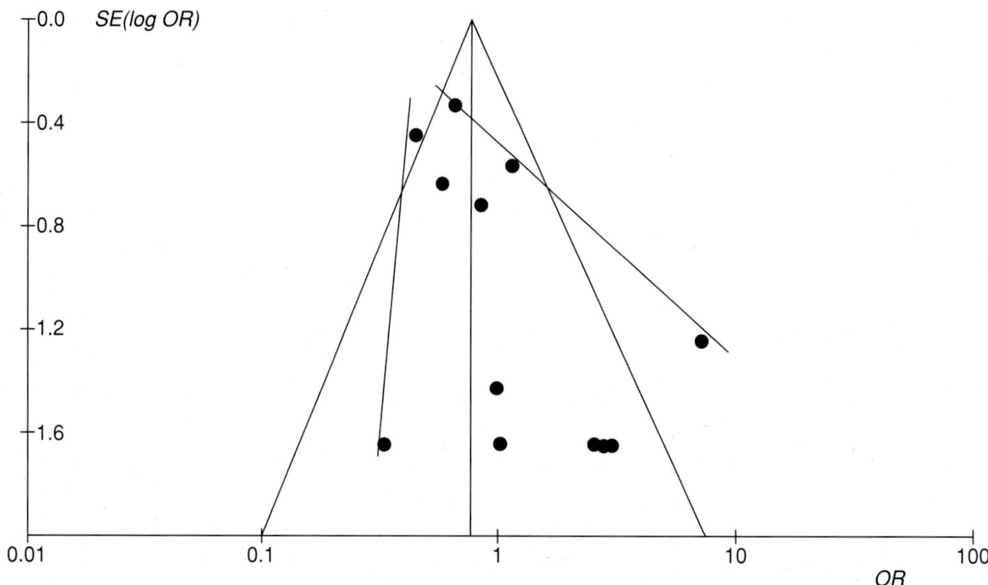

Figure 2.3 An example of a funnel plot demonstrating publication bias.

by using suitable statistical methods (i.e., multivariate analysis, stratification, or matching). Randomized trials eliminate confounders if the sample sizes are adequate, but confounding variables should still be screened for potential confounding.

Chance is the probability that two unrelated events will seem related by random occurrence or vice versa. Chance can take two forms. *Type I error* is the conclusion that a true association between variables exist when in reality there is no difference. *Type II error* is the probability of failing to find an association when one actually exists (Table 2.2). If multiple comparisons are being performed, it is important to adjust for multiple tests in order to not inflate the type I error.

METHODS FOR CONTROLLING SELECTION BIAS

Selection bias can be controlled in the design or analysis phase of the study. In the design phase, selection bias can be controlled by randomization, restriction, or matching. *Randomization* involves the random assignment of patients into each arm of the study; with appropriate design, each patient has an equal chance of being in each arm of the study. *Restriction* involves limiting which patients are eligible for the study (i.e., inclusion and exclusion criteria). *Matching* involves intentionally selecting patients who are similar to one another in each known confounder, but who are different in the outcome of interest in order to determine important associated risk factors for that given outcome (i.e., case-control study design).

In the analysis phase of the study, stratification, simple adjustment, or multivariate techniques can be used to adjust for confounders. *Stratification* involves comparing subgroups of patients; for example, comparing operative versus nonoperative fracture care, one may opt to stratify by severity. *Simple adjustment* involves adjusting effect measures for strata of patients by some confounder. *Multivariate analysis* allows for adjustment by multiple factors at once.

TABLE 2.1
AGE AND GENDER BY IMPLANT TYPE

Factor	Cemented	Uncemented	P value
Age	67	66	.48
Gender (% female)	56	54	.45

Example of potential confounders in which there is no evidence of association between independent factors that are also associated with the outcome of interest (longevity of implant).

TABLE 2.2
THE RELATIONSHIP BETWEEN TYPE I AND TYPE II ERROR

	Study Shows Association	Study Shows No Association
True association	Study is accurate ($p = 1 - \alpha$)	Type II error ($p = \beta$)
No association	Type I error ($p = \alpha$)	Study is accurate ($p = 1 - \beta$)

A WORD ABOUT CAUSALITY

Most often in epidemiological studies, we observe associations not causes. For causality to be assigned, a number of factors, first described by Sir Bradford Hill, must be satisfied.

1. *Temporality*: Cause precedes effect
2. *Strength*: Large effect size (relative risk, odds ratio, hazard ratio)
3. *Dose response*: Larger dose, higher/more likely effect
4. *Reversibility*: Reduction in exposure associated with decreased disease
5. *Consistency*: Repeatedly observed by different researchers in time and space
6. *Biologic plausibility*: Reasonable based on current knowledge
7. *Specificity*: One cause, one effect
8. *Analogy*: Similar cause and effect exist for a similar disease/exposure pair

Often we do not observe causality but we do recognize associations.

STUDY DESIGN AND EVIDENCE-BASED MEDICINE

Overview

Evidence-based medicine is the conscientious usage of the most convincing literature to make decisions in the care of individual patients. The best information is attained through epidemiologic and scientific studies from which inferences are made. The more rigorous the design and the more diligent the control of error, the more meaningful a specific study is. An outline of the levels of evidence is presented Table 2.3.

Observational Versus Experimental Studies

The more thorough one is in controlling for confounding and bias, the more confident one can be in drawing conclusions and making inferences about the general population. Broadly, research can be divided into observational and experimental research. The majority of orthopaedic research is observational. ***Descriptive observational studies*** include case reports, case series, and cross-sectional studies; these studies are easy to perform but somewhat vulnerable to bias due to lack of controls. ***Case studies*** are reports of individual patient treatment and outcomes. ***Case series*** are a number of patients (>1) who had similar treatment but without controls with whom to compare them. ***Cross-sectional studies*** are a snapshot in time that can determine what the prevalence of a disease is and the demographic or personal medical characteristics of patients who tend to present with a disease they have. These studies are unable to demonstrate causality; however, these can show strong associations and can often lay the groundwork for more sophisticated prospective or experimental designs.

Analytic observational studies are often retrospective but can provide useful information regarding associations predictive of an outcome of interest. ***Case-control studies*** are studies in which cases are chosen by outcome, and a similar set of controls without that outcome are chosen to determine if there are certain factors that are associated with the disease. In case-control studies, cases are chosen by dependent variable (failure of fixation, success, or disease of interest), so this type of design is particularly useful and

TABLE 2.3
LEVELS OF EVIDENCE

Level*	Therapeutic	Prognostic	Diagnostic
I	High-quality RCT, narrow confidence intervals, >80% follow-up	High-quality prospective study where all patients enrolled at same point in disease, 80% follow-up	Testing of previously developed diagnostic criteria with consecutive patients with gold standard reference
II	Lesser-quality RCT <80% follow-up, no blinding, improper randomization, etc.	Retrospective study, untreated controls from an RCT, lesser-quality prospective study (e.g., patients enrolled at different points in their disease, <80% follow-up)	Development of diagnostic criteria on consecutive patients with universally applied gold standard
III	Case-control study, retrospective comparative study	Case-control study	Study of nonconsecutive patients without gold standard
IV	Case series	Case series	Case-control study
V	Expert opinion	Expert opinion	Expert opinion

RCT, randomized clinical trials
*A systematic review of any level of evidence is equal to that level of evidence. Data from *Clinical Orthopaedics and Related Research* (http://www.clinorthop.org/library/Downloads/levels_oe.doc).

efficient when the disease of interest is rare. ***Cohort studies*** are studies in which the groups are chosen by the exposure or treatment and subsequently followed to observe an outcome of interest. These studies may be prospective or retrospective. In cohort studies, exposure is monitored, and then patients are followed for outcome, so they are useful in cases where the exposure is rare or of particular interest to the researcher. In this manner, exposure may be assessed statistically to determine the risk of subsequent disease or outcome development. ***Meta-analysis*** is used when there are a number of similar studies describing the same phenomenon, or analyzing the same treatment, disease, or outcome, but each individual study is of insufficient power to stand alone. Meta-analysis may also be used to analyze the state of current knowledge, or to trace changes in practice over time. Analytic observational studies are useful because there is no preset allocation of treatment groups, they are often easier and cheaper to perform than prospective studies, and, if done properly, can make inferences about causality. These studies can also provide background information for designing experimental or future prospective observational studies.

Observational studies can be prospective or retrospective depending on the line of inquiry. In ***retrospective*** studies, the inquiry begins with the outcome of interest and attempts to elucidate a risk factor or exposure that may be associated with that outcome. Prospective studies begin typically with the exposure of interest and follow patients over time to determine outcomes. It should be noted that a study that starts with an exposure or treatment may be retrospective if patients with that treatment in the past are reviewed for outcomes that are already documented (Fig. 2.4)

The prime example of an ***experimental study*** is the ***randomized clinical trial***. These studies are ideal for evaluating treatment efficacy but tend to be expensive and time and labor intensive.

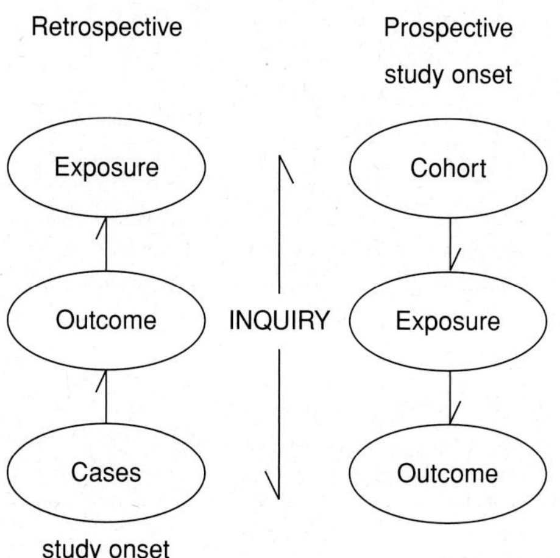

Figure 2.4 Direction of inquiry for prospective and retrospective studies.

DESCRIPTION OF STUDY TYPES

A *case series* is a retrospective observational descriptive account of a group of patients with an interesting treatment, condition, or constellation of symptoms. These studies are typically useful for hypothesis generation, or to show feasibility or safety of a treatment. A new technique can be described with outcomes of that technique. This type of study typically may provide the framework for more sophisticated studies. An example of this type of study was John Charnley's description of the usage of methyl methacrylate cement for securing components in total hip arthroplasty. This paper helped convince surgeons of its utility, safety, and effectiveness. Case series are inexpensive, useful to describe novel treatments and complication rates, and provide background data for future studies. However, because no control group exists, they are vulnerable to confounding and bias. Inferences that can be drawn are limited because there is no hypothesis being tested. Case series provide level IV evidence.

A ***cross-sectional study*** is an observational/descriptive technique that is essentially a "snapshot" in time of a population. One may ascertain the distribution of an outcome or risk factor in a population. Population-based normative data can also be generated using cross-sectional studies. These studies are quick, data that may be extrapolated to a larger population can be gained, and associations may be observed. In addition, baseline information on demographics, normative characteristics, or baseline disease data can be collected. A cross-sectional study can provide information on ***prevalence*** of a disease, but not on ***incidence***. Prevalence is equal to the total number of cases at a time divided by the total population at risk, whereas incidence is equal to the number of new cases that develop divided by the population or sample at risk over that time period. Sampling error may limit the external validity of these studies. Cross-sectional studies are typically level IV evidence of demography, epidemiology, or normative values to be used for power calculations, or as baseline data preferably in prospectively designed studies.

A ***case-control study*** is a retrospective observational/analytical study in which patients with a given outcome (cases) are compared with patients who lack that outcome (controls), to determine associations with the outcome of interest. The outcomes of interest are typically rare, and results are often reported as an odds ratio, or the odds of a case being exposed compared to the odds of a control being exposed to the same factor. For example, suppose we wanted to compare patients with nonunions to patients with united fractures for exposure to nonsteroidal anti-inflammatory drugs (NSAIDs). This could be done through a case-control design. The case-control model is efficient for rare outcomes and is inexpensive. Weaknesses of this model include difficulty in finding appropriate controls and incomplete medical records. Controls should be matched, or multivariate analysis should be conducted to adjust for confounding. Significant bias in the form of recall, reporting, or sampling bias can exist. These studies are typically level III or IV evidence depending on the sophistication of the study design and analysis.

Prospective cohorts are observational analytical studies that follow a population with a specific exposure or treatment over time to identify outcomes of interest. The Framingham Heart study is one of the more famous cohort studies that investigated the risk factors for heart disease. Cohorts can estimate disease incidence, evaluate a disease's course or natural history, and identify risk factors. The cohort study has the ability to identify nested case-control studies within the cohort (i.e., an interim outcome is identified and studied). The power of the study increases with increasing disease frequency (number of patients with the outcome of interest). Cohorts are however expensive and labor intensive, often require multiyear grants and a comprehensive data collection system, and are susceptible to bias, error, confounding, and loss of follow-up. Typically, the effect measure is reported as a relative risk, that is, the risk of an exposed individual to develop the disease compared with the risk of the unexposed individual to develop the disease. Typically, prospective cohorts are level II to III evidence depending on sophistication, data collection method, and rate of follow-up.

Randomized clinical trials (RCTs) are experimental studies that involve usage of concurrent (RCT), sequential (crossover), or historical controls. The gold standard RCT is the randomized double-blind, placebo-controlled trial. RCTs require a protocol that establishes eligibility (inclusion and exclusion criteria), sample size (a power analysis), randomization (to minimize bias and confounders), blinding (to minimize performance, detection, and interviewer bias), stopping rules, monitoring for compliance, safety assessment, and intention to treat analysis to minimize nonresponder bias. Although these studies are the gold standard of biomedical research, these are extremely expensive and logistically difficult. Ethically, these studies require the optimal treatment to be truly unknown. The level of evidence is I or II depending on the above listed factors, type of randomization, and patient retention (>90% for level I). Randomized clinical trials have excellent internal validity, because the result occurred under ideal experimental conditions. It is also important to note that if inclusion and exclusion criteria are too stringent, a clinical trial may have very poor external validity (may be poorly generalizable to the population as a whole).

In addition to observational and experimental studies, reviews are another form of research. Expert opinion is level V evidence, but it is a form of review based on expert experience. ***Systematic reviews*** (level IIa and IIIa) are an evidence-based summary of the literature that uses a complete search and critical analysis of the study. If the studies involved are level III evidence, then the systematic review is also level III. ***Meta-analysis*** is the process by which qualitative methods are applied to compile the results of several independent studies to produce summary statistics. A true meta-analysis contains only those studies that are homogeneous with respect to inclusive criteria and outcomes of interest. Forest plots can show the summary effects of data collected from multiple studies. Q tests can be used to assess for heterogeneity of studies in clinical treatment, methodology, or measured effect. Lastly, publication bias should be investigated. Funnel plots are useful to detect general publication bias; other special tests can be used to detect publication bias by date or geographic location.

HYPOTHESIS TESTING

The classic approach to determine ***statistical significance*** is to compare observed findings with expected findings. This comparison allows one to determine if an outcome could have occurred simply by chance. The comparison between treatments or between a risk factor and an outcome typically takes on the null hypothesis that there is no difference between treatments or there is no association between a risk factor (independent variable) and a condition (dependent variable). The alternative hypothesis states that there is a true difference between the groups. Type I error exists if one finds no difference/association when there truly is one, and a type II error exists if one finds a difference where none exists (Table 2.2). Where multiple hypotheses exist, one must adjust the type I error to account for that number of multiple tests, otherwise the type I error will cumulatively increase with increasing numbers of hypotheses.

P values are the probability of an event occurring by chance alone; these values are the result of the statistical test that is performed. The p value is a measure of the strength of the evidence in favor of the null hypothesis. If $p > \alpha$, then the null hypothesis may be rejected. P values do not provide units, are not a measure of the strength of an association, and there is little inherent precision to a p value. Similarly, the p value does not convey practical significance but rather an observed probability based on the sample studied. ***Confidence intervals*** are constructed around a mean, and if the result is statistically significant, the intervals do not overlap or, in the case of odds ratios, do not include one. These confidence intervals are based on the alpha levels determined at study onset. These values are more precise than p values because these provide a range of values. Alpha is the probability of concluding that two things are different when in fact they are not. The lower the α, the more rigorous the criteria are for rejecting the null hypothesis, and the less likely a researcher is to conclude that there is a difference when that difference was the result of chance alone. The most common α is 0.05; at that level, the probability of making a type I error (concluding there is a difference when there is none is 1 in 20). β is the probability of making a type II error, that is, concluding there is no difference when in fact there is. ***Power*** is $1-\beta$. When a study demonstrates that there is a significant difference,

TABLE 2.4
STATISTICAL TESTS AND SETTINGS OF USE

Type of Data	Number of Groups	Independent	Paired
Continuous normal	2	Student's *t* test	Paired *t* test
Continuous not normal	2	Mann–Whitney *U* test	Wilcoxin signed rank test
Continuous normal	>2	ANOVA	Repeated-measures ANOVA
Continuous not normal	>2	Kruskal–Wallis test	Friedman test
Ordinal	2	Mann–Whitney *U* test	Wilcoxin signed rank test
Ordinal	>2	Kruskal–Wallis test	Friedman test
Nominal	2	Fisher test	McNemar test
Nominal	>2	Pearson chi square	Cochran Q test
Survival	2/>2	Log-rank statistic	Conditional logistic regression

ANOVA, analysis of variance.

there is a potential to make a type I error, and when there is no difference, there is a possibility of making a type II error. That possibility is increased if the study is underpowered, and so if a study shows no difference, a power analysis should be reported. Statistical tests are ways of determining the probability of making a type I error (Table 2.4).

Specific statistical tests can be used to measure association or difference. The following tests determine the significance of a difference:

- Chi-square (X^2) test compares observed versus expected proportions.
- Fisher's exact test compares proportions for a small number of observations (where there is a cell with <5).
- Mann-Whitney *U* test compares median values.
- Student's *t* test compares mean values.
- ANOVA compares two or more means.

The following tests are used to describe or measure agreement:

- Regression coefficient: Association between an independent and dependent variable;
- Pearson's *r*: Association between two variables; and
- Cohen's kappa: A measure of agreement between or within observers, values range from 0 (completely chance) to 1 (perfect agreement).

Power analysis is essential to determine how many patients are necessary to detect the difference a researcher is interested in. If the researcher sets the difference at the minimum clinically important difference, if no difference is detected, it is safe to say that there is no clinically important difference between groups. The elements of a power analysis are the type I error rate that is acceptable, the type II error rate that is acceptable, the variance of the expected mean, the sample size, and an entity called the delta (effect size). ***Delta*** is the minimum detectable change. In many cases, the variance will be unknown, and an effect size is estimated on the basis of what the researcher considers to be clinically important. In general, post hoc power analysis should be avoided, because at the end of the study, the power has already been determined by the number of patients enrolled.

Clinical significance is distinct from statistical significance. A study can find a statistically significant result, but the magnitude of difference, or the parameter studied, may not matter practically or clinically. If a study has a large sample size, a statistical difference may be detected, but that difference may not be clinically important. For example, suppose two techniques for measuring leg lengths following total hip arthroplasty are available, and the two methods differ by 0.1 mm, but because of the number of patients or precision of instruments, the statistical difference is found to have a p value of .001. It could be said that the difference between these two methods is highly statistically significant but do not demonstrate clinically important differences.

Measures of Effect

Other tests are used to give information about the association between variables. Unadjusted tests include probability, odds, odds ratio, relative risk, and hazard ratio. ***Probability*** takes the form of a value between 0 and 1 and represents the likelihood of an event happening on the basis of the number of events over the number of trials; for example, tossing a coin should have a probability of 0.5. ***Odds*** are the probability of observing an event in a trial over the probability of not observing that event; for a coin toss, odds would be equal to 0.5/0.5 or 1. The ***odds ratio*** represents the odds of exposure to a risk factor between a case group and a control group. The relative risk represents the incidence of disease in an exposed population over the incidence of disease in an unexposed population. The ***hazard ratio*** compares two groups in terms of the risk of an event occurring in a particular period of time. Hazard ratios can be calculated with Kaplan–Meier survival analysis. Many

TABLE 2.5
UNIVARIATE AND MULTIVARIATE ANALYSIS

Outcome	Univariate	Multivariate
Continuous	Pearson's *r*	Linear regression
Binary	Odds ratio	Logistic regression
Time series	Hazard ratio (Kaplan Meier)	Cox regression

of the measures of association or effect measures can be adjusted to take into account multiple confounders. This process is called ***multivariate analysis*** (Table 2.5). Multivariate analysis often involves complicated procedures and post hoc analysis, and performance of these tests should involve someone familiar with their execution.

TEST CHARACTERISTICS

Often times in medicine, it is beneficial to develop a test to diagnose a condition. When developing such a test it is often compared to a "gold standard." Gold standard tests typically have excellent ability to diagnose conditions but are often expensive, invasive, or otherwise inconvenient; for example, the gold standard for diagnosing meniscus tears is arthroscopy, but arthroscopy is invasive and is not always indicated. It is therefore desirable to find an alternative test. These alternative tests are often compared to the gold standard for sensitivity, specificity, positive predictive value, and negative predictive value. ***Sensitivity*** is the ability of a test to detect a condition when it is present; thus, mathematically, it is the number of true positives over the number of true positives plus false negatives (or all positive tests). ***Specificity*** is the ability of a test to not falsely assign a well person as sick; thus, mathematically, it is the number of true negatives over all negative tests (true negatives plus false positives). ***Positive predictive value*** is the probability of having the disease with a positive test; it is therefore represented by true positives over all positive tests. ***Negative predictive value*** is the probability of not having the disease with a negative test, and it is therefore equal to true negatives over all negative tests. Sensitivity and specificity are often a trade off; for example, suppose the fasting level of blood sugar necessary to diagnose diabetes was dropped to 80, then the sensitivity would be nearly 100%, we would diagnose 100% of diabetes, but we would falsely diagnose more patients; thus, the specificity would drop this paradox and can be represented graphically with a ***receiver operator curve*** (Fig. 2.5). An example of this is where it is desirable to figure out how many white blood cells in a total joint constitute an infection. If the cutoff is too low, too many people will have needless surgery; if it is too high, too many infections will be missed. In addition, it is important to note that positive predictive value will be low if the prevalence is low

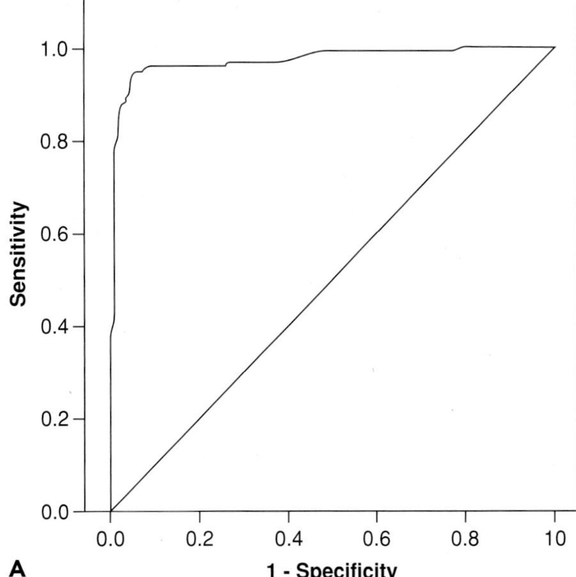

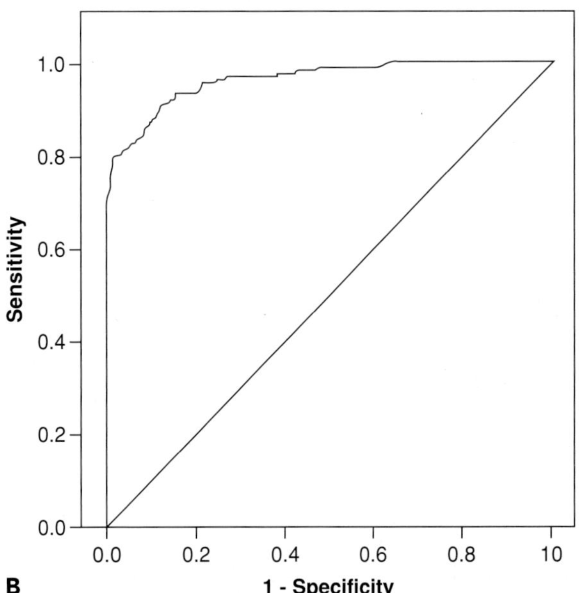

Figure 2.5 Reciever operating curves for predicting periprosthetic infection. An area under the curve of 1 demonstrates an ideal test with a 100% sensitivity and specificity, whereas an area under the curve of less than 0.5 indicates that the diagnostic has poor discriminatory value. **(A)** The cutoff value for optimal accuracy in diagnosis of PJI was 1100 cells/L for fluid leukocyte count. **(B)** The cutoff value for optimal accuracy for fluid neutrophil differential was 64%. When both tests yielded results below their cutoff values, the negative predictive value of the combination increased to 99.6%, whereas if both tests were greater than their cutoff values the positive predictive value improved to 100%. (*Redrawn with permission from* Parvizi J, Ghanem E, Sharkey P, Aggarwal A, Burnett SJ, Barrack RL. Diagnosis of infected total knee: findings of a multicenter database. *Clin Orthop Relat Res.* 2008;466(11):2628–2633.)

even if sensitivity and specificity are high, because it is likely that any positive will be a false positive. This is the rationale behind selective screening. Suppose, we wanted to screen everyone for lung cancer with a chest x-ray. The prevalence of lung cancer in the general population is relatively low, so any positive result would likely be a false positive. If we restrict the screening tool to smokers with hemoptysis, the predictive value would get much higher because the prevalence in that population would be higher.

HEALTH OUTCOMES RESEARCH

The American Academy of Orthopaedic Surgeons and other organizations have created ***musculoskeletal outcomes instruments*** to collect standardized patient data to assess and compare treatment modalities and regimens. These instruments have been validated, and many have normative scores available for the purposes of power analysis and comparison. Examples of such scores include the Hip Society Score, the Knee Society Score, the DASH, Pediatric Outcomes Data Collection Instrument, and the ASES (American Shoulder and Elbow Surgeons) subjective shoulder scale. ***General health outcome*** instruments measure general health and well-being, the most common is the SF-36. ***Visual analog scales*** can be used to measure patient satisfaction, pain, and general outcome.

RECOMMENDED READINGS

Abel U, Koch A. The role of randomization in clinical studies: myths and beliefs. *J Clin Epidemiol.* 1999;52;487–489.

Benson K, Hartz AJ. A comparison of observational studies and randomized controlled trials. *N Engl J Med.* 2000;342:1878–1886.

Bernstein J, McGuire K, Freedman KB. Statistical sampling and hypothesis testing in orthopaedic research. *Clin Orthop Relat Res.* 2003;413:55–62.

Bernstein J. Evidence-based medicine. *J Am Acad Orthop Surg.* 2004; 12(2):80–88.

Freedman KB, Back S, Bernstein J. Sample size and statistical power of randomized controlled trials in orthopaedics. *J Bone Joint Surg Br.* 2001;83(3):397–402.

Hunsacker FG, Cioffi DA, Amadio PC, Wright JG, Caughlin B. The American Academy of Orthopaedic Surgeons outcomes instruments: normative values from the general population. *J Bone Joint Surg Am.* 2002;84(2):208–215.

Kocher MS, Zurakowski D. Clinical epidemiology and biostatistic: a primer for orthopaedic surgeons. *J Bone Joint Surg Am.* 2004; 86-A(3):607–620.

Imaging in Orthopaedic Surgery

3

Turner Vosseller ***John N. Delahay***

This chapter will offer a brief introduction into the major imaging modalities used in orthopaedic surgery. The most basic medium of imaging remains plain radiography, which can provide a wealth of information quickly for relatively little cost. In the past 30 years, the imaging repertoire available to the orthopaedic surgeon has expanded greatly, with the advent and widespread availability of computed tomography (CT) scans and magnetic resonance imaging (MRI). Ultrasonography, nuclear scintigraphy, and bone densitometry are also commonly used in the evaluation of musculoskeletal disease. Finally, a brief discussion of safety and radiation exposure to the orthopaedic surgeon is included.

PLAIN RADIOGRAPHY

As stated above, plain radiography is the most commonly used imaging test in the evaluation of orthopaedic trauma and musculoskeletal pain. It gives excellent visualization of the osseous anatomy as well as some indirect information about the surrounding soft tissues. Because of their ease of acquisition and low cost, plain x-rays are almost always the first step in the imaging workup, and diagnostic errors can occur when they are omitted.

When evaluating plain x-rays, it is important to remember that the image is a two-dimensional representation of a three-dimensional structure. On a single x-ray view, displacement of a fracture in only two out of the three possible planes of displacement is visualized. For example, an anteroposterior (AP) view of the wrist demonstrates displacement in the medial lateral plane and the superior–inferior plane but does not provide any information regarding displacement in the AP plane. In order to evaluate displacement in the AP plane, a second film that is orthogonal to the first must be obtained. A lateral view of the wrist will demonstrate the AP displacement as well as superior–inferior displacement.

For the distal joints and extremities, obtaining the two orthogonal views is easily accomplished by rotating either the extremity or the x-ray beam 90 degrees. For the more proximal joints, such as the hip and shoulder, this is not possible, so special radiographic views have been developed to provide the necessary information. In addition to these views, a number of special techniques have been developed to better visualize structures that are not well seen on routine AP and lateral radiographs. The following sections contain a description of many of these special views used in the evaluation of each of the major anatomic regions of the body. Illustrations of many of the techniques described, as well as example radiographs, are contained in the later chapters in this book that cover the orthopaedic subspecialties. The reader is also encouraged to seek out other texts that are dedicated specifically to orthopaedic imaging for more detailed descriptions of radiographic positioning and techniques.

Cervical Spine

The routine trauma series of the cervical spine includes a ***lateral view***, an ***AP view***, and an ***open mouth odontiod view***. The lateral view is improved by pulling down on the patient's arms; traction should never be placed on the head. A ***swimmer's view*** may be necessary if the entire cervical spine down to the C7-T1 disk space is not visualized on the lateral view. This view is obtained with one of the patient's arms raised and the other at the patient's side. Soft-tissue swelling can be indicative of injury in the absence of obvious bony deformity. The general rule is 6 mm of soft-tissue swelling at C2 and 22 mm of soft-tissue swelling at C6 is indicative of pathology.

The utility of trauma oblique views, performed with the patient supine, is arguable, and they are not routinely obtained to "clear" the cervical spine. They may be effective in high-risk settings, in which a better evaluation of the articular pillars and the C2 segment can be made. Oblique views are most useful if a trauma table with an articulated C-arm is available, or if they are done upright, which is possible only in low-risk cases.

Lateral views of the cervical spine in flexion and extension are of very limited utility in trauma. They may provide added confidence in clearing low-risk cases, particularly when equivocal findings are noted on the preliminary evaluation or when patients report pain that is out of proportion with normal x-ray findings. Flexion and extension views are contraindicated when the patient's level of consciousness is altered. In cases in which the clinical suspicion of instability or ligamentous laxity is high, MRI is a better and safer test than flexion and extension radiographs.

The pillar view is an AP projection taken with the x-ray tube angled approximately 25° in a caudal direction. This view better visualizes the articular pillars and lamina of the lower cervical spine, which are at particular risk in hyperextension/compression injuries. A pillar view may be useful when the standard AP view suggests possible malalignment of the pillars.

With the increasing availability, speed, and utility of CT evaluation in traumatized patients, the threshold to perform CT should be low in high-risk patients, particularly if routine radiographs are suboptimal or suspicious, and the patient is already going to CT for evaluation of the head or body.

Shoulder

A *true AP* of the shoulder (Grashey view) takes into account the fact that the coronal plane of the glenohumeral joint is angled about 40° medially to the coronal plane of the body (Fig. 3.1). Therefore, the x-ray beam is angled about 40° medially so that it is perpendicular to the glenohumeral joint line (Fig. 3.2). Often the evaluation of the shoulder not

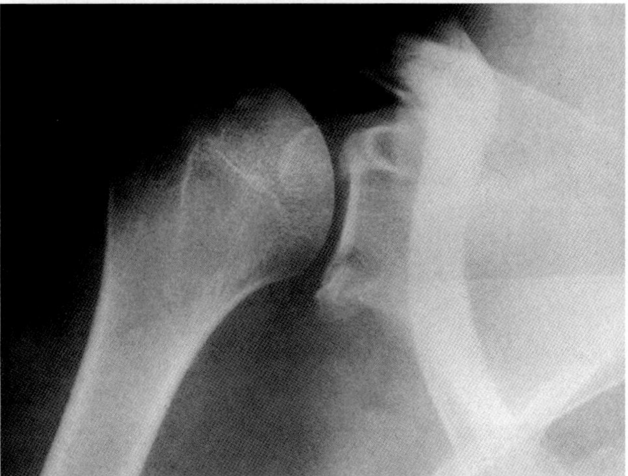

Figure 3.1 A true anteroposterior (AP) of the shoulder showing an anteroinferior glenoid fracture. Note the visualization of the glenohumeral joint space afforded by this view. (*Reprinted with permission from* Bucholz RW, Heckman JD, Court-Brown C, et al. *Rockwood and Green's Fractures in Adults*. 6th ed. Philadelphia, PA: Lippincott Williams & Wilkins, 2006.)

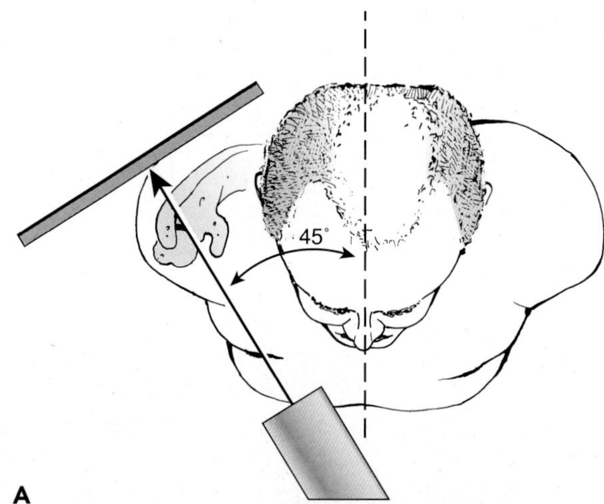

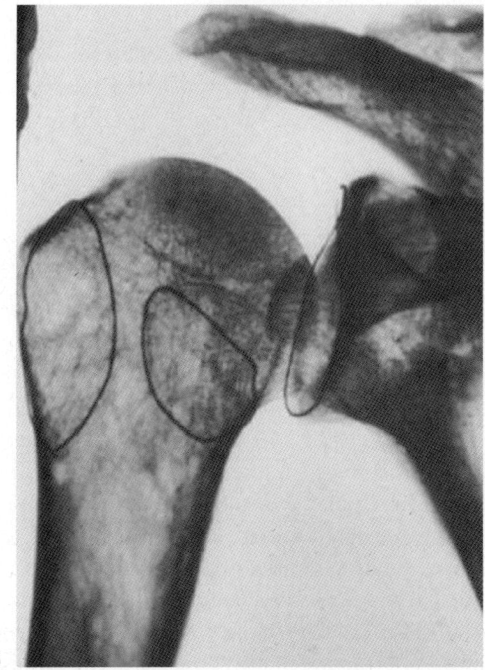

Figure 3.2 **A.** The true AP view of glenohumeral joint requires the beam to be angled 45 degrees from the sagittal plane. **B.** True AP view shows the joint in profile and the tuberosities are outlined. (Reprinted with permission from Bucholz RW, Heckman JD, Court-Brown C, et al. *Rockwood and Green's Fractures in Adults*, 6th ed. Philadelphia, PA: Lippincott Williams & Wilkins, 2006.)

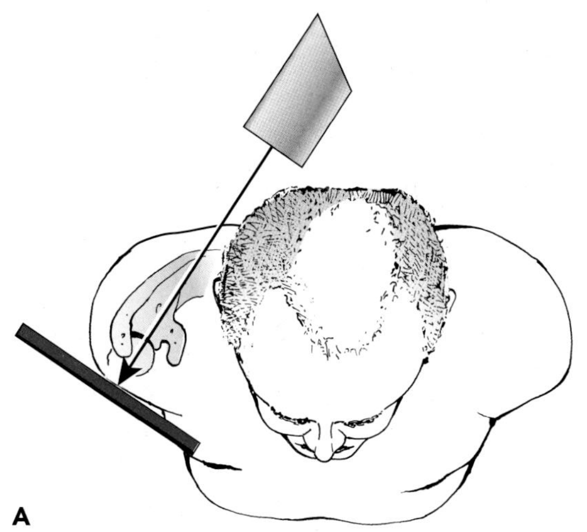

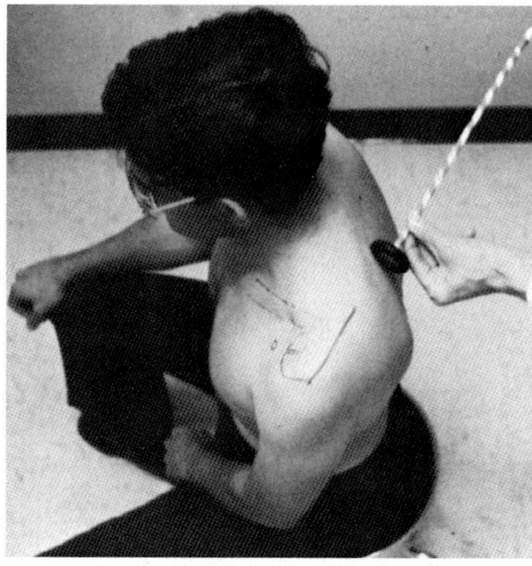

Figure 3.3 Technique for obtaining a scapula lateral, also known as the "Y-view, x-ray." With the cassette placed on the lateral aspect of the shoulder **(A)**, the x-ray beam is directed parallel to the plane of the scapula **(B)**. (*Reprinted with permission from* Bucholz RW, Heckman JD, Court-Brown C, et al. *Rockwood and Green's Fractures in Adults.* 6th ed. Philadelphia, PA: Lippincott Williams & Wilkins, 2006.)

initiated by the orthopaedic surgeon begins with an "AP" of the shoulder in internal and external rotation. In fact, this AP is an anteroposterior view of the chest, not a true AP of the shoulder. While these views can be useful to visualize calcifications within the tendons of the rotator cuff, they provide little information about the glenohumeral joint as there is overlap of the humeral head on the glenoid.

The ***axillary view*** is orthogonal to the true AP and evaluates the glenohumeral joint and the relative positions of the humeral head and the glenoid fossa in the axial plane. This x-ray is performed with the arm fully abducted and the x-ray beam aimed at the axilla. This view is especially helpful in the evaluation of the dislocated shoulder and must be obtained to confirm reduction. Often, it is difficult to get the patient to abduct sufficiently to obtain an axillary lateral view due to pain. In this setting, a Velpeau axillary view can be obtained with the patient leaning backward over the cassette and the x-ray shot from superior to inferior. Along with the true AP and the axillary lateral, the third view that completes the routine evaluation of the shoulder is the transscapular or ***scapular Y view*** (Fig. 3.3). This view can act as an adjuvant to the axillary lateral view to further assess anterior or posterior displacement of the humeral head in the setting of dislocation. The humeral head should be visualized within the glenoid fossa between the coracoid process anteriorly and the scapular spine posteriorly.

A modification of the axillary view is the ***West Point view***, which improves detection of an anteroinferior glenoid rim fracture after dislocation. The patient is positioned prone with the arm abducted 90° and the central ray angled 20° to 30° cephalad and 25° to 30° medially. The Stryker or ***"notch" view*** is used to visualize Hill-Sachs defects in the humeral head. It is obtained with the patient supine, the arm flexed, and the palm placed on top of the head with the central ray directed 10° cephalad (Fig. 3.4). ***Zanca*** (or ***apical oblique***) and ***serendipity*** views image the lateral and medial clavicle, respectively, with 10° to 40° of cephalic tilt (Fig. 3.5).

Hand and Wrist

The routine wrist series consists of ***postero-anterior (PA)***, ***lateral***, and ***oblique*** views. Traction x-rays can be useful in distal radial fractures to better define fracture anatomy, especially in intra-articular fractures. The lateral view is

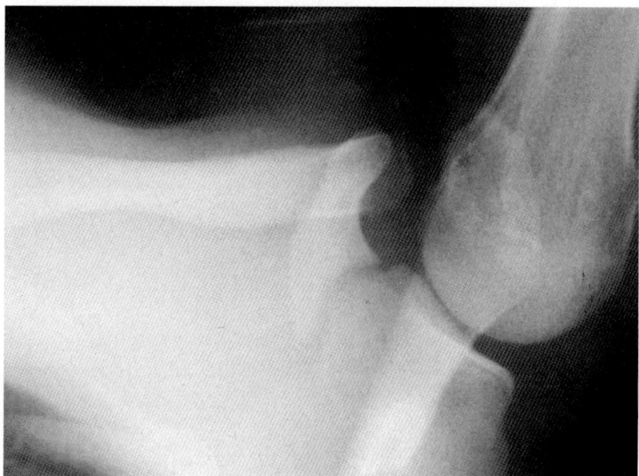

Figure 3.4 A fracture of the base of the coracoid is best seen on a Stryker notch view. (*Reprinted with permission from* Bucholz RW, Heckman JD, Court-Brown C, et al. *Rockwood and Green's Fractures in Adults.* 6th ed. Philadelphia, PA: Lippincott Williams & Wilkins, 2006.)

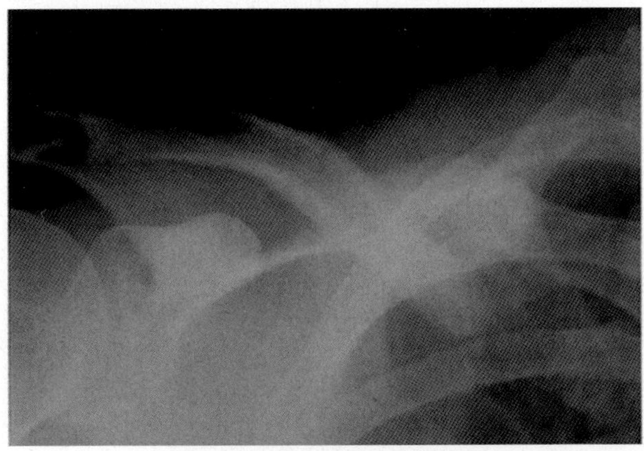

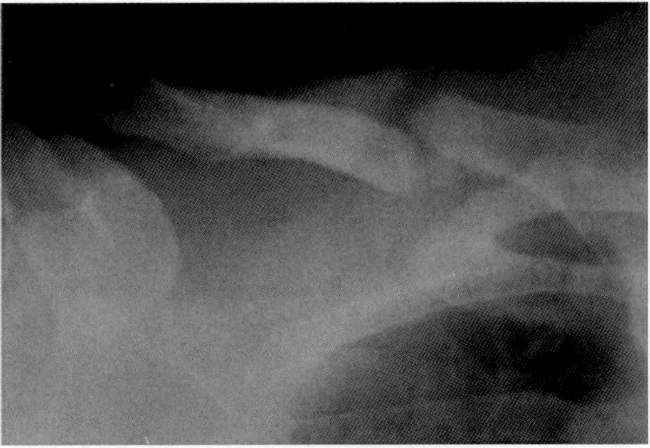

Figure 3.5 A true anteroposterior (AP) radiograph **(A)** commonly obscures the fracture pattern. An apical oblique view **(B)** is helpful to better demonstrate the fracture pattern. (Reprinted with permission from Bucholz RW, Heckman JD, Court-Brown C, et al. *Rockwood and Green's Fractures in Adults*, 6th ed. Philadelphia, PA: Lippincott Williams & Wilkins, 2006.)

used to evaluate for dislocation, malalignment, or intercalated segment instability. The adequacy of the lateral view can be evaluated by looking for the distal pole of the scaphoid to be in line with the hook of the hamate. A lateral view with the wrist angulated approximately 20° off the cassette allows for a look at the radiocarpal joint space, taking into account the radial inclination. Specific views of the scaphoid should be obtained in the setting of trauma. This view is done in the PA projection, with the wrist ulnarly deviated and with slight cephalad angulation of the beam, which elongates the waist of the scaphoid. However, one must keep in mind that a scaphoid fracture can have normal radiographs initially. A ***clenched fist view*** can be used to evaluate for scapholunate widening and is typically done in supination with ulnar deviation. Views of the opposite side can be obtained for comparison. A ***carpal tunnel view***, obtained by hyperextending the hand and directing the beam 30° above the horizontal axis is used to visualize the hook of the hamate and the pisiform.

Pelvis and Hip

The ***standard AP view*** of the pelvis is taken with the patient supine and the feet internally rotated approximately 15° in order to get a true coronal view of the femoral necks. The internal rotation is necessary to counteract the 15° of anteversion present in the femoral neck. In the setting of acetabular fracture, ***Judet views*** are obtained. These x-rays are 45° oblique views of the pelvis. The obturator oblique shows the anterior column and the posterior rim of the acetabulum and can be identified by the O of the obturator foramen on the x-ray (Fig. 3.6). The "Spur sign" seen on the obturator oblique is pathognomonic of a both column acetabular fracture. The iliac oblique shows the posterior

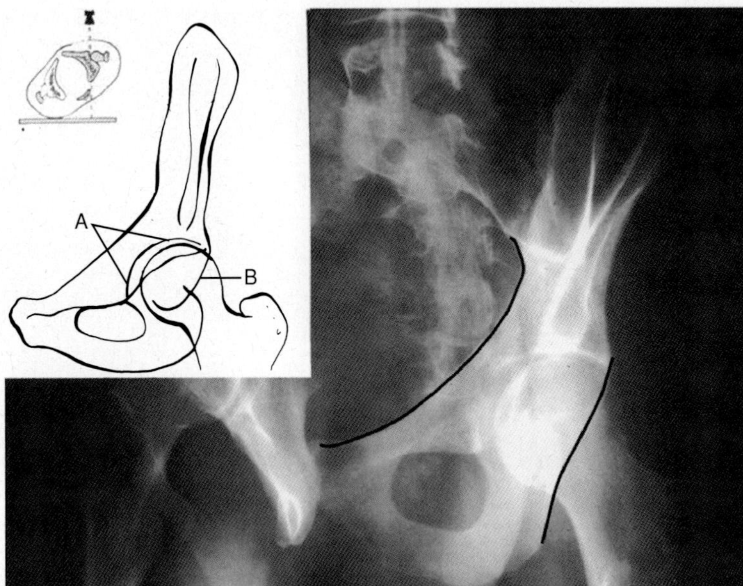

Figure 3.6 Radiographic lines of the acetabulum on the obturator oblique x-ray. **A:** Iliopectineal line. **B:** Posterior rim. Note also the view of the obturator foramen as well as the ischial ramus. (*Reprinted with permission from* Bucholz RW, Heckman JD, Court-Brown C, et al. *Rockwood and Green's Fractures in Adults*. 6th ed. Philadelphia, PA: Lippincott Williams & Wilkins, 2006.)

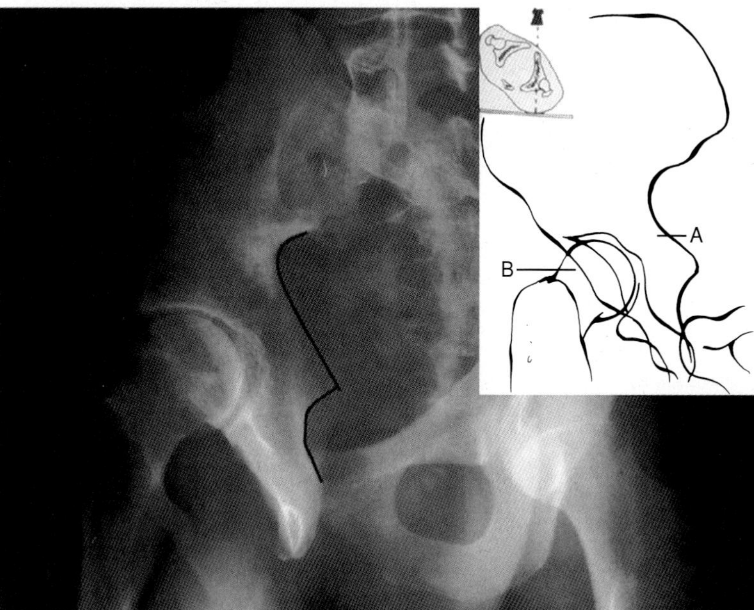

Figure 3.7 Radiographic lines of the acetabulum on the iliac oblique x-ray. **A:** Posterior border of the innominate bone. **B:** Anterior rim. (*Reprinted with permission from* Bucholz RW, Heckman JD, Court-Brown C, et al. *Rockwood and Green's Fractures in Adults.* 6th ed. Philadelphia, PA: Lippincott Williams & Wilkins, 2006.)

column and the anterior rim of the acetabulum and can be identified by the *en face* view of the iliac wing (Fig. 3.7). Major pelvic ring disruptions may be further assessed with ***inlet*** (beam angled 20° caudally) and ***outlet*** (beam angled 20° cephalad) ***views***. The inlet view depicts the degree of AP displacement across the pelvic ring. The outlet view depicts superoinferior displacement and nicely depicts pubic ramus fractures that can be missed on the routine AP (Fig. 3.8). The sacroiliac joints are best assessed using coned down AP views with a cephalad beam angulation of 30°, a view termed the ***Ferguson view***. Oblique projections may be of some benefit, but they are difficult to optimize.

Routine evaluation of the hip includes an AP view in internal rotation as above, as well as a ***frog leg lateral view*** with the hip abducted and externally rotated. In this way the requisite two orthogonal views are obtained without turning the patient. For trauma patients a groin lateral view of the hip can be obtained with an angled beam aimed at the groin, with the contralateral hip flexed out of the beam. Thus, a lateral view of the hip is obtained without moving the injured hip.

Knee

The full series of radiographs in the evaluation of knee pathology involves an AP view, a lateral view with 20° to 35° of flexion, and a view of the patellofemoral joint. In the evaluation of osteoarthritis, the ***AP views*** should be weight-bearing. In fact, AP weight-bearing views of the knee in 30° of flexion are more sensitive for early joint space loss. Internal and external oblique 45° views can be helpful in the setting of proximal tibial fracture to help evaluate fracture lines (Fig. 3.9). A ***tunnel view*** or intercondylar notch view is obtained with the knee flexed 45° and the beam angled along the axis of the tibial plateau. This view allows for evaluation of loose bodies and osteochondritis dissecans lesions.

Evaluation of the patellofemoral joint is done to look for arthrosis, malalignment, or subluxation. The ***sunrise view*** of the patella is acquired with the patient prone and the knee in greater than 90° flexion, providing an axial view of the patella. It does not depict patellar subluxation or malalignment, which must be assessed at lesser degrees of flexion. Another patellofemoral view is the ***Merchant view*** in which the patient is supine and the knee is flexed to 45° with the beam 30° from the horizontal. The sulcus angle can be measured on this radiograph as the angle subtended by the trochlea, while the congruence angle is a measure of patellar seating within the trochlea. The congruence angle averages −6° (arbitrarily defined as negative, i.e., 6° medial to a zero reference line that bisects the sulcus angle); a more positive congruence angle is indicative of patellar subluxation.

Foot and Ankle

Routine radiographic assessment of the ankle begins with AP, lateral, and mortise views. ***Mortise view*** is an AP view obtained with the foot in 15° to 20° of internal rotation. This view takes into account the fact that the fibula sits posterior to the tibia in the coronal plane and thus allows an assessment of the lateral gutter of the ankle joint. The mortise view will depict talar shift and ligamentous widening of the syndesmosis. The medial clear space and the tibiofibular clear space both serve as measures of lateral talar shift and can be measured on the mortise view. The

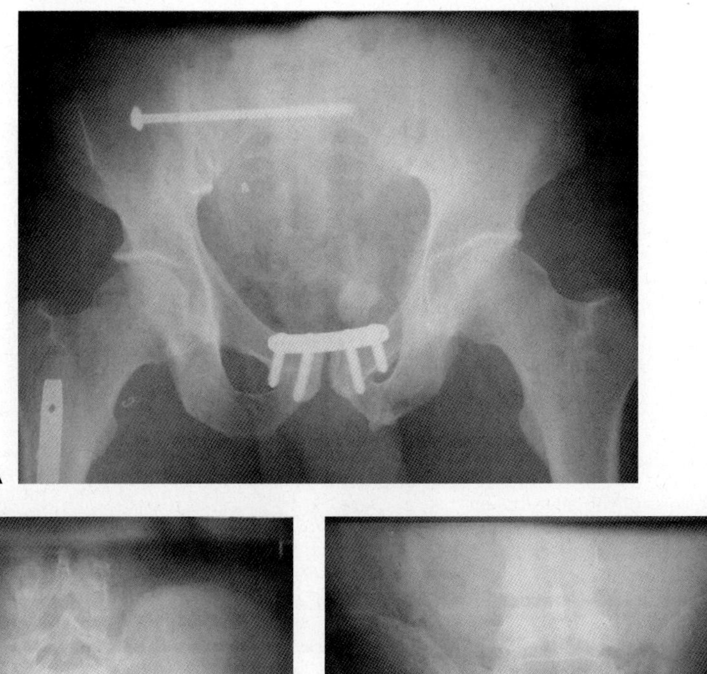

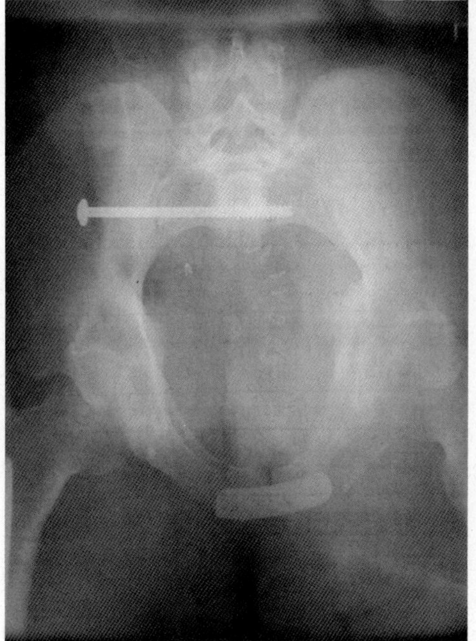

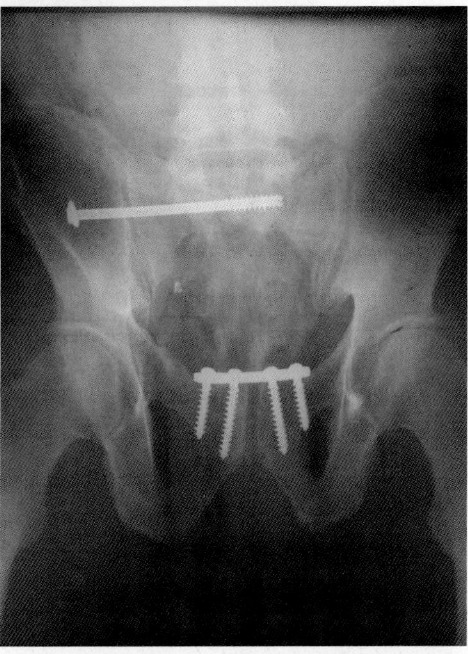

Figure 3.8 **A:** Postoperative anteroposterior (AP) view of a right vertical shear pelvic injury. Fixation was achieved with a right iliosacral screw in conjunction with symphyseal plating. **B:** Inlet view. **C:** Outlet view. (*Reprinted with permission from* Bucholz RW, Heckman JD, Court-Brown C, et al. *Rockwood and Green's Fractures in Adults.* 6th ed. Philadelphia, PA: Lippincott Williams & Wilkins, 2006.)

medial clear space is used as a marker of lateral talar shift and should be less than 4 mm as measured on a mortise view of the ankle. The tibiofibular clear space is measured from the medial border of the fibular to the incisura fibularis on the tibia on an AP view and should measure less than 6 mm.

Standard projections of the foot include AP, lateral, internal oblique, and external oblique. Non–weight-bearing views are adequate for assessing anatomy but do not view the foot in a physiologic position and are therefore suboptimal. The internal oblique complements the AP and lateral and especially evaluates the lateral tarsometatarsal articulations. Tarsal coalitions, especially calcaneonavicular, can also be seen on oblique views.

Special views of the hindfoot can provide more information. The ***Broden view*** provides a reliable image of the posterior facet of the subtalar joint and is used to evaluate intra-articular calcaneal fractures. It is obtained with the ankle in neutral dorsiflexion, the leg internally rotated 30°, and the x-ray beam centered over the lateral malleolus. ***Canale and Kelly*** described a talar neck view for evaluation of talar neck fractures. This view is obtained with the ankle in maximal equinus with the foot pronated 15° and centered 15° cephalad (Fig. 3.10). An axial view of the calcaneus, the ***Harris-Beath view,*** allows analysis of the medial and posterior facets of the subtalar joint, as well as an assessment of the alignment of the heel. Finally, the ***Cobey view*** depicts heel position and axis relative

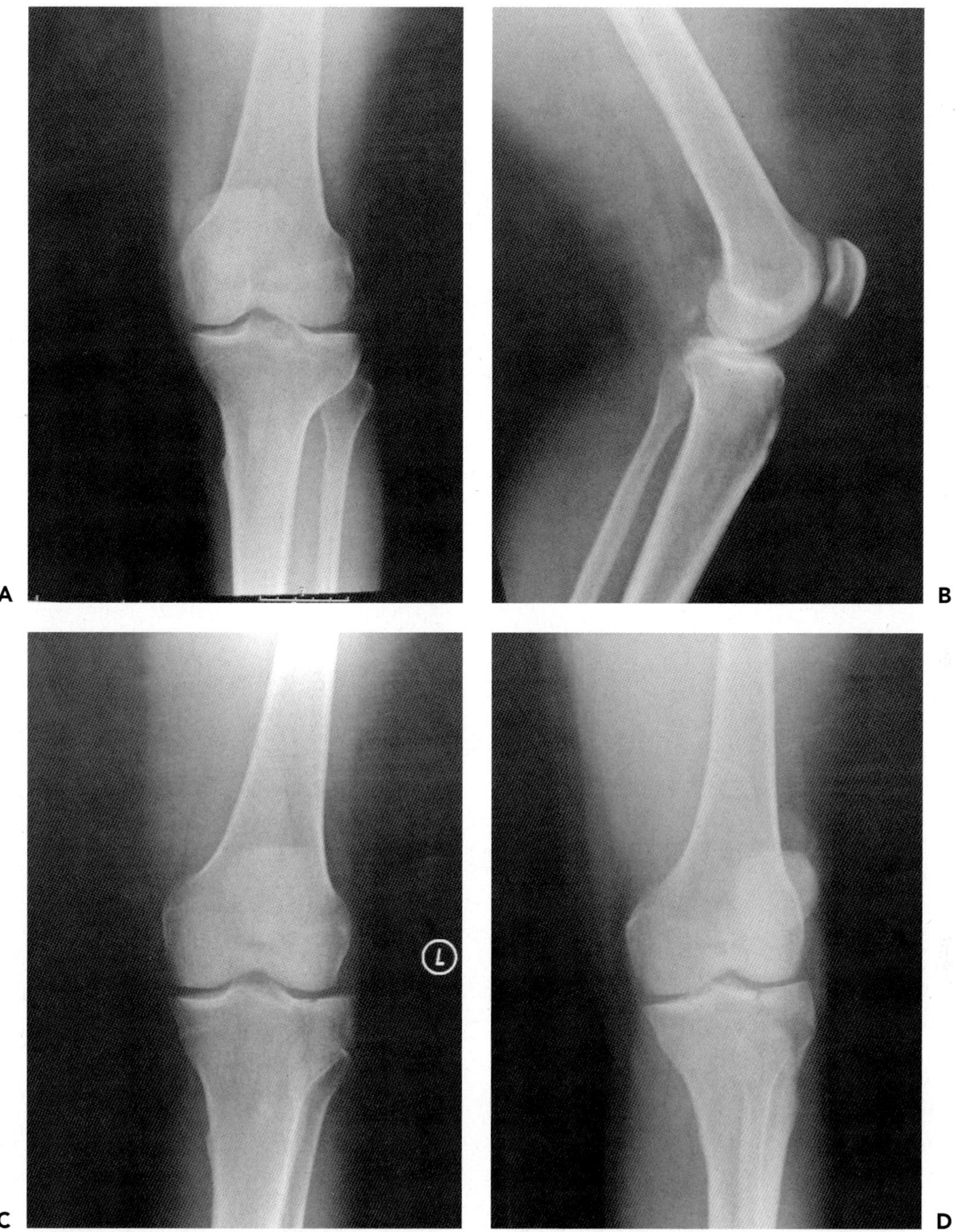

Figure 3.9 Standard radiographic trauma series. Internal oblique view **(A)**, a lateral view **(B)**, an anterior-posterior **(C)**, and an external rotation oblique **(D)** reveal a minimally displaced split fracture of the lateral plateau. (Reprinted with permission from Bucholz RW, Heckman JD, Court-Brown C, et al. *Rockwood and Green's Fractures in Adults*, 6th ed. Philadelphia, PA: Lippincott Williams & Wilkins, 2006.)

to the main tibial axis. It is performed PA with the patient standing on a platform with the beam angled 20° caudally.

CONVENTIONAL ARTHROGRAPHY

Intra-articular needle placement under fluoroscopic guidance can be performed for purposes of contrast injection, fluid aspiration, or instillation of steroid or analgesic medication. Conventional arthrography has been largely replaced by MRI, but it is still a useful tool for diagnosing full-thickness rotator cuff tears of the shoulder and for evaluating the interosseous ligaments and triangular fibrocartilage complex of the wrist in patients unable to undergo MRI scan. The basic principle is that contrast is injected into one compartment and should not extravasate outside

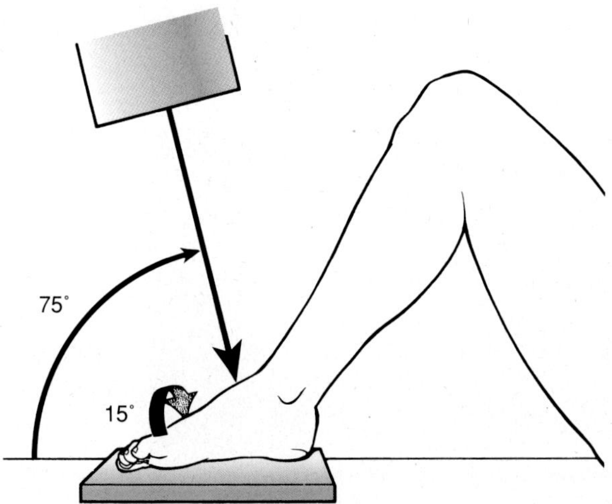

Figure 3.10 Canale and Kelly view of the foot. The correct position of the foot for x-ray evaluation of the foot is shown. (*Reprinted with permission from* Bucholz RW, Heckman JD, Court-Brown C, et al. *Rockwood and Green's Fractures in Adults.* 6th ed. Philadelphia, PA: Lippincott Williams & Wilkins, 2006.)

of that compartment unless there is a disruption of the tissue that defines the compartment. For example, in the shoulder dye injected into the glenohumeral joint should not enter the subacromial space unless there is a tear of the rotator cuff allowing communication between the two areas.

Contrast arthrography is not generally used for diagnosing loosening of arthroplasty components. However, fluoroscopic needle placement and aspiration are still important as part of the workup for deep infection in painful joint replacements. Arthrography and tenography can be used in the foot and ankle to help localize pathology and guide injection of steroid and local anesthetic. Using contrast helps to confirm proper positioning of the needle and can identify any anomalous connection between joints or between joints and tendon sheaths that may exist.

C-arm fluoroscopy is an important tool for guiding needle injection of the disk and facet joints in an effort to determine specific pain sources in both the preoperative spine patient and patients with failed back surgery. Epidural injections and nerve blocks using long-acting steroids can also be performed under fluoroscopy as therapeutic procedures.

COMPUTED TOMOGRAPHY

CT is a technique that generates cross-sectional images that are reconstructed from multiple digital radiographic projections or views. These views are combined through the method of "back-projection" to generate the cross-sectional image. Recent advances in CT include the development of helical or spiral scanners, which allows continuous unidirectional tube motion. Ultimately, this allows for more rapid acquisition of images, covering large body areas in a relatively short period of time. This rapid acquisition has facilitated CT evaluation of the trauma patient.

The helical CT also generates a three-dimensional projectional data set, allowing retrospective reconstruction of cross-sectional images at arbitrary locations throughout the data set. These reconstructions do not come at the cost of a higher radiation dose to the patient. Newer multi-detector array CT will not only allow retrospective reconstruction of images at variable scan collimation but also dramatically increase scan acquisition speed. Thinner scan sections can be achieved at reduced radiation dose.

CT is extremely helpful in clarifying the pattern and severity of traumatic bony injuries and hence may be very helpful in preoperative planning. Compared with plain radiography, CT more accurately depicts the relationship and degree of comminution of fracture fragments. It is particularly helpful in the evaluation of articular fractures, pelvic and acetabular fractures, and calcaneal fractures. In articular fractures, joint surface depression and step-off, as well as identification of the different pieces into which the joint surface is fractured, allow for better understanding of the fracture pattern and therefore a more accurate approach to reconstruction (Fig. 3.11). Indeed, the most commonly used classification of calcaneal fractures (Sanders' classification) is based on the coronal cut of the CT scan (Fig. 3.12).

Although CT is chiefly used for problem solving and preoperative planning in cases of skeletal trauma, it can also be used as an important and necessary adjunct for diagnosis in skeletal areas that are difficult to evaluate with routine radiography, such as the spine and calcaneus. Instability or subluxation of the distal radioulnar joint (DRUJ) or sternoclavicular joint is difficult to diagnose by radiography but can be accurately assessed with a fast, limited CT protocol. CT is now widely used in most trauma settings for clearing the cervical spine and, in many cases, has supplanted plain radiography in this purpose. Many of these patients get a CT as a routine part of their general surgical trauma evaluation, so it is both cost-effective and efficient to add a cervical CT while the patient is already in the scanner.

CT can be done after intra-articular administration of dilute iodinated contrast medium or air to produce a CT arthrogram. The utility of CT arthrography is seen in a few settings. It can be useful in the shoulder in defining instability lesions of the capsulolabral ligamentous complex. CT arthrography is ideally suited to the evaluation of calcified loose bodies within a joint. It also allows evaluation of the joint surface for chondral defects and tears, though less accurately than MR arthrography. CT arthrography can also provide information about the stability of chronic osteochondral lesions.

In the oncologic setting, CT is often helpful in characterizing bony lesions and evaluating the extent of cortical

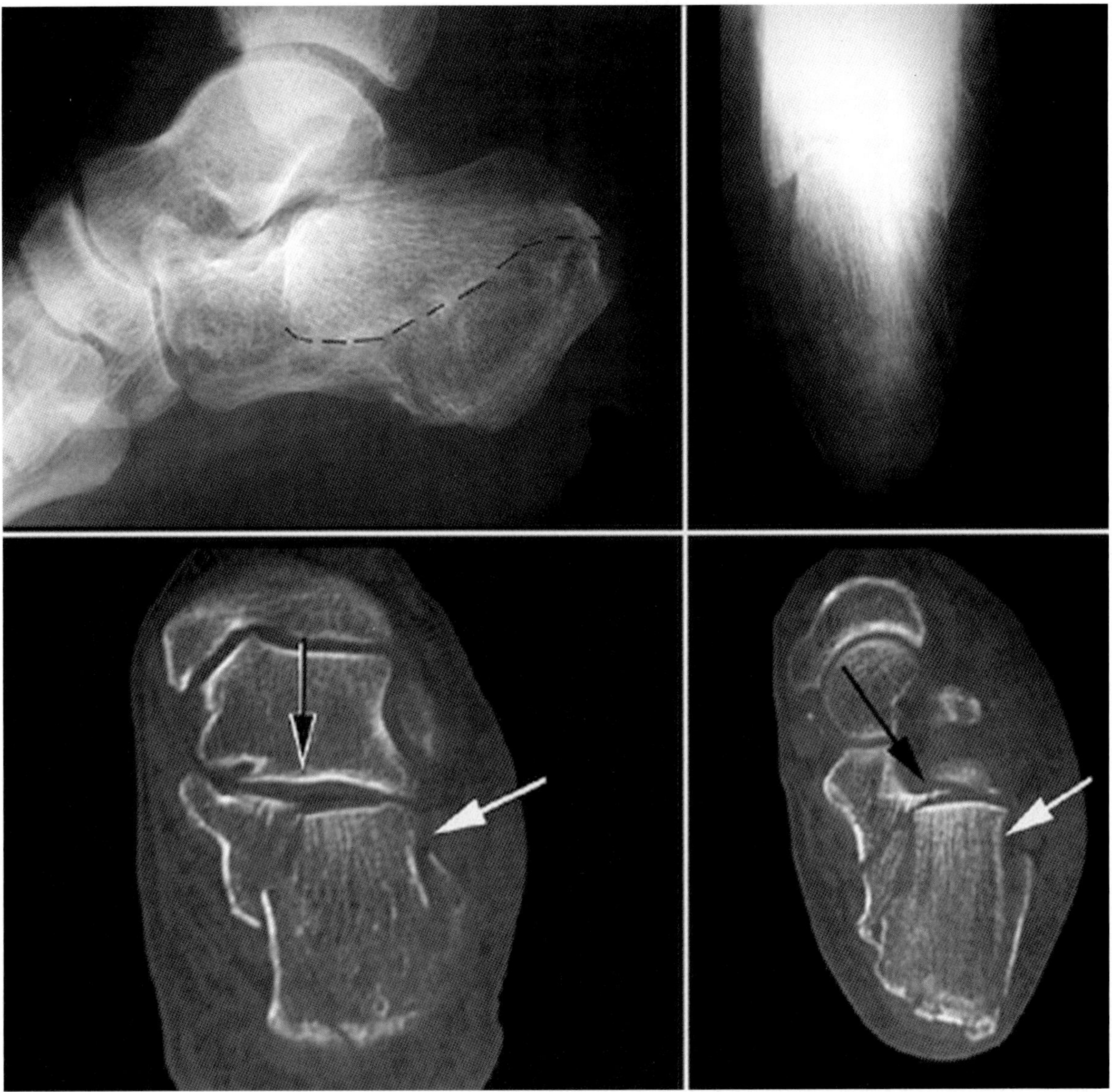

Figure 3.11 True intra-articular tongue fracture (Type IIB). Plain radiographs are unable to indicate whether the fracture involves the posterior facet. Semi-coronal and transverse CT scans verify intra-articular displacement. Note *black arrows* indicating intra-articular fracture, and *white arrows* indicating the intact lateral wall component typical of tongue fractures. (Reprinted with permission from Bucholz RW, Heckman JD, Court-Brown C, et al. *Rockwood and Green's Fractures in Adults,* 6th ed. Philadelphia, PA: Lippincott Williams & Wilkins, 2006.)

bone destruction. By depicting lesion mineralization and patterns of bone destruction, CT may narrow the differential diagnosis. CT is less effective than MRI at showing the extent of marrow involvement and the soft-tissue component of the tumor. CT can show soft-tissue extension, as well as possible involvement of neurovascular structures, although these components are better imaged by other means. In the case of extraskeletal disease, the use of intravenous contrast is usually helpful. Contrast can enhance the CT delineation of soft-tissue extension. Moreover, when performed as an angiogram, it can help to delineate the proximity of vascular structures. CT is also well suited to the fast and accurate guidance of needle biopsy procedures.

MAGNETIC RESONANCE IMAGING

MRI has emerged as the most versatile and powerful means of diagnostic imaging. It was developed as an offshoot of technology initially developed for nuclear magnetic resonance (NMR). It is based on the detection of radiofrequency signals emanating from hydrogen nuclei as they resonate within a strong, static magnetic field. These signals,

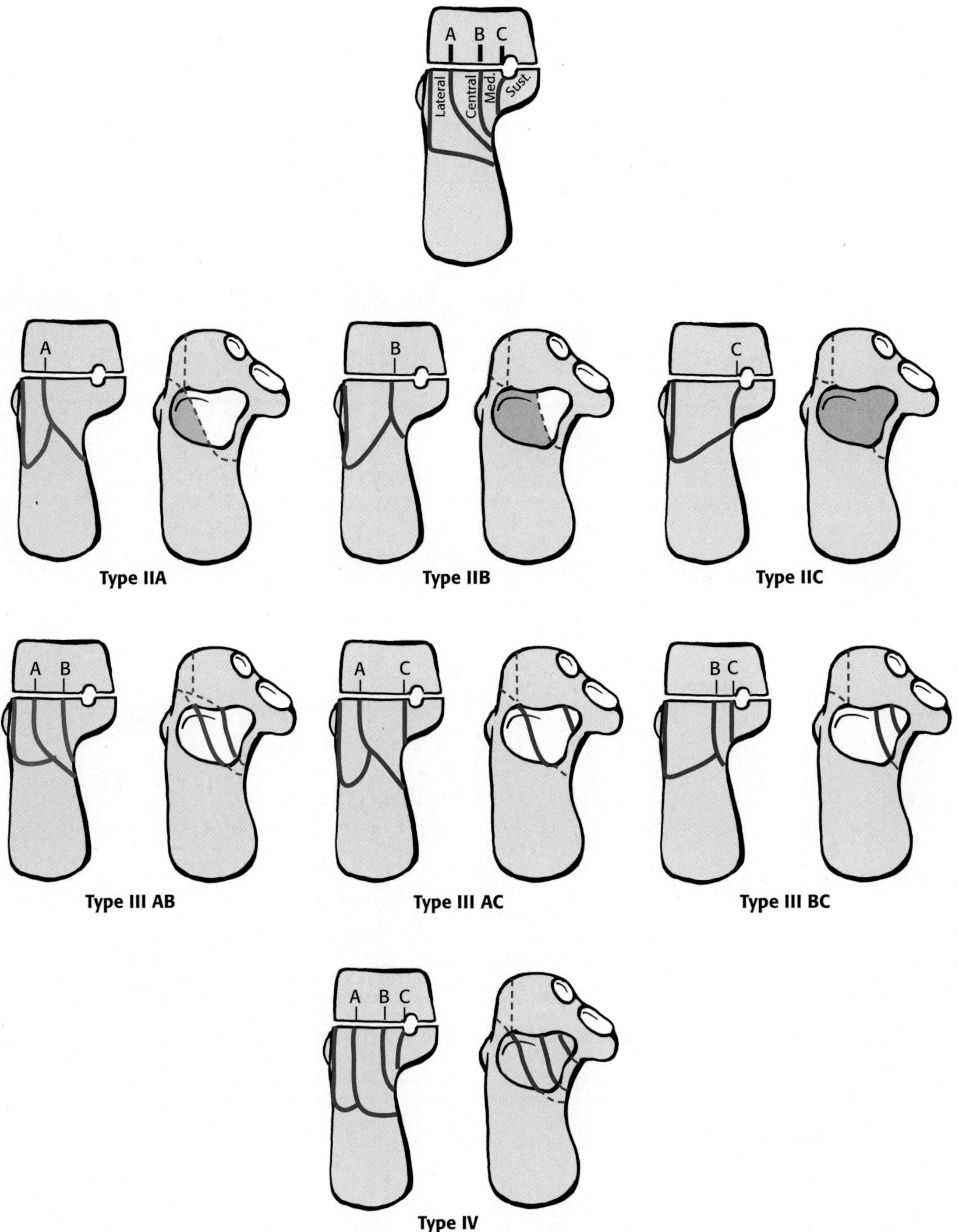

Figure 3.12 Sanders' computed tomography (CT) scan classification of calcaneal fractures. (From Sanders R. Current concepts review—displaced intra-articular fractures of the calcaneus. *J Bone Joint Surg Am.* 2000;82:233.) (*Reprinted with permission from* Bucholz RW, Heckman JD, Court-Brown C, et al. *Rockwood and Green's Fractures in Adults.* 6th ed. Philadelphia, PA: Lippincott Williams & Wilkins, 2006.)

similar in frequency to FM radio signals, are generated by hydrogen nuclei after their selective and carefully timed radio frequency excitation. Radiofrequency signal strength is determined chiefly by the number of resonating protons per tissue voxel, or proton density, and by the two relaxation constants, T1 and T2. The so-called T1-weighted images favor proton species with short T1 relaxation constants, such as the aliphatic hydrogen nuclei in fat. T2-weighted images favor proton species with a long T2 relaxation constant, such as the hydrogen nuclei in free water. Because of the large magnetic fields required for MRI scanning, patients with pacemakers or other metallic devices or foreign bodies are unable to undergo scans.

MRI innovation continues at a rapid pace, and newer MRI techniques are both faster and higher in resolution. For orthopaedic imaging, the resolution requirements are currently most important, but MRI can now generate information about tissue physiology, such as the diffusability of water molecules, the relative perfusion of organs, and the circulating blood volume within tissues. Spectroscopic information from MRI can also measure and map biochemical markers of tissue structure and function. The utility of these functional MR tools for orthopaedic applications remains to be explored.

Resonating proton signals are larger and, correspondingly, image fidelity and resolution are improved at higher magnetic fields. One point five- and three-tesla scanners are considered "high field" units and are typically of a closed-bore, tunnel-like design. These high-field designs are more likely to result in claustrophobia for the patient and their 55- to 60-cm bore diameter is commonly unable to accommodate very broad or obese patients. Open MRI designs usually employ a sandwich arrangement of permanent magnets and are usually of 0.3 tesla or lower field strength. These units are less claustrophobia inducing and can accommodate larger patients. The "open" feature confers the additional advantage that patients can be positioned such that the imaging area of interest is at "isocenter," or the most homogenous portion of the magnetic field. The lower field strength of open magnet designs can be compensated for by longer scan times, but these units are still limited in their ability to image small parts at high resolution.

Intravenous, paramagnetic contrast agents are chelates of gadolinium and are routinely administered for MRI of the central nervous system. The indications for intravenous MRI contrast material for musculoskeletal imaging are more limited. An intravascular agent does provide information about blood flow and capillary permeability or leakage within specific tissues of interest. This material is occasionally helpful in characterizing mass lesions with MRI. Contrast enhancement may also be beneficial in outlining reactive or inflammatory tissues surrounding abscesses. Finally, contrast material enhancement may be of value in surveillance for recurrence of tumor after surgery or radiotherapy.

Direct intra-articular injection of either saline or a dilute solution of saline and a paramagnetic MRI contrast agent is known as MRI arthrography. This technique optimizes delineation of synovial joints and their supporting structures. MRI arthrography is most commonly used in the evaluation of instability lesions of the shoulder. It may also be of value in the evaluation of the acetabular labrum of the hip.

The high-contrast resolution of MRI offers a considerable advantage over CT for the evaluation of soft tissues. MRI is also extremely useful for evaluation of the marrow space, due to the fat content of the marrow that generates a high MRI signal, at least on T1-weighted images. Pulse sequences that suppress fat signal are often useful in evaluation of the marrow, given that pathologic changes will show up as an area of high signal against the dark, fat-suppressed, marrow signal. Fat-suppressed imaging, particularly the STIR (short tau inversion recovery) technique, is especially sensitive to edema or inflammation whether in bone or soft tissue, and is also quite effective at delineating disease extent in the case of neoplasia. MRI evaluation of supporting connective tissue structures requires high spatial resolution and an appropriately tailored examination that targets the specific structures of interest.

MRI is the best noninvasive test for the evaluation of the joint surface (Fig. 3.13). Traumatic chondral tears as well as advanced chondral loss are easily imaged, typically with some form of T2-weighted imaging. Low-grade chondromalacia is also diagnosed accurately with high-resolution techniques. The initial changes of chondromalacia are difficult to visualize on MRI. When MRI is performed with intravenous contrast material enhancement, it is much more sensitive than radiography for the detection of early bone erosion in the case of inflammatory arthritis. This increased sensitivity may have implications for evaluating new therapies for rheumatoid arthritis.

Unlike hyaline cartilage, the fibrocartilaginous meniscus of the knee is low in signal intensity on most MRI sequences. Meniscal derangement appears as zones of increased signal against the normal, low signal fibrocartilage of the meniscus. Assessment of the knee for possible meniscal derangement is one of the most common reasons a musculoskeletal MRI is ordered. With modern MRI, the sensitivity and specificity of MRI for meniscal tear are each over 90% (Fig. 3.14). MRI also provides information about the orientation of the tear and the presence of displacement (Fig. 3.15). It must be remembered, however, that MRI findings must be correlated with clinical symptoms, as the incidence of meniscal tears has been proven to be high in older patients in the absence of symptoms. As in other areas of the body, MRI should be used as a confirmatory test to confirm a clinical suspicion based on history and physical examination findings.

Fibrocartilaginous supporting structures in other joints, that is, the labrum of the shoulder and the hip, can also be evaluated by MRI. These structures, however, are less easily evaluated than the meniscus of the knee. MR arthrography is superior to conventional MR for the evaluation of the labrum of the shoulder, especially in the setting of instability. MR arthrography can help identify the spectrum of instability lesions including Bankart lesions, humeral avulsion of the glenohumeral labrum (HAGL), anterior labroperiosteal sleeve avulsion (ALPSA), and glenoid labrum articular disruption (GLAD) lesions (Fig. 3.16).

MRI is effective at diagnosing acute ligamentous injuries. It has a specificity and sensitivity of over 95% in the

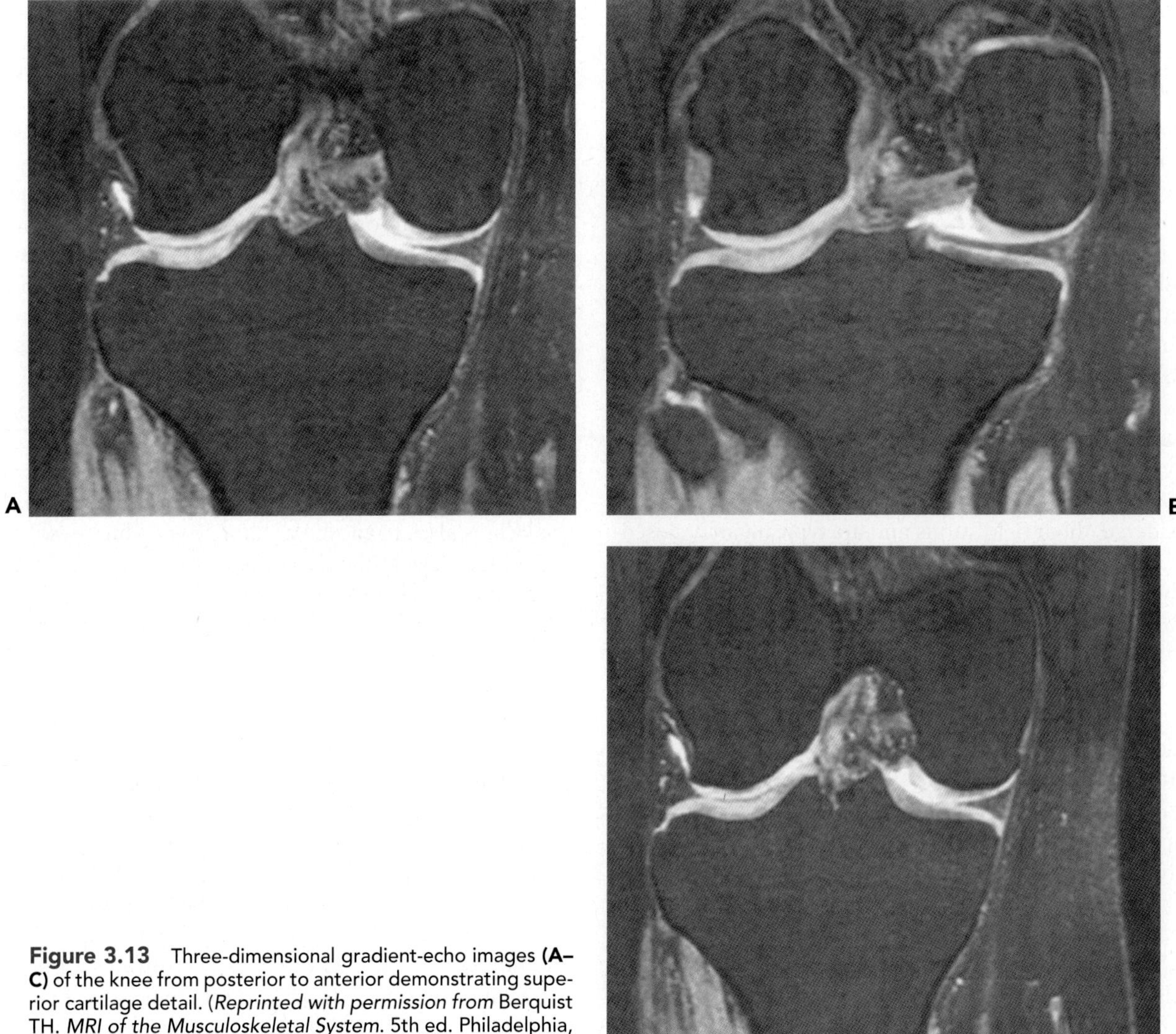

Figure 3.13 Three-dimensional gradient-echo images **(A–C)** of the knee from posterior to anterior demonstrating superior cartilage detail. (*Reprinted with permission from* Berquist TH. *MRI of the Musculoskeletal System.* 5th ed. Philadelphia, PA: Lippincott Williams & Wilkins, 2006.)

evaluation of anterior cruciate ligament (ACL) ruptures. The characteristic bone bruise pattern seen in MR images is a bone bruise on the posterior lateral tibia with a corresponding bruise on the femoral condyle. It is similarly useful in evaluating acute ligamentous injuries in other locations. However, it is less useful in the evaluation of the chronically insufficient ligament.

The multiplanar imaging capability and high soft-tissue contrast of MRI makes it ideally suited to the evaluation of the spine. Spinal canal and foraminal stenosis, as well as alterations in spinal alignment, can be accurately assessed. The intervertebral disk is clearly depicted, with the nucleus pulposus being higher in signal intensity than the annulus fibrosis and the posterior longitudinal ligament. Disk protrusions, extrusions, and sequestrations can be differentiated (Fig. 3.17). The role for CT myelography continues to diminish as MRI techniques improve. In cases of major trauma and suspected instability, MRI is a safer and more effective test for ligamentous spinal injury and potential instability than traditional flexion and extension radiographs. T2 STIR images are especially effective for evaluating ligamentous spinal injury.

MRI is quite sensitive for tendon disruptions if studies are performed with sufficient spatial resolution. This application is useful in the staging of impingement in the shoulder with tendonosis within the rotator cuff tendons. It can show the spectrum from tendonosis to partial-thickness and ultimately full-thickness tears, although it can be difficult to differentiate tendonosis from partial-thickness tearing. Short echo times are especially useful in the imaging of tendonosis wherever it may occur in the body, although MRI is more useful in making these distinctions in the larger rotator cuff and the Achilles tendon (Fig. 3.18).

MRI is sensitive in detecting muscle sprains and tears. In suspected cases of hamstring injury, for example, MR evaluation may be of some prognostic value, particularly in elite athletes in whom the size of injuries, the extent of intramuscular fluid collections, and the presence of hemorrhage can

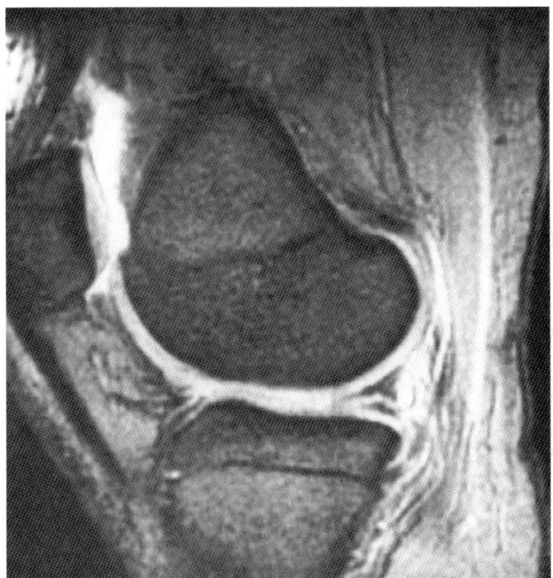

Figure 3.14 Sagittal gradient-echo image demonstrating a horizontal cleavage tear in the posterior horn. (*Reprinted with permission from* Berquist TH. *MRI of the Musculoskeletal System*. 5th ed. Philadelphia, PA: Lippincott Williams & Wilkins, 2006.)

be delineated. MRI is also sensitive to other physiologic and pathologic changes in muscle. Transient changes in muscle signal are seen on MRI immediately after exercise, likely related to shifts in muscle water compartmentalization. For reasons that are not well understood, MRI, and particularly STIR sequences, are very sensitive to muscle alterations that occur very early in denervation states and neuropraxia and thus may serve as a useful adjunct to electrodiagnostic studies. These MRI signal changes occur very early and precede electromyographic changes. Finally, MRI effectively maps the often heterogeneous changes seen in inflammatory myopathies. This capability may contribute to more effective, image-guided muscle biopsy for diagnosis of these often complex and confusing disease entities.

Although cortical bone itself does not produce an MRI signal, the cellular and fatty elements in bone marrow do, and thus, MRI has become a powerful tool in diagnosing infiltrative, inflammatory, and traumatic conditions of bone. Fairly specific MRI changes are seen in avascular necrosis of bone, in which zones of necrotic marrow become demarcated by reactive tissue and edema that exhibit abnormal MRI signals relative to normal marrow (Fig. 3.19). These changes are evident within weeks of the ischemic event, and the MRI findings are more specific and seen with greater resolution than they are with bone scan.

Similarly, the marrow reactions to both stress and trauma create alterations in the bone marrow signal that make MRI a very sensitive means to diagnose fractures, both of the fatigue and traumatic variety. In many cases, MRI will visualize the fracture or fatigue zone as a low signal line, which confers greater specificity in diagnosis compared with bone scan. MR, like bone scan, is very sensitive for bony injury short of frank fracture (Fig. 3.20). These lesions can be referred to as "bone bruises or stress reactions," depending on where they are in the body. MRI allows for multiplanar imaging and high resolution, which

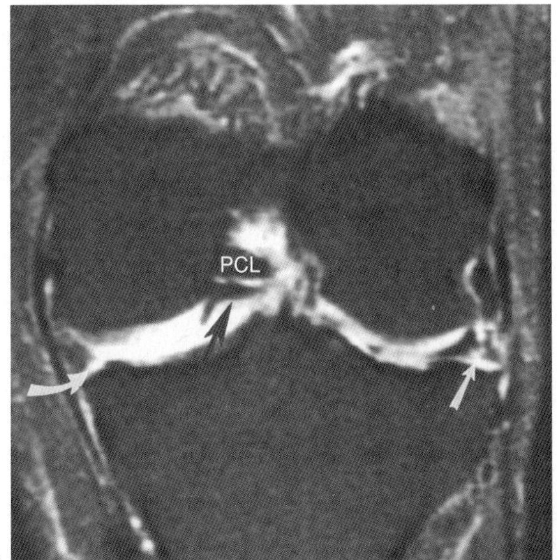

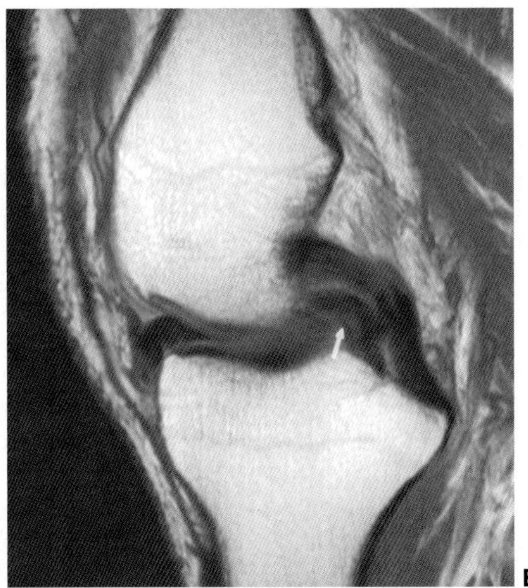

Figure 3.15 Coronal fat-suppressed T2-weighted image **(A)** demonstrating a medial tear (*curved arrow*) with a large displaced fragment (*black arrow*) that gives the appearance of two posterior cruciate ligaments (PCLs). There is also a complex tear of the lateral meniscus (*white arrow*) and loss of articular cartilage. Sagittal proton density-weighted image **(B)** demonstrating a medial meniscal tear with a large displaced fragment (*small arrow*), resulting in a double-PCL sign. (*Reprinted with permission from* Berquist TH. *MRI of the Musculoskeletal System*. 5th ed. Philadelphia, PA: Lippincott Williams & Wilkins, 2006.)

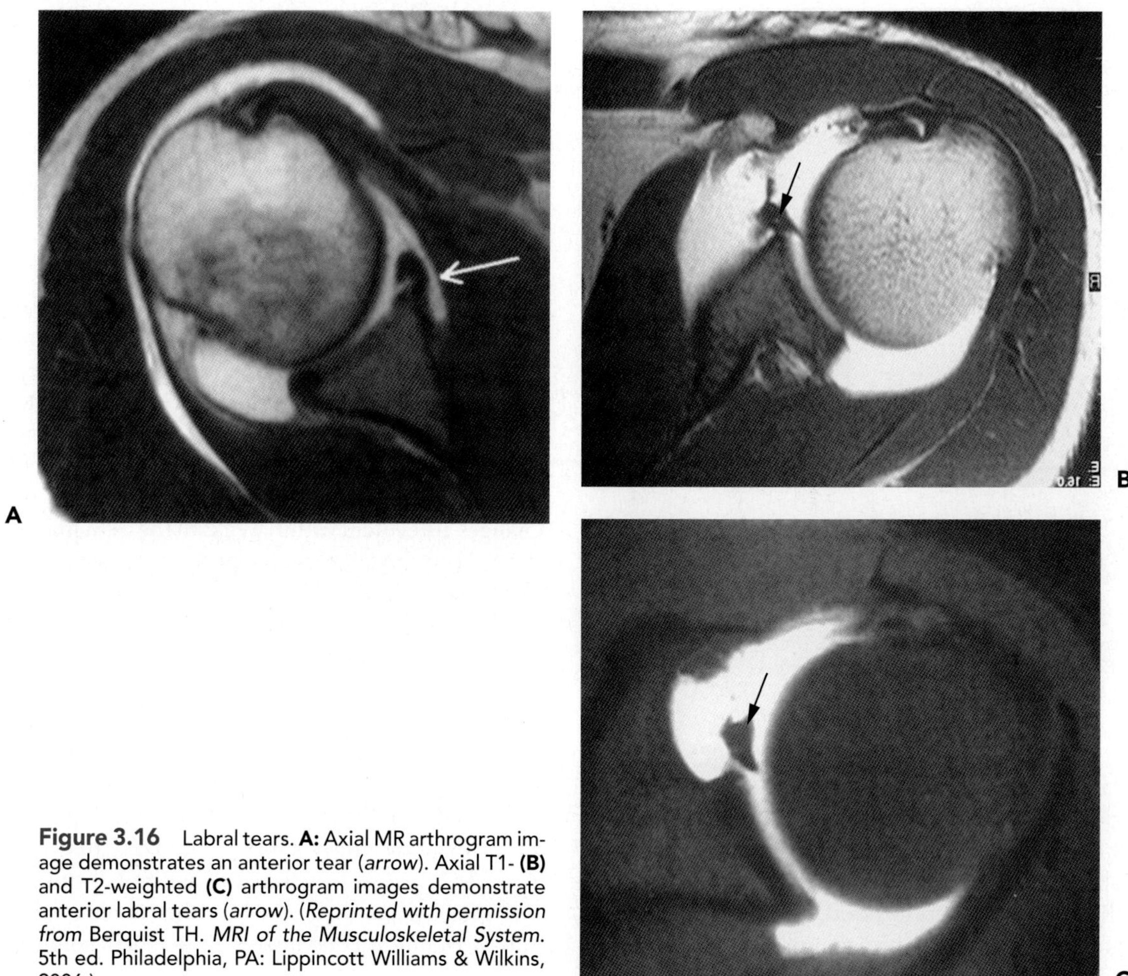

Figure 3.16 Labral tears. **A:** Axial MR arthrogram image demonstrates an anterior tear (*arrow*). Axial T1- **(B)** and T2-weighted **(C)** arthrogram images demonstrate anterior labral tears (*arrow*). (*Reprinted with permission from* Berquist TH. *MRI of the Musculoskeletal System.* 5th ed. Philadelphia, PA: Lippincott Williams & Wilkins, 2006.)

once again provides a superior evaluation compared with bone scintigraphy.

The sensitivity of MRI to marrow edema and soft-tissue inflammation makes MRI an effective test for osteomyelitis. The use of intravenous contrast material is not essential but may aid in identifying areas of necrosis or abscess formation. The high resolution will often make MRI a more useful preoperative study than bone scan (Fig. 3.21). Bone scan does have the advantage that it can survey larger areas, whereas MRI is best used in a fashion directed by history and physical examination. The utility of MRI and bone scan both is decreased if there has been prior recent trauma or surgery that might impart alterations in bone marrow physiology, mimicking those of infection.

MRI is very sensitive for detecting marrow replacement that occurs in metastatic and primary tumors of bone. It is more sensitive and specific for metastatic disease to bone than either CT or bone scan. MRI accurately defines the extent of disease in the marrow space and delineates extraosseous extension of tumor (Fig. 3.22). Although the signal characteristics of tumors are not usually specific, MRI is quite effective in distinguishing cystic masses from solid masses and identifies the presence of secondary aneurysmal bone cyst components and tumor necrosis.

MRI is not usually used to diagnose diffuse marrow diseases such as leukemia and myeloma. These infiltrative diseases can be difficult to detect by MRI. Signal characteristics on normal MRI sequences may not reliably distinguish these marrow infiltrates from normal hematopoietic or red marrow. The pattern or extent of marrow cellularity (i.e., the replacement of normal yellow marrow) is more telling than the infiltrates themselves.

MRI is the modality of choice for the imaging evaluation of suspected soft-tissue tumors. The utility of MRI is primarily in lesion detection and delineation, which aids management and surgical or biopsy planning. MRI has a higher sensitivity for soft-tissue masses than does CT (Fig. 3.23). Although MRI features are not usually specific for one histologic diagnosis, MR does often contribute information that may significantly narrow the differential diagnosis. Occasionally, specific diagnoses can be made with confidence based on MRI, particularly in the case of vascular origin or fat-containing tumors. The use of intravenous contrast material may aid in the identification of tumor necrosis and the confirmation of the cystic nature of certain

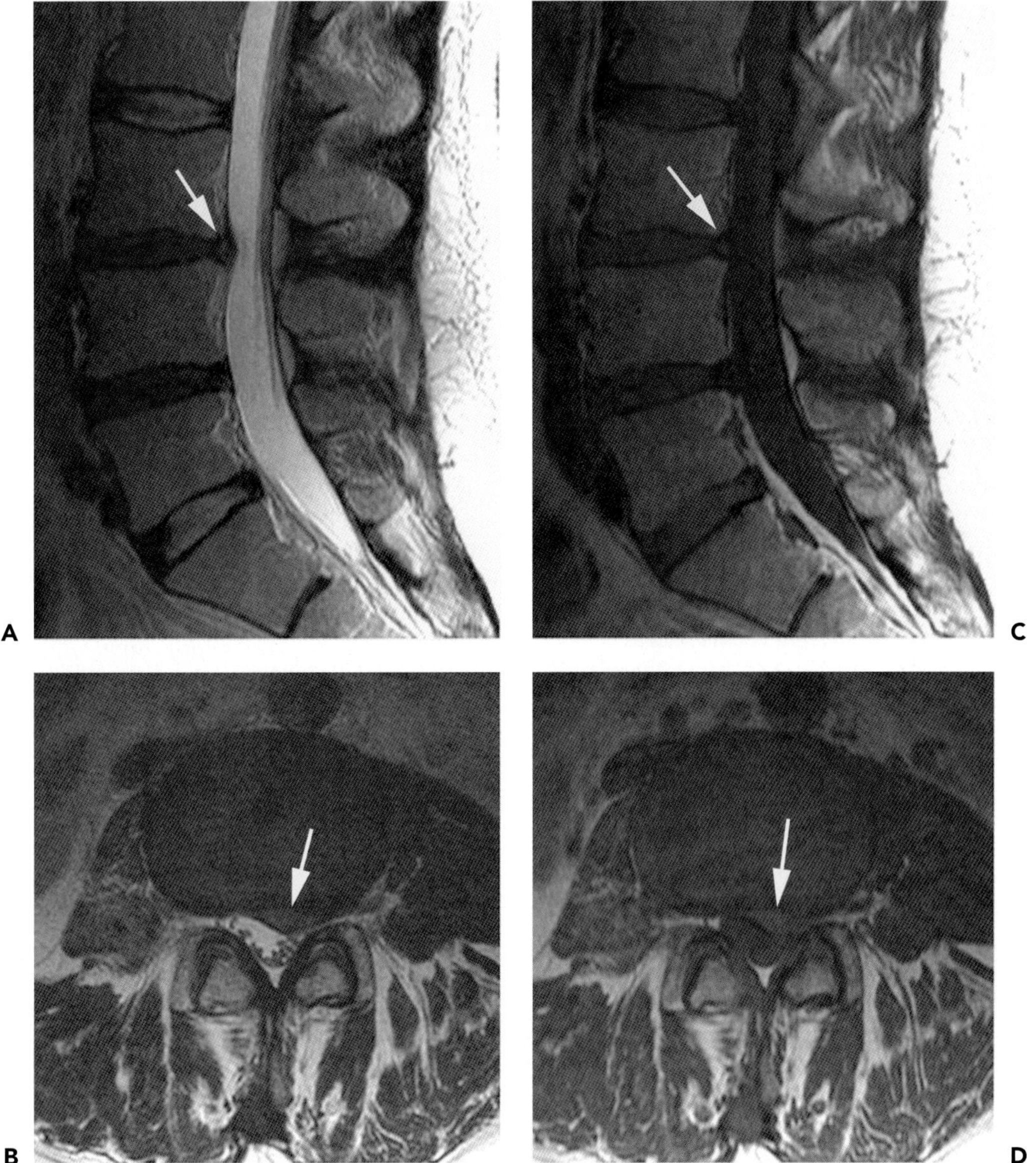

Figure 3.17 Lumbar disc protrusion. L3 disc herniation with the base of the herniation wider than the distance away from the parent disc. The protrusion is evident principally as a distortion of the cerebrospinal fluid–containing thecal sac on the T2-weighted images (**A** and **B**) and as effacement of the epidural fat on the T1-weighted images (**C** and **D**). (*Reprinted with permission from* Berquist TH. *MRI of the Musculoskeletal System*. 5th ed. Philadelphia, PA: Lippincott Williams & Wilkins, 2006.)

lesions. It is not, however, essential to the MRI evaluation of mass lesions.

ULTRASONOGRAPHY

Ultrasound has the distinct advantages of being semi-portable, easily tolerated, and relatively inexpensive. With new transducer technology, ultrasound can surpass MRI and CT in spatial resolution and can be effectively used in the imaging of small and superficial body parts. The main drawback to ultrasound is that the quality of the images is extremely dependent on the skill of the technician performing the ultrasound. Furthermore, most orthopaedists are not able to interpret ultrasound images on their own, so they must rely on the radiologists report.

Common examples of the clinical application of high-resolution ultrasound include the diagnosis of Morton's neuroma and ganglion cysts. Ultrasound is well suited to the evaluation of tendonopathy and reliably detects ruptures of tendons. Common clinical applications include evaluation of the Achilles tendon and the rotator cuff.

Ultrasound can be used to evaluate ligamentous structures, although a working knowledge of anatomy is a prerequisite. In this setting it has the advantage of allowing for dynamic evaluation as opposed to the static images

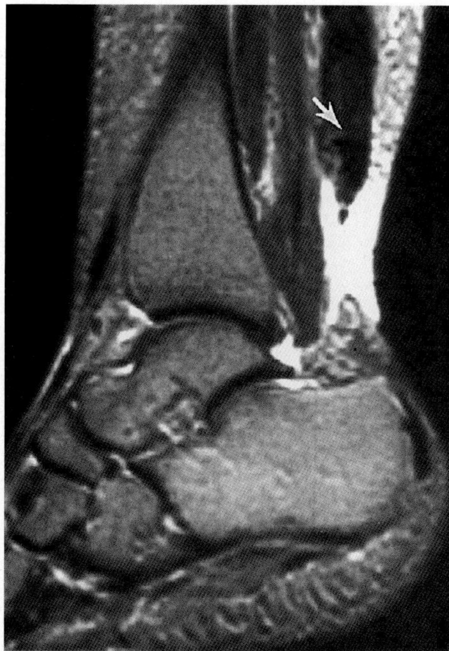

Figure 3.18 Complete Achilles tendon tear. Sagittal T2-weighted image of the ankle demonstrates high signal intensity with thickening and retraction of the proximal fragment (*arrow*) commonly seen with complete tears. (*Reprinted with permission from* Berquist TH. *MRI of the Musculoskeletal System*. 5th ed. Philadelphia, PA: Lippincott Williams & Wilkins, 2006.)

produced by traditional imaging techniques. For example, ultrasound can be used to assess disruption of the ulnar collateral ligament of the thumb metacarpal-phalangeal joint, the so-called Gamekeeper's thumb, by imaging the ligament, as a deforming force is applied to the thumb. As a real-time imaging modality, ultrasound is also well suited for imaging guided biopsies. It can also be used effectively to identify foreign bodies not seen on x-ray.

Ultrasound has perhaps been underutilized in the evaluation of soft-tissue mass lesions. It is particularly effective in determining the vascularity of lesions, particularly with the advent of real-time color Doppler imaging technology. Power Doppler display is analogous to the circulating blood volume, and it is highly sensitive to low-velocity flow. With this enhancement ultrasound can accurately assess the vascularity of lesions and can identify hyperemia around inflammatory masses.

Ultrasound can be used in more than one setting in pediatric patients. A short ultrasound evaluation may be useful in excluding the presence of a joint effusion and possibly obviating needle aspiration. Also, ultrasound is the imaging modality of choice in the evaluation of infants with suspected developmental dysplasia of the hip. Ultrasound allows both a static evaluation and a dynamic evaluation to assess for potential dislocation, dislocatability, and subluxability of the hip. Ultrasound can be performed with a Pavlik harness in place, and it can also be used to follow the maturation of the hip joint until the capital femoral epiphysis can be seen radiographically when it begins to ossify at 12 to 18 months of age.

NUCLEAR SCINTIGRAPHY

The specificity of nuclear medicine studies is determined by the radiopharmaceutical agent that is administered. Selective uptake of radiopharmaceutical agents occurs in tissues in a temporally predictable fashion. The radiotracer portion of the radiopharmaceutical is typically a gamma-emitting

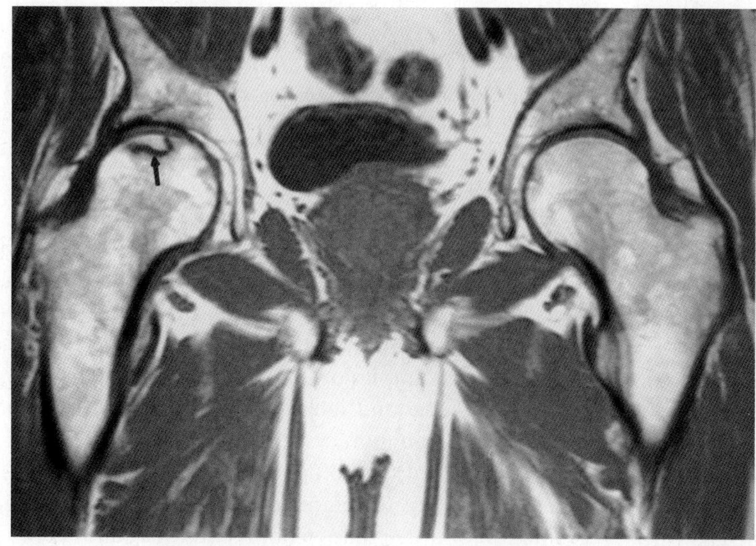

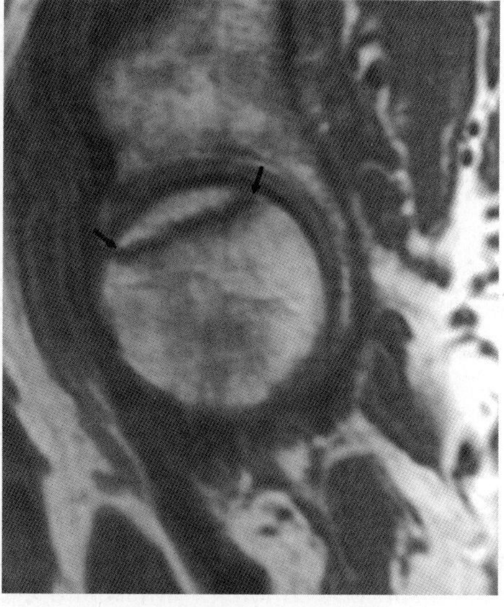

Figure 3.19 SE 500/10 images of the hips in a patient with early AVN on the right. Radiographs were normal. **A:** Coronal image demonstrating a small linear subchondral defect (*arrow*). **B:** Sagittal image of the right hip more clearly defines the extent of involvement (*arrows*). (*Reprinted with permission from* Berquist TH. *MRI of the Musculoskeletal System*. 5th ed. Philadelphia, PA: Lippincott Williams & Wilkins, 2006.)

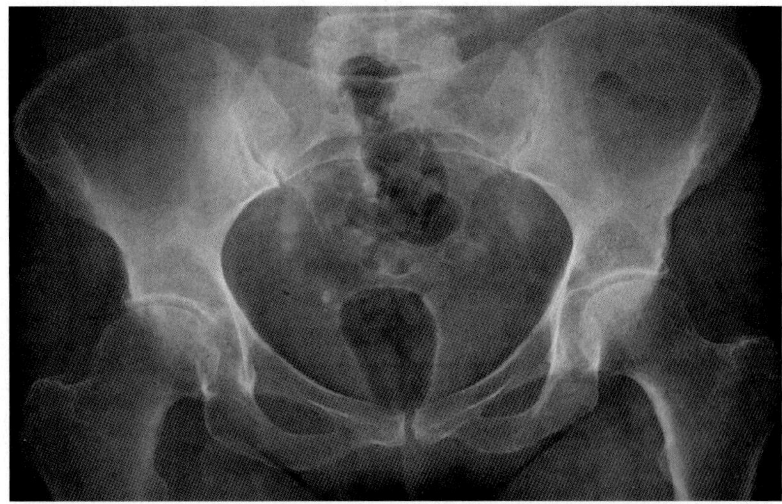

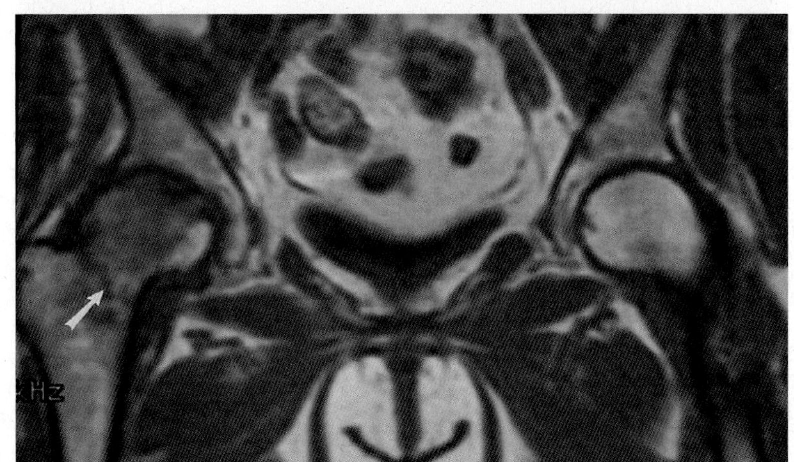

Figure 3.20 Patient with right hip pain and normal radiograph **(A)**. Coronal T1-weighted image **(B)** demonstrates decreased signal intensity due to edema and a fracture at the base of the femoral neck (*arrow*). (*Reprinted with permission from* Berquist TH. *MRI of the Musculoskeletal System*. 5th ed. Philadelphia, PA: Lippincott Williams & Wilkins, 2006.)

isotope, and the distribution of the radiopharmaceutical is imaged by a gamma (scintillation) camera. These cameras have large faces and can scan large areas of the body quickly to produce planar images. Gamma cameras can also be designed to rotate around the patient to collect multiple views, which can then be reconstructed into tomographic or cross-sectional images in various planes. This application is referred to as SPECT (single photon emission computed tomography) imaging. Technetium-99 m (^{99m}Tc) is the radioisotope used most commonly for clinical scintigraphy because of its inexpensive production from portable generators, convenient half-life of 6 hours, and a principle photon energy of 140 keV, which is well suited to detection by gamma cameras.

Skeletal scintigraphy, or bone scan, is the nuclear medicine examination most commonly performed for the evaluation of orthopaedic problems. Imaging commences approximately 2 to 4 hours after the intravenous administration of the radiopharmaceutical, which is usually ^{99m}Tc-methylene diphosphonate (MDP). The MDP bone scan is highly sensitive for a diversity of bony abnormalities, images the entire skeletal system, and is well tolerated by patients. Image acquisition requires 30 to 40 minutes. The uptake of ^{99m}Tc-MDP is determined by both the osteoblastic activity of bone and the blood flow to the bone. MDP uptake is diminished in osteoporosis and in patients who are on bisphosphonate therapy.

The most common application of skeletal scintigraphy is in detecting metastatic disease, for which the sensitivity approaches 95%. Metastatic disease causes altered bone metabolism that subsequently effects a focal increase in uptake of MDP. Metastatic disease is detected much earlier on bone scans than on radiography (Fig. 3.24). Bone density has to change by 30% to 50% before a plain radiograph will depict infiltrative disease; therefore, bone scanning is the most appropriate means to establish metastatic disease in most cases. However, certain aggressive and purely osteolytic tumors, such as multiple myeloma, may not produce increased uptake on bone scan, or they may present as photon-deficient or "cold" areas that can be overlooked. Consequently, multiple myeloma is staged with a radiographic skeletal survey.

Occasionally, after effective chemotherapy, metastatic bone lesions may exhibit increased osteoblastic activity that

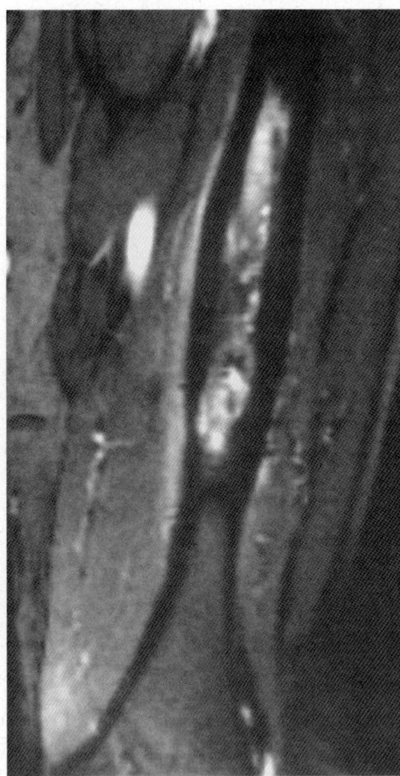

Figure 3.21 Osteomyelitis in the left femur. Coronal STIR sequence shows subtle thickening of the cortex with increased signal intensity in the marrow and adjacent soft tissues. (*Reprinted with permission from* Berquist TH. *MRI of the Musculoskeletal System.* 5th ed. Philadelphia, PA: Lippincott Williams & Wilkins, 2006.)

manifests as increased activity on follow-up bone scans and is known as the "flare" phenomenon. Therefore, increased uptake in this setting should not be interpreted as a sign that metastatic disease has progressed. With advanced and diffuse metastatic disease (typically secondary to prostate or breast carcinoma), the bone scan may show such diffusely increased bone activity that it assumes a pseudonormal appearance, known as a "superscan." This scan may be recognized by noting the diminished or absent renal tracer activity that also characterizes most of these cases.

Bone scintigraphy is of limited value in imaging primary bone neoplasms. The area of uptake may not reflect the true tumor margins, and soft-tissue involvement will not be appreciated. Bone scans are not reliable in distinguishing malignant from benign lesions, although the pattern of uptake may reflect the aggressiveness of the lesion. In evaluating what is presumed to be a solitary bone lesion, a bone scan is mainly useful in excluding multifocal disease or unsuspected metastatic disease.

Clinical history and examination are important in interpreting bone scans, as tracer uptake is highly nonspecific. Sites of bony trauma and degenerative joint disease will routinely appear as incidental, focal areas of increased radiotracer uptake on bone scan. Bone scans are therefore good studies in detecting occult and stress fractures. About 80% of occult fractures are seen at 24 hours after fracture and 95% by 3 days. The greatest tracer uptake is seen approximately 7 days after fracture. Bone scans will revert back to normal at about 1 year after fracture. Stress fractures and stress reactions appear as focal increased areas of tracer uptake, while the related entity of shin splints appears as a more diffuse area of increased tracer localization.

Avascular necrosis, regardless of cause, can be readily identified on bone scan, although the appearance depends on the time course of the disease process. Because of the decreased blood flow to the site, recently infarcted bone will appear photopenic. Depiction of the infarcted, photopenic areas requires spatial resolution, possibly requiring SPECT imaging. Later in the disease process, healing and new bone formation will appear as increased activity about the area of infarction. This presentation can be difficult to distinguish from arthrosis.

Osteomyelitis, especially in its acute form, can be diagnosed by bone scanning much more readily than with plain radiography. Radiotracer uptake will generally be increased at sites of osteomyelitis within the first 24 hours of infection, while radiographic change occurs later in the disease process. Dynamic multiphase imaging heightens the specificity of bone scan by better differentiating osteomyelitis from cellulitis or septic arthritis. The first phase (flow phase) consists of dynamic acquisition of images over the area of interest every 2 to 5 seconds for the first 1 to 3 minutes after injection and reflects regional blood flow. In the second phase, static images are obtained during the first 10 to 20 minutes after injection after adequate recirculation of tracer; this phase is known as the "blood pool or tissue phase" and reflects circulating blood volume. For the third, or delayed, phase, images are obtained 2 to 4 hours after injection, at which point substantial clearance of soft tissue and blood pool activity has occurred. Increased activity on all three phases of bone-scan imaging is seen in osteomyelitis, whereas cellulitis is abnormal on only the first two phases. However, a positive three-phase bone scan is not entirely specific for osteomyelitis and can be seen in inflammatory arthritis, gout, acute fracture, reflex sympathetic dystrophy, and neuropathic joint disease. The sensitivity of the three-phase bone scan may also be decreased in cases of severe peripheral vascular disease and in the diabetic foot.

Gallium-67 citrate had traditionally been used in conjunction with technetium to increase the specificity of diagnosis for osteomyelitis. More recently, scanning with labeled leukocytes has largely supplanted gallium scanning in the scintigraphic evaluation of osteomyelitis and soft-tissue abscesses. Gallium still has use in a few settings, however. Gallium can be useful to evaluate potential disk space and vertebral infections. It can also be used in the evaluation of pediatric patients in that gallium is not as fully taken up by the growth plate as is technetium. Gallium is also useful for staging and assessing progression in patients with lymphoma.

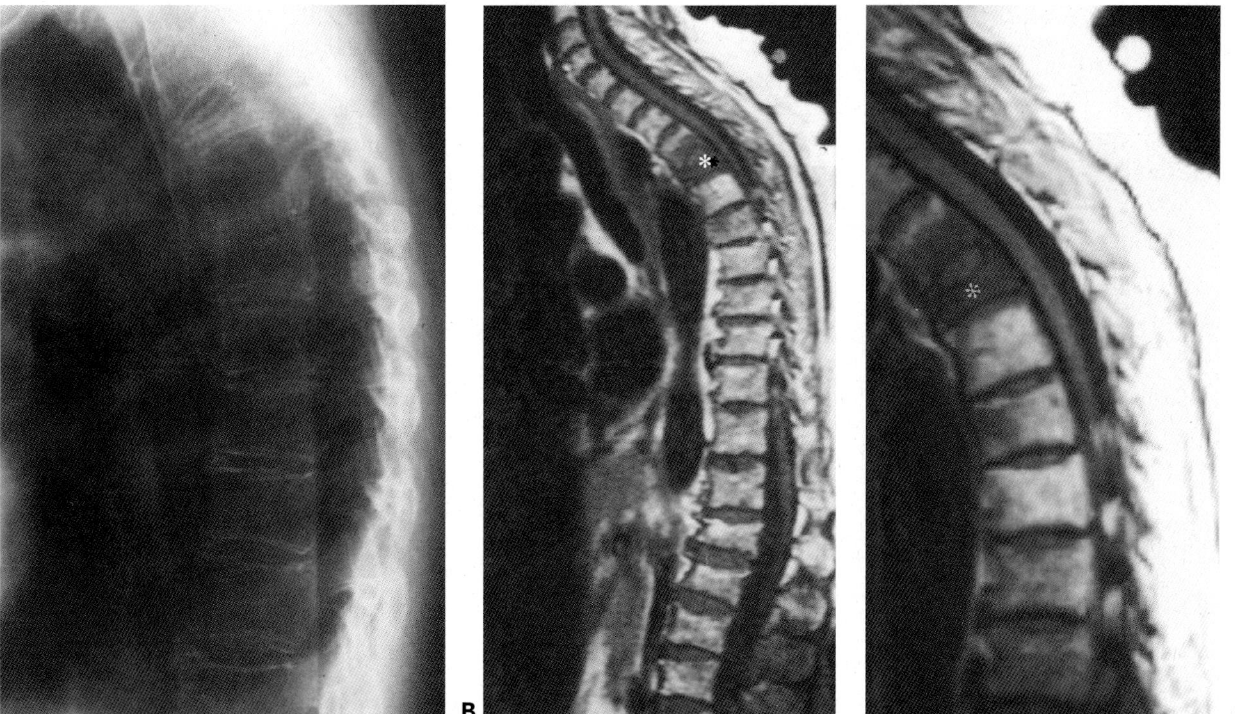

Figure 3.22 Pathologic compression fracture of the T4 vertebral body in a 73-year-old woman being evaluated for metastatic disease after identification of a lung carcinoma. **A:** Lateral thoracic spine radiograph shows marked compression fracture of the T4 vertebral body. No other lesions are seen. **B:** Large field of view T1-weighted (500/15) SE MR image of the spine shows the fracture at T4 (*asterisk*) and as partial replacement of the marrow in the T3 vertebral body and T6 vertebral body. **C:** Corresponding small field of view lateral T1-weighted (500/15) image shows areas of marrow replacement to better advantage. Transpedicular biopsy of the T4 lesion revealed multiple myeloma. (*Reprinted with permission from* Berquist TH. *MRI of the Musculoskeletal System*. 5th ed. Philadelphia, PA: Lippincott Williams & Wilkins, 2006.)

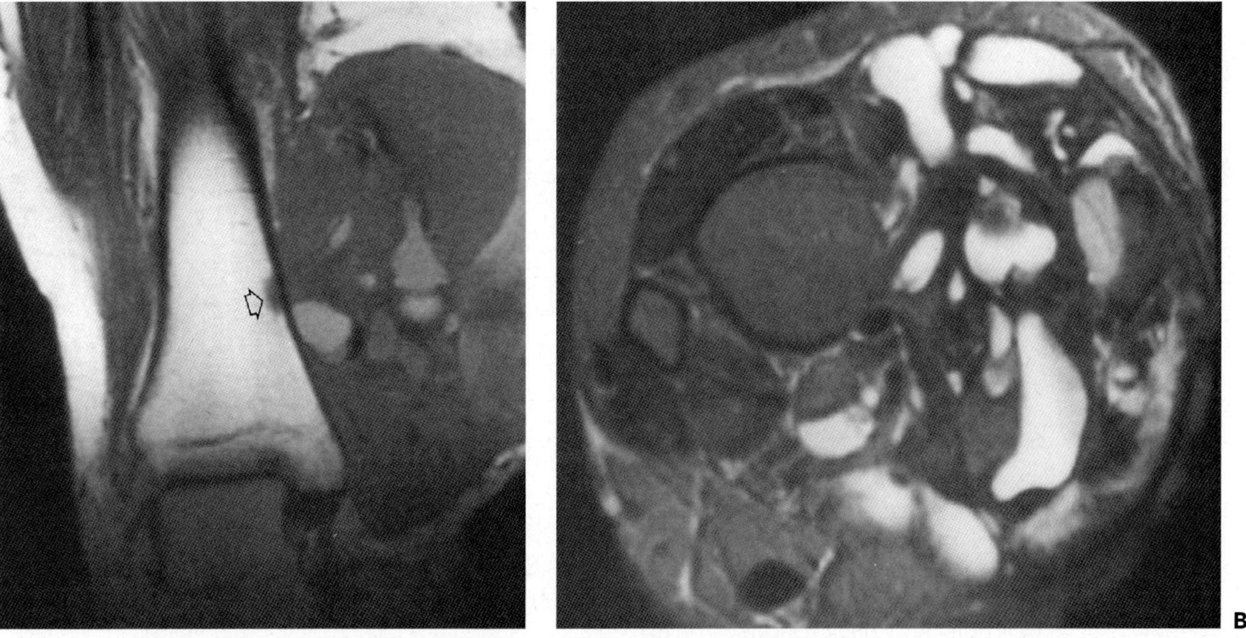

Figure 3.23 Synovial sarcoma in the ankle of a 37-year-old woman. Coronal T1-weighted (600/20) **(A)** and axial T2-weighted (2,000/80) **(B)** SE MR images show a large well-defined mass, with a complex signal intensity compatible with previous hemorrhage. Note subtle area of bone invasion in **A** (*open arrow*). (*Reprinted with permission from* Berquist TH. *MRI of the Musculoskeletal System*. 5th ed. Philadelphia, PA: Lippincott Williams & Wilkins, 2006.)

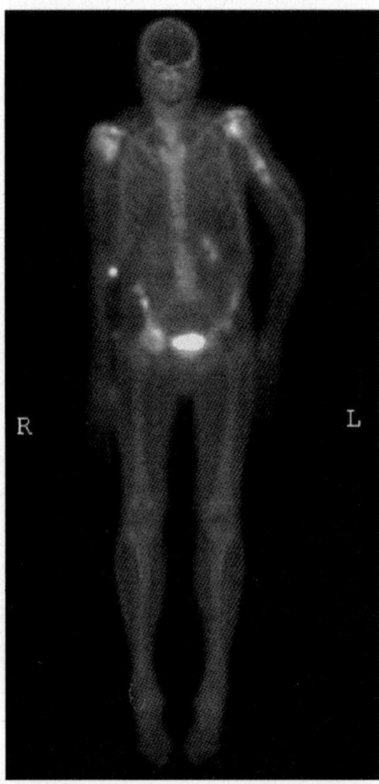

Figure 3.24 Radionuclide bone scan demonstrates abnormal radiotracer uptake within the midshaft of the left humerus, right iliac crest, and right acetabulum, which is suspicious for bone metastasis. Increased uptake within the shoulder joints is related to osteoarthritis. (Reprinted with permission from Chew F, Roberts C, *Musculoskeletal Imaging: A Teaching File*, 2nd ed. Philadelphia PA: Lippincott Williams & Wilkins, 2006.)

Leukocyte scintigraphy (i.e., white blood cell scan) has largely replaced gallium scanning for the assessment of complicated osteomyelitis. A white blood cell scan is performed by separating white blood cells from approximately 50 mL of whole blood. These cells are then labeled with either indium-111 oxine or ^{99m}Tc hexamethylpropylenamine oxime (HMPAO). The labeled cells are then reintroduced into the patient. Scanning is usually performed at about 6 and 12 hours after the injection. Technetium is preferable to gallium for this purpose because the shorter half-life of technetium permits a larger dose to be used. This more favorable dosing allows for a higher count rate and therefore a higher resolution image.

Labeled white cell studies have proven to be effective in diagnosing infection about total joint arthroplasties and internal fixation hardware. Regular bone scanning is somewhat limited for this indication, although it can give some information about prosthetic loosening. Localization of white blood cells around orthopaedic implants is not entirely diagnostic of infection, and, indeed, localization can occur in the absence of infection. However, if the white blood cell scan is correlated with a technetium colloid marrow scan, the diagnostic capability is enhanced. If the white blood cell scan shows strong uptake and the marrow scan does as well, then the white cell accumulation is deemed physiologic. White cell localization with a negative marrow scan is indicative of infection. The accuracy of white blood cell scanning for osteomyelitis is lower in the spine, and it may also be diminished after antibiotic therapy and in cases of chronic osteomyelitis.

The availability of whole-body positron emission tomography (PET) imaging is increasing. In particular, fluorine-18-fluorodeoxyglucose PET (FDG-PET) imaging has gained acceptance for its ability to effectively stage tumors and evaluate for recurrent neoplasia. This imaging technique, which identifies sites of increased glucose utilization, is also an alternative method to diagnose osteomyelitis in complicated clinical settings.

BONE DENSITOMETRY

Osteoporosis is increasingly being recognized as a major public health problem, with huge attendant health care costs and morbidity rates. Bone densitometry studies are increasingly used to assess fracture risk and to guide treatment decisions. Guidelines for the use of this imaging modality continue to evolve.

The technique that is most commonly used for osteoporosis screening is dual energy x-ray absorptiometry (DEXA). Routine DEXA screening is performed on the lumbar spine and the hip. The dual-energy feature of this examination permits separate calculation of x-ray attenuation from bone and from soft tissue. In this way the bone mineral content can be derived from a two-dimensional projection technique. Modern DEXA scanners utilize a fan-beam x-ray source and are thus quite fast (<5 minutes for image acquisition).

The advantages of DEXA over traditional methods of osteoporosis imaging are the extremely low radiation dose (<5 mrad), high precision, and relatively low cost. Measured bone mineral density from DEXA examinations is most commonly expressed as a standard deviation from the mean bone density of healthy young control subjects (*T* score), or, less important, as a standard deviation from the mean for age- and sex-matched control subjects (*Z* score). A *T* score between -1 and -2.5 indicates osteopenia, whereas a *T* score of less than -2.5 is diagnostic of osteoporosis. Various regions of interest are reported for the hip, but the bone mineral content of the femoral neck is probably the most precise and, therefore, the most useful measurement.

RADIATION EXPOSURE CONSIDERATIONS

One further subject that must be broached in this review is that of radiation exposure to the orthopaedic surgeon. Radiographic visualization is a necessary part of many orthopaedic procedures, and many orthopaedic surgeons are poorly educated about the perils of radiation exposure and steps that can be taken to avoid potentially harmful radiation exposure. Radiation safety and protection largely falls under the jurisdiction of the U.S. Food and Drug Administration (USFDA), which typically follows the advice of advisory bodies such as the National Council on Radiation Protection and Measurements (NCRP) and the International Commission on Radiological Protection (ICRP). These advisory bodies periodically review the scientific literature and make recommendations regarding radiation safety and protection.

There are various units used to measure radiation exposure, but the SI unit is Gray. Gray is a unit of measurement defined as 1 Joule (J) of energy deposited in 1 kg of material. However, the unit most commonly used in the literature, and that which is used to define exposure limits, is the rem. One milliGray (mGy) is equal to 100 millirems (mrem).

To put exposures in perspective, the minimum dose that causes skin erythema is approximately 2 to 3 Gray. Death occurs in 10 to 24 hours after exposures of 6 to 10 Gray. Of greater practical concern are the risks associated with low-level radiation exposures, and these are estimated from mathematical and statistical models. The incremental lifetime risk of cancer (usually leukemia or lymphoma) is estimated to be approximately 0.1% per 0.01 Gray. Expressed differently, if 100,000 people each received a dose of 0.01 Gray, approximately two new cases of cancer would be anticipated per year, based on a life expectancy of about 75 years.

In the terms of an orthopaedic surgeon, the primary way to decrease radiation effects is to minimize exposure, both by using radiation only when necessary and by wearing appropriate shielding. Hands are at the greatest risk for exposure. Using a regular C-arm, exposure rates for an orthopaedic surgeon are estimated to be as high as 20 mrem per minute to the torso and 30 mrem per minute to the hands. If a given intramedullary rod procedure requires 5 minutes of fluoroscopy, then the exposure dose to the surgeon is 100 mrem for the torso and 150 mrem for the hands. Protection of the torso can reduce that exposure to 10 mrem, but the hand exposure remains. The current NCRP guideline allows 5 rem of exposure to the torso and 50 rem exposure to the hand yearly. Using these numbers, an orthopaedic surgeon would thereby be limited to only 333 cases with this degree of exposure in one year. While these guidelines are just that (i.e., not law), one must realize the serious and potentially detrimental nature of radiation exposure and must not take it lightly.

As stated above, the best way to minimize risk is to avoid exposure and wear shielding. Other ways to accomplish this goal include using a mini C-arm, inverting the C-arm, and increasing one's distance from the C-arm. Using a mini-C-arm, average radiation dose to the hand in a given case is 20 mrem. The radiation dose with the mini-C-arm is typically about 10% of that of the dose with the regular C-arm. One must remember, however, that typically one works much closer to the beam when using a mini-C-arm and also closer to the scatter created. Tremains et al. noted that the radiation dose to the patient and the surgeon is significantly less if the C-arm is inverted. With the regular C-arm, studies have shown that only those within 6 ft of the beam need to wear protective shielding, as the dose precipitously drops off the further one gets away from the beam. This distance for the mini-C-arm is 3 ft. Despite these facts, it is probably best for those who are often in the setting of fluoroscopy to use protection every time.

RECOMMENDED READINGS

Domb BG, Tyler W, Ellis S, McCarthy E. Radiographic evaluation of pathological bone lesions: current spectrum of disease and approach to diagnosis. *J Bone Joint Surg Am.* 2004;86-A(suppl 2): 84–90.

Grissom L, Harcke HT, Thacker M. Imaging in the surgical management of developmental dislocation of the hip. *Clin Orthop Relat Res.* 2008;466(4):791–801.

Sanders TG, Miller MD. A systematic approach to magnetic resonance imaging interpretation of sports medicine injuries of the knee. *Am J Sports Med.* 2005;33(1):131–148.

Sanders TG, Morrison WB, Miller MD. Imaging techniques for the evaluation of glenohumeral instability. *Am J Sports Med.* 2000; 28(3):414–434.

Shindle MK, Foo LF, Kelly BT, et al. Magnetic resonance imaging of cartilage in the athlete: current techniques and spectrum of disease. *J Bone Joint Surg Am.* 2006;88(suppl 4):27–46.

Electrodiagnostic Testing

4

Michael K. Kuo

INTRODUCTION

Electrodiagnostic medicine is "a specific area of medical practice in which a physician integrates information obtained from the clinical history, observations from physical examination, and scientific data acquired from recording electrical potentials from the nervous system and muscle to diagnose, or diagnose and treat diseases of the central, peripheral, and autonomic nervous systems, neuromuscular junctions, and muscle." Electrodiagnostic testing typically consists of two components, nerve conduction studies (NCS) and electromyography (EMG).

It is critical that electrodiagnostic testing be used as an extension of a focused history and physical examination. The history and examination is used to formulate an initial differential diagnosis. Based on this differential diagnosis, specific nerves and muscles are examined with NCS and EMG. The techniques used as well as the specific nerves and muscles examined are initially determined by this differential diagnosis. The early NCS and EMG findings will determine what additional testing is required and will further narrow the differential diagnosis. The electrodiagnostic impression is determined not only by the test results but also by the clinical information. Relying solely on the electrodiagnostic data to formulate an impression frequently leads to misdiagnosis. For example, normal NCS and EMG for a patient with a clinical lumbar radiculitis does not rule out a lumbar nerve root source for the patient's symptoms. The diagnostic limitations of NCS and EMG make clinical correlation crucial.

Electrodiagnostic testing is used as a tool for diagnosing neuromuscular disorders. Although information can be obtained regarding the central nervous system, electrodiagnostic testing is primarily used to diagnose peripheral nervous system and muscle disorders. Anatomically this may include anterior horn cells, sensory and motor roots, brachial and lumbosacral plexuses, peripheral nerves, neuromuscular junctions, and muscles. In addition to diagnosis, electrodiagnostic testing can help with localization, determining severity, and prognosis. For example, a patient with hand numbness can be diagnosed with a median neuropathy with NCS and EMG. The testing can further localize the lesion to the wrist or forearm, determine which nerve fiber types are involved (motor/sensory), verify how much axon loss versus demyelination has occurred, and give a prognosis based on this information.

NERVE CONDUCTION STUDIES

NCS involve the induction of a propagating action potential along a peripheral nerve and the subsequent recording of this electrical waveform. The induction is performed with a brief electrical stimulus from a stimulator probe applied to the surface of the skin overlying the peripheral nerve to be examined. The recording is performed by placing recording electrodes over a more distal portion of the peripheral nerve or over a muscle that is innervated by the nerve. The waveforms produced have parameters that can provide information regarding the location of the injury and type of pathology involved (axon loss vs. demyelination).

Basic NCS include *motor NCS* and *sensory NCS*. *Late responses* (F-waves and H-reflexes) can provide additional information regarding proximal portions of tested peripheral nerves. *Repetitive nerve stimulation (RNS) studies* are useful for diagnosing neuromuscular junction disorders.

Patient Preparation

In preparing for NCS, patients are instructed to avoid skin creams and lotions as surface electrodes may not fasten securely to the skin. There are no absolute contraindications for NCS, although these are not recommended in patients with external cardiac pacemakers. In patients with implanted cardiac pacemakers, NCS can be performed as long as stimulation near the thorax is avoided. In patients with central lines, stimulation over the central line site is not recommended as the electrical impulse could travel to the heart via the catheter.

Sensory NCS

Sensory NCS are performed by placement of recording electrodes over the nerve to be examined. There are two recording electrodes, an active electrode and a reference electrode. As both electrodes record electrical waveforms, attention to electrode placement is vital. The active electrode is placed over the nerve. The reference electrode is placed distally on the nerve 3 to 4 cm from the active electrode. An electrical stimulus from the stimulator probe is applied to the nerve at a measured distance from the active electrode.

The electrical waveform produced is known as the *sensory nerve action potential* (SNAP). The SNAP waveform represents the summation of the individual sensory action potentials stimulated. The waveform has the following parameters: *onset latency, peak latency, amplitude, duration,* and *conduction velocity* (Fig. 4.1). Normal values are available for latencies at defined distances and amplitudes for specific sensory nerves.

Conduction velocity is calculated by dividing the distance traveled by the electrical stimulus by the onset latency. This simple calculation cannot be used with respect to motor NCS as will be discussed later. Normal conduction velocities tend to be greater than 48 m per second for upper limb studies and greater than 39 m per second for lower limb studies.

Motor NCS

Motor NCS are performed by placement of the active electrode over the motor endplate, usually the center of the muscle belly. The reference electrode is placed distally over an inactive point such as the tendon insertion. The peripheral nerve is stimulated at a measured point proximally.

The waveform produced is known as the *compound muscle action potential* (CMAP). The CMAP is the summated electrical activity from depolarization of muscle fibers under the active electrode. The most common parameters analyzed include *onset latency, amplitude, duration,* and *conduction velocity* (Fig. 4.2). Normative data are available for latencies and amplitudes.

The complexity of the motor onset latency makes measurement of motor conduction velocities less straightforward than measurement of sensory conduction velocities. Simply dividing the distance traveled by the electrical stimulus by the onset latency will not produce an accurate conduction velocity because of the variability in the neuromuscular junction time. To calculate a motor conduction velocity, the nerve must be stimulated at two different sites, distal and proximal. The onset latency from the distal stimulation is subtracted from the onset latency of the proximal stimulation. This "subtracts" out the neuromuscular transmission time, as well as the latency of activation, leaving the action potential time between the two stimulation points. The conduction velocity is calculated by dividing the

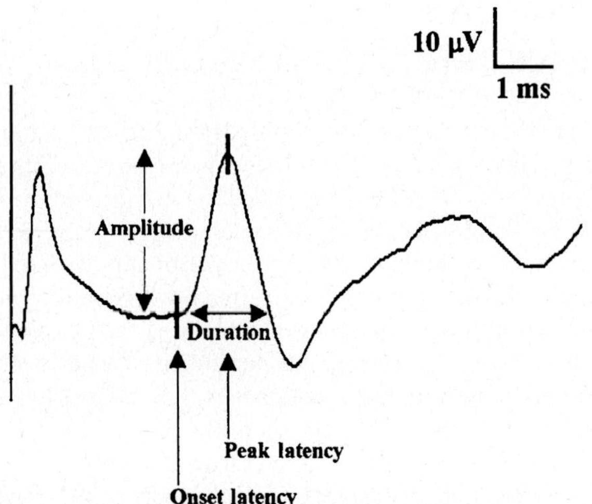

Figure 4.1 Sensory nerve action potential (SNAP). The SNAP is usually biphasic or triphasic in configuration. Latencies are measured in ms. Amplitudes are measured in μV. (*From* Preston DC, Shapiro BE. *Electromyography and Neuromuscular Disorders.* 2nd ed. Philadelphia, PA: Elsevier, Butterworth-Heinemann, 2005, *with permission.*)

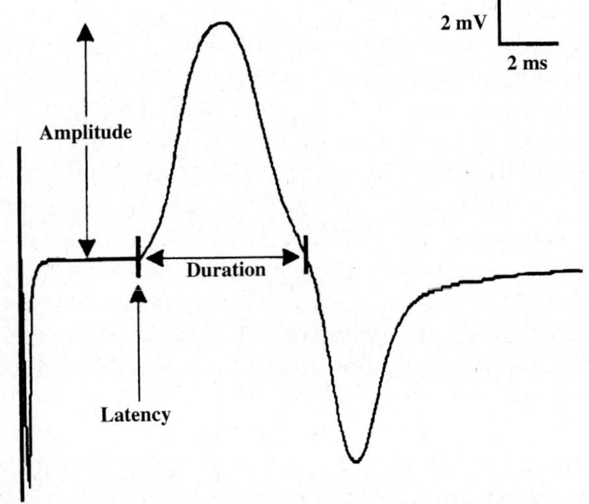

Figure 4.2 Compound muscle action potential (CMAP). The CMAP is biphasic. Latencies are measured in ms. Amplitudes are measured in millivolt. (*From* Preston DC, Shapiro BE. *Electromyography and Neuromuscular Disorders.* 2nd ed. Philadelphia, PA: Elsevier, Butterworth-Heinemann, 2005, *with permission.*)

distance between the two stimulation points by the action potential time between the points. Normal conduction velocities tend to be greater than 48 meters per second for upper limb studies and greater than 39 meters per second for lower limb studies.

Late Responses

In addition to sensory and motor conduction studies, *late responses* can be obtained to assess the proximal portions of the nerves. Late responses include *F-waves* and *H-reflexes.* Theses waveforms involve an action potential traveling proximally to the spinal cord and then distally to the recording electrodes.

F-waves only involve motor neurons. They are late motor responses that occur after the CMAP. They were first noted in the foot muscles, hence the name, F-wave. F-waves can be elicited from any nerve that has motor axons. Active and reference electrodes are placed the same way as for a motor conduction study. An electrical stimulus is applied to the nerve distally. A supramaximal stimulus is used. A CMAP (also known as the *M-wave*) is produced when the action potential travels from the stimulation site distally to the recording electrodes. The F-wave is produced from the action potential that is traveling in the opposite direction. This action potential travels to the anterior horn cells at the spinal cord. A small proportion of the anterior horn cells will "backfire," resulting in an action potential that will travel back down the nerve to the recording electrodes, and produce an F-wave (Fig. 4.3).

F-waves tend to be small (1% to 5% of CMAP amplitude). They also vary in latency. For this reason, at least 10 F-waves are obtained and the fastest waveform (F-wave minimum, or F-wave min) is chosen. Normative data are available for specific nerves and different leg lengths (heights). F-waves are usually performed bilaterally, and side-to-side differences are evaluated. Normal side-to-side differences are less than 2.0 ms for the upper limbs and less than 4.0 ms for the lower limbs.

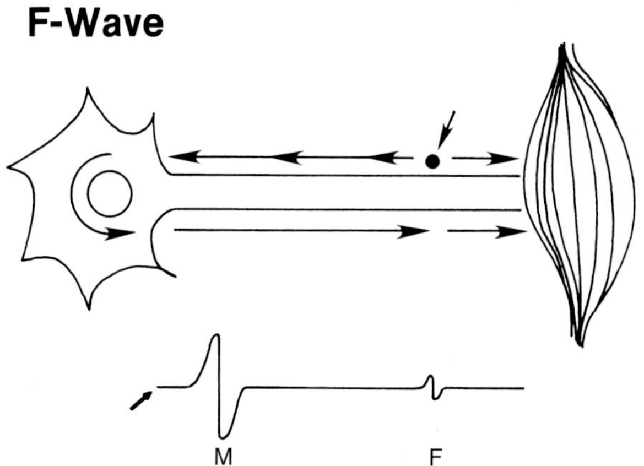

Figure 4.3 F-wave. The course of the depolarization following stimulation (dot) is shown by the arrows. Initially, depolarization travels both directly to the muscle fibers, producing the M-wave, and in a retrograde fashion up the axon to the neuron, where the excitation of the neuron causes "backfiring" in a small percentage of neurons (randomly occurring), resulting in an action potential returning back down the axon to produce the delayed F-wave. The trace below shows a recording of the M-wave and F-wave. (*From* Pease WS, Lew HL, Johnson EW. *Johnson's Practical Electromyography.* 4th ed. Philadelphia, PA: Lippincott Williams & Wilkins, 2007, *with permission.*)

Although F-waves are used to assess the more proximal portions of the nerves, their diagnostic utility is limited. While they are helpful in diagnosing generalized neuropathic processes that may affect proximal nerve segments such as polyneuropathies and polyradiculopathies (i.e., Guillain-Barré Syndrome), they are of minimal use with radiculopathies and plexopathies. F-wave limitations are related to multiple factors. F-waves require only a few intact fast fibers for the F-wave min response to be normal. As most muscles are innervated by two or more nerve roots, single nerve root abnormalities usually result in a normal F-wave min. Since F-waves involve only motor fibers, a sensory radiculopathy will result in a normal F-wave min. F-waves test long segments. Unless the pathology is severe, the abnormalities may be "diluted out" because of the long distance assessed.

Since F-waves involve not only the proximal nerve segment but also the distal, an abnormal F-wave min alone will not localize the lesion. For example, a patient with a median neuropathy at the wrist can have a delayed median F-wave due to slowing of the F-wave across the carpal tunnel. On the other hand, an abnormal F-wave with normal *distal* motor conduction studies does suggest a proximal lesion. For instance, if the median motor conduction studies are completely normal, but the median F-waves are delayed or absent, this would suggest a lesion more proximally.

Hoffman first described the H-reflex in 1918. This is a late response that has sensory afferent and motor efferent components, and is thus a true reflex. In adults, the H-reflex is typically obtained with stimulation of the tibial nerve while recording over the gastrocnemius/soleus muscle. For the tibial H-reflex, the active electrode is placed over the gastrocnemius muscle (the point that bisects the line from popliteal fossa to the medial malleolus). The reference electrode is placed over the Achilles tendon. An electrical stimulus is applied to the tibial nerve at the popliteal fossa. The optimal stimulus is a *long-duration, submaximal* stimulus. This type of stimulus will selectively activate Ia afferent sensory fibers. The action potential will travel along the sensory nerve to the spinal cord, traverse a synapse to the motor neuron, travel down the motor nerve to the recording electrodes, and produce the waveform known as the "H-reflex" (Fig. 4.4). The type of stimulus is vital. Too small a stimulus will not produce a response. Too high a stimulus will extinguish the H-reflex and produce an F-wave.

Unlike the F-wave, the H-reflex tends to be larger (can be as large as the CMAP) and is of constant latency. For this reason, it is not necessary to obtain 10 or more waveforms. As with the F-wave, the H-reflex can be used to assess

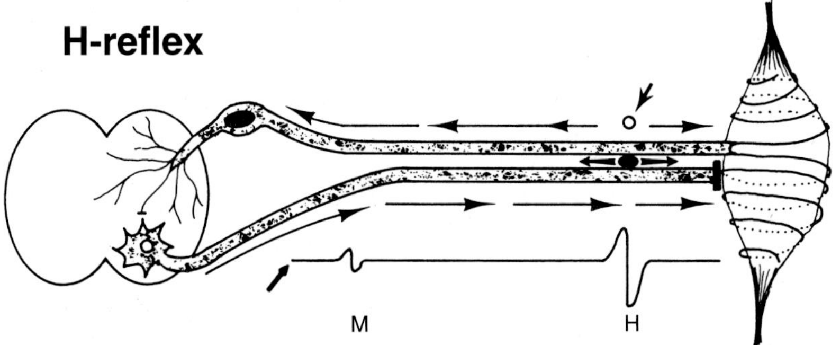

Figure 4.4 H-reflex. The response is obtained with stimulation (open dot) of the afferent sensory fiber **(top)**. A long-duration, low-amplitude stimulus selectively activates the sensory afferents. A few motor fibers are usually activated as well, producing a rudimentary M-wave. The action potential travels along the sensory fiber **(top)** to the spinal cord, synapses with the motor neuron, and then travels back down the motor fiber **(bottom)** to the muscle, producing the H-reflex. (*From* Pease WS, Lew HL, Johnson EW. *Johnson's Practical Electromyography*. 4th ed. Philadelphia, PA: Lippincott Williams & Wilkins, 2007, *with permission*.)

the proximal portions of the nerve. Its diagnostic utility is similar to that of F-waves with respect to polyneuropathy and polyradiculopathy. Uniquely, the H-reflex can be used to evaluate S1 radiculopathies as the tibial H-reflex is primarily made up of S1 fibers. The limitations of the H-reflex are similar to those of the F-wave, although one advantage of the H-reflex is that it involves sensory as well as motor fibers. F-waves only involve motor fibers. A S1 sensory radiculopathy may result in an abnormal tibial H-reflex, whereas the rest of the electrodiagnostic testing will be normal. As with F-waves, performing bilateral studies is the standard. A side-to-side difference of greater than 1.5 ms is considered abnormal. Normal values for H-reflex latencies are dependent on age and leg length.

Repetitive Nerve Stimulation

RNS is primarily used to assess neuromuscular junction disorders. The technique is similar to a motor conduction study, except that in this study 5 to 10 successive supramaximal stimulations are applied. Multiple CMAPs are produced and usually displayed on the same baseline. In normal subjects, RNS at 2 to 3 Hz will produce CMAP waveforms with constant amplitude (Fig. 4.5). In a patient with a neuromuscular junction disorder, a gradual reduction in the CMAP amplitude is often seen, and this is known as a "decrement." This decrement can be accentuated using exercise or high-frequency RNS. Exercise (10 to 15 second isometric contraction) or high-frequency RNS (20 to 50 Hz) results in calcium build-up at the axon nerve terminal. When RNS at 2 to 3 Hz is performed immediately after exercise or high-frequency RNS, the CMAP amplitude enlarges temporarily. This is known as "facilitation." The RNS at 2 to 3 Hz is repeated every 1 minute for 5 to 6 minutes. In a patient with a neuromuscular junction disorder, the decrement will be noticeably accentuated, known as "postexercise exhaustion" (Fig. 4.6). The pattern of the decrement, facilitation, and postexercise exhaustion can help determine whether the neuromuscular junction disorder is postsynaptic (i.e., myasthenia gravis) or presynaptic (i.e., Lambert-Eaton myasthenic syndrome).

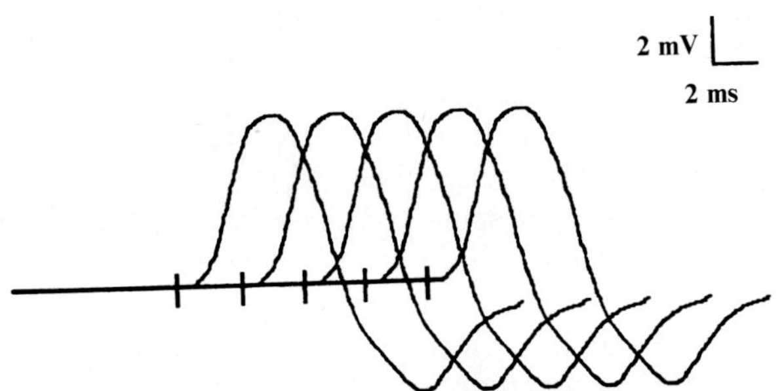

Figure 4.5 Repetitive nerve stimulation (RNS) at 3 Hz in a normal subject. In this example, five successive motor nerve stimulations were performed and recorded. In normal subjects, the amplitude should change minimally or not at all. (*From* Preston DC, Shapiro BE. *Electromyography and Neuromuscular Disorders*. 2nd ed. Philadelphia, PA: Elsevier, Butterworth-Heinemann, 2005, *with permission*.)

NCS PITFALLS

Electrodiagnostic medicine is wrought with pitfalls, some related to inherent limitations of the testing itself and also to technical factors. As noted previously, NCS and EMG should be used as an extension of a focused history and physical examination. Too frequently, testing is now being performed by technicians without electrodiagnostic physicians' direct supervision or involvement. This often results in excessive testing and erroneous diagnoses. The limitations of NCS and EMG vary depending on the specific disease processes and diagnoses being evaluated.

With respect to technical factors, there are many. Today's automated electrodiagnostic equipment requires minimal instrumentation adjustments. Although this improves the ease of testing, one must be careful as normative data are based on specific NCS and EMG techniques using specific instrument settings and electrode placement. Performing testing using different filter settings, sweep speeds, and sensitivity can affect the waveform morphology and/or the measurement of the waveform parameters. Attention needs to be made with respect to active and reference electrode placement in accordance with the NCS technique described.

For NCS, distance measurements are performed with a simple tape measure. Care must be taken to make precise measurement to reduce latency and calculated conduction

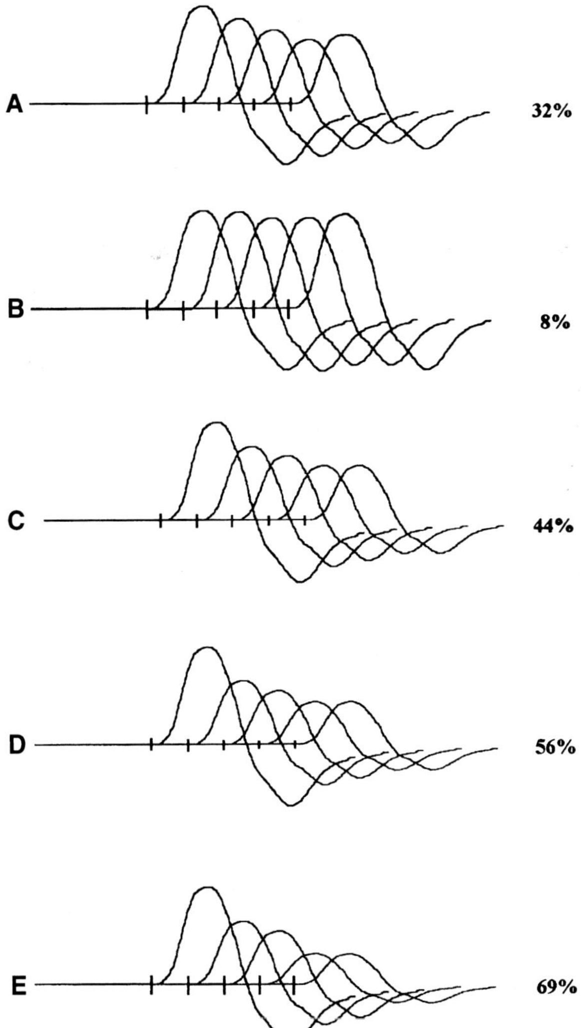

Figure 4.6 Postexercise facilitation and exhaustion in a patient with myasthenia gravis. Three-Hz RNS is performed. **A:** Decrement of compound muscle action potential (CMAP) amplitude at rest. **B:** Postexercise facilitation. Decrement of CMAP immediately following 10 seconds of maximal voluntary exercise has repaired toward normal. **C–E:** Postexercise exhaustion. Decrements of CMAP 1, 2, and 3 minutes after the previous exercise. Decrement becomes progressively more marked over the baseline decrement. *(From* Preston DC, Shapiro BE. *Electromyography and Neuromuscular Disorders.* 2nd ed. Philadelphia, PA: Elsevier, Butterworth-Heinemann, 2005, *with permission.)*

velocity errors. Over shorter interstimulus distances, measurement errors produce significantly higher conduction velocity calculation errors.

Physiologic factors such as age, temperature, limb length/height, and anomalous innervations influence NCS and EMG. With respect to age, newborns have nerve conduction velocities one-half of normal adult conduction velocities. At the age of 3 to 5 years, conduction velocities reach adult values. After the age of 50 years, conduction velocities drop 1 to 2 m per second per decade because of loss of large axons and segmental demyelination/remyelination. With advancing age, nerve conduction amplitudes decline as well. Compared with 18- to 25-year-olds, SNAP amplitudes can be reduced by one-half in 40- to 60-year-olds, and by two-thirds in 70- to 88-year-olds. This is of particular importance with lower limb SNAP amplitudes as they are normally small to begin with. For example, normal sural and superficial peroneal SNAP amplitudes may be as small as 6 to 10 uV. A 2- to 3-uV response in an 80-year-old subject may be difficult to record because of limitations of the instrumentation.

Temperature greatly affects NCS. As nerve temperatures decline, latencies become prolonged, and conduction velocities decline. This occurs because of slowing of sodium channel *activation*. For every 1°C drop in temperature, conduction velocity drops approximately 1 to 2.4 m per second depending on the nerve tested. Declining temperatures also result in slowed sodium channel *inactivation*, resulting in increased SNAP and CMAP amplitudes. Although correction factors can be used to calculate the corresponding latency, conduction velocity, or amplitude at a specific temperature, this adds further calculation error to the testing and is not recommended. The best technique is to warm the cold limb to the appropriate temperature before performing the NCS. Warming methods include hydroculator packs, running the limb under warm tap water, infrared lamps, hairdryers, etc. As the direct nerve temperature is difficult to assess, surface skin temperatures are used. Optimal surface skin temperature is at least 32°C for the upper limbs and at least 30°C for the lower limbs. The temperature should be monitored throughout the testing and recorded on the electrodiagnostic report. Overdiagnosis, particularly when evaluating polyneuropathy, can occur if adequate temperatures are not maintained.

Limb length affects conduction velocity. Longer lower limbs (greater height) tend to have slower conduction velocities. The reduction in conduction velocity is thought to be due to declining axon diameters at uniform distances from the anterior horn cell. Upper limb length does not seem to affect conduction velocity; however, lower limb conduction velocities tend to be slower than uppers, also likely due to smaller axon diameters in the lower limbs compared with the uppers.

Anomalous innervation may lead to NCS and EMG misdiagnosis. These anomalous innervations are more appropriately termed "anatomical variants" as the more common ones can occur in up to 30% of the population. In the upper limbs, the *Martin-Gruber anastomosis* is autosomal dominant with incidence up to 34% and is bilateral in up to 68%. It involves a connection of median motor fibers to ulnar motor fibers in the forearm. The anatomic connection usually occurs through a branch of the median nerve, the anterior interosseous nerve. The anastomosis supplies the first dorsal interosseous muscle (95% to 100% of the time), hypothenar muscles (41% to 61% of the time), and adductor pollicis (14% of the time). Clinically, a patient with a complete ulnar lesion at the elbow may continue to have good hand function if the Martin-Gruber anastomosis occurs.

The *Riche–Cannieu anomaly* occurs in up to 77% of people. It involves an anatomical connection of the median and ulnar nerves in the hand between the recurrent branch of the median nerve and the deep branch of the ulnar nerve. The percentage of median nerve fibers involved is quite variable. With this variant, it is clinically possible to have an "all ulnar hand." In this case, a patient with complete severance of the median nerve at the wrist may continue to have abductor pollicis brevis and opponens pollicis function.

At the lower limbs, the *accessory deep peroneal nerve* has an incidence up to 28% and when present is bilateral up to 57% of the time. Normally, the extensor digitorum brevis (EDB) muscle is innervated by the deep peroneal nerve. In subjects with the variant, the superficial peroneal nerve gives off a branch (accessory deep peroneal nerve) to innervate the EDB. Clinically, a patient with a complete deep peroneal nerve lesion may have a normal EDB EMG and normal EDB function.

ELECTROMYOGRAPHY

Needle EMG involves the use of a fine needle electrode to record electrical activity from muscles. The most commonly used EMG needles are either *concentric* or *monopolar*. Standard concentric needle electrodes consist of a hollow, stainless steel cannula with a central platinum or nichrome silver wire. The wire is the active electrode and the cannula serves as the reference electrode. Monopolar needle electrodes consist of a solid stainless steel needle that is Teflon coated except the tip. The monopolar needle serves as the active electrode. A separate reference electrode, typically a surface electrode, is required. The recording surface area of a monopolar needle is larger than that of a concentric, resulting in recorded motor unit action potentials (MUAPs) with larger amplitudes, longer durations, and more polyphasia. Monopolar needles are associated with more interference and background noise but tend to be less expensive than concentric needles. Both concentric and monopolar needles are available in different lengths and various gauges (23 to 30 gauge). The majority of electromyographers use sterile disposable EMG needles, although some use nondisposables and sterilize them before each use.

Patient Preparation

In general, the needle EMG tends to be more uncomfortable than the NCS. It is recommended that the patient be aware that some discomfort or pain may occur during testing; however, most patients are able to tolerate the procedure without problem. Patient tolerability for electrodiagnostic testing is reliant on numerous factors, including the individual's pain tolerance as well as the examiner's technique and ability to keep the patient distracted. Analgesic or anxiolytic medications prior to testing can be used but are rarely necessary. Topical analgesics are of limited benefit as the majority of discomfort is related to the needle insertions in the muscle and not the skin puncture. There are no absolute contraindications for performing needle EMG; however, relative contraindications include coagulopathy (bleeding risk) and lymphedema (infection risk).

Needle Electromyographic Technique

Typically, the NCS are performed before the needle EMG, although in some cases the needle EMG may be more useful than the NCS and thus performed first. The muscles to be examined via needle EMG are determined by the history and physical examination (and the NCS findings if already performed). The basic steps in needle EMG are (a) insertional activity, (b) muscle at rest to assess for spontaneous activity, and (c) minimal to moderate muscle contraction to assess MUAPs. The electrical activity is evaluated not only visually on the display monitor but also by sound from the EMG speaker.

Insertional Activity

Insertional activity and *muscle at rest* are usually evaluated in same sequence. The needle electrode is inserted into the targeted muscle while the muscle is at rest. The patient's limb may have to be repositioned to relax it adequately. The needle is then quickly inserted further in 0.2 to 2 mm increments with a several second pause between insertions. The needle movement mechanically depolarizes muscle fibers while moving through the muscle. This depolarization is recorded as bursts of electrical activity that stop abruptly after needle movement has stopped. Normal insertional activity has a duration of less than 300 ms after needle movement cessation. Increased insertional activity has a duration greater than 300 ms after needle movement and can occur in muscle denervation or myopathy but can be a normal variant. Decreased insertional activity is either the absence or a significant reduction of the electrical bursts with needle movement. This can occur when the needle is not in muscle, but instead in fat or scar tissue. Minimally, the needle electrode is inserted into four different regions of the muscle at three different depths.

Muscle at Rest

When the needle is being inserted, insertional activity is assessed. When needle movement has stopped, the muscle at rest can be assessed. Electrical activity that is not due to needle movement or voluntary muscle contraction is called *spontaneous activity*.

Spontaneous activity can be normal in the form of *miniature endplate potentials* (MEPPs) and *endplate spikes*. These potentials can be seen when the needle electrode is placed close to the muscle's endplate region. As these potentials are normal, and the majority of other types of spontaneous activity suggest pathology, it is critical to be able to identify MEPP and endplate spikes. MEPP are thought to originate from spontaneous release of single quanta of acetylcholine at the presynaptic nerve terminal. MEPP have small amplitudes and duration, are irregular, and sound like a "seashell." Endplate spikes are mechanically produced by needle movement at the endplate region, resulting in a subthreshold endplate potential. These spikes are larger than MEPPs; they are rapid and irregular and sound like "sputtering fat on a frying pan."

Other types of spontaneous activity frequently suggest pathology. This spontaneous activity includes fibrillation potentials, positive sharp waves, complex repetitive discharges (CRDs), myotonic discharges, myokymic discharges, fasciculations, cramps, and tremors. Each waveform has a distinct appearance and sound.

Fibrillation potentials and *positive sharp waves* are often observed together. Although they have different appearances, their clinical significance is thought to be similar. Fibrillations are usually biphasic or triphasic (initial downward deflection), of short duration, of 20 to 1000 uV amplitude, and usually have regular rhythm. They sound like "rain on a tin roof." The amplitude of a fibrillation potential tends to diminish with time. For example, fibrillation size in the first month can be up to 1000 uV. After one year, the size is usually less than 100 uV. Positive sharp waves are usually biphasic (large initial downward deflection, followed by long upward deflection), have less than 1000 uV amplitude, and are regular (Fig. 4.7). Fibrillations and positive sharp waves can occur in both neuropathic and myopathic processes. In a neuropathic process with motor axon loss and Wallerian degeneration, muscle fibers become denervated. The denervated muscle fibers can spontaneously produce action potentials from single muscle fibers. These are known as "fibrillation potentials." There is controversy on the origin of positive sharp waves, but most believe they are similar to fibrillations except that they require deformation of a muscle fiber by the needle electrode.

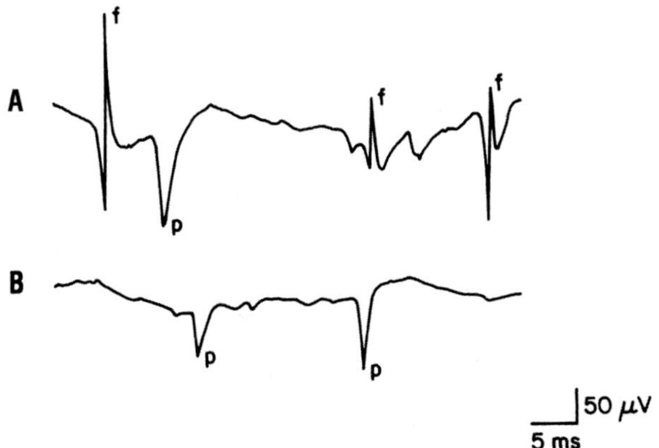

Figure 4.7 Fibrillation potentials and positive sharp waves. **A:** Biphasic and triphasic fibrillation potentials (f) recorded in denervated muscles. **B:** Positive sharp waves (p) recorded form the same muscle. (*From* Dumitru D, Amato AA, Zwarts M. Electrodiagnostic Medicine. 2nd ed. Philadelphia, PA: Hanley & Belfus, 2002, *with permission.*)

Fibrillations and positive sharp waves can also occur in primary muscle disease. In a myopathic process that results in segmental muscle necrosis, portions of the muscle fiber may lose connection from the terminal axon and become "denervated." Other myopathic processes that involve significant inflammation and muscle fiber splitting can result in similar denervation of single muscle fibers. Metabolic processes that affect muscle can make the resting muscle membrane potential unstable and also produce fibrillations and positive sharp waves without denervation.

CRDs are high-frequency discharges that characteristically start and stop abruptly. They are made up of a run of multiple spikes that repeat regularly at a rate of 20 to 150 Hz. CRDs are thought to occur from ephaptic conduction along damaged muscle tissue. They are seen in muscles where there has been chronic denervation and reinnervation, such as certain myopathies and chronic neuropathies. They distinctly have a "motorboat or motorcycle" sound.

Myotonic discharges are seen in myotonic disorders, certain myopathies, and occasionally in chronic neuropathies. They originate from alterations with the muscle membrane ion channels. Characteristically, they wax and wane with respect to amplitude and frequency, giving them a "dive bomber" type sound.

Clinical myokymia is seen as a rippling movement of the skin. *Myokymic discharges* occur as rhythmic bursts of discharges at a frequency of 0.1 to 10 Hz. The bursts are made of a single motor unit firing up to 60 Hz. The rhythm is very regular, producing a sound that has been described as "marching soldiers." Myokymic discharges likely originate from ephaptic conduction along damaged axons. Limb myokymia is classically seen in radiation-induced plexopathy. As expected, the incidence of radiation plexopathy increases with the dose of radiation delivered. The onset of radiation plexopathy varies from a few months to several years after exposures. Facial myokymia is most commonly seen in brainstem neoplasm, multiple sclerosis, and Bell's palsy.

Fasciculations are clinically visible as spontaneous intermittent contractions of muscle. *Fasciculation potentials* appear as normal MUAPs but are very irregular. Voluntarily activated MUAPs fire in a regular fashion and not any slower than 4 to 5 Hz. Fasciculations fire at frequencies between 0.1 and 10 Hz, but usually less than 2 Hz. They can be benign and found in the normal population, particularly following fatigue, heavy exercise, or caffeine. Pathological fasciculations are seen in motor neuron disease such as amyotrophic lateral sclerosis, as well as lower motor neuron diseases. There is no reliable way to distinguish "benign" from "malignant" fasciculations. However, finding fasciculation potentials with other types of abnormal spontaneous activity (i.e., fibrillations and positive sharp waves) and abnormal voluntary MUAPs would suggest that observed fasciculation potentials are pathological.

Cramps are sustained muscle contractions lasting seconds or minutes. They can be normal, or induced by electrolyte imbalances, metabolic disorders, or ischemia. *Cramp discharges* on needle EMG appear as multiple motor units firing in synchrony at 40 to 60 Hz. They usually have an abrupt onset and cessation but can fire irregularly in a sputtering fashion, especially just before termination.

A tremor can occur during voluntary muscle contraction but also can occur spontaneously with the muscle at rest. *Tremor* on needle EMG appears as synchronous bursts of MUAPs. Tremor sounds similar to myokymia ("marching soldiers"); however, the individual bursts within a tremor are composed of many different motor units, whereas myokymic bursts are made up of the same motor unit firing repetitively.

Minimal to Moderate Contraction to Evaluate Motor Unit Action Potentials

Motor units are assessed with needle EMG. A motor unit consists of an anterior horn cell, its peripheral nerve, and all single muscle fibers innervated by that nerve. After assessing for spontaneous activity, voluntary MUAPs are evaluated. A MUAP represents the summated electrical activity of all single muscle fibers belonging to one motor unit that are close enough to the needle electrode to be recorded. The needle is positioned in the targeted muscle and the patient is asked to slightly contract the muscle. The needle position is adjusted so that the recording surface of the electrode is very close to the muscle fibers of the MUAPs being assessed. This is noted by a short MUAP rise time or MUAPs that sound crisp and sharp. MUAP *parameters* and *recruitment* are then assessed.

Commonly assessed MUAP parameters include *amplitude, duration,* and *phases* (Fig. 4.8). As noted previously, the range of normal for these parameters is different with monopolar versus concentric needles. *Amplitude* is measured from the highest peak to the lowest peak (maximum peak-to-peak distance). MUAP amplitude is affected not only by the number of muscle fibers in the motor unit but also by the distance of the needle from the muscle fibers being recorded, the diameter of the muscle fibers, and the synchrony of muscle fiber firing. MUAP amplitudes typically are greater than 100 uV and less than 3 mV. Abnormal MUAP amplitudes occur in neuropathic and myopathic processes and are time dependent.

Duration best reflects the number of muscle fibers within a motor unit. Normal duration is 5 to 15 ms. Short-duration MUAPs are classically seen in myopathic disorders.

Most MUAPs have two to four phases. A *phase* is defined as the segment of the waveform above or below the baseline. The total number of phases can be easily visualized or determined by counting the number of baseline crossings and adding one. The number of phases is dependent on the synchrony of muscle fiber firing within a MUAP. A MUAP with more than four phases is considered *polyphasic.* Normal muscles can have 15% to 35% polyphasic MUAPs depending on needle type. Higher percentages of polyphasia may signify muscle denervation with reinnervation or myopathic processes.

MUAP recruitment is assessed with mild to moderate contraction of the muscle. Recruitment can be *normal, decreased,* or *increased.* Normal recruitment occurs temporally as well as spatially. When a muscle is initially contracted, a MUAP will start firing regularly at approximately 5 Hz. With increased contraction, that MUAP will fire faster. When the MUAP reaches a frequency of about 10 Hz, a second MUAP will start firing at approximately 5 Hz. With further contraction, the first MUAP will fire around 15 Hz, the second MUAP at 10 Hz, and the third MUAP at 5 Hz. The maximal

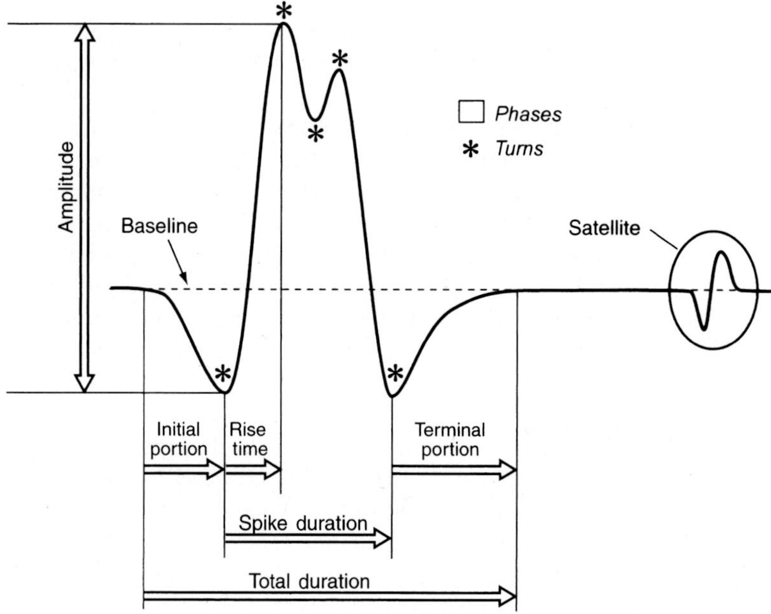

Figure 4.8 Motor unit action potential (MUAP) parameters. (*From* Dumitru D, Amato AA, Zwarts M. *Electrodiagnostic Medicine.* 2nd ed. Philadelphia, PA: Hanley & Belfus, 2002, *with permission.*)

	Motor Unit Recruited		
1st (A)	2nd (B)	3rd (C)	4th (D)
A (5 Hz)			
A (10 Hz)	B (5 Hz)		
A (15 Hz)	B (10 Hz)	C (5 Hz)	
A (20 Hz)	B (15 Hz)	C (10 Hz)	D (5 Hz)

Figure 4.9 Normal motor unit action potential (MUAP) recruitment. MUAP A begins firing stably at about 5 Hz. With a minimal increase in force of muscle contraction, MUAP A increases its firing rate to 10 Hz and MUAP B begins firing at 5 Hz. With further contraction, MUAP A fires at 15 Hz, MUAP B fires at 10 Hz, and new MUAP C begins firing at 5 Hz. The same process continues as MUAP D is activated. (*From* Dumitru D, Amato AA, Zwarts M. *Electrodiagnostic Medicine.* 2nd ed. Philadelphia, PA: Hanley & Belfus, 2002, *with permission.*)

firing rate for a MUAP is about 30 to 50 Hz. This sequence of events is known as "normal MUAP recruitment" (Fig. 4.9).

Reduced recruitment occurs in neuropathic disorders. Reduced MUAP recruitment will be seen as a "few MUAPs firing rapidly" instead of the normal pattern. In a neuropathic disorder, either axon loss or demyelination can cause dysfunction of certain MUAPs. With muscle contraction, the first MUAP will fire regularly at 5 Hz. With further contraction, the first MUAP will increase in frequency to 10 Hz. This is when the second MUAP should come in. In a neuropathic disorder, this second MUAP, and potentially the third MUAP (etc.), will not fire. The first MUAP keeps increasing its firing frequency though. It may reach 20 to 30 Hz before the next MUAP fires (if another one fires at all) (Fig. 4.10).

Increased or *early* recruitment occurs in myopathic disorders. In myopathic disorders, the MUAPs may be intact; however, the muscle fibers are dysfunctional. In this case, the patient contracts the muscle, the first MUAP fires at 5 Hz, but the force produced by this MUAP is much less than that anticipated due to the myopathic process. For this reason, the second MUAP will fire immediately with the first. The second MUAP also produces much less force than expected, so the third MUAP activates immediately as well (and the fourth, fifth, etc. may do the same). This is seen as multiple different MUAPs firing simultaneously despite minimal contraction (Fig. 4.11).

	Motor Unit Recruited		
1st (A)	2nd (B)	3rd (C)	4th (D)
A (20 Hz)			
A (25 Hz)	0	0	
A (30 Hz)	0	0	D (20 Hz)

Figure 4.10 Neuropathic or reduced recruitment. In this case, motor unit action potential (MUAP) B and C are not present due to a neuropathic process. MUAP A begins firing at 20 Hz because MUAP B and C are not available. When motor unit A fires at 30 Hz, MUAP D finally becomes activated at 20 Hz. With neurogenic recruitment, fewer motor units are firing at higher than anticipated rates. (*From* Dumitru D, Amato AA, Zwarts M. *Electrodiagnostic Medicine.* 2nd ed. Philadelphia, PA: Hanley & Belfus, 2002, *with permission.*)

		Motor Unit Recruited		
1st (A)	2nd (B)	3rd (C)	4th (D)	5th (E)
A (15 Hz)	B (15 Hz)	C (15 Hz)	D (15 Hz)	E (15 Hz)

Figure 4.11 Myopathic or increased recruitment. A random loss of muscle fibers results in each motor unit containing a smaller complement of muscle fibers. For a given force output, therefore, more individual units must fire earlier and faster than normal. With initial muscle contraction, multiple motor units fire immediately. *From* Dumitru D, Amato AA, Zwarts M. *Electrodiagnostic Medicine.* 2nd ed. Philadelphia, PA: Hanley & Belfus, 2002, *with permission.*)

Single-Fiber Electromyography

Standard needle EMG evaluates MUAPs. A MUAP represents the summated electrical activity of all single muscle fibers belonging to one motor unit that are close enough to the needle electrode to be recorded. Single-fiber EMG (SFEMG) can evaluate the electrical activity from individual muscle fibers. A SFEMG needle electrode is made up of stainless steel cannula with a central platinum wire similar to a standard concentric needle; however, the wire exits through a side port of the cannula, resulting in a very small recording surface (25 μm). This allows the needle to record from single muscle fibers. *Fiber density* and *jitter* are analyzed with SFEMG, which has been used to better understand motor units in myopathy and neuropathy. Diagnostically, it is primarily used to assess neuromuscular junction disorders. This technique is technically demanding and not routinely performed by the majority of electrodiagnosticians.

Fiber density is the number of single muscle fibers from the same motor unit within the uptake of the needle electrode. In normal human muscles, very few muscle fibers from the same motor unit are adjacent to each other. In conditions with muscle denervation followed by reinnervation by collateral sprouting, more muscle fibers from the same motor unit can end up adjacent to each other. This results in increased fiber density, which can be assessed by SFEMG. Normative values for fiber density exist for various muscles and age groups. With advancing age, especially after the sixth decade, fiber density gradually increases because of denervation/reinnervation.

Jitter is the time variation between single muscle fiber potential pairs. The variability is normally between 5 and 60 microseconds. The SFEMG needle is positioned in a muscle (usually the extensor digitorum communis), so that two different single muscle fiber action potentials can be recorded at the same time. Approximately 50 to 100 time intervals per pair and 20 different pairs are recorded. Normal values are available for specific muscles and age groups. In patients with neuromuscular junction disorders, the time variability between the two single muscle fiber action potentials (jitter) increases. Increasing jitter can result in failure of neuromuscular transmission and absence of the second muscle fiber action potential of the pair. This is known as "blocking."

SFEMG is the most sensitive test in the diagnosis of myasthenia gravis (MG). As SFEMG is technically demanding, it is best used if RNS and acetylcholine antibody test results are normal in a patient with suspected MG. Although increased jitter is quite sensitive in testing for neuromuscular junction disorders, it is not specific. It can also be seen in neuropathic and myopathic disorders.

NERVE REACTION TO INJURY

Regardless of the cause of injury, there are two basic pathophysiologic responses to nerve injury: *demyelination* or *axon loss*. With a nerve injury causing focal demyelination only, the damage stays at the site of injury. The nerve proximal and distal to the injury site remains normal. Across the site of injury, a phenomenon known as "conduction block" occurs. Conduction block is failure of a nerve impulse to propagate through a portion of structurally intact axon. With axon loss, Wallerian degeneration will occur. The axon dies from the point of injury and then will, over the next several days, die distally, resulting in denervation of muscle or skin. These processes can be assessed with NCS and EMG.

A common classification scheme for peripheral injuries is the Seddon classification. It divides nerve injuries into *neurapraxia, axonotmesis,* and *neurotmesis. Neurapraxia* involves focal demyelination (conduction block) only. If neurapraxia is very short lived, it is thought to occur from focal ischemia. As no axon damage has occurred, no Wallerian degeneration will follow. Recovery tends to be spontaneous

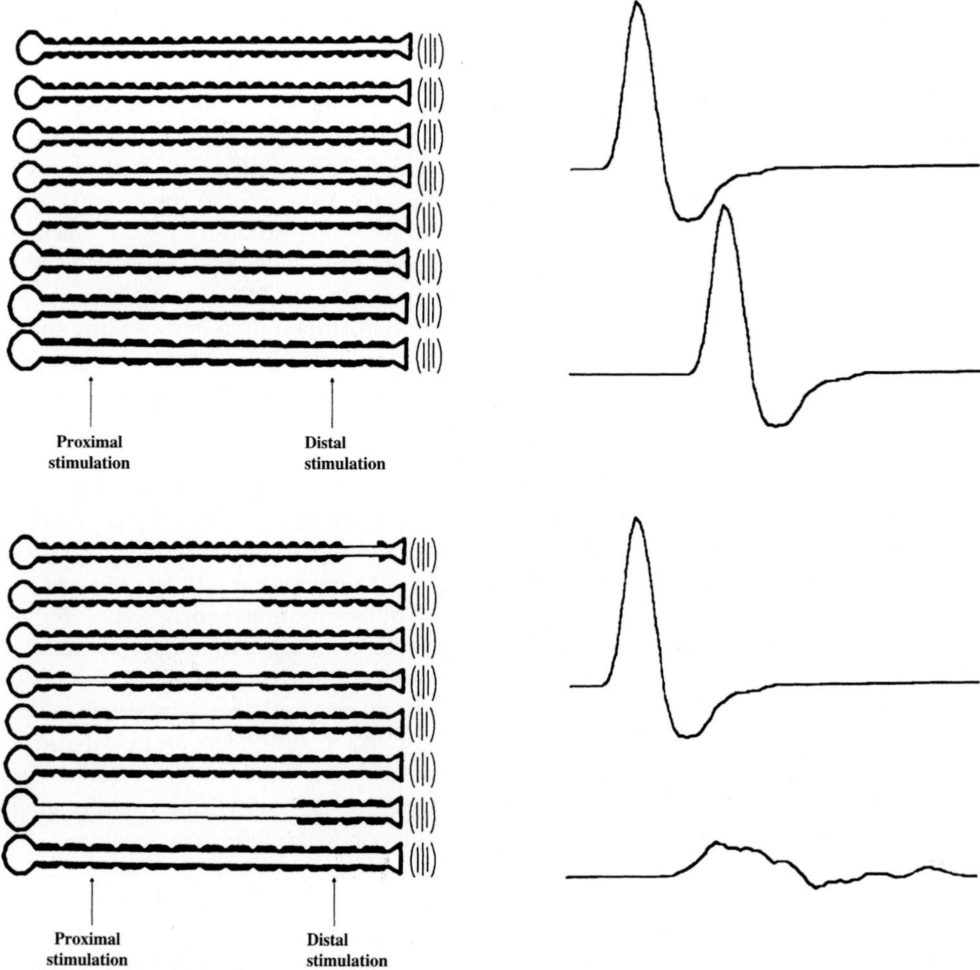

Figure 4.12 Conduction block. In a normal motor nerve **(top),** the compound muscle action potential (CMAP) amplitude and morphology usually is similar between distal and proximal stimulation sites. When focal demyelination has occurred **(bottom),** the distal CMAP amplitude and morphology remains the same; however, the proximal CMAP drops in amplitude and the area becomes dispersed. (*From* Preston DC, Shapiro BE. *Electromyography and Neuromuscular Disorders.* 2nd ed. Philadelphia, PA: Elsevier, Butterworth-Heinemann, 2005, *with permission.*)

(hours to months). With *axonotmesis*, there is axon loss with a variable amount of supporting tissue damage. Wallerian degeneration occurs. The success of axon recovery depends on the amount of intact supporting tissues. *Neurotmesis*, also known as a complete injury, involves severance of the nerve (axons and supporting tissue structures). Wallerian degeneration occurs. Prognosis for recovery is very poor.

Neurapraxic lesions involve focal demyelination. On motor and sensory NCS, this is seen as a blockage of nerve impulses across the lesion site. The amplitude of the response is much smaller when testing across the lesion site, then compared with testing distally. This is known as "conduction block." Alternatively, focal demyelination may result in slowing of conduction velocity across the lesion site. The following figures demonstrate the effect of conduction block on a motor nerve conduction study. For example, testing the median motor nerve typically requires placement of the active electrode over the thenar eminence. A distal stimulation over the median nerve at the wrist and a proximal stimulation over the nerve at the antecubital space are performed. Normally, the CMAP amplitudes produced from the distal and proximal stimulation sites are about the same. If focal demyelination occurs between the two stimulation sites, conduction block may occur (Fig. 4.12). Any nerve impulse that has to pass through the area of focal demyelination will demonstrate conduction block. Nerve impulses that do not have to pass through the injury site will be normal (Fig. 4.13). On needle EMG, neurapraxic lesions will immediately demonstrate reduced MUAP recruitment. Abnormal spontaneous activity, such as fibrillations and positive sharp waves, will not be seen, as Wallerian degeneration will not occur.

With axonotmesis, Wallerian degeneration occurs over a 3- to 9-day period. The axons die at the site of injury, and then distally. On NCS, the amplitudes of the responses will be decreased at all stimulation sites (Fig. 4.14). On needle EMG, decreased MUAP recruitment will be seen immediately after injury. Abnormal spontaneous activity such as fibrillations and positive sharp waves will be seen around day 7 to day 10.

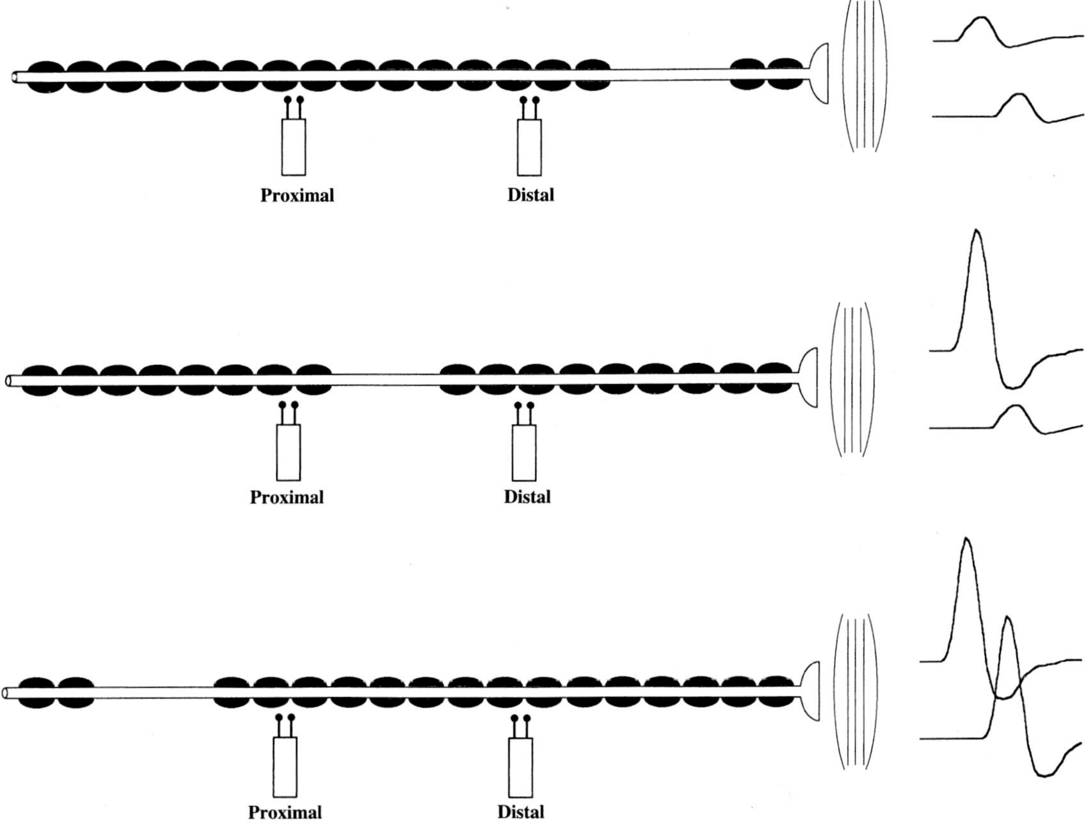

Figure 4.13 Conduction block location and stimulation site. In these examples, a typical motor conduction study is performed with stimulating a nerve distally and proximally and recording from a muscle. **Top:** If a conduction block is present between the usual distal stimulation and the muscle, the CMAP amplitudes will be low at both distal and proximal stimulation sites. **Middle:** If a conduction block is present between the distal and proximal stimulation sites, a normal CMAP amplitude will be recorded distally, while a reduced CMAP amplitude will occur proximally. **Bottom:** If a conduction block is proximal to the most proximal stimulation site, the nerve remains normal distally; thus, both proximal and distal stimulation sites produce normal CMAP amplitudes. (*From* Preston DC, Shapiro BE. *Electromyography and Neuromuscular Disorders*. 2nd ed. Philadelphia, PA: Elsevier, Butterworth-Heinemann, 2005, *with permission*.)

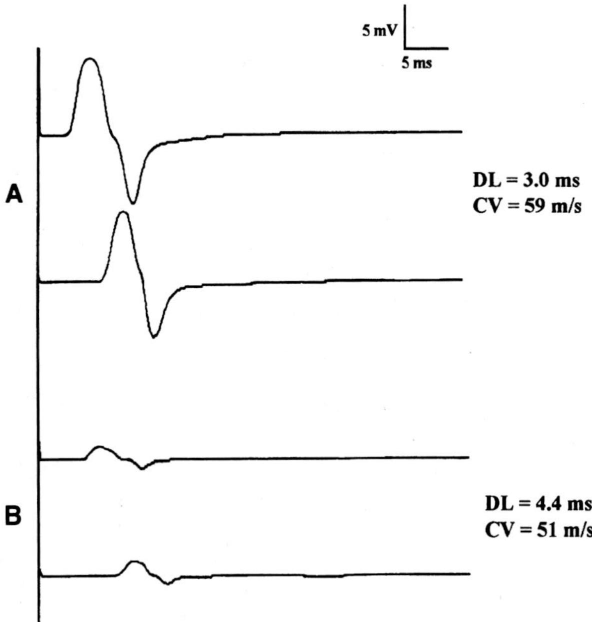

Figure 4.14 Axon loss. **A:** Normal motor nerve conduction studies (NCS) with distal and proximal stimulation sites producing normal compound muscle action potential (CMAP) amplitudes. **B:** With axon loss lesions, if enough time has occurred for Wallerian degeneration, CMAP amplitudes will decline at all stimulations sites. Caveat: Notice how this pattern of abnormality could also represent conduction block distal to the most distal stimulation site (see Fig. 4.13, **Top**). (*From* Preston DC, Shapiro BE. *Electromyography and Neuromuscular Disorders.* 2nd ed. Philadelphia, PA: Elsevier, Butterworth-Heinemann, 2005, *with permission.*)

In complete lesions (neurotmesis), the nerve is completely severed. Wallerian degeneration occurs over a 3- to 9-day period. The motor and sensory NCS will be absent both proximal and distal to the injury site. On needle EMG, no active MUAPs will be recruited from the tested muscle. Fibrillations and positive sharp waves will be seen around day 7 to day 10.

Timing of the electrodiagnostic study is crucial in evaluating nerve injuries. Although evidence for focal demyelination or conduction block can be seen immediately after nerve injury, the findings for axon loss and Wallerian degeneration occur over a 3- to 9-day period. For this reason, the electrodiagnostic findings for neurapraxia (focal demyelination) versus axonotmesis/neurotmesis (axon loss) may look identical during the first few days of injury. In the following illustrations, nerve conductions performed immediately after injury look the same for severe neurapraxia versus neurotmesis. The difference is noted by day 7 to day 10. No response is produced with distal stimulation for the neurotmetic lesion. The distal response remains normal at all times for the neurapraxic lesion (Figs. 4.15 and 4.16). Optimally, performing testing immediately after injury will give a baseline that can be compared with testing at the 10- to 14-day point. From a practical standpoint, waiting to test at the 10- to 14-day point after injury would be sufficient. If testing for a radiculopathy, waiting for 4 to 5 weeks

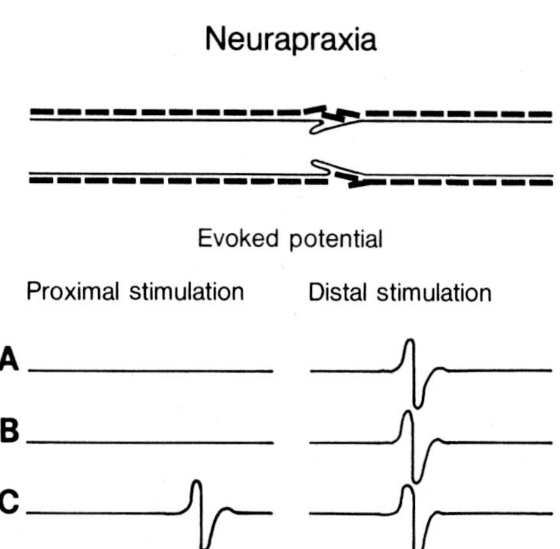

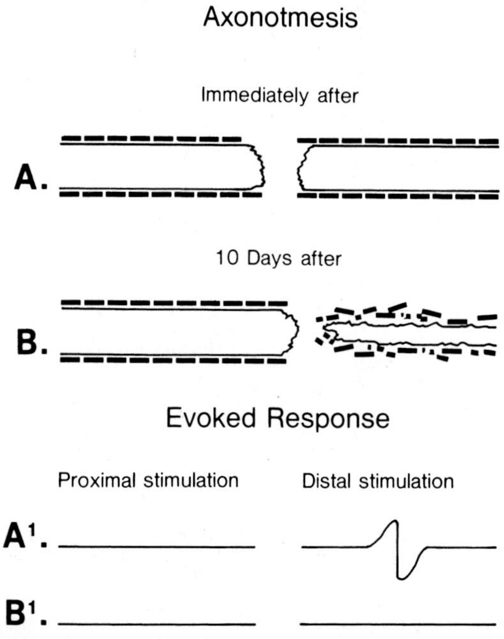

Figure 4.15 Neurapraxia. In this example, focal demyelination (conduction block) has occurred between the distal and proximal stimulation sites. **A:** Immediately after injury, the distal amplitude is normal, the proximal amplitude is absent. At this time, it is too early to tell if this is due to conduction block versus axon loss. **B:** 7 to 10 days after injury. Enough time has elapsed for Wallerian degeneration to occur if axon loss is present. The distal amplitude remains normal; thus, no axon loss has occurred. The proximal amplitude is still absent signifying 100% conduction block. **C:** Several weeks after injury. There has been partial recovery of the conduction block. The distal amplitude remains normal. The proximal amplitude is reduced but improved. (*From* Pease WS, Lew HL, Johnson EW. *Johnson's Practical Electromyography.* 4th ed. Philadelphia, PA: Lippincott Williams & Wilkins, 2007, with permission.)

Figure 4.16 Neurotmesis or severe axonotmesis. In this example, nerve severance or severe axon loss has occurred between distal and proximal stimulation sites. **A^1:** Immediately after injury, the distal amplitude is normal, but the proximal amplitude is absent. This is the same pattern of response seen in Figure 4.15 A. It is too early to tell if this abnormal response is due to conduction block versus axon loss. **B^1:** 7 to 10 days after injury, the distal response is now absent due to Wallerian degeneration from severe axon loss. The proximal response remains absent. (*From* Pease WS, Lew HL, Johnson EW. *Johnson's Practical Electromyography.* 4th ed. Philadelphia, PA: Lippincott Williams & Wilkins, 2007, *with permission.*)

is recommended, as evidence for muscle denervation after Wallerian degeneration can be seen at the paraspinal muscles at day 7 to day 10, but may not be apparent in distal limb muscles for 4 to 5 weeks.

Nerve conduction testing after injury as outlined above will provide information regarding the type of lesion and amount of axon loss versus demyelination present. For severe injuries, serial testing every 2 to 3 months, over a period 6 months, may be necessary to determine if a complete lesion is present. For milder injuries, waiting too long after injury to test may result in electrodiagnostic findings that are normal or minimally abnormal, due to remyelination and collateral sprouting or axon regrowth.

The amount of nerve recovery after injury depends on the severity of injury. As expected, purely neurapraxic lesions have the best prognosis with recovery usually within 3 months. Axon loss lesions recover more slowly requiring collateral sprouting and/or axon regeneration. In collateral sprouting, nearby intact axons give off axon "sprouts" to reinnervate muscle or skin that has been previously denervated. Axon regeneration is a slower process, requiring growth of axons at the site of injury to eventually reach the target end organ. Axon regeneration occurs at an approximate rate of 1 mm per day or 1 inch per month. The effectiveness of axon regeneration is dependent on the amount of intact supporting tissue that is left. For motor fiber recovery after axon loss, reinnervation needs to occur within 18 to 24 months. Beyond that time, too much muscle fiber atrophy and fibrosis has occurred, making reinnervation impossible. Although sensory fibers do not have this problem of end organ degeneration, severe sensory nerve injuries rarely recover fully likely due to inability of the sensory axons to reach the skin.

COMMON CLINICAL APPLICATIONS

Electrodiagnostic testing is used as a tool for diagnosing neuromuscular disorders. Although information can be obtained regarding the central nervous system, the majority of NCS and EMGs are used to diagnose peripheral nervous system disorders. Anatomically this may include anterior horn cells, sensory and motor roots, brachial and lumbosacral plexuses, peripheral nerves, neuromuscular junctions, and muscles.

Mononeuropathies

The most common mononeuropathies are median neuropathy at the wrist, ulnar neuropathy at the elbow, radial neuropathy at the humerus, and peroneal neuropathy at the fibular head.

Median neuropathy at the wrist is the most common of all mononeuropathies. Clinically, it manifests as carpal tunnel syndrome. Patients typically complain of numbness in a median nerve distribution, pain at the hand and wrist (and frequently more proximally into the forearm). Nocturnal symptoms commonly wake patients up at night. Difficultly with fine manipulation may occur because of loss of sensory or motor function. In severe cases, atrophy of median-innervated thenar muscles will occur. On examination, the finding of sensory loss in a median nerve distribution, thenar atrophy/weakness, a Tinel's sign over the median nerve at the wrist, and positive Phalen's maneuver can be seen.

Electrodiagnostic testing for median neuropathy at the wrist is quite sensitive. The goal is not only to localize the lesion to the median nerve at the wrist but also to determine the amount of demyelination or axon loss. Many nerve conduction study methods exist for assessing carpal tunnel syndrome. The typical testing includes standard median motor and sensory testing. The ulnar motor and sensory nerves are usually performed as well to rule out a polyneuropathy. Other protocols involve comparison tests between median versus ulnar or median versus radial conductions. The mixed (sensory and motor) palmar studies comparing ulnar versus median conductions across the wrist are also popular and considered quite sensitive. The most common finding with median neuropathy at the wrist is slowing of conduction velocity or a delay of latency across the wrist. Less commonly, a drop in amplitude across the wrist occurs. Both findings suggest focal demyelination. On needle EMG, if there is significant motor fiber involvement, reduced recruitment can be seen. If motor axon loss is present, fibrillations and positive sharp waves may be present. The testing should attempt to confirm a median neuropathy at the wrist, determine its severity, and rule out other neuromuscular causes for the patients' symptoms, such as a proximal median nerve lesion, brachial plexopathy, or cervical radiculopathy.

The second most common mononeuropathy is *ulnar neuropathy* at the elbow. This neuropathy usually occurs with stretching or compression of the ulnar nerve at the ulnar groove or just distal to the groove at the cubital tunnel. Clinically, patients complain of numbness in an ulnar distribution, weakness with grip and pinch, and frequently pain at the elbow and forearm. On examination, weakness of the ulnar innervated flexor digitorum profundus to the fourth and fifth digits can be noted if the patient tries to make a fist. Weakness with the ulnar innervated adductor pollicis can be noted by having the patient pinch a piece of paper between the thumb and the index finger (Froment's sign). Sensory loss at the fifth digit and the ulnar portion of the fourth digit may be detected and a Tinel's sign over the ulnar nerve at the elbow may also be present.

In a significant ulnar neuropathy at the elbow, sensation loss will also occur over the dorsal ulnar hand. This part of the hand is innervated by the dorsal ulnar cutaneous nerve, a branch of the ulnar nerve. As this branch comes off the ulnar nerve several centimeters proximal to the wrist and does not pass through Guyon's canal at the wrist, it is not affected by ulnar neuropathies at the wrist but can be affected by an ulnar neuropathy at the elbow. If significant sensory loss is noted in the medial forearm, this suggests a lesion more proximal to the elbow. The sensation to the medial forearm is provided by the medial antebrachial cutaneous nerve, which comes off the medial cord of the brachial plexus; thus should be spared in an ulnar neuropathy at the elbow.

Electrodiagnostic testing for ulnar neuropathy at the elbow tends to be less sensitive than testing for median neuropathy at the wrist. This is due to technical limitations of the studies available. Milder lesions may not be detectable by testing. Severe injuries will demonstrate electrodiagnostic abnormalities, but exact localization of the injury may be difficult. Standard testing includes ulnar sensory, dorsal ulnar cutaneous, and ulnar motor conductions. The median sensory and motor conductions are commonly performed as well to rule out a polyneuropathy or plexopathy. The finding of ulnar nerve slowed conduction velocity or a drop in amplitude across the elbow help to localize the lesion there. Unfortunately, the error in measurement and calculating the conduction velocity across the elbow is quite high, even with optimal elbow positioning. A drop in motor amplitude (conduction block) is useful for localizing the lesion, but it is often not seen. A drop in sensory amplitude across the elbow is difficult to call abnormal as normal temporal dispersion causes a drop in sensory amplitudes with more proximal stimulation. Needle EMG may be normal in milder cases. In more severe cases, needle EMG will demonstrate decreased MUAP recruitment and fibrillations/positive sharp waves in ulnar innervated forearm and hand muscles. As there are no ulnar-innervated muscles above the elbow, the EMG may only be able to conclude that an ulnar neuropathy exists proximal to the takeoff to the flexor carpi ulnar muscle. The goals of electrodiagnostic testing for ulnar neuropathy at the elbow include localizing the lesion, determining the degree of demyelination versus axon loss, and ruling out other etiologies such as brachial plexopathy or cervical radiculopathy.

The most common entrapment site for the *radial nerve* is at the humeral spiral groove. This nerve is quite susceptible to compressive forces and fractures as it wraps around the mid humerus. Patients can present with a wrist drop and numbness in a superficial radial sensory distribution. On examination, elbow extension should be normal as the triceps receive innervation from the radial nerve proximally to the spiral groove. The exception would be triceps' weakness secondary to direct muscle trauma to the triceps muscle at the time of injury. Radially innervated muscles distal to the spiral groove such as the brachioradialis, and finger/wrist extensors can be weak. Grip strength may seem weak, but this is due to lack of mechanical advantage from loss of the wrist extensors.

Electrodiagnostic testing includes radial motor studies with stimulation at the forearm, elbow, below spiral groove, and above spiral groove. A drop in motor amplitude across the spiral groove signifies conduction block. A drop in conduction velocity is less useful, due to error in measurement. The superficial radial sensory nerve can be abnormal if there has been significant axon loss. Needle EMG will demonstrate decreased MUAP recruitment. If motor axon loss is present, fibrillations and positive sharp waves can be seen in radially innervated muscles distal to the spiral groove. Goals are to localize the lesion to the radial nerve at the spiral groove, rule out radial neuropathy at the axilla, radial neuropathy at the forearm (posterior interosseous neuropathy), and rule out brachial plexopathy or cervical radiculopathy.

Peroneal neuropathy (or *fibular neuropathy*) most commonly occurs at the fibular head. The nerve is susceptible to compression and stretching there. Patients typically present with a foot drop and numbness at the lateral calf and dorsum of the foot. At the fibular head, the common peroneal nerve divides into deep and superficial branches. The clinical presentation will vary depending on how much each branch is affected. Electrodiagnostic testing commonly includes peroneal motor conductions at the ankle, below the fibular head, and above the fibular head. The superficial peroneal nerve is tested with stimulation at the lateral calf and will be abnormal in lesions with significant axon loss. The tibial motor and sural sensory conductions are usually obtained to rule out polyneuropathy or more proximal neuropathy. Needle EMG would include peroneal innervated muscles of the lower limb. To rule out a more proximal lesion, testing tibial innervated muscles and sciatic innervated hamstring muscles is useful. The short head of the biceps is particularly useful as it is innervated by the peroneal portion of the sciatic nerve but above the fibular head. Abnormalities at this muscle would place the lesion more proximal to the fibular head (sciatic nerve, lumbosacral plexus, or lumbosacral radiculopathy).

Polyneuropathies

Polyneuropathy or generalized peripheral neuropathy is commonly assessed by electrodiagnostic studies. The differential diagnosis for polyneuropathy is vast. The goal of electrodiagnostic testing is to confirm the presence of a polyneuropathy and to classify it into a subcategory to narrow the differential diagnosis. Specifically, the testing should help determine whether the polyneuropathy is diffuse or multifocal, involves sensory and/or motor fibers, and primarily involves axonal loss and/or demyelination. Polyneuropathy can be subdivided by electrodiagnostic testing into the following categories: (a) uniform demyelinating, mixed sensorimotor, (b) segmental demyelinating, motor greater than sensory, (c) axon loss, motor greater than sensory, (d) axon loss, sensory, (e) axon loss, mixed sensorimotor, and (f) mixed axon loss, demyelinating, sensorimotor.

For instance, acute inflammatory demyelinating polyneuropathy (AIDP) or Guillain-Barré syndrome would fall under the segmental demyelination, motor greater than sensory polyneuropathy category. With segmental demyelination, prominent conduction block and abnormal temporal dispersion is seen. Although demyelination is the main disease process, secondary axon loss can occur. This is important to note as pure axon loss or pure demyelination rarely occurs. Late responses such as F-waves and H-reflexes are frequently useful in assessing polyneuropathies as they evaluate the more proximal portions of the nerves. Late responses are particularly useful in AIDP, as they are frequently absent early in the course of the disease while the rest of the electrodiagnostic testing remains within normal limits.

Most uniform demyelinating polyneuropathies are hereditary. Hereditary motor sensory neuropathy (HMSN) I or Charcot-Marie-Tooth disease falls under this category. The predominant finding is decreased conduction velocities without conduction block or abnormal temporal dispersion.

The majority of polyneuropathies are primarily axonal. The axon loss mixed sensorimotor polyneuropathy is the largest category of polyneuropathy; hence the more difficult type of polyneuropathy to determine the cause. Causes for axonal polyneuropathies include alcoholism, heavy metals, toxins, pharmaceuticals, connective tissue diseases, endocrine disorders, and nutritional deficiencies such as B_{12}, folate, or thiamine. NCS reveal reduced amplitudes. Slowing of conduction velocity can occur because of loss of fast conducting axons; however, conduction velocity does not drop below 75% of normal. If motor axon loss is present, needle EMG may show fibrillations/positive sharp waves and abnormal MUAPs.

A caveat regarding electrodiagnostic testing and polyneuropathies is the small-fiber polyneuropathy. Standard electrodiagnostic testing assesses large fiber nerves. All motor nerves are large diameter fibers; however, sensory fibers can be large or small. For this reason, patients with small-fiber polyneuropathy may have normal electrodiagnostic studies. Fortunately, from a diagnostic standpoint, most polyneuropathies will affect large and small fibers. However, common causes of polyneuropathy such as diabetes mellitus and alcoholism, which usually affect both large and small fibers, can also manifest predominantly as a small-fiber polyneuropathy.

Radiculopathies

Radiculopathies are disease processes involving the nerve roots and most commonly caused by compression from intervertebral discs and/or osseoligamentous structures. Although electrodiagnostic testing tends to be sensitive for detecting mono- and polyneuropathies, it is less sensitive for detecting radiculopathies, particularly milder ones. The reduced sensitivity is due to the natural course of radiculopathies and anatomical considerations.

Sensory NCS are classically normal in radiculopathies. The majority of radiculopathies involve lesions proximal to the sensory dorsal root ganglion (DRG). Damage to sensory nerve roots proximal to the DRG will result in normal sensory nerve conductions, despite clinical sensory loss. For example, a complete lesion (severance) of the left C6 sensory root proximal to the DRG will present as loss of sensation at the C6 dermatome that includes the thumb. Wallerian degeneration will occur at the injury site and distally to the DRG; however, as the sensory cell bodies in the DRG remain intact, the sensory axons from the DRG and distally will not be affected. Median and radial sensory nerve conductions to the thumb will remain normal, despite the clinical sensory loss.

Motor NCS are usually normal in radiculopathies. The cell bodies for the motor nerves are located at the anterior horn of the spinal cord. Damage to motor roots causing axon loss will result in Wallerian degeneration and muscle denervation. Severe axon motor axon loss may cause a drop in CMAP amplitude. Less significant axon loss will result in relatively normal motor amplitudes as the majority of muscles have multi-root innervation. Conduction velocities remain normal.

The needle EMG is the most sensitive part of the electrodiagnostic study in assessing radiculopathy. Motor root lesions with axon loss can produce needle EMG abnormalities such as fibrillations/positive sharp waves, reduced MUAP recruitment, and MUAP waveform abnormalities. The goal is to find needle EMG abnormalities in a myotomal pattern, preferably in muscles innervated by different peripheral nerves, and to find paraspinal muscle abnormalities. For example, an acute C6 radiculopathy could be diagnosed with fibrillations/positive sharp waves at the following muscles: cervical paraspinal, biceps (musculocutaneous, C5-C6), deltoid (axillary, C5-C6), brachioradialis (radial, C5-C6), pronator teres (median, C6-C7). Normal rhomboid (dorsal scapular, C5), extensor carpi ulnaris (radial, C7-C8), and abductor pollicis brevis (median, C8-T1) would further support the C6 pathology.

There are several pitfalls when diagnosing radiculopathy with electrodiagnostic testing. Unless there is significant involvement of motor roots, the needle EMG will be normal. Focal demyelination at a motor nerve root will not result in Wallerian degeneration. Only if there is enough demyelination to cause conduction block will MUAP recruitment be affected. Abnormal spontaneous activity such as fibrillations and positive sharp waves will not occur unless motor axon loss occurs.

Another pitfall has to do with the number of abnormal muscles on needle EMG. Frequently, even if there is motor axon loss, only a few muscles of the affected myotome will be abnormal, making localization to a single root difficult. Often, even the paraspinal muscles will be normal. In this case, a plexopathy cannot be completely ruled out.

The majority of patients who present with radicular symptoms complain of pain and sensory symptoms, but no motor complaints. Pain fibers are small sensory fibers that cannot be assessed with routine electrodiagnostic studies. Damage to sensory roots tends to occur proximal to the DRG and will not cause abnormal sensory conductions. If there is no motor involvement, motor conductions and EMG will be normal. Thus, the majority of patients with this presentation will have normal electrodiagnostic testing.

Cervical and lumbar radiculopathies are frequently assessed with electrodiagnostic testing. Thoracic radiculopathies are not common. Testing for thoracic radiculopathies is more difficult due to the limited muscles that can be assessed: thoracic paraspinal, intercostal, and rectus abdominus.

Timing affects the electrodiagnostic assessment of radiculopathy. Decreased MUAP recruitment can be seen early; however, detecting motor axon loss in the form of fibrillations and positive sharp waves may take several weeks. Wallerian degeneration typically occurs in 7 to 10 days. Although needle EMG findings of fibrillations and positive sharp waves in the paraspinal muscles may be seen at day 10 to day 14 , it may take 4 to 5 weeks for these findings to occur in distal muscles. Hence, testing too early will produce limited findings. Optimal timing is 4 to 5 weeks. Testing too late will also produce limited findings due to reinnervation.

Late responses, such as F-waves, seemingly would be useful as they assess the more proximal segments of the nerve; however, they tend to have a low diagnostic yield in radiculopathy. As described earlier in this chapter, H-reflexes can be useful in suspected S1 radiculopathy.

Despite the pitfalls, electrodiagnostic testing remains an important tool in diagnosing radiculopathies. Spinal imaging for assessing radiculopathy is known to have high false-positive rates. Electrodiagnostic testing has much lower false-positive rates and is the only diagnostic tool able to evaluate the physiologic function of nerves and muscles. In addition to confirming a diagnosis of radiculopathy and determining its severity, electrodiagnostic testing will rule out other causes for patients' symptoms such as mononeuropathies and polyneuropathies.

Plexopathy

Brachial and lumbosacral plexopathies are assessed with electrodiagnostic testing in a similar fashion as radiculopathies. The major difference is plexus lesions typically occur distal to the DRG. Therefore, unlike radiculpathies, plexus lesions with sensory axon loss will result in abnormal sensory nerve conductions. For instance, a patient with a significant upper trunk plexopathy classically will have clinical sensory loss at the lateral forearm and the thumb. Median and radial sensory NCS are expected to be abnormal, unlike our previous example of a C6 radiculopathy. If significant motor axon loss has occurred, motor NCS may reveal decreased amplitudes in muscles innervated by the damaged portion of the plexus. The needle EMG can show evidence for abnormal spontaneous activity (fibrillations and positive sharp waves) and/or abnormal MUAPs. Paraspinal muscles should be normal, unlike radiculopathy.

The pitfalls for diagnosing plexopathy with electrodiagnostic testing are similar to those for diagnosing radiculopathies. The needle EMG is by the far the best way to diagnose and localize a plexus lesion. In a patient with suspected plexopathy only with sensory deficits, the testing may only show abnormal sensory nerve conductions, making localization of the plexus injury difficult. If motor nerve damage occurs, but no axon loss, localization will rely on abnormal MUAP parameters and recruitment, which is more subtle to evaluate than abnormal spontaneous activity. Late responses such as F-waves and H-reflexes have not been found to be of significant utility with diagnosing plexopathy, due to limitations previously discussed.

Other Clinical Applications

Electrodiagnostic testing is used to evaluate other disease processes including myopathies, neuromuscular junction disorders, and motor neuron diseases. The specifics of testing for these disorders go beyond the scope of this chapter and can be further reviewed with the recommended readings listed later.

CONCLUSION

Electrodiagnostic testing used properly as an extension of the clinical history and examination can be an invaluable way to assess neuromuscular disorders. The electrodiagnostic medicine physician must have a strong knowledge base in the disease processes being tested so that the clinical information and the electrodiagnostic data can be used appropriately. Attention to detail with respect to instrumentation and testing technique, is required to reduce errors. Anatomical variations and electrodiagnostic testing limitations need to be recognized. Improper use of electrodiagnostic testing will lead to misdiagnosis. Optimal use of electrodiagnostic testing can provide a definitive diagnosis, narrow the differential diagnoses by confirming or ruling out certain types of pathology, help localize and determine the severity of lesions, and provide guidance with treatment plans and prognosis.

REFERENCE

1. AANEM Nomenclature Committee. AANEM glossary of terms in electrodiagnostic medicine. *Muscle Nerve*. 2001;24(suppl 10):S10–S11.

RECOMMENDED READINGS

Donofrio PD, Albers JW. AAEM minimonograph #34: polyneuropathy: classification by nerve conduction studies and electromyography. *Muscle Nerve*. 1990;13:889–903.

Kincaid JC. AAEM minimonograph #31: the electrodiagnosis of ulnar neuropathy at the elbow. *Muscle Nerve*. 1998;11:1005–1015.

Landau ME, Diaz MI, Barner KC, Campbell WW. Changes in nerve conduction velocity across the elbow due to experimental error. *Muscle Nerve*. 2002;26:838–840.

Robinson LR. AAEM minimonograph #28: traumatic injury to peripheral nerves. *Muscle Nerve*. 2000;23:863–873.

Stevens JC. AAEM minimonograph #26: the electrodiagnosis of carpal tunnel syndrome. *Muscle Nerve*. 1997;20:1477–1486.

Wilbourn AJ, Aminoff MJ. AAEM minimonograph #32: the electrodiagnostic examination in patients with radiculopathies. *Muscle Nerve*. 1998;21:1612–1631.

Musculoskeletal Infections

5

Andrew F. Kuntz John L. Esterhai

INTRODUCTION

Musculoskeletal infections are devastating problems that require significant time and resources for proper treatment. As a group, infections of the bones, joints, and surrounding soft tissues are common and have the potential to cause significant morbidity. Treatment requires proper diagnosis and aggressive treatment. Surgical intervention and antibiotic therapy are the mainstays of successful eradication of infection. Delayed or incomplete treatment can result in chronic pain, deformity, functional impairment, and in the worst case, loss of limb or even death. Fortunately, the later are rare and arrest of infection is typically achievable with appropriate treatment.

PATHOGENESIS OF INFECTION

The human body possesses many defenses against the multitude of pathogens that can cause infection. On the most basic level, these defense mechanisms include physical barriers, innate immunity, and the adaptive immune response. In concert, these systems protect the body against microscopic and macroscopic pathogens. However, a breakdown in any one of these defenses can result in the clinical picture of infection.

The skin and mucous membranes serve as a primary barrier to infection, blocking the entry of pathogens into the bloodstream and soft tissues. Even though these physical barriers are extremely effective in preventing infection, they are certainly not absolute. When infectious material does violate the skin or mucus membranes, the innate immune system is activated. Responsible for the signs and symptoms of acute inflammation, activation of the innate immune system involves recruitment of phagocytic cells, such as neutrophils and macrophages, as well as the initiation of the complement system. The innate immune system is also responsible for activation of the adaptive immune system. It is the adaptive immune system that enables the host to tailor the immune response to a specific pathogen through the involvement of T-cells and B-cells. The adaptive immune system is also responsible for immunological memory.

Despite this complex series of interconnected defenses, resistance against pathogens is not perfect, as any one of these mechanisms can fail or become overwhelmed. The ability of a microorganism to overcome a host defenses is known as "virulence." Each and every organism has differing degrees and means of virulence. The goal of this chapter is not to review the virulence of different microorganisms. However, it is critical to understand that infection in any tissue requires an inoculation of a pathogen or microorganism into a tissue with a subsequent interaction between the inoculum and the host tissue. In many cases of infection, it is necessary to understand the virulence of the offending pathogen in order to properly and definitively treat the infection.

In addition to the virulence of a pathogen, local and systemic host factors play a role in the development of infection. Systemic host factors such as renal and liver disease, malignancy, diabetes mellitus, malnutrition, alcoholism, rheumatologic disease, and immune system dysfunction all increase the risk of infection. Local tissue factors such as decreased vascularity and neuropathy can also be favorable to the development of infection. Both blunt and penetrating trauma can result in compromise of local soft tissues as well as formation of dead space and hematoma. The presence of implants not only adversely affects phagocytosis but also allows for adherence of microbes with subsequent biofilm formation. Finally, intravenous drug use results in recurrent episodes of bacteremia, with a corresponding increased risk of local and systemic infection.

Staphylococcus aureus is the most common causative organism of musculoskeletal infections. Over recent years, *S. aureus* resistant to treatment with the antibiotic methicillin (methicillin-resistant *Staphylococcus aureus* or MRSA) has become increasingly more common. Initially seen only in health care–acquired situations, MRSA is now frequently acquired in the community as well, with more than 1% of community members testing positive for the bacteria. Recent outbreaks of community-acquired MRSA skin infections have been reported among athletes, military recruits, and children. With the increasing prevalence of MRSA in the community and hospitals, musculoskeletal infections due to MRSA are also more common. This presents a specific challenge to the treating physician as MRSA bacteria have a large number of defense mechanisms. First, an increased number of surface proteins facilitate adherence to host tissues and foreign material such as orthopaedic implants. In addition, cell–cell interactions between bacteria allow for quorum sensing and the rapid production of a protective glycocalyx layer. As a result, MRSA-related infections can be extremely difficult to treat, with up to hundred times greater antibiotic resistance than other bacteria.

ANTIBIOTICS

Antibiotic therapy is paramount in the treatment of musculoskeletal infections. In order for antibiotic treatment to be effective, an appropriate regimen must be selected. Typically, antibiotic therapy begins with broad coverage, in order to treat the most common pathogens. Once culture and sensitivity data are available, the antibiotic regimen should be tailored to the specific infection. This approach requires knowledge of the microorganisms typically responsible for specific infections, as well as the mechanism of action and spectrum of activity for common antibiotics.

Antibiotics can be broadly categorized into six groups on the basis of their mechanism of action. The first group of antibiotics includes those with activity against the bacterial cell wall. Within this group, penicillins and cephalosporins comprise a subgroup of antibiotics collectively referred to as "β-lactam antibiotics." These antibiotics inhibit bacterial peptidoglycan synthesis via interaction with penicillin-binding proteins on the bacterial cell membrane. The spectrum of activity for the various β-lactams is quite broad, although certain antibiotics within the subgroup have a narrow spectrum of coverage. β-lactamase inhibitors are a subgroup of cell wall active antibiotics that are available in combination with certain penicillin antibiotics. The combination of the two types of antibiotics improves coverage against both gram-positive and gram-negative organisms. Vancomycin is another antibiotic in this group, interfering with insertion of glycan units into the cell wall. Vancomycin has activity against Enterococcus species, *Staphylococcus aureus,* and *Staphylococcus epidermidis.* It is the antibiotic of choice for MRSA and is commonly substituted for penicillin or cephalosporin antibiotics in patients with allergies to the β-lactams. Overall, this broad group of antibiotics includes the most commonly used antibiotics in orthopaedics. Cell wall active antibiotics are routinely used as antibiotic prophylaxis in the perioperative period and for definitive treatment of musculoskeletal infections.

The second group of antibiotics includes those active against bacterial ribosomes. Within this group, clindamycin binds to the 50 S-ribosomal subunit, inhibiting dissociation of peptidyl-tRNA from the ribosome during translocation. Macrolide antibiotics (erythromycin, clarithromycin, etc.) function in a very similar manner. Aminogylcosides (gentamycin, tobramycin, etc.) bind to cytoplasmic ribosomal RNA, thereby inhibiting bacterial protein synthesis. The tetracyclines (tetracycline, doxycycline, etc.) also inhibit bacterial synthesis, but via interaction with 70S- and 80S-ribosomes. Together as a group, these antibiotics provide activity against a broad spectrum of pathogens. Clindamycin is unique among all antibiotics in that it achieves the highest antibiotic concentration in bone, which is nearly equal to serum concentrations following intravenous administration.

Rifampin alone comprises the third group due to its unique mechanism of action. It inhibits RNA synthesis in bacteria and has a spectrum of action against many gram-positive and gram-negative bacteria. Rifampin is rarely used alone, as bacterial resistance to rifampin develops rapidly.

The fluoroquinolones (ciprofloxacin, levofloxacin, etc.) inhibit DNA gyrase. All antibiotics in this group have excellent gram-negative coverage. Certain antibiotics within the group offer gram-positive and atypical bacteria coverage. Unique to the fluoroquinolones is the excellent serum antibiotic concentrations achieved following oral administration. As a result, treatment with these antibiotics is often associated with decreased cost of treatment and length of hospitalization.

Antimetabolites are another group of antibiotics, with trimethoprim-sulfamethoxazole being the most common drug in this group. Trimethoprim-sulfamethoxazole is a combination of two antimetabolites most effective when given together in fixed combination. Trimethoprim binds to bacterial dihydrofolate reductase, interfering with folic acid synthesis. Sulfamethoxazole, a sulfonamide, inhibits bacterial dihydrofolate synthetase, which is also necessary for the synthesis of folic acid. Therefore, the two antimetabolites act synergistically to prevent the production of folic acid, inhibiting bacterial development. Trimethoprim-sulfamethoxazole is a broad-spectrum antibiotic that has excellent coverage against gram-negative organisms and certain gram-positive bacteria as well.

The final group of antibiotics includes the reducing compounds. Metronidazole is the most common antibiotic

TABLE 5.1
ANTIBIOTIC GROUPS AND MECHANISMS OF ACTION

Antibiotic Groups and Subgroups	Mechanism of Action
Cell wall active	
β-lactams	Bind to penicillin-binding proteins on bacterial cell membrane to inhibit peptidoglycan synthesis
Vancomycin	Interferes with insertion of glycan subunits into the cell wall
Ribosome active	
Clindamycin	Binds to 50S-ribosomal subunit, inhibiting dissociation of peptidyl-tRNA from the ribosome during translocation
Macrolides	Same as clindamycin
Aminoglycosides	Bind to cytoplasmic ribosomal RNA to inhibit bacterial protein synthesis
Tetracyclines	Bind to 70S- and 80S-ribosomes to inhibit bacterial protein synthesis
Rifampin	Inhibits bacterial RNA synthesis
Fluoroquinolones	Inhibit bacterial DNA gyrase
Antimetabolites (Trimethoprim-sulfamethoxazole)	Inhibits folic acid synthesis
Reducing compounds (Metronidazole)	Inhibits anaerobic DNA synthesis via free radical damage to bacterial DNA

in this group. Following uptake by anaerobic bacteria, metronidazole is reduced to a free radical, which, in turn, damages bacterial DNA and inhibits DNA synthesis, ultimately resulting in cell death. Metronidazole is lethal only for strict anaerobic bacteria that lack protective enzymes. For this reason, metronidazole is used nearly exclusively for the treatment of infections caused by anaerobic bacteria. Table 5.1 reviews the common antibiotic groups and their mechanisms of action.

In addition to antibiotics' use in the treatment of established musculoskeletal infections, these are routinely used to prevent infections. Prophylactic antibiotics should be administered within 1 hour before orthopaedic surgery and for varying lengths of time postoperatively to reduce the incidence of local and systemic infection. In most instances, including when orthopaedic hardware is implanted, a first-generation cephalosporin given 1 hour preoperatively and for 24 hours postoperatively is sufficient prophylaxis. Antibiotics are also routinely given in the setting of open fractures to prevent osteomyelitis and local soft-tissue infection. Generally accepted guidelines include the administration of a first-generation cephalosporin to any patient with an open fracture. In the setting of a type III open fracture, an aminoglycocide should also be given. The data regarding the need for an aminoglycocide for a type II open fracture is mixed. Patients with grossly contaminated open fractures should also be covered by the addition of penicillin.

Despite the critical role antibiotics play in the prevention and treatment of musculoskeletal infections, their use must be monitored closely, and limited to appropriate situations only, in order to minimize the development of antibiotic resistance. Acquired antibiotic resistance is mediated by bacterial plasmid DNA. Subtherapeutic dosages, treatment courses that are too short, and the use of ineffective antibiotics can all lead to resistance. Resistance is easily transmitted, which may, in turn, increase the difficulty of treating infection by limiting the spectrum of effective antibiotics. In recent years, antibiotic resistance has been increasing, due to all of the reasons previously outlined.

DIAGNOSIS OF INFECTION

The evaluation and workup of infection should always begin with a though history and physical examination. Once an adequate history has been obtained and a detailed physical examination performed, radiographic and laboratory studies can aid in the diagnosis of infection and identification of the causative pathogen. An understanding of the application and limitations of the various imaging modalities and laboratory studies helps in the selection of appropriate tests and the practice of cost-effective medicine.

IMAGING

Radiographs are relatively inexpensive and are excellent in showing bony anatomy, bone changes such as resorption and periosteal reaction, and in some cases soft-tissue swelling. Radiographs are extremely helpful in evaluation for the presence and configuration of orthopaedic hardware. Lucency at the bone-implant interface can be a sign of infection, but it can also represent aseptic loosening. Radiographs effectively demonstrate fractures and tumors that can mimic infection on clinical presentation.

Computed tomography (CT) is excellent for more detailed evaluation of the musculoskeletal system, as well as for the assessment of three-dimensional anatomy. CT is useful in many situations, but it is particularly important when evaluating for fracture union in the setting of infection, and in the determination of the size of a lesion or collection in soft tissues or bone.

Magnetic resonance imaging (MRI) is useful for detecting marrow changes during the early stages of infection. It has a sensitivity that approaches 100% when used for the detection of osteomyelitis. In the setting of osteomyelitis, local edema and hyperemia result in increased signal on T2-weighted images and decreased marrow signal on T1-weighted images. However, these findings can be difficult to interpret after acute trauma, repeated injury (such as in the patient with peripheral neuropathy), or in the presence of stainless steel orthopaedic hardware. MRI is also 97% sensitive and 92% specific in the detection and diagnosis of septic arthritis. It is important to remember that some patients, such as those with a pacemaker or a recently placed inferior vena cava filter or aneurysm clip, are unable to undergo MRI.

Ultrasound is less commonly used in the evaluation of an orthopaedic infection. However, an ultrasound study can be performed relatively quickly, is inexpensive, provides real-time information, and does not subject the patient to radiation. Ultrasound can be very useful in detecting fluid collections or bone surface changes, such as in the presence of an abscess or periostitis.

Other imaging modalities are also useful in the workup of musculoskeletal infections. Bone scintigraphy with technetium Tc-99m phosphate allows for identification of anatomic areas of increased perfusion and osteoblast activity. In the typical three-phase bone scan, the initial phase demonstrates perfusion of the radionuclide into the tissues, with increased blood flow and tracer distribution in regions of infections. The second, or intermediate, phase is recorded approximately 15 minutes after radionuclide injection and demonstrates the presence of tracer in the extracellular space. The final phase, the third or delayed phase, is recorded between 2 and 4 hours after initial injection and correlates with osteoblastic uptake of the radionuclide. Uptake in a specific region during the second phase that is then absent during the third phase is typically consistent with superficial cellulitis and not osteomyelitis. Leukocyte scans with indium-111–labelled leukocytes are useful in distinguishing infectious from noninfectious etiologies. The two technologies, leukocyte scans and bone scans, can be used in combination to increase the sensitivity and specificity when evaluating for infection. A much newer technique, positron emission tomography (PET) with F-18 fluorodeoxyglucose, has become favorable in the evaluation of chronic musculoskeletal infection due to 100% sensitivity and 88% specificity.

LABORATORY STUDIES

Laboratory studies are also useful in the evaluation and management of musculoskeletal infection. Elevation of the peripheral white blood cell (WBC) count with a predominance of polymorphonuclear leukocytes is suggestive of infection. However, in greater than half of patients with musculoskeletal infection, an elevated WBC count is not observed. Therefore, the erythrocyte sedimentation rate (ESR) and C-reactive protein (CRP) are the more commonly used markers of infection and inflammation. Both ESR and CRP are markers of acute inflammation. CRP begins to rise within 6 hours of onset of infection and returns toward normal approximately 1 week after initiation of successful treatment. In contrast, the ESR becomes elevated during the first 2 days of infection but does not normalize until roughly 3 weeks after eradication of infection. As a result, the CRP is more commonly used for diagnosis of acute infection and for monitoring the response to treatment. It is important to remember that surgical intervention also results in elevation of both the ESR and the CRP.

Tissue and fluid specimens from the site of infection should be evaluated by culture and gram stain. Overall, gram stain results in identification of a specific organism in only one-third of cases. However, gram stain can be extremely specific and is often used to guide initial antibiotic selection. The gold standard in diagnosis of infection is tissue culture. Unfortunately, inadequate sampling, errors in handling and processing, and effects of previously administered antibiotics can all result in incomplete and false-negative culture results.

Molecular genetics may be the future diagnostic technique of choice. The use of polymerase chain reaction (PCR) to detect bacterial DNA without the need for in vitro culture could allow for earlier diagnosis and decrease the false-negative rate from previous antibiotic administration. However, concerns regarding false-positive results stemming from the extreme sensitivity of this technique remain unresolved.

ADULT INFECTIONS

Osteomyelitis

In strict definition, *osteomyelitis* refers to inflammation of bone or bone marrow. Since this inflammation is always the result of infection, the term "osteomyelitis" implies infection of bone or its marrow contents. In the adult population, osteomyelitis most commonly results from contiguous spread from local infection, trauma, or after a surgical procedure such as open reduction and internal fixation. Hematogenous spread is far less common, but it does occur and is most frequently encountered in intravenous drug users. Infection with any bacteria can cause osteomyelitis; however, *Staphylococcus aureus* is the most common pathogen.

Classification

Osteomyelitis can be classified on the basis of patient age (pediatric or adult), causative organism, pathogenesis (contiguous spread, traumatic, hematogenous), anatomic location, or duration of symptoms (acute, subacute, chronic). These variables can be used individually or in combination for categorization. There are also a number of named classification systems that focus on various clinical aspects of osteomyelitis, but no one system is universally accepted. The most commonly used classification system for adult osteomyelitis is the Cierny–Mader staging system, which is based on the anatomic location of infection within the bone and the physiologic status of the host (Table 5.2).

TABLE 5.2
CIERNY–MADER STAGING SYSTEM OF ADULT OSTEOMYELITIS

Anatomic type
- Stage 1: Medullary osteomyelitis
- Stage 2: Superficial osteomyelitis
- Stage 3: Localized osteomyelitis
- Stage 4: Diffuse osteomyelitis

Physiologic class
- A host: Healthy
- B host:
  - Bs: Systemic compromise
  - Bl: Local compromise
  - Bls: Local and systemic compromise
- C host: Treatment worse than the disease

Factors affecting immune surveillance, metabolism, and local vascularity
- Systemic factors (Bs): Malnutrition, renal or hepatic failure, diabetes mellitus, chronic hypoxia, immune disease, extremes of age, immunosuppression or immune deficiency
- Local factors (Bl): Chronic lymphedema, venous stasis, major vessel compromise, arteritis, extensive scarring, radiation fibrosis, small-vessel disease, neuropathy, tobacco abuse

Reprinted with permission from Cierny G, Mader JT, Pennick H. A clinical staging system of adult osteomyelitis. *Contemp Orthop.* 1985;10:17–37.

Presentation

The clinical presentation of osteomyelitis is extremely variable. Host status, chronicity of infection, anatomic location, and the offending pathogen(s) all factor in to the clinical picture of each individual case. In general, systemic symptoms can include fever, chills, night sweats, and malaise. However, the absence of any or all of these symptoms does not preclude a diagnosis of osteomyelitis. A myriad of local symptoms may also exist. Pain, erythema, warmth, and swelling are the most common local indicators of osteomyelitis. A draining sinus tract may serve as the cause of, or result from, an underlying bone infection. When the lower extremity is involved, a limp, pain with weight-bearing, or an inability to bear weight may also be associated with osteomyelitis.

History and Physical Examination

A thorough history should focus on the location, severity, and chronicity of local and systemic symptoms. A history of previous musculoskeletal surgery, open fracture, or infection (including a history of osteomyelitis) must always be investigated. Current and previous medications including antibiotics, as well as drug allergies, should be obtained. Vital signs should always be part of every physical examination, as fever, tachycardia, and hypotension can all indicate systemic illness or, in the worst case, septic shock related to hematogenous spread of infection. A detailed physical examination should focus on local symptoms by evaluating for erythema, warmth, swelling, and tenderness to palpation. Evaluation of the skin and soft tissues must include careful inspection for localized fluctuance and draining sinuses. In the setting of prior fracture, bone stability and tenderness at the fracture site are assessed in order to determine clinical fracture union. With confirmed or suspected osteomyelitis adjacent to a joint, the presence of an effusion or pain with range of motion may indicate spread of infection into the joint resulting in septic arthritis.

Diagnostic Studies

As previously mentioned, both imaging and laboratory studies are used in combination to make the diagnosis of osteomyelitis. However, the only way to make a definitive diagnosis is with tissue culture. This can be achieved through surgical biopsy or needle aspiration in some cases. However, the combination of history and physical examination, imaging, and basic laboratory studies are often sufficient to raise suspicion for the diagnosis of osteomyelitis and initiate empiric antibiotic therapy.

Differential Diagnosis

The clinical presentation of osteomyelitis can be very similar to the presentation of tumors or fractures. Therefore, these diagnoses must always be considered when suspicion for infection is raised. Once the diagnosis of osteomyelitis has been made, the differential diagnosis of causative pathogens is extensive. Overall, *Staphylococcus aureus* is the most common causative organism. In the setting of chronic osteomyelitis, *Staphylococcus epidermiditis, Pseudomonas aeruginosa, Serratia marcescens,* and *Escherichia coli* are also common causative organisms. Microbacteria, fungi, and less virulent pathogens must be considered in the immunocompromised host.

Treatment

Successful treatment of osteomyelitis involves an aggressive, multifaceted approach. In cases of acute hematogenous osteomyelitis (AHO), antibiotic therapy alone can be successful, with surgical debridement reserved for refractory scenarios. However, cases of chronic and nonhematogenous osteomyelitis typically require soft-tissue and bony debridement in conjunction with systemic and local antibiotic therapy for successful results. When limb salvage is the goal of treatment, wound management as well as treatment of fracture nonunions, bony defects, and skeletal instability must follow initial surgical debridement and initiation of antibiotic therapy. Successful treatment of osteomyelitis can be prolonged and associated with significant morbidity. Therefore, amputation should remain a treatment option in the most complex and limb-threatening situations.

Adequate surgical debridement of nonviable bone and soft tissue is paramount in successful treatment of osteomyelitis. Debridement must proceed until viable, bleeding tissue is confirmed at the surgical margins. In the

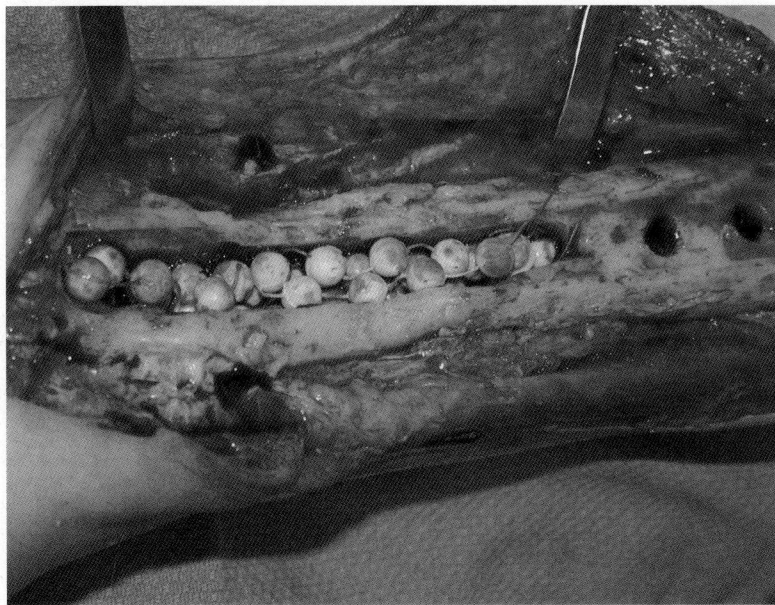

Figure 5.1 Antibiotic beads placed in a trough of bone following removal of a plate for infection. Here the beads provide no structural support but help in local delivery of antibiotic. (*Reprinted with permission from* Bucholz RW, Heckman JD, Court-Brown C, et al. *Rockwood and Green's Fractures in Adults*. 6th ed. Philadelphia: Lippincott Williams & Wilkins, 2006.)

presence of nonhost materials such as orthopaedic implants, removal of all foreign materials is typically necessary for cure. This is due to the rapid formation of biofilms by the infecting bacteria. Biofilms are resistant to host defenses and antibiotic penetration and, therefore, typically require hardware removal for effective treatment. However, in the setting of a healing fracture, the decision to retain or remove hardware can be difficult. In the acute setting, prior to the diagnosis of a nonunion, rigid internal fixation may be retained in order to maintain fracture stability. If the fracture goes on to union but infection persists, the implant should be removed. In the setting of a nonunited fracture and loose hardware, all loose implants should be removed. Fracture reduction and stability should be maintained by another method such as external fixation. Whether hardware is present or not, adequate and aggressive debridement must include sending a sufficient amount of local tissue for pathology evaluation and laboratory culture with antibiotic sensitivity analysis. Although thorough debridement can be devastating to limb function and stability, inadequate debridement is likely to result in treatment failure.

Early initiation of systemic antibiotic therapy is also critical to the successful treatment of osteomyelitis. Broad-spectrum, empiric treatment should be started as early as possible, with subsequent antibiotic therapy tailored to a specific organism on the basis of wound biopsy and culture results. The standard of care for adult osteomyelitis is 4 to 6 weeks of intravenous antibiotics. However, oral therapy can have a role in limited situations. Only antibiotics with good soft-tissue bioavailability such as linezolid and the fluoroquinolone antibiotics are commonly used in an oral regimen. Regardless of the route of antibiotic administration, the surgical wound and the ESR and CRP should be monitored over time to determine the success of treatment.

In addition to systemic antibiotic treatment, local delivery of antibiotics has also been shown to be very successful. The use of antibiotic-impregnated polymethylmethacrylate (PMMA) cement allows for delivery of high concentrations of antibiotic to local tissues with a reduced risk for systemic side effects and toxicity. Vancomycin, tobramycin, and cefepime are all commonly used in this manner as these drugs are available in powder form and unaffected by the high temperatures generated during setting of the cement. PMMA can serve a dual purpose of providing structural support in the presence of a bone defect as well as allowing for local delivery of antibiotics. Antibiotic-impregnated PMMA can also be fashioned into small beads, which can then be packed into the soft tissues, allowing for local antibiotic delivery without providing structural support (Fig. 5.1).

Following successful surgical debridement and initiation of antibiotic therapy, management of both surgical and nonsurgical wounds must begin early. Definitive wound management depends on the status of the local soft tissues. When possible, primary closure or delay primary closure of a wound is preferred. When primary closure is not possible, either local or free muscle flap coverage should be considered. Benefits of muscle flaps include the reestablishment of a physical barrier to infection from outside sources as well as the elimination of dead space, which results in increased local delivery of systemic antibiotics. Before committing to transfer of a muscle flap, the viability and status of the muscle to be used must be adequately assessed. Transfer of damaged and nonviable muscle will only increase the risk of local infection, instead of providing the benefits of a viable muscle flap.

The final stage of treatment for osteomyelitis involves addressing bone defects that result from infection and/or surgical debridement. Typically, bone defects are addressed

6 to 8 weeks after the final surgical debridement or tissue coverage procedure. At that point in time, antibiotic therapy has been completed and, in the setting of a muscle flap, incorporation of the flap has been achieved. Bone defects can be filled with auto- or allograft. However, autograft remains the gold standard in the setting of previous infection. When a bone defect is greater than 6 cm, treatment options include vascularized bone grafting and distraction osteogenesis.

With appropriate, stepwise treatment, limb salvage for osteomyelitis can result in successful outcomes. However, the treatment can be very long, with significant social, financial, and medical demands. Therefore, limb amputation should be considered and discussed in the most difficult cases. When considered early, amputation may offer a less costly treatment option, with a more rapid return to function.

Septic Arthritis

Similar to adult osteomyelitis, septic arthritis in the adult population can result from hematogenous or adjacent tissue spread or direct inoculation of the joint following trauma or surgery. Hematogenous spread of bacteria is most common. Immunocompromised hosts, including those with rheumatoid arthritis, systemic lupus erythematous, or human immunodeficiency virus, and those taking chronic immunosuppressive medications, are at increased risk and susceptibility to joint infection. Intravenous drug abusers are at an increased risk as well, due to repeated episodes of bacteremia. Single joint involvement is most common, although multifocal infection is not rare. Overall, the knee is the most commonly affect joint.

All healthy joints possess several unique defenses to infection. The synovial fluid in a healthy joint is significantly bactericidal. In addition, synoviocytes have phagocytic potential, allowing for removal of bacteria and other pathogens from the intra-articular environment. These defense mechanisms are altered in patients with rheumatoid arthritis and lupus, resulting in an increased risk of infection. Previously damaged joints are also more susceptible to infection, due in part to synovial neovascularity and increased synovial adhesion factors, both of which increase the chance for hematogenous bacterial spread and joint seeding.

Following joint inoculation, activation of the innate immune response results in local recruitment of polymorphonuclear leukocytes. The resultant release of enzymes from the recruited inflammatory cells, synoviocytes, and bacteria initiates degradation of glycosaminoglycans in the articular cartilage. The end result is destruction of intra-articular cartilage. A large joint effusion can also cause a rise in intra-articular pressure, resulting in the potential for reduced blood flow and aseptic necrosis. This cascade of events begins early after infection and requires urgent attention and treatment in order to avoid joint destruction.

Classification

There is no specific classification system in place for septic arthritis. Infections can be grouped on the basis of route of inoculation, pathogen involved, and chronicity of infection. In adult septic arthritis, the most common classification is to divide nongonococcal from gonococcal arthritis. In young, sexually active adults, the most common causative pathogen is *Neisseria gonorrhoeae*. Otherwise, *S. aureus* is the most common pathogen. Periprosthetic infections represent a separate class of septic arthritis and will be discussed later in the chapter.

Presentation

The classic clinical presentation is one of a painful, erythematous joint with a significant effusion. Patients typically hold the affected joint motionless. When a joint of the lower extremity is involved, the patient may present with the inability to bear weight on the involved limb. Systemic symptoms of fever, chills, and malaise may be present. Just as with osteomyelitis, host status, chronicity of infection, anatomic location, and offending pathogen all factor in to the clinical presentation.

History and Physical Examination

The history of present illness should focus on the current symptoms as well as the patient's overall medical history and any precipitating factors. The patient should be questioned regarding previous surgeries, trauma to the affected joint, and any previous joint aspirations. Pre-existing joint pain must be fully explored. A history of gout or pseudogout, rheumatoid arthritis, lupus, or any other systemic illness must be investigated as well. A history of outdoor activity or tick bite should also be sought to evaluate for the possibility of Lyme disease (see Chapter 11). Likewise, any history of human or animal bite should be elucidated. A thorough social history should include the patient's sexual activity, given the high prevalence of gonococcal arthritis in the young, sexually active adult. Finally, the patient's list of medications should be reviewed for any immunosuppressive agents that may impair the defense against infection or medications that may predispose the patient to gout.

The most common findings on physical examination are erythema and warmth associated with a joint effusion and significant pain with joint motion. In the immunocompetent host, micromotion pain or pain with even the slightest movement of the joint should be considered septic arthritis until proven otherwise. However, it is very important to remember that in the elderly or immunocompromised patient, these signs and symptoms may be diminished.

Evidence of previous surgery or trauma to the affected joint is important to investigate. A thorough physical examination should also evaluate other joints for similar signs of infection. In nongonococcal arthritis, monoarticular involvement occurs in 85% to 90% of cases. Polyarticular involvement is more common in cases of gonococcal, viral, Lyme, and reactive arthritis. Polyarticular arthralgias, fever, and dermatitis are most common in gonococcal arthritis. Septic bursitis, most commonly olecranon and prepatellar bursitis, can mimic septic arthritis, with diffuse swelling, erythema, and warmth located about a joint. However, pain with range of motion is not as dramatic with septic bursitis as it is with septic arthritis. Finally, indications of previous gouty arthritis, such as the presence of soft-tissue tophi, should be sought, although their presence does not rule out the diagnosis of septic arthritis.

Diagnostic Studies

Although typically of minimal use, x-rays are often obtained during the evaluation and workup of septic arthritis. X-rays may reveal the presence of a foreign body following a traumatic injury, or chondrocalcinosis and juxta-articular erosions that could signify chronic or previous gouty arthritis. In the setting of chronic septic arthritis, x-rays may reveal joint space narrowing or complete joint space obliteration with arthrofibrosis. However, in acute septic arthritis, the most common findings on x-ray are joint effusion and soft-tissue swelling.

CT is more likely than x-ray to reveal an effusion; however, CT is otherwise of minimal help. MRI, on the other hand, is excellent for evaluation of soft-tissue edema. Therefore, MRI is the imaging modality of choice for evaluation of a joint effusion and surrounding soft-tissue swelling. This is especially true for evaluation of the spine and small joints of the hands and feet. Ultrasound may reveal an effusion when a larger joint such as the elbow, hip, or knee is involved. Ultrasound can be very useful when used to guide a needle aspiration of a joint.

Systemic laboratory markers of inflammation will be elevated in the setting of septic arthritis. ESR and CRP cannot be used to make a diagnosis of septic arthritis but are commonly used to monitor clinical improvement following treatment. An elevated systemic WBC count is present only in 50% of patients with septic arthritis. Similarly, blood cultures are rarely useful, being positive for the causative organism in 50% of patients with nongonococcal arthritis and in only 10% of those with gonococcal arthritis.

When gonococcal arthritis is suspected, a mucosal surface culture should be performed. In the setting of acute gonococcal arthritis, cervical samples are positive for gonococcus bacteria in more than 90% of women and urethral samples are positive in up to 75% of men. Pharyngeal specimens are less reliable than specimens obtained from the primary source of infection, such as the urethra or cervix. Positive culture from any mucosal membrane is much less common with chronic and disseminated gonococcal infections. PCR analysis of cervical, vaginal, urethral, and urine specimens allows for screening of the asymptomatic patient and can be used in conjunction with tissue culture.

The gold standard in the diagnosis of septic arthritis remains arthrocentesis with analysis of the synovial fluid. Joint fluid should be sent for WBC count with differential, crystal analysis, gram stain, and culture. Diagnosis of septic arthritis is confirmed when the synovial fluid WBC count is greater than 50,000 cells per mm^3, with a differential of greater than 75% polymorphonuclear cells. It is critical to remember that a cell count lower than this does not preclude a diagnosis of septic arthritis, as the immunocompromised host may not be capable of mounting such an immune response. A diagnosis of gout or pseudogout can be made when crystal analysis reveals negatively or positively birefringent crystals, respectively. Gram stain of the synovial fluid may not be diagnostic for a specific organism but can be used to tailor initial antibiotic therapy. Synovial fluid culture is most important, but positive only in 90% of patients with nongonococcal arthritis and in 25% of patients with gonococcal arthritis. Previous administration of antibiotics can result in false-negative culture results. PCR techniques can also be used to amplify and detect bacterial DNA present in the synovial fluid. However, these tests are not currently part of standard synovial fluid analysis.

Differential Diagnosis

The differential diagnosis of septic arthritis is broad. As previously mentioned, septic bursitis can closely resemble intra-articular infection. However, careful examination, use of appropriate imaging, and mindful aspiration of the bursa and not the joint (or vice versa) will confirm the diagnosis of one versus the other. The clinical presentation of crystalline arthropathy can also be identical to that of septic arthritis. Joint aspiration with crystal analysis is typically required to confirm a diagnosis of gout or pseudogout. Reactive arthritis is an autoimmune condition that closely mimics septic arthritis. The classic triad of arthritis, especially if it is polyarticular, conjunctivitis, and urethritis, and a history of previous viral or bacterial infection should raise the suspicion of reactive arthritis. In the case of reactive arthritis, joint aspiration may reveal an elevated WBC count, similar to that seen in septic arthritis, but gram stain and culture are negative. Once the diagnosis of septic arthritis is made, the differential diagnosis of causative organisms is extensive. Clinical history and synovial fluid culture are then used to determine the pathogen and dictate definitive treatment.

Treatment

Surgical treatment is the standard of care for nongonococcal septic arthritis. Joint arthrotomy with irrigation and debridement has traditionally been the treatment of choice. However, arthroscopic irrigation and debridement are common for larger, easily accessible joints. Regardless of the method of surgical intervention, treatment aims to relieve joint pressure through evacuation of effusion, and remove bacteria, inflammatory mediators, and enzymes via copious irrigation. Early treatment with this approach can minimize cartilage damage. When infection involves intra-articular hardware or allograft material, removal of the nonhost material is often required. In the setting of chronic or recurrent infections, complete synovectomy is often performed. When surgical intervention is not possible, due to the patient's comorbidities or other extenuating circumstances, serial joint aspirations can be effective. Serial aspirations should not be considered for septic arthritis of the hip or small joints.

In addition to surgical decompression and joint lavage, antibiotic therapy must be started early, typically once joint fluid cultures have been collected. When systemic antibiotics have to be started prior to surgical intervention, an attempt should be made to obtain adequate joint fluid via arthrocentesis before antibiotic administration. Otherwise, culture results may be falsely negative. In the healthy adult, therapy typically begins with a third-generation cephalosporin to treat for both *S. aureus* and *N. gonorrhoeae*. Antibiotic therapy can then be adjusted on the basis of culture results. A minimum of 4 weeks of antibiotic therapy is standard for nongonococcal arthritis.

The treatment of acute gonococcal arthritis varies significantly from nongonococcal septic arthritis. Following joint aspiration and confirmation of gonococcal infection, intravenous antibiotic therapy with a third-generation cephalosporin is initiated. Once clinical improvement is noted, typically 24 to 48 hours after antibiotic initiation, antibiotic therapy is changed to an oral third-generation cephalosporin. Oral antibiotics are continued for a minimum of 1 week or until the resolution of symptoms. Patients with large joint effusions may require a longer course of antibiotics until the effusion has resolved, but surgical drainage is rarely required. Patients with chronic or disseminated gonococcal infections require intravenous antibiotics for 4 to 6 weeks and should be monitored closely for evidence of endocarditis and meningitis. All patients should also be tested for *Chlamydia* infection and treated as necessary, due to a coinfection rate that approaches 50%.

PEDIATRIC INFECTIONS

Osteomyelitis

Pathogenesis

Unlike adult osteomyelitis, osteomyelitis in the pediatric population is most commonly acute in presentation and hematogenous in origin. Infection due to trauma, surgery, or spread from a local site is less common. Similarly, subacute and chronic presentations of osteomyelitis are less common than in adults. Pediatric osteomyelitis usually occurs in the metaphysis of long bones, especially the femur and the tibia. In the metaphyseal region, end-arteries transition into large venous sinusoids and circulation is significantly slowed; this allows blood-borne organisms to migrate through vessel walls and deposit in the porous cancellous bone (Fig. 5.2). In addition, the metaphysis has a relative lack of phagocytic cells, making it easier for bacteria to establish a clinical infection. Once formed, purulence can spread through the cancellous bone and eventually rupture through the thin metaphyseal cortex, creating a subperiosteal abscess (Fig. 5.3). Increasing pressure under the periosteum can cause ischemia to the underlying cortical bone, which may become necrotic. The dead bone that results from this process is known as a "sequestrum." Since the overlying periosteum remains viable, new bone

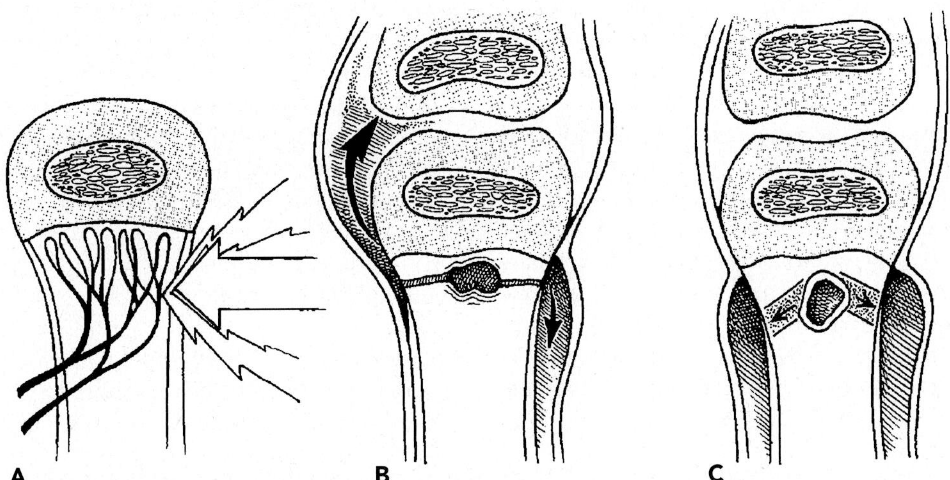

Figure 5.2 **(A)** In the metaphysis, a low flow state is present as end arteries transition into venous lakes; this allows bacteria to migrate through vessel walls. This region is also relatively deficient in phagocytic cells. **B:** Once established, the infection will eventually track through the porous metaphyseal cortical surface and elevate the surrounding periosteum. If the metaphysis is intra-articular (see section on septic arthritis), the infection can break into the joint and cause a septic arthritis. **C:** The elevated periosteum lays down new bone initially (involucrum), and the dead bone becomes a sequestrum. *(Reproduced with permission from* Dormans JP, Drummond DS. Pediatric hematogenous osteomyelitis: new trends in presentation, diagnosis, and treatment *J Am Acad Orthop Surg.* 1994;2:333–341.)

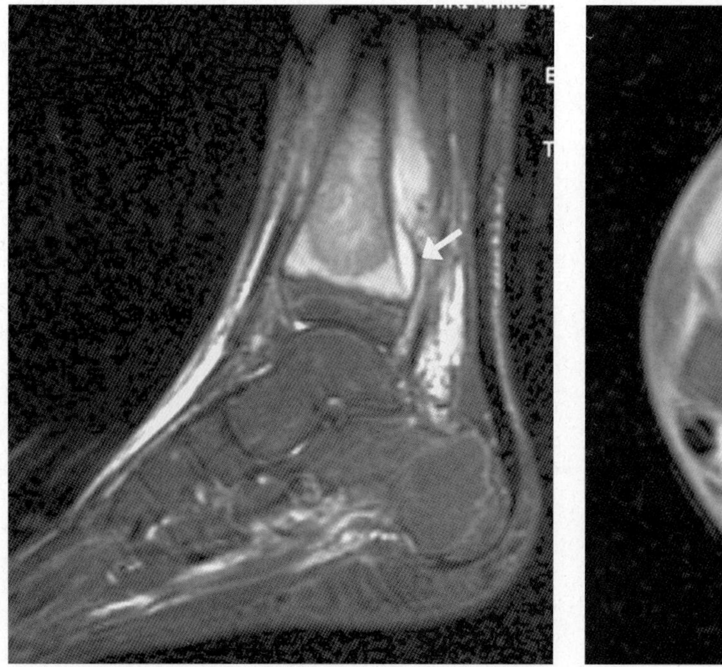

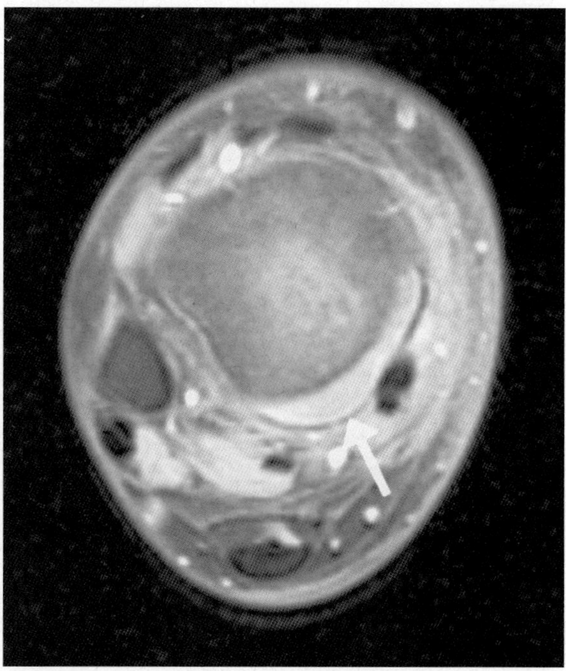

Figure 5.3 **(A)** Sagittal and **(B)** axial MRI (magnetic resonance imaging) images demonstrating osteomyelitis of the distal tibia with a large posterior subperiosteal abscess. (*Courtesy of Wudbhav Sankar, MD.*)

can be formed around the sequestrum, which is known as the "involucrum."

A unique aspect of osteomyelitis in the neonate results from the presence of arteries that traverse the physis, allowing for spread of bacteria and infection from the metaphysis to the epiphysis. As a result, adjacent joint infection occurs in one-third of all cases of metaphyseal osteomyelitis in this population.

In AHO, males are more commonly affected than females, with the lower extremities involved more frequently than the upper extremities. Pediatric osteomyelitis is also slightly more common in the warmer months. As in adults, *S. aureus* is the most common pathogen. In the neonatal population, group B *streptococci* and gram-negative infections are also common. *Streptococcus pneumonia* and *Streptococcus pyogenes* are also common in children younger than 3. Infection from *Salmonella* species is common in children with sickle cell disease. Immunocompromised children are more susceptible to fungal infections and other less virulent pathogens. Because of an effective vaccination program, infection with *Haemophilus influenza* type B, once extremely common, is now rarely encountered.

Classification

Osteomyelitis in children is generally classified by the chronicity of symptoms. As mentioned, acute osteomyelitis is the most common presentation. Subacute osteomyelitis is caused by a similar mechanism but usually involves a less virulent pathogen. Patients often have mild to moderate symptoms for several weeks or months before the diagnosis is made. Most respond to antibiotics and surgery is rarely necessary. Chronic osteomyelitis refers to patients who have had long-standing infections and have developed bone necrosis. These areas are often walled off from the rest of the circulatory system by new bone and granulation tissue. As a result, antibiotic penetrance is markedly diminished and most require repeated surgical debridements to eradicate the infection.

Presentation

Children with acute osteomyelitis classically present with pain, fever, and refusal to bear weight on the involved extremity. In the neonatal population, presentation can be much more subtle, making diagnosis a challenge. The differential diagnosis for pseudoparalysis of a limb in the neonate must always include osteomyelitis until infection is definitively excluded.

History and Physical Examination

A careful and detailed history must be obtained from the child and care provider. Attention should focus on complaints of systemic illness such as fever, chills, or malaise. A history of recent bacterial or viral infection at any site including the respiratory and gastrointestinal systems is important to obtain. Likewise, any history of surgery or trauma must be noted. A thorough medical history should always be included in any workup, including details of contact with sick individuals. In children old enough to cooperate, a history of acute onset of symptoms with localized bone pain is most common. In these patients, the pain is usually severe enough to limit activity and use of the affected limb.

Physical examination becomes easier with increasing age of the child. The approach to the child with osteomyelitis must be slow and gentle, since significant pain is common. The most common finding on physical examination is point tenderness to palpation of the osteomyelitic region. Swelling may be localized or involve the entire extremity. Erythema and warmth at the site of infection may signal spread of the infection to the local soft tissues and potential abscess development. If the affected bone is subcutaneous, redness and warmth at the skin may result from the osteomyelitis alone.

Diagnostic Studies

Similar to the workup of adult osteomyelitis, both laboratory and imaging studies are routine in the evaluation of pediatric osteomyelitis. In the setting of AHO, the most common finding on plain radiographs is soft-tissue swelling. Focal osteopenia and periosteal changes including elevation, thickening, and new bone formation can also be observed but are not typically present until later in the course of disease. It is important to remember that these radiographic changes lag behind clinical symptoms by up to 2 weeks, both at clinical presentation and after appropriate treatment has been initiated. Lytic lesions are typically not evident until more than 50% of the bone matrix has been destroyed.

CT is not commonly necessary in the diagnosis of pediatric osteomyelitis. While ultrasound may be helpful to localize an abscess, MRI is the most common imaging modality for the evaluation of osteomyelitis in children. Both the high sensitivity and specificity of MRI and the absence of exposure to radiation have increased the use of MRI in this population. Because of its superior soft-tissue resolution, MRI is extremely useful for differentiating cellulitis from osteomyelitis and for ruling out the presence of a neoplasm. In addition to its diagnostic utility, MRI allows accurate localization of subperiosteal and soft-tissue abscess, which is extremely helpful in guiding surgical treatment.

Although the use of bone scans has been somewhat replaced by MRI, this modality is still useful especially when the site of infection is unclear. Acute osetomyelitis generally demonstrates increased uptake on all three phases. In certain cases, a "cold" scan can be evidence of severe and/or chronic osteomyelitis. The biggest limitation of bone scanning, however, is a relative lack of specificity since a "hot" scan can be caused by trauma, tumor, or even disuse.

Laboratories studies routinely ordered for evaluation of pediatric osteomyelitis include a peripheral WBC count with differential, ESR, and CRP. On clinical presentation, an elevated CRP will be present in greater than 95% of children with AHO. Elevation of the ESR above 40 mm per hour is also common. Elevation of the peripheral WBC count is much less reliable, with an elevated result observed only in 50% of cases. Blood cultures can be helpful but are negative in roughly half the patients. The most reliable way to obtain a definitive diagnosis is with bone aspiration or surgical culture, which reveal the causative organism in up to 85% of cases.

Differential Diagnosis

A broad differential must be kept in mind when evaluating a child with suspected osteomyelitis. While the clinical presentation may be clearer in the older child, in the neonate and young child, symptoms are often vague and studies may be nondiagnostic. Fracture and tumor can commonly present in a very similar manner and therefore must be excluded during the workup. Septic arthritis must also be excluded. In children with sickle cell anemia, bone infarction must be differentiated from acute osteomyelitis.

Treatment

Antibiotics should be initiated early, preferably after bone aspiration or surgical culture has been performed. Initial antibiotic therapy should be directed at the most common pathogen for the child's age group. Because *S. aureus* is common in every age group, antibiotic therapy should always provide coverage for this organism. Both oral and intravenous antibiotic regimens have been proven successful, depending on the clinical presentation and the responsible organism. The most common course of antibiotics is 4 to 6 weeks.

In patients with AHO, prompt initiation of antibiotic therapy may prevent the need for surgical intervention. Surgical incision and drainage is indicated if an abscess develops or if the child fails to respond to medical therapy alone. With appropriate antibiotic treatment, roughly 50% of patients do not require surgery due to the lack of abscess formation. In cases of late presentation, chronic osteomyelitis, septic arthritis of the adjacent joint, or nonhematogenous origin, surgical treatment is often necessary.

Septic Arthritis

Pathogenesis

Septic arthritis in children is often caused by similar pathogens as for osteomyelitis, but patients generally present more rapidly with more severe symptoms. Joint infections in the pediatric population are typically due to hematogenous spread, although spread from an adjacent infection and direct inoculation from surgery or trauma can occur. As discussed in the previous section, contiguous spread from adjacent metaphyseal osteomyelitis in neonates is possible due to blood vessels that traverse the physis. In children, septic arthritis can be caused by adjacent metaphyseal osteomyelitis in the elbow, shoulder, hip, and ankle since a portion of the metaphysis is contained within the capsule for these joints. Overall, the knees and hips are the most commonly involved joints in all age groups.

Classification

There is no specific classification system of septic arthritis in children. Infections are typically classified as acute or chronic and by the mechanism of infection. The age of the patient is also useful to consider.

Presentation

Clinical presentation is very similar to that of osteomyelitis, although symptoms are often more severe. Like other infections, the most common clinical symptoms on presentation are fever, pain, and refusal to move the involved joint. Older patients, in particular, are more likely to verbalize their pain as associated with motion of the involved joint. Thus, pseudoparalysis is a common presentation, as is the refusal to bear weight when a lower extremity joint is involved.

History and Physical Examination

The child and the caregiver should be questioned regarding the onset of symptoms and the presence of constitutional symptoms. Symptoms associated with rheumatic fever and poststreptococcal arthritis, such as migratory arthritis, painful subcutaneous nodules, rash and/or carditis, should be specifically questioned. A history of trauma, including bite and puncture wounds, should be investigated. In addition to these specific questions, a thorough medical and surgical history should always be obtained.

Physical examination typically reveals a painful, erythematous, and swollen joint. The hallmark physical finding is severe pain with even micro-motion of the affected joint. When the lower extremity is involved, the inability to bear weight is common. In the setting of hip joint infection, the extremity is typically held in a position of slight flexion, with more pronounced abduction and external rotation. This position maximizes the volume of the hip joint, thereby reducing irritation of the joint capsule that results from the joint effusion.

Diagnostic Studies

Diagnostic studies are the same as those discussed for osteomyelitis in the child. Once again, elevation of the peripheral WBC count is present only in 50% of patients. However, the ESR and CRP are elevated in more than 90% of patients with septic arthritis. Any child suspected of having a septic joint should have his or her joint aspirated to make the definitive diagnosis. Synovial fluid should be sent for WBC count, gram stain, culture, and crystal analysis. Similar to the adult population, elevation of the joint fluid WBC count above 50,000 cells per mm^3 is highly suggestive of septic arthritis. Some children, however, may manifest lower cell counts. Therefore, an evaluation of the gram stain and culture are very important for determining the appropriate treatment.

Plain radiographs of the affected joint may reveal an effusion with or without surrounding soft-tissue swelling. Radiographs should be carefully reviewed to evaluate for the presence of adjacent osteomyelitis. With a large enough effusion, joint subluxation or dislocation may occur. As with osteomyelitis, MRI is an extremely useful tool for evaluating septic arthritis. Although joint aspiration is generally sufficient to make the diagnosis, MRI allows visualization of the adjacent bone and soft tissues and can therefore rule out a coexisting osteomyelitis or soft-tissue abscess. In the setting of a suspected septic arthritis, ultrasonography is most useful to guide arthrocentesis, especially when the hip is involved. Bone scans are helpful for multiple joint involvement and can also be used to localize monoarticular disease when the site of infection is not clinically apparent.

Differential Diagnosis

The differential diagnosis for septic arthritis includes osteomyelitis and joint effusion caused by inflammatory arthropathy including rheumatic fever, poststreptococcal arthritis, and juvenile rheumatoid arthritis. Lyme disease is a septic arthritis of sorts but is nonpyogenic and rarely requires surgical treatment (see Chapter 11). When the hip is involved, the most important condition to consider in the differential diagnosis for septic arthritis is transient synovitis (see Chapter 11). According to a study by Kocher et al. in 1999, four signs and symptoms can be used to differentiate these two conditions. When a child presents with a fever, inability to bear weight, a peripheral WBC count greater than 12,000 cells per mm^3, and an ESR greater than 40 mm per hour, the diagnosis is septic arthritis more than 99% of the time. When only three of these signs or symptoms are present, the probability of septic arthritis drops to 93%. Septic arthritis is the correct diagnosis in 40% and 3% of patients when only two or one variable is present, respectively.

Treatment

Septic arthritis should be considered a surgical emergency, and irrigation and drainage in the operating room is the gold standard of treatment. Both open and arthroscopic techniques have been proven successful, but surgery must be accomplished urgently in order to avoid damage to the articular cartilage. Urgent treatment is even more important for septic arthritis of the hip in order to avoid necrosis of the femoral head that can result from the increased intra-articular pressure created by the joint effusion. Similar to adult septic arthritis, serial aspiration of easily accessible joints may be appropriate in select scenarios.

In addition to surgical decompression, early antibiotic therapy must be initiated. Once synovial fluid has been obtained for culture, empiric antibiotic therapy should begin. Culture and sensitivity results can then be used to tailor antibiotic therapy as they become available. A minimum of three weeks of treatment is routine, with the potential for conversion from intravenous to oral antibiotics as clinical improvement is observed.

PERIPROSTHETIC INFECTIONS

With the number of joint arthroplasties performed each year exceeding one million in the United States alone, the complications of these procedures pose a significant burden on both the affected individual and the health care system. One devastating complication of joint replacement surgery is periprosthetic infection. The incidence of periprosthetic infection is roughly 1% for all forms of arthroplasty. Infection results from direct inoculation or hematogenous spread of the offending organism. Direct inoculation can occur at the time of surgery, in the early postoperative period in the setting of a draining wound, or at any time following joint replacement due to trauma to the joint. Hematogenous spread can occur at any time but is most common in the two years following placement of the arthroplasty. It is theorized that the increased infection rate during this period is related to the relative hypervascularity of the synovium that results from surgery and incomplete host mechanical protection of the components.

Classification

Periprosthetic infections are commonly classified on the basis of the duration of symptoms. Acute infections can occur in the immediate postoperative period or at any time remote from arthroplasty due to acute hematogenous spread. Acute infections in the postoperative period are defined as those presenting within 4 weeks of the initial surgery. Acute hematogenous infections are those in which symptoms have persisted for less than 2 to 4 weeks in a previously well-functioning, asymptomatic joint. Chronic infections are those that have persisted for longer than 4 weeks. This classification is important in determining the appropriate treatment.

Presentation

The presentation of a periprosthetic infection can be identical to septic arthritis of a native joint. Local symptoms may include pain, drainage, and decreased range of motion. Systemic symptoms may also be present, but their absence does not exclude the diagnosis of infection. In many cases, pain is the only symptom. Infection must also be considered as the cause of failure in any failed arthroplasty.

History and Physical Examination

When periprosthetic infection is on the differential diagnosis, history should first focus on the duration of symptoms. Truly acute infections must be differentiated from chronic and acute-on-chronic processes. Often, the history is the only way to make this determination. When an acute hematogenous infection is suspected, a source of bacteremia such as a recent dental or urologic procedure, infection at a remote site, or even penetrating trauma at another site should be sought. The history of wound healing and appearance is important when a chronic infection is being considered. Any history of wound drainage or delayed wound healing should raise the suspicion for infection originating during the original perioperative period.

Erythema, edema, pain, and decreased range of motion are all common findings on physical examination. Although wound drainage in the immediate postoperative period may increase the risk of infection, it is not a definite sign of infection. However, wound drainage at any other point following arthroplasty is highly concerning for infection. Chronically draining wounds must be inspected thoroughly for the presence of sinus tracts that may communicate directly with the joint and prosthesis.

Diagnostic Studies

The diagnostic workup for a periprosthetic infection should always begin with basic laboratory tests including WBC count, ESR, and CRP. Infection can essentially be ruled out when the ESR, CRP, and peripheral WBC count are all normal. However, when any one of these laboratory values is elevated or when clinical suspicion indicates, joint aspiration should be performed. The aspirate must be sent for cell count and culture. Unlike septic arthritis in a native joint, the cutoff value for diagnosing infection based on the number of leukocytes in the joint fluid aspirate is lower. Based on newer data, the cutoff value has been proposed as low as 1,700 WBCs per microliter of joint aspirate. However, 2,500 cells per microliter is currently the most commonly accepted value. In the absence of previously administered antibiotics, positive culture results carry up to 86% sensitivity and 94% specificity for infection. When antibiotics have been administered prior to aspiration, negative culture results do not indicate the absence of infection. Although joint fluid is often sent for gram stain analysis, the results from such a procedure have very low sensitivity and specificity as wear debris can be misinterpreted as bacteria. When preoperative testing fails to confirm a diagnosis of infection, intra-operative frozen section analysis of the periprosthetic tissue and implant membranes should be performed. Although criteria for diagnosing infection based on frozen section analysis has not been definitively established, more than five neutrophils per high-powered field is routinely regarded as suggestive of infection.

Other serum markers and laboratory techniques have been proposed and investigated recently in order to find more sensitive and specific tests for diagnosing periprosthetic infection. However, none are routinely used at this point. One promising serum marker is interlukin-6 (IL-6), a factor produced by monocytes and macrophages. Although the serum IL-6 level can be elevated in the setting of infection, inflammatory arthropathy, or recent surgery, values normalize within 48 hours of operation and are not elevated in the presence of aseptic loosening. Molecular biology techniques have also been investigated. PCR has been used to detect the presence of bacteria, most commonly by identifying the 16S rRNA gene conserved by nearly all bacterial species. Unfortunately, use of PCR has resulted

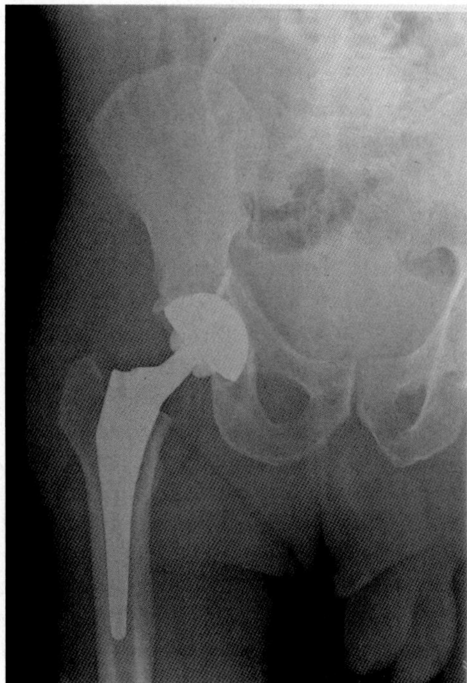

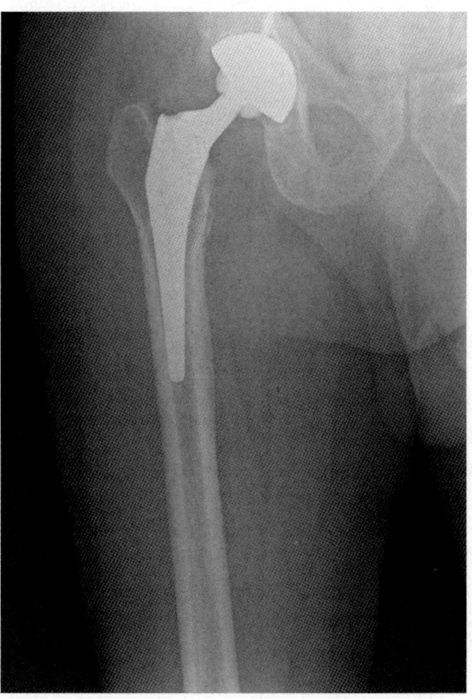

Figure 5.4 Radiographs in a patient status post right total hip arthroplasty. At initial follow-up, radiographs show **(A)** a well-fixed acetabular component with no evidence of loosening. One year later, radiographs demonstrate **(B)** lucency around the entire acetabular component. Further workup confirmed the diagnosis of infection.

in a high rate of false-positive results and identification of bacteria not responsible for clinical infection.

Aside from laboratory studies, several imaging modalities can be used in the workup and diagnosis of periprosthetic infection. Although routinely ordered, plain radiographs of an infected joint are often normal but help to exclude a diagnosis of implant wear, implant failure, or periprosthetic fractures, all of which can mimic infection in clinical presentation. Periosteal reaction and osteolysis and bone resorption in the absence of implant wear are two potential findings on x-ray that, when present, should raise suspicion for infection. Lucency around a previously well-fixed prosthesis may indicate infection but must be differentiated from aseptic loosening (Fig. 5.4). Bone scintigraphy can serve as an excellent screening test due to the high predictive value of a negative result. However, false positives are not uncommon and significantly reduce the sensitivity of this modality. FDG-PET (fluorodeoxyglucose-positron emission tomography) imaging is a newer modality that is not widely available. Early data regarding the use of FDG-PET in the diagnosis of periprosthetic infections show promise for the ability to distinguish aseptic prosthetic loosening from infection.

Differential Diagnosis

Although *S. aureus* is the most common pathogen in periprosthetic infections, the differential diagnosis for potential causative organisms is quite broad, and the possible source and mechanism of infection is even greater. Periprosthetic infection must always be considered in the patient with a persistently painful or a failed joint prosthesis. The presentation of periprosthetic infection, aseptic loosening, prosthesis wear, and prosthesis failure can be very similar. Therefore, each should be considered and workedup when any of the others is considered as the cause of a problematic prosthesis.

Treatment

Because of the morbidity of periprosthetic infections, every effort should be made to prevent their occurrence. Prior to joint replacement surgery, patients should undergo routine assessment to ensure good dental hygiene and the absence of indolent infection, such as a urinary tract infection. Antibiotics are always given immediately prior to surgery and during the acute postoperative period. Wounds that continue to drain following joint arthroplasty should be managed carefully. Following joint replacement surgery, patients must be informed of the need for single-dose antibiotic prophylaxis prior to any dental or surgical procedure. Previous recommendations for antibiotic prophylaxis only during the first 2 years following joint arthroplasty have been changed and now indicate the need for prophylaxis for as long as the prosthesis remains in place.

When prevention of infection fails, successful treatment always involves surgical irrigation and debridement of the involved joint and the administration of intravenous antibiotics for 4 to 6 weeks. Definitive treatment depends on the chronicity of the infection, host response to the infection, stability of the prosthesis, quality of the local soft tissues, and the virulence of the causative organism.

Treatment of acute infections typically begins with irrigation and debridement of the joint, and exchange of any accessible modular components, such as the polyethylene liner. Well-fixed components can be maintained, although implant retention may lower the rate of successful treatment due to the presence of an otherwise undetectable biofilm. Intravenous antibiotic therapy is initiated after cultures of the synovial fluid have been obtained. Broad-spectrum antibiotic therapy should be initiated but appropriately narrowed once culture and sensitivity results are available. Persistence of the infection despite appropriate intervention necessitates further evaluation as to the source of the infection and treatment as if the infection were chronic.

Chronic infections are also treated with joint irrigation and debridement. However, when symptoms of infection have been present for more than 4 weeks, it is unlikely that the infection will be eradicated without implant removal. In the United States, two-stage exchange arthroplasty is most common and associated with 90% to 95% success rates. Two-stage exchange arthroplasty involves resection of the implants and placement of an antibiotic-impregnated spacer (Fig. 5.5). Intravenous antibiotics are then administered for 6 weeks. Following a full course of antibiotic therapy, patients are monitored for an additional 2 to 6 weeks off antibiotics, to ensure that signs and symptoms of infection do not recur. At that point, if the WBC count, ESR, and CRP are normal, and bone stock is adequate, a new prosthesis can be placed. Although single-stage exchange arthroplasty is associated with lower rates of eradication of infection (70% to 85%), this procedure is associated with lower patient morbidity and may be considered in a very select patient population.

When reimplantation of a prosthesis is not possible, resection arthroplasty or arthrodesis may be considered. Circumstances that may preclude reimplantation include multiple failed previous exchange arthroplasties, the presence of an organism resistant to treatment, inadequate bone stock, compromised local soft tissues, and a severely ill or compromised patient. Either resection arthroplasty or arthrodesis may be considered for joints of the upper extremity while arthrodesis is most common for the knee, and resection is typically preferred for the hip. In the patient too ill to undergo surgery or a patient with a limited life expectancy, chronic antibiotic suppression may also be considered. When all other treatment options have failed, amputation of the involved extremity may be the only option for eradication of infection.

NECROTIZING FASCIITIS

Although necrotizing fasciitis is one of the least common soft-tissue infections, it is associated with significant morbidity and mortality. Prompt diagnosis and initiation of appropriate treatment are critical for patient survival. When

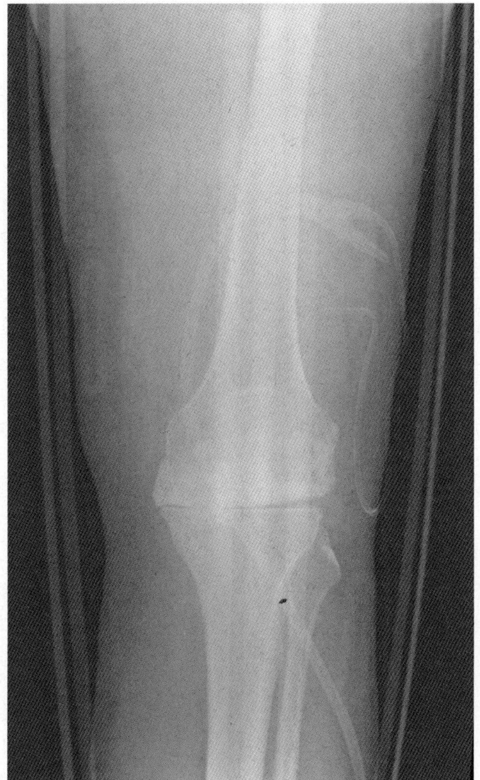

A

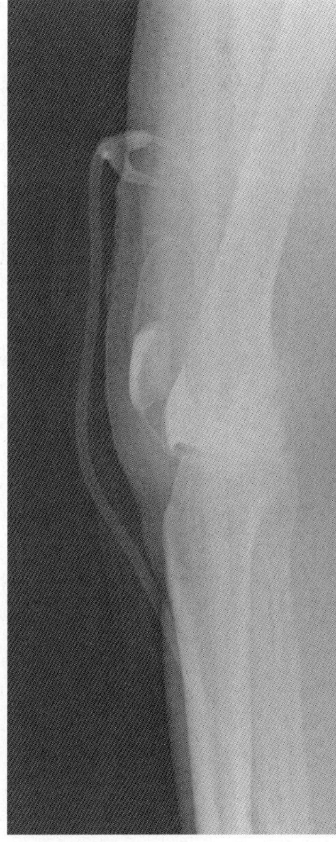

B

Figure 5.5 **(A)** Anteroposterior (AP) and **(B)** lateral radiographs demonstrating an antibiotic spacer in a knee after explantation of an infected knee arthroplasty.

surgical intervention is delayed, mortality as high as 75% has been reported.

Classification

Gram stain and culture results can be used to classify necrotizing fasciitis into one of three groups. Type 1 infections are most common, accounting for 80% to 90% of all cases. In this type of necrotizing fasciitis, gram stain and cultures reveal a polymicrobial infection, involving anaerobic and non–group A streptococcus bacteria. Wound cultures typically reveal the presence of four to five bacteria species. Type 1 infections are associated with abdominal and perineal wounds and frequently affect the immunocompromised host. Type 2 infections are most common in the extremities and result from the presence of group A β-hemolytic streptococci species. *Staphylococcus* species are the most common second species present when infection is not due to group A β-hemolytic streptococci alone. Type 3 infections often result from exposure to seawater or marine animals and are characterized by the presence of the gram-negative rod marine vibrios.

Presentation

Prompt and correct diagnosis of necrotizing fasciitis can be made extremely difficult because of its often benign initial presentation. The most common presentation is quite similar to that of cellulitis with a localized region of inflammation, swelling, and erythema. Necrotizing fasciitis is often differentiated from cellulitis by a disproportionate level of pain and rapid progression of signs and symptoms. Commonly, regions of skin induration and erythema expand rapidly, at a rate of greater than 1 cm per hour, despite the administration of intravenous antibiotics. Classic signs of necrotizing fasciitis appear later and consist of blister and bullae formation, skin discoloration and sloughing, and crepitus due to the presence of gas in the soft tissues. Bullae and blisters may initially drain serosanguineous fluid but later become hemorrhagic. As the fascia and overlying superficial fat necrose, the classic "dishwater pus" and foul-smelling drainage become obvious. In addition, the intense pain observed early in the course of the disease may give way to localized anesthesia, as cutaneous nerve endings are destroyed. Fever and chills may present early, but symptoms of systemic shock, including hypotension, tachycardia, and altered mental status, are common later. Renal and hepatic failure, coagulopathy, and acute respiratory distress syndrome can all ensue.

History and Physical Examination

A proper history and physical examination will result in heightened clinical suspicion for necrotizing fasciitis, which is critical for early initiation of treatment. Although necrotizing fasciitis most commonly results from an injury to the affected site, the patient may not recall such an injury. Any lesion that allows bacteria to breach the skin can result in necrotizing fasciitis. Blunt and penetrating trauma, surgical incisions, burns, insect bites, and ulcers have all been implicated as the cause of infection, but in up to 45% of infections, the portal of bacteria entry is not evident. Physical examination findings are quite varied and related to the many potential signs and symptoms described in the previous section. Infection typically begins in the extremities but can rapidly spread to the trunk. Involvement of the trunk and perineal region is associated with significantly higher morbidity and mortality.

Diagnostic Studies

Basic laboratory studies should include a complete blood cell count, comprehensive metabolic panel, and coagulation studies. Anemia, thrombocytopenia, hyponatremia, hypocalcemia, azotemia, hypoproteinemia, hypoalbuminemia, and hyperbilirubinemia are all common. ESR, CRP, and creatinine kinase values are typically elevated. Laboratory values may be normal in early infection but become progressively more abnormal as the disease progresses. Several models have been developed to help diagnose necrotizing fasciitis and distinguish it from other soft-tissue infections. In one simple model developed by Wall et al., simultaneous hyponatremia, with a serum sodium level of less than 135 mmol per liter, and leukocytosis, with elevation of the WBC count to greater than 15,400 cells per microliter, is 90% sensitive for necrotizing fasciitis. However, this model should only be used to rule out the diagnosis of necrotizing fasciitis as both the specificity and the positive predictive value are low, at 76% and 26%, respectively. The Laboratory Risk Indicator for Necrotizing Fasciitis (LRINEC) is another commonly used model that combines the results of six common laboratory studies (CRP, WBC count, hemoglobin, sodium, creatinine, and glucose) to predict the probability of necrotizing fasciitis. The positive predictive value of this model is 92% when used to detect early cases of disease.

In addition to laboratory studies, radiographic evaluation is critical in making a timely diagnosis. Plain films are most often normal, even in the presence of disease, but are helpful for detecting gas in the soft tissues when present. CT is very useful in the evaluation of a suspected patient. Common findings in the presence of disease include gas in the soft tissues, fascial thickening, and stranding and attenuation of the subcutaneous fat. However, a negative CT does not rule out the diagnosis. A CT scan can also be extremely helpful in delineating the extent and margins of soft-tissue involvement. The sensitivity of MRI is greater than 90%; however, MRI is of a lesser priority in the evaluation of patient due to the amount of time required to obtain a meaningful study.

Differential Diagnosis

Necrotizing fasciitis is most commonly misdiagnosed as cellulitis. As previously mentioned, early stages of necrotizing fasciitis may be nearly identical to cellulitis, so adequate clinical suspicion should result in further workup to definitively confirm or exclude the more serious condition. Other diseases that may be confused with necrotizing fasciitis include erysipelas, lymphangitis, gas gangrene, and acute febrile neutrophilic dermatosis.

Treatment

Successful treatment relies on prompt diagnosis with subsequent surgical debridement and initiation of broad-spectrum antibiotic therapy. Surgical intervention should be appropriately aggressive, with removal of all involved skin, fascia, and muscle during the initial debridement. The resulting wound must be evaluated on a daily basis for further progression of the infection and tissue necrosis. Repeat debridement is often necessary until a stable, viable wound is achieved. Between debridements, the wound should be covered with sterile dressings to promote healing and decrease the risk of secondary infection. In some circumstances, limb amputation is required initially in order to preserve the patient's life. Following appropriate surgical debridement, the resulting wound(s) and soft-tissue defect(s) may require skin grafting or free tissue transfer for definitive coverage and closure. It is important to remember that surgical intervention is the only treatment for necrotizing fasciitis proven to reduce mortality.

Antibiotic therapy must be initiated as soon as necrotizing fasciitis is suspected and microbial cultures are obtained. Initial empiric therapy should include coverage for gram-positive, gram-negative, and anaerobic organisms. Broad-spectrum empiric coverage typically includes clindamycin in combination with imipenem, meropenem, ampicillin/sulbactam, or piperacillin/tazobactam. The antibiotic regimen can be tailored to culture and sensitivity results once available. Although antibiotic therapy is critical to successful treatment, it can never be used as the sole intervention. Antibiotics can help reduce the systemic effects of the infection and decrease bacterial load but cannot eradicate the infection alone. This is due to limited antibiotic delivery to the site of infection, which results from poor vascularity of the fascia that is further compromised by the infection itself.

In addition to surgical debridement and antibiotic administration necessary for successful treatment, supportive care with appropriate fluid resuscitation and blood pressure maintenance are often needed in the septic patient. Nutritional support is critical in all patients due to the loss of fluid, electrolytes, and protein through the often large surgical wound(s). Adjunctive therapy with intravenous immunoglobulin G, recombinant human-activated protein C, and hyperbaric oxygen have all been reported to improve outcomes but have yet to become standard in treatment protocols.

SUMMARY

Musculoskeletal infections affect patients of all ages, can involve any anatomic region in the body, and result from any one of an infinite number of etiologies. Successful treatment relies on proper and timely diagnosis followed by antibiotic therapy, surgical intervention, or both. Careful attention must be given to infections in the setting of fractures and the presence of orthopaedic hardware. Given the morbidity of musculoskeletal infections and the treatment required for successful eradication, future research must focus on prompt and accurate diagnosis as well as prevention.

RECOMMENDED READINGS

Bauer TW, Parvizi J, Kobayashi N, Krebs V. Current concepts review: diagnosis of periprosthetic infection. *J Bone Joint Surg Am*. 2006;88:869–882.

Bellapianta JM, Ljungquist K, Tobin E, Uhl R. Necrotizing fasciitis. *J Am Acad Orthop Surg*. 2009;17:174–182.

Cierny G III, DiPasquale D. Treatment of chronic infection. *J Am Acad Orthop Surg*. 2006;14:S105–S110.

Dormans JP, Drummond DS. Pediatric hematogenous osteomyelitis: new trends in presentation, diagnosis, and treatment. *J Am Acad Orthop Surg*. 1994;2:333–341.

Mader JT, Wang J, Calhoun JH. Antibiotic therapy for musculoskeletal infection. *J Bone Joint Surg Am*. 2001;83:1878–1890.

Patel A, Calfee RP, Plante M, et al. Methicillin-resistant *Staphylococcus aureus* in orthopaedic surgery. *J Bone Joint Surg Br*. 2008;90:1402–1406.

Metabolic Bone Diseases

6

Aasis Unnanuntana **_Brian P. Gladnick_**
Benjamin McArthur **_Moira McCarthy_** **_Joseph M. Lane_**

INTRODUCTION

Metabolic bone disease encompasses a group of disorders that impair balances between bone formation and bone resorption or defects in mineralization of bone. Theoretically, any disease affecting bone cells, collagen, noncollagenous protein, or mineral deposition could adversely affect bone and, therefore, constitute disease involving bone metabolism. The most common and perhaps most important metabolic bone disease is osteoporosis. Other significant metabolic bone diseases include rickets and osteomalacia, renal osteodystrophy, and Paget's disease of bone. This chapter will provide basic knowledge of factors that lead to the development of metabolic bone disease, along with an overview of metabolic bone disorders that are commonly encountered during clinical practice.

MINERAL HOMEOSTASIS AND ENDOCRINE FUNCTION IN BONE

Calcium is the most abundant mineral in human body. Calcium accretion begins during the third trimester of fetal life, increases throughout childhood, adolescence, and adulthood before peaking in early adulthood and declining thereafter. The rate of decline is approximately 1% to 2% per year. The total body calcium is exchanged in the remodeling process mediated by osteoblasts and osteoclasts. Ninety-nine percent of the total body calcium is stored in skeleton, leaving approximately 1% to circulate in the extracellular fluid. It is this 1% that controls and regulates the body function. The extracellular concentration of calcium is generally 10^5-fold greater than intracellular concentration of calcium. Forty percent of the circulating calcium is bound to albumin, 45% is in the active, free, ionized form, and 15% is bound to phosphate and other inorganic ions. Abnormalities in the serum protein concentrations alter the amount of calcium in the extracellular fluid. Therefore, it is important to calculate the corrected serum calcium level when the circulating albumin is abnormal in order to get an accurate estimate of the free calcium, or one can directly measure the actual free, ionized calcium.

Calcium in the skeleton exists as a hydroxyapatite crystal in the mineral phase of bone. The crystal contributes to the mechanical properties of bone and also serves as a calcium and phosphate reservoir that can be rapidly mobilized to support numerous biological systems if needed. The biological actions of calcium are attributed to the ionized fraction, which is readily exchangeable with pools of calcium in bone, blood, and intracellular sites. Calcium regulates a number of essential cell functions such as intracellular signaling and neuromuscular activity including muscle contraction.

Calcium is primarily absorbed in the duodenum and proximal jejunum and is controlled principally by 1,25-dihydroxy-vitamin D. Gastric acid is necessary for the absorption of calcium. Despite calcium intake of 400 to 1500 mg per day, the net calcium absorption from the intestine is between 200 and 400 mg per day. The systems of absorption and excretion are tightly coupled and regulated by the ionized serum calcium concentration. The kidneys filter between 8 to 10 g of calcium per day, of which only 2% to 3% is excreted. Most of the filtered calcium is reabsorbed through passive mechanisms in the proximal tubules with the remainder being reabsorbed in the loop of Henle and the distal convoluted tubules. These processes are highly regulated, and certain drugs that affect renal tubule physiology may alter calcium homeostasis. For example, thiazide diuretics reduce the excretion of urine calcium, and thus increase its serum concentration. Alternatively, loop diuretics enhance the excretion of calcium and therefore decrease the level of serum calcium.

Similar to calcium, 85% of the 600 g of phosphorus in the body is stored in bone. Phosphorus is important for structural proteins, enzymes, transcription factors, high-energy stores such as ATP, and nucleic acids. Daily phosphate anion loads are between 500 and 1000 mg. Phosphate anions are absorbed passively through the small intestine. 1,25-dihydroxy-vitamin D activates active transport of phosphate, resulting in absorption of up to 90% of the intestinal phosphate. Renal excretion of phosphate is dependent on the daily phosphate load. Parathyroid hormone (PTH) regulates serum phosphate concentrations by decreasing its reabsorption from the proximal tubule.

Calcium–phosphate homeostasis is achieved by the coordination among three organs: intestine, kidneys, and skeleton. Calcium balance becomes positive during skeletal growth in childhood and adolescent, pregnancy, and lactation. Conversely, negative balance may occur with high rates of bone remodeling during estrogen deficiency and with some disorders such as hyperthyroidism or primary hyperparathyroidism. The regulation of calcium–phosphate homeostatic system to maintain its balance is mediated primarily by parathyroid hormone (PTH), vitamin D, and calcitonin. On a larger time scale, these hormones control ionized calcium or phosphate levels through changes in intestinal absorption or kidney excretion. However, on the more immediate time scale they act on bone.

Parathyroid Hormone

PTH, produced by the chief cells of parathyroid gland, plays a major role in calcium homeostasis. The actions of PTH are directly through bone and kidneys and indirectly through stimulation of 1-hydroxylation of 25-hydroxy-vitamin D to 1,25-dihydroxy-vitamin D. In bone, PTH stimulates the release of calcium and phosphate. In the kidney, it produces the reabsorption of calcium and inhibits that of phosphate. In addition, PTH increases the activity of the renal 1α-hydroxylase, thereby enhancing the synthesis of 1,25-dihydroxy-vitamin D, which, in turn, increases the intestinal absorption of calcium and phosphate. As a result of these three actions, serum calcium rises, while serum phosphate declines. Generally, there are three main physiological regulators of PTH secretion and synthesis: extracellular calcium, phosphate ions, and 1,25-dihydroxy-vitamin D. Among the three regulators, extracellular calcium concentration is the most important physiological regulator of the secretion of PTH.

The action of PTH on bone is complex and partially understood. PTH activates its receptor, which is expressed on stromal cells and osteoblasts. Once activated, the expression of M-CSF and RANKL is increased, which subsequently enhances the formation of osteoclasts from the precursor cells and increases the activity of the existing mature osteoclasts. Therefore, increased secretion of PTH associated with primary hyperparathyroidism leads to an increase in osteoclast cell number and activity. Paradoxically, intermittent PTH administration leads to increased amounts of trabecular bone. This anabolic activity of PTH, however, is not well understood. Depending on the dose of PTH given, the mode of administration (intermittent or continuous), and the specific target site (trabecular or cortical bone), the net effects of PTH on bone can be either anabolic or catabolic.

Vitamin D

When exposed to sunlight, cutaneous cholesterol (7-dehydrocholesterol or provitamin D_3) absorbs solar radiation and transforms itself into previtamin D_3, which rapidly undergoes an isomerization process to vitamin D_3. Vitamin D_3 is then translocated from the skin into the circulation, where it is bound to vitamin D–binding protein. Vitamin D is also found in food. The major natural sources of vitamin D are oily fish such as salmon and mackerel, fish liver oils, and cod liver oil. There are two types of vitamin D: vitamin D_2 and vitamin D_3. Vitamin D_2 derives from yeast and plants, whereas vitamin D_3 is found in oily fish and cod liver oil and also made in the skin. Vitamin D_2 is approximately 30% as effective as vitamin D_3 in maintaining vitamin D status.

Once vitamin D enters the circulation, it is transported and metabolized by liver to 25-hydroxy-vitamin D (Fig. 6.1). It is 25-hydroxy-vitamin D that clinicians use to determine the status of vitamin D whether deficiency, sufficiency, or intoxicated. Because the liver has a large capacity to produce 25-hydroxy-vitamin D, more than 90% of the liver tissue has to be injured before it is unable to make an adequate quantity of 25-hydroxy-vitamin D, which is transported to the kidneys where the enzyme 1α-hydroxylase metabolizes 25-hydroxy-vitamin D to 1,25-dihydroxy-vitamin D, which is an active form of vitamin D. This hydroxylation step is activated by PTH but repressed by calcium as well as by the active form of vitamin D itself. In addition, the active form of vitamin D activates the 24-hydroxylase enzyme in the kidney, which creates 24,25-dihydroxy-vitamin D, an inactive form of vitamin D.

The major function of 1,25-dihydroxy-vitamin D for bone mineralization process is to maintain blood levels of calcium and phosphorus in the normal range for proper mineralization. 1,25-dihydroxy-vitamin D, however, does not have a direct effect in the mineralization process. There are several additional roles of this active vitamin D including increased bone-specific alkaline phosphatase,

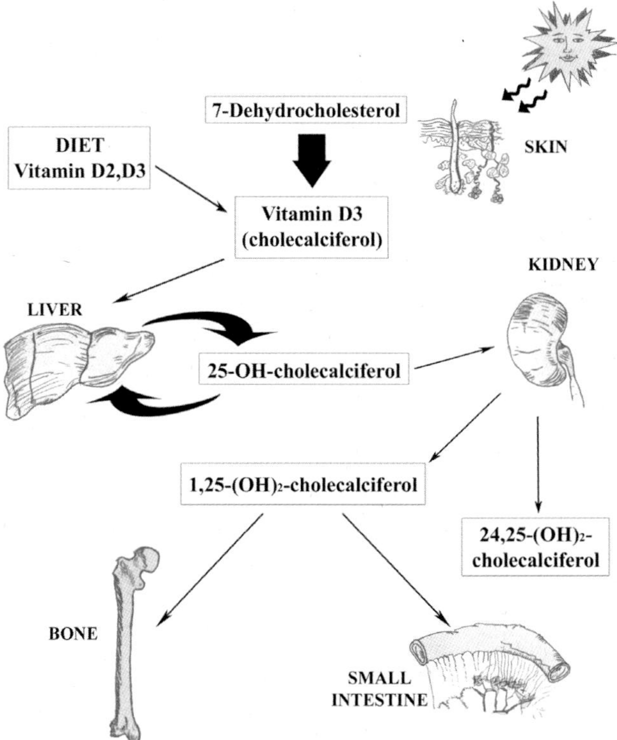

Figure 6.1 Vitamin D metabolism. After undergoing photoconversion in the skin, Vitamin D is metabolized first in the liver and then in the kidney. The target end organs of the active vitamin D, 1,25-dihydroxy-vitamin D, are the intestine and bone. (Adapted from Brinker MR, O'Connor DP. Basic Sciences: Bone. In: Miller MD, ed. *Review of Orthopaedics*, 5th ed. Philadelphia, PA: Saunders, an imprint of Elsevier, 2008:20.)

osteocalcin, and osteonectin and altered proliferation and apoptosis of skeletal cells. Nonskeletal roles for vitamin D involve cancer prevention, facilitated muscle function, and enhancement of the immune system.

Vitamin D deficiency can be caused by a variety of conditions and disorders such as excessive sunscreen use, clothing of all sun-exposed areas, obesity, aging, and some medications. A sunscreen with a sun protection factor (SPF) of 8 reduced vitamin D production by 95%. It is, therefore, recommended to consider exposing body parts (hands, face, and arms) to a suberythemal degree of sunlight (an amount that would cause mild pinkness to the skin) 2 to 3 times a week before applying sunscreen lotion. Increased vitamin D deposition in body fat is the cause of vitamin D deficiency in obesity. Some medications such as anticonvulsants, glucocorticoids, and rifampicin enhance the catabolism of 25-hydroxy-vitamin D and thus cause vitamin D insufficiency.

Calcitonin

Calcitonin is a peptide that is secreted by thyroid C cells. It consists of 32 amino acids and acts against osteoclasts in their resorptive function. Calcitonin is metabolized by many organ systems, including the kidney, liver, bone, and even the thyroid gland. The secretion of calcitonin is regulated by serum calcium. When serum calcium rises acutely, there is an increase in secretion of calcitonin. Conversely, an acute decline in serum calcium leads to a corresponding decrease in serum calcitonin level. If hypercalcemia is severe or prolonged, the C cells, however, exhaust their secretory reserve. Because of its properties, there are applications to use calcitonin for various disorders that are characterized by increased bone resorption such as Paget's disease, osteoporosis, and hypercalcemia of the malignancy. In addition, calcitonin has been used as a tumor marker for medullary thyroid carcinoma (MEN type II).

BONE STRENGTH, BONE MINERAL DENSITY, AND BONE QUALITY

Bone strength reflects the integration of two main factors: bone density and bone quality. Bone mineral density (BMD) has been shown to correlate well with bone strength as a whole; however, there are still some limitations. For instance, it does not distinguish the specific attributes of the three dimensions of bone quality such as the size and shape of the bone, the cortical and trabecular components, and the microarchitecture or intrinsic property of the bone matrix. In addition, it represents only a static parameter, which provides no information regarding bone turnover in an individual patient. Currently, there has been an increasing interest in another determinant of bone strength: bone quality. Bone quality is a function of the structural and material properties of bone. The structural properties include its geometry and microarchitecture, whereas the material properties include its mineral and collagen components. In general, bone undergoes continuous renewal by the process of coupled bone resorption and formation, so-called "bone remodelling." This process, therefore, influences both BMD and bone quality and consequently affects the whole bone strength (Fig. 6.2).

Bone Turnover or Bone Remodelling

Bone turnover is the principal factor that controls both the quality and the quantity of bone. An imbalance between bone resorption and bone formation ultimately results in a net loss or gain of the bone tissue. High bone turnover leads to thinning of the bone structure, resulting in abnormal bone microarchitecture and reduced bone mineralization. Conversely, low bone turnover results in hypermineralization and accumulation of microdamage, which leads to increased bone fragility.

Bone turnover can be assessed by combined calcium balance and isokinetic studies, which are time consuming and expensive; by tetracycline-based histomorphometry, which is an invasive technique; or by biochemical bone markers. The measurement of biochemical bone markers has several advantages including that it is generally available, can be assessed serially, and can measure changes in bone turnover over a short time interval. Thus, the measurement of

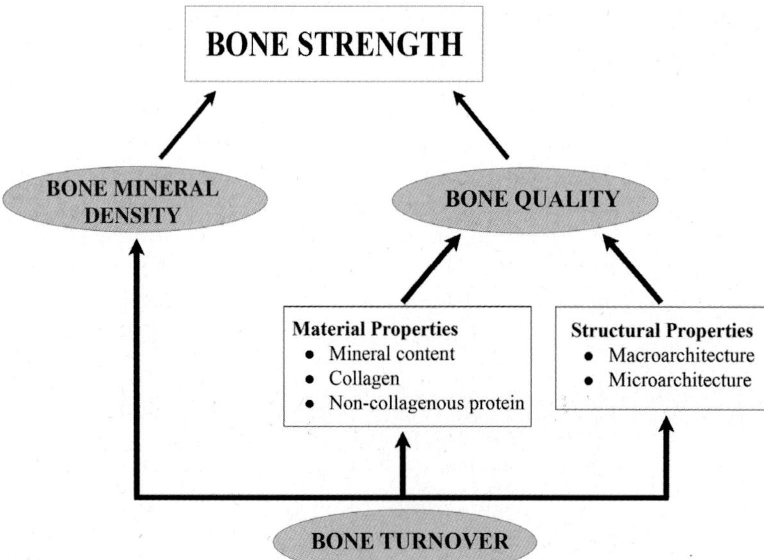

Figure 6.2 Bone strength is a function of bone mineral density (BMD) and bone quality. The bone turnover rate affects both BMD and bone quality and subsequently contributes to overall bone strength.

biochemical bone markers represents a significant advance in the evaluation and treatment of patients with metabolic bone diseases.

A biochemical bone marker can be categorized as a bone formation marker or a bone resorption marker. Each of the markers represents a product that is released during either bone formation or bone resorption (Table 6.1). During bone formation, osteoblasts produce type I collagen, which is their major synthetic product. Carboxyterminal propeptide and aminoterminal propeptide of type I collagen, known as PICP and PINP, respectively, are cleaved from the newly formed collagen molecule and, therefore, can be used as the indices to indicate type I collagen biosynthesis. Osteoblasts also secrete a variety of noncollagenous proteins, two of which are used clinically as markers of osteoblast activity: bone-specific alkaline phosphatase and osteocalcin. It is these noncollagenous products that are most useful as markers for bone formation. Although alkaline phosphatase is derived from several tissues, the two most common sources are liver and bone. The utilization of tissue-specific monoclonal antibodies allows for the differentiation between liver and bone isoform; however, the bone isoform has 10% to 20% cross-reactivity with the liver isoform.

TABLE 6.1
BIOCHEMICAL MARKERS OF BONE TURNOVER

Bone Formation Markers	Bone Resorption Markers
Serum	Serum
▪ Bone-specific alkaline phosphatase	▪ Tartrate-resistant acid phosphatase
▪ Osteocalcin	▪ N-telopeptide of collagen cross-links (NTx)
▪ Carboxyterminal propeptide of type I collagen (PICP)	▪ C-telopeptide of collagen cross-links (CTx)
▪ Aminoterminal propeptide of type I collagen (PINP)	
	Urine
	▪ Free and total pyridinolines (Pyd)
	▪ Free and total deoxypyridinolines (Dpd)
	▪ N-telopeptide of collagen cross-links (NTx)
	▪ C-telopeptide of collagen cross-links (CTx)

(Adapted from Camacho P. Biochemical markers of bone turnover. In: Favus MJ, ed. *Primer on the Metabolic Bone Diseases and Disorders of Mineral Metabolism.* 6th ed. Washington, DC: American Society for Bone and Mineral Research, 2006:127.)

During osteoclast-mediated bone resorption, the collagen structure within bone is degraded. This collagen degradation product is used as an indicator for bone resorption. In general, collagen molecules in bone matrix are staggered to form collagen fibrils by covalent cross-links. These cross-links consist of pyridinolines (Pyd) and deoxypyridinolines (Dpd). Pyd and Dpd cross-links occur at two intermolecular sites in collagen molecule: amino-terminal-telopeptide and carboxy-terminal-telopeptide. As part of this degradation process, cross-linked collagen peptides from both the amino-terminal-telopeptide (NTx) and the carboxy-terminal-telopeptide (CTx) are released and achieve measurable concentrations in both serum and urine (Fig. 6.3). Therefore, when osteoclasts resorb bone, they release a variety of collagen breakdown products into the circulation that are further metabolized by liver and kidney. These include free Pyd, free Dpd, NTx, and CTx. In addition to these markers, serum tartrate-resistant acid phosphatase (TRAP) has been used to evaluate bone resorption. TRAP is a lysosomal enzyme that is present in osteoclasts. It is released into the circulation when bone is being resorbed. TRAP, however, is not entirely specific

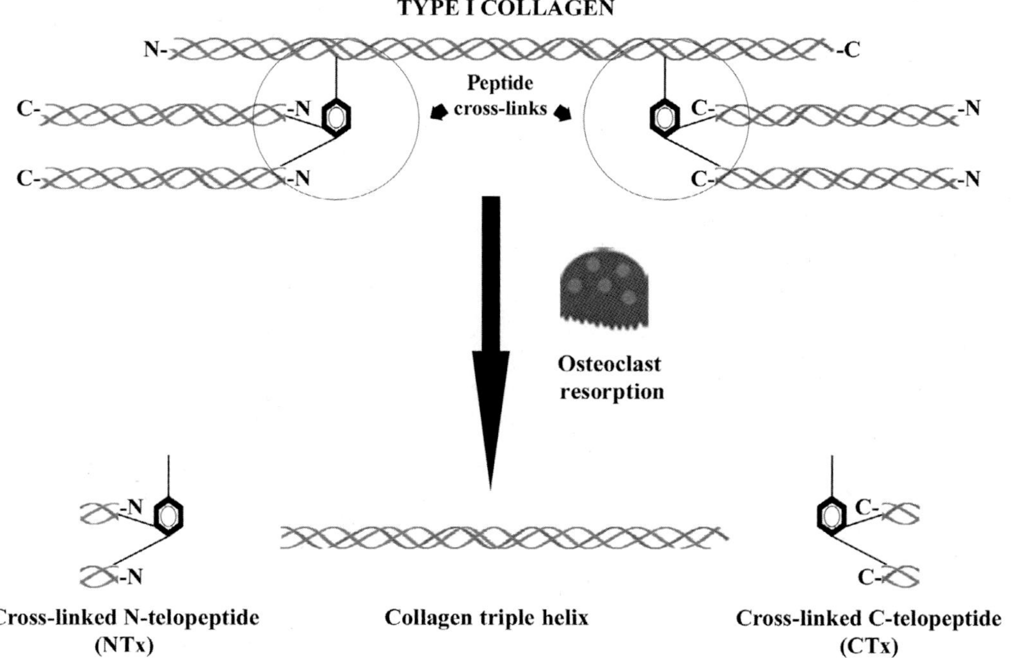

Figure 6.3 The collagen molecule is a triple helix consisting of two pro-α1(I) chains and a single pro-α2(I) chain. The collagen triple helix is cross-linked to adjacent molecules at the amino(N)- and carboxy(C)- terminals (as circled in the figure). During osteoclast-mediated resorption of bone, the collagen molecule is degraded, releasing these cross-linked N-telopeptides (NTx) and cross-linked C-telopeptides (CTx). NTx and CTx are specific for bone resorption. (Adapted from Unnanuntana A, Gladnick BP, Donnelly E, Lane JM. The assessment of fracture risk. *JBJS Am.* 2010; 92:749.)

for the osteoclasts, and the enzyme is relatively unstable in frozen samples.

Bone Material Property

Bone is a composite material, consisting of minerals, proteins, water, cells, and other macromolecules (lipids, sugars, etc). Although bone cells are the principal regulators of bone metabolism, bone matrix and minerals have a function in the control of the cell-mediated process. Therefore, the inorganic and organic components of the bone have both structural and regulatory properties.

The degree of mineralization of bone tissue, which reflects the mineral property of bone, influences not only the mechanical resistance of bones but also the BMD measured by dual-energy X-ray absorptiometry (DEXA). Similar to the mineral content, collagen and other extracellular matrices are important constituents of the bony composition. The noncollagenous proteins are not as abundant as collagen, but they provide for the regulation of mineralization, which reflects bone strength. The degree of mineralization of bone tissue can be determined by tetracycline-labeled transiliac bone biopsy, Fourier transformed infrared spectroscopy (FTIR), and phosphorus-31 solid-state nuclear magnetic resonance spectroscopy (31P solid-state NMR). The FTIR technique can examine the relative amount of minerals and matrix content, collagen maturity, and the arrangement of apatite and organic matrix, whereas the 31P solid-state NMR imaging can be used to measure quantitatively the mass of hydroxyapatite. These two techniques, however, are not widely used in clinical practice.

Bone Structural Property

The structural properties of bone can be divided into macroarchitecture and microarchitecture. The macroarchitecture, or bone geometry, refers to the size and shape of the bone. Microarchitecture describes the general connectivity of the trabeculae, the mean thickness of individual trabeculae, the mean spacing between trabeculae, and the number of the trabeculae. Changes in the geometry can influence the load and stresses to the bone and, therefore, affect bone strength. At the microarchitectural level, horizontal trabeculae form a network connecting various trabeculae, strengthening the bone against compressive forces in the same way as cross-struts of a three-legged chair contribute to the stability of the chair (Fig. 6.4). Destruction of these connecting trabeculae, which is seen in postmenopausal osteoporosis, results in increased fragility of the skeleton.

Measurement of bone geometry (macroarchitecture) can be done from the plain radiographs, whereas measurement of microarchitecture is obtained from bone biopsy. Bone biopsy yields various histomorphometric parameters that involve the quantitative analysis of undecalcified bone. The parameters of skeletal remodelling are expressed in terms of trabecular volume/tissue volume, trabecular number, trabecular separation, and marrow star volume (a measure of porosity). Currently, these parameters can

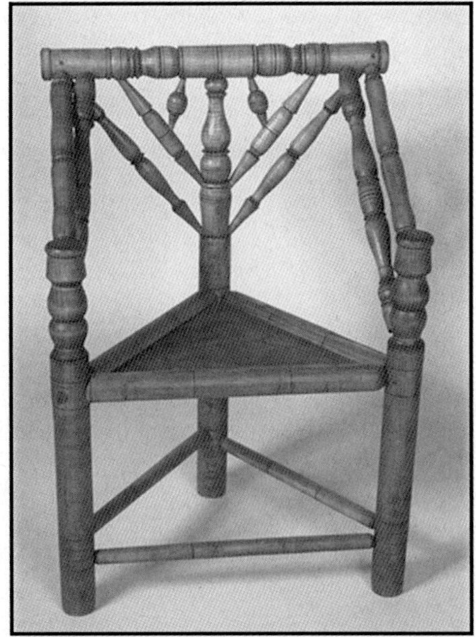

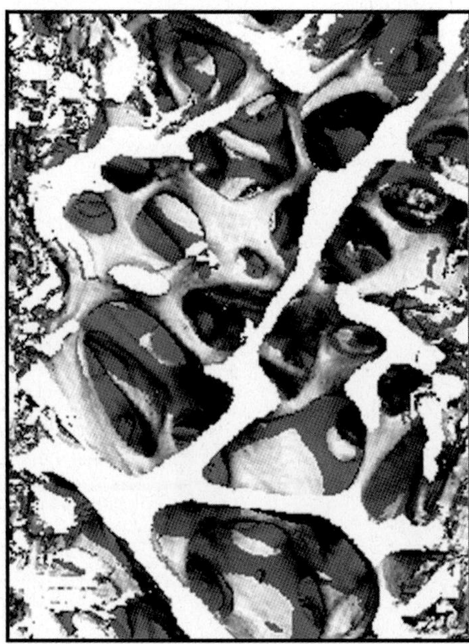

Figure 6.4 The cross-struts of a three-legged chair are important in providing the stability of the chair. Similarly, the horizontal trabeculae provide structural support to the bone.

be obtained by using three-dimension microcomputed tomography or high-resolution magnetic resonance imaging.

METABOLIC DISORDERS OF BONE

OSTEOPOROSIS

Osteoporosis is a condition characterized by decreased bone mass, microarchitectural deterioration, and ultimately increased bone fragility resulting in an increased risk of fracture. It is the most prevalent metabolic bone disease and is a source of significant morbidity and mortality as well as tremendous cost. Current estimates suggest that osteoporosis affects more than 200 million people worldwide, and the problem continues to grow. It is projected that the worldwide incidence of hip fractures will increase from 1.26 million in 1990 to 2.6 million by 2025 and 4.5 million by 2050.

Epidemiology

In the United States alone, an estimated 10 million people older than 50 are affected and another 34 million are at risk. The fracture incidence among affected Americans is approximately 1.5 million per year. Of these, approximately 700,000 are vertebral fractures, 300,000 are hip fractures, and 200,000 are wrist fractures. Women are affected more commonly than men. In addition, men are noted to have a relatively later onset of disease, up to one decade on average. The lifetime probability of hip fracture is 14% in Caucasian women and 5% to 6% in Caucasian men. Other ethnic groups can vary considerably in terms of their incidence of fracture. African Americans have a considerably lower rate of fracture than do Caucasians, with only 3% and 6% for men and women, respectively. The risk of fracture in Mexican American women has been noted to be intermediate, greater than that of African Americans but less than that of Caucasians.

There is significant morbidity and mortality associated with low-energy fractures. Vertebral fractures may be a source of chronic and disabling pain. Approximately one-third of patients with hip fractures are discharged to nursing homes, and the 1-year mortality rate among patients with hip fracture is approximately 20%. Thus, orthopaedic surgeons must be increasingly suspicious of this disease in certain patient demographics, achieve a firm understanding of the pathogenesis of osteoporotic bone and the conditions that result in bone fragility, and become familiar with the current strategies for diagnosis, prevention, and treatment of osteoporosis.

Classification

Osteoporosis is classically divided into two categories, primary and secondary. Primary osteoporosis is the result of predictable physiologic changes in BMD, which can result in clinical disease in some patients. It may be one of two types. Type I, or postmenopausal osteoporosis, is associated with the relative estrogen deficit seen in postmenopausal women. The lack of estrogen seen in the years following menopause is associated with an accelerated rate of bone loss. This is the most common form of osteoporosis in the general population, and it is from this subgroup that most of our current data on osteoporosis are derived. Type II, or senile osteoporosis, is seen in men and women alike older than 70. It is the result of age-related decline in BMD, which is common to both men and women beginning in midlife. While women undergo accelerated BMD loss in the perimenopausal years, the rate of loss declines

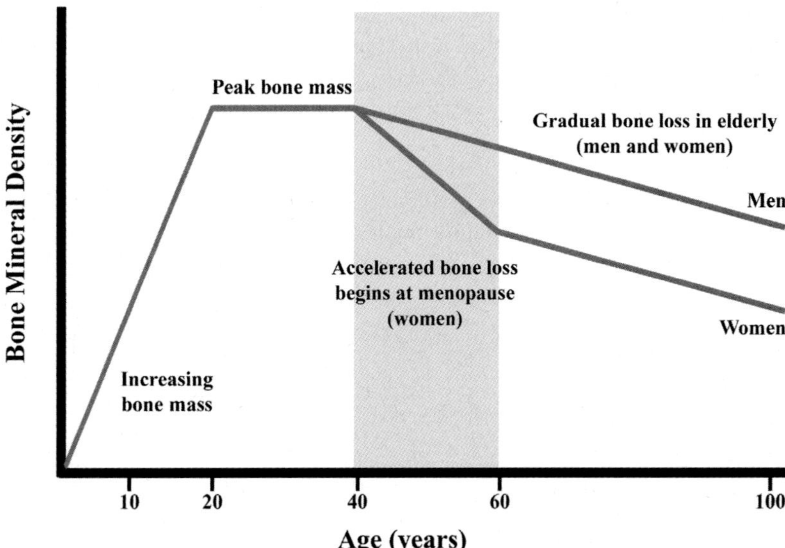

Figure 6.5 Bone mineral density (BMD) steadily increases from birth until it peaks during the third decade. With age, BMD gradually decreases in both men and women; however, women experience accelerated bone loss during the first few years after menopause.

in the years that follow and by the age of 60, men and women have similar rates of decline (Fig. 6.5).

Secondary osteoporosis is defined by the presence of some pre-existing disease process or other causative factor that causes a secondary decline in BMD (Table 6.2). Approximately 20–30% of osteoporotic women and 66% of osteoporotic men have their osteoporosis secondary to some underlying condition. Therefore, patients with secondary osteoporosis must be identified because definitive treatment of the underlying cause is necessary to prevent further bone loss, and thus lower the risk of fracture.

TABLE 6.2
CAUSES OF SECONDARY OSTEOPOROSIS

Hormone excess
- Parathyroid (primary or secondary)
- Thyroid
- Cortisol

Hormone deficiency
- Estrogen (premenopausal or postmenopausal)
- Testosterone

Diseases
- Inflammation (rheumatoid arthritis, ulcerative colitis)
- Tumor or malignancy (multiple myeloma, lymphoma)
- Collagen vascular disease
- Renal osteodystrophy
- Others (liver diseases, immobilization)

Drugs
- Corticosteroids
- Thyroxine
- Alcohol
- Anticonvulsants (barbiturates, phenytoin)
- Anticoagulants (heparin, coumadin)
- Antimetabolites (methotrexate, cyclosporin)

(From Yue J, Guyer R D, Johnson JP, et al. *The Comprehensive Treatment of the Aging Spine: Minimally Invasive and Advanced Techniques*, Philadelphia, PA: Elseiver 2010 with permission).

Osteoporosis may also be categorized into two forms based on bone turnover rate: low-turnover and high-turnover osteoporosis. The *low-turnover* state describes a situation in which normal bone homeostasis is altered by decreased osteoblast activity; however, the osteoclast activity remains normal. Low BMD in this setting, therefore, is a result of reduced bone formation. Conversely, the *high-turnover* state is characterized by increased activity of both osteoblasts and osteoclasts. However, osteoclasts are activated to a greater extent. The bone remodeling process is shifted toward bone resorption, resulting in an imbalance of bone turnover that causes osteoporosis. High-turnover osteoporosis is the most common form and appears at menopause, whereas low-turnover osteoporosis occurs following drug interventions including chemotherapy, steroids, and prolonged bisphosphonate use.

Diagnosis

To date, DEXA is considered the gold standard in the measurement of BMD and diagnosis of osteoporosis. DEXA scanning as a part of osteoporosis screening typically involves scans of the hip, lumbar spine, and occasionally the distal radius. Results for a given patient are compared to the average values for age-matched controls and young normal patients at their peak BMD, and from these comparisons the *Z*-scores and *T*-scores are derived, respectively. *T*-scores between 1 and 2.5 standard deviations below the norm (between −1 to −2.5) are diagnostic for osteopenia, while scores equal to or below −2.5 are diagnostic for osteoporosis. For patients younger than 35, diagnosis of osteoporosis is dependent only on the *Z*-score. A *Z*-score of less than −1.5 is significant in that it may be indicative of a secondary cause of osteoporosis.

Early detection of osteopenia and osteoporosis with DEXA screening is an important means of reducing the risk of fracture and associated morbidity. However, universal screening is neither practical nor feasible. The International Society for Clinical Densitometry (ISCD) advocates DEXA screening for any patient who is

1. a female aged 65 or older;
2. a postmenopausal female younger than 65 who has clinical risk factors for fracture, such as low body mass index, prior fracture, or use of a high-risk medication;
3. a woman during the menopausal transition with clinical risk factors for fracture;
4. a male aged 70 years or older;
5. a male aged 70 years or younger with clinical risk factors for fracture;
6. an adult with a history of a fragility fracture;
7. an adult with an illness known to cause bone loss or low BMD;
8. an adult taking a medication known to cause bone loss or low BMD;
9. any patient being considered for pharmacologic treatment of bone loss;
10. any patient currently being treated for low BMD in order to monitor the treatment effect; or
11. any patient not receiving therapy in whom evidence of bone loss would lead to pharmacologic treatment.

In addition to these guidelines, it is important to take into account other factors that may increase a patient's propensity for low BMD or fracture. Patients with poor general health, alcoholism, dementia, frailty, recent discontinuation of estrogen replacement therapy, or long-term history of estrogen deficiency should be considered for DEXA scanning even if they do not fit into the ISCD criteria.

Evaluation for Osteoporosis

Once diagnosed with osteoporosis, a complete medical history should be obtained with particular attention to the risk factors for osteoporosis. The physical examination should be performed particularly of the spine region. Height should be measured and compared with the greatest known height to determine height loss, which is an indicator of vertebral compression fractures. Balance and walking gait should be observed in each individual. The assessment of functional balance is performed by using the single limb stance test and the 6-minute walking test.

As osteoporosis is a clinically silent condition, diagnostic imaging modalities such as plain radiographs, computed tomography (CT), or magnetic resonance imaging (MRI) may often be the first study available for patients who present with a fragility fracture. Two-thirds of vertebral fractures are clinically silent and are diagnosed only after diagnostic imaging is employed. Thin cortices and generalized decrease in radio-opacity are two major indicators of decreased bone density and, when seen in a patient with a low energy fracture, should alert clinicians to the likely diagnosis of osteoporosis.

Laboratory Investigations

In addition to diagnostic imaging, some routine tests should be performed to obtain baseline values as part of the initial workup. These include complete blood cell count with differential, urinalysis, and blood chemistry profiles with serum calcium and phosphate. Because vitamin D deficiency is very common among elderly populations, with a prevalence of approximately 50%, all elderly patients should be tested for vitamin D deficiency by measuring levels of 25-hydroxy-vitamin D. If low, adequate vitamin D supplementation is encouraged. Vitamin D deficiency, as defined by a serum 25-hydroxy-vitamin D of less than 20 ng per mL, is associated with poor muscle function as well as mineralization defects. Markers of bone turnover are important to indicate the status of bone metabolism. Measurement of bone markers is helpful for following a patient's response to treatment over time. Therefore, it is advisable to get a baseline value as part of the initial workup.

When secondary osteoporosis is suspected on the basis of clinical findings or because the patient is relatively young and presented with fragility fracture, specific tests should be considered to evaluate contributing causes that may require additional medical attention. These include basic laboratory investigation of a complete blood cell count with differential, erythrocyte sedimentation rate, serum calcium and phosphate levels, liver function tests, thyroid-stimulating hormone level, testosterone level in men, and a serum protein electrophoresis if myeloma is considered (Table 6.3). When abnormalities are detected, the patient should be referred to a specialist for further evaluation and specific treatment.

Assess for Risk of Falls and Fracture Risk

Certain comorbidities associated with the aging population may predispose a patient to falls, such as unsteady gait, use of sedative or hypnotic medications, and impaired visual or neuromuscular function. By identifying patients at particularly high risk for falls early in the course of treatment, it is possible to prevent a subsequent fracture. It is well recognized that the fracture rate is highest among osteoporotic patients (T-score −2.5 or below). However, a much larger proportion of patients reside in the range of osteopenia (below −1.0 to above −2.5). Consequently, more total fractures occur in this osteopenic group (55% of hip fractures). To adjust for the disparity, a new vehicle called the Fracture Risk Assessment Tool (FRAX) has been developed that adds additional risk factors to the calculation and offers a better assessment of fracture risk than DEXA scanning alone. This instrument calculates the patient's 10-year fracture risk on the basis of (a) age, (b) sex, (c) weight, (d) height, (e) previous fracture, (f) parent with a fractured hip,

TABLE 6.3
LABORATORY INVESTIGATIONS FOR SECONDARY OSTEOPOROSIS

Medical Diseases	Diagnostic Study
Endocrine	
■ Hyperparathyroidism	Serum calcium, serum phosphate, parathyroid hormone levels
■ Hyperthyroidism	TSH, T3, free T4
■ Hypogonadism	LH, FSH, estrogen, testosterone (men)
■ Diabetes	Blood glucose
GI disorders	
■ Crohn's disease, ulcerative colitis	CBC, ESR, CRP, serum albumin, colonoscopy
Liver disease	
■ Primary biliary cirrhosis, chronic active hepatitis	Liver function test, antimitochondrial antibody, antibody for hepatitis A, B, and C
Bone marrow disorders	
■ Multiple myeloma, leukemia, lymphoma	CBC with differential, serum calcium, serum protein electrophoresis
Collagen vascular disease	
■ Osteogenesis imperfecta, Ehlers–Danlos syndrome, Marfan syndrome	Genetic testing for collagen defects
Others	
■ Rheumatoid arthritis	CBC, ESR, CRP, rheumatoid factor
■ Renal failure	BUN, creatinine

TSH, thyroid-stimulating hormone; LH, luteinizing hormone; FSH, follicle-stimulating hormone; CBC, complete blood cell count; ESR, erythrocyte sedimentation rate; CRP, c-reactive protein; BUN = blood urea nitrogen. (From Yue J, Guyer R D, Johnson JP, et al. *The Comprehensive Treatment of the Aging Spine: Minimally Invasive and Advanced Techniques*, Philadelphia, PA: Elseiver 2010 with permission).

(g) current smoking, (h) use of glucocorticoids (i) presence of rheumatoid arthritis, (j) secondary osteoporosis (k) alcohol use (≥3 drinks/day), and (l) BMD at the femoral neck area. Calculated risk may serve as a helpful guide in therapeutic decision making for patients at risk of fracture. FRAX models for the United States, United Kingdom, and a number of other countries are available on the Internet at http://www.shef.ac.uk/FRAX/index.htm.

Treatment

Nonpharmacologic Treatment

A multidisciplinary approach is critically important in the management of osteoporosis. Nonpharmacologic treatment is used concurrently with pharmacologic therapy to optimize fracture risk reduction. Thus, every patient should be considered for nonpharmacologic management. Commonly used nonpharmacologic treatments include, but are not limited to, calcium and vitamin D supplementation, fall prevention, and balance and exercise programs.

A negative calcium balance or suboptimal levels of 25-hydroxy-vitamin D must be addressed first before any pharmacologic intervention is undertaken since these represent a constant impetus for bone demineralization and decreased bone density and strength. The recommended daily calcium requirement is between 1200 and 1500 mg per day. In addition to encouraging dietary sources of calcium, calcium supplementation can be carried out with a number of formulations, the most common of which are calcium carbonate and calcium citrate. Absorption of calcium carbonate is dependent upon gastric pH and can be compromised in patients taking proton pump inhibitors, while calcium citrate is absorbed at all pH levels. In addition, calcium citrate binds to oxalate, reducing its intestinal absorption, and citrate in urine inhibits crystal formation, thus reducing the incidence of kidney stones.

The current recommended dosages of vitamin D_3 from the Institute of Medicine are 200 to 600 IU per day. However, many experts consider these recommendations to be too low, and suggest that the minimum adult intake should be 1000 to 2000 IU per day. The appropriate amount of vitamin D intake should be evaluated by monitoring 25-hydroxy-vitamin D level and serum PTH. For patients with markedly low levels of vitamin D, 50,000 international units of vitamin D_2 can be taken orally once a week or every other week for 6 to 8 weeks, followed by a maintenance dose of 1000 to 2000 IU of vitamin D_3 per day. Toxicity is rare even if a dosage of 10,000 IU per day is given for up to 5 months.

Pharmacologic Treatment

The pharmacologic agents currently available are commonly divided into two groups: antiresorptive and anabolic. Antiresorptive agents have been developed to address the high-turnover state. These include estrogen, selective estrogen receptor modulators (SERMs), calcitonin, and bisphosphonates. The anabolic agent, parathyroid hormone, provides active building of bone mass and has been suggested to treat the low-turnover state.

Estrogen

Estrogen is an anti-osteoporotic agent that has been shown to increase bone mass and thus decreases the risk of vertebral and hip fracture by approximately 30% to 40% as compared with patients taking placebo. Estrogen, however, has been found to increase rates of stroke and deep vein thrombosis, while combined estrogen and progesterone therapy is associated with increased risks of cardiovascular disease, breast cancer, dementia, and gall bladder disease. As a consequence, estrogen is mainly used in the early postmenopausal period to treat postmenopausal syndrome and then lowered to the lowest dose that effectively controls symptomatology. The risks associated with estrogen formulations preclude their use as primary agents in the treatment of osteoporosis.

Selective Estrogen Receptor Modulators

Selective Estrogen Receptor Modulators (SERMs) are a class of agents that bind to estrogen receptors. They have a significant effect on breast tissue and bone cells; however, they act as antagonists in the other receptor sites. Of the SERMs currently being used for clinical settings, only raloxifene has been approved for the prevention and treatment of osteoporosis. Early data suggest that raloxifene decreases the risk of breast cancer by 70%, which has made raloxifene a preferred agent among osteoporotic patients with breast cancer risk. Although raloxifene has been shown to reduce the risk of vertebral fracture, there was no significant reduction in the overall risk of nonvertebral fracture. In addition, by stimulating estrogen receptors, raloxifene increases the risk of pulmonary emboli and thrombophlebitis and may cause profound postmenopausal symptoms. Therefore, clinicians must weigh the benefits of the reduced risks of vertebral fracture and invasive breast cancer against the increased risks of venous thromboembolism and fatal stroke when considering this agent for osteoporosis management.

Calcitonin

Calcitonin is available as both a parenteral injection and a nasal spray. The intranasal spray is the most commonly used formulation due to its superior compliance and ease of use. Calcitonin reduces the risk of vertebral fracture; however, there is only a modest increase in BMD. In addition, calcitonin treatment shows no benefit for reducing the risk of hip and other nonvertebral fractures. There is some data suggesting the analgesic effect of calcitonin. Although there is a hypothesis that calcitonin-induced analgesia may be mediated by increased beta-endorphins and may directly affect pain receptors in the central nervous system, the exact mechanism is still unknown. Therefore, the current indication for calcitonin treatment is for alleviating painful vertebral compression fractures. It should be discontinued as soon as pain has been controlled, since other pharmacologic agents are more effective in preventing future fractures.

Bisphosphonates

Bisphosphonates have been a mainstay of osteoporosis treatment for the past 30 years. The chemical structure of this class of drugs is closely related to that of inorganic pyrophosphate (PPi), a common byproduct of numerous synthetic reactions, which has been shown, in vivo, to have a high affinity for hydroxyapatite and an associated inhibitory effect on calcification. The bisphosphonates share this high affinity for hydroxyapatite and as a result are rapidly absorbed and retained in bone. Once there, they inhibit bone resorption by inducing osteoclast apoptosis.

Bisphosphonates have been proven effective for the reduction of fracture risk in patients with osteoporosis and a number of other metabolic bone diseases. Data from the Fracture Intervention Trial, a multicenter randomized control study, revealed a relative reduction in risk of 47% for hip fractures and 55% for clinical vertebral fractures in patients taking alendronate when compared to placebo. Their efficacy and ease of use have led to widespread use of these agents as first-line therapy for osteoporosis and osteopenia. Both oral and intravenous formulations are available (Table 6.4). While oral administration may be more convenient, intravenous administration is often utilized for patients with severe gastrointestinal complaints after oral intake, a history of severe gastroesphageal reflux or peptic ulcers, or disorders that compromise absorption such as short bowel syndrome or Crohn's disease.

Adverse effects of bisphosphonates include flu-like symptoms, especially with intravenous administration, severe gastroesophageal reflux, and, rarely, osteonecrosis of the jaw. Furthermore, by inhibiting bone remodeling, bisphosphonates slow fracture healing and should be avoided or discontinued in the setting of acute fracture. In addition, there has been a growing concern over the years regarding the potential for bisphosphonates to induce a frozen bone syndrome wherein prolonged oversuppression of bone remodeling results in deleterious effects on bone quality, which may culminate in low-energy fractures (Fig. 6.6). Several reports in the literature make reference to an association between long-term alendronate use and atraumatic or low-energy femoral shaft fractures. Although a causal relationship has not been demonstrated, these findings, in combination with animal studies demonstrating reduced repair and accumulation of microdamage in animals treated with alendronate, suggest that impaired bone turnover may put patients at risk for low-energy fractures.

Nonetheless, bisphosphonates remain one of the most potent agents available for the reduction of fracture risk in osteoporotic patients. One solution that has been adopted

TABLE 6.4
BISPHOSPHONATES RECOMMENDED TO TREAT OSTEOPOROSIS

Generic Name	Trade Name	Recommended Dose	Route of Administration	Instructions
Alendronate	Fosamax	10 mg/d 70 mg/wk	Oral	Oral bisphosphonates: take with 8 oz of water and wait at least 30 min in an upright position before eating or drinking anything
Risedronate	Actonel	5 mg/d 35 mg/wk 75 mg/2 wk 150 mg/mo	Oral	
Ibandronate	Boniva	150 mg/mo 3 mg/3 mo	Oral Intravenous	Intravenous bisphosphonates: infusion over 15 to 45 min and coadministration with Benadryl and Tylenol
Zoledronic acid	Reclast	5 mg/y	Intravenous	

All bisphosphonates: precaution in patients with severe renal insufficiency or hypocalcemia.

by many clinicians is to monitor the effect of antiresorptive therapy through the use of serum or urine markers of bone turnover such as NTx. Regular monitoring of NTx levels may allow the clinician to titrate anti-resorptive therapy to a desired level of action and prevent oversuppression of bone turnover by halting administration of antiresorptive medications in patients already in a low-turnover state.

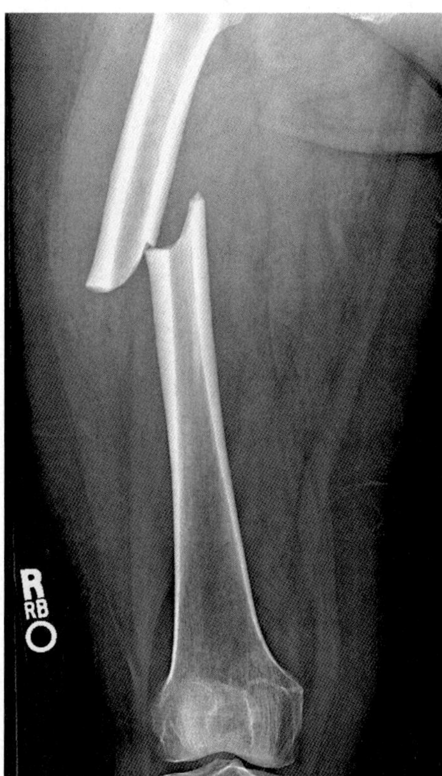

Figure 6.6 Plain radiograph anteroposterior view showing femoral shaft fracture. Fracture after prolonged treatment with bisphosphonates is characterized by **(A)** simple or transverse fracture; **(B)** beaking of the cortex on one side; **(C)** hypertrophied diaphyseal cortices; and **(D)** result from minimal or no trauma.

Teriparatide

Teriparatide, a recombinant fragment of human PTH, represents a relatively new and powerful agent for the treatment of osteoporosis. It is the only anabolic agent approved for the treatment of osteoporosis in the United States. Teriparatide is administered as a daily subcutaneous injection. While continuous administration of PTH, as seen in primary hyperparathyroidism, results in increasing bone resorption, by mechanisms that remain unclear, the administration of low-dose intermittent PTH in the form of teriparatide acts as a powerful inducer of bone formation. While cost is currently a major limiting factor in the use of teriparatide as a first-line therapy for osteoporosis, it remains an important agent for the treatment of patients with following conditions:

1. patients with low-turnover osteoporosis;
2. patients who have been on bisphosphonates and still have fragility fracture;
3. patients with declining bone densities while taking bisphosphonates

Teriparatide has been associated with osteogenic sarcoma when given in extremely high doses to laboratory rats. As such, its use is contraindicated for any pediatric patient or a patient with a history of recent radiation therapy, as both may be associated with an increased incidence of osteogenic sarcoma. Teriparatide should be discontinued after 2 years of treatment. After that, bisphosphonate therapy should be initiated to maintain its results.

RICKETS AND OSTEOMALACIA

Rickets is a clinical condition in which there is inadequate mineralization of the growing skeleton, and thus by definition occurs solely in children. Conversely, osteomalacia is a defect of mineralization that occurs after cessation of the skeletal growth. While important distinctions exist between these two diseases, they arise from similar etiologies and thus there is much overlap between the clinical, radiographic, and histologic presentations of each. Rickets and osteomalacia have a relatively higher prevalence in populations that receive limited sunlight throughout the year, or wear cultural attire that precludes ultraviolet exposure to the skin, especially in parts of Asia and the Middle East. In United States, it is estimated that 25% of elderly people have chronically low levels of vitamin D because of undernourishment and low exposure to sunlight. In addition, the absorption of vitamin D from the gastrointestinal tract is reduced in this particular age group.

Etiology of Rickets and Osteomalacia

Bone mineralization depends on the presence of calcium, phosphate, and alkaline phosphatase enzyme. Therefore, any condition that reduces the availability of serum calcium, phosphate, or alkaline phosphatase enzyme will result in rickets or osteomalacia (Table 6.5). Although there are a number of causes for rickets and osteomalacia, most of them share similar histologic changes, as well as clinical and radiographic appearances.

Nutritional rickets and osteomalacia are the oldest and best known forms of hypocalcemic disorders; however, the prevalence rate has now been greatly reduced in developed countries. Low levels of vitamin D results in decreased absorption of calcium across the intestinal tract, causing a decline in the concentration of serum calcium. This reduced serum calcium triggers a compensatory increase in the synthesis and secretion of PTH by the parathyroid glands. PTH secretion may elevate the serum calcium concentration back to normal by three major mechanisms: (a) increasing calcium reabsorption in the proximal tubule of the kidney; (b) stimulating the hydroxylation of 25-hydroxy-vitamin D to the more active 1,25-dihydroxy-vitamin D (which facilitates intestinal absorption of calcium); and (c) enhancing the osteoclast-mediated resorption of bone. The increased parathyroid activity reduces serum phosphate as a result of decreased tubular reabsorption of phosphate. This results in hyperphosphaturia and hypophosphatemia. The bone changes are related to a decrease in the available calcium and phosphate needed to synthesize calcium hydroxyapatite and a secondary hyperparathyroidism, which causes osteoclastic destruction of the existing bony structure. Low levels of vitamin D may also occur in persons with inadequate dietary intake, gastrointestinal malabsorption (celiac sprue, status post gastrectomy, and chronic pancreatitis), or chronic low exposure to sunlight. Certain anticonvulsants may accelerate the catabolism of vitamin D in the liver, causing decreased levels in the serum.

There are two forms of vitamin D–resistant rickets secondary to inherent defects of the vitamin D metabolic pathway, designated as type 1– and type 2–dependent rickets. Type 1–dependent rickets refers to a deficiency of the 1α-hydroxylase enzyme that converts 25-hydroxy-vitamin D to 1,25-dihydroxy-vitamin D, whereas type 2–dependent rickets is an inherent defect in the vitamin D intracellular receptor. As a result of this end organ insensitivity in type 2–dependent rickets, the circulating level of 1,25-dihydroxy-vitamin D is exceedingly high. Interestingly, there is evidence that certain tumors may secrete a factor that causes renal proximal tubule derangement, resulting in reduced vitamin D synthesis or phosphate deficiency, which can also lead to skeletal demineralization.

While vitamin D deficiency is the primary etiology of rickets and osteomalacia, other less common causes of skeletal demineralization exist. X-linked hypophosphatemia is the most common inherited etiology for rickets. The disease causes isolated renal phosphate wasting, leading to hypophosphatemia. The specific treatment for this condition is oral administration of phosphate. Renal tubular abnormalities such as renal tubular acidosis and Fanconi syndrome cause renal wasting of mineral contents including phosphate and, therefore, result in a vitamin D–resistant form of rickets/osteomalacia. Finally, a deficiency in alkaline phosphatase enzyme produces abnormal mineralization of bone and thus creates clinical features that overlap with rickets in the child and osteomalacia in the adult.

TABLE 6.5
CAUSES OF RICKETS AND OSTEOMALACIA

Low serum calcium
Nutritional rickets
- Vitamin D deficiency
- Dumping syndrome
- Chronic liver disease
- Chronic bowel disorder
- Anticonvulsant medications

Vitamin D–resistant rickets
- Type 1–dependent (1α-hydroxylase deficiency)
- Type 2–dependent (end organ insensitivity to vitamin D)

Renal tubular acidosis
Low serum phosphate
X-linked hypophosphatemia
Low serum alkaline phosphatase
Hypophosphatasia

Clinical Presentation

The developing skeleton requires an abundant source of calcium and phosphate in order to properly mineralize during periods of rapid bone growth. In children with rickets, the process of mineralization cannot keep pace with the production of new osteoid. The result is a relatively demineralized skeleton that lacks the compressive strength of normal bone, and subsequently develops considerable deformity in a predictable pattern. Weight-bearing bones

TABLE 6.6
BIOCHEMICAL CHANGES IN RICKETS AND OSTEOMALACIA

	Biochemical Changes							
Etiology	Ca^{2+}	PO_4^{3-}	AP	PTH	25-OH-Vit D	1,25-OH_2-Vit D	Urine Ca^{2+}	Associated Findings
Nutritional rickets								
▪ Vitamin D deficiency	N, ↓	↓	↑	↑	↓	↓	↓	Low diet, chronic bowel disease (i.e., Crohn's disease)
▪ Dietary phosphate deficiency	N	↓	↑	N	N	N	N	Phosphate-binding antacid abuse, aluminum toxicity
Type 1 dependent	↓	↓	↑	↑	N	↓↓	↓	No alopecia
Type 2 dependent	↓	↓	↑	↑	N, ↑	↑↑	↓	Alopecia, with near-total loss of body hair
X-linked hypophosphatemia	N	↓	↑	N	N	N	N	Decreased renal tubular absorption of phosphate
Hypophosphatasia	↑	↑	↓↓	N	N	N	↑	Failure to thrive, early loss of teeth, craniosynostosis

Ca^{2+}, calcium; PO_4^{3-}, phosphate; AP, alkaline phosphatase; PTH, parathyroid hormone; 25-OH-Vit D, 25-hydroxy-vitamin D; 1,25-OH_2-Vit D, 1,25-dihydroxy-vitamin D; ↑, increase; ↓, decrease; N, normal. (Adapted from Mankin HJ. Metabolic bone disease. In: Jackson DW, ed. *Instructional Course Lectures*, volume 44. American Academy of Orthopaedic Surgeons, 1995:10.)

are the most noticeably affected, such as the forearms in infants learning to crawl. Older children who walk may suffer varus or valgus deformity of the lower extremity. Children may be irritable and complain of bone pain, dental caries, muscle aches, and weakness exacerbated by activity.

Mineralization is of particular importance at the epiphyseal plate, where a zone of calcification precedes the replacement of cartilage by newly forming bone. Patients with rickets cannot efficiently calcify the cartilage in this region, resulting in a marked profusion of cells in the noncalcified zone of hypertrophy. This presents clinically as a widening of the epiphyses, most noticeably in the wrists, elbows, knees, and ankles. Other common findings on physical examination that result from bony demineralization include shortness of stature, frontal bossing, a softening of the skull, prominence of the costochondral junctions (the so-called rachitic rosary), and a thoracic kyphosis.

The clinical presentation of adults with osteomalacia is similar in many respects to that of children with rickets. Bone pain, muscle aches, and weakness are typical complaints. Osteomalacic patients may also present with polyarthralgias, which may be mistaken for rheumatoid arthritis. Osteomalacia occurs by definition after the skeleton has already matured; therefore, some of the characteristic findings in rickets (bowing deformities of the limbs, widening of the epiphyses) are not necessarily found in osteomalacic patients.

Laboratory Investigations

A variety of etiologies may cause the skeletal demineralization typical of rickets and osteomalacia, and each is associated with a characteristic set of biochemical derangements (Table 6.6). Depending on the primary metabolic insult, the patient may have abnormal serum concentrations of calcium, phosphate, alkaline phosphatase, PTH, or vitamin D. In nutritional deficiencies, 25-hydroxy-vitamin D is the most reliable marker. Recognition of these patterns is helpful in making the diagnosis and in directing subsequent management of the patient's metabolic deficiency.

Radiographic Features

Plain radiographs of the patient with suspected osteomalacia or rickets are helpful in characterizing the extent of skeletal demineralization. Patients with rickets classically show widening of the epiphyseal plates, with cupping and flaring of the distal ends of the long bones. Cortical thinning is apparent, and a "ground-glass" appearance of the cancellous bone may be present secondary to the layers of unmineralized osteoid being deposited around the bony trabeculae. Focal depositions of unmineralized osteoid may also be apparent on plain radiographs as radiolucent areas extending perpendicularly across the cortex. These "pseudofractures" are known as "Looser's lines" and tend to occur on the concave aspect of long bones, at the medial femoral neck, inferior to the lesser trochanter, on the ischial and pubic rami, at the posterior aspect of the rib, on the clavicles, and at the lateral aspect of the scapulae (Fig. 6.7). In cases where the presence of Looser's line is questionable, a bone scan may be helpful in identifying the cortical mineral defect. Looser's lines are characteristic of both rickets and osteomalacia and may propagate into a true fracture if the patient is left untreated. Bone scan and MRI can detect fractures not visible on radiographs.

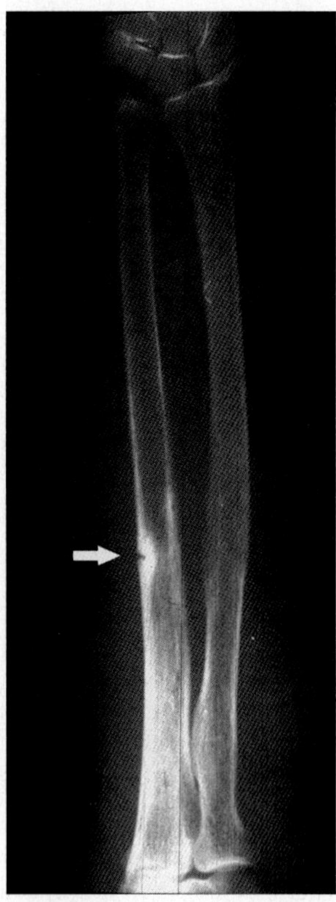

Figure 6.7 Plain radiograph of the ulna of a patient with rickets showing pseudofracture at the medial border of the diaphysis, also known as Looser's line, umbauzonen, or Milkman's pseudofracture. (*Courtesy of Bernard Ghelman, MD.*)

Plain radiographs in osteomalacia often look normal, and unless a Looser's line is identified the patient may be misdiagnosed with osteoporosis. Some characteristic radiographic findings commonly found in osteomalacia include an overall reduction in bone density, and a coarsening of the trabeculae, or a ground glass appearance to the spine.

Treatment

A treatment strategy for the patient with rickets or osteomalacia should be selected to address the underlying etiology of skeletal demineralization. In patients with nutritional rickets, calcium and vitamin D supplementation is appropriate. A common dosing regimen is ergocalciferol 50,000 IU one to two times per week, with 1,000 to 1,500 mg of calcium per day. The treatment should last from 6 months up to 1 year. If the patient has a syndrome of gastrointestinal malabsorption, an injectable form of vitamin D should be considered. Patients with dependent rickets should be carefully studied and treated with 1,25-dihydroxy-vitamin D for both type 1– and type 2–dependent forms. However, treatment with high doses of vitamin D produces a variable clinical response in type 2–dependent patients. The specific treatment for patients with X-linked hypophosphatemia is oral administration of phosphate and the active form of vitamin D. Those with oncogenic causes of skeletal demineralization should have their tumors completely removed, even if benign. Patients with renal tubular acidosis or other renal tubular abnormalities that causes loss of bone mineral content can be treated with phosphate replacement and supplemental vitamin D. Electrolyte imbalances need monitoring and treatment, and the underlying renal disease should also be treated if possible. Finally, the provider should consider changing any drugs or other medical interventions that may cause iatrogenic skeletal demineralization.

RENAL OSTEODYSTROPHY

Renal osteodystrophy is a pathologic bone condition in which the primary cause of the disorder is chronic renal failure. Because of the advent of modern medical treatment, patients with chronic renal disease are living longer and are more physically active. Therefore, the chance of this group of patients presenting to the orthopaedic community either for elective surgery or in an emergency trauma situation increases.

Pathophysiology

Kidneys are the vital organs for regulating calcium homeostasis. The proximal convoluted tubule is the site that produces 1,25-dihydroxy-vitamin D. This hormone is a prime regulator of intestinal calcium absorption and provides the feedback mechanism to inhibit PTH synthesis. In addition, kidneys serve as the primary route for excretion of waste products including phosphate, aluminum, and other toxic agents. Therefore, chronic renal failure results in a significant rise in blood urea nitrogen, creatinine, and phosphate. The injury to renal tissue creates a reduced tubular mass, which interrupts 1,25-dihydroxy-vitamin D synthesis. This leads to a drop in serum calcium, which causes a marked increase in serum PTH and resulting secondary hyperparathyroidism. The bone pathology, therefore, shows signs consistent with both rickets or osteomalacia and hyperparathyroidism (Fig. 6.8).

The pathophysiology of renal osteodystrophy is subdivided into two groups: high turnover and low turnover. The high-turnover state is the classic form of this disease. This form of renal osteodystrophy is associated with high PTH. Serum levels of PTH may be 5 to 10 times above the upper level of normal in patients with secondary hyperparathyroidism. In the presence of elevated PTH levels, bone turnover remains high and thus increases the activity of both osteoblasts and osteoclasts. Conversely, the low-turnover state is associated with normal to low serum PTH. The pathogenesis of low-turnover renal osteodystrophy is complex and includes a large number of factors such as aluminum-based phosphate binder and peritoneal

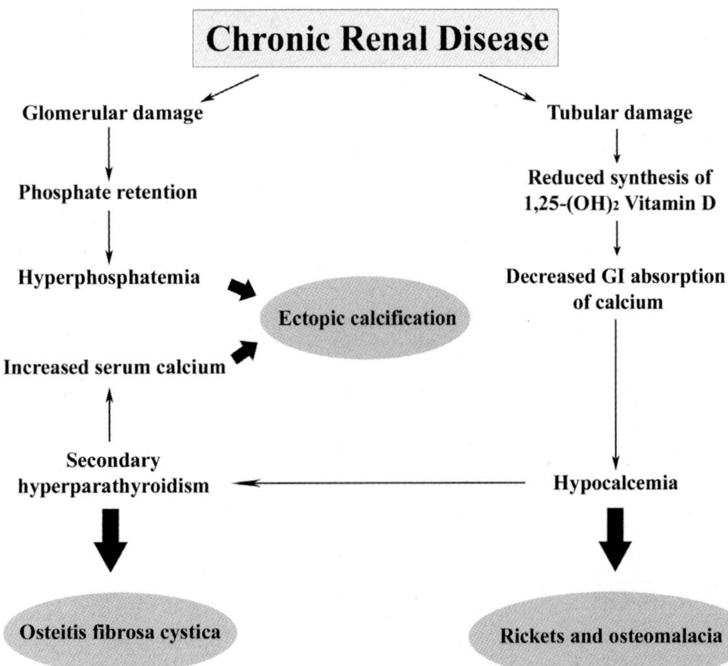

Figure 6.8 The pathophysiology of renal osteodystrophy. The skeletal presentation in patients with renal osteodystrophy shows changes consistent with both rickets and osteomalacia and osteitis fibrosa cystica, which is an antiquated term for hyperparathyroidism. (Adapted from Mankin HJ. Metabolic bone disease. In: Jackson DW, ed. *Instructional Course Lectures*, volume 44. American Academy of Orthopaedic Surgeons, 1995:15.)

dialysis. It is also believed that changes in a variety of growth factors and cytokines could directly impact the bone formation rate.

Clinical Presentation

The clinical manifestations of renal osteodystrophy are diverse and nonspecific. Bone pain is usually diffuse and may be associated with weight-bearing positions. Proximal muscle weakness is also relatively common. Children with renal osteodystrophy may manifest with linear growth failure, deformities of the long bones, slipped capital femoral epiphysis, and fractures. The elevation of both serum calcium and phosphate levels leads to extraskeletal calcification. These include periarticular calcification, vascular calcification of medium and small arteries (Monckeberg's sclerosis), and calcification of the visceral organs such as lungs, heart, kidneys, or skeletal muscle. Some patients may present with ischemic necrosis of the skin (calciphylaxis), which is a rare condition with catastrophic consequences.

Radiographic Features

Generally, the imaging studies of patients with renal osteodystrophy show changes consistent with both rickets/osteomalacia and hyperparathyroidism. In its severe form, hyperparathyroid bone disease may predominate and manifest as subperiosteal or subchondral erosions. The classic sites of subchondral resorption are at the distal clavicle, sacroiliac joints, and pubic symphysis, while subperiosteal resorption occurs along the medial border of the proximal tibia, the radial border of the middle phalanges, and at the tufts of the distal phalanges (Fig. 6.9). Brown tumor, which is a lytic area with a marked decrease in cortical structure, can also be found (Figs. 6.10 and 6.11). In some patients, the cancellous bone adjacent to the vertebral

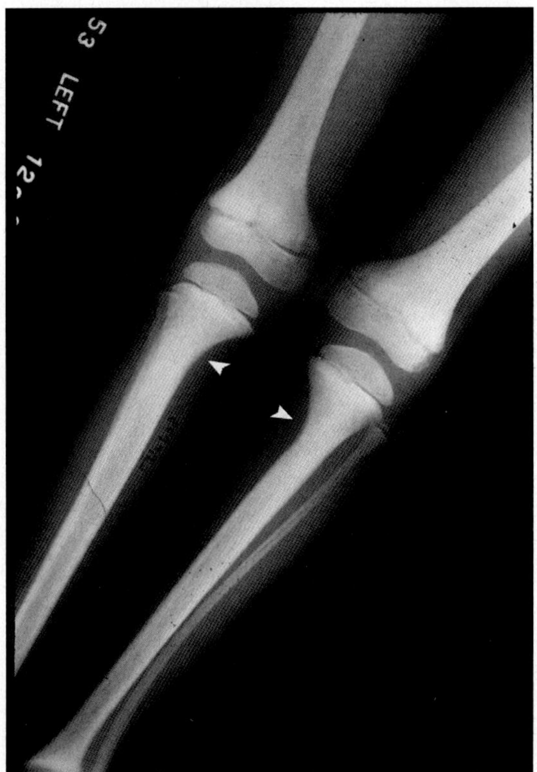

Figure 6.9 Anteroposterior radiograph of the right and left tibia, showing subperiosteal resorption at the medial border of the proximal tibia (*arrowheads*). (*Courtesy of Bernard Ghelman, MD.*)

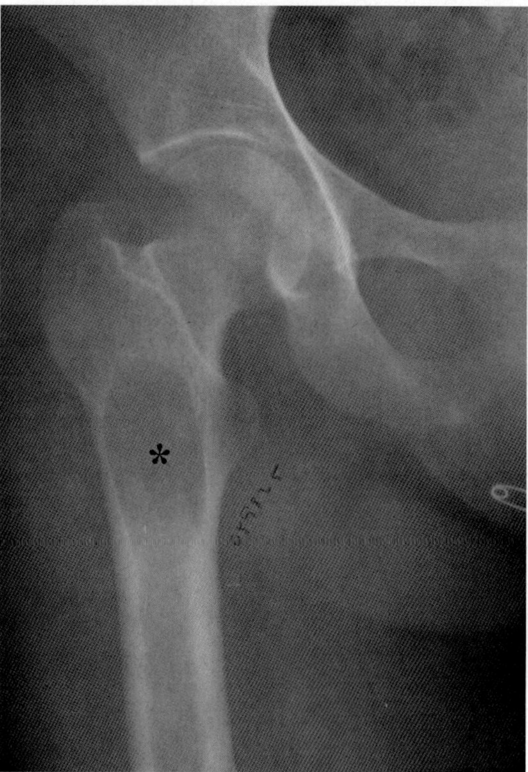

Figure 6.10 Anteroposterior radiograph of the right hip showing a well-demarcated lytic lesion in the proximal femur. The cortices are thin on both sides but remain intact. This localized area of bone destruction is known as brown tumor. Treatment of underlying hyperparathyroidism results in the resolution of these lesions. (*Courtesy of Bernard Ghelman, MD.*)

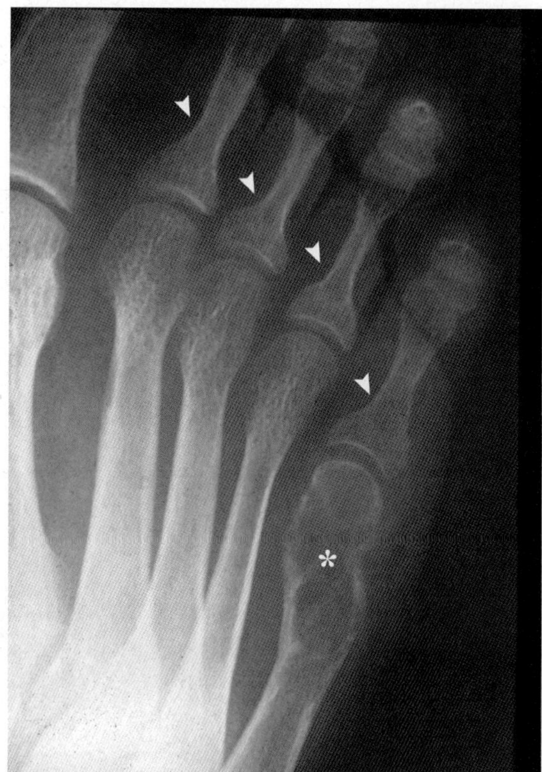

Figure 6.11 Radiograph of the right foot in a patient with hyperparathyroid bone disease showing brown tumor of the distal metaphysis of the fifth metatarsal (*asterisk*), and subperiosteal resorption of the second, third, fourth, and fifth proximal phalanges (*arrowheads*). (*Courtesy of Bernard Ghelman, MD.*)

endplates condenses into radiopaque bands, giving a distinct striped appearance of alternating lucent and opaque bands known as "rugger jersey" spine (Fig. 6.12).

Treatment

The treatment of renal osteodystrophy is dependent on the renal disease. The goals are to maintain serum levels of calcium and phosphorus as close to normal as possible, to avoid aluminum and iron toxicity, and to prevent the development of parathyroid hyperplasia or, if secondary hyperparathyroidism has already developed, to reduce the serum PTH level to acceptable value. Dietary restriction of phosphorus can help in regulating serum phosphate levels and thus preventing soft-tissue calcification. Active vitamin D sterols (1,25-dihydroxy-vitamin D) are important to correct vitamin D deficiency and to control hyperparathyroidism. Recently, a new agent for the treatment of hyperparathyroidism, cinacalcet hydrochloride, which blocks PTH actions, has been introduced and seems to be extremely useful in decreasing the levels of PTH. In situations where serum PTH remains excessively high, surgical removal of parathyroid tissue may also be required.

PAGET'S DISEASE

Paget's disease of bone (also known as osteitis deformans) is a localized disorder of bone remodeling. The disease process is initiated by increases in bone resorption, with subsequent compensatory increases in new bone formation. Because of the rapid bone turnover rate, the affected bone loses its control of the bony structure and thus results in disorganized mosaic pattern of woven and lamellar bone. Although most patients are asymptomatic, those affected with this disease may experience a variety of clinical symptoms and signs depending on the severity, number, and location of the affected skeletal sites. The clinical presentation includes bone pain, secondary osteoarthritis, bone deformity, and complications from bony compression to the adjacent soft-tissue structure, such as neural tissue surrounding the pagetoid bone.

Epidemiology and Etiology

Paget's disease is the second most common metabolic bone disease after osteoporosis with most series describing a slight male predominance. The prevalence rate of the disease is dependent on geographic area. Among all populations, Caucasians, especially people from England,

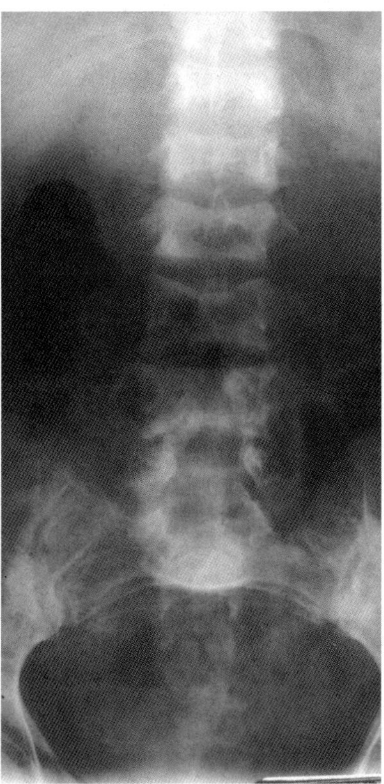

Figure 6.12 Anteroposterior radiograph of the lumbosacral spine demonstrates sharply defined thick bands of sclerosis of both the superior and inferior vertebral endplates, giving a horizontal striped appearance, or so-called rugger jersey (football sweater) spine. (*Courtesy of Bernard Ghelman, MD.*)

Australia, and New Zealand, have much higher prevalence rates than the native Americans, Scandinavians, Africans, Indians, or Asians. Paget's disease has been reported at a rate as high as 3% to 4% in Australia and New Zealand, whereas the prevalence rate was approximately 0.3% of the population in Norway and Sweden. To date, the etiology of this disorder is still unclear. There are several hypotheses for the pathophysiology of Paget's disease including genetic predisposition and slow viral infection. Several studies showed that 15% to 30% of patients with Paget's disease have positive family history of this disorder. Because of the documented frequency of familial history with Paget's disease, there is a suggestion that this disease is transmitted as an autosomal dominant trait. The other intriguing hypothesis is a possible relationship between Paget's disease and viral infection such as parvomyxoviruses (measles, mumps, and parainfluenza). Although some literature suggests the possibility of animal-related infection or chronic infection from respiratory syncytial virus, the conclusion was not borne out from additional studies.

Pathology

Paget's disease is a disorder in which bone is synthesized and degraded at rapid rates but generally equal. Therefore, the overall bone turnover is equivalent. The histopathologic finding is dependent on the stage of the disorder to affected bone. The early phase is dominated by increased bone resorption by activated osteoclasts, resulting in a lytic lesion that is appreciated radiographically as "blade of grass" lesion in long bone or "osteoporosis circumscripta" in skull. These osteoclasts are more numerous and contain more nuclei than do normal osteoclasts. In order to respond to the increased bone resorption, osteoblasts are recruited to the affected area. During this blastic phase, because of the nature of rapid turnover, the newly deposited collagen fibers are laid down in a disorganized pattern, creating a more primitive woven bone. This results in an irregularity of contour of the new trabeculae and cortices. In addition, the bone marrow is infiltrated by the osteoclasts, osteoblasts, and blood vessels between the trabeculae, creating the hypervascular state of the bone.

Over time, the hypervascularity and hypercellularity process extinguishes by itself, leaving the end result of a sclerotic, enlarged, mosaic pattern. This is a sclerotic phase or a so-called burned out Paget's disease in which neither bone formation nor resorption takes place. Generally, all phases can be seen at the same time in different areas of the patients with Paget's disease.

Clinical Presentation

Paget's disease is most commonly diagnosed in individuals older than 50. Many patients, therefore, have Paget's disease for a period of time before the diagnosis is made. It may present as a monostotic lesion, which affects only one bone, a portion of bone, or a polyostotic lesion, which involves two or more bones. The most common areas of involvement include the pelvis, femur, spine, skull, and tibia. Upper extremities, hand, and feet are less commonly affected. In general, most patients with Paget's disease are asymptomatic and the diagnosis is made when abnormal blood chemistry such as an elevated alkaline phosphatase is noted or when an incidental finding from the radiographs is found. The development of symptoms or complications of Paget's disease is influenced by area of involvement, the extent of metabolic activity, and the effect of pagetoid bone to the adjacent structure.

Bone pain, either mild or severe, is probably the most common symptom. Bone pain may be associated with a high-turnover state when there is hypervascularity at the area of involvement. Bowing deformity especially of the femur and tibia are common and can lead to secondary osteoarthritis from alteration of the mechanical axis and abnormal gait pattern. Paget's disease of the vertebral bodies can produce signs and symptoms similar to spinal stenosis, while Paget's disease of the skull may affect cranial nerves, causing cranial nerves palsies in cranial nerves II, VII, VIII. Increased blood supply to the affected bone results in a large amount of cardiac output and, if prolonged and untreated, may impair left heart function and lead to high-output left heart failure. Paget's sarcoma is a rare and devastating complication with an incidence of less than 1%. The malignant transformation is typically located in the femur, pelvis, humerus, and skull.

Diagnosis

When Paget's disease is suspected, the diagnostic evaluation includes a thorough medical history, physical examination, laboratory investigations, and imaging studies. Patients with Paget's disease usually show elevated serum bone-specific alkaline phosphatase levels, which indicate increased osteoblast activity, whereas high concentration of NTx or CTx in the urine reflects increased bone resorption. Although these findings are not specific, the utility of these markers is primarily to assess the response of treatment and to follow the course of disease over time.

The findings from plain radiographs include four important findings: (a) the width and sometimes length of involved bone are greater than normal; (b) the cortices are wider; (c) the trabeculae in the medullary canal are coarse but disorganized; and (d) the medullary bone often contains lytic areas of various sizes (Fig. 6.13). Generally, the characteristic findings from plain radiograph and clinical features of Paget's disease can eliminate other differential diagnoses.

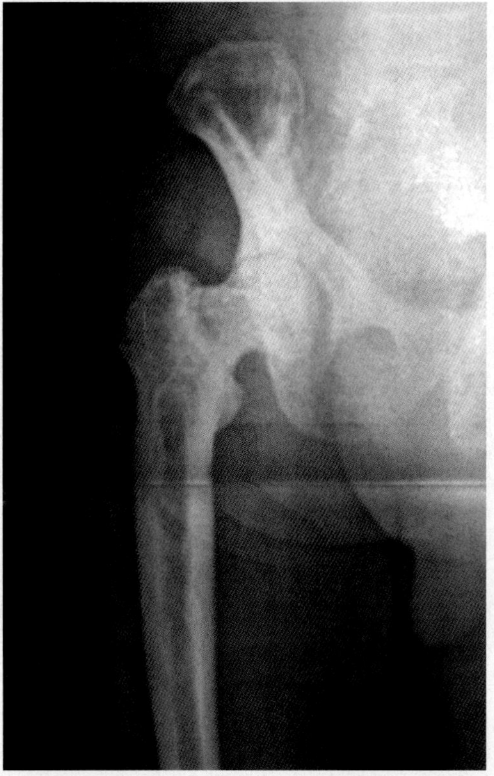

Figure 6.13 Anteroposterior radiograph of the right proximal femur in a patient with Paget's disease. Note the increased width of the femoral shaft, markedly thickened cortices, coarse but disorganized trabeculae, and small lytic areas within the medullary canal.

Treatment

Patients who are asymptomatic can be treated conservatively by serial follow-up with radiographs, bone scan, and assays for bone markers. There is no clear indication for treating this group of patients. Two logical recommendations for treatment of Paget's disease are to relieve symptoms and to prevent future complications. It is still inconclusive whether asymptomatic patients with active disease (elevated alkaline phosphatase) should be treated. In this setting, medical treatment may prevent the patients from developing later problems or complications, especially in the younger patient for whom many years of coexistence with the disease is likely. However, there is no clinical study to prove that disease suppression reduces the progression of bone deformity. Specific therapeutic agents available in the United States for treatment of Paget's disease include bisphosphonates and calcitonin.

The action of bisphosphonates is principally by altering calcium metabolism and inhibiting osteoclast activity. Currently, four bisphosphonates have been recommended as the first- line drugs of treatment: alendronate, risedronate, pamidronate, and zoledronic acid. The dosage for treatment of Paget's disease, however, is higher and more frequent than that recommended for treatment of postmenopausal osteoporosis. Studies showed that patients treated with intravenous bisphosphonates have a remission in their symptoms and a marked change in their biochemical profiles. In addition, bisphosphonate therapy has been shown to reduce arthritis difficulty, spinal canal narrowing, hearing loss, and fracture rates.

Calcitonin has been shown to be effective in Paget's disease for more than 30 years. However, only the injectable formulation is approved by the FDA for treatment of Paget's disease. The improvement of clinical signs and symptoms is noted in a few weeks, and the reduction of serum alkaline phosphatase is usually observed after 3 to 6 weeks of treatment. The initial starting dose is 100 IU everyday. Once the patient observes the symptomatic benefits from medication, the dose should be reduced to 50 to 100 IU every other day. Because new generation bisphosphonates offer greater efficacy and are easier to use, calcitonin is now reserved for patients who cannot tolerate or have contraindications to bisphosphonate therapy.

Patients who develop osteoarthritis, fractures, or spinal stenosis may need to be treated with surgical intervention. However, surgery in these patients may be complicated by excessive blood loss, high-output cardiac failure, heterotopic bone formation, or loosening of the implant. Therefore, patients need careful attention during the pre- and postoperative period. It is recommended to give bisphosphonates before an elective surgery. The goal is to reduce hypervascularity associated with active disease, which will reduce the amount of blood loss and potential complication from left heart failure.

SUMMARY

Metabolic bone diseases are a group of disorders that occur as a result of changes in osteoblast and osteoclast function. The osteoblast and osteoclast play a major role to maintain structural and material properties of bone, control the synthesis of bone matrix, and regulate mineral metabolism as well as the mineralization process. Thus, an alteration of these cell functions results in a variety of clinical disorders. An understanding of the pathogenesis of such diseases and an attempt to define the cause of the patient's acute problem is the key for treatment. This requires a thorough medical history, physical examination, imaging studies, and appropriate laboratory investigations. Orthopaedic surgeons should be aware of these biologic and biochemical disorders and familiar with their clinical presentation. The ultimate success in treatment of the orthopedic manifestations of these disorders often necessitates direct correction of the underlying disease process.

RECOMMEND READINGS

Holick MF. Vitamin D deficiency. *N Engl J Med*. 2007;357(3):266–281.

Lin JT, Lane JM. Osteoporosis: a review. *Clin Orthop Relat Res*. 2004;(425):126–134.

Mankin HJ, Mankin CJ. Metabolic bone disease: an update. In: Ferlic DC, ed. *Instructional Course Lectures*. Rosemont, IL: American Academy of Orthopaedic Surgeons, 2003:769.

Reginato AJ, Coquia JA. Musculoskeletal manifestations of osteomalacia and rickets. *Best Pract Res Clin Rheumatol*. 2003;17(6):1063–1080.

Siris ES, Jacobs TP, Canfield RE. Paget's disease of bone. *Bull N Y Acad Med*. 1980;56(3):285–304.

Rheumatology and Immunology for the Non-Rheumatologist

7

Daniel J. Clauw *Jacob N. Ablin*

THE IMMUNE SYSTEM

Overview

The immune system serves many vital functions, including defense against foreign organisms and surveillance against tumors. But function, or dysfunction, of the immune system also plays a significant role in many rheumatic diseases. In some cases, the damage caused by the immune system is an inevitable consequence of killing invading microorganisms (e.g., polymorphonuclear [PMN] cells attacking bacteria in a septic joint). In other instances, hyperactivity of the immune system is the primary problem, as occurs in autoimmune disorders where "self" antigens are recognized as foreign, such as rheumatoid arthritis (RA) or systemic lupus erythematosus (SLE). In yet other settings, an initial injury can be followed by an inflammatory response that is responsible for continued symptoms (e.g., tendinitis or bursitis).

Thus, to understand the diagnosis and management of rheumatic disorders, it is crucial to understand the basic organization of the immune system. The focus of this review is to introduce the basic concepts of immunology and immunopathology as they relate to rheumatic disorders. As with any attempt to make an extremely complex system simple, important details are necessarily omitted, and the reader is encouraged to consult more detailed reviews of these subjects for this information.

The immune response can be divided into two broad categories: specific and nonspecific. The nonspecific immune response includes mucosal barriers of defense, some types of immune cells, and the alternative pathway of complement activation. The specific immune response involves a sophisticated afferent system to recognize self from non-self. After the immune system has distinguished self from non-self, there is a set of specific effector agents that acts to target and destroy external agents, hopefully with the least damage possible to host tissues. Defects in the function of this system lead to most of the classic autoimmune disorders.

Components of the Immune System

General Concepts

During fetal development, hematopoietic cells move from the yolk sac to the bone marrow and other tissues to begin differentiating into lymphoid and myeloid cell lines. Myeloid cells are widely distributed in many tissues, whereas lymphoid cell lines concentrate in hematopoietic organs such as the thymus, spleen, lymph nodes, and bone marrow. The development of lymphoid cells is particularly complex. Although all lymphoid cells are produced in the bone marrow, one type of cell line migrates to the thymus (the "T" cell) for further development. The thymus plays a crucial role, being particularly important for the development of the ability to recognize self from non-self (tolerance) by these cell lines. Mature T lymphocytes then direct the immune role of self-recognition and regulate both cell- and antibody-mediated (humoral) immunity.

During early development, cells that will eventually become B cells (a name derived from the involvement of a bursa in this process in birds) mature independent of the thymus. These cells develop cell surface markers such as surface immunoglobulins (Igs), and their major function is to produce antibodies.

An important concept for understanding the function of both T and B cells is the process of clonal expansion. In early development, the immune system has cells that could theoretically respond to virtually any possible antigen. The subsequent interaction of the individual with the environment will largely determine which of these cell lines are stimulated to expand and replicate (i.e., clonal expansion) and which are deleted (because they react with self-antigens). This latter concept that describes the loss of reactivity to self-antigens is termed *immune tolerance.*

Another basic distinction important for understanding the way in which the immune system functions in sickness and in health is that between the innate and the adaptive immune response. The innate immune response is a phylogenetically more ancient system designed primarily for combating infectious agents. This response is characterized by not being dependent on previous exposure to antigen to respond. These cells recognize fixed pathogen-associated molecular patterns. This rapid response mechanism is, however, limited in its ability to react to novel threats. The adaptive immune system, on the other hand, functions through selection and mutation of the immune cells to mount a highly targeted response to a previously encountered antigen.

Antigen-Presenting Cells

This class of cells has many roles both in the innate and the adaptive immune response. In the latter, the first step is the interaction between antigen and antigen-presenting cells (APCs). There are a number of cell types that are capable of acting as APCs, including B cells, tissue macrophages, and site-specific cells such as dendritic cells in the skin or Kupffer cells in the liver. In general, these cells first "process" antigen by internalizing protein and digesting the protein into peptides, and then "present" these peptides on the cell surface for recognition by another class of lymphocytes known as *T cells,* through an interaction with specific T cell receptors (TCRs).

T Cells

T cells (particularly the CD4+ subset of T cells, also called *helper T cells*) are responsible for the recognition of antigens on APC cells in a T-cell–dependent antibody response. When the immune system is functioning properly, T cells will respond to foreign antigens but not to self-antigens. This process occurs primarily in the thymus and involves the positive selection of clones of cells that respond to foreign antigens and the elimination of clones that respond to self-antigens. In addition, rapid cell death (apoptosis) of activated T cells must occur at the termination of the immune response to prevent undue accumulation of hazardous immune cells.

When a CD4+ T cell binds to an antigen on an APC, several processes occur. The T cell becomes "activated" and expresses a different set of cell surface receptors and subsequently produces a number of soluble molecules (cytokines) that can cause both local and distant effects on immune and nonimmune functions. A prominent function of these cytokines is to attract new macrophages to the tissue. These new macrophages that were not involved in the initial antigen presentation are more effective at phagocytosis and microorganism killing.

The other major class of T cells is the CD8+ (T suppressor) cell. T suppressor cells have quite different functions than their CD4+ counterparts, having no role in the humoral antibody process but instead being responsible for T-cell killing. This mechanism of direct cell killing is particularly important in defense against viruses and intracellular organisms. Cytotoxic T cells can kill infected cells by the excretion of perforin, a protein capable of drilling holes in the cell membrane, or by ligands that activate death receptors such as Fas or tumor necrosis factor-alpha (TNF-α) receptor. These cells have specificity for antigens associated with the major histocompatibility complex (MHC) class I products, the HLA-A, B, and C antigens, in contrast to the class II product specificity of CD4+ cells (Fig. 7.1).

In addition, the CD4+ and CD8+ cells play an essential role in regulating the overall function of the immune system. Immunoregulatory cytokines including interleukins (ILs) 2, 4, 5, 7, 9, 10, 11 and gamma interferon (IFN) are released by T-lymphocyte subsets and exert both positive and negative effects on the overall activity of the inflammatory response.

Within the classic autoimmune disorders, some are characterized by a relative excess of activity of CD4+ cells

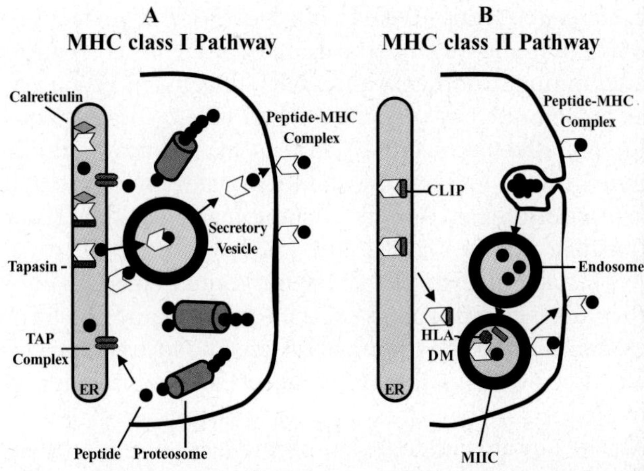

Figure 7.1 Antigen processing by mononuclear phagocytes. **(A)** Major histocompatibility complex (MHC) class I pathway. **(B)** MHC class II pathway. (*Reprinted with permission from* Koopman WJ, Moreland LW. *Arthritis and Allied Conditions: A Textbook of Rheumatology*. 15th ed. Philadelphia, PA: Lippincott Williams & Wilkins, 2005.)

(e.g., SLE, RA), whereas others (e.g., ankylosing spondylitis, reactive arthritis) are characterized by a relative CD8+ excess. This runs in parallel to our understanding of the immunogenetic risk factors for these types of disorders. For example, the seronegative spondyloarthropathies (SSs) (e.g., ankylosing spondylitis) are strongly associated with the presence of the HLA-B27 (or related haplotypes, e.g., B7, Bw22, B42) haplotypes, and CD8+ cells have specificity for these MHC I products. In contrast, the immunogenetic risk for developing disorders such as SLE or RA is conferred by certain MHC class II haplotypes (e.g., HLA DR4), again in parallel with the more prominent role of CD4+ cells in the pathogenesis of these disorders. This phenomenon of reciprocal roles of CD4 and CD8 cells also appears to be evident when persons with autoimmune disorders become infected with the human immunodeficiency virus (HIV). The lowering of the CD4+ count associated with this disease frequently leads to an improvement in CD4+–dependent disorders such as SE or RA but a marked worsening of CD8+–dependent disorders such as the SSs. Different types of antigens also elicit different types of immunologic responses. For example, some antigens, such as mycobacterium and fungi, elicit exclusively a cell-mediated response, whereas most pathogens elicit a mixed response.

B Cells

Once activated, the major function of the B cell is to produce antibodies. This activation can occur via a T-cell–dependent or a T-cell–independent mechanism. In the T-cell–dependent system, the CD4+ cell is activated via an interaction with a specific APC. Some antigens are capable of directly interacting with B cells, independent of T cells, and lead to a less-specific Ig response. A small proportion of B cells will develop into long-lived memory cells, retaining the information and the capacity to respond rapidly upon reexposure to a previously encountered antigen. After such reexposure, such cells can develop into plasma cells—large, terminally differentiated cells that have the capacity to specifically produce large amounts of antibody.

Immunoglobulins

Igs are the product of activated mature B cells. There are nine classes of Igs, each of which consists of two heavy chains and two light chains. For each type of Ig, there is a constant region that is largely responsible for the physiologic functions of the Ig molecule (e.g., complement activation) and a variable domain that is largely responsible for the antigen specificity of that particular Ig. Each of the subclasses of Ig serves different functions (Table 7.1).

Autoantibodies are Igs directed against self-antigens. The two most commonly considered autoantibodies are antinuclear antibodies (ANAs) and rheumatoid factor (RF). ANAs are antibodies directed against various components of the cell nucleus. These antibodies are a serological hallmark of autoimmune disease such as SLE, in which they are present in 99% to 100% of patients. Several factors need, however, to be considered before ordering this test. First, a substantial percentage of the general population (as high as 30%) will have a "positive" result for this assay using newer, more sensitive techniques. Because of the low specificity of this test, it should be ordered only when there is a high pretest probability that the person has a disease characterized by a positive ANA. If this test is found to be positive, then further testing for extractable nuclear antigens can be considered (e.g., anti-Ro [SSA], anti-La [SSB], anti-Sm, anti-RNP, anti-dsDNA) since these are much less commonly present as false-positive tests in normal individuals.

TABLE 7.1
SELECTED BIOLOGIC PROPERTIES OF CLASSES AND SUBCLASSES OF IMMUNOGLOBULINS

	IgG				IgA				
	1	2	3	4	1	2	IgM	IgD	IgE
Percentage of total (%)	65	20	10	5	90	10			
Complement fixation	++	+	++	−	−	−	++	−	−
Complement fixation (alternative)			+	+	+/−	+/−			
Placental passage	+	+	+	+	−	−	−	−	−
Fixing to mast cells or basophils	−	−	−	−	−	−	−	−	+
Binding to									
Macrophages	+	±	+	±	−	−	−	−	−
Neutrophils	+	+	+	+	+	+	−	−	−
Platelets	+	+	+	+	−	−	−	−	−
Lymphocytes	+	+	+	+	−	−	+	−	−
Reaction with *Staphylococcus A*	+	+	−	+	−	−	−	−	−
Half-life (days)	23	23	8–9	23	6	6	5	3	2.5
Synthesis mg/kg/day	25	?	3.5	?	24	?	7	0.4	0.02

+, Positive; ++, Highly positive; −, Negative; ±, Equevical.

RFs represent a heterogeneous group of antibodies directed against the Fc portion of IgG. As with ANA, this test should be ordered only in persons with a high pretest probability of RA, since while approximately 80% of persons with RA will have a positive value, RF will also be present in some normal individuals and in a proportion of patients with a variety of other disorders, including viral and bacterial infections, other rheumatic diseases, and lymphoproliferative diseases. Although the rate of false positive RF is lower for RF than for ANA, ordering this test in persons without evidence of synovitis or elevated inflammatory indices will lead to far more false positives than true positives.

Antibodies directed against cyclic citrullinated peptides (anti-CCPs) have been found in serum of many RA patients; a specificity rate as high as 98% has been reported for this antibody.

However, it is important to recognize that the serum levels of RF, anti-CCPs, and ANA *do not correlate with the level of disease activity*, so that once these tests are ordered and known to be positive, there is little value of following these values longitudinally in an individual patient.

PMN Leukocytes: Neutrophils

The cells most active in the initial stages of an inflammatory response are neutrophils. Neutrophils may be attracted to the site of inflammation by many factors, including proinflammatory cytokines (e.g., TNF-α, IL-1, IL-6, IL-8) released by mononuclear immune cells, immune complexes, and components of the complement cascade. Once present, a neutrophil will attempt to phagocytose individual particles or microorganisms by internalizing and then digesting the foreign material. Alternatively, in some settings, the neutrophils degranulate and release the contents of their lysosomal enzymes such as matrix metalloproteinases (MMPs), elastase, and lysozyme into the tissue environment, a process that can be responsible for extensive tissue damage. A related toxic effect of neutrophils, both to microorganisms and tissues involved in inflammation, is the release of oxygen free radicals. After activation, neutrophils rapidly undergo programmed cell death (apoptosis), which is critical for controlling the inflammatory response.

Eosinophils are a specialized class of PMN cells mainly found within tissue. These cells are mainly activated by IgA and IgE antibodies and play an important role in the body's defense against helminthic and parasitic infections, on the one hand, and in atopic and allergic reactions on the other hand.

Monocyte/Macrophages

Monocytes are circulating unstimulated macrophages. In addition to the previously described role of these cells as APCs, macrophages also play a vital role in control of the inflammatory response. It has been estimated that there are more than 100 products produced and released by macrophages, including cytokines, complement components, coagulation factors, and bioactive lipids such as cyclooxygenase and lipoxygenase products.

These cells are typically attracted to sites of inflammation through the activity of chemoattractant molecules (chemokines) and carry specific membrane receptors for these signals. Monocytes and macrophages also carry multiple receptors for components of the complement system. These cells appear to participate in many additional roles besides combating infectious agents. For example, scavenger macrophages participate in uptake of cholesterol particles combating development of atherosclerotic plaque while uptake and clearance of apoptotic cells in the circulation by macrophages is a homeostatic function, which prevents the development of autoimmune reactions to these dying cells.

Complement

The complement system consists of a series of proteins that are involved in mediating a variety of inflammatory effects. As with other components of the immune system, this system is vital in protecting the organisms against infection (particularly bacterial pathogens) but can be responsible for tissue damage in rheumatic disorders.

Three separate pathways of complement activation have been identified: the classical pathway, the alternative pathway, and the lectin pathway (LP) (Fig. 7.2). Although these

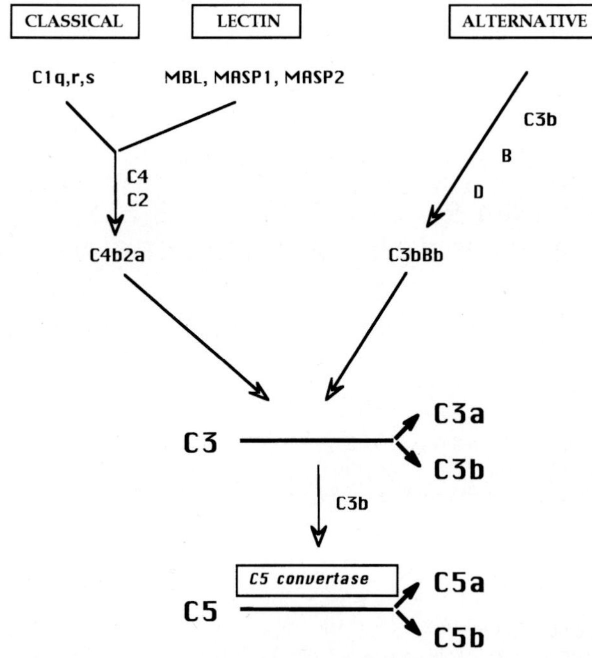

Figure 7.2 Complement activation pathways. (*Reprinted with permission from* Koopman WJ, Moreland LW. *Arthritis and Allied Conditions: A Textbook of Rheumatology.* 15th ed. Philadelphia, PA: Lippincott Williams & Wilkins, 2005.)

pathways are activated in different manners, the terminal event in all sequences is the cleavage of C3 to C3a and C3b. Activation of the complement system is closely regulated by inhibitory enzymes such as C1 inhibitor, which act to prevent excessive and dangerous activation of the complement cascade. A number of components of the complement cascade are responsible for the biological consequences of activation. C3a and several other products of the classical complement cascade act as anaphylatoxins. These substances lead to mast cell and basophil degranulation, releasing a variety of mediators responsible for smooth muscle contraction, local edema, and increased vascular permeability. C3b begins a series of steps leading to the formation of membrane attack complex (MAC) that is capable of leading to damage or death of a number of different cell types via insertion into the cell membrane. In addition to being a major part of the innate immune response, the complement system also participates in adaptive (humoral) immunity. Thus, IgM and IgG activate complement, leading to opsonization and lysis of cells. Complement also plays an important role in apoptotic cells uptake and clearance.

Homozygous deficiencies of complement may lead either to an increased incidence of infection (especially of organisms such as *Neisseria* that are killed by MAC) or to autoimmune disorders. The paradoxical development of autoimmune disorders in individuals with hereditary complement deficiencies has been perplexing since many autoimmune diseases are characterized by complement consumption. The best supported theory for this phenomenon is that complement is vital for normal clearance of immune complexes in the circulation and that these deficiency states are characterized by ineffective immune complex clearance and subsequent complement activation. Patients deficient in specific components of the complement classical pathway may suffer from an extremely high prevalence of SLE (up to 90% in C1q deficiency).

Complement measurements can sometimes be useful in assessing an individual for the presence of, or activity of, an autoimmune disorder. The CH50 is an assay of total hemolytic complement activity and is a useful screening test if a homozygous complement deficiency is suspected. Assays for individual complement levels (C3 and C4 are the most available commercially) can sometimes be helpful to assess for activity of autoimmune disorders characterized by complement consumption (e.g., immune complex-mediated disorders such as SLE, RA, cryoglobulinemia). However, in many instances, these values are difficult to interpret since complement is produced in increased quantities by the liver as an acute phase reactant. Thus, in many autoimmune disorders characterized by complement consumption, a normal plasma value can still occur because of increased liver synthesis. Measurement of complement activation fragments (such as C3a and C5a) may be more specific, not being influenced by inherited deficiencies. However, these tests are more costly and less frequently available in clinical use.

Immunoregulation and Immunopathology

Immunoregulation involves a tenuous balance of reacting to pathogens without harming the host. There are several levels of immunoregulation, beginning in early development with establishment of tolerance. Once the organism can appropriately identify self-antigens, the response to these challenges must be appropriate to the potential danger of the challenge. An inflammatory response that is not localized to the area of infection, or that persists after the infection has been cleared, will cause undue damage to the organism.

Classically, four types of specific immunopathologic mechanisms have been identified:

Type I

IgE Mediated

The combination of an IgE antibody binding to the Fc receptor of a basophil or mast cell and an antigen binding to that antibody leads to stimulation of these cells. Products contained in basophilic granules include histamine, serotonin, bradykinins, and other substances. This type of reaction is most prominent in allergic diseases.

Type II

Direct Antibody-Mediated Effects on Cells

Autoantibodies binding to self-antigens on a cell or tissue can cause complement fixation and/or direct cytotoxic killing of that particular cell. An example occurs in some types of hemolytic anemia, where red blood cells (RBCs) are destroyed when autoantibodies bind to cell surface antigens. This type of reaction is relatively uncommon.

Type III

Immune Complex Formation

In contrast to type II reactions, where antibody binds to antigens on a cell or tissue surfaces, in this instance, soluble antigens bind to antibodies in the circulation. These immune complexes may bind to cell surface receptors or activate complement and cause an inflammatory process in the tissue(s) where they are deposited. Many classic systemic autoimmune disorders, such as SLE, are characterized by the presence of circulating and tissue immune complexes. However, it remains unclear how much of the disease process is actually caused by these immune complexes.

Type IV

Direct Cell Injury

Several types of immune cells, including both T cells and CD8+ cells, can cause direct cell injury, whereas other types of cells such as CD4+ cells can affect cell injury by attracting other types of cells. This mechanism is probably operative in a number of autoimmune and other rheumatic disorders.

EVALUATION OF THE PATIENT WITH ARTHRITIS

History

The important elements of the history in the patient with suspected arthritis are the same as for other orthopaedic problems, although there is more of an emphasis on certain features. These include elucidating the pattern and timing of joint involvement, differentiating inflammatory from noninflammatory processes, and determining whether extraarticular symptoms are present or absent.

The pattern of involvement can be particularly helpful when evaluating the patient with arthritis. Examples of such patterns are whether the arthritis is monoarticular or polyarticular (Tables 7.2 and 7.3). Although this distinction is rarely absolute, as with any clinical pearl, it can be helpful.

Another critical point in the evaluation of the patient with joint pain is how the symptoms began. Extremely rapid onset of symptoms (e.g., over seconds), especially if accompanied by trauma, suggests a mechanical process (e.g., fracture, loose body). Acute onset of symptoms over hours or days may occur in a number of types of arthritis and is especially common in inflammatory arthropathies (e.g., infectious, crystal-induced). The onset of symptoms is less helpful if the process is chronic or evolves over days to weeks, since this can occur with many different forms of arthritis.

Both the history and physical examination are helpful in differentiating whether the patient is suffering from an inflammatory or noninflammatory arthritis. Elements of the history that suggest an inflammatory process include prominent morning stiffness; improvement with exercise or activity (or worsening by prolonged immobility); or a history of warmth, redness, or swelling of the affected region(s). Pain that is worse after exercise or activity, on the other hand, is suggestive of a noninflammatory arthritis.

The presence or absence of nonarticular features can also be helpful in diagnosing the patient with arthritis. Nonarticular features are commonly seen in a number of conditions, especially systemic autoimmune disorders, where the joint is but one tissue that is being targeted by the inflammatory process.

Although the patient who presents with the complaint of joint pain may indeed have a process localized to the joint, it is equally important to recognize the plethora of periarticular or nonarticular syndromes that frequently may present in this manner, such as fibromyalgia, tendinitis, bursitis.

TABLE 7.2

DIFFERENTIAL DIAGNOSIS OF INFLAMMATORY MONOARTHRITIS

A. Crystal-induced

1. Gout—male, lower extremity, previous attack, nocturnal onset, precipitated by medical illness or surgical procedures, response to colchicine, hyperuricemia, sodium urate crystals in joint fluid with neutrophils predominating, and WBC count 10,000–60,000/mm^3
2. Pseudogout—elderly patient, knee or other large joint, previous attack, precipitated by medical illness or surgical procedure, flexion contractures, chondrocalcinosis on radiography, calcium pyrophosphate dihydrate crystals in joint fluid with neutrophils predominating, and WBC count 5,000–60,000/mm^3
3. Calcific tendinitis, bursitis, or periarthritis—extraarticular, tendon or capsule of larger joints, previous attack in same or other area, calcification on radiography, chalky or milky material aspirated from area, neutrophils with phagocytosed ovoid bodies microscopically

B. Palindromic rheumatism

Middle-aged or elderly male, sudden onset, little systemic reaction, previous attacks, may be positive rheumatoid factor, little or no residual chronic joint inflammation, residual olecranon bursal enlargement, joint fluid rarely obtained, fibrin deposition on biopsy

C. Infectious arthritis

1. Septic—severe inflammation, primary septic focus, drug or alcohol abuse, joint fluid with neutrophils predominating, WBC count 50,000–300,000/mm^3 (pus), infectious agents identified on smear and culture, or bacterial antigens identified in joint fluid
2. Tubercular—primary focus elsewhere, drug or alcohol abuse, marked joint swelling for long period, joint fluid with neutrophils predominating, acid-fast organisms on smear and culture
3. Fungal—similar to tuberculosis
4. Viral—antecedent or concomitant systemic viral illness, joint fluid can be of inflammatory or noninflammatory type, either mononuclear cells or neutrophils may predominate

D. Other

1. Tendinitis—as in A.3, but without radiologic calcification, antecedent trauma including repetitive motion
2. Bursitis—as mentioned earlier, but inflamed area is more diffuse, antecedent trauma
3. Juvenile rheumatoid arthritis—one or both knees swollen in preteen or teenager without systemic reaction, no erosions, mildly inflammatory joint fluid with some neutrophils, and no depression in synovial fluid $C'H_{50}$ levels.

WBC, white blood cell.

(*Reprinted with permission from* Koopman WJ, Moreland LW. *Arthritis and Allied Conditions: A Textbook of Rheumatology*. 15th ed. Philadelphia, PA: Lippincott Williams & Wilkins, 2005.)

TABLE 7.3
DIFFERENTIAL DIAGNOSIS OF INFLAMMATORY POLYARTHRITIS

A. RA

1. Seropositive—female patient, symmetric joint and tendon involvement, synovial thickening, joint inflammation "in phase," nodules, weakness, systemic reaction, erosions on radiogram, rheumatoid factor present, $C'H_{50}$ level depressed in joint fluid that has 5,000–30,000 WBC/mm^3 and approximately 50%–80% neutrophils, possible occurrence in children
2. Seronegative—either sex, symmetric joint and tendon involvement, joint inflammation "in phase," more bony reaction radiographically (sclerosis, osteophytes, fusion, periostitis), rheumatoid factor absent, $C'H_{50}$ not depressed in joint fluid that has 3,000–20,000 WBC/mm^3 and approximately 20%–60% neutrophils, more asymmetric than in seropositive cases, some cases probably are adult juvenile RA

B. Collagen vascular disease

1. Systemic lupus erythematosus—female patient, symmetric joint distribution identical to RA, hair loss, mucosal lesions, rash, systemic reaction, visceral organ or brain involvement, leukopenia, positive STS, no erosions radiographically, noninflammatory joint fluid with good viscosity and mucin clot and 1,000–2,000 WBC/mm^3, mostly small lymphocytes, serum $C'H_{50}$ often depressed, ANA titer elevated, antinative human DNA antibody titer increased, anti-SM antibody increased, anti-SSA (Ro) subset (subacute cutaneous lupus)
2. Scleroderma—tight skin; Raynaud phenomenon; resorption of digits; dysphagia; constipation; lung, heart, or kidney involvement; symmetric tendon contractures; little or no synovial thickening; radiographic calcinosis circumscripta; positive ANA with speckled or nucleolar pattern; anti-SCL-70 (systemic); and anticentromere antibodies (CREST syndrome)
3. Polymyositis (dermatomyositis)—proximal muscle weakness in pelvic and pectoral girdles, tender muscles, rash, typical nailbed and knuckle pad erythema, symmetric joint involvement, EMG showing combined myopathic and denervation pattern, muscle biopsy abnormal, elevated serum creatinine phosphokinase level
4. Mixed connective tissue disease—swollen hands, Raynaud phenomenon, tight skin, symmetric joint and tendon involvement, possible evidence of joint erosions radiographically, positive ANA speckled pattern, anti-RNP antibody increased, strong response to corticosteroid therapy in anti-inflammatory doses
5. Polyarteritis nodosa—symmetric involvement, diverse clinical picture of systemic disease, histologic or angiographic diagnosis

C. Rheumatic fever

Young (2–40 years of age), sore throat, group A streptococci, migratory arthritis, rash, pancarditis or pericardial involvement, elevated ASO titers, joint inflammation responds dramatically to aspirin treatment, often no cardiac findings in adults

D. Juvenile RA

Symmetric joint involvement, rash, fever, absence or rheumatoid factor, radiographic periostitis, erosions late, possibly beginning or recurring in an adult, ANA-positive pauciarticular girls may develop iridocyclitis, B27-positive boys with possible fusion of sacroiliac and spinal joints

E. Psoriatic arthritis

Asymmetric boggy joint and tendon swelling, skin or nail lesions not always prominent or may follow arthritis, DIP joints may be prominently involved, radiologic periostitis or erosions, no rheumatoid factor, $C'H_{50}$ level usually not depressed in inflammatory joint fluid with neutrophilic predominance

F. Reactive arthritis

Male patient, homosexual and/or sexually promiscuous, urethritis, iritis, conjunctivitis, asymmetric joints, lower extremity, nonpainful mucous membrane ulcerative lesion, balanitis circinata, keratoderma blennorrhagica, weight loss, $C'H_{50}$ increased in serum and in joint fluid with 5,000–30,000 WBC/mm^3, macrophages in joint fluid with three to five phagocytosed neutrophils ("Reiter" cell), possible sequela of enteric infections or urethritis, syndrome may be incomplete and may affect females

G. Gonorrheal arthritis

Migratory arthritis or tenosynovitis finally settling in one or more joints or tendons, either sex, primary focus urethra, female genitourinary tract, rectum, or oropharynx, skin lesions, vesicles, gram-negative diplococci on smear but not on culture of vesicular fluid, positive culture at primary site, blood, or joint fluid

H. Polymyalgia rheumatica

Elderly patient (>50 years), symmetric pelvic or pectoral girdle complaints without loss of strength, morning stiffness of long duration, prominent fatigue, weight loss, possible joint involvement, especially of shoulders, sternoclavicular joint, knees, sedimentation rate elevated, fibrinogen and [- and T-globulin elevation, anemia, complete response to low doses (10–20 mg) prednisone, serum CPK level normal, elevated alkaline phosphatase (liver) level

I. Crystal-induced

1. MSU crystals (gout)—symmetric arthritis, flexion contractures, history of acute attacks, tophi, out-of-phase joint inflammation, systemic corticosteroid treatment for RA, hyperuricemia, MSU crystals in joint fluid
2. CPPD crystals (pseudogout)—symmetric arthritis, MCP flexion contractures, as well as of wrist, elbow, shoulder, hip, knees, and ankles, prior acute attacks (sometimes), out-of-phase joint inflammation, CPPD crystals in joint fluid
3. BCP crystals (Milwaukee shoulder)

J. Other amyloid arthropathy, peripheral arthritis of inflammatory bowel disease, tuberculosis, SBE, viral or spirochetal arthritis

ANA, antinuclear antibody; ASO, antistreptolysin O; BCP, basic calcium phosphate; CPK, creatinine phosphokinase; CPPD, calcium pyrophosphate dihydrate disease; CREST syndrome, calcinosis, Raynaud phenomenon, esophageal involvement, sclerodactyly, and telangiectasia; DIP, dorsal interphalangeal; EMG, electromyography; MCP, metacarpophalangeal; MSU, monosodium urate; RA, rheumatoid arthritis; RNP, ribonucleoprotein; SBE, subacute bacterial endocarditis; STS, serologic tests for syphilis; WBC, white blood cell.

(*Reprinted with permission from* Koopman WJ, Moreland LW. *Arthritis and Allied Conditions: A Textbook of Rheumatology.* 15th ed. Philadelphia, PA: Lippincott Williams & Wilkins, 2005.)

Physical Examination

Both a general physical examination and a musculoskeletal examination are important in the patient who presents with arthritis. As noted earlier, there are a plethora of nonarticular features that can accompany arthritis.

In the musculoskeletal examination, the goal of the evaluation is to (1) determine the extent of involvement, (2) localize the anatomic structure(s) involved, and (3) determine whether the process is inflammatory or noninflammatory. To determine the extent of involvement, it is important to perform a generalized examination of the joints and soft tissues, even if the patient presents with a localized complaint. The patient with a systemic inflammatory process will very frequently present with the complaint of pain in a single joint. Limiting the focus to that joint will lead to an improper diagnosis and ineffective treatment.

The best manner to localize the anatomic structure(s) involved is to perform the musculoskeletal examination by palpating with firm pressure (enough to blanch the examiner's fingernail) over both joints and soft tissues, first in regions of the body where the person is not complaining of pain and finally in the affected region. This type of examination accomplishes several objectives. One is to assess the patients' overall pain threshold. If individuals have tenderness over bones and soft tissues in a number of regions in the body, they may suffer from a generalized disturbance in pain processing (e.g., fibromyalgia) rather than a process localized to a specific region. This type of examination also will detect whether periarticular structures (e.g., tendon insertions, bursae) are involved. Second, this procedure identifies individuals who may have more than one process that is coexpressed and responsible for symptoms (e.g., the patient with osteoarthritis [OA] of the hip or knee and concurrent trochanteric or anserine bursitis involving those same regions, respectively).

Using the above-mentioned technique, special attention is paid to the joints, and in particular, examining the joint for evidence of synovitis. To the unskilled examiner, an enlarged joint represents "arthritis." But with experience, palpation of enlarged joints can differentiate the firm and less painful bony proliferation secondary to osteophytes (as occurs with Heberden and Bouchard nodes in the distal interphalangeal [DIP] and proximal interphalangeal [PIP] joints of the hands in OA) from the tender, "boggy" swelling seen in chronic inflammatory arthritis due to synovial proliferation and/or joint effusions.

Diagnostic Testing

Again, the evaluation of the patient with arthritis parallels that of the patient with other orthopaedic problems, although certain points bear emphasis. Perhaps, the most important point to emphasize is that the history and physical examination typically yield far more useful information than do laboratory studies. This can be stated in two different ways: (1) if you do not have a good idea of the correct diagnosis before ordering the laboratory tests, it is unlikely that such testing will be helpful and (2) it is rarely appropriate to perform an extensive laboratory evaluation when a person initially presents with a joint pain.

There are several reasons for the strong note of caution regarding diagnostic testing in patients who present with joint pain. Unfortunately, there are virtually no diagnostic tests that can be ordered in this setting that function well as screening tests; most of the laboratory studies done in the evaluation of persons with joint pain have a relatively low positive or negative predictive value unless they are ordered in the appropriate setting. Luckily, in most rheumatic disorders, it is not necessary to make a definitive diagnosis before initiating treatment. This combination of poor diagnostic utility of frequently ordered tests, and the fact that treatments can be initiated before diagnoses are established, is somewhat unusual when compared with other fields of medicine.

A suggested diagnostic approach to patients with joint pain is to first consider whether patients may have an infection or malignancy causing their symptoms. It is important to recognize that it is unusual for persons who are not immunocompromised (e.g., HIV infection, malignancy) or without some recent surgical event or trauma to a joint to develop septic arthritis. The exceptions to this are disseminated gonococcal infection, Lyme disease, and tuberculous arthritis, which can occur in persons with intact immune systems and no other risk factors. If a septic joint is suspected, then the study of choice is to perform an arthrocentesis and synovial fluid analysis. If a malignancy is suggested, for example, because of weight loss or other systemic symptoms, then imaging studies of the involved region should be performed immediately, followed by a biopsy in most settings.

Once those individuals with infection and malignancy have been identified, the next consideration is whether they may have a life-threatening (or organ-threatening) autoimmune disorder. These individuals will rarely present with nonspecific symptoms and mild impairment but instead will appear and feel very ill. In this setting, the workup should be guided by the presenting symptoms, with particular attention to detecting organ involvement (e.g., cardiopulmonary, central nervous system [CNS], renal) that may require specific and aggressive intervention. This is also the setting where extensive diagnostic testing for the presence of autoantibodies, complement, and other studies (e.g., antineutrophil cytoplasmic antibodies for systemic vasculidities) is likely to be helpful in rapidly establishing a diagnosis and initiating aggressive treatment.

If the history and physical examination suggest that a person may suffer from a systemic autoimmune disorder, then a general set of screening laboratory studies can be helpful. A reasonable choice would include a complete blood cell (CBC) count, renal and hepatic studies, urinalysis, and screen for acute phase reactants. The most

TABLE 7.4
USE OF GROSS ANALYSIS, MUCIN CLOT TEST, AND TOTAL AND DIFFERENTIAL LEUKOCYTE COUNTS IN THE CLASSIFICATION OF SYNOVIAL FLUIDS

Criteria	Normal	Noninflammatory (Group I)	Inflammatory (Group II)	Purulent (Group III)
Volume (mL) (knee)	<4	Often >4	Often >4	Often >4
Color	Clear to pale yellow	Xanthochromic	Xanthochromic to white	White
Clarity	Transparent	Transparent	Translucent to opaque	Opaque
Viscosity	Very high	High	Low	Very low
Mucin clot[a]	Good	Fair to good	Fair to poor	Poor
Spontaneous clot	None	Often	Often	Often
Leukocytes per mm^3	<50	<3,000	3,000–50,000	50,000–300,000
Polymorphonuclear leukocytes (%)	<25	<25	>70	>90

[a]A bedside test for indicating viscosity of synovial fluid – the more viscous and "stringy" the fluid is when it is dripped the more normal.
(*Reprinted with permission from* Koopman WJ, Moreland LW. *Arthritis and Allied Conditions: A Textbook of Rheumatology.* 15th ed. Philadelphia, PA: Lippincott Williams & Wilkins, 2005.)

commonly ordered tests that assess acute phase reactants are the erythrocyte sedimentation rate (ESR) and the C-reactive protein (CRP). As noted previously, tests for ANA and RF, and for other autoantibodies, should generally be reserved for persons with objective features suggesting autoimmune disorders or in whom this initial screening indicates abnormalities. The ESR is a nonspecific measure of inflammation that is inexpensive and easy to measure, but the results of this test must be interpreted with caution. The rate at which RBCs sediment in anticoagulated blood depends on many factors but in most settings is closely related to the plasma concentration of acute phase proteins, with fibrinogen being the most important. Although a Westergren sedimentation rate of greater than 20 mm/h is generally considered to be abnormal, there are many factors, such as normal aging, that may cause mild elevations in this value. Other noninflammatory factors that can influence the ESR including anemia (elevated), polycythemia (decreased), pregnancy (elevated), drugs (heparin and valproic acid level elevated), or changes in shape of RBC (decreased). Very high the ESRs (e.g., more than 100 mm/h) are typically seen only in inflammatory disorders, infection, and malignancy.

The CRP is a single plasma protein that is produced in the liver in response to various types of tissue injury. The advantage of measuring this protein instead of the ESR is that there are fewer noninflammatory stimuli that cause an elevation of the CRP, and this value will rise and fall more rapidly in response to inflammatory stimuli. The normal CRP value is less than 1 mg/dL. Values between 1 and 10 mg/dL are seen in a variety of inflammatory states, whereas values above 10 mg/dL are usually (but not always) indicative of infection.

Synovial Fluid Analysis

The aspiration of an involved joint and analysis of extracted synovial fluid can be particularly helpful in assessing the person with arthritis. In addition to a CBC count and a differential count, the appearance and viscosity of the fluid should be assessed, and the protein and glucose concentration in the fluid should be determined. Gram staining and culture are useful for the diagnosis of septic arthritis, whereas examining the fluid under a polarizing microscope allows detection of crystals responsible for crystal-induced arthropathy, for example, gout and pseudogout. Tables 7.4 and 7.5 indicate how this information can be used, together with the history, physical examination, and other diagnostic tests, in assessing the patient with arthritis.

RHEUMATOLOGIC DISORDERS

A brief overview of a number of rheumatic disorders that may present with orthopaedic problems is given in the following section. Space constraints severely limit both the breadth and depth of this section, and the reader should refer to several excellent rheumatology textbooks for a more extensive overview of these and other rheumatologic disorders.

Rheumatoid Arthritis

RA is the most common form of chronic, systemic inflammatory arthritis. It is estimated that 1% to 2% of the population worldwide suffers from this disorder. Population-based studies may overestimate the prevalence of "true" RAs, as many people identified in such studies may have self-limited forms of inflammatory arthritis (e.g., postviral arthritis) or do not have inflammatory arthritis at all. Nonetheless, this is likely the most common autoimmune rheumatic disease. As with most autoimmune disorders, women are affected more commonly than men, with a ratio of approximately 2.5 to 1. RA can strike at any age, from the youth to the elderly. As with most autoimmune disorders,

TABLE 7.5
EXAMPLES OF RHEUMATIC CONDITIONS PRODUCING DIFFERENT TYPES OF SYNOVIAL FLUID

Noninflammatory (Group I)	Inflammatory[a] (Group II)	Purulent[a] (Group III)	Hemorrhagic (Group IV)
Osteoarthritis	Rheumatoid arthritis	Bacterial infections	Trauma, especially fracture
Early rheumatoid arthritis	Reactive arthritis	Tuberculosis	Neuroarthropathy (Charcot joint)
Trauma	Crystal synovitis, acute (gout, pseudogout, other)	Pseudosepsis	Blood dyscrasia (e.g., hemophilia)
Osteochondritis dissecans	Psoriatic arthritis		Tumor, especially villonodular synovitis or hemangioma
Osteonecrosis pigmented	Arthritis of inflammatory bowel disease		Chondrocalcinosis
Osteochondromatosis	Viral arthritis		Anticoagulant therapy
Crystal synovitis; chronic or subsiding acute (gout and pseudogout)	Rheumatic fever		Joint prostheses
Systemic lupus erythematosus[b]	Behçet disease		Thrombocytosis
Polyarteritis nodosa[b]	Fat droplet synovitis		Sickle cell trait or disease
Scleroderma disease	Some bacterial infections, e.g., coagulase-negative *Staphylococcus, Neisseria, Borrelia, Moraxella*		Myeloproliferative
Amyloidosis (articular)			Milwaukee shoulder syndrome
Polymyalgia rheumatica			
High-dose corticosteroid therapy			

(*Reprinted with permission from* Koopman WJ, Moreland LW. *Arthritis and Allied Conditions: A Textbook of Rheumatology.* 15th ed. Philadelphia, PA: Lippincott Williams & Wilkins, 2005.)

the cause of RA is unknown. Genetic risk factors play some role, in that monozygotic twins show an 11-fold risk over dizygotic twins, and the majority of individuals who develop this disorder have the HLA DR4 and/or DR1 epitope.

Specific "susceptibility cassettes," or shared epitopes on the β chains of DR, such as DRB*0401, DRB*0404, DRB*0101, and DRB*1402, carry the greatest association with RA. But genetic factors play a relatively small overall role, since even individuals with a positive family history of RA and one of the putative HLA epitopes have a low *absolute* risk of developing this disorder. It has long been suspected that the combination of these genetic immune risk factors and subsequent exposure to infectious agents lead to the development of disease. However, no infectious agents have currently been clearly identified as being causal in RA.

The hallmark of RA is the presence of a chronic polyarticular, inflammatory arthritis. This can begin either abruptly or more indolently and can begin in small or large joints. The presence of inflammatory arthritis can be documented by the finding of synovitis on examination, the finding of inflammatory (white blood cell [WBC] count $>$2,000 cells/mm^3) synovial fluid, or the radiographic appearance of characteristic erosions (not present until later in the course of the illness). If the diagnosis of RA is made primarily on the basis of the physical examination, then it must be clear that synovial proliferation is present there, not just tenderness over the joint.

The 1987 revised American Rheumatism Association criteria for the classification of RA include some of the most important clinical features of this disorder (Table 7.6). Although prolonged morning stiffness occurs in nearly all cases of RA, this is observed in a number of other inflammatory and noninflammatory disorders and is not specific for this diagnosis. Three of the criteria are related to the fact that RA usually involves the small joints of the hand and typically is relatively equally distributed on both sides of the body (i.e., symmetric). The joints initially and ultimately involved in RA are listed in Figure 7.3.

In patients with polyarticular inflammatory arthritis, laboratory and radiographic testing can be helpful to make a specific diagnosis. RF is found in approximately 80% of persons with RA. The presence of RF is helpful because it makes it much more likely that RA is the most likely diagnosis, and RA patients who are RF positive are more likely to have severe disease as well as extraarticular features such as rheumatoid nodules, interstitial lung disease, and Felty syndrome. But once RF is found to be positive, there is no reason to order the test sequentially, because the titer does not correlate with disease activity. Anti-CCPs may be positive earlier than RF in the course of the disease or may be the only positive serological finding in patients who remain RF negative. These antibodies appear to be more specific than RF and also predict an erosive course of RA.

Another test that is helpful in this setting is testing for the IgM titer for parvovirus infection (especially if patients have been exposed to ill children), since an acute parvovirus infection in adults can cause an inflammatory arthritis that resembles RA but remits in several months. In areas that are endemic for Lyme disease, Lyme titers may be a helpful test, especially in those with a history of a tick bite or rash or those with mono- or oligoarticular large joint involvement.

Early in RA, radiographs are not likely to show the characteristic erosions seen late in the disease. The most common radiographic finding in early RA is a normal radiograph, with soft tissue swelling. Periarticular osteopenia is

TABLE 7.6

1987 AMERICAN COLLEGE OF RHEUMATOLOGY REVISED CRITERIA FOR THE CLASSIFICATION OF RHEUMATOID ARTHRITIS (TRADITIONAL FORMAT)[a]

Criterion	Definition
Morning stiffness	Morning stiffness in and around the joints, lasting at least 1 hour before maximal improvement
Arthritis of three or more joints	At least three joint areas simultaneously with soft tissue swelling or joint fluid observed by a joint areas physician; the 14 possible areas are (right or left): PIP, MCP, wrist, elbow, knee, ankle, and MTP joints
Arthritis of hand joints	At least one area swollen in a wrist, MCP, or PIP joint
Symmetric arthritis	Simultaneous involvement of the same joint areas on both sides of the body (bilateral involvement of PIP, MCP, or MTP acceptable without perfect symmetry)
Rheumatoid nodules	Subcutaneous nodules over bony prominences or extensor surfaces, or in juxtaarticular regions, observed by a physician
Serum rheumatoid factor	Abnormal amount of serum rheumatoid factor by any method for which the result has been positive in <5% of control subjects
Radiographic changes	Erosions or unequivocal bony decalcification localized in or most marked adjacent to the involved joints (osteoarthritis changes excluded), typical of rheumatoid arthritis on posteroanterior hand and wrist radiographs

MCP, metacarpophalangeal; MTP, metatarsophalangeal; PIP, proximal interphalangeal.
[a]For classification purposes, a patient is said to have rheumatoid arthritis if four of seven criteria are satisfied. Criteria 1 to 4 must have been present for at least 6 weeks. Patients with two clinical diagnoses are not excluded.
(*From* Arnett FC, Edworth SM, Bloch DA, et al. The American Rheumatism Association 1987 revised criteria for the classification of rheumatoid arthritis. *Arthritis Rheum.* 1988;31:315–324, with permission.)

the next most common finding. The involvement of certain joints by RA bears special mention. Cervical spine involvement is relatively common and is the source of significant morbidity and mortality. The most serious involvement involves C1 (particularly the transverse ligament) and C2 (especially the odontoid process), leading to C1–C2 instability. This should be considered in patients with established RA who present with neck pain and/or myelopathic symptoms or findings. Patients with longstanding RA who are undergoing surgery that involves intubation should be screened for this complication. These patients should have flexion–extension radiographs of the cervical spine taken, and those with a preodontoid space of greater than 5 mm, an inadequate space available for the cord, or instability should be considered for surgical intervention.

Hand involvement is very common in RA. Although the DIP joints are rarely involved in this disorder, nearly all other hand joints are commonly involved. The

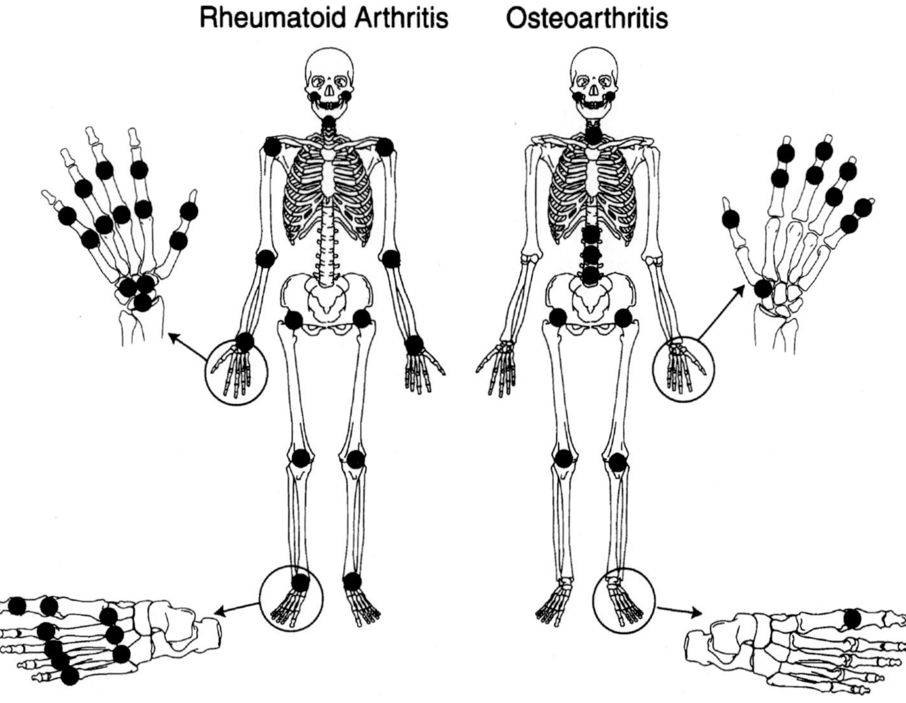

Figure 7.3 The joint distribution of the two most common forms of arthritis—rheumatoid arthritis (RA) and osteoarthritis (OA)—are compared and contrasted. Joints involved in these arthritides are noted by the black circles over involved joint areas. (*Reprinted with permission from* Koopman WJ, Moreland LW. *Arthritis and Allied Conditions: A Textbook of Rheumatology.* 15th ed. Philadelphia, PA: Lippincott Williams & Wilkins, 2005.)

characteristic deformities seen in the digits (e.g., swan-neck deformity, boutonniere deformity, and ulnar deviation at the metacarpophalangeal [MCP] joints) are due to a combination of joint destruction and laxity of ligaments and tendons. Tenosynovitis commonly can lead to clinical symptoms in RA, especially "trigger fingers" when the flexor tendons of the digits are involved.

Extraarticular manifestations of RA are also common, especially in persons with a positive serum RF. Rheumatoid nodules most commonly occur on the extensor surfaces of the arm in the olecranon region but can occur nearly anywhere in the body, particularly on other extensor surfaces. The formation of nodules can become accelerated in persons with RA given methotrexate.

There are a variety of forms of pulmonary disease in RA. As with many cardiopulmonary manifestations in patients with autoimmune disorders, this occurs in nearly all RA patients in autopsy series but is less commonly clinically apparent. Interstitial fibrosis preferentially involving the basilar regions is most commonly seen. Pleural involvement, nodules in the lung (especially fulminant in coal miners and termed Caplan syndrome), and bronchiolitis obliterans are also seen.

Cardiac involvement, which may include pericarditis, myocarditis, and cardiac conduction defects (perhaps due to rheumatoid nodules involving the conduction system), can be seen in RA. Vasculitis may also occur in persons with RA, and in this setting, it is termed *rheumatoid vasculitis*. This can involve both small- and medium-sized vessels of the skin, peripheral nerves, and visceral organs. Felty syndrome is the combination of RA, splenomegaly, ischemic leg ulcers, and neutropenia. These persons also commonly exhibit lymphadenopathy and thrombocytopenia, and sometimes splenectomy is necessary for effective treatment.

The natural history of RA has become better understood recently and has led to consideration of different treatment paradigms. It has become increasingly clear that much of the joint damage in RA occurs in the first several years of the illness. Thus, old "pyramid" treatment strategies that slowly added one drug at a time have been replaced by more aggressive paradigms. Also, in the past, RA had been considered an indolent, debilitating disorder characterized by a slow progressive course, with eventual remission in some patients. It is now clear that patients with RA have significantly increased mortality and die 10 to 15 years earlier than expected. This excess mortality appears to be multifactorial, including an increased risk of infections, cardiovascular disease, and pulmonary and gastrointestinal (GI) complications.

There is no unanimity on exactly how to treat RA, but nearly all persons without a contraindication to taking nonsteroidal anti-inflammatory drugs (NSAIDs) will benefit from taking this class of medication. It is unusual for RA to be controlled with this agent alone, and in milder disease, a logical step is to add hydroxychloroquine (200 mg twice daily). The principal concern with this agent is retinal toxicity. Hence, twice-yearly ophthalmologic examinations are typically recommended. For patients with more aggressive disease or those who fail hydroxychloroquine, weekly methotrexate is a logical next choice. This medication is typically given orally once weekly, beginning at 7.5 mg per week and escalating as high as 20 mg or more per week. Folic acid is typically coadministered at 100 mg/d to help avoid GI toxicity. Short-term side effects of this medication include diarrhea, nausea, fatigue, and stomatitis, whereas the more serious toxicities are liver disease and hypersensitivity pneumonitis. Leflunomide, which acts as an antipyrimidine agent, is of similar effectivity (and toxicity). When and where to use corticosteroids in the chronic treatment of RA remains controversial, with some data suggesting that long-term, low-dose (e.g., <10 mg/d of prednisone) is both helpful and relatively free of side effects.

The treatment of RA has been revolutionized over the last decade due to the introduction of biologic anticytokine medications into common clinical use. Three medications that act by neutralizing the activity of TNF-α have been introduced (infliximab, etanercept, and adalimumab). These agents, which are administered by the intravenous or subcutaneous route, have proven extremely effective in cases refractory to conventional medications. Since these drugs inhibit a major component of the immune system, their use may expose the patient to infection with pathogens such as *Mycobacterium tuberculosis*. Prior infection with this pathogen must, therefore, be ruled out before initiating such treatment.

Another biologic agent that has been recently introduced for the treatment of RA is rituximab, which acts by targeting B-cell lymphocytes, which express the CD20 antigen. This medication, originally developed for the treatment of B-cell malignancies, can bring about long-term clinical remission (lasting up to 1 year) after a single infusion. Introduction of additional classes of biological agents, including inhibitors of IL-1, IL-6, and so on, is likely to further improve the management of RA.

Osteoarthritis

OA likely represents a number of different pathologic processes, all characterized by progressive loss of articular cartilage and new bone formation in the subchondral region (sclerosis) and the joint margins (osteophytes). OA is the most common joint disease, affecting the majority of people (in some site) older than 65 years and nearly all people older than 80 years. Although increasing age is the single largest risk factor for OA, other genetic and environmental factors play a role, especially for certain joints. For example, genetic factors play a significant role in OA of the hands, especially in women. In the knee, genetic factors play a minor role. For this joint, obesity decreased muscle strength in the quadriceps and a history of major knee trauma are the most consistently identified risk factors. Although major trauma to any joint can lead to OA and certain occupations have an increased incidence of OA, use in general, and even mild overuse, is not a risk factor for OA.

The precise pathologic mechanisms leading to OA are unclear. Most believe that this disease process is a result of an interaction between abnormal biology of cartilage and bone and/or abnormal forces being applied to the joints. With respect to biology, one of the earliest changes seen in OA is *increased* cartilage thickness. This early increase in thickness is likely due to increased water content of the cartilage due to disruption of the collagen network. Chondrocytes respond to this process by increasing proteoglycan synthesis. This early phase of cartilage hypertrophy is followed by loss of cartilage and a decrease in proteoglycan synthesis. In the early stages of cartilage loss, small crevices or clefts develop in cartilage, and with continued time and use, these clefts deepen and widen, whereas chondrocytes cluster, forming "clones" of cells. Finally, there is complete loss of cartilage and bone denudation. Bone responds in a number of ways to the cartilage changes that occur in OA. Appositional bone growth occurs in the exposed subchondral regions, leading to sclerosis. At the joint margins, bone and cartilage grow and lead to osteophyte formation. Abnormal forces can lead to the development of OA, even if biology is normal. The examples of OA caused by trauma or repetitive activities are evidence of this phenomenon. Once OA has begun, whether the initial problem is biological or mechanical, abnormal forces usually play a role. This is particularly true in weight-bearing joints.

The diagnosis of OA is based on appropriate symptoms and radiographic findings. The most common symptom of OA is pain. The pain is frequently deep, aching, and poorly localized. Early in the course of the illness, pain will typically occur primarily with use of the affected joint, whereas later in the disease, pain may occur even at rest. Because OA is not an inflammatory condition, there is minimal (i.e., less than 30 minutes) morning stiffness. Other symptoms may include crepitus, limitation of motion, and "giving way" of joints.

Plain radiographs remain the "gold standard" for diagnosing OA, although there are several caveats necessary to interpret this information correctly. The classic findings in OA are joint space narrowing (in many cases asymmetric), sclerosis of subchondral bone, and formation of marginal osteophytes and cysts. Studies that have compared the results of radiographs with the findings on arthroscopy have demonstrated that mild changes of OA may be visualized via arthroscopy or on magnetic resonance imaging (MRI) examination before any radiographic abnormalities are present. This is not of substantial clinical consequence because most of these persons are asymptomatic. A larger problem with interpreting radiographs is that a minority of people with radiographic evidence of OA will be symptomatic. The reason for this disparity between radiographic changes and the presence of pain and disability is not clear, and this discrepancy is not seen only in OA but also in nearly any chronic pain condition. Nonetheless, this points out that treatments such as those described for nonanatomic pain syndromes such as fibromyalgia should be considered for nonmechanical mechanisms that may be operative in many patients who present with pain and are found to have OA and in patients in whom there is a poor relationship between symptoms and pathology.

The management of OA is primarily nonsurgical, until very late in the disease. Several nonpharmacologic therapies have been shown to be effective in randomized controlled trials, including patient education, weight loss (in persons who are obese, particularly for the knee), strengthening exercises (again especially for the knee), and aerobic exercise. Topical applications of heat or cold can be a helpful adjunct in some patients. The use of various orthotics, including insoles, braces, heel lifts, and splints can be of significant use in the appropriate situations. Likewise, the use of a cane can improve pain originating from hip OA. Other nonpharmacological strategies for combating pain in OA such as spa therapy, acupuncture, and transcutaneous electrical nerve stimulation may offer pain relief to OA patients, although they are less well–evidence-based. The Arthritis Foundation has established many of these programs and is a valuable resource for this type of patient information.

In persons who do not respond to nonpharmacologic therapy, acetaminophen is often effective. In patients who fail acetaminophen alone, topical capsaicin cream or intraarticular corticosteroids can be considered, especially for the knee joint. If these treatments are ineffective, then use of low-dose NSAIDs, followed by high-dose NSAIDs, is a reasonable option (see "Pharmacologic Therapy"). Several new therapies for OA of the knee have recently emerged, and their place in the treatment algorithm remains unclear. Multiple small, randomized controlled trials studies have suggested that glucosamine and chondroitin sulfate may be effective in relieving pain in OA of the knee. Large-scale studies are now being conducted to confirm these findings. Several intraarticular hyaluronic acid preparations for the use in knee OA are available. These products must be given with a series of injections and were shown to be more effective than sham injection and the use of acetaminophen. This treatment modality may be most effective in those who have a contraindication to using an NSAID or those who have failed a trial of several NSAIDs.

The use of narcotic analgesics is usually reserved for severe cases of OA that fail to obtain satisfactory relief from other medications and treatment modalities. Careful patient selection is important due to the side effects of these medications (particularly in elderly patients). The outstanding progress made over recent years in the treatment of inflammatory joint disease such as RA highlights the relative paucity of options currently available for influencing the actual process of cartilage degradation, which is the hallmark of OA. A number of treatments have been studied for this indication, including tetracyclines, growth factor and cytokine manipulation, and the use of diacerein, a drug that inhibits the synthesis of IL-1β and is in use for treatment of OA in Europe. None of these modalities are currently available in the United States.

Fibromyalgia and Regional Soft Tissue Rheumatism

Fibromyalgia is the second most common rheumatic condition in the United States, after OA. It affects approximately 2% of the population: women much more than men. In the classic form, this condition is characterized by widespread musculoskeletal pain and diffuse soft tissue tenderness. The American College of Rheumatology criteria for this illness require that persons have pain throughout the entire body, as well as in 11 of 18 "tender points," but many persons with the clinical diagnosis of fibromyalgia will exhibit pain only in few regions of their body or have less than 11 tender points.

A diagnosis of fibromyalgia should be suspected when a person presents with multifocal pain with no evidence of inflammation or damage to peripheral structures on physical examination and/or further diagnostic workup. Other clinical features that occur commonly in the setting of fibromyalgia are fatigue, insomnia, memory or concentration difficulties, headaches, and irritable bowel symptoms. It is also common to find a lifetime history of chronic pain in localized regions of the body, such as the neck or back and temporomandibular joint.

A strong familial association has been observed in fibromyalgia, and evidence shows that there is a significant genetic underpinning for this syndrome. At the same time, a large number of environmental stimuli, including infection (viral and other), physical trauma, and stress can act as triggers for the development of fibromyalgia in genetically predisposed individuals.

Routine laboratory testing will be normal in this condition, and imaging studies will either be normal or detect abnormalities of uncertain clinical significance (e.g., mild degenerative changes, bulging discs).

There is considerable evidence that the pain in fibromyalgia occurs because of a disorder in the central nervous system processing of sensory stimuli, and thus, this condition typically does not respond to analgesics that act primarily in the periphery, such as acetaminophen, NSAIDs. Thus, the central nervous system fails to properly attenuate incoming painful stimuli at the level of the spinal cord, and alterations in levels of pain-related neurotransmitters, such as norepinephrine, serotonin, and substance P are observed in the cerebrospinal fluid of fibromyalgia patients. Medications that act by manipulating the concentration of these neurotransmitters in the central nervous system, for example, norepinephrine–serotonin reuptake inhibitors, are most effective in alleviating the pain of fibromyalgia.

Low doses of tricyclic drugs such as cyclobenzaprine (Flexeril) and amitriptyline (Elavil) given at bedtime can be effective analgesics in this setting. These drugs should be initiated at very low doses (e.g., 10 mg), given several hours before bedtime and escalated slowly (e.g., 10 mg every 1 to 2 weeks). The maximum dose is 40 mg of cyclobenzaprine, or approximately 70 mg of amitriptyline, but side effects of dry eyes and mouth, morning sedation, constipation, and weight gain often prevent dose escalation. Tramadol (Ultram), which acts both as a weak opioid and as a reuptake inhibitor, can also be used for pain relief. Antiepileptic drugs, which are widely used in the treatment of various chronic pain conditions, have been proven to be effective in fibromyalgia. In a randomized, double-blinded, placebo-controlled trial, pregabalin (Lyrica) demonstrated efficacy against pain, sleep disturbances, and fatigue as compared with placebo in fibromyalgia. Pregabalin has been the first medication to gain the U.S. Food and Drug Administration (FDA) approval for the treatment of fibromyalgia, whereas gabapentin, an older antiepileptic drug used for treatment of postherpetic neuralgia, appears to be of similar efficacy.

Dual reuptake inhibitors, which act by elevating levels of norepinephrine and serotonin in the CNS, are gaining rapid popularity in the treatment of fibromyalgia. Most recently, duloxetine (Cymbalta) and milnacipran (Savella) have gained FDA approval for this indication, and additional dual reuptake inhibitors are likely to be introduced in the near future.

Low-impact aerobic exercise can be particularly useful, but as with the tricyclic drugs, this should be started very slowly and increased very gradually. Cognitive behavioral therapy or other structured pain management programs are also very beneficial, particularly for combating the negative functional aspects of fibromyalgia.

Seronegative Spondyloarthropathies

The four classic SSs are ankylosing spondylitis, reactive arthritis, inflammatory bowel disease–associated arthropathy, and psoriatic arthritis. These disorders are considered together because they share an immunologic predisposition (HLA-B27) that leads to both (1) similar articular features (an inflammatory arthritis involving the axial skeleton), and (2) common extraarticular features (e.g., inflammatory eye disease, cardiac conduction defects, aortic valve disease). Even the approximately 80% of individuals who are HLA-B27–positive do not develop a SS have an independent risk of developing the classic extraarticular features seen in this spectrum of illness.

Ankylosing Spondylitis

Ankylosing spondylitis is the prototypical disease in this category. The characteristic features of this illness are shown in Table 7.7. The earliest joint involved in most persons with this disorder is the sacroiliac joint. Clinically, these individuals will complain of indolent onset of morning stiffness and pain involving the low back, which typically improves with exercise. Other characteristic features of the pain seen

TABLE 7.7

CLASSIFICATION CRITERIA FOR ANKYLOSING SPONDYLITIS

Amor Classification for Spondyloarthropathies[a]
Clinical systems/past history (score). Requires a score of 6 for spondyloarthropathy
Lumbar/dorsal pain at night; morning stiffness (1)
Asymmetrical oligoarthritis (2)
Buttock pain (1)
Sausage-like toe/digit (2)
Heel pain/enthesopathy (2)
Iritis (2)
Nongonococcal urethritis/cervicitis <1 mo (1)
Acute diarrhea <1 mo (1)
Psoriasis, balanitis, IBD (2)
Radiologic findings (2)
Sacroiliitis (bilateral grade 2 or unilateral grade >2)
Genetic background (2)
HLA-B27 positive
Family history of AS, REA, IBD, psoriasis, or uveitis
Response to treatment (2)
Clear-cut improvement (within 48 h) with NSAIDs
European Spondyloarthropathy Study Group Criteria for Spondyloarthropathies[b]
1. Inflammatory spinal pain
2. Synovitis (symmetric or predominantly lower limbs)
One or more of the following (in addition to criterion 1 or 2):
Alternate buttock pain, sacroiliitis enthesopathy, positive family history, psoriasis, IBD, urethritis/cervicitis/diarrhea <1 month prior
Modified New York Criteria[c]
Low-back pain of 3 months' duration improved by exercise and not relieved by rest
Limitation of lumbar spine in sagittal and frontal planes
Chest expansion decreased relative to normal values for age and sex
Bilateral sacroiliitis, grade 2–4[d]
Unilateral sacroiliitis, grade 3–4[d]
Definite AS if unilateral grade 3 or 4 or bilateral grade 2–4 sacroiliitis and any clinical criteria

AS, ankylosing spondylitis; IBD, inflammatory bowel disease; NSAID, nonsteroidal anti-inflammatory drug; ReA, reactive arthritis.
[a]Amor B, et al. *Rev Rhum Mal Osteoartic.* 1990;57:85–89.
[b]Dougados M, van der Linden S, Juhlin R, et al. The European Spondyloarthropathy Study Group preliminary criteria for the classification of spondyloarthropathy. *Arthritis Rheum.* 1991;34:1218–1227.
[c]van der Linden S, Valkenburg HA, Cats A. Evaluation of diagnostic criteria for ankylosing spondylitis. *Arthritis Rheum.* 1984;27:361–367.
[d]Grading of radiographs: 0 = normal; 1 = suggestive; 2 = minimal sacroiliitis; 3 = moderate sacroiliitis; 4 = complete ankylosis.
(*From* Dawes PT. Stoke ankylosing spondylitis spine score. *J Rheumatol.* 1999;26:993–996.)

TABLE 7.8

FEATURES OF INFLAMMATORY BACK PAIN

Younger age at onset of pain (peak 26 y)
Pain and early morning stiffness of the spine
Improvement with exercise/activity
Insidious in onset
Symptoms lasting for more than 3 mo
Spinal mobility and deep breathing may be restricted
Radiographic evidence of sacroiliitis or ankylosis

Reprinted with permission from Koopman WJ, Moreland LW. *Arthritis and Allied Conditions: A Textbook of Rheumatology*, 15th ed. Philadelphia: Lippincott Williams & Wilkins, 2005.

in ankylosing spondylitis, as well as the symptoms that help differentiate mechanical back disease from inflammatory back disease, are shown in Table 7.8.

On physical examination, individuals with sacroiliac involvement will usually demonstrate limited motion in this area of the body. The most commonly performed test to demonstrate this is the modified Schober test. In this test, a mark is made on the skin overlying the spine where an imaginary line would connect the left and right posterior iliac spines. Another dot is placed 10 cm higher, and the patient is asked to maximally flex forward. The distance in normal individuals should increase to at least 15 cm, and if not, it suggests that there is some limitation of motion in this region.

The classic radiographic findings of ankylosing spondylitis include sacroiliitis, enthesopathy (periostitis at tendon and ligament insertions), and ankylosis (fusion) (Figs. 7.4 and 7.5). Early cases of sacroiliitis that cannot be detected by conventional radiography are visible on gadolinium-enhanced MRI examination. In the spine, the initial change seen is a loss of concavity of vertebral bodies due to enthesopathic disease, eventually followed by fusion, leading to the classic "bamboo spine." It is important to differentiate this finding from that of diffuse idiopathic skeletal hyperostosis, in which the hyperostoses are thicker and typically only involve the right side of the thoracic spine. In addition to an inflammatory arthritis involving the axial skeleton, patients with ankylosing spondylitis may also develop peripheral joint involvement. Female patients may be more likely than male patients to have primarily peripheral joint involvement and isolated cervical involvement.

The extraarticular manifestations of ankylosing spondylitis are similar to those that can occur in other seronegative arthropathies. Inflammatory anterior eye disease (uveitis or iritis) typically presents with unilateral eye pain, photophobia, and blurred vision. Cardiac conduction defects may occur in up to 7% of patients with long-standing disease and aortic insufficiency in 10% of patients with chronic disease. Interstitial lung disease in this illness has an unusual predilection for the upper lobes. Neurologic involvement is rare but can be catastrophic, usually when a patient with a fused spine is involved in trauma, and may present with paresis.

Laboratory testing is generally unhelpful, except in some cases to rule out other disorders. Inflammatory indices such as an ESR and a CRP may be elevated. In persons with inflammatory peripheral arthritis, an RF (which will be negative, thus the term *seronegative spondyloarthropathy*)

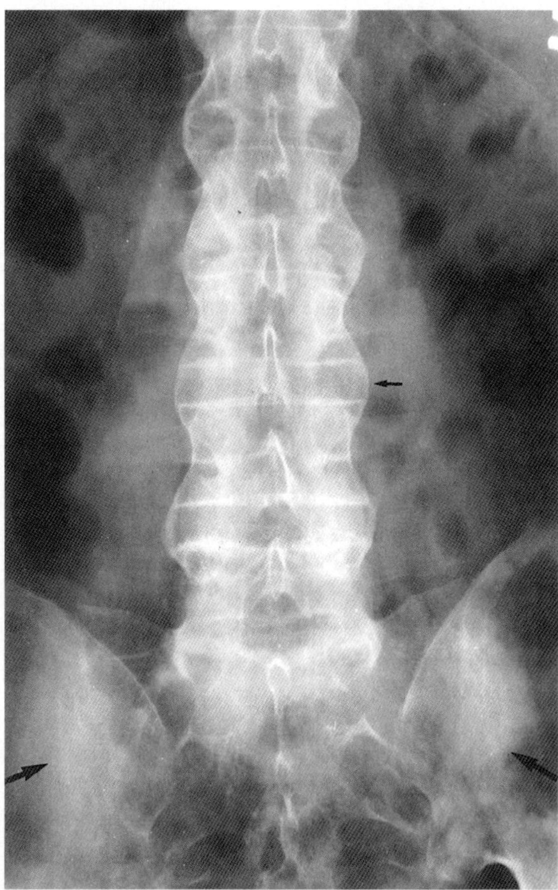

Figure 7.4 Anteroposterior radiograph of the upper pelvis and lumbar spine. Both sacroiliac joints (*large arrows*) are fused (grade IV sacroiliitis), and there are bilateral, symmetric syn-desmophytes (*small arrow*), resulting in the typical "bamboo" appearance of ankylosing spondylitis. (*Reprinted with permission from* Koopman WJ, Moreland LW. *Arthritis and Allied Conditions: A Textbook of Rheumatology*. 15th ed. Philadelphia, PA: Lippincott Williams & Wilkins, 2005.)

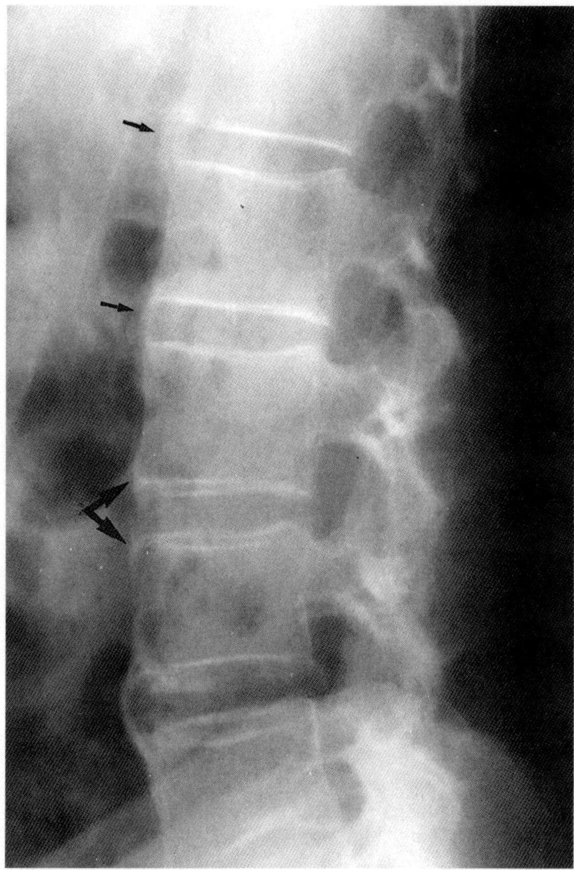

Figure 7.5 Lateral radiograph of the lumbar spine in ankylosing spondylitis with "shiny corners" or Romanus lesions (*large arrows*) due to marginal erosions of vertebral bodies and typical marginal syndesmophytes (*small arrows*). (*Reprinted with permission from* Koopman WJ, Moreland LW. *Arthritis and Allied Conditions: A Textbook of Rheumatology*. 15th ed. Philadelphia, PA: Lippincott Williams & Wilkins, 2005.)

is useful. Testing for HLA-B27 is rarely indicated, because this haplotype is seen in approximately 6% of Caucasians (lesser percentages of Asians and African Americans) and only approximately 20% of those who are positive will develop this disorder.

The first-line treatment of SSs is with NSAIDs. There is some evidence, primarily anecdotal, that indomethacin is the most effective of the commonly used NSAIDs, especially when given at a dose of 150 mg/d. Patients should be encouraged to remain active and to routinely perform stretching exercises to maintain chest expansion, cervical extension, and lumbar flexion. Sulfasalazine is typically a slow-acting antirheumatic drug (SAARD) chosen to control symptoms of this illness unresponsive to NSAID. This drug is typically begun at 1,000 mg twice daily, with the maximum dose being a total of 4 g/d. Sulfasalazine has been shown to be effective for controlling peripheral polyarticular synovitis in ankylosing spondylitis, but it does not appear to be of use in treating the axial involvement.

Anti–TNF-α medications are extremely effective in the treatment of ankylosing spondylitis. Both infliximab, a chimeric monoclonal anti–TNF-α antibody (3–5 mg/kg every 6–8 weeks after an initial saturation phase), and etanercept, a 75-kD TNF-α receptor fusion protein (25 mg subcutaneously two times each week), are in current use and lead to significant improvement in signs and symptoms.

Reactive Arthritis

Reactive arthritis (formerly Reiter disease) is classically described by the clinical triad of arthritis, urethritis, and conjunctivitis. Since the initial description, it has become clear that there are several variations on this theme, with some individuals having only two of three manifestations (i.e., incomplete reactive arthritis), and others having colitis instead of urethritis. This syndrome typically develops in a genetically susceptible host following infection of the genitourinary or GI tract with organisms such as *Chlamydia*, *Salmonella*, *Shigella*, *Yersinia*, or *Campylobacter*; hence the term *reactive* arthritis.

The arthritis that occurs in reactive arthritis is typically asymmetric and oligoarticular, with a predilection for the large joints of the lower extremities. Occasionally, the synovial fluid cell counts in this disorder can be very high, in the range normally only seen in septic arthritis. In addition to the joint involvement, inflammation of tendinous insertion into bone is common, such as the Achilles tendon or plantar fascia. Another characteristic finding related to the presence of an enthesopathy is the finding of a "sausage digit," a diffusely swollen toe or finger due to the presence of both synovitis and enthesopathy. In addition to the peripheral arthritis that accompanies the acute illness, some persons with reactive arthritis will develop a spondyloarthropathy similar to ankylosing spondylitis. This process is typically less symmetric than ankylosing spondylitis and the syndesmophytes are usually larger.

Other clinical features are commonly seen on initial presentation. Urethritis is more likely to be symptomatic in men than in women, and involvement of other portions of the urogenital tract (e.g., cystitis, prostatitis) may also occur. Eye disease is most commonly conjunctivitis, but uveitis and iritis may also be seen. There are a variety of distinctive mucocutaneous features that can be seen, including stomatitis, keratoderma blennorrhagica, circinate balanitis, and nail changes.

In the patient who presents with the classic triad of findings, the diagnosis is straightforward. With atypical presentations, other diagnosis must be considered including gonococcal arthritis, Lyme disease, rheumatic fever, and crystal-induced arthropathies. The similarities and differences between reactive arthritis and gonococcal arthritis are particularly important.

Just as with the other SSs, NSAIDs are the treatment of choice, and indomethacin is the drug most frequently used. COX-2 inhibitors such as celecoxib are equally effective as conventional NSAIDs. Anecdotal evidence suggests that the acute phase of this illness is less responsive to systemic corticosteroids than other types of inflammatory arthritis, but topical corticosteroids may be helpful for extraarticular features. Because of the infectious triggers of this illness, antibiotics may be appropriate in cases where active infection is evident. There is no evidence to justify prolonged antibiotic treatment beyond this indication. Some patients with reactive arthritis will have an acute self-limited course, but many will develop chronic symptoms. These patients with chronic disease may benefit from the addition of sulfasalazine. As in ankylosing spondylitis, however, sulfasalazine is effective only for the peripheral joint involvement in reactive arthritis, not for axial disease (e.g., sacroiliitis).

The biological anti–TNF-α infliximab and etanercept have a dramatic effect in reactive arthritis, and their use should be strongly considered in severe cases, particularly with axial involvement.

Psoriatic Arthritis

Psoriatic arthritis shares many features with reactive arthritis, and in some instances, these two conditions are indistinguishable. The presence of psoriasis is necessary for the diagnosis of psoriatic arthritis (although in some instances, the arthritis antedates the rash). Only approximately 5% of individuals with psoriasis develop psoriatic arthritis. Axial skeleton involvement and extraarticular features are similar in psoriatic arthritis and reactive arthritis. One distinctive feature of psoriatic arthritis is more extensive involvement of the DIP joints and the relationship between this feature and nail pitting. Only approximately 20% of persons with psoriasis have nail pitting, but 80% of persons with psoriatic arthritis have nail pitting. Other unusual articular features seen in some patients with psoriatic arthritis are resorption of the tufts of the distal phalanges, peripheral joint ankylosis, and characteristic "pencil-in-cup" deformities.

Enteropathic Arthritis

Enteropathic arthritis is the term commonly used to describe the arthritides associated with inflammatory bowel diseases. The two main forms of enteropathic arthritis are: (1) acute episodes of peripheral oligoarticular arthritis that resemble reactive arthritis and are typically associated with flares of the colitis, and (2) an axial spondyloarthropathy that is closely related to HLA-B27 positivity and follows a slow, indolent course that is largely independent of the bowel disease.

Crystal-Induced Arthropathies

There are three types of crystal-induced arthropathies that will be discussed: (1) gout, (2) calcium pyrophosphate deposition disease (CPDD), and (3) hydroxyapatite deposition disease (HADD). It is important to recognize that nearly any crystalline or particular substance that can somehow be introduced into the joint or soft tissues (e.g., injected steroid, fragments from prostheses, plant thorns) can lead to a localized inflammatory response.

Gout

Although "gout" refers to the disease process that occurs when monosodium urate crystals deposit in various tissues in the body, only the articular manifestations will be emphasized. The serum uric acid concentration primarily determines whether monosodium urate crystals will deposit in tissues. Purine metabolism is largely genetically determined, but male gender, increased age, increased body weight, high-purine diet, diabetes, hypertension, alcohol, and other drugs (e.g., diuretics, cyclosporine) will raise serum concentration of uric acid. The higher the serum uric acid concentration, the more likely an individual will develop gout. It is important to recognize that only a small percentage of hyperuricemic individuals ever develop gout.

Rheumatic features of gout include some combination of acute attacks of monoarticular or polyarticular arthritis and more indolent changes caused by accumulation of uric acid crystals (tophi). The first metatarsophalangeal (MTP) joint of the foot is the most commonly involved joint during a first attack of gout. Other peripheral joints in the lower extremity (e.g., other MTP joints, mid foot, ankle, and knee) are next most commonly involved, followed by peripheral joints in the hand (e.g., DIP, PIP, MCP, and wrist). The predilection for peripheral joints farthest from the body core is likely due to temperature. Uric acid solubility decreases considerably as temperature decreases, and thus in the setting of a high serum (and thus tissue) uric acid level, crystal formation and deposition occur in these cooler areas of the body. For this same reason, acute gout is rarely seen in the axial skeleton. This temperature-related decrease in solubility may also explain why acute gout attacks frequently occur at 2:00 AM OR 3:00 AM in the morning, abruptly awakening an individual from sleep. During this period, a person's core body temperature falls slightly because of diurnal changes, and the inactivity of the extremity also contributes to decreased blood flow and cooler peripheral temperatures.

An acute gout attack will usually begin as a monoarticular process, which may become polyarticular with chronicity. Men are much more likely to be affected than women, largely because at any given age, men have higher serum uric acid levels. Postmenopausal women may develop gout, but even then this usually occurs because of other risk factors (e.g., alcohol or medication use). During an acute attack, a person may be febrile, and there is typically an acute inflammatory response evident over the involved region. This inflammatory response is so pronounced that it is common for the skin overlying an attack to desquamate after the attack has subsided. The acute inflammatory response can also resemble cellulitis, especially when it occurs in the mid or hind foot or in the dorsum of the wrist. In addition to articular involvement and soft tissue inflammation, an acute bursitis can sometimes occur, especially in the olecranon region.

When a 50-year-old man presents with an acute onset of MTP joint arthritis, the diagnosis of gout is straightforward. In many settings, other clinical information is necessary to establish the diagnosis. The presence of tophi is helpful. Tophi may occur in various locations in the body, including the helix of the ear, fingers, or olecranon region. Laboratory testing is not typically useful. Most people with gout will have an elevated uric acid level during an acute attack, but some will not. Many persons will exhibit leukocytosis or elevations in inflammatory indices, but these will not help differentiate the patient with gout from those with other types of inflammatory or septic arthritis. Radiographs during an acute attack will typically be normal or will reveal only soft tissue swelling; with chronic tophaceous disease, radiographs will show evidence of sclerotic marginal erosions, typically with preservation of the joint space until late in the disease.

The detection of monosodium urate crystals in the joint fluid is the most definitive way to establish the diagnosis of gout. Uric acid crystals are thin, needle-shaped crystals that are approximately the same length as a leukocyte and, in fact, may be seen inside leukocytes. Under a polarizing microscope, the crystals will appear bright yellow and blue, depending on the axis of polarization. This is in contrast to calcium pyrophosphate dihydrate crystals that are pleomorphic in both size and shape, are less intensely birefringent, and thus appear pale yellow and blue.

The management of gout can be divided into treatment of the acute attack and prophylaxis against future attacks. The goal in treating the acute attack is to inhibit the ability of WBCs to phagocytize the crystals. The most effective drugs in this setting are NSAIDs, and indomethacin is a preferred agent because of the rapid onset of action and potent anti-inflammatory properties. Any other NSAID, including COX-2 inhibitors, can also be used, but those with a rapid onset of action are preferred. Colchicine can also be helpful during an acute attack of gout, although the GI intolerance of this medication frequently limits the effectiveness. Classically, the patient is instructed to take 0.6 mg tablet once hourly until the attack subsides, until side effects occur, or until a total of 10 tablets are taken. Colchicine, and to a lesser extent NSAIDs, is much more effective when treatment is begun rapidly. The reason for this is likely that these anti-inflammatory regimens (especially colchicine) act in part by inhibiting chemotaxis of leukocytes to the joint, and once this has occurred, these agents are much less effective. In persons with contraindications to colchicine (renal or hepatic impairment) or NSAIDs, corticosteroids can be effectively used to treat acute gout attacks. These can be administered intra-articularly, or systemically, if there is monoarticular involvement. When these are given systemically, the person typically needs to receive treatment for several days to avoid a rebound effect (alternatively, a single intramuscular dose of a depot form of corticosteroids can be given).

When persons have frequent attacks of gout, or when there is evidence of tophaceous (or extraarticular) disease, therapy directed toward lowering serum uric acid level should be initiated. A low purine diet, or avoiding alcohol use, is sometimes all that is necessary to lower serum uric acid level. If behavioral modifications are ineffective, then either uricosuric drugs or allopurinol can be used. These drugs should not be used in the setting of an acute attack, as this can paradoxically precipitate a worsening of the attack. Probenecid is the most commonly used uricosuric drug, and it can be started at 500 mg/d and increased to 2 g/d. This drug is effective only in persons with relatively normal renal function; it should not be used in those with a history of nephrolithiasis, and patients must be counseled to maintain a high fluid intake. Allopurinol is a drug that inhibits the enzyme xanthine oxidase, thus inhibiting the production of uric acid. It can be used as an alternative for uricosuric treatment, e.g., in patients with impaired renal function or nephrolithiasis. Allopurinol can be given beginning at doses ranging from 100 mg (in the elderly or those with impaired renal function) to 300 mg once daily. The principal concern with this drug is hypersensitivity reaction, so patients must be warned to stop this medication immediately if they develop a rash or pruritus. Approximately 5% of individuals taking allopurinol will develop a pruritic maculopapular rash that resolves when the medication is stopped. However, a small percentage of these patients will go on to develop a serious and sometimes fatal hypersensitivity reaction reminiscent of a Stevens–Johnson reaction.

Currently, there are no adequate alternatives for those patients who fail to maintain normal serum levels of uric acid under treatment with uricosuric medication and/or allopurinol (or for patients intolerant for these drugs). A number of novel medications are, however, under development, including the xanthine oxidase inhibitor febuxostat and the enzyme–drug uricase, which catalyzes conversion of uric acid to the more soluble compound allantoin. Rasburicase, a recombinant form of uricase, currently in use for the prevention of tumor lysis syndrome in hematological malignancies, has also been suggested for short-term therapy in refractory cases of gout. An alternative approach to prophylaxis against gout attacks is to use a low dose of colchicine (e.g., 0.6 mg twice daily in persons with normal renal and hepatic function) or an NSAID chronically.

Calcium Pyrophosphate Deposition Disease

CPPD crystals can be deposited in a number of articular structures including cartilage, synovium, tendons, and ligaments. In most cases, there is no clear reason why a person has CPPD deposition (i.e., idiopathic), whereas in other instances, this occurs as a hereditary disorder or secondary to another disease process (Table 7.9). Having CPPD is not necessarily associated with any disease, as a significant percentage of persons with this finding will be asymptomatic. For instance, it is estimated that nearly 50% of individuals have CPPD of the knees by the time they reach age 80. In other instances, CPPD deposition is associated with disease. The disease processes commonly seen in association with CPPD include episodes of acute or chronic inflammatory arthritis (pseudogout) and an accelerated chronic degenerative arthritis (pseudo-OA).

TABLE 7.9

CONDITIONS PROBABLY ASSOCIATED WITH CALCIUM PYROPHOSPHATE DIHYDRATE CRYSTAL DEPOSITION

Aging
Amyloidosis
Familiar hypocalciuric hypercalcemia
Gout
Hemochromatosis
Hemosiderosis
Hyperparathyroidism
Hypomagnesemia
Hypophosphatasia
Hypothyroidism
Neuropathic joints
Trauma, including surgery

(*Reprinted with permission from* Koopman WJ, Moreland LW. *Arthritis and Allied Conditions: A Textbook of Rheumatology.* 15th ed. Philadelphia, PA: Lippincott Williams & Wilkins, 2005.)

CPDD is diagnosed with a combination of appropriate clinical findings, radiographs, and synovial fluid analysis (Fig. 7.6). The joint distribution of CPDD overlaps somewhat with similar disorders (e.g., Gout, OA), but the overall pattern of involvement can be helpful in differentiating these disorders. The knees, hips, symphysis pubis, and wrist are all common locations for CPPD deposition, and radiographs of these regions will commonly show the typical chondrocalcinosis (i.e., calcification of cartilage). In the knee, chondrocalcinosis may be seen in either the tibiofemoral joint or the patellofemoral joint, with the latter sometimes being preferentially involved. Another clinical clue to the presence of CPPD is more aggressive destruction of the joint than would otherwise be expected in OA. Synovial fluid analysis identifying the characteristic rod-shaped (and pleomorphic) crystals of CPPD is helpful.

The treatment of CPDD depends somewhat on the mode of presentation. If CPDD is secondary to a metabolic disorder, then this obviously should be addressed. If CPPD presents as pseudogout, the treatment is very similar to that of gout noted earlier. Both NSAIDs and corticosteroids can be used to manage acute attacks, and colchicine is even somewhat efficacious, although less so than for gout. Both NSAIDs and colchicine can be used to prophylax against acute attacks of pseudogout and for the pseudo-OA presentation.

Hydroxyapatite Deposition Disease

Hydroxyapatite may be deposited in soft tissues, periarticular structures, or joints. As with other crystal deposition syndromes, hydroxyapatite deposition may either occur as an asymptomatic finding or be associated with disease. Soft tissue calcification usually occurs as a result of illnesses such as scleroderma, dermatomyositis, and chronic renal insufficiency. In some instances where the calcification is extensive and causes troublesome symptoms, surgical intervention is necessary. Much more commonly, hydroxyapatite may be deposited in the periarticular tissues. This usually occurs at tendon insertions, especially in the shoulder, hands, hip, and knee. When symptomatic, this can be treated with NSAIDs or corticosteroid injections, although the use of crystalline steroid preparations may in some instances exacerbate the problem. HADD involving the joints is uncommon. McCarty and colleagues coined the term "Milwaukee shoulder" to describe an aggressive degenerative process affecting the entire shoulder region, primarily affecting older women. A similar process may uncommonly affect other joints.

Systemic Lupus Erythematosus

SLE is the prototypic systemic autoimmune disorder. A systemic response by the body against various self-antigens

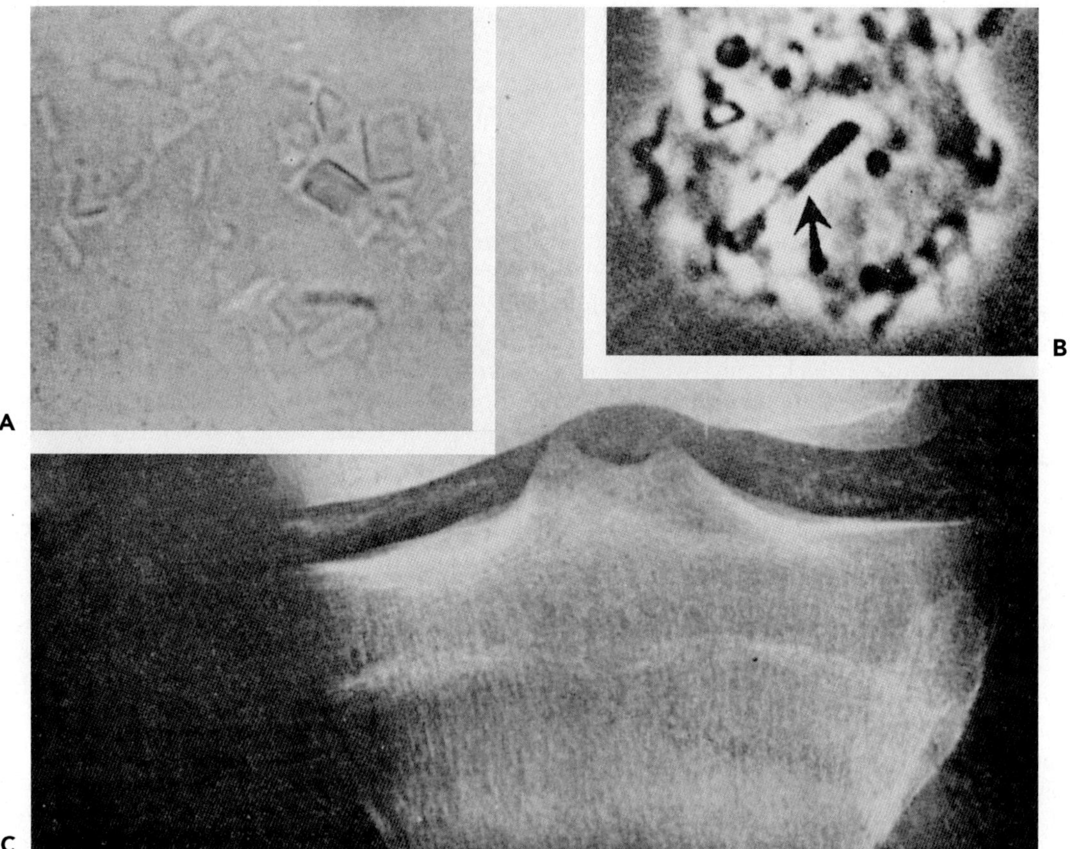

Figure 7.6 **(A)** Weakly birefringent monoclinic and triclinic calcium pyrophosphate dihydrate disease (CPPD) microcrystals in synovial fluid removed from a chronically symptomatic knee (polarized light, original magnification 1,250). **(B)** Phagocytosed crystal (*arrow*) in a polymorphonuclear leukocyte (phase contrast, original magnification 1,250). **(C)** Anteroposterior radiograph of the knee, showing typical punctate and linear deposits of CPPD in the menisci and articular hyaline cartilage. (*Reprinted with permission from* Koopman WJ, Moreland LW. *Arthritis and Allied Conditions: A Textbook of Rheumatology*. 15th ed. Philadelphia, PA: Lippincott Williams & Wilkins, 2005.)

leads to inflammation, immune complex deposition, and damage to blood vessels throughout the body. Women are affected approximately five times more commonly than men, and the peak incidence is in the third and fourth decade of life.

SLE can affect nearly any organ or tissue in the body. Table 7.10 lists the frequency of clinical symptoms, laboratory findings, and diagnostic certainty in this disorder. The musculoskeletal features bear special emphasis, because these are the manifestations that may bring the patient to an orthopaedist. Nearly all patients with this illness eventually have either arthralgias or arthritis. The main difference from RA or other types of inflammatory arthritis is that there is little synovitis or joint destruction seen in SLE, although the joints may be very painful.

Some patients with SLE develop ulnar deviation of the fingers, swan-neck deformities, and other changes that appear very similar to those seen in RA. On examination, however, these deformities are all reducible, and this entity has been termed "Jacoud arthropathy." This seems to occur because of tendon laxity rather than destruction of

TABLE 7.10
PRESENTING AND CUMULATIVE SYMPTOMS/SIGNS OF SYSTEMIC LUPUS ERYTHEMATOSUS

Symptom/Sign	Percentage with Manifestation	Cumulative Percentage
Malar (butterfly) rash	30	56
Discoid lupus	14	27
Photosensitivity	29	54
Arthritis	40	70
Proteinuria	21	53
Seizures	4	10
Psychosis	2	5
Pericarditis	6	18
Pleurisy	16	38
Leukopenia	18	46
Thrombocytopenia	9	20

(*Reprinted with permission from* Koopman WJ, Moreland LW. *Arthritis and Allied Conditions: A Textbook of Rheumatology*. 15th ed. Philadelphia, PA: Lippincott Williams & Wilkins, 2005.)

joints, and radiographs will reveal normal joints. Another orthopaedic problem encountered relatively frequently in SLE is avascular necrosis (AVN). Corticosteroid therapy is probably the major reason for this complication, although AVN has been noted in SLE patients who were not treated with steroids (especially those with a positive anticardiolipin antibody).

The diagnosis of SLE is based on a combination of clinical and laboratory features. The ACR diagnostic criteria for SLE are helpful in this setting (Table 7.11). Patients who have four or more of these features are likely to have SLE. The ANA element of the criteria is particularly important, because nearly all patients with SLE will have a positive ANA.

The treatment of SLE is based on the symptoms and the site of involvement. Generally, skin and musculoskeletal involvement is treated nonaggressively with NSAIDs, topical corticosteroids, and/or hydroxychloroquine. Hematologic involvement, serositis, and severe constitutional symptoms are usually managed with corticosteroids, typically with "steroid-sparing" drugs (e.g., azathioprine, methotrexate, hydroxychloroquine) given concurrently to minimize the long-term complications of the steroids. Renal and central nervous system involvement is treated very aggressively, in many instances with both corticosteroids and cytotoxic drugs such as cyclophosphamide and cyclosporine. Mycophenolate mofetil, a drug widely used to prevent rejection of allografts, is currently used in some cases as a less toxic alternative to cyclophosphamide in lupus nephritis.

TABLE 7.11

THE 1997 REVISED AMERICAN COLLEGE OF RHEUMATOLOGY CRITERIA FOR SYSTEMIC LUPUS ERYTHEMATOSUS

1. Malar rash: Fixed malar erythema, flat or raised
2. Discoid rash: Erythematous raised patches with keratotic scaling and follicular plugging; atrophic scarring may occur in older lesions
3. Photosensitivity: Skin rash as an unusual reaction to sunlight, by patient history or physician observation
4. Oral ulcers: Oral or nasopharyngeal ulcers, usually painless, observed by physician
5. Arthritis: Nonerosive arthritis involving two or more peripheral joints, characterized by tenderness, swelling, or effusion
6. Serositis
   a. Pleuritis (convincing history of pleuritic pain or rub heard by physician or evidence of pleural effusion) OR
   b. Pericarditis (documented by ECG or rub or evidence of pericardial effusion)
7. Renal disorder
   a. Persistent proteinuria >0.5 g/d or $>3+$ OR
   b. Cellular casts of any type
8. Neurologic disorder
   a. Seizures (in the absence of other causes)
   b. Psychosis (in the absence of other causes)
9. Hematologic disorders
   a. Hemolytic anemia
   b. Leukopenia ($<4,000/mm^3$ on two or more occasions)
   c. Lymphopenia ($<1,500/mm^3$ on two or more occasions)
   d. Thrombocytopenia ($<100,000/mm^3$ in the absence of offending drugs)
10. Immunologic disorder
    a. Anti-dsDNA OR
    b. Anti-Smith (anti-Sm) OR
    c. Positive finding of antiphospholipid antibodies based on
       i. An abnormal serum level of IgG or IgM anticardiolipin antibodies, OR
       ii. A positive test result for lupus anticoagulant using a standard method, OR
       iii. A false-positive serologic test for syphilis known to be positive for ≥ 6 mo and confirmed by *Treponema pallidum* immobilization or fluorescent treponemal antibody absorption test
11. Antinuclear antibody: An abnormal titer of ANA by immunofluorescence or an equivalent assay at any time and in the absence of drugs known to be associated with "drug-induced lupus syndrome"

ANA, antinuclear antibody; dsDNA, double-stranded deoxyribonucleic acid; ECG, electrocardiogram.
(*Reprinted with permission from* Koopman WJ, Moreland LW. *Arthritis and Allied Conditions: A Textbook of Rheumatology.* 15th ed. Philadelphia, PA: Lippincott Williams & Wilkins, 2005.)

Polymyalgia Rheumatica

Polymyalgia rheumatica (PMR) is a common disorder occurring almost exclusively in persons older than 50 years and characterized by stiffness and pain in the proximal muscles. The onset may be abrupt or indolent. Patients will have prominent "gelling" whenever they are inactive for prolonged periods. In some persons, there is swelling and/or synovitis of the hands associated with this condition. In a subset of individuals, PMR coexists with temporal arteritis, which can be associated with visual symptoms, headaches, jaw claudication, and alopecia. Patients with these symptoms or with temporal artery tenderness on palpation should have a temporal artery biopsy(s) to determine whether temporal arteritis is present because more aggressive treatment regimens are used for this subset of patients. Doppler examination of the temporal arteries is a useful diagnostic adjunct.

In the appropriate clinical setting, the diagnosis of PMR is confirmed by finding a markedly elevated ESR. Other diagnoses that should be considered are fibromyalgia and hypothyroidism. Another diagnostic test is treatment with intermediate doses of corticosteroids, usually 20 mg of prednisone per day for several weeks with a rapid taper to 5 to 10 mg/d. In patients who do not respond rapidly and completely to corticosteroids, the diagnosis should be questioned. Typically, patients will need to stay on corticosteroids at least 1 to 2 years and sometimes much longer.

Infectious Arthritis

Bacterial Agents

Septic arthritis from common pathogens is covered in detail in infection chapter of this book. Such processes usually occur in an immunocompromised host or as the result of bacteremia or direct bacterial inoculation of a joint. But there are a few types of infectious (or postinfectious arthritis) that can occur without such risk factors. Rheumatic fever and gonococcal infections are specific examples.

The arthritis associated with rheumatic fever does not occur because the joint is infected with the causative organism but rather because of an immunologic reaction to the group A streptococcus organism. For reasons that are unclear, only pharyngeal infections with this organism are associated with rheumatic fever. The classic manifestations of rheumatic fever are described by the Jones criteria and may follow the pharyngitis by several days to weeks. The major clinical findings include polyarthritis, carditis, chorea, erythema marginatum, and subcutaneous nodules; minor findings include fever, arthralgia, and previous rheumatic fever. The arthritis associated with rheumatic fever is unique in that this is one of the few arthritides that is truly migratory, that is, the arthritis moves from one joint to the next. Large peripheral joints are most commonly involved. The onset is typically abrupt and severe, with coexistence of myalgia and fever. Although this disorder is uncommon in adults, the articular features may predominate the clinical picture, with an absence of extraarticular features. Also, in adults the arthritis may be more "additive" than migratory and be less responsive to salicylates or NSAIDs than it is in children. Gonococcal arthritis can follow a gonococcal infection involving the urethra, cervix, pharynx, or rectum. Typically, an individual will initially experience several days of fevers, chills, multiple skin lesions, and polyarthralgias or tenosynovitis. If untreated in this stage, it will typically progress to involve just a few joints or tendons. Individuals with such a clinical picture should be started immediately on an antibiotic such as ceftriaxone and should have cultures taken of all orifices, any affected synovium, and any skin lesions. These cultures should be plated at the bedside on Thayer–Martin media or chocolate agar. Persons in the early phase are most likely to have positive blood cultures, whereas those in the later phase are more likely to have positive synovial or skin lesion cultures.

Nonbacterial Agents

Less commonly, joints (or soft tissue structures) can become infected with nonbacterial agents such as tuberculosis or fungi. With the exception of tuberculosis, which can cause a septic arthritis in persons with normal immune function, most persons who have joint infections with these types of organisms have an underlying defect in immune function.

Viral Agents

Nearly all viral agents can lead to the development of a postviral arthritis in a small percentage of affected individuals. It appears as though the most common cause of postinfectious arthritis in persons who seek medical attention is that associated with parvovirus B19 infections. This virus is common in children, leading to Fifth disease, or erythema infectiosum. In affected children, cutaneous manifestations predominate, with the characteristic "slapped cheeks" appearance, as well as a serpiginous rash affecting the torso or extremities. Adults who develop this infection have less prominent cutaneous features and more prominent articular features. The articular features closely resemble those of RA, so closely in fact that up to 50% of these persons will meet criteria for the diagnosis of RA. The diagnostic test of choice is an IgM titer for parvovirus B19, which will be positive at the time joint symptoms begin and last approximately 2 months. Although this illness typically has a self-limited course and is not associated with joint damage, these patients are quite uncomfortable and debilitated and may need treatment with NSAIDs or even low-dose steroids for several months.

Rubella, hepatitis B, and hepatitis C are additional examples of viral agents capable of causing arthralgia and arthritis. HIV infection is associated with a wide range of musculoskeletal manifestations. These patients suffer from a high prevalence of seronegative forms of arthritis including psoriatic arthritis and reactive arthritis as well as from a peripheral arthritis similar to other forms of viral arthritis.

Lyme Disease

Lyme disease is a multisystem illness caused by the tick-borne spirochete *Borrelia burgdorferi.* The characteristic lesion develops within days to weeks of a bite by an infected tick. This lesion is termed *erythema chronicum migrans* and evolves into an annular lesion with a central clearing. Once the organism becomes hematogenously spread, a variety of manifestations can occur, including similar annular lesions in other regions of the body, fever, lymphadenopathy, myalgia, arthralgia, and fatigue. This early phase, even if treated, typically evolves into an intermediate phase, characterized by arthritis, cardiac, and/or neurological involvement. The true arthritis of Lyme disease (in contrast to the arthralgia and myalgias that occur early) develops months after the exposure. This will usually begin as intermittent episodes of inflammatory arthritis involving the large joints and, over years, will progress to become a constant monoarticular or oligoarticular arthritis involving large joints. The knees are frequently involved, and in severe cases, joint erosions and damage may occur.

PHARMACOLOGIC THERAPY

Overview

The basic principle of pharmacologic therapy for any disorder is to use the least toxic and least expensive medication for the illness being treated. This is particularly true for the rheumatic diseases, where there are several relatively nontoxic and inexpensive drugs (e.g., acetaminophen, over-the-counter [OTC] NSAIDs) available that are effective for many conditions.

Two important factors need to be considered when choosing the most appropriate pharmacologic therapy for a patient with a rheumatic problem. The first is whether the problem is local or systemic in nature, and the second is whether the process is inflammatory or noninflammatory. For local problems, topical analgesics or injections may be considered instead of systemic therapy. For noninflammatory conditions, analgesics such as acetaminophen can be considered instead of NSAIDs or other potentially more toxic regimens.

Analgesics

Acetaminophen is an effective and safe analgesic for many noninflammatory rheumatic conditions. For example, in OA, several randomized controlled trials have suggested that this compound is as effective as either the OTC or prescription strength of NSAIDs. The principal toxicity of acetaminophen is hepatic, although this typically occurs in persons either consuming concurrent hepatotoxins (especially alcohol) or exceeding the recommended dose. Tramadol is a moderate-strength analgesic that can be considered in persons who require an analgesic but do not respond to acetaminophen. Finally, narcotics can be effective in both the short- and long-term management of pain, although both tolerance and addiction are potential problems.

NSAIDs

The NSAIDs represent one of the most commonly prescribed classes of drugs. Aspirin is the original and prototypical NSAID. These drugs all act largely by inhibiting cyclooxygenase, the enzyme that transforms arachidonic acid into prostaglandins, prostacyclin, and thromboxane; the clinical relevance of the effects of NSAIDs on lipid metabolism, granulocyte migration, and bradykinin synthesis is less well understood. Although there are now dozens of NSAIDs available, the newer drugs in this class are not necessarily more effective than older ones or even aspirin, but they are generally better tolerated (Table 7.12). The main differences among NSAIDs are (1) half-life, (2) relative potency at the prescribed dose, (3) tolerability, and (4) cost.

When considering the appropriate NSAID, several factors should be considered in regard to the medication's half-life. If a drug is to be used to treat an acute inflammatory conditions (e.g., an attack of gout), a drug with a short half-life and rapid onset of action, such as indomethacin, should be considered. On the other hand, when prescribing NSAIDs for elderly patients, which comprise the subset of NSAID users that develop nearly all of the major GI bleeds and death from this class of drugs, compounds with long half-lives should generally be avoided.

With respect to potency, there again are several factors to consider. The first is that for most NSAIDs, the recommended prescription dose has an anti-inflammatory effect, and one-half to one-third of that dose (the dose that is typically available OTC) has an analgesic effect. One of the most important principles in prescribing this class of drugs is to use the lowest dose possible, because the gastric and renal side effects of these compounds are directly related to the ability of these compounds to block cyclooxygenase. Thus, if one chooses to treat a noninflammatory condition such as OA with this class of drugs, a dose lower than the typical prescription dose usually will be just as efficacious and safer. It is difficult to directly compare the relative potency of one NSAID versus another, because there are no established in vitro assays that predict the relative potency of this class of compounds. But generally, NSAIDs that have been marketed more recently are tested and released at relatively less potent doses than older compounds.

Tolerability is an important issue with respect to NSAIDs and should not be confused with toxicity. There is a general misconception that when a person takes an NSAID and develops dyspepsia, heartburn, or other GI side effects, this person may be developing peptic ulcer disease (PUD). Innumerable studies have demonstrated that there is little relationship between the *symptoms* (i.e., tolerability) that persons develop when they consume an NSAID and the development of PUD. Most persons who develop a major GI bleed from NSAIDs have no symptoms that antedate the bleed, and in fact *symptomatic* persons taking NSAIDs are actually *less likely to have a peptic ulcer* than asymptomatic persons. The reason for this appears to be that the tolerability of an NSAID may be influenced by local factors such as acidity in the GI tract (and thus is improved by taking antacids or H2 blockers, or by enteric coating of tablets), whereas the development of PUD is due to a systemic effect of the NSAID on the production of prostaglandins in the stomach. For this reason, NSAIDs that are administered parenterally are just as likely to cause PUD as orally administered compounds. Misoprostol, a prostaglandin analog, is currently approved as prophylaxis against NSAID-induced gastropathy.

COX-2 inhibitors are a class of NSAIDS developed specifically for prevention of GI side effects. Since cyclooxygenase 1(COX-1) is the enzyme responsible for maintaining gastric epithelial integrity while COX-2 is the major enzyme involved in inflammation, theoretically, compared with nonspecific COX-1/COX-2 inhibitors (traditional NSAIDs), COX-2–specific drugs maintain anti-inflammatory efficacy without damaging the GI tract (Fig. 7.7). These medications still must be used with caution, however, in the presence of renal impairment and cardiovascular disorders. Indeed, while COX-2 inhibitors have gained tremendous popularity over the last decade, serious concerns have arisen regarding their adverse cardiovascular profile, leading to the withdrawal of one of the most popular medications in this group, rofecoxib (Vioxx).

TABLE 7.12
CHARACTERISTICS OF CURRENTLY APPROVED NONSTEROIDAL ANTI-INFLAMMATORY DRUGS (NSAIDS)

Drug (Trade Names)	Indications and Uses	Formulations	Daily Dose	Metabolism	Half-life	Other Considerations
Salicylates						
Aspirin	Arthralgia, dental pain, dysmenorrhea, fever, headache, JRA, migraine, mild pain, myalgia, OA, RA, prevention and treatment of cardiovascular thrombosis	Numerous	Variable, depending on indication; maximum (adults) 2.4–5.4 g/d in four or more divided doses	Hepatic and renal	Acetylsalicylic acid 15–30 min; salicylate 2–30 h	Dose in children body weight <25 kg is 60–90 mg/kg/d. Serum salicylate levels may need to be monitored at higher doses.
Choline magnesium trisalicylate (Trilisate)	Fever, JRA, mild to moderate pain, OA, RA	Solution Tablets	3 g/d in divided doses	Hepatic and renal	Low dose 2–3 h; high dose 15–30 h	Dose in children <37 kg is 50 mg/kg/d Serum salicylate levels may need to be monitored at higher doses.
Salsalate (Disalcid)	Mild to moderate pain OA, RA	Capsules Tablets	2–4 g daily divided dose	Hepatic and renal	1 h	Serum salicylate levels may need to be monitored at higher doses.
Nonselective NSAIDs						
Naproxen (Naprosen, Anaprox)	Ankylosing spondylitis, arthralgia, bursitis, dental pain, dysmenorrhea, fever, gout arthritis, headache, JRA, mild to moderate pain, myalgia, OA, RA, tendinitis	Tablet Extended-release tablet Suspension	500–1,000 mg b.i.d.	Hepatic and renal	10–20 h	Dosage in children aged >2 y is 10–15 mg/kg/d in two divided doses. Naproxen may falsely elevate urinary 17-ketosteroid concentrations and interfere with 5-hydroxyindoleacetic acid determination. Discontinue 72 h before testing.
Flurbiprofen (Ansaid)	Arthralgia, mild-moderate pain, miosis inhibition, myalgia, OA, RA	Tablets Ophthalmic solution	50–100 mg b.i.d. or t.i.d.; maximum 300 mg/d	Hepatic	3–9 h	
Diclofenac (Voltaren, Arthrotec)	Actinic keratoses, allergic conjunctivitis, ankylosing spondylitis, arthralgia, corneal ulcer, dysmenorrhea, headache, keratoconjunctivitis, migraine, mild to moderate pain, myalgia, OA, postoperative ocular inflammation, RA	Tablets Tablets (combination with misoprostol) Ophthalmic solution Topical solution	50–100 mg b.i.d.; maximum 225 mg/d	Hepatic	1–2 h	Cholestyramine reduced bioavailability of diclofenac Diclofenac/misoprostol combination contraindicated in pregnancy because of abortifacient effect of misoprostol
Sulindac (Clinoril)	Ankylosing spondylitis, arthralgia, bursitis, gouty arthritis, moderate pain, OA, RA, tendinitis	Tablets	150–200 mg b.i.d.	Hepatic	8–16 h	Nonindicated use in JRA 2–4 mg/kg/d suggested
Oxaprozin (Daypro)	Moderate pain, OA, RA	Tablets	600–1200 mg q.d.	Hepatic	36–92 h	Nonindicated use in JRA of 10–20 mg/kg/d reported

Diflunisal (Dolobid)	Mild to moderate pain, OA, RA	Tablets	500–1,000 mg b.i.d.	Hepatic	8–12 h 68–138 h in severe renal disease	50% increase in acetaminophen plasma concentration following administration of diflunisal Diflunisal is a salicylic acid derivative, association with Reye syndrome not known. Avoid in children Diflunisal may falsely elevate serum salicylate levels
Piroxicam (Feldene)	Arthralgia, headache, moderate pain, myalgia, OA, RA	Capsule	20 mg q.d.	Hepatic with enterohepatic recirculation	50 h	Particular caution in high-risk individuals
Indomethacin (Indocin)	Ankylosing spondylitis, arthralgia, bursitis, gouty arthritis, moderate pain, myalgia, OA, patent ductus arteriosus, RA, severe pain, tendinitis	Capsules Extended-release capsules Suspension Suppositories Parenteral	25–50 mg t.i.d. to q.i.d.	Hepatic Some enterohepatic recirculation	Biphasic: 1 h initial; 2.6–11.2 h in second phase Prolonged half-life in neonates and premature neonates	Increased serum aminoglycoside concentrations in neonates; monitor aminoglycoside levels closely in all patients Indomethacin augments the hypothalamic—pituitary–adrenal axis response to dexamethasone Possible false-normal results in patients with depressed response
Ibuprofen (Motrin)	Arthralgia, dental pain, dysmenorrhea, fever, headache, JRA, migraine, mild to moderate pain, myalgia, OA, RA	Numerous	Adults: 400–800 mg t.i.d. to q.i.d. Children: 5–10 mg/kg	Hepatic	2–4 h	Safety demonstrated in children 6 mo of age and older
Fenoprofen (Nalfon)	Arthralgia, mild to moderate pain, myalgia, OA, RA	Tablets Capsules	300–600 mg t.i.d. to q.i.d.; maximum 3,200 mg/d	Hepatic Enterohepatic recirculation	2.5–3.0 h	Aspirin can decrease fenoprofen plasma concentrations by 50% and reduce half-life. Phenobarbital can decrease plasma concentrations of fenoprofen. Monitor barbiturate levels after initiation or withdrawal of fenoprofen. Elevated free and total triiodothyronine plasma concentrations by some methods
Etodolac (Lodine)	Arthralgia, bone pain, dental pain, mild pain, moderate pain, myalgia, OA RA	Tablets Extended release tablets	600–1,200 mg daily	Hepatic	6–7 h	
Ketoprofen (Orudis)	Arthralgia, dental pain, dysmenorrhea, fever, headache, mild to moderate pain, myalgia, OA, RA	Capsules Extended release capsules Tablets	75 mg t.i.d. or 50 mg q.i.d.	Hepatic	1.1–4 h	Increased plasma concentration of ketoprofen when administered with probenecid.

(continued)

TABLE 7.12
(Continued)

Drug (Trade Names)	Indications and Uses	Formulations	Daily Dose	Metabolism	Half-life	Other Considerations
Ketorolac (Toradol)	Allergic conjunctivitis, arthralgia, moderate pain, myalgia, ocular pain, ocular pruritus, photophobia, postoperative ocular inflammation	Tablets	30 mg i.m. or i.v. every 6 h; maximum 120 mg/d; do not use for more than 5 days	Hepatic	Biphasic; terminal phase 4–6 h	Elimination half-life of ketorolac is doubled during administration with probenecid. Concomitant use should be avoided.
		Parenteral (i.m. or i.v.) Ophthalmic solution	10 mg p.o. every 4–6 h; maximum of 40 mg daily for 5 days			Parenteral ketorolac can enhance the muscle relaxant effect of nondepolarizing skeletal muscle relaxants. Caution with concomitant use.
Meclofenamate, mefenamic acid (Ponstel)	Arthralgia, dysmenorrhea, mild to moderate pain, OA, RA	Capsule	50–100 mg t.i.d. to q.i.d.; maximum 400 mg/d Mefenamic acid: 250 mg every 6 h for 7 days; maximum 1,250 mg/d	Hepatic	2 h	Mefenamic acid may cause false-positive test result for urinary bile.
Meloxicam (Mobic)	OA	Tablets	7.5–15 mg q.d.	Hepatic	15–30 h	Cholestyramine may increase clearance meloxicam. No platelet inhibition at indicated doses.
Nabumetone (Relafen)	Moderate pain, OA, RA	Tablets	1,000 mg q.d.; maximum dose of 2,000 mg q.d.	Hepatic	24 h	
Tolmetin (Tolectin)	Arthralgia, JRA, moderate pain, myalgia, OA, RA	Tablets Capsules	400 mg t.i.d. to q.i.d.; maximum dose 2,000 mg/d	Hepatic	Biphasic: initial 1–2 h; terminal 5 h	Dosage in children age 2 y and above 5–7 mg/kg/dose p.o. every 6–8 h. False-positive reaction for proteinuria on acid precipitation test; no effect on urine dipstick test for protein.
Selective COX-2 inhibitors						
Celecoxib (Celebrex)	Bone pain, dental pain, dysmenorrhea, FAP, headache, moderate to severe pain, OA, RA	Capsules	100–200 mg b.i.d.; 400 mg b.i.d. in FAP	Hepatic	11 h	Reduce dose by 50% in setting of moderate liver dysfunction. Fluconazole inhibits celecoxib metabolism in the liver. Use lowest celecoxib dose with concomitant fluconazole.
Rofecoxib (Vioxx)	Bone pain, dental pain, dysmenorrhea, headache, mild to moderate pain, OA, RA	Tablet Suspension	12.5–25 mg q.d.; 50 mg q.d. for 5 days for pain	Hepatic	17 h	
Valdecoxib (Bextra)	Dysmenorrhea, OA, RA	Tablet	10 mg q.d.; 20 mg q.d. as needed for dysmenorrhea	Hepatic	8–11 h	

b.i.d., twice daily; FAP, familial adenomatous polyposis; i.m., intramuscularly; i.v., intravenously; JRA, juvenile rheumatoid arthritis; OA, osteoarthritis; p.o., by mouth; q.d., daily; RA, rheumatoid arthritis; t.i.d., three times daily.

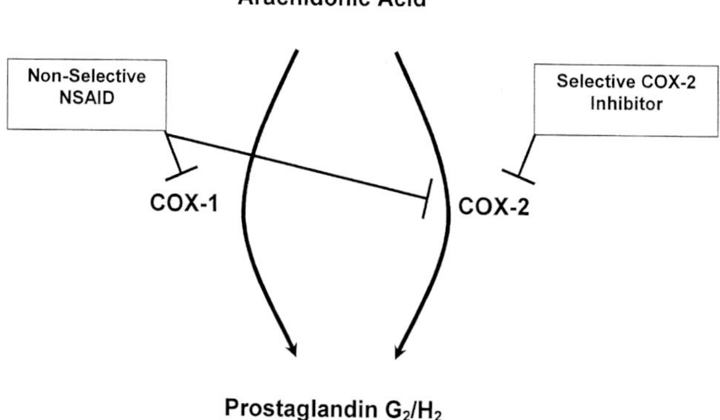

Figure 7.7 Prostaglandin synthesis pathway with sites of nonsteroidal anti-inflammatory drug inhibition. (*Reprinted with permission from* Koopman WJ, Moreland LW. *Arthritis and Allied Conditions: A Textbook of Rheumatology.* 15th ed. Philadelphia: Lippincott Williams & Wilkins, 2005.)

A difficult issue in clinical practice is to decide which patients who are prescribed NSAIDs should also receive prophylaxis against PUD. It is first important to understand which persons are at increased risk of developing this complication. The factors that place a patient at higher risk of developing a GI bleed include a history of PUD, chronic use of antacids or H2 blockers, cigarette smoking, alcohol use, anticoagulant use, concomitant corticosteroid therapy, and being older than 65 years. The more of these risk factors persons have, the more likely they are to develop a major GI bleed. But arguably, the most important risk factor is being elderly. Although elderly persons taking NSAIDs are only approximately 1.5 times as likely to develop a GI bleed as a younger person, nearly all of the mortality from NSAID-associated GI bleeds occurs in persons older than 65 years. The reason for this appears to be that younger persons tolerate GI bleeds better than the elderly, who commonly will develop a myocardial infarction, stroke, or some other major medical event in association with a GI bleed.

The coagulation effects of NSAIDs are also widely misunderstood in clinical practice. Aspirin *irreversibly* binds to cyclooxygenase, so that the inhibition of platelet function that occurs after consuming aspirin lasts until all of the platelets that were exposed to the drug die (approximately 2 weeks). But all other NSAIDs *reversibly* bind to cyclooxygenase, so the antiplatelet effects of these drugs last only while they are in the circulation (i.e., several half-lives). There is no need to stop nonaspirin NSAIDs more than a few days before a surgical procedure to avoid the antiplatelet effects of these drugs.

By far, the most common renal side effect of the NSAIDs is a reversible decline in renal function. This almost always occurs in persons who have diminished baseline renal blood flow, for example, in patients with low cardiac output states, renal artery stenosis, or preexisting renal disease. The reason for the selective occurrence of this side effect in these persons is likely that vasodilatory prostaglandins are produced only by the kidney as a compensation for low renal blood flow. Administering these medications in this setting will decrease local prostaglandin synthesis in the kidney, decrease renal blood flow, and worsen renal function. In some instances, this decline in renal function can be permanent, so NSAIDs should be prescribed with caution in this setting. Concomitant use of angiotensin-converting enzyme inhibitors may exacerbate the reduction in renal function, so extreme care must be exercised when prescribing NSAIDs together with these medications.

Corticosteroids

Because of the potent anti-inflammatory effects of corticosteroids, these drugs are useful for the treatment of a number of local and systemic inflammatory conditions. A thorough review of the mechanism(s) of actions of these drugs is not possible, but these drugs likely act by a variety of mechanisms, including interference with cell adhesion and migration into inflammatory sites; interruption of cell–cell communication; impairment of prostaglandin, leukotriene, and neutrophil superoxide production; and impairment of antigen opsonization and immune complex clearance.

The short-term use of systemic corticosteroids is relatively well tolerated, even at higher doses. Uncommon but serious side effects in this setting may include AVN, psychosis or lesser mood disturbance, hyperglycemia, hypertension, and electrolyte disturbances. In contrast, the long-term uses of corticosteroids, even at low doses, are associated with a plethora of side effects, including osteoporosis, accelerated atherosclerosis, infections, cataracts, skin changes, and others. Because of this, and because of the fact that steroids represent by far the most effective medications to bring inflammatory processes under rapid control, most clinicians attempt to use high doses initially for short periods, followed by as rapid a taper as possible, either with complete discontinuation or to chronic regimens (e.g., less than 7.5 mg of prednisone per day or alternate day dosing) that minimize toxicity.

Another significant problem with chronic steroid usage is suppression of the hypothalamic–pituitary–adrenal (HPA) axis. This can occur with as little as 1 week of high-dose steroid treatment and occurs in nearly all people who receive chronic corticosteroid treatment. This is important because persons with a suppressed HPA axis need to receive exogenous steroids when exposed to stressors, such as undergoing a major surgical procedure. There is no "correct" regimen in this setting, but administering 100 mg of hydrocortisone parenterally on call to the operating room, and 50 mg every 6 hours for 24 hours, then 25 mg every 6 hours for another 24 hours, is more than sufficient in this setting (less aggressive regimens may also be used).

TABLE 7.13
SLOW-ACTING ANTIRHEUMATIC, DISEASE-MODIFYING, AND CYTOTOXIC DRUGS

Drugs	Class	Mechanism of Action
Hydroxychloroquine	Antimalarial	Interferes with intracellular function dependent on acidic microenvironment
Sulfasalazine	Antimicrobial	Exact mechanism unknown
Methotrexate	Antimetabolite	Purine inhibition
Leflunomide	Antimetabolite	Pyrimidine inhibition
Cyclophosphamide, chlorambucil	Alkylating cytotoxics	Active metabolites alkylate DNA
Azathioprine, 6-Mercaptopurine	Purine analog cytotoxics	Inhibit purine synthesis
Cyclosporine, Tacrolimus (FK506)	Calcineurin inhibitors	Inhibit calcium-dependent T-cell activation and interleukin-2 (IL-2) production
Sirolimus (rapamycin)	Non–calcineurin-binding macrolide immunoregulator	Blocks IL-2– and growth factor–mediated signal transduction
Mycophenolate mofetil	Purine synthesis inhibitor	Mycophenolic acid inhibits inosine monophosphate dehydrogenase

SAARDs and Disease-Modifying and Cytotoxic Drugs

Table 7.13 lists a number of SAARDs and cytotoxic drugs that are used in the management of patients with autoimmune disorders. These medications are commonly used in a variety of settings, sometimes as single agents in less aggressive disease (e.g., hydroxychloroquine in mild RA, sulfasalazine in reactive arthritis) or as steroid-sparing drugs (to minimize the usage of long-term steroids) in illnesses such as SLE, vasculitis. As noted earlier, the biological medications, such as anti–TNF-α medications, are becoming increasingly common for the treatment of a large number of rheumatologic disorders, such as RA, AS, and other SSs.

The main reason that the practicing orthopaedist needs to be aware of these medications is because of their effects on wound healing and infections (especially perioperative). Although it is commonly felt that many of these drugs (e.g., high-dose corticosteroids, methotrexate) may increase the rate of perioperative infections, the data to support this are largely anecdotal. Nonetheless, most clinicians will attempt to stop methotrexate for 1 week prior to, and 2 weeks after, major surgical procedures. With respect to corticosteroids, there is typically an attempt to get the patient to the lowest dose possible prior to surgery.

RECOMMENDED READINGS

Clauw DJ. Fibromyalgia: update on mechanisms and management. *J Clin Rheumatol.* 2007;13(2):102–109.
Drazen JM. COX-2 inhibitors—a lesson in unexpected problems. *N Engl J Med.* 2005;352(11):1131–1132.
Felson DT, Lawrence RC, Dieppe PA, et al. Osteoarthritis: new insights, I: the disease and its risk factors. *Ann Intern Med.* 2000;133(8):635–646.
O'Dell JR. Therapeutic strategies for rheumatoid arthritis. *N Engl J Med.* 2004;350(25):2591–2602.
Olsen NJ, Stein CM. New drugs for rheumatoid arthritis. *N Engl J Med.* 2004;350(21):2167–2179.
Rahman A, Isenberg DA. Systemic lupus erythematosus. *N Engl J Med.* 2008;358(9):929–939.
Rice PA. Gonococcal arthritis (disseminated gonococcal infection). *Infect Dis Clin North Am.* 2005;19(4):853–861.
Schumacher HR. Crystal-induced arthritis: an overview. *Am J Med.* 1996;100(2A):46S–52S.
van Vollenhoven RF. Corticosteroids in rheumatic disease: understanding their effects is key to their use. *Postgrad Med.* 1998;103(2):137–142.

Overview of Musculoskeletal Neoplasms

8

Atul F. Kamath   Harish S. Hosalkar   Richard D. Lackman

INTRODUCTION

Tumors of the musculoskeletal system may present initially with nonspecific symptoms, making it hard to distinguish neoplastic manifestations from other common disorders. While bone and soft-tissue tumors are rare, it is critically important that the orthopaedist include these entities in the differential diagnosis to avoid overlooking these potential serious conditions.

This chapter presents a systematic method for evaluating tumors of the musculoskeletal system. It also presents a brief overview of the distinguishing characteristics, pathology, and treatment of several of the most common entities.

BONE TUMORS

Patient Evaluation

In the evaluation of a patient with a bone tumor, there are several areas where data can be gathered that impact upon the differential diagnosis. These include the history, physical examination, and review of imaging studies. Ultimately, it may be determined that histologic confirmation is required at which time careful evaluation of lesional tissue will confirm a specific diagnosis.

The history associated with the presence of a musculoskeletal tumor defines the clinical context of the lesion. Age, sex, duration of symptoms, presence and quality of pain, history of trauma, weight loss, smoking history, and history of prior malignancy are all important historical factors. Critical to the early diagnosis of a skeletal tumor is an appreciation of the fact that the early symptoms associated with skeletal neoplasms mimic all types of ordinary musculoskeletal disorders. Any pain that extends beyond the expected duration associated with a tentative diagnosis should raise the suspicion of an underlying tumor. Night pain is another red flag again leading to the supposition of an occult lesion although many nonneoplastic conditions may also cause pain at night.

One of the most disorienting parts of a history in a patient with an occult tumor is a history of trauma. Frequently, patients will experience some mild trauma to the affected area and then notice pain that would probably not have occurred in the absence of an underlying lesion. This is frequently not clear to the patient however who directly attributes the local symptoms and findings to the traumatic event. The history related in this way frequently fools a treating physician who then follows the local lesion until it becomes obvious that the true nature of the lesion goes well beyond a minor trauma. An example of this is the story related by a waiter who kicked a kitchen door to open it while carrying a heavy tray. The door was stuck and did not move, resulting in an apparent calf injury. When the pain did not resolve, a compartment syndrome was suspected and it was not until several months later that tissue was obtained which revealed an underlying lymphoma. Similar is the history of an elderly female on full-dose warfarin for a mechanical heart valve who bumped her thigh on a kitchen table and found out months later that the large anterior thigh mass was a soft-tissue sarcoma and not a simple hematoma.

Imaging

Plain radiographs offer detailed information for bone lesions, as well as some potentially important information for soft-tissue lesions. It is estimated that about 30% to 40% of the bone must be destroyed before the changes can be seen in plain radiographs. It is useful to ask the following when evaluating plain radiographs of bony lesions: Where is the lesion located in the bone? What is the lesion doing to the bone? How is the bone reacting to the lesion? What is the periosteal response?

A lesion's margin with adjacent medullary bone may suggest an indolent versus an aggressive process. Any lesion that is stable and recognized by the bone as foreign will be "walled off" by dense sclerotic bone, implying a very slow growing or static lesion. However, lesions not recognized as foreign will not generate surrounding sclerosis despite being present for extended periods. A benign enchondroma, for example, elicits no surrounding bone response because it is not considered "foreign." Multiple myeloma is a malignant tumor but still elicits no response in the marrow, as plasma cells are a normal part of marrow and hence not recognized as foreign.

Marrow response to a lesion is the most sensitive for characterizing aggressive lesions. Marrow surrounding a lesion may demonstrate a geographic (e.g., in multiple myeloma), moth-eaten (e.g., in giant cell tumor), or permeative (e.g., in osteosarcoma) appearance based on the degree and nature of the offending lesion. The cortex exists as a more gross marker of malignant damage to bone, including endosteal scalloping, cortical thinning or expansion, and of course gross cortical destruction. The pattern of periosteal reaction itself is also an indicator of the biologic activity of a lesion. A lesion may elicit no reaction for one of two reasons: either the tumor is not permeating the periosteum (e.g., in giant cell tumor) or the periosteum does not recognize the tumor cells as foreign (e.g., in lymphoma).

Although no single periosteal reaction is unique for a given tumor, a continuous periosteal reaction indicates a long-standing (slow-growing) benign process. An interrupted reaction, on the other hand, is commonly seen in malignant tumors. In these malignant tumors, the periosteal response may appear in an onionskin (lamellated) or sunburst pattern. Codman's triangle, a classic reactive periosteal cuff at the periphery of the tumor, may also be seen. Some unique radiographic findings that point toward specific differential diagnoses are listed in Table 8.1.

TABLE 8.1

DIFFERENTIAL DIAGNOSES ASSOCIATED WITH SPECIFIC RADIOGRAPHIC FINDINGS

- Sclerotic soap bubble lesion in the anterior cortex of the shaft of the tibia: adamantinoma versus cortical fibrous dysplasia
- Sclerotic lesion with a central lytic nidus: osteoid osteoma versus stress fracture versus infection. Since many stress fractures or stress reactions involve intramedullary edema, they can mimic lymphomas. Sequential MRI (magnetic resonance imaging) scans will demonstrate healing of a stress reaction but no healing of a lymphoma that may appear stable or progressive.
- Cauliflower exophytic lesion: cauliflower osteochondroma versus secondary chondrosarcoma arising in an osteochondroma. Remember to measure the thickness of the cartilage cap.
- Multiple lesions in bone: metastases, myeloma, enchondromas, histiocytosis, fibrous dysplasia, nonossifying fibromas
- Lytic lesion in the humeral shaft in a child with no periosteal reaction: simple bone cyst
- Lytic lesions in the sacrum: chordoma, chondrosarcoma, giant cell tumor, metastasis, myeloma
- Calcified lesion on the surface of a bone: osteochondroma, periosteal osteosarcoma, parosteal osteosarcoma, myositis ossificans, periosteal chondroma, periosteal chondrosarcoma
- Aggressive meta-epiphyseal lesion in young patients (<30 years): osteosarcoma, Ewing sarcoma, infection, aneurysmal bone cyst, giant cell tumor
- Aggressive meta-epiphyseal lesion in older patients (>30 years): osteosarcoma, chondrosarcoma, metastasis, adult round cell tumors, giant cell tumor
- Lytic lesion in the epiphysis of a child with edema seen on MRI: chondroblastoma versus infection

Computed Tomography

The major value of a CT scan is to show fine detail in bone. This includes bone formation as well as bone destruction. In addition, CT scans are the best study to see whether or not soft-tissue calcification is present. It is not optimal for looking for the extent of a permeative lesion in bone or soft-tissue extension from a bone lesion. CT may be particularly helpful in difficult imaging areas, such as the pelvis, sacrum, and vertebrae.

Magnetic Resonance Imaging

For bone-forming tumors, magnetic resonance imaging (MRI) scans are excellent for showing the extent of a lesion in bone, the presence and extent of edema within or around bone, and the presence or absence of an associated soft-tissue component. MRI is the study of choice for any soft-tissue lesion. The addition of contrast to an MRI scan can also help elucidate areas of cyst formation, which do not contrast enhance (but may show rim enhancement), from areas of solid tumor which frequently enhance. One exception to this are chondroid lesions, such as low-grade chondrosarcoma, which may also show rim enhancement with little internal enhancement and thus mimic a cyst.

One must always be careful in differentiating between edema in bone and tumor in bone. For example, lymphoma frequently presents as high signal in marrow and must be in the differential of traumatic marrow lesions such as stress fracture. A lesion suspected to represent edema in bone should be followed by MR imaging to resolution, and a lack of resolution should suggest the need for a biopsy.

Technetium Bone Scan

Bone scans are most useful when utilized as a skeletal survey tool to look for the total number of lesions present or when a singular lesion is suspected but not seen on initial x-ray. Most active lesions that either form bone or generate a bone reaction are hot, whereas some lytic lesions that engender no bone reaction may be normal or cold (e.g., myeloma).

Positron Emission Tomography

Positron emission tomography, or PET imaging, represents another tool in the diagnostic armamentarium. Based on radionucleotide tracing of metabolic activity, it can be used in the diagnosis and sequential evaluation of bone and soft-tissue tumors. The role of PET imaging in musculoskeletal oncology continues to evolve.

Biopsy

Not all lesions require a biopsy, as many benign and inactive lesions may be diagnosed via imaging studies alone. The ideal biopsy is one that provides all tissues needed to establish a histologic diagnosis without affecting subsequent treatment options. Current biopsy options include both open and needle techniques. In most locations, the carefully performed open biopsy is still the gold standard, while needle biopsy techniques are gaining in popularity. The advantage of a needle biopsy is that it minimizes tissue contamination in the local tissues surrounding a tumor. Needle techniques also minimize the need for anesthesia and can frequently be done outside an operating room, minimizing expense. Problems associated with needle biopsies include sampling error and a frequent inability to obtain sufficient tissue to make a definitive histologic diagnosis.

Another question that arises, especially with open biopsy, concerns who should perform the biopsy. Not all musculoskeletal biopsies can be performed by orthopaedic oncologists, and so how does one decide whether to perform a biopsy locally in the context of a general orthopaedic practice or to refer the biopsy to a subspecialty trained surgeon? In general, if a surgeon sees a patient and knows from the initial imaging studies that this is a lesion that he or she would not treat primarily, then the biopsy is best referred to the treating surgeon.

For example, if a community orthopaedic surgeon sees an adolescent with an obvious osteosarcoma of the femur that would not be appropriate to treat locally, then that biopsy is best referred to the oncologist who will perform the definitive treatment. The same may be true for a large deep mass thought to most likely represent a soft-tissue sarcoma. Regardless of who performs the biopsy, Table 8.2 lists several fairly simple rules that must be adhered to rigorously in order to avoid subsequent problems.

TABLE 8.2
GUIDELINES FOR BIOPSY

1. Make a small incision over the lesion in a manner that does not contaminate neurovascular structures.
2. The incision should be in line with a reasonable resection incision and typically should be longitudinal (not transverse) on the extremities.
3. In dealing with sufficiently large anatomic structures such as in the thigh or leg, it is better to go through one structure than between two, which would contaminate both.
4. Utilize minimal retraction so as to minimize adjacent tissue contamination with tumor.
5. Always make a small hole in a tumor capsule, especially if there is no tourniquet above the lesion, in order to minimize bleeding, which can be substantial.
6. Never use an Esmarch bandage over a tumor, as it could rupture the tumor into surrounding tissues.
7. Obtain a frozen section on the tissue obtained to make certain that you have diagnostic material.
8. If a drain is necessary, bring it out a short distance from either end of the incision inline with the incision so that the drain tract can be easily excised with a subsequent resection incision.
9. Perform a meticulous, watertight closure to prevent oozing and to promote primary healing of the biopsy to facilitate further treatment.

Staging

Staging of a patient with a suspected malignant tumor is mandatory prior to definitive treatment. Fully characterizing a lesion and its differential diagnosis prior to surgical biopsy prevents making wrong decisions that may alter the eventual outcome and management. Staging studies for bone and soft-tissue sarcomas usually includes a CT scan of the chest and an MRI of the primary lesion. Other studies such as a CT scan of the abdomen and pelvis or a technetium bone scan may also be indicated, depending on the specific diagnosis and the propensity of the tumor in question to metastasize to areas other than the lung. The Musculoskeletal Tumor Society adopted the Enneking Surgical Staging System for bone sarcomas (Table 8.3). A whole bone, a joint, or a functional muscle group with a fascial boundary is each considered a separate compartment in this staging system.

TABLE 8.3
ENNEKING SURGICAL STAGING SYSTEM FOR BONE SARCOMAS (1986)

Stage	Grade	Site
I	Low	A: Intracompartmental B: Extracompartmental
II	High	A: Intracompartmental B: Extracompartmental
III	Any grade with regional or distant metastasis	Any

TABLE 8.4
RADIOGRAPHIC DIFFERENTIAL DIAGNOSES OF BONE LESIONS

Bone-Forming Tumors	Cartilage-Forming Tumors	"Third List"
■ Osteoid osteoma ■ Osteoblastoma ■ Osteochondroma ■ Osteosarcoma ■ Blastic metastases ■ Paget's disease	■ Osteochondroma ■ Chondromyxoid Fibroma ■ Chondroblastoma ■ Enchondroma ■ Chondrosarcoma	■ Infection ■ Metastasis ■ Round cell tumors ■ Ewing sarcoma ■ Lymphoma ■ Myeloma ■ Neuroblastoma ■ Fibrous dysplasia ■ Nonossifying fibroma ■ Simple bone cyst ■ Aneurysmal bone cyst ■ Eosinophilic granuloma (histiocytosis) ■ Giant cell tumor ■ Stress fracture ■ Metabolic condition ■ Hemangioma

Differential Diagnosis

It is only through intellectual discipline and diligence that early diagnoses can be accomplished. The easiest way to assemble a complete differential is to have memorized or available a reasonable list of common lesions to review as you contemplate each set of x-rays. Without such mental organization, it is difficult or impossible to assemble a comprehensive differential diagnosis of a particular lesion. Table 8.4 contains a list of common neoplasms found in bone separated into bone-forming lesions, cartilage-forming lesions, and a "third list" of miscellaneous lesions. By going through these lists each time an x-ray is reviewed, one can make sure to include most relevant lesions in a specific differential diagnosis. Primary bone tumors can also be classified based on their direction of differentiation (Table 8.5).

TABLE 8.5
CLASSIFICATION OF MUSCULOSKELETAL TUMORS BASED ON ORIGIN

Bone tumors
- **Bone origin:** osteoid osteoma, osteoblastoma, osteosarcoma
- **Cartilaginous origin:** osteochondroma, chondroblastoma, chondromyxoid fibroma, enchondroma, periosteal chondroma, chondrosarcoma
- **Fibrous origin:** nonossifying fibroma, fibrous dysplasia, osteofibrous dysplasia, desmoplastic fibroma, fibrosarcoma
- **Miscellaneous:** unicameral bone cyst, aneurysmal bone cyst, giant cell tumor, Langerhans cell histiocytosis, Ewing sarcoma

Musculoskeletal manifestations of leukemia
Bone lymphomas
Metastatic tumors: neuroblastoma, retinoblastoma, hepatoblastoma, lung, renal, prostate, breast, thyroid

The anatomic location of a bone tumor is also helpful in narrowing the differential diagnosis, as most tumors have a predilection for certain bone and even certain locations within those bones. Within a bone, a tumor may be epiphyseal, metaphyseal, or diaphyseal, and central or eccentric. Table 8.6 classifies the common bone lesions based on anatomic location.

In order to include or exclude lesions in a differential diagnosis it is imperative that the orthopaedist have a clear

TABLE 8.6
COMMON LOCATIONS OF BONE TUMORS

Epiphysis Pelvis
- Chondroblastoma, Ewing sarcoma
- Brodie's abscess of the epiphysis, osteosarcoma
- Giant cell tumor, osteochondroma
- Fibrous dysplasia, metastasis

Metaphysis, fibrous dysplasia
- Any tumor, anterior elements of spine

Diaphysis, Langerhans cell histiocytosis
- Fibrous dysplasia, leukemia
- Osteofibrous dysplasia, adamantinoma metastatic
- Langerhans cell histiocytosis, giant cell tumor
- Ewing sarcoma, posterior elements of spine
- Leukemia, lymphoma, aneurysmal bone cyst
- *Occasional diaphyseal*, osteoblastoma
- Osteoid osteoma, osteoid osteoma
- Unicameral bone cyst, rib

Multiple fibrous dysplasia
- Leukemia (metastasis), Langerhans cell histiocytosis
- Multiple hereditary exostoses, Ewing sarcoma
- Langerhans cell histiocytosis, metastasis
- Polyostotic fibrous dysplasia
- Enchondromatosis

image of each archetype lesion as well as an appreciation of the variability possible within the range of presentations. It is also important to keep in mind that not all bone forming tumors will show obvious bone formation on an x-ray and the same is true of chondroid lesions, which also may show no obvious chondroid calcification on plain x-ray. The following sections present the various types of bone tumors. Each section describes the incidence, clinical presentation, diagnostic workup, and brief treatment plan for each type of tumor. These sections do not attempt to present all possible lesions; rather, there is a focus on more common lesions, on the spectrum of disease, and on the underlying diagnostic themes. Radiographic images are included to demonstrate the classic appearance of these lesions. The benign tumors of the bone for each of the three categories outlined in Table 8.4 are presented first, followed by malignant lesions.

BENIGN BONE LESIONS

Bone Forming

Osteoid Osteoma

Osteoid osteoma (Fig. 8.1) is a common benign bone tumor that affects mostly children and young adults. Osteoid osteomas are associated with a classic pattern of constant pain, especially night pain, which is relieved very effectively but for short periods with prostaglandin inhibiting drugs, such as aspirin and other nonsteroidal anti-inflammatory drugs (NSAIDs). The femur, tibia, and posterior spine are the most common sites.

The lesions appear as a small lytic nidus often with a "target" appearance surrounded by significant sclerosis. The "nidus" may be small and difficult to find on x-ray; it usually appears as a small focus (3 to 5 mm in diameter) surrounded by significant sclerosis. CT scans with fine cuts (i.e., 1 mm) are the study of choice for finding the lesion. Bone scintigraphy shows focal intense uptake. If NSAID use is not tolerated or significant pain persists, surgical treatment, including excision or radiofrequency ablation, may be used. If the lesion is in a location where RFA or surgical excision is excessively hazardous or morbid, medical treatment with long-term NSAIDs is reasonable and most lesions become asymptomatic via spontaneous regression within 4 years.

Osteoblastoma

Osteoblastoma is most often seen in the posterior elements of the spine or in the meta-diaphyseal region of long bones. Radiographically, osteoblastoma appears more lytic and destructive than osteoid osteoma. The nidus is usually 1 to 2 cm or occasionally larger and has a less sclerotic surrounding bone. Histologically, osteoblastoma is nearly identical to osteoid osteoma, showing excessive osteoblastic activity and osteoid formation with numerous giant cells in a vascular fibrous stroma. Marginal resection or curettage and bone grafting usually provide an acceptable long-term result, though recurrence is not uncommon.

Osteochondroma (Exostosis)

Osteochondromas (Fig. 8.2) are formed by radial growth of bone during childhood such that the lesion grows out

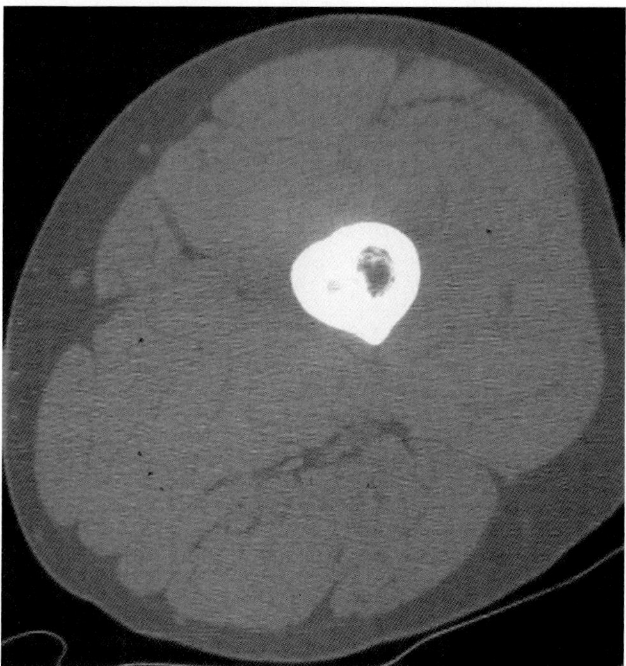

A

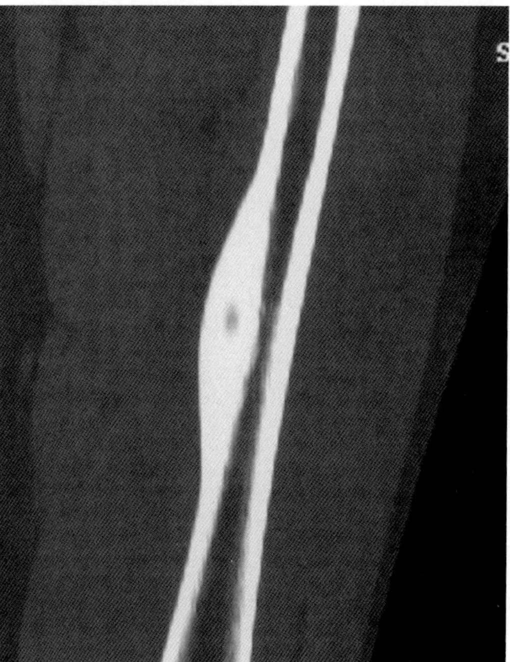

B

Figure 8.1 Osteoid osteoma. Axial and coronal CT (computed tomography) images demonstrating the classic nidus with surrounding sclerosis of an ostoid osteoma.

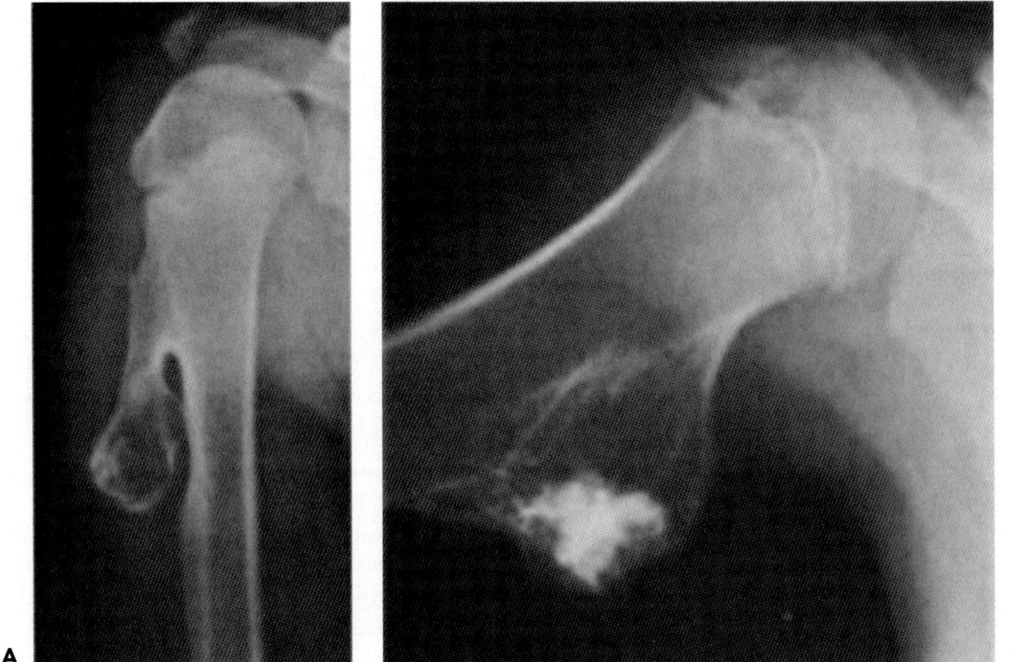

Figure 8.2 Pedunculated **(A)** and sessile **(B)** osteochondromas of the proximal humerus. (*Reprinted with permission from* Greenspan A, Remagen W. *Differential Diagnosis of Tumors and Tumor-like Lesions of Bones and Joints.* Philadelphia, PA: Lippincott-Raven, 1998:148.)

away from the bone at an angle from the adjacent growth plate. The cortex of the bone is continuous with the cortex of the lesion, and the medullary canals are also continuous. This stands in contrast with parosteal osteosarcoma, for example, which grows on the surface of an intact cortex. These lesions can be sessile (broad based) or pedunculated (narrow based). Those that grow out of the flat bones or the proximal femurs can be very large and take on a "cauliflower" appearance. Secondary chondrosarcomatous degeneration should be suspected in any osteochondroma in an adult, which grows or has a large (greater than 2.5 cm) and growing cartilage cap. Pain is also concerning in terms of potential malignant transformation but also occurs commonly in benign osteochondromas due to pressure on adjacent structures. Multiple hereditary exostoses is a rare, autosomal dominant disorder characterized by multiple osteochondroma throughout the body; malignant degeneration is more common in this inherited condition than in solitary lesions (up to 28% vs. less than 1%, respectively) Treatment in most cases is observation. Surgery may be indicated for pain, deformity, or malignant degeneration.

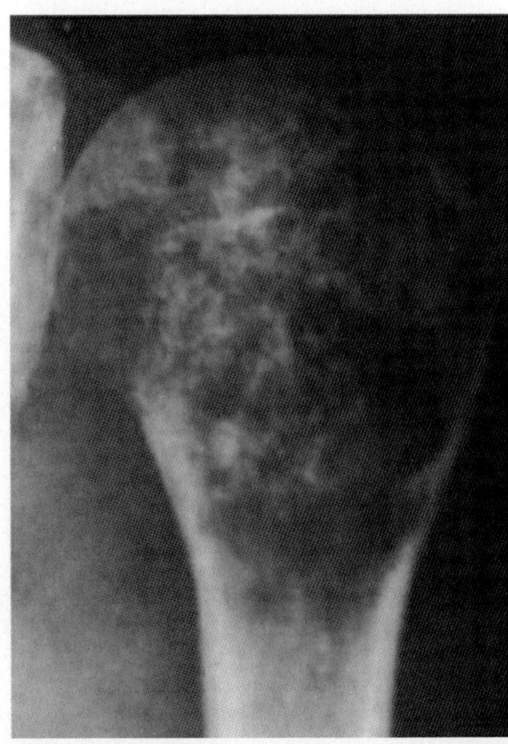

Figure 8.3 An enchondroma is a nest of cartilage tissue typically in the metaphysis of a long bone that is usually encountered as an incidental finding. (*Reprinted with permission from* Greenspan A, Remagen W. *Differential Diagnosis of Tumors and Tumor-like Lesions of Bones and Joints.* Philadelphia, PA: Lippincott-Raven, 1998:124.)

Chondroid Forming

Enchondroma

Enchondroma (Fig. 8.3) is a nest of cartilage tissue typically in the metaphysis but occasionally diaphyseal that is usually encountered as an incidental finding. Enchondromas are most common in the short tubular bones of the hands and in the femur and humerus. These lesions tend to be noncalcified or minimally calcified in young adults and usually show an increase in calcification but not an increase in size with follow-up over many years. The calcification has a typical stippled or "popcorn" pattern. Enchondroma scan be difficult to distinguish from low-grade chondrosacromas, both radiographically and histologically.

The hallmarks of chondrosarcoma include more aggressive radiographic factors, such as intralesional lysis, endosteal scalloping, cortical thinning, erosion, or expansion; clinically, pain distinguishes chondrosarcomas from benign enchondroma. Multiple enchondromas are rare but exist in Maffucci's syndrome (multiple enchondromas associated with systemic hemangiomas) or Ollier's disease (multiple enchondromas, typically on one side of the body). These patients have a higher rate of malignant degeneration to chondrosarcoma than do those with solitary enchondromas.

Chondroblastoma

Chondroblastoma (Fig. 8.4) typically presents as a painful lytic lesion in the epiphysis of a child, with significant edema seen on MRI scan. In adolescents it can occasionally grow across an old epiphyseal line to involve the adjacent metaphysis. The most common locations are the distal femur, proximal tibia, and proximal humerus. The picture of a painful epiphyseal lytic lesion with abundant edema may cause this lesion to be confused with infection or even osteochondritis dessicans. Malignant degeneration is extremely rare. Treatment consists of intralesional curettage and bone grafting.

"Third List"

Aneurysmal Bone Cyst

Aneurysmal bone cyst (ABC) (Fig. 8.5) is a nonneoplastic reactive condition that is usually found in the first three decades of life. ABCs occur in bone as a primary *de novo* lesion, or they may occur in association with other vascular tumors, such as giant cell tumor, Ewing sarcoma, osteosarcoma, or metastatic renal cell carcinoma. Primary lesions usually occur in the metaphyses of long bones, especially in the femur and tibia, but they may also be seen in the posterior spine. Patients typically present with pain and swelling. The classic radiographic finding is an eccentric, lytic, ballooning expansion within the metaphysis. Lesions frequently have a delicate rim of expanded cortical bone, which may be best seen on CT scan; fluid–fluid levels within the lesion are usually seen on MRI scans. Typical histologic features are blood-filled spaces without endothelial lining. Not all lesions require treatment as they sometimes reach an inactive state. Treatment is curettage and bone grafting, with a reasonably high rate of local recurrence (25% or more). In light of the vascular nature of these lesions, embolization has also been reported as a helpful adjuvant or as primary treatment for lesions of the spine where surgery may carry significant morbidity.

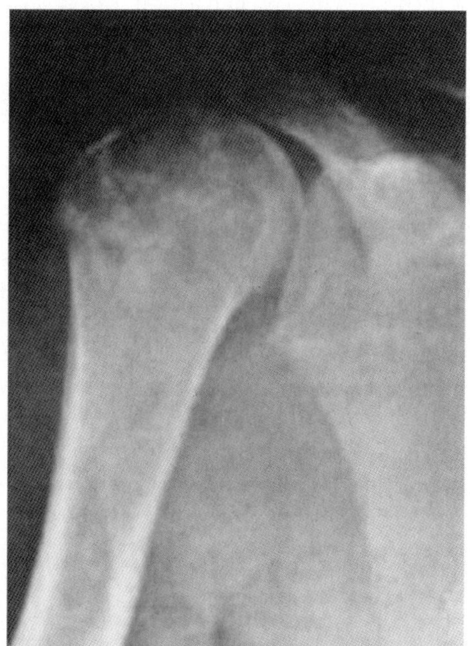
A

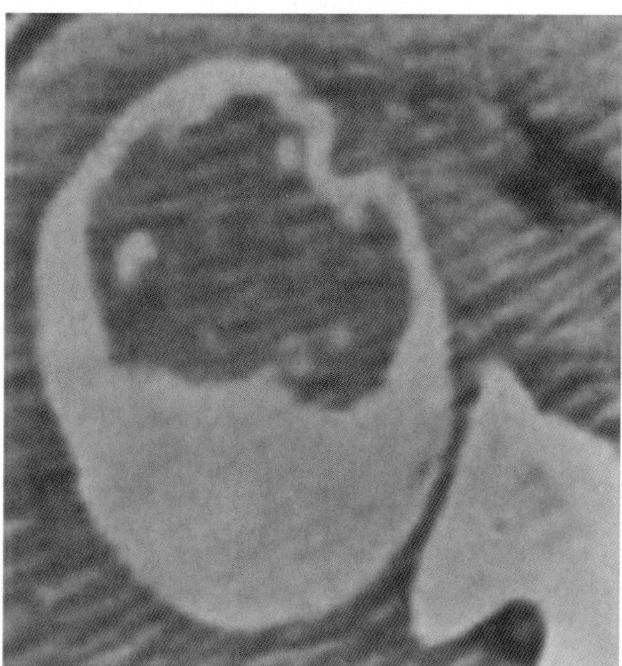
B

Figure 8.4 Chondroblastoma. **A:** Radiograph of lesion in proximal humeral epiphysis. **B:** CT (computed tomography) shows the calcifications clearly. (*Reprinted with permission from* Greenspan A, Remagen W. *Differential Diagnosis of Tumors and Tumor-like Lesions of Bones and Joints.* Philadelphia, PA: Lippincott-Raven, 1998:161.)

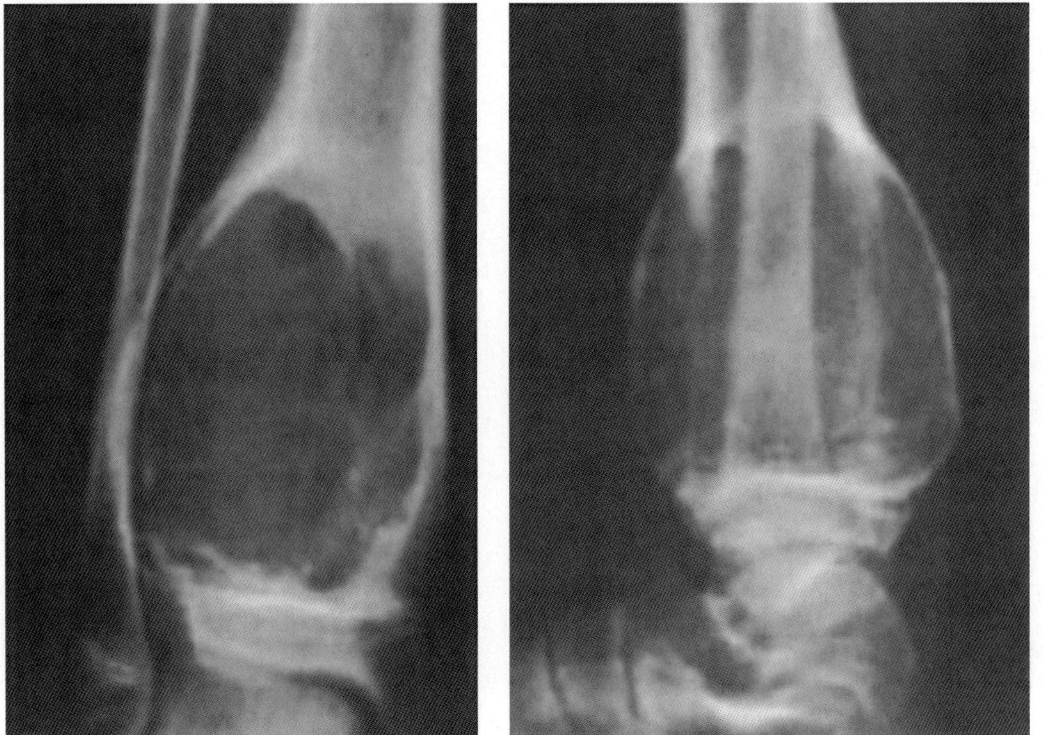

Figure 8.5 Anteroposterior (AP) and lateral radiographs demonstrating an aneurismal bone cyst of the distal tibia. (*Reprinted with permission from* Greenspan A, Remagen W. *Differential Diagnosis of Tumors and Tumor-like Lesions of Bones and Joints*. Philadelphia, PA: Lippincott-Raven, 1998:331.)

Simple Bone Cyst

Simple bone cyst (Fig. 8.6), or unicameral bone cyst, is a common lesion that presents in the first two decades of life. Simple bone cysts are a frequent cause of pathologic fracture in children and are frequently asymptomatic until fracture. The lesions occur almost exclusively in the metaphases of long bones, especially in the proximal humerus, proximal femur, and proximal tibia. Radiographically, they appear as a central, full-width lytic area with symmetric cortical thinning and slight expansion of the bone. Unlike ABCs, they are rarely wider than the width of the adjacent physeal plate. The fallen leaf sign—signifying a piece of cortical bone that fell into the intramedullary cyst as a result of fracture—is often seen. Simple bone cysts usually heal without intervention by the time of skeletal maturity, allowing for observation in most cases. Larger lesions or those in weight-bearing locations can be treated with repeated aspiration and injection with methylprednisolone, bone marrow or bone substitute, or with curettage and bone grafting.

Eosinophilic Granuloma

Also known as solitary Langerhan's cell histiocytosis (LCH), eosinophilic granuloma (Fig. 8.7 A+B) is the most benign member of a group of disorders of the reticuloendothelial system, including Hand–Schuller–Christian and Letterer–Siwe syndromes. LCH is a self-limiting process that can lead to focal destruction of bone. It is most prevalent in the first and second decades, with half of patients younger than 10 years. Lesions are most common in the skull, although virtually any bone may be affected; vertebral involvement occurs in approximately 10% to 15% of cases. The most common appearance is a well-circumscribed marrow lesion with no periosteal reaction. Larger lesions may demonstrate a moth-eaten pattern with some sclerosis. Occasionally, a periosteal reaction is produced in accordance with the inflammatory nature of the lesion. In the spine, LCH often presents as complete collapse of the vertebral body without spine deformity, which is classically referred to as "vertebra plana." While LCH is the most common cause of vertebra plana, malignant neoplasms and occasionally infections may mimic this appearance. Treatment of symptomatic lesions includes curettage and bone grafting. Local steroid injections have also been used. Chemotherapy is recommended in cases of disseminated LCH.

Nonossifying Fibroma

Nonossifying fibroma (Fig. 8.8), or metaphyseal fibrous defect, is a benign lesion left behind by the growth plate in the course of endochondral ossification. As such, it is never seen in the epiphysis. It is commonly seen in the lower extremity of children as an eccentric metaphyseal lesion with a geographic margin and surrounding sclerosis. As growth of the patient continues and external remodeling occurs, lesions that were previously intramedullary in the metaphysis become intra-cortical in the meta-diaphysis. When this occurs, cortical thinning is seen as the remodeling bone grows into the lesion. While most of these

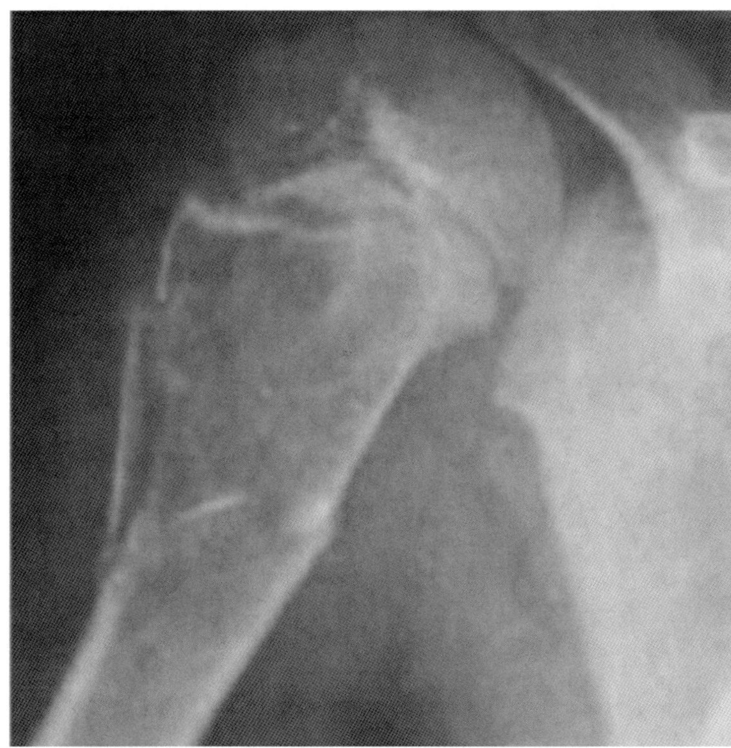
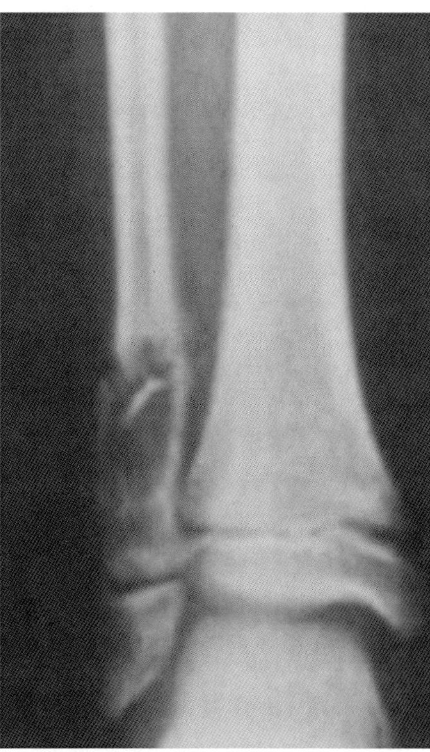

Figure 8.6 Simple bone cyst: "fallen fragment". **A:** Pathologic fracture of proximal humeral diaphysis. **B:** Radiolucent lesion in the distal diaphysis of the fibula. (*Reprinted with permission from* Greenspan A, Remagen W. *Differential Diagnosis of Tumors and Tumor-like Lesions of Bones and Joints.* Philadelphia, PA: Lippincott-Raven, 1998:325.)

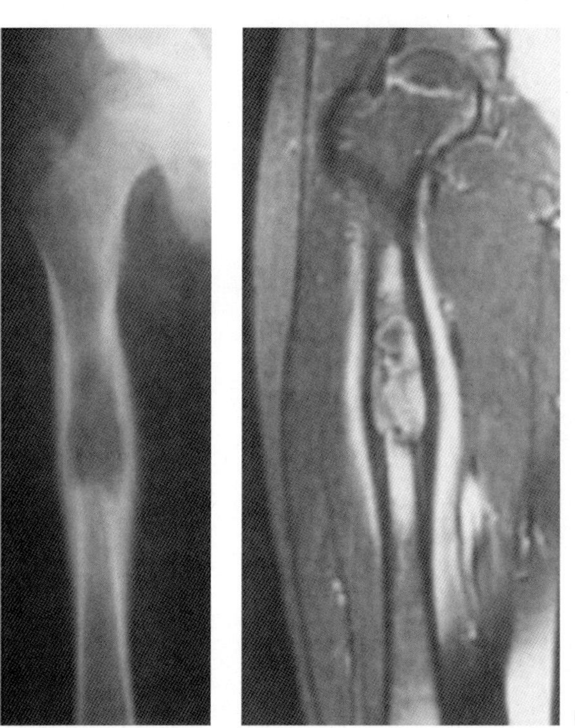

Figure 8.7 Anteroposterior (AP) x-ray **(A)** and coronal MRI (magnetic resonance imaging) **(B)** scan demonstrating an eosinophilic granuloma. (*Reprinted with permission from* Greenspan A, Remagen W. *Differential Diagnosis of Tumors and Tumor-like Lesions of Bones and Joints.* Philadelphia, PA: Lippincott-Raven, 1998: 251.)

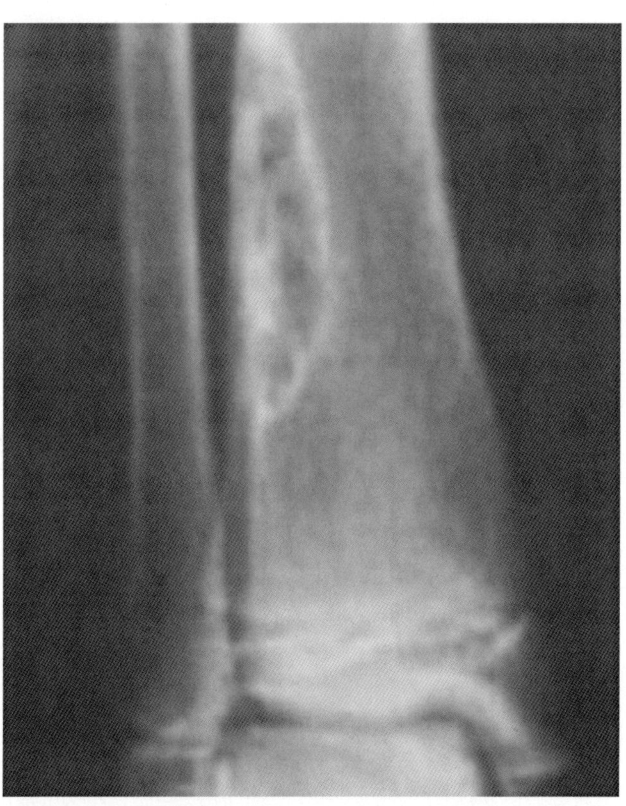

Figure 8.8 A nonossifying fibroma of the distal tibia. (*Reprinted with permission from* Greenspan A, Remagen W. *Differential Diagnosis of Tumors and Tumor-like Lesions of Bones and Joints.* Philadelphia, PA: Lippincott-Raven, 1998:207.)

lesions are asymptomatic, incidental findings requiring only observation, larger lesions may cause mechanical pain. In this small percentage of patients, curettage and bone grafting may be needed to stop the symptoms.

Giant Cell Tumor

Giant cell tumors (Fig. 8.9) are benign but locally aggressive lesions that occur in the juxta-articular regions of skeletally mature individuals. The most common locations are about the knee; the distal femur and proximal tibia account for about 50% of all cases. The distal radius, pelvis, and sacrum can also be involved. Pain is common, and pathologic fracture can occur. Despite its benign classification, the tumor can metastasize to the lungs in approximately 2% of cases. Located at the metaphyseal–epiphyseal junction, these lesions appear on radiographs as lytic, juxta-articular lesions with moth-eaten margins and cortical thinning but usually no periosteal reaction. Histologically, the lesion is composed of multinucleated giant cells and mononuclear stromal cells, such that the nuclei in both cell populations are identical. Currently, most lesions are treated with aggressive intra-lesional surgery; this includes the creation of a large cortical window, followed by curettage and burring. Adjuvants, such as phenol or liquid nitrogen, are popular, but

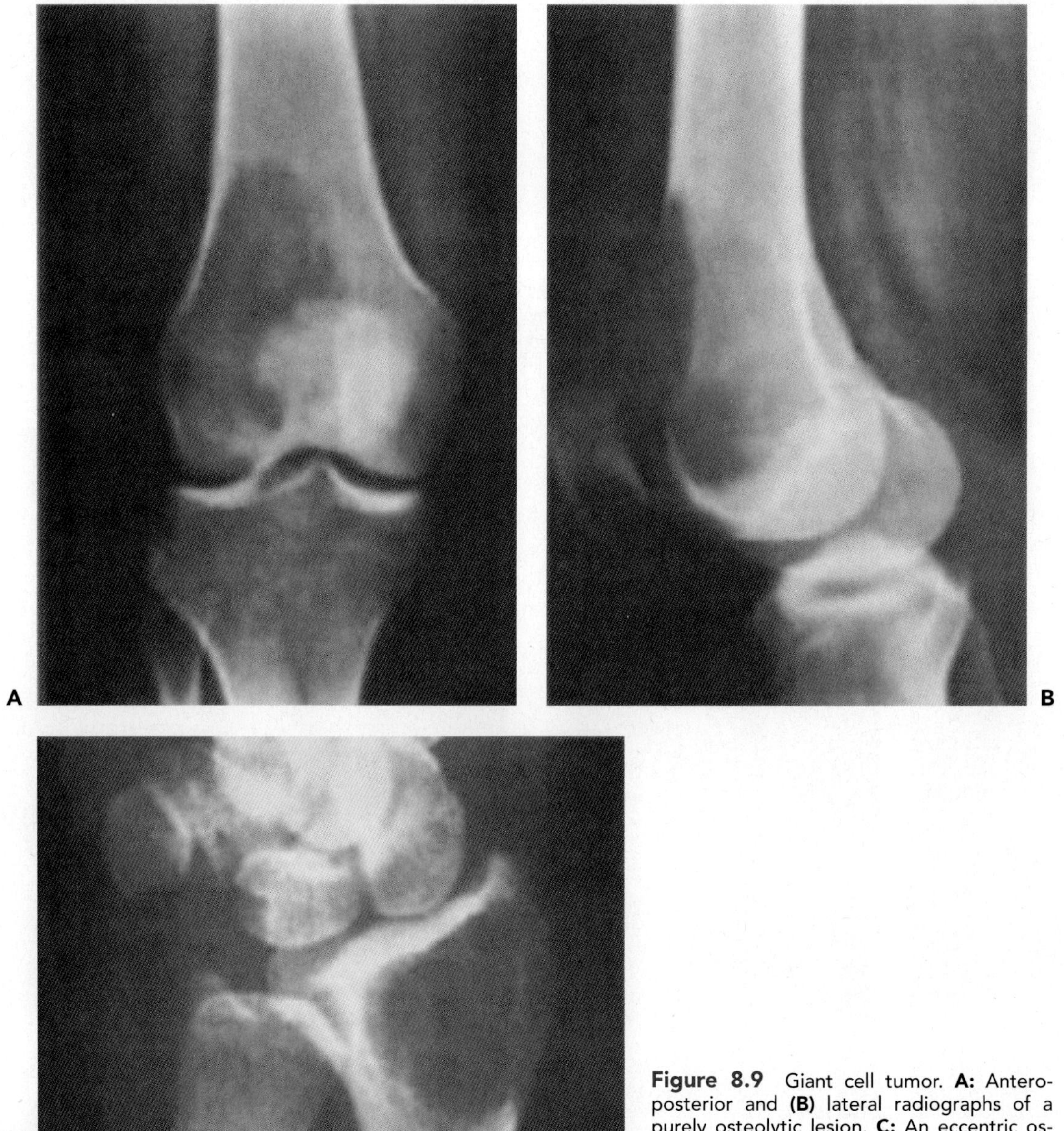

Figure 8.9 Giant cell tumor. **A:** Anteroposterior and **(B)** lateral radiographs of a purely osteolytic lesion. **C:** An eccentric osteolytic lesion. (*Reprinted with permission from* Greenspan A, Remagen W. *Differential Diagnosis of Tumors and Tumor-like Lesions of Bones and Joints.* Philadelphia, PA: Lippincott-Raven, 1998:313.)

little data exist concerning their contribution beyond that of a well-executed intra-lesional procedure. Packing with bone cement or bone graft is then performed to reconstitute the cavity. This approach has been shown to reduce recurrence rates to 6% to 15%. Embolization has been employed for treatment of sacral giant cell tumors as a minimal morbidity primary line of therapy. Close follow-up for recurrent disease and pulmonary involvement is important.

Fibrous Dysplasia

Fibrous dysplasia (Fig. 8.10) is a disturbance in bone-forming processes that causes arrest in the woven state. It is most commonly diagnosed in the second or third decade. Virtually any bone may be involved, but the proximal femur is the most common location. Other areas that are frequently involved include the tibia, pelvis, humerus, radius, and ribs. Monostotic disease is frequently an incidental radiographic finding in an asymptomatic patient. Polyostotic disease tends to remain unilateral rather than bilateral. Classic fibrous dysplasia occurs as a long lesion in a long bone with ground glass appearance, medullary calcification, and cortical thinning without periosteal reaction. However, fibrous dysplasia has a broad spectrum of appearance, ranging from a very long lesion in a long bone to a small eccentric lytic lesion with surrounding sclerosis. As such, fibrous dysplasia should be included in the differential of every benign-appearing lesion in bone. The typical histologic appearance is metaplastic woven bone scattered through a benign fibrous tissue stroma. Often, the woven trabeculae are disorganized and have been described as having a "Chinese letter" appearance. McCune–Albright syndrome is a polyostotic disorder manifested by brownish skin lesions and endocrine abnormalities resulting in precocious puberty. Fibrous dysplasia can very rarely convert to malignancy, most commonly osteosarcoma, although this occurs less than 0.5% of the time. Surgery is indicated when the patient has progressive deformity, large lesions with pain, nonunion, failure of nonsurgical therapy, or malignancy.

Hemangioma

Hemangiomas (Fig. 8.11) of the spine are common, occurring in approximately 10% of all adults and are notably more common in vertebral bodies than in the posterior elements. Hemangiomas typically contain trabecular condensations surrounded by abnormal vascular channels, which are more lucent on plain films and CT and give the vertebral body vertical striations on plain films. This appearance is popularly referred to as a "jail house" vertebra; the appearance on axial CT images resembles "polka-dots." Most spinal hemangiomas are incidental findings and require no treatment. Symptomatic hemangiomas usually respond well to conservative surgical procedures. Selective arterial embolization is usually safer and more effective treatment than radiation. Anterior resection and fusion are reserved for pathologic collapse and neural compromise or refractory cases.

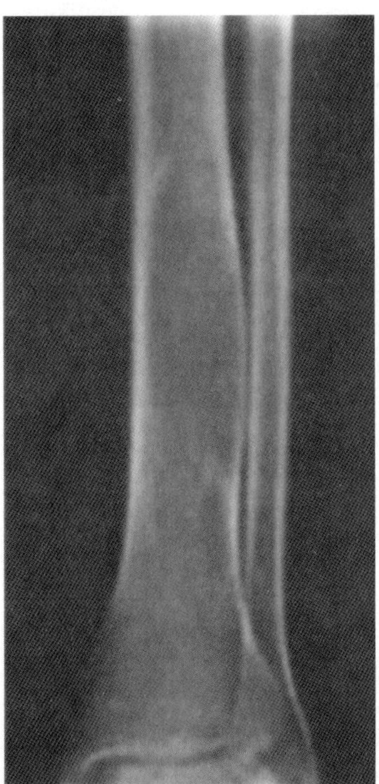

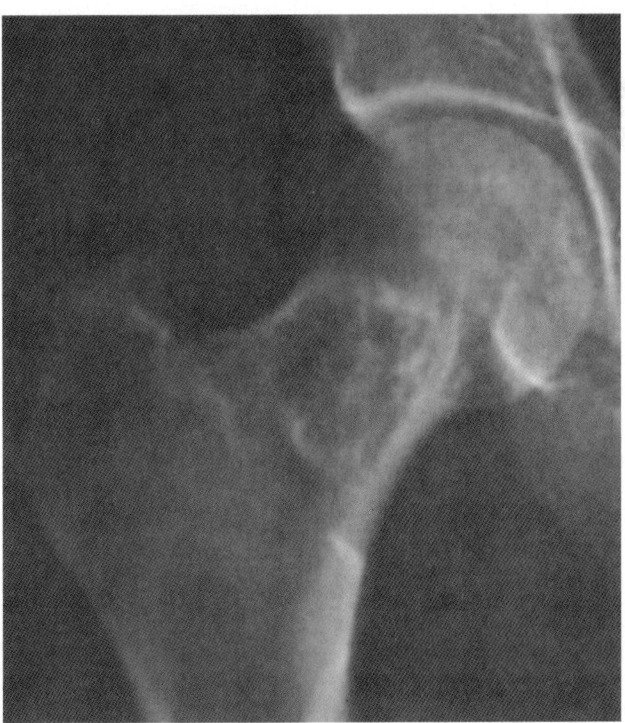

Figure 8.10 Fibrous dysplasia of the diaphysis of the tibia **(A)** and femoral neck **(B)**. (*Reprinted with permission from* Greenspan A, Remagen W. *Differential Diagnosis of Tumors and Tumor-like Lesions of Bones and Joints.* Philadelphia, PA: Lippincott-Raven, 1998:217.)

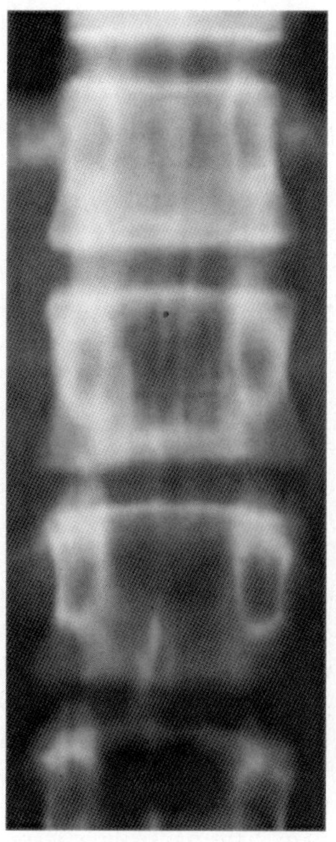

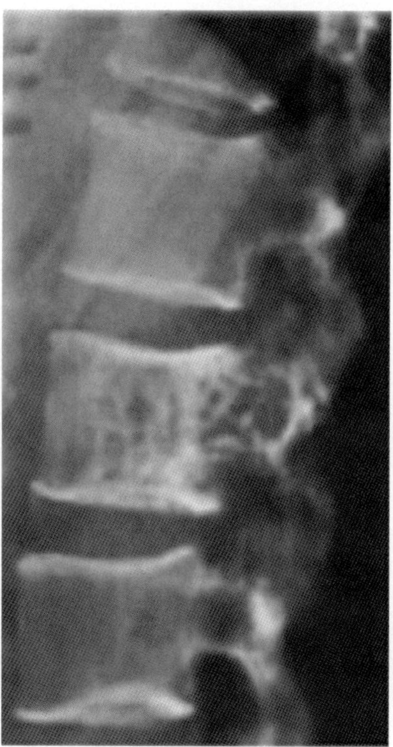

Figure 8.11 Anteroposterior (AP) **(A)** and lateral **(B)** radiographs demonstrating the classic "jail house" vertebra of hemangioma. (*Reprinted with permission from* Greenspan A, Remagen W. *Differential Diagnosis of Tumors and Tumor-like Lesions of Bones and Joints.* Philadelphia, PA: Lippincott-Raven, 1998:291.)

MALIGNANT BONE LESIONS

Bone Forming

Osteosarcoma

The classic form of osteosarcoma (Fig. 8.12) is seen most often in the second and third decades. The majority of lesions are in the metaphyses of the long bones, with 50% found about the knee. Males are at higher risk. Most patients have symptoms of pain before a mass is noticed. Radiographically, these are permeative, metaphyseal lesions with soft-tissue extension and new bone formation. Periosteal reaction is common and frequently the new neoplastic bone takes on a sunburst or "hair on end" appearance as the tumor continues to expand into the soft tissue. Chest CT scans are essential for evaluation of pulmonary metastasis. Histologically, there is a presence of neoplastic woven bone in association with a malignant spindle cell stroma. Common subtypes of osteosarcoma are listed in Table 8.7. Chemotherapy is given preoperatively to reduce tumor burden and to kill malignant cells in the reactive zone and in micrometastases. This also causes the tumor to "heal in," during which time it shrinks and loses its vascularity, thus facilitating wide resection. Tumor necrosis due to chemotherapy is a prognostic indicator. Wide margin surgical resection and reconstruction using segmental replacement endoprostheses or allografts can then be performed. Adjuvant chemotherapy is given after resection. Currently, with the use of chemotherapy and surgery, survival rates are typically in the range of 65% to 75%. Secondary osteosarcoma arises most frequently from prior radiated fields or in the context of long-standing Paget's disease.

Chondroid Forming

Chondrosarcoma

Malignant cartilage tumors are primarily tumors of adulthood and old age. About 85% of chondrosarcomas (Fig. 8.13) are low-grade. Findings associated with chondrosarcoma include intralesional lysis, endosteal scalloping, cortical thinning or expansion, and pain. Most will show chondroid calcification, but high-grade lesions may take on a purely lytic appearance. Chondrosarcomas are very resistant to radiation and chemotherapy. Furthermore, they tend to recur locally and require complete surgical resection with a wide margin to achieve cure. The treatment of low-grade is somewhat controversial, as some prefer aggressive intralesional curettage and adjuvant therapy with phenol or liquid nitrogen while others prefer wide excision. For intermediate and high-grade chondrosarcoma, wide-margins are required.

Other Lesions

Ewing Sarcoma

Ewing sarcoma (Fig. 8.14) is an undifferentiated tumor characterized by the t(11;22) translocation in 90% of cases. It occurs primarily in patients between 5 and 25 years of age with a male predominance. Twenty percent of patients will have associated systemic symptoms, such as fever, chills, and a high erythrocyte sedimentation rate and white blood

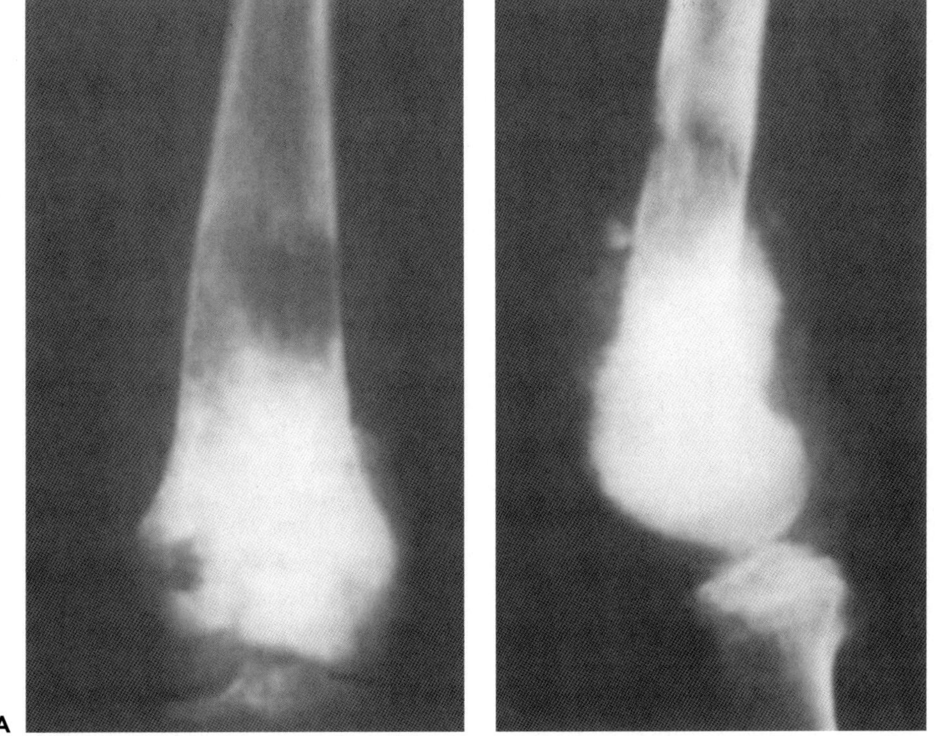

Figure 8.12 Anteroposterior (AP) **(A)** and lateral **(B)** x-rays of the distal femur demonstrating the aggressive nature of conventional osteosarcoma. (*Reprinted with permission from* Greenspan A, Remagen W. *Differential Diagnosis of Tumors and Tumor-like Lesions of Bones and Joints.* Philadelphia, PA: Lippincott-Raven, 1998:65.)

cell count; this clinical picture may mimic osteomyelitis. Ewing sarcoma classically presents as a diaphyseal, permeative lesion with "onion skin" periosteal reaction and a large associated soft-tissue mass. The most common locations are the femur, pelvis, tibia, and humerus. Histologically, Ewing sarcoma consists of small round cells arranged in sheets. The natural history is of an aggressive disease with approximately 20% of patients exhibiting metastases on presentation. Those with locally resectable disease fair well, but those with advanced metastatic disease have at best a 30% survival rate at 5 years. Excision of lung metastases, if possible, can improve survival. Treatment is typically preoperative chemotherapy, wide surgical excision, and adjuvant chemotherapy. In cases where resection results in positive margins, postoperative radiation is possible as this tumor is radiosensitive. Radiation may also replace surgical resection in areas where wide surgical excision is not feasible.

TABLE 8.7
SUBTYPES OF OSTEOSARCOMA

- **Parosteal osteosarcoma:** A low-grade variant that occurs on the cortical surface of long bones, usually near the location of the metaphysis. It accounts for less than 5% of all osteosarcomas and occurs more often in females. The most common sites are the distal femur, proximal tibia, and proximal humerus. Treatment is wide surgical resection, which is often curative.
- **Periosteal osteosarcoma:** A surface-based osteosarcoma arising in long bones, typically in the diaphyses, and low to intermediate in grade. It accounts for less than 2% of all osteosarcoma. The most common sites are the distal femur, proximal tibia, and proximal humerus. It grows from under the periosteum, giving rise to the typical radiographic appearance of a sunburst-type lesion over a depressed cortical base. Treatment is wide surgical resection, with adjuvant chemotherapy for more advanced, higher grade lesions.
- **Hemorrhagic osteosarcoma (telangiectatic):** This is a high-grade variant that is extremely lytic and destructive. On radiographs, it resembles an aneurysmal bone cyst. Histologically, there is hemorrhage with malignant stromal cells and giant cells. Treatment is similar to classic osteosarcoma with similar outcomes.
- **Secondary osteosarcoma:** Secondary osteosarcoma may arise from many benign conditions including fibrous dysplasia, giant cell tumor, osteoblastoma, osteochondroma, Paget's disease, and chronic osteomyelitis. Radiation-induced osteosarcoma can result after any significant radiation exposure, typically greater than 30 Gray. The average delay in onset is approximately 15 years but can vary widely. This subtype carries a poor prognosis with very high rates of metastasis.

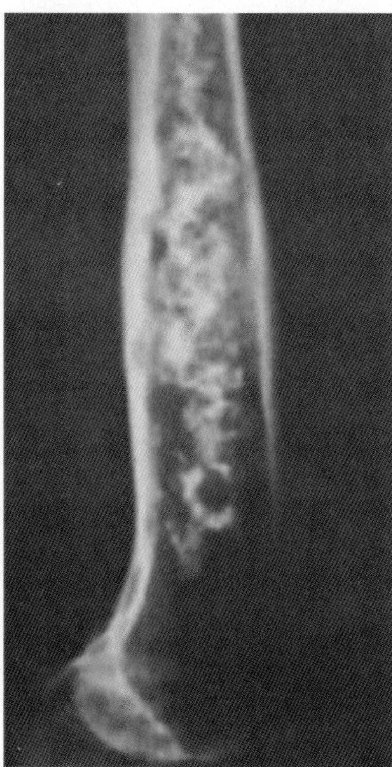

Figure 8.13 Lateral radiograph of the distal femur demonstrating a calcified chondrosarcoma. (*Reprinted with permission from* Greenspan A, Remagen W. *Differential Diagnosis of Tumors and Tumor-like Lesions of Bones and Joints.* Philadelphia, PA: Lippincott-Raven, 1998:176.)

Primary Lymphoma of Bone

Lymphoma may present as an isolated tumor within bone or as a systemic disease. Primary lymphomas of the bone (Fig. 8.15) account for 3% of all malignant bone tumors. These patients typically have none of the general constitutional complaints so commonly associated with systemic lymphoma, even when lesions are extensive.

Lymphoma is typically a very permeative but minimally destructive lesion. The usual progression is that lymphomas fill up the medullary canal and then grow into the surrounding soft tissues while causing little destruction of the bone itself. Plain radiographs may be unremarkable, while MRI scans show marrow replacement and often an associated soft-tissue mass. Surgical intervention is typically reserved for select cases to prevent or treat pathologic fracture; primary treatment centers on radiation and multiagent chemotherapy.

Plasmacytoma and Multiple Myeloma (Plasma Cell Tumor)

Solitary myeloma is one of many B-cell lymphoproliferative diseases, which also include multiple myeloma. True solitary myeloma is relatively rare, accounting for only 3% of all plasma cell neoplasms. Monoclonal proteins are more often absent or undetectable in solitary myeloma compared with multiple myeloma. Diagnostic criteria for solitary myeloma include a solitary lesion on skeletal survey, histologic confirmation, and bone marrow plasmacytosis. Treatment of choice in solitary plasmacytoma is radiation. Surgical intervention is typically reserved for decompression of neural structures in the case of spinal involvement and stabilization when the long bones are involved. MRI provides the earliest indication of local recurrence, and serum protein electrophoresis has proven to be the best indicator of dissemination. The primary treatment for disseminated myeloma is systemic chemotherapy.

Chordoma

Chordoma (Fig. 8.16) is a low-grade, relatively uncommon malignancy of the spine typically found in patients in their fourth to sixth decade. Chordomas routinely localize to the midline, arise from primitive notochord remnants, and are primarily found in the sacro-coccygeal area or at the base of the skull. Chordomas grow slowly with few early symptoms, frequently reaching considerable size before diagnosis. Many patients, however, have a long history of mild aching perineal pain or numbness, which should be a sign of a potential pelvic tumor compressing the sacral plexus. Often chordomas can be palpated directly on rectal examination. Surgical resection with wide margins is the only curative procedure. Since the tumor is a low-grade lesion, growth is slow and recurrence and eventual metastases are common.

SOFT-TISSUE TUMORS

Clinical Presentations

Most soft-tissue tumors present with pain and/or a mass. It is also remarkable that soft-tissue masses including sarcomas can reach tremendous size and yet cause minimal or no symptoms. Many patients falsely assume that because the lesion is painless it must also be harmless. This is obviously not the case but is often responsible for long delays in diagnosis on the part of the patient or, less frequently, the physician. Ironically, the lesions in soft tissue that are most commonly painful are the benign soft-tissue tumors, including desmoid tumors, hemangiomas, benign nerve sheath tumors, and soft-tissue infections.

Radiographic Evaluation

Most soft-tissue masses are seen poorly or not at all on plain x-rays; however, those that show calcification will be more apparent. The most common lesion to present with soft-tissue calcification is myositis ossificans, but synovial sarcoma can present in a similar manner. Myositis typically exhibits histologic peripheral maturation and an associated "egg shell" calcification, while malignant soft-tissue

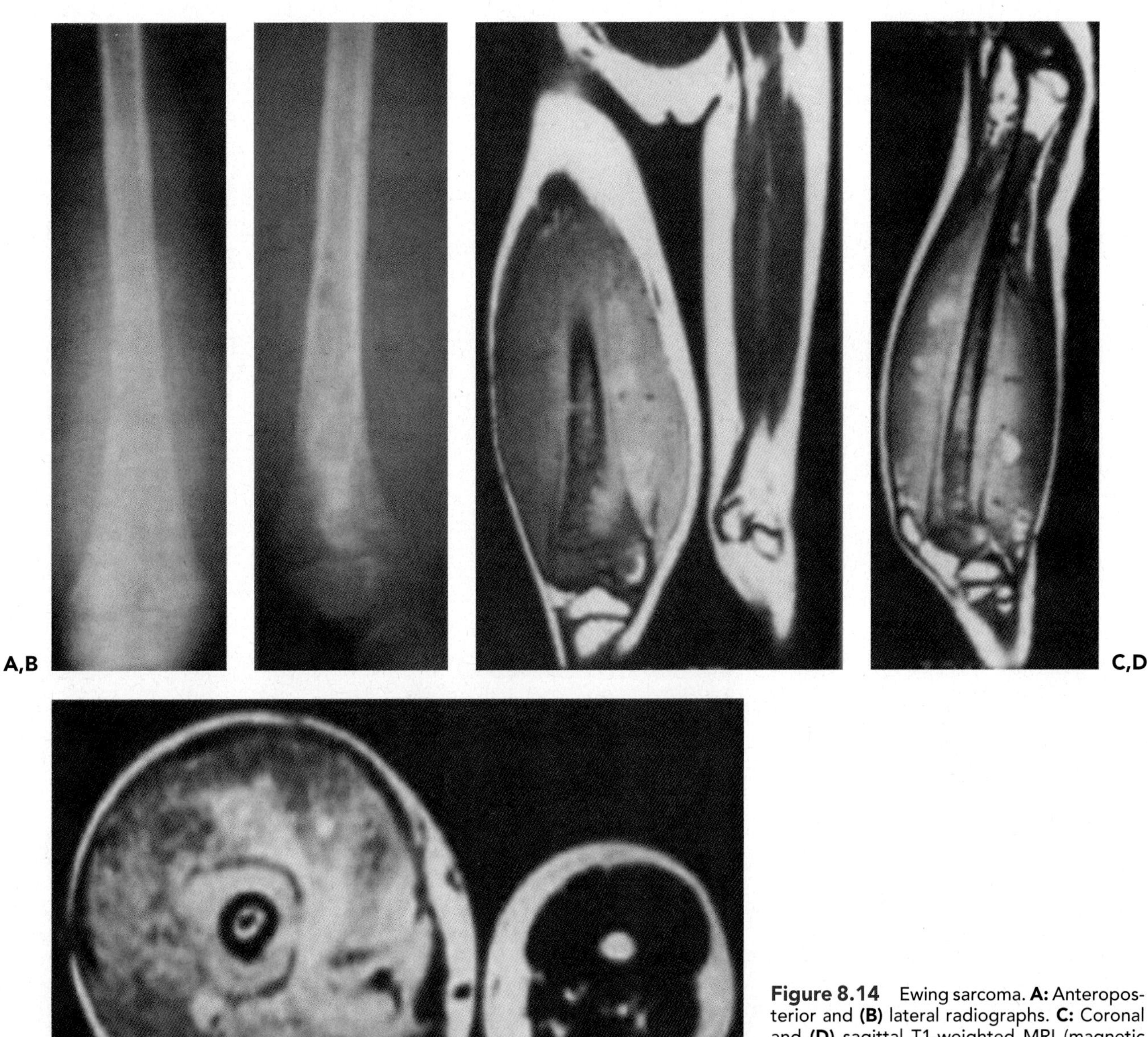

Figure 8.14 Ewing sarcoma. **A:** Anteroposterior and **(B)** lateral radiographs. **C:** Coronal and **(D)** sagittal T1-weighted MRI (magnetic resonance imaging). **E:** Axial T2-weighted MRI. (*Reprinted with permission from* Greenspan A, Remagen W. *Differential Diagnosis of Tumors and Tumor-like Lesions of Bones and Joints.* Philadelphia, PA: Lippincott-Raven, 1998:260.)

tumors are usually less organized, so any calcification is more random.

The classic MRI finding in most soft-tissue tumors is a lesion that is well circumscribed and low signal (dark) on T1, and high signal (bright) on T2, fat-suppressed T2, or short tau inversion recovery (STIR) sequences. Such a lesion would support benign tumor, malignant tumor, abscess, cyst, or hematoma in the differential diagnosis. Most soft-tissue sarcomas are very distinct, while often showing a bit of edema in the compartment in which they occur. On the contrary, many benign lesions are poorly marginated on MRI scans; these include desmoid tumors, hemangiomas, inflammation, injury, and infection. This is the opposite of what is seen in bone, where benign lesions tend to be well marginated, and malignant tumors tend to be poorly marginated.

Differential Diagnosis

As in the case of bone lesions, soft-tissue tumors can be quite confusing when approached as a large number of unrelated topics. Again, a systematic approach to the diagnosis of these lesions reveals a limited number of clinical presentations. Histologically, however, they do form a large and diverse group with fewer trends than those found in bone tumors.

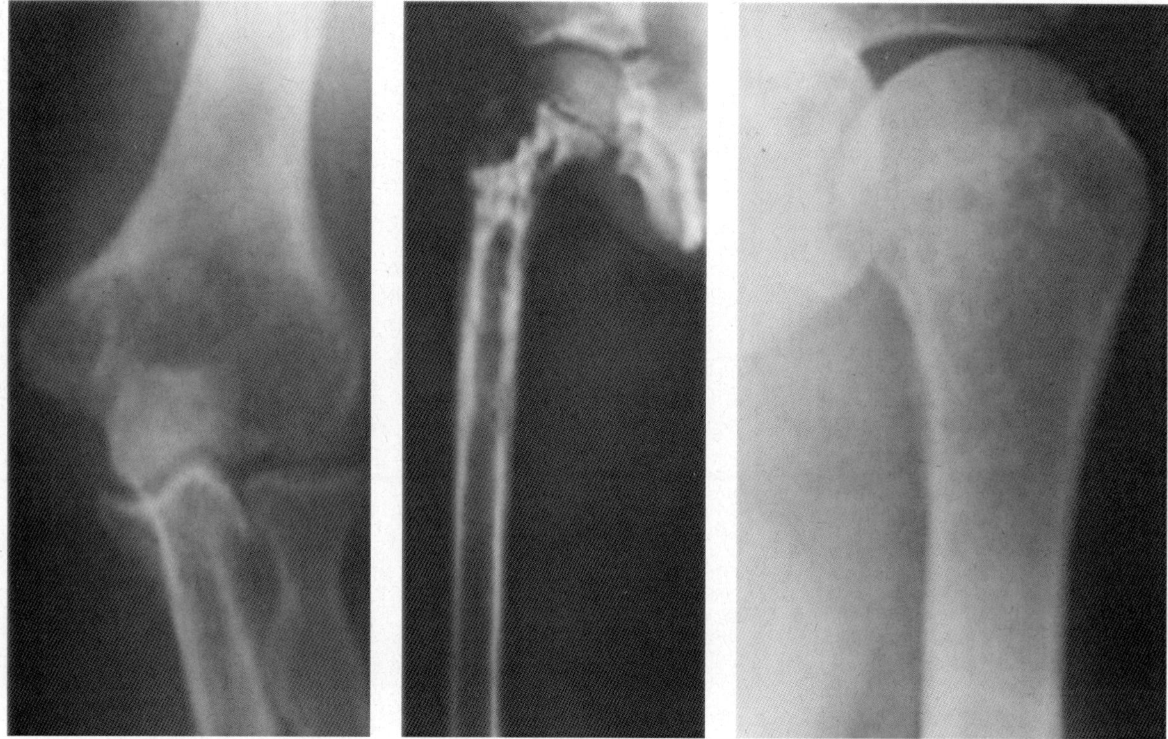

Figure 8.15 Multiple radiographs demonstrating the variable appearance of primary lymphoma of the bone. (*Reprinted with permission from* Greenspan A, Remagen W. *Differential Diagnosis of Tumors and Tumor-like Lesions of Bones and Joints.* Philadelphia, PA: Lippincott-Raven, 1998:268.)

FATTY TUMORS

Lipoma

This is one of the few diagnoses that can be made confidently on the basis of MRI and clinical findings alone. Benign lipomas appear as masses of uniform fat density and parallel the appearance of normal subcutaneous fat on all sequences: bright on T1 and T2 sequences and dark on fat-suppressed T2 and STIR sequences. Therefore, a mass seen on MRI as a uniform fat density with no interstitial markings is diagnostic of benign lipoma. Histologically, lipomas consist of mature fat cells with no atypia. Without symptoms, these lesions can be monitored. If excision is warranted, marginal resection has a low recurrence rate. Several lipoma variants exist, including fibrolipoma, angiolipoma, spindle cell lipoma, and hibernoma. These lesions have a different appearance from simple lipoma and frequently require biopsy to establish a definitive diagnosis.

Atypical Lipoma

Continuing along the spectrum of fatty tumors, this benign tumor has also been labeled "well differentiated liposarcoma" and "lipoma-like well differentiated liposarcoma," especially when found in the retroperitoneum. This is a fat-containing lesion characterized by lobules of fat signal on MRI with surrounding layers of fibrous tissue demonstrating thin layers of high signal that enhance with the use of intravenous contrast. Histologically, lobules of normal fat are seen surrounded by fibrous bands containing lipoblasts and atypical cells. These lesions are very invasive into surrounding tissue, and local recurrence following excision is common. While atypical lipomas do not metastasize, they do carry a 10% risk of malignant transformation, usually to high-grade liposarcoma. Myxoid liposarcoma and pleomorphic liposarcoma exist at the far end of the fatty tumor spectrum, representing two variants with aggressive, malignant features.

FIBROUS

Desmoid Tumor (Fibromatosis)

Desmoid tumors are an uncommon group of benign soft-tissue neoplasms with aggressive local behavior. They appear on MRI scans as dense fibrosis, typically remaining dark on T1, T2, and fat-suppressed T2 sequences. Unlike most soft-tissue tumors, they are poorly marginated and often have a stellate margin on MRI, reflecting their extreme invasiveness into surrounding tissues. They are frequently painful and demonstrate an increased incidence in women following pregnancy. Histologically, desmoid tumors are composed of benign-appearing spindle cells

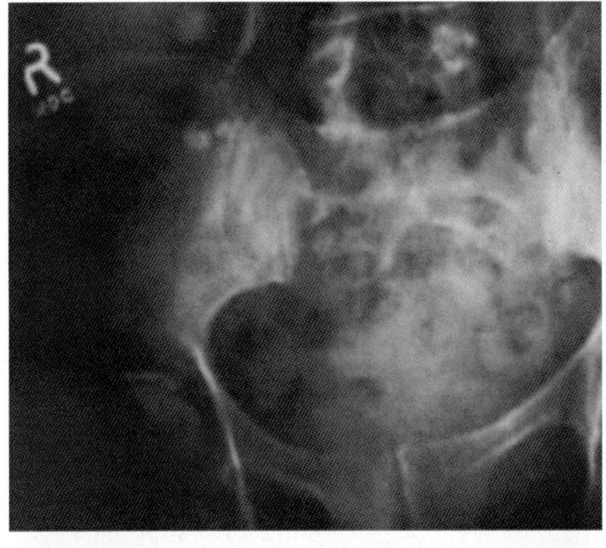

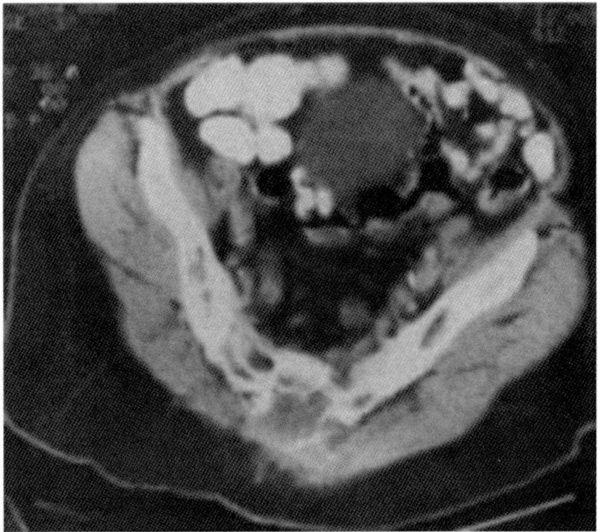

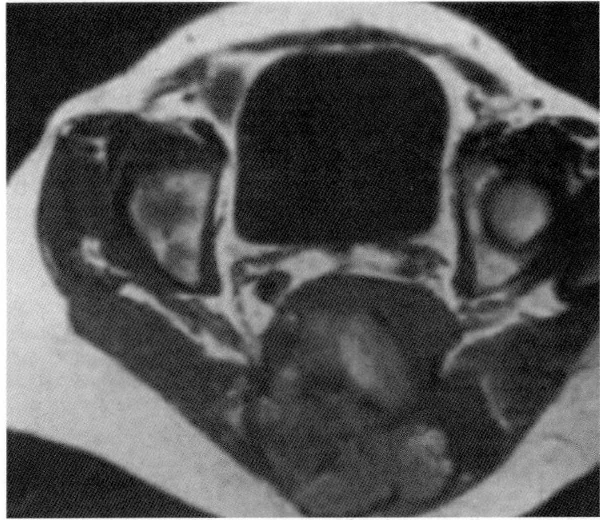

Figure 8.16 Anteroposterior (AP) radiograph **(A)**, axial CT (computed tomography) scan **(B)** and axial T-1 weighted MRI (magnetic resonance imaging) scan **(C)** demonstrating a chordoma. This tumor of notochord remnants occurs almost exclusively in the sacrum or at the base of the skull. (*Reprinted with permission from* Greenspan A, Remagen W. *Differential Diagnosis of Tumors and Tumor-like Lesions of Bones and Joints.* Philadelphia, PA: Lippincott-Raven, 1998:355.)

interspersed amid a background of abundant collagen fibers. While desmoid tumors are benign, they are very aggressive locally and have a tremendous ability to invade local tissues at a considerable distance from the primary tumor. Surgery has historically been the mainstay of treatment but has a very high failure rate and considerable associated morbidity. Therefore, nonsurgical treatments such as low-dose chemotherapy and radiation therapy have also been popular, either as sole treatment or as part of a multidisciplinary treatment regimen.

Fibrosarcoma

Fibrosarcoma is a rare soft-tissue sarcoma. Clinically, it appears as a typical soft-tissue malignancy usually presenting as a painless mass. MRI findings are typical for the group of soft-tissue sarcomas demonstrating dark signal on T1 and bright signal on fat-suppressed T2 sequences, along with contrast enhancement. Histologically, fibrosarcomas present a unique picture of malignant spindle cells arranged in a herringbone pattern with marked cellularity and moderate atypia. Local control is usually achieved with a combination of wide marginal excision and adjuvant or neo-adjuvant radiation therapy. As chemotherapy has progressed, so has enthusiasm for its use as an adjuvant in patients with large (>5 cm), high-grade soft-tissue sarcomas that demonstrate reasonable medical risk for this therapy.

MYXOID

Myxoma

Benign myxomas are typically seen within skeletal muscle, where they usually present as a painless mass. They do demonstrate a fairly typical appearance on MRI scanning: they are usually darker than muscle on T1 and uniformly bright on fat-suppressed T2 views, with some edema usually along the inferior and superior aspects. This is, however, not diagnostic for benign myxoma and can be seen with other soft-tissue masses, both benign and malignant. Treatment is marginal excision and recurrence is rare.

Low-Grade and High-Grade Fibromyxosarcoma

These lesions extend the spectrum of myxoid soft-tissue tumors and represent grades of atypia and cellularity. These lesions are noted for their heterogeneity, and sampling error in biopsy can be a problem. Histologically, they are comprised of loose myxoid tissue showing atypical cells in a loose matrix. Higher grade lesions show more cellularity, atypia, and necrosis.

NEURAL

Benign Schwannoma

This is a benign tumor found in peripheral nerves, most commonly in spinal roots and in the major nerves of the extremities. On MRI imaging, schwannomas demonstrate a typical soft-tissue tumor pattern showing low signal on T1 and high signal on fat-suppressed T2 sequences. Since they occur commonly within peripheral nerves, they typically have a fusiform shape and are long in the longitudinal axis of the extremity. Histologically, the lesion is described as having dense Antoni A (compact spindle cells, often in a whorl-like pattern) and loose Antoni B (less cellular and orderly) areas. Verucae bodies exhibit typical patterning of spindle cells. Malignant transformation is extremely rare. Most of these lesions are symptomatic and demonstrate a positive Tinel's sign (shooting pain with percussion of the lesion). In light of this, most lesions require surgical excision. Since these lesions frequently occur within the neural sheath of major nerves, excision of the lesion should be carried out in such a manner as to protect the nerve of origin as much as possible.

Neurofibroma

Solitary neurofibroma is a benign, fibrotic, fusiform tumor arising from a peripheral nerve; the nerve of origin may be too small to recognize. It occurs most commonly in the third to sixth decades. The lesion is usually asymptomatic except for the presence of a mass. Treatment is excision. In neurofibromatosis, or Von Recklinghausen's disease, small café au lait spots appear in the first few years of life, along with multiple neurofibromas, which develop later. The neurofibromas appear as soft pedunculated nodules in the skin or as firm or soft masses in the deeper tissues. Malignant degeneration of these neurofibromas in Von Recklinghausen's disease is much more common (3% to 5% of patients) than in the solitary variant. When indicated, definitive treatment for benign neurofibromas is excision.

BENIGN SYNOVIAL PROLIFERATIVE DISORDERS

Synovial Chondromatosis

This is a benign, uncommon disorder characterized by metaplastic proliferation of cartilaginous nodules in the synovial membrane of joints. Typically diagnosed in the third to fifth decade, it is most often found in the knee, followed by the hip, shoulder, and elbow. Pain and swelling are the most common complaints, but joint effusion, tenderness, and limited range of motion occur. The radiographic findings range from simple joint effusion to multiple radiopaque joint bodies, depending on the degree of calcification of the cartilaginous nodules. MRI may show the calcifications as signal void on T2-weighted images, with a high-signal intensity background of inflamed, hyperplastic synovium. Clinically, synovial chondromatosis may appear as distinct osteochondral bodies in the synovium or as masses of confluent cartilage. Synovectomy, either open or arthroscopic, with removal of the lesion is the treatment of choice, although recurrence is common.

Pigmented Villonodular Synovitis

Pigmented villonodular synovitis (PVNS) is a locally destructive fibrohistiocytic proliferation, which affects joints, bursae, and tendon sheaths. Clinically, PVNS is a slowly progressing process that causes pain and joint swelling, often with limited range of motion. The knee is the most common location. More than half of patients present with a bloody joint effusion. Thus, a patient with bloody effusion of the knee without trauma is suggestive of this diagnosis. On radiographs a soft-tissue density is often present in the affected joint. This is sometimes interpreted as a joint effusion, but it is denser because of the hemorrhagic fluid and lobulated synovial tissue. Calcifications are rare. PVNS appears dark on T1, T2 and fat-suppressed T2 sequences due to the presence of hemosiderin pigment; gradient echo sequences are often helpful in characterizing the lesion. PVNS frequently occurs also outside of a joint in association with tenosynovial tissue. In these cases, the lesion is termed "giant cell tumor of tendon sheath," but it is histologically identical to PVNS. Treatment for PVNS consists of synovectomy. While arthroscopic procedures have less morbidity than open procedures, they probably carry a higher risk of recurrence.

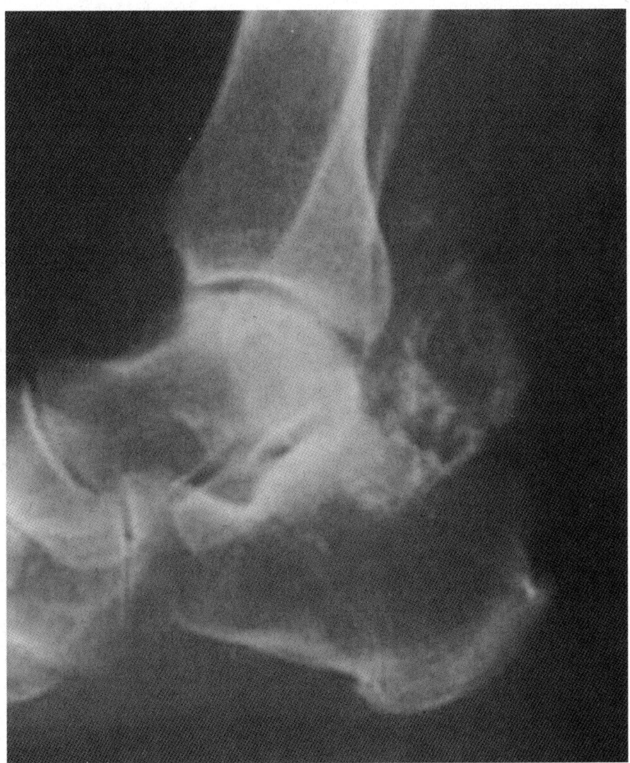

Figure 8.17 Lateral radiograph of the ankle demonstrating a calcified soft-tissue mass which is characteristic of synovial cell sarcoma. (*Reprinted with permission from* Greenspan A, Remagen W. *Differential Diagnosis of Tumors and Tumor-like Lesions of Bones and Joints.* Philadelphia, PA: Lippincott-Raven, 1998:410.)

OTHER

Synovial Sarcoma

Despite its name, this lesion does not arise from synovium. It comprises 8% to 10% of soft-tissue sarcomas and typically occurs before the age of 50. The most common sites are around the knee and foot. Most of these tumors occur in an extra-articular location, but very rarely may be intra-articular. The radiologic features of synovial sarcoma (Fig. 8.17) include a soft-tissue mass often close to a joint. Soft-tissue calcifications are present in about 15% of cases and may present with a slight amount of calcification or show diffuse calcification to the extent that the lesion mimics mature myositis ossificans. Synovial sarcoma can also develop significant cystic areas mimicking a synovial cyst or diffuse hemorrhage mimicking a hematoma. Histologically the classic pattern is a biphasic picture of malignant spindle cells in association with areas of columnar epithelium. In these cases, the malignant stromal cells are positive for vimentin (a mesenchymal marker) but also show cytokeratin positivity in the epithelial cells. Treatment is the same as for most soft-tissue sarcomas and has been described in the section on fibrosarcoma.

Malignant Fibrous Histiocytoma

Malignant fibrous histiocytoma (MFH) is the most common soft-tissue sarcoma of adulthood. Similar to other soft-tissue malignancies, it usually presents as a painless deep soft-tissue mass. Histologically, it is composed of atypical spindle cells in a whorled or cartwheel configuration. In accordance with its high-grade status, it is a very cellular tumor with significant atypia and necrosis. MFH is basically a diagnosis of exclusion as it is a tumor that fits no other more specific tumor type.

BASIC TREATMENT PRINCIPLES

In treating musculoskeletal tumors, there are basically three modes of treatment available: surgery, radiation therapy, and chemotherapy. In rare cases, modalities such as radiofrequency ablation or embolization may also be available. In order to understand how surgery fits into this scenario, it is critical to understand the oncologic surgical margins that can be obtained. The terms used for these margins in contemporary treatment were popularized by Enneking and are defined as intra-lesional, marginal,

TABLE 8.8
TREATMENT MATRIX FOR BONE AND SOFT-TISSUE SARCOMAS

	Sarcoma Treatment Modalities	
	Radio Resistant	**Radio Sensitive**
Low grade	Surgery ▪ Chondrosarcoma ▪ Chordoma ▪ Adamantinoma	Surgery + radiation ▪ Low-grade soft-tissue sarcomas
High grade	Surgery + chemotherapy ▪ Osteosarcoma ▪ Ewing sarcoma ▪ Other high-grade bone sarcomas	Surgery + radiation + chemotherapy ▪ High-grade soft-tissue sarcomas

wide, and radical. For the most part, benign tumors of bone, such as giant cell tumor, osteoblastoma, chondroblastoma, and chondromyxoid fibroma, are treated with intra-lesional surgery. Benign lesions in soft tissue, such as lipoma, schwannoma, and myxoma, are treated with simple marginal excision. Table 8.8 demonstrates a general treatment matrix for bone and soft-tissue malignancies.

RECOMMENDED READING

Lewis VO. What's new in musculoskeletal oncology. *J Bone Joint Surg Am*. 2007;89(6):1399–1407.

Sim FH, Frassica FJ, Frassica DA. Soft-tissue tumors: diagnosis, evaluation, and management. *J Am Acad Orthop Surg*. 1994;2(4):202–211.

Weber K, Damron TA, Frassica FJ, Sim FH. Malignant bone tumors. *Instr Course Lect*. 2008;57:673–688.

Principles of Sports Medicine

9

F. Winston Gwathmey Jr.   Joseph M. Hart   Mark D. Miller

INTRODUCTION

Medicine and sports share a common origin in ancient Greece. Hippocrates, universally regarded as the father of medicine, was also among history's first sports physicians. The leading athletes of his time participated in the Olympic Games, and he was proficient at treating their injuries, dressing their wounds, splinting fractures, and stitching lacerations. The Hippocratic method for reducing a shoulder dislocation remains in use into modern times. When Galen was appointed physician for the gladiators of Pergamum, he arguably became history's first team physician. His athletes frequently sustained traumatic wounds inflicted by heavy weapons and wild animals, and in the management of these injuries, he gained invaluable insight into the function of muscles, nerves, and blood vessels.

In modern times, the proliferation of organized sports in society has stimulated the evolution of sports medicine and has established the physician as an integral member of the athletic community. Physician involvement in the modern Olympic Games reflects this developing role. Prior to 1924, the U.S. Olympics team traveled without a physician or other health care provider. In 2008, a team of 61 health care professionals representing multiple specialties including orthopaedics, cardiology, obstetrics and gynecology, internal medicine, emergency medicine, and pediatrics traveled to Beijing with the Olympics athletes.

Sports medicine is a field dedicated to the prevention and treatment of athletic injuries and diseases and encompasses multiple disciplines collectively involved in the care of athletes. The athlete represents a unique patient as success in sports directly correlates with strength, conditioning, and physical and mental well-being. To provide optimal care, a comprehensive approach involving physicians, athletic trainers, therapists, and nutritionists is required. The inherent diversity of the athletic population presents challenges to the health care provider as patients may range from the youth soccer player to the elderly golfer and from the recreational runner to the high-level collegiate or professional athlete. The conditions and injuries that affect this population vary substantially with age, gender, sport, and level of performance. Consequently, the method of diagnosis and treatment must be tailored to each patient and each situation.

The degree of physician involvement in the care of athletes also depends upon the physician, the sport, and the level of performance. For the majority of athletes, the general practitioner plays the role of sports physician. For high-level athletic organizations and institutions, the daily health and training demands require dedicated physicians responsible for coordinating the care of the players on the team. These physicians provide care for athletes across the entire spectrum of their participation and may be their only doctor in many cases.

This chapter address many of the issues specific to the care of athletes, including the role of the team physician, ethical issues in sports medicine, preparticipation evaluation, athletic event coverage, common athletic injuries, medical conditions effecting athletes, the care of the female athlete, principles of athletic rehabilitation, the pharmacology of sports medicine, and athletic nutrition.

THE TEAM PHYSICIAN

The role of team physician requires a broad understanding of medicine as it applies to the athlete and the ability to quarterback a team of health care providers, which include athletic trainers, physical therapists, nutritionists, dieticians, and other health care specialists. It is important for the team physician to involve the coaches and parents to facilitate communication and to ensure that appropriate training regimens and precautions are implemented to prevent injuries.

Dr. Frank McCue, the long-time team physician at the University of Virginia, outlines the three A's of being a team physician: *availability*, *affability*, and *ability*. *Availability* is imperative to providing optimal care for the athlete, and the team physician must be accessible throughout the season and off-season. Injuries occur without warning and the physician must be at hand to direct care, especially for emergencies. Responsibilities include game coverage, evaluation on the sidelines and in the training room, and athlete clinics.

The team physician must possess *affability* to forge strong relationships with the players, coaches, parents, trainers, and other health care providers. Developing trust within these relationships strengthens the physician–patient interaction and optimizes care.

At the foundation of serving as team physician is the *ability* to diagnose and treat athletic injuries. The physician must understand the rules and physical requirements particular to the sport to address the conditions that may arise from participation. Often the team physician is the primary care provider for the athlete, and thus a broad understanding of the medical conditions that afflict this patient population is crucial to ensure proper treatment.

ETHICS IN SPORTS MEDICINE

Since the earliest interaction between sports and medicine, the disparate objectives of the athlete who desired victory and the physician who sought good health have stimulated conflict. Hippocrates and Galen criticized the immoderate athletic lifestyle and felt that the strenuous training, excessive diets, and obsession with winning constituted unhealthy and dangerous behavior. The timelessness of these concerns is reflected in many of the challenges that face the modern sports physician. It would seem that sports promote healthy lifestyle, but the demands of training, the insatiable desire to win, and the urge to play through injury are often detrimental to health, both in the short and long term.

The sports physician must recognize the immense pressure athletes face to play and perform. Athletes strive to achieve in their sports, sometimes at the risk of endangering their health. Excessive training and dieting as well as the temptations of performance-enhancing substances are commonplace among athletes at every level. In addition, a third party is introduced into the doctor–patient relationship in the form of the team or organization. A team relies upon its athletes to succeed, and the goals of the team may interfere with the best interests of the players. Collegiate and professional teams endure the expectations of the administration, media, and fans. Clear communication between the health care team and the coaching staff is important to alleviate undue stress on the athlete and to establish a realistic understanding of an athlete's capability to participate.

The team physician should also be aware of the social and financial influences of athletics. The ability to perform on the athletic field may provide athletes with an opportunity to attend college on a scholarship or engage in a lucrative career as a professional athlete. These motivations may compel players to abuse performance-enhancing drugs or engage in other illegal or unhealthy behavior.

PREPARTICIPATION EVALUATION

The preparticipation evaluation is the key to the prevention of sports-related disease and injury. The objective of this assessment is to screen potentially disabling or life-threatening disorders and identify conditions that predispose to injury or illness. It also serves to determine the general health of the athlete and provides an entry point into the health care system for adolescents. All athletes participating in organized high school, college, and professional sports are required to undergo this systematic assessment before being cleared to play.

Ideally, the preparticipation evaluation should take place 6 weeks before the start of the sports season so that issues that arise may be addressed prior to participation. For practical purposes, a complete evaluation need be performed only upon entry to a higher level of participation, while an interim health questionnaire and limited, focused examination suffices in subsequent years. The objectives and focus of the evaluation shift as athletes get older. Among younger athletes, screening preexisting medical and congenital conditions that affect participation takes precedence. The likelihood of discovering a serious preexisting condition diminishes as athletes advance and undergo yearly assessments. At higher levels, the physician may concentrate on age- or sport-specific issues, and previous injuries and concerns related to training and play should be addressed.

The preparticipation evaluation may take place either in the physician's office on an individualized basis or in a mass screening setting such as a high school gymnasium. While the office has the advantage of fostering the doctor–patient relationship, most physicians have limited time available, especially during the time of year that most evaluations need to be completed. The mass screening venue allows for evaluation of a larger number of athletes quickly and introduces the ability to utilize a collaboration of health care providers with condition-specific training. In addition, direct access to the coaching and athletic training staff is afforded by performing evaluations at the athlete's school.

Health Questionnaire

A health questionnaire should be completed carefully in advance by the athlete with input from parents and the primary care provider. The questionnaire identifies the majority of potential problems and should focus on developmental and medical, family, social, allergies, medications, and immunization history. The review of medical history should address recent illnesses, neurological deficits and prior head injuries, heart and lung conditions, musculoskeletal problems, loss of organs, previous heat illness, substance or supplement abuse, and, in the female athlete, disordered eating and menstrual abnormalities. The cardiovascular portion of the history is especially important as heart disease is implicated in 95% of sudden deaths in athletes younger than 30 years. A prior occurrence of exertional chest pain or syncope, exercise-associated fatigue, heart murmurs, arrhythmia, history of elevated blood pressure, or a family history of premature death or disability secondary to cardiovascular disease should raise red flags and need to be explored. The medical history questionnaire should be carefully reviewed by a health care professional and appropriate workup for any concerning elements of the history must be undertaken prior to participation.

Physical Examination

Once the medical history has been obtained, the athlete should undergo a thorough but focused physical examination. Recording and tracking the height, weight, and body mass index of each athlete may identify disordered eating, steroid use, or obesity. Vital signs should be taken, and irregularities in pulse rate, blood pressure, or respiratory rate warrant further workup.

HEENT: The physical examination generally starts with the head, eyes, ears, nose, and throat. Poor vision, strabismus, astigmatism, refractive errors, and anisocoria should prompt referral. Eye protection is required for athletes with corrected vision less than 20/40, absence of one eye, or history of eye trauma or surgery.

Cardiovascular: According to the American Heart Association, the cardiovascular examination should include blood pressure measurement, auscultation for murmurs, palpation of lower extremity pulses, and assessing for stigmata of Marfan syndrome. Electrocardiography is indicated for any abnormal heart rhythm and may identify potentially lethal arrhythmias. Murmurs should be assessed in standing and supine positions, and cardiology referral is recommended for significant systolic murmur (>3/6), any diastolic murmurs, and all murmurs amplified by standing or Valsalva maneuver.

Lungs: The lung examination should focus on detection of abnormal breath sounds, use of accessory respiratory muscles, and presence of cough. Asthma is among the most common conditions facing young athletes and is characterized by chest tightness, wheezing, and shortness of breath. Exercise-induced bronchospasm is not reliably detected during preparticipation screening, and any athlete who reports asthma-like symptoms after exertion should undergo formal testing.

Gastrointestinal/Gastrourinary: The abdominal examination should be performed with patient supine with knees flexed. The physician should assess for organomegaly, masses, abdominal distension, or tenderness. A male testicular examination is not routine but may be indicated if the patient discloses a history of undescended or absent testicle, pain, swelling, mass, or hernia.

Musculoskeletal: The musculoskeletal examination should screen for muscular or bone abnormalities and reassess prior injuries. The neurological examination may be integrated into this portion of the evaluation and any unexplained weakness, paresthesias, or focal deficits indicate further workup. For the general participant, a 14-point musculoskeletal screening examination may be performed (Table 9.1). More elaborate joint-specific and sport-specific examination techniques may be used to augment the musculoskeletal examination, especially in the event of a previous injury. All positive findings necessitate more detailed evaluation to prevent new injuries and ensure that prior injuries and conditions have been fully rehabilitated prior to participation.

Clearance to Play

The culmination of the preparticipation evaluation is the decision on clearance to play. A physician must carefully review all elements of the preparticipation evaluation to determine whether participation is safe both for athletes and their teammates in the context of the sport in which they will be participating. As the physical demands and degree of contact vary among sports, the American Academy of Pediatrics has classified sports on the basis of contact (Table 9.2). An athlete precluded from engaging in a heavy-contact sport may be allowed to participate in a limited or noncontact sport. Treatable conditions should be addressed expeditiously and reassessed prior to clearance. Once all issues are reviewed, the physician should submit the final decision that the athlete may participate without restrictions, participate only after undergoing further evaluation or rehabilitation, participate with restrictions, or may not participate in the specific sport because of clearly defined disqualifying conditions. In the event that the athlete and physician do not agree about clearance issues, a written consent or legal waiver signed by the athlete and the parent should be obtained. A second opinion may also be sought by the athlete.

TABLE 9.1
THE 14-POINT MUSCULOSKELETAL SCREENING EXAMINATION

Examination	Assessment
1. Stand facing examiner	General appearance, habitus, symmetry
2. Look at ceiling, floor, and over both shoulder and touch ears to shoulders	Cervical spine range of motion
3. Shrug shoulders against resistance	Trapezius strength
4. Abduct shoulders against resistance	Deltoid strength
5. Full internal and external rotation of shoulders	Shoulder range of motion
6. Flex and extend elbows	Elbow range of motion
7. Pronate and supinate	Elbow and wrist range of motion
8. Spread fingers, clench fist	Hand/finger range of motion; deformities
9. Stand with back to examiner	Symmetry of trunk, upper extremities
10. Extend back with knees straight	Pain suggests spondylolysis or spondylolisthesis
11. Flex back with knees straight	Thoracic and lumbar spine range of motion; curvature; hamstring flexibility
12. Examine lower extremities; contract/relax quadriceps	Symmetry and alignment of lower extremities
13. "Duck walk" four steps	Hip, knee, ankle range of motion, strength, balance
14. Stand on toes, then on heels	Symmetry, calf strength, balance

(*Adapted from* McKeag D, Moeller JL, eds. *American College of Sports Medicine's Primary Care Sports Medicine.* 2nd ed. Philadelphia, PA: Lippincott Williams & Wilkins, 2007.)

TABLE 9.2
CLASSIFICATION OF SPORTS BY CONTACT

Contact/Collision	Limited Contact	Noncontact
Basketball	Adventure racing	Badminton
Boxing	Baseball	Bodybuilding
Cheerleading	Bicycling	Bowling
Diving	Canoeing or kayaking (white water)	Canoeing or kayaking (flat water)
Extreme sports	Fencing	Crew or rowing
Field hockey	Field events	Curling
Football, tackle	High jump	Dance
Gymnastics	Pole vault	Field events
Ice hockey	Floor hockey	Discus
Lacrosse	Football, flag or touch	Javelin
Martial arts	Handball	Shot put
Rodeo	Horseback riding	Golf
Rugby	Martial arts	Orienteering
Skiing, downhill	Racquetball	Power lifting
Ski jumping	Skating	Race walking
Snowboarding	Ice	Riflery
Soccer	In-line	Rope jumping
Team handball	Roller	Running
Ultimate Frisbee	Skiing	Sailing
Water polo	Cross-country	Scuba diving
Wrestling	Water	Swimming
	Skateboarding	Table tennis
	Softball	Tennis
	Squash	Track
	Volleyball	
	Weight lifting	
	Windsurfing or surfing	

(*From* Rice SG. American Academy of Pediatrics Council on Sports Medicine and Fitness: medical conditions affecting sports participation. *Pediatrics.* 2008;121(4):841–848.)

GAME COVERAGE

Preparedness

Preparation for game-day must take place long before the first whistle. The physician should be in communication with the administration and athletic training staff about all issues pertaining to the health and safety of the athletes. The responsibilities of the members of the health care team should be clearly defined, as well as the chain of command for game-day issues such as clearance to play, emergencies, environmental concerns, and playing conditions. An efficient and rehearsed emergency response plan should be in place prior to the start of the season and should be verified with the athletic trainer and emergency personnel prior to each practice and game. The establishment of a network of other health care providers including primary care providers, specialists, and athletic trainers facilitates prompt treatment and thorough follow-up.

The physician covering a sporting event from the sidelines should be familiar with the common conditions and injuries that arise from participation and should be prepared for all potential causes of on-field emergencies (Table 9.3). The medical equipment and supplies available on the sideline should consist of general medical essentials and reflect the risks specific to the sport. Contact sports such as football require consideration for impact injuries, whereas endurance sports such as long-distance running necessitate treatment strategies for fatigue and dehydration. Supplies for sport-specific protective equipment such as the face mask removal tool for football helmets should be readily available. The American College of Sports Medicine provides recommendations for contents of the medical bag and on-site medical supplies (Tables 9.4 and 9.5).

TABLE 9.3

POTENTIAL ON-FIELD EMERGENCIES

Traumatic	Medical
Head injury	Cardiac event
Spinal cord injury	Cerebrovascular accident
Cardiac tamponade	Bronchospasm
Cardiac contusion	Anaphylaxis
Commotio cordis	Pulmonary embolism
Hemothorax	Hyperventilation
Tension pneumothorax	Spontaneous pneumothorax
Pulmonary contusion	Hypoglycemia
Flail chest	Hyponatremia
Splenic rupture	Dehydration
Ruptured viscus	Heatstroke
Fracture	Hypothermia
Dislocation	Lightning
Blood loss	Drug/medication overdose

TABLE 9.4

RECOMMENDED CONTENTS OF A MEDICAL BAG

- Airway
- Alcohol/povidone–iodine swabs
- Bandage scissors, bandages, sterile/nonsterile, Band-aids
- Blood pressure cuff
- Cricothyrotomy kit
- Dental kit (e.g., cyanoacrylate, Hank solution)
- Epinephrine 1:1,000 in a prepackaged unit
- Eye kit (e.g., blue light, fluorescein stain strips, eye patch pads, cotton tip applicators, ocular anesthetic and antibiotics, contact remover, mirror)
- Flashlight
- Gloves
- Large bore (14–16 G) Angiocath for tension pneumothorax
- List of emergency numbers
- Local anesthetic/syringes/needles
- Mouth-to-mouth mask
- Nasal packing material
- Oto-ophthalmoscope
- Prescription pad
- Rectal thermometer
- Reflex hammer
- Short-acting β-agonist inhaler
- Skin staple applicator
- Small mirror
- Stethoscope
- Supplemental oral and parenteral medications
- Suture set/steri-strips
- Tongue depressors
- Topical antibiotics
- Wound irrigation materials (e.g., sterile normal saline, 10–50 cc syringe)

TABLE 9.5

ON-SITE MEDICAL SUPPLIES

- ACLS drugs and equipment
- Automated external defibrillator
- Blanket
- Cervical collar
- Crutches
- Extremity splints
- Face mask removal tool (for sports with helmets)
- Ice
- Ice immersion for events with risk of heat illness
- Mouth guards
- Oral fluid replacement
- Plastic bags
- Sideline concussion assessment protocol
- Sling psychrometer and temperature/humidity activity risk chart
- Slings
- Spine board and attachments
- Tape cutter
- Telephone

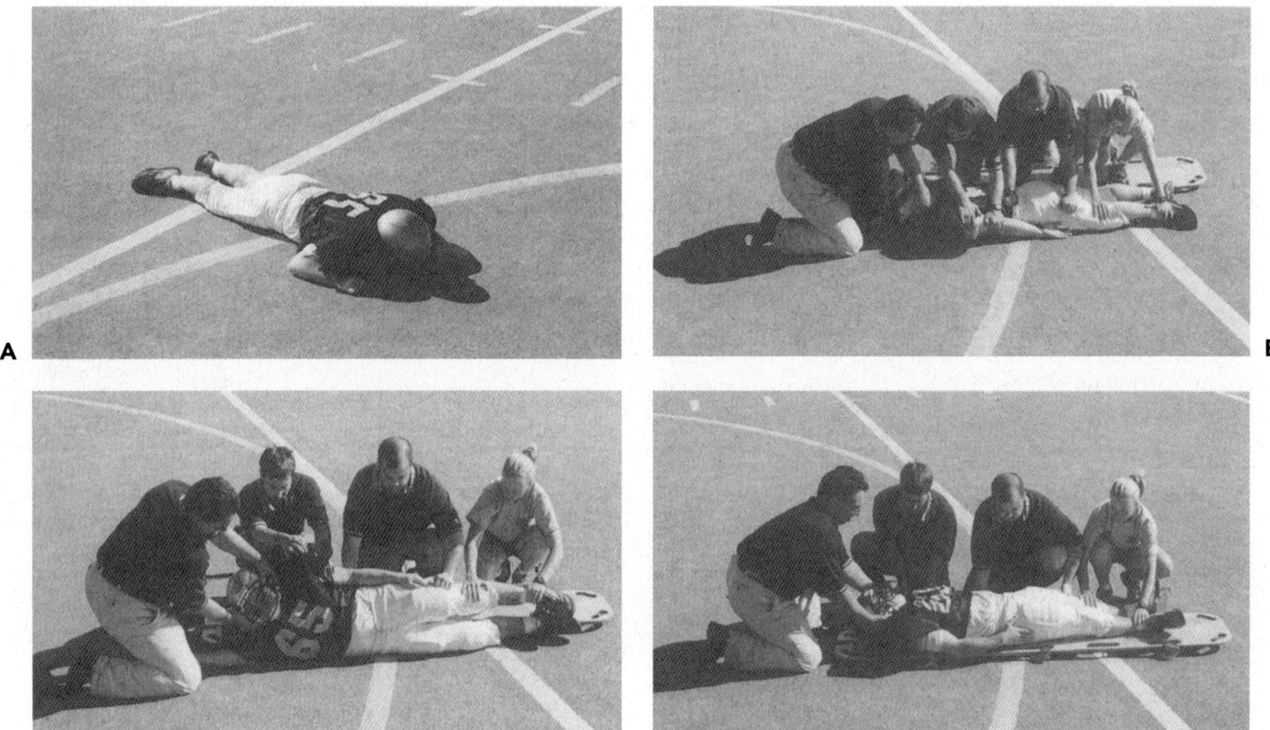

Figure 9.1 **(A-D)** The logroll technique should be used when spine injury is suspected. (*Reprinted with permission from* Garrett WE, Kirkendall DT, Squire DL. *Principles and Practice of Primary Care Sports Medicine*. Philadelphia, PA: Lippincott Williams & Wilkins, 2000.)

Approach to the Injured Athlete

When an athlete goes down during play, the initial assessment should take place immediately on the field. Serious injury must be completely excluded before moving the athlete or removing any equipment. In the event of serious injury, basic life support protocol, including a primary survey, should be initiated to manage potentially life-threatening conditions. Cervical immobilization should be maintained until spinal cord injury has been ruled out, especially if the athlete was involved in a collision or demonstrates neurological deficits or altered mental status. A spine injury should be presumed in all unconscious patients. The prone athlete may be logrolled to the supine position (Fig. 9.1). In football players, the face mask should be removed as soon as possible to obtain access to the airway, but the helmet absolutely must not be removed until cervical spine injury is excluded (Fig. 9.2). If the primary survey reveals any concerning issues or if the athlete is unstable, the prearranged emergency response plan should be activated promptly and the athlete should be transported to a hospital.

The predominance of injuries sustained on the field of play are not life-threatening and do not necessarily merit such attention. In most cases, once serious injury has been excluded and after a focused examination, the player may be helped off the field so that play can resume. Evaluation of the injury and a complete secondary survey may then proceed in a more controlled setting on the sideline. Injuries should be fully evaluated and treated in the context of the sport before allowing reentry into the game. The team physician should be involved in all injuries or conditions where the ability to participate is in question. Provisional management such as bandaging or taping may allow return to play, but the injured player should be reassessed in sport-specific activity before final clearance. Decisions about participation should be clearly communicated to the player and coaching staff to prevent any confusion. Any athlete who expresses hesitancy about returning to play should be held out until concerns are addressed. All injuries and conditions should be documented so that they receive appropriate follow-up and rehabilitation, and the player's family and primary care provider should be informed and involved in decisions pertaining to continuing care.

COMMON ATHLETIC INJURIES

The kinetic energy inherent to sports puts the body at risk of injury. Collision with another player is responsible for the majority of significant injuries sustained in sports, but other objects such as the ground, goalposts, walls, and stands may inflict harm as well. Noncontact injury mechanisms are pervasive regardless of sport and represent a larger

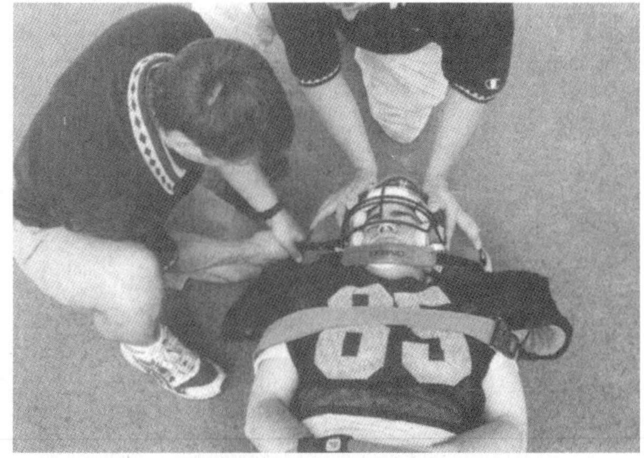

A

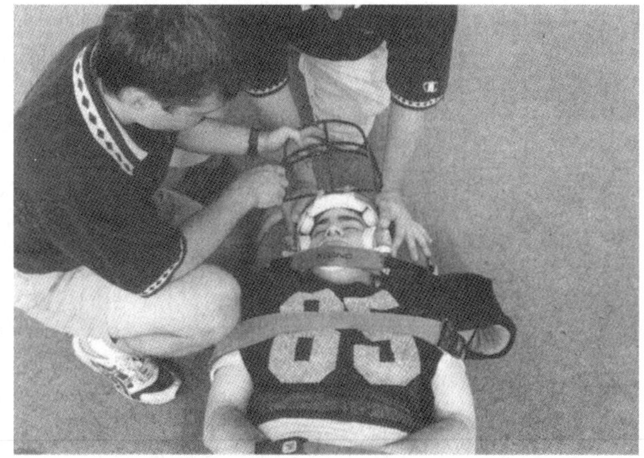

B

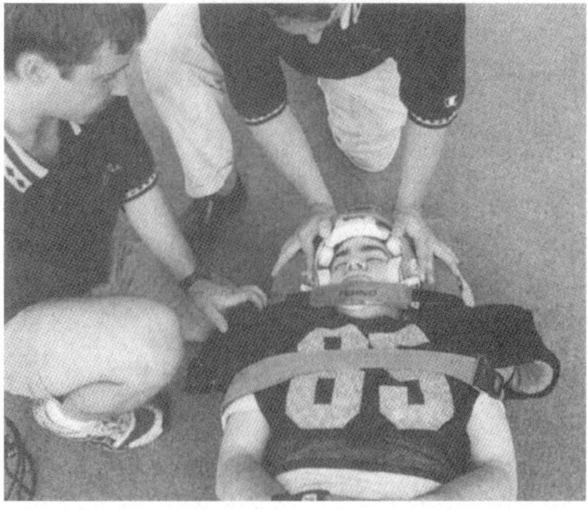

C

Figure 9.2 **(A-C)** A bolt cutter or face mask removal tool should be used to remove the face mask as soon as possible to provide access to the player's airway. (*Reprinted with permission from* Garrett WE, Kirkendall DT, Squire DL. *Principles and Practice of Primary Care Sports Medicine*. Philadelphia, PA: Lippincott Williams & Wilkins, 2000.)

proportion of training and practice injuries than in-game injuries. The lower extremity accounts for more than half of all sports-related injuries, with the ankle or knee representing the most frequently injured joint. The distribution of injury during competition and training by body part as reported by the National Collegiate Athletic Association is illustrated in Figure 9.3.

HEAD INJURIES

More than 300,000 sports-related head injuries were treated in U.S. emergency departments in 2007, with cycling and football comprising the most frequently implicated sports. The risk of head injury increases with the amount of energy to which an athlete is exposed. Despite rule modifications and advances in helmet design and other protective equipment, the force of impact seen in some sports such as football, boxing, and rugby approaches that of motor vehicle accidents. Any athlete who exhibits signs and symptoms to include headache, loss of consciousness, altered mental status, cranial nerve dysfunction, or worsening symptoms should be considered to have a significant traumatic brain injury and should undergo a thorough neurological evaluation along with serial examinations.

Concussion

Concussion is the most common head injury sustained by athletes and is characterized by a transient posttraumatic impairment of cerebral neural function. Generally, the result of a direct blow to the head either by another player, an object, or the ground, initial signs and symptoms of concussion may include loss of consciousness, confusion, amnesia, vision or balance dysfunction, nausea, or headache while persistent effects include memory or cognitive deficits, sleep disturbance, and emotional lability. Frequently, teammates may identify a player who is demonstrating concussive symptoms. The sideline interview is the most effective method of detecting impairment, and the Standardized Assessment of Concussion (SAC) permits documentation of symptoms for serial examination (Fig. 9.4).

The goal of management is to minimize postconcussive syndrome symptoms and prevent second-impact syndrome. Postconcussive syndrome is characterized by persistence of concussion symptoms secondary to cerebral metabolic derangements and neurotransmitter dysfunction. Athletes with prolonged postconcussive syndrome should not be allowed to participate in any exertional activities and may require neuroimaging or expert consultation. Second-impact syndrome is a rare but catastrophic sequela

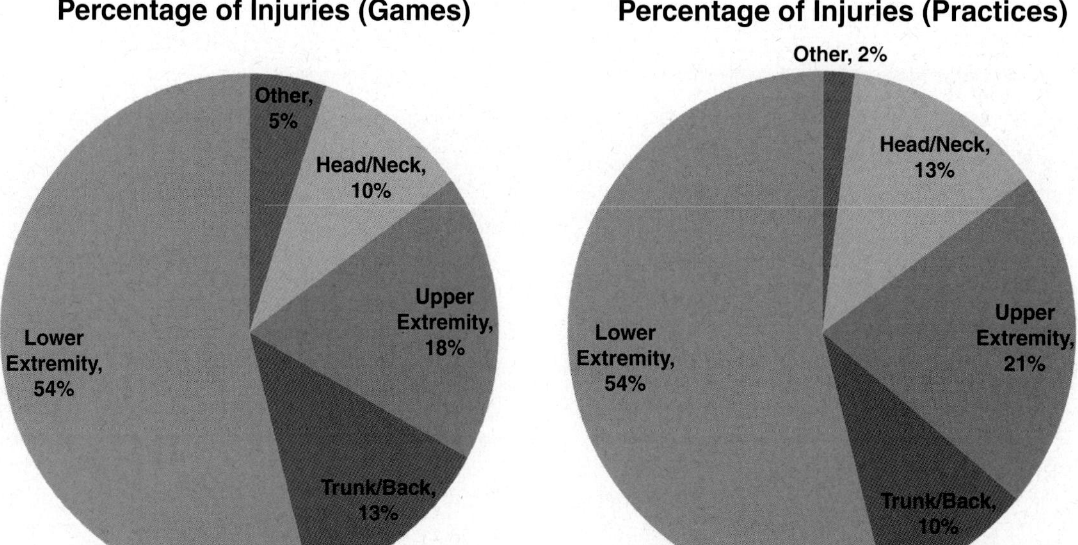

Figure 9.3 **(A)** Percentages of injuries by body part during competition for 15 sports, National Collegiate Athletic Association 1988–2004. **(B)** Percentages of injuries by body part during training/practice for 15 sports, National Collegiate Athletic Association 1988–2004. (*Data from* Hootman JM, Dick R, Agel J. Epidemiology of collegiate injuries for 15 sports: summary and recommendations for injury prevention initiatives. *J Athl Train.* 2007;42(2):311–319.)

1) ORIENTATION:

Month: ______	0	1
Date: ______	0	1
Day of week: ______	0	1
Year: ______	0	1
Time (within 1 hr): ______	0	1
Orientation Total Score ______	/	5

2) IMMEDIATE MEMORY: (all 3 trials are completed regardless of score on trial 1 & 2; total score equals sum across all 3 trials)

List	Trial 1		Trial 2		Trial 3	
Word 1	0	1	0	1	0	1
Word 2	0	1	0	1	0	1
Word 3	0	1	0	1	0	1
Word 4	0	1	0	1	0	1
Word 5	0	1	0	1	0	1
Total						

Immediate Memory Total Score ______ / 15

(Note: Subject is not informed of delayed recall testing of memory)

NEUROLOGIC SCREENING:

Loss of Consciousness: (occurrence, duration)

Retrograde & Posttraumatic Amnesia: (recollection of events pre- and post-injury)

Strength:

Sensation:

Coordination:

3) CONCENTRATION:

Digits Backward (If correct, go to next string length. If incorrect, read trial 2. Stop after incorrect on both trials.)

4-9-3	6-2-9	______	0	1
3-8-1-4	3-2-7-9	______	0	1
6-2-9-7-1	1-5-2-8-6	______	0	1
7-1-8-4-6-2	5-3-9-1-4-8	______	0	1

Months in Reverse Order: (entire sequence correct for 1 point)

Dec-Nov-Oct-Sep-Aug-Jul
Jun-May-Apr-Mar-Feb-Jan ______ 0 1

Concentration Total Score ______ / 5

EXERTIONAL MANEUVERS
(when appropriate):

5 jumping jacks — 5 push-ups
5 sit-ups — 5 knee bends

4) DELAYED RECALL:

Word 1	0	1
Word 2	0	1
Word 3	0	1
Word 4	0	1
Word 5	0	1
Delayed Recall Total Score ______	/	5

SUMMARY OF TOTAL SCORES:

ORIENTATION ______	/	5
IMMEDIATE MEMORY ______	/	15
CONCENTRATION ______	/	5
DELAYED RECALL ______	/	5
OVERALL TOTAL SCORE ______	/	30

Figure 9.4 Standardized Assessment of Concussion testing permits documentation of symptoms for serial examination. (*Reprinted with permission from* McCrea M. Standardized mental status testing on the sideline after sport-related concussion. *J Athl Train.* 2001;36(3):274–279.)

TABLE 9.6
CANTU AND AMERICAN ACADEMY OF NEUROLOGY GRADING SYSTEMS FOR CONCUSSION

Grade	Cantu	AAN
1 (Mild)	▪ No LOC, PTA <30 min, PCS <24 h ▪ *First concussion:* RTP if asymptomatic for 1 wk ▪ *Second concussion:* RTP in 2 wk if asymptomatic for 1 wk ▪ *Third concussion:* Terminate season; RTP next season if asymptomatic	▪ No LOC, transient confusion; symptoms resolve in <15 min. ▪ *First concussion:* RTP if asymptomatic for 15 min ▪ *Second concussion:* RTP if asymptomatic for 1 wk
2 (Moderate)	▪ LOC <1 min or PTA ≥30 min or PCS ≥24 h *and* <7 d ▪ *First concussion:* RTP if asymptomatic for 2 wk ▪ *Second concussion:* RTP in 1 mo if asymptomatic for 1 wk ▪ *Third concussion:* Terminate season; RTP next season if asymptomatic	▪ No LOC, transient confusion; symptoms persist for >15 min. ▪ *First concussion:* RTP if asymptomatic for 1 wk ▪ *Second concussion:* RTP if asymptomatic for 2 wk
3 (Severe)	▪ LOC ≥1 min or PTA ≥24 h or PCS ≥7 d ▪ *First concussion:* No RTP for at least 1 mo; must be asymptomatic for >1 wk ▪ *Second concussion:* Terminate season; RTP next season if asymptomatic ▪ *Third concussion:* Consider no further contact sports	▪ Any LOC ▪ *First concussion:* Transport to hospital; if LOC brief, may RTP if asymptomatic for 1 wk; for prolonged LOC (>1 min), RTP if asymptomatic for 2 wk ▪ *Second concussion:* RTP if asymptomatic for 1 mo

AAN, American Academy of Neurology; LOC, loss of consciousness; PTA, posttraumatic amnesia; PCS, postconcussive syndrome; RTP, return to play.
(*Adapted from* Patel DR, Greydanus DE, Luckstead EF Sr. The college athlete. *Pediatr Clin North Am.* 2005;52(1):25–60, vii–viii.)

of recurrent head trauma prior to resolution of concussion symptoms distinguished by a secondary loss of cerebrovascular autoregulation that results in increased intracranial pressure from excessive blood flow. A preventable condition, second-impact syndrome is associated with 50% mortality and 100% morbidity, typically from cerebral edema and herniation, which may result from seemingly minor contact.

Given the potential complications, clearing an athlete to play after a concussion presents a difficult clinical decision. Regardless of how benign they appear, all concussions require an observation period of at least 15 to 20 minutes. During this time, the athlete should be monitored closely, and deterioration of mental status, development of focal deficits, seizure activity, or vital sign lability should prompt immediate transfer to a hospital. If the athlete appears to be improving, the physician should then repeat the SAC evaluation looking carefully for memory or cognition deficits. No athlete actively demonstrating symptoms should be allowed to play. The presence of a headache should not be discounted. Return to play may be considered after complete resolution of symptoms after the period of observation, and the athlete should be exerted prior to reentry to ensure that no symptoms reemerge. If symptoms recur later in the game, the player should be removed from play and be closely observed.

More severe concussions such as those with loss of consciousness or persistent symptoms typically disqualify the athlete from participation for the remainder of the day of injury, and return to play is based on severity and duration of symptoms. Multiple grading systems including the Cantu and American Academy of Neurology grading systems have been developed to classify the severity of a concussion and provide a general outline on when to allow return to play (Table 9.6). Accurately grading a concussion acutely may be difficult, and each athlete should be managed on an individual basis. Regardless of the grade, concussions associated with abnormal computed tomography (CT) or magnetic resonance imaging (MRI) scans should preclude return to play for the remainder of the season.

Intracranial Hemorrhage

Clinical deterioration and development of focal deficits may be manifestations of severe traumatic brain injury. A direct blow to the head may cause a *cerebral contusion,* in which cerebral parenchymal blood vessels are violated, resulting in bruising and internal bleeding. Patients may show focal symptoms such as partial paralysis, cranial nerve involvement, or labile vital signs. A high-velocity impact to the temple may fracture the skull, disrupting the middle meningeal artery to cause an *epidural hematoma.* In this injury, blood accumulates in the potential space between the skull and the dura mater, and the characteristic clinical sequence begins with a brief loss of consciousness, followed by a lucid interval, and culminates in rapid deterioration of neurologic function. The bridging veins traversing the subdural space are vulnerable to acceleration-/deceleration-type forces. An injury to these vessels results in a *subdural hematoma,* and neurological consequences may appear immediately or develop over the course of several days or weeks. Symptoms are generally progressive and range from

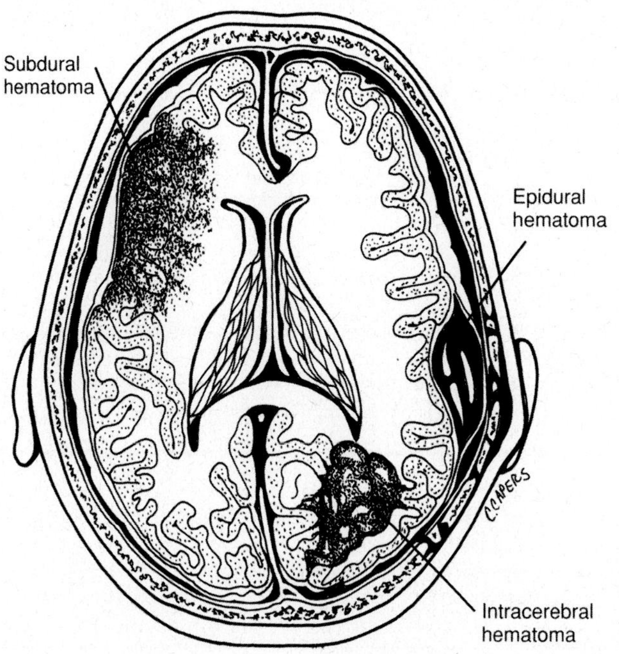

Figure 9.5 Types of intracranial hemorrhage: epidural hematoma occurs when blood accumulates in the epidural space usually due to injury of the middle meningeal artery. Subdural hematoma results from damage to bridging veins between the brain and dura. Intracerebral hematoma occurs deep within the brain. (*Reprinted with permission from* Baker CL, Flandry F, Henderson JM. *The Hughston Clinic: Sports Medicine Book*. Philadelphia, PA: Williams & Wilkins, 1995.)

mild alteration in level of consciousness to coma or major focal neurological deficit. Suspected intracranial bleeding mandates immediate transport to a hospital where further evaluation and treatment should take place (Fig. 9.5).

FACIAL INJURY

Because of the abundant vascularity of the face, facial injuries are frequently associated with profuse bleeding and significant swelling. Closed head injury and cervical spine injury should be considered with all facial traumas. Facial lacerations are common and bleeding may be controlled with direct pressure. Universal precautions should be maintained when managing any bleeding. Following thorough irrigation, small lacerations may be closed with an adhesive bandage, whereas larger wounds may require stitches. Simple anterior nasal bleeds involving disruption of the Kiesselbach venous plexus in the anterior nose may be controlled with direct pressure or a vasoconstrictive nasal spray such as oxymetazoline or phenylephrine. Posterior epistaxis in which brisk nasopharyngeal bleeding occurs from injury to the sphenopalatine artery or other larger vessel may not respond to nasal spray and warrants nasal packing and transfer to the hospital for further management (Fig. 9.6).

Nasal fractures compose the majority of facial fractures and usually are associated with epistaxis, soft tissue swelling, septal hematoma, and obvious nasal deformity. Depending on the degree of displacement, conservative or surgical management may be indicated.

Eye injuries also occur frequently in sports and may result in long-term morbidity. Sports-related eye injuries are a leading cause of adolescent blindness, and 90% of these injuries may be avoided with protective eyewear. Significant eye injury may present with photophobia, partial or complete vision loss, double vision, or eye pain. *Corneal abrasion* may occur with direct trauma such as a finger to the eye

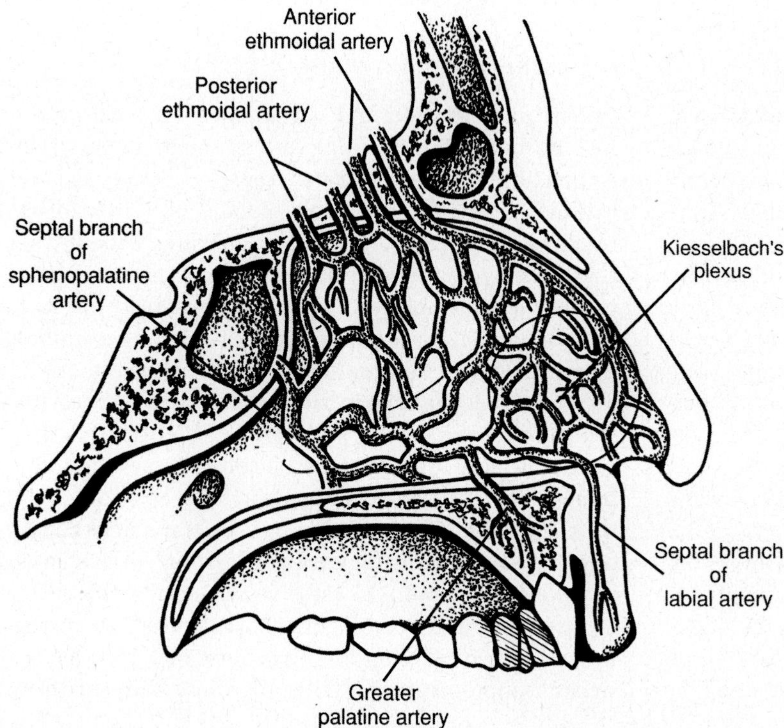

Figure 9.6 Vascularity of the nasal cavity. (*Reprinted with permission from* Baker CL, Flandry F, Henderson JM. *The Hughston Clinic: Sports Medicine Book*. Philadelphia, PA: Williams & Wilkins, 1995.)

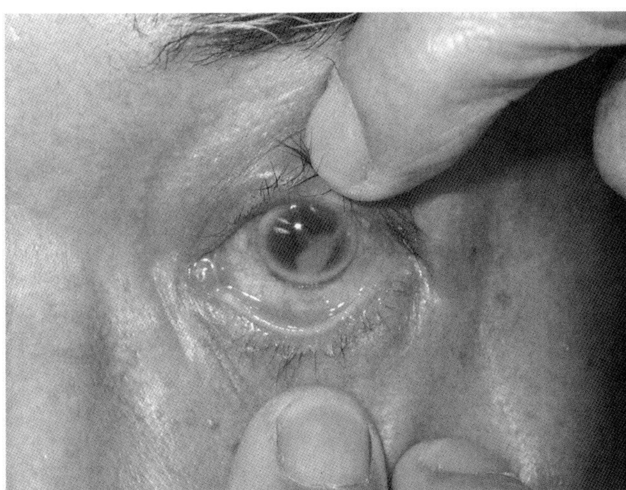

Figure 9.7 Fluorescein-stained central corneal abrasion. (*Reprinted with permission from* Greenberg MI, Hendrickson RG, Silverberg M, et al., eds. *Greenberg's Text-Atlas of Emergency Medicine.* Philadelphia, PA: Lippincott Williams & Wilkins, 2004.)

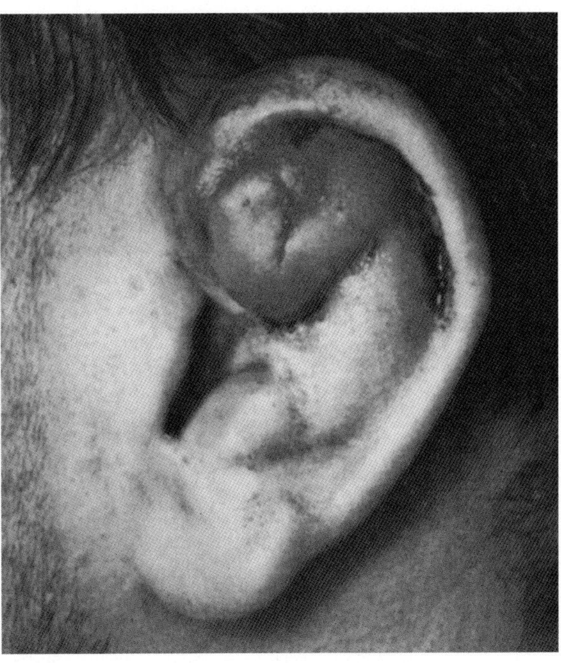

Figure 9.8 Cauliflower ear. (*Reprinted with permission from* Greenberg MI, Hendrickson RG, Silverberg M, et al., eds. *Greenberg's Text-Atlas of Emergency Medicine.* Philadelphia, PA: Lippincott Williams & Wilkins, 2004.)

(Fig. 9.7). Athletes may complain of photophobia and sensation of a foreign object. Diagnosed with fluorescein stain, athletes with significant abrasions may require antibiotics and an eye patch. Periorbital contusion or "black eye" generally may be treated with conservative management involving ice to control swelling and observation. Athletes who sustain a black eye should undergo a thorough ophthalmologic examination to ensure that the eye is not injured and the orbit is not fractured. More serious eye injuries should be referred to an ophthalmologist.

The cauliflower ear, commonly seen in boxers and wrestlers, represents the consequences of recurrent ear trauma (Fig. 9.8). Auricular hematomas develop between the skin and underlying cartilage and should be treated with ice to reduce swelling. Severe swelling may cause cartilage breakdown, and fluid accumulation may necessitate aspiration.

Mouth guards should be worn by athletes participating in contact sports to prevent dental injury. In the event of dental injury, bleeding may be controlled with direct pressure. Loose teeth should be gently pushed back into their normal position, and fractured or avulsed teeth should be located and placed into Hank solution, milk, or sterile saline. An avulsed tooth should be handled by the crown to prevent root injury. Athletes who sustain a dental injury should be referred to a dentist for further care.

SPINE

According to the National Spinal Cord Injury Statistical Center, sports-related spinal cord injuries accounted for approximately 7.4% of all spinal cord injuries since 2005, with almost 25% of spinal cord injuries in patients younger than 15 years and 15% of those in patients between 15 and 30 years. The incidence of catastrophic spinal cord injuries in sports ranges from 0.5 to 2.5 in 100,000. Diving, bicycling, and football are among the sports most commonly implicated in spinal cord injury, and the cervical spine is the most frequently involved.

Cervical Spine

Neck pain, focal neurological deficits, loss of consciousness, or abnormal reflexes may signify a spinal cord injury and should be systematically documented. Spine precautions consisting of in-line immobilization and logrolling must be maintained for all unconscious athletes and all those suspected of sustaining a cervical spine injury. Players should not be transported until proper immobilization is in place. Cervical collars, backboards, and stretchers are essential equipment and should be readily available for any sporting event in which a spinal cord injury is a possibility. The helmet of football players must not be removed. Removing a football helmet without the shoulder pads produces unacceptable motion in the cervical spine and may compromise the cord. The player should be transported to the hospital, immobilized on a spine board with helmet and pads in place. The face mask should always be removed from the helmet as soon as possible to ensure access to the airway. If the airway needs to be secured, the cervical spine may be protected with the jaw-thrust and chin-lift maneuver. The head-tilt maneuver should be avoided.

A methodical radiographic analysis should begin with anteroposterior, lateral, and oblique plain radiographs and

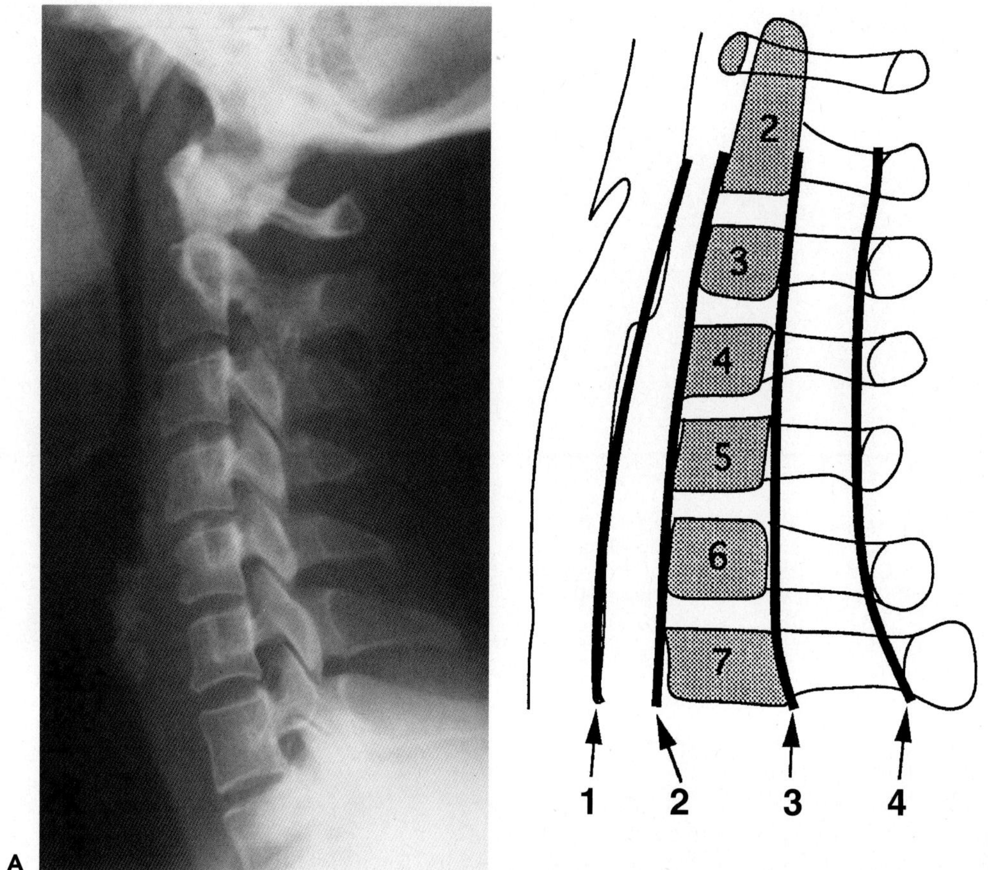

Figure 9.9 The lateral cervical spine radiograph should be examined for alignment and evidence of instability. (*Reprinted with permission from* Brant WE, Helms CA, eds. *Fundamentals of Diagnostic Radiology*. 3rd ed. Philadelphia, PA: Lippincott Williams & Wilkins, 2007.)

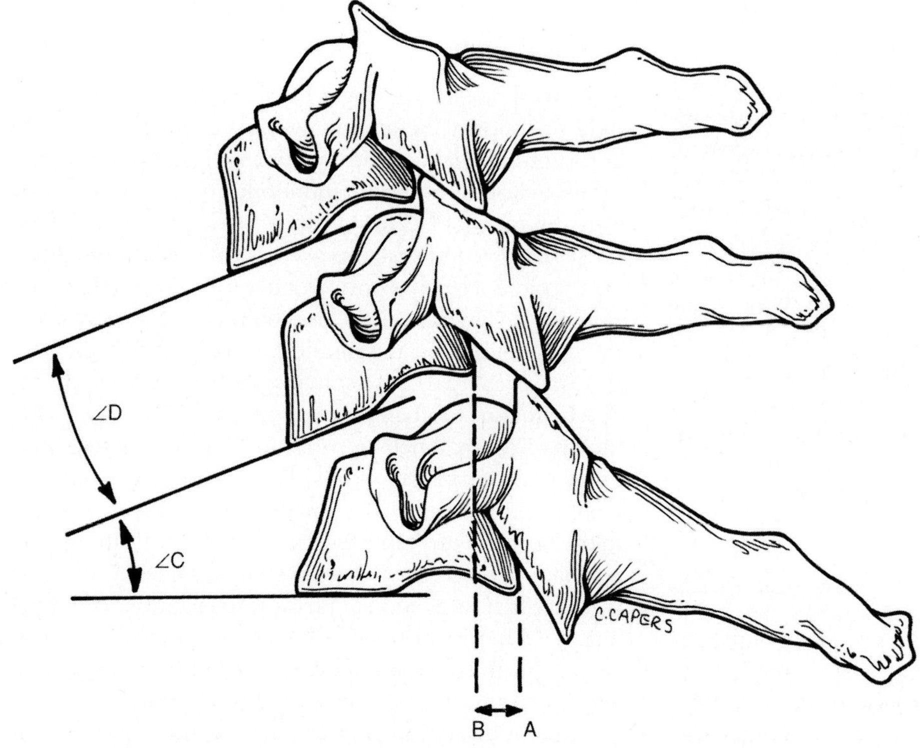

Figure 9.10 Instability is indicated by translation of more than 3.5 mm (distance between **A** and **B**) or junctional kyphosis of more than 11 degrees (difference between angle **C** and **D**). (*Reprinted with permission from* Baker CL, Flandry F, Henderson JM. *The Hughston Clinic: Sports Medicine Book*. Philadelphia, PA: Williams & Wilkins, 1995.)

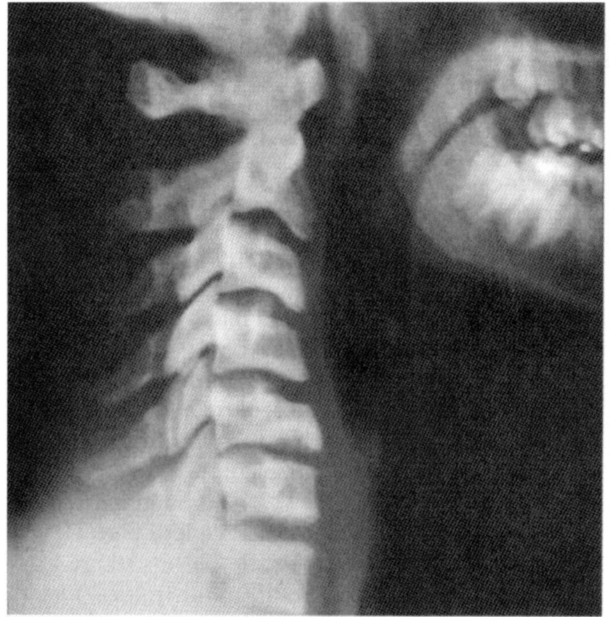
A

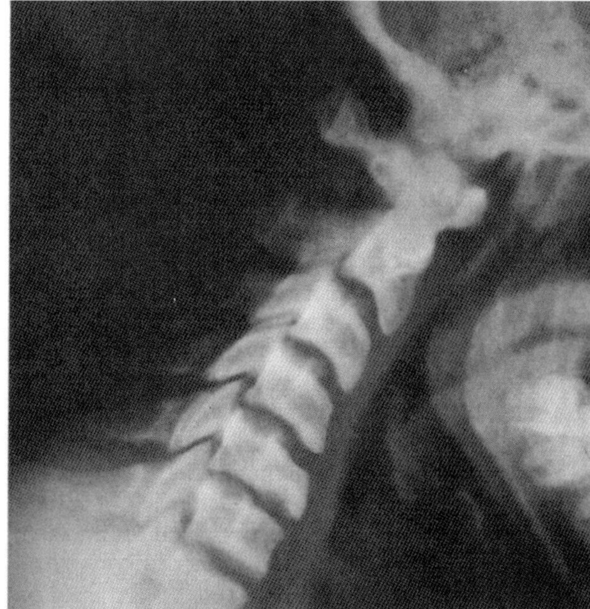
B

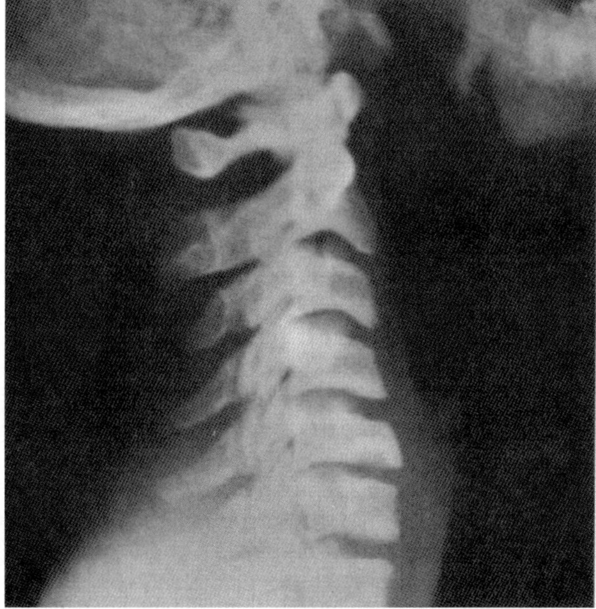
C

Figure 9.11 Spear tackler's spine involves cervical stenosis and loss of lordosis and is associated with increased risk of spinal cord injury. This condition prohibits contact sports. (*Reprinted with permission from* Garrett WE, Speer KP, Kirkendall DT, eds. *Principles and Practice of Orthopaedic Sports Medicine*. Philadelphia, PA: Lippincott Williams & Wilkins, 2000.)

must include the cervicothoracic junction (Fig. 9.9). Vertebral deformity, soft tissue swelling, loss of lordosis, step-offs, or splaying of posterior elements signify spinal injury. Instability is indicated by junctional kyphosis of more than 11 degrees or anteroposterior translation greater than 3.5 mm (Fig. 9.10). The space available for the cord between C3 and C7 averages approximately 17 mm in adults. Relative and absolute stenosis are present if the canal narrows to less than 13 mm and 10 mm, respectively, and represents a relative or absolute contraindication to contact sports depending upon presence of symptoms. Spear tackler's spine is an entity that involves cervical stenosis and loss of lordosis typically seen in football players and prohibits participation in contact sports (Fig. 9.11). Fractures may be further elucidated by CT scans with reconstructions, and an MRI study to assess soft-tissue, ligamentous, or disc pathology is indicated for neurological deficits, radiculopathy, or myelopathy. A referral to a spine surgeon is indicated for any abnormalities.

Guidelines for participation in sports for a number of cervical spine conditions are outlined in the Torg guidelines (Table 9.7).

Minor Neck Injuries

The majority of cervical spinal cord injuries are self-limited sprains characterized by persistent neck pain and limited range of motion with no neurological symptoms.

TABLE 9.7

GUIDELINES FOR ATHLETES WITH CERVICAL SPINE ABNORMALITIES

No Contraindication to Contact Sports

- Asymptomatic cervical stenosis
- Klippel–Feil type 2 anomaly with full range of motion with no evidence of instability
- Spina bifida occulta
- Healed, stable nondisplaced fractures without sagittal malalignment
- Asymptomatic disc herniations treated conservatively in the past
- After a healed one-level anterior or posterior cervical fusion in asymptomatic patient

Relative Contraindications to Contact Sports for Asymptomatic Patients

- Cervical stenosis with one episode of cord neuropraxia
- Prior upper cervical spine fracture
- Healed, stable minimally displaced fracture of the body without sagittal malalignment or canal compromise
- Healed, stable fracture of the posterior elements
- Minimal residual facet instability after surgical or conservative treatment of cervical disc disease
- After a healed two- or three-level cervical fusion

Absolute Contraindications to Contact Sports

- Cervical stenosis
  - With one episode of cord neuropraxia and MRI evidence of cord injury
  - With one episode of cord neuropraxia associated with instability or neurologic symptoms lasting for more than 36 h
  - With multiple episodes of cord neuropraxia
- Odontoid anomalies
- Atlantooccipital fusion
- Atlantoaxial instability
- Atlantoaxial rotatory fixation
- Certain Klippel–Feil anomalies
- Spear tackler's spine
- Subaxial spinal instability
- Acute fracture of either the body or posterior elements
- Healed fracture with residual sagittal malalignment or canal compromise
- Continued pain, abnormal neurological findings, or limited motion from a healed cervical fracture
- Symptomatic acute soft or chronic disc herniation
- After any fusion in the presence of congenital stenosis

MRI, magnetic resonance imaging.
(*Adapted from* Torg JS, Guille JT, Jaffe S. Injuries to the cervical spine in American football players. *J Bone Joint Surg Am.* 2002;84-A(1):112–122.)

Immobilization with a cervical collar should continue until resolution of acute symptoms at which time dynamic flexion and extension radiographs may be obtained. Radiographic evidence of instability warrants further investigation of ligamentous injury with MRI. Treatment of sprains consists of conservative management including anti-inflammatories and physical therapy. An athlete may return to play once symptoms subside if there are no radiographic abnormalities.

Stingers and Transient Quadriplegia

Sports-related neck injuries with self-limited neurological symptoms include stingers and transient quadriplegia. A temporary unilateral upper extremity burning dysesthesia with associated motor weakness, a *stinger* or *burner* is usually the result of traction or direct trauma to the brachial plexus or momentary foraminal compression of a nerve root from neck extension or lateral flexion (Fig. 9.12).

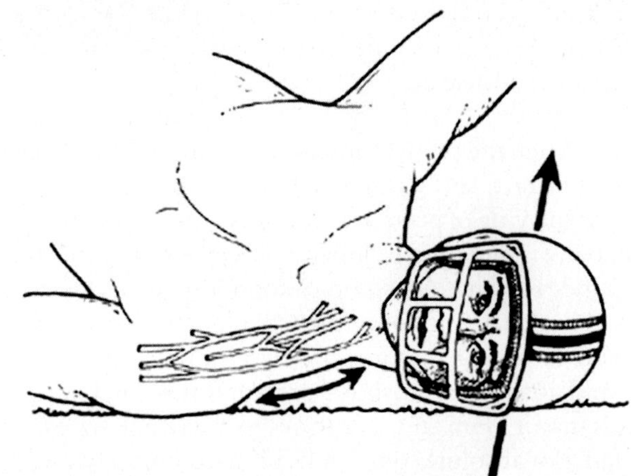

Figure 9.12 A stinger or burner may result from traction on the brachial plexus. (*Reprinted with permission from* Fu FH, Stone DA, eds. *Sports Injuries: Mechanisms, Prevention, Treatment.* 2nd ed. Philadelphia, PA: Lippincott Williams & Wilkins, 2001.)

Approximately half of all collision-sports athletes will experience a stinger at some point during their career. The typical complaint is a painful sensation that radiates from the neck to fingertips after a lateral blow to neck or shoulder. The effects of a stinger are short-lived, and generally, return to play is permissible if symptoms resolve. Persistent or recurrent symptoms preclude from play and require further workup.

Transient quadriplegia is less common, affecting approximately 1.3 in 10,000 athletes, but entails a more serious injury than a stinger. Usually a result of hyperextension often accompanied by axial loading of the neck, transient quadriplegia is characterized by bilateral symptoms that may include burning, paresthesias, loss of sensation, and/or weakness in the arms and/or legs. The severity of symptoms may range from mild paresthesias to complete paralysis and may persist for up to 36 hours. Athletes with transient quadriplegia, especially those with symptoms for more than 36 hours, should receive imaging of the cervical spine.

All athletes with symptoms of cord neuropraxia should be presumed to have a spine injury and spine precautions should be maintained until appropriate evaluation has taken place. Determination of return to play for these types of injuries presents a challenge to the sports physician. No athlete should be allowed to play with neurological deficit, painful range of motion of neck, or pain on axial loading of spine. Instability, disc disease, congenitally fused segments, and canal stenosis predispose athletes to transient quadriplegia, and careful consideration of these potentially dangerous conditions should be made before allowing return to play.

Thoracolumbar Spine

Thoracolumbar spine injuries and conditions also affect the athletic population. While the majority of these injuries are minor, severe injuries may occur, and proper management is important to prevent further injury. The thoracolumbar spine may be controlled with logrolling and placing the athlete on a backboard. Neurological function may be assessed by examining motor and sensory function in the extremities, and deficits prompt more thorough evaluation.

The most common etiology of low back pain is *lumbar strain*, a condition characterized by point tenderness in the paraspinal musculature of the low back and pain with motion. Strains generally respond to rest, activity modification, therapy, and symptomatic treatment. Radicular symptoms may develop if a nerve root is compressed or irritated, usually from a bulging disc. Low back pain with radiculopathy also tends to improve with conservative treatment. Athletes with persistent or progressive symptoms should be referred to a spine surgeon.

In some athletes such as gymnasts and football players, repetitive lumbar hyperextension produces impaction of the inferior articular facet upon the pars interarticularis, leading to *spondylolysis* (Fig. 9.13). In this condition in which a defect develops in the pars, the athlete may complain of low back pain exacerbated by extension and paraspinal muscle spasm and hamstring tightness. Bilateral pars defects may lead to *spondylolisthesis* or slippage of the vertebra. Diagnosis is confirmed by oblique radiographs of the lumbar spine or single-photon emission CT scan. Athletes with suspected spondylolysis or spondylolisthesis should be referred to a spine surgeon.

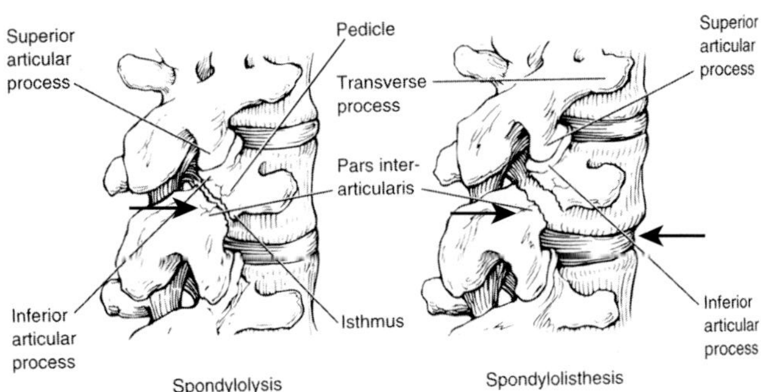

Figure 9.13 Spondylolysis **(A)** is a stress fracture of the pars interarticularis that may result from repetitive hyperextension of the lumbar spine. Spondylolisthesis **(B)**, or slippage of the vertebra, may occur with bilateral pars fractures. (*Reprinted with permission from* Anderson MK, Hall SJ, eds. *Sports Injury Management*. Baltimore, MD: Williams & Wilkins, 1995.)

THORACIC INJURY

Athletes involved in high-speed or contact sports are vulnerable to injuries of the chest wall and intrathoracic organs. *Rib fractures* constitute the majority of chest wall injuries, most commonly resulting from blunt trauma, although noncontact and overuse mechanisms may also cause rib fracture. Usually involving the midaxillary region of ribs 4 through 9, rib fractures are associated with local pain and tenderness and pain on deep inspiration. An isolated rib fracture typically may be treated expectantly, but sternal fractures, pneumothorax, flail chest, and fractures of the first rib constitute more serious injury and require further management.

Although protected by the chest wall, the intrathoracic organs are vulnerable to high-energy trauma. Cardiac contusion manifests as a dull chest pain after blunt chest wall trauma and should be evaluated by electrocardiography due to the risk of associated dysrhythmia. *Commotio cordis* is a lethal ventricular arrhythmia resulting from a direct blow to the chest, precisely corresponding to the repolarization phase of the contracting heart. Most commonly described in youth baseball, commotio cordis must be treated with cardiopulmonary resuscitation and early defibrillation to prevent almost certain death. Basic life support training and accessibility of automated external defibrillators are vital to preventing cardiac-related morbidity and mortality.

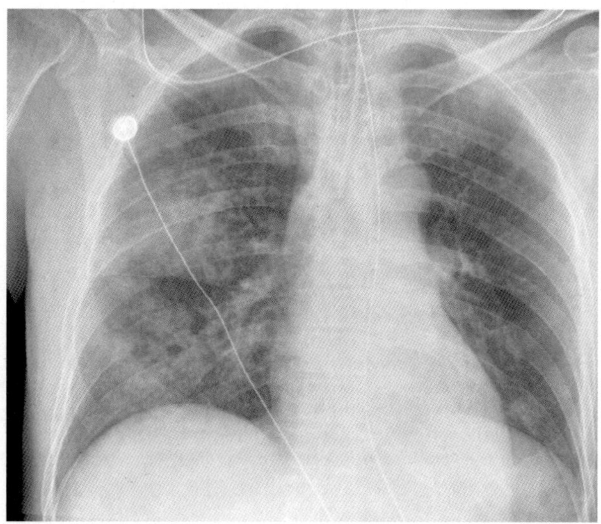

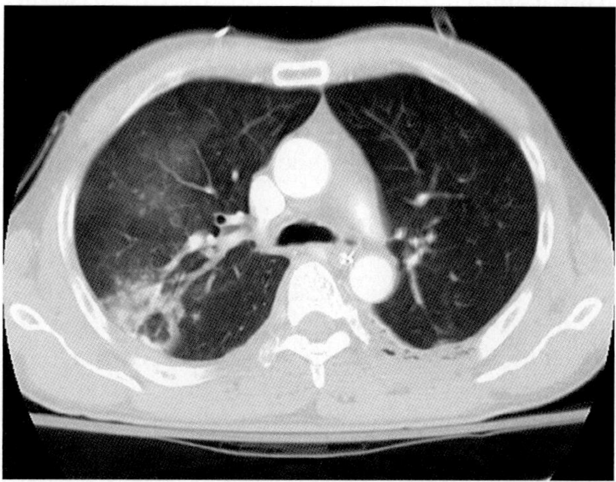

Figure 9.14 Right-sided pulmonary contusion as demonstrated on chest radiograph **(A)**, and axial computed tomography scan **(B)**. (*Reprinted with permission from* Greenberg MI, Hendrickson RG, Silverberg M, et al., eds. *Greenberg's Text-Atlas of Emergency Medicine*. Philadelphia, PA: Lippincott Williams & Wilkins, 2004.)

Acute onset of shortness of breath may signify pulmonary injury. Transient dyspnea after a blow to the chest or abdomen is due to a brief diaphragmatic spasm that spontaneously remits. This is referred to by the colloquial phrase "getting the wind knocked out of you" and generally requires no further management once symptoms subside. *Pulmonary contusion* may occur in blunt chest wall trauma and often accompany rib fractures (Fig. 9.14). Pulmonary contusions resolve with time, but the physician should be aware of possible complications such as pneumonia or respiratory distress. Sudden onset of dyspnea, pleuritic chest pain, and decreased breath sounds are characteristic of *pneumothorax*, a potentially serious condition in which the lung partially or completely collapses. Pneumothorax may be the result of impact or may occur spontaneously, and athletes exhibiting symptoms should be placed on oxygen and transported to a hospital for management. *Tension pneumothorax* is a medical emergency characterized by dyspnea, tachycardia, neck vein distension, and tracheal deviation. Decreased breath sounds and tympany to percussion identify the affected side. If suspected, the athlete may decompensate quickly, and large-bore needle decompression into the second intercostal space at the midclavicular line of the affected side may be life-saving.

ABDOMINAL INJURY

A sudden increase in intra-abdominal pressure from a direct blow may disrupt the diaphragm or intra-abdominal organs (Fig. 9.15). Athletes who sustain abdominal trauma may initially have a normal abdominal examination, and serial examinations for development of tenderness, rigidity,

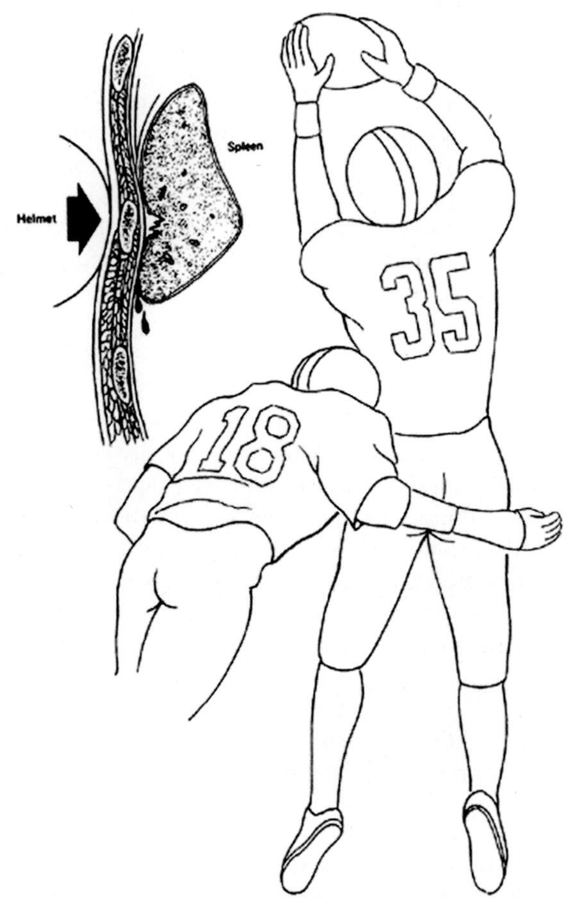

Figure 9.15 Athletic collision may cause intra-abdominal injury. Bleeding may be slow and symptoms may develop insidiously. (*Reprinted with permission from* Fu FH, Stone DA, eds. *Sports Injuries: Mechanisms, Prevention, Treatment*. 2nd ed. Philadelphia, PA: Lippincott Williams & Wilkins, 2001.)

and distension may be required to detect a serious intraabdominal injury. A ruptured viscous is a surgical emergency, and an athlete who suffers a significant bowel injury needs to be transferred immediately to a hospital for urgent management. The poor visceral sensory innervation delays onset of symptoms from intraabdominal injury, and nonspecific symptoms such as diffuse abdominal pain, nausea, diarrhea, or hypotension may appear insidiously. Development of such symptoms in the context of abdominal trauma warrants further workup.

Splenic injury presents with nausea, left upper quadrant tenderness or referred left shoulder pain (Kehr sign) after a blow to the abdomen. Small capsular lacerations may heal without becoming clinically apparent, but large lacerations may progress to splenic rupture, resulting in intraabdominal hemorrhage and hemodynamic instability. Splenic enlargement is a feature of mononucleosis, and athletes with active or resolving mononucleosis should be restricted from contact until the spleen has returned to normal size.

Right upper quadrant pain with radiation to the right shoulder may indicate a *hepatic injury* and should be evaluated with liver function tests and CT. Periumbilical or back pain along with nausea may be manifestations of *pancreatic injury* and patients should be monitored closely for development of pancreatitis.

Positioned posteriorly in the abdomen, the kidneys are vulnerable to direct blows to the back. *Renal contusion* is usually accompanied by flank tenderness and gross or microhematuria. Diagnosis is confirmed by urinalysis, intravenous pyelogram, or renal ultrasound. CT scan with contrast may be obtained to detect more serious injuries to the kidney such as lacerations, bleeding, or ureteral injuries. Extensive bleeding with renal fracture or vascular pedicle injury requires urgent surgery. Because of the risk of kidney injury, athletes with one kidney deserve special consideration when determining clearance to play.

MUSCULOSKELETAL INJURY

Approximately 75% of injuries sustained in college athletics involve the extremities, with ankle sprains accounting for almost 15% of all sports-related injuries. Evaluation of a suspected extremity injury should include inspection for deformity, lacerations, abrasions, bruising, swelling, and neurovascular status. The range of motion and stability of the involved joint should be noted, and associated injuries should be explored. Extremity injuries may occur in conjunction with spinal cord injuries, and cervical immobilization and spine precautions should be maintained until spinal cord injury is excluded. Soft tissue injuries compose the overwhelming majority of musculoskeletal extremity injuries sustained in sports. For most of these injuries, initial management involves protection, rest, ice, compression, and elevation (PRICE).

Orthopaedic Emergencies

Few extremity injuries constitute emergencies, but these should be identified and addressed promptly when assessing a downed athlete. Fractures of the pelvis or femur, fractures associated with vascular injuries, penetrating trauma, and open fractures may jeopardize hemodynamic stability or threaten an extremity, and the physician should immediately provide provisional treatment while the emergency response plan is initiated. Typically the result of a high-energy mechanism, the physician should maintain a high index of suspicion for concomitant head, spine, intrathoracic, or intraabdominal injury when evaluating these injuries. Vital signs and the condition of the affected extremity should be monitored closely, and the athlete should be transferred to a hospital as soon as possible.

Active bleeding should be controlled with direct compression and elevation of the injured extremity. Universal precautions should be maintained while treating a bleeding athlete. Open fractures should be irrigated copiously with saline before dressing and splinting. Joint dislocations should be reduced as soon as possible to prevent neurovascular compromise and osteonecrosis. Some dislocations, such as shoulder dislocations, may be reduced on the field acutely prior to onset of muscle spasm. Irreducible dislocations necessitate prompt transfer to a hospital where sedation and muscle relaxants may be administered. A neurovascular examination before and after reduction should be documented, and changes in pulses or neurological status demand urgent attention.

Compartment Syndrome

Compartment syndrome occurs because of elevated pressure within a fascial compartment that attenuates blood flow and may occur following injury, with exercise, or a constricting bandage or splint. Involving the leg or forearm in most cases, compartment syndrome is a clinical diagnosis based on observed tightness of a compartment, paresthesias, pain on passive stretch of muscles that traverse the compartment, and pain out of proportional to physical examination findings. Symptoms generally develop gradually, and once diagnosed, emergent fasciotomy is needed to prevent tissue necrosis. Pallor, paralysis, and pulselessness are late signs and signify that damage has already occurred.

Exertional compartment syndrome is activity-related pain that occurs when exercising muscle swells, becoming constricted to the point of ischemia by the unyielding fascia. Pain is generally quickly alleviated by rest. Measurement of compartment pressures before and after exercise is diagnostic, and treatment involves fasciotomy of the affected compartments. Compartment pressures of more than

15 mm Hg at rest, more than 30 mm Hg 1 minute after exercise, and/or more than 20 mg Hg 5 minutes after exercises are considered diagnostic of exertional compartment syndrome.

Muscular Injury

Muscles are injured by direct trauma, overuse, or overstretch. A *contusion* is caused by direct impact, which compresses the muscle against the underlying bone. Most commonly affecting the anterior thigh and biceps, contusions may be prevented with appropriate padding and usually respond to conservative management of a short period of immobilization followed by range-of-motion exercises and strengthening. Repeated trauma or inadequate rehabilitation may result in *myositis ossificans*, in which calcification develops in the muscle, resulting in ectopic bone formation. *Delayed-onset muscular soreness* develops 24 to 72 hours after vigorous activity and is most frequently seen at the start of the training when the athlete is not accustomed to intense exercise. This condition is self-limited and pain may be alleviated with rest and nonsteroidal anti-inflammatory drugs (NSAIDs).

Gradual onset of symptoms distinguishes muscular soreness from *muscular strain*, which is an overstretching injury to the muscle, characterized by immediate pain and loss of function. Ranging in severity from mild disruption of muscle fibers to complete tears, strains or "pulled muscles" most often affect the myotendinous junction of muscles that cross two joints such as the hamstrings or quadriceps and during eccentric contraction. Symptoms include localized tenderness, swelling, weakness, and painful motion. Prevention of strains entails adequate stretching and conditioning, and treatment consists of PRICE. Once the acute pain and swelling has improved, emphasis should be shifted to strengthening and rehabilitation. Reinjury is common despite seemingly sufficient therapy, and chronic muscle strains may persist for several months.

Ligamentous Injury

The static stabilizers of joints, ligaments may be disrupted under excessive tension from extremes in joint motion. Minor damage to the fibers of a ligament is designated a *sprain* and is characterized by local pain and tenderness, swelling, and pain on joint range of motion. The most commonly sprained joint, the ankle is typically injured when athletes plant their foot awkwardly and roll or twist the ankle. Treatment of minor sprains is symptomatic and includes PRICE. Activity should be restricted to allow the ligament to heal, a process that may take up to 6 weeks. Protected range of motion is implemented to prevent stiffness. The recurrence rate after return to play is high due to attenuation of fibers and compromise of joint proprioception. Athletes may benefit from wrapping or bracing the injured joint. *Partial* or *complete ligament tears* represent more severe injuries. In addition to pain and swelling around the joint, these injuries are associated with joint laxity or instability. Plain radiographs should be obtained to check for osseous injury as avulsion fractures have a similar clinical picture. Stress radiographs or MRI may assist in diagnosis.

The severity and location of the tear guide treatment. A more conservative approach may be appropriate if fiber continuity is maintained. Complete tears imply that all fibers are disrupted, and the ligament may not heal properly if the ends are not approximated. In general, intraarticular structures such as the anterior cruciate ligament (ACL) of the knee will not heal because of the ineffectiveness of the fibrin clot in the intraarticular environment. These ligaments frequently require reconstruction when torn. Extraarticular structures such as the medial collateral ligament of the knee may heal with conservative management. These types of generalizations do not dictate treatment, and each athlete and ligament injury should be evaluated individually. Factors such as the joint involved, severity of symptoms, sport played, and level of competition must be considered in developing a management strategy. Conservative therapy consists of a period of immobilization and symptomatic treatment followed by therapy and rehabilitation. Surgical treatment involves primary repair or reconstruction using autograft or allograft. Return-to-play determination should be made on an individual basis and should take into account the resolution of symptoms and the strength and stability of the joint.

Stress Fractures

Stress fractures result from repetitive insults to normal bone, which progressively disrupt internal trabeculae, eventually leading to cortical weakness. The tibia, metatarsals, and fibula of track-and-field athletes and military recruits are most commonly involved (Fig. 9.16). This pattern of presentation reflects the pathophysiology behind these overuse injuries. The weight-bearing bones of endurance athletes sustain cyclic trauma with inadequate recovery. This repetitive stress accumulates to overcome the capacity of the bone to remodel. Upper extremity stress fractures may also occur in sports such as baseball and tennis, which expose the bones of the arms or hands to similar types of recurrent loads.

Stress fractures present with localized pain exacerbated by the offending activity and transiently relieved by rest. Pain may persist after cessation of activity and at night as the fracture evolves. Plain radiographs are unreliable during the early stages of stress fracture but may show periosteal reaction, trabecular discontinuity, or a linear band of sclerosis. Advanced imaging modalities such as MRI or bone scan are useful to establish a definitive diagnosis. Treatment generally entails activity modification to avoid the excessive forces upon the bone, although immobilization and non–weight-bearing on the injured extremity may be indicated. For high-risk stress fractures such as those on the

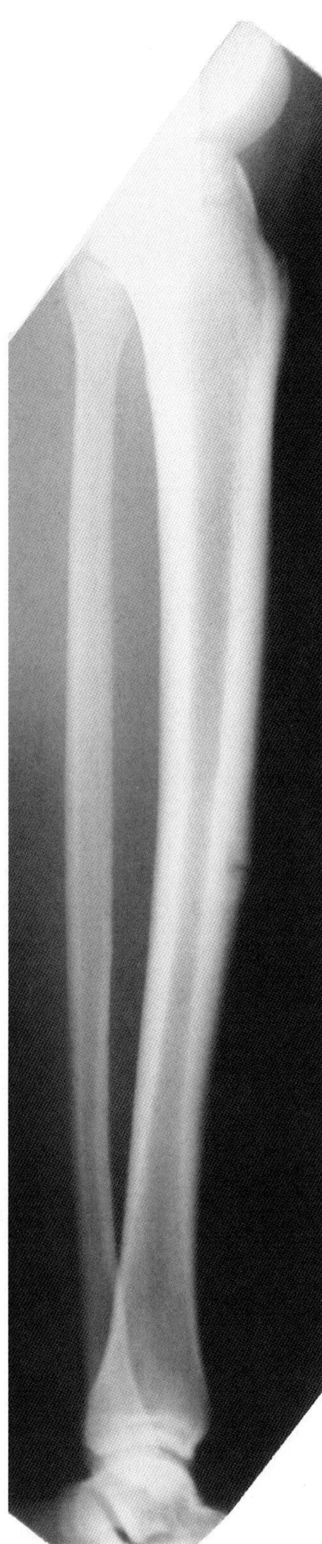

Figure 9.16 The lateral radiograph of the left tibia of a collegiate track athlete demonstrating cortical thickening and the dreaded black line of a stress fracture. (*Reprinted with permission from* Bucholz RW, Heckman JD, Court-Brown CM, eds. *Rockwood and Green's Fractures in Adults*. 6th ed. Philadelphia, PA: Lippincott Williams & Wilkins, 2006.)

tension side of the femoral neck, prophylactic fixation may prevent further propagation or displacement.

MEDICAL CONDITIONS

Cardiovascular Disease

Sudden death in an athlete, although rare, is a devastating event that is most commonly related to cardiac causes. The cardiovascular screening portion of the preparticipation evaluation is crucial to preventing the potentially severe outcomes of cardiovascular dysfunction or disease. *Hypertrophic cardiomyopathy* is implicated in more than one quarter of sudden cardiac deaths in athletes (Fig. 9.17). Affecting 1 of 500 athletes, this condition is usually asymptomatic and may initially present as sudden death due to dynamic outflow obstruction or ventricular arrhythmia. Hypertrophic cardiomyopathy is inherited as an autosomal dominant trait, and family history of sudden death, especially in a relative younger than 45 years, should raise concern. Physical examination findings may include a late systolic murmur that increases in intensity on standing or with Valsalva maneuver and decreases with squatting. The affected athlete may report dyspnea on exertion, chest pain, palpitations, or syncopal episodes. If suspected, the athlete should be prohibited from play and referred to a cardiologist. Echocardiography is diagnostic.

Marfan syndrome has been identified as a risk factor for sudden death in the athlete due to acute dissection of the aortic root. A constellation of physical examination findings including tall stature, arachnodactyly, and lens dislocations distinguishes this condition and should be recognized during the preparticipation evaluation. Athletes with Marfan syndrome should undergo a thorough cardiovascular evaluation before being cleared to play.

A number of additional cardiovascular conditions with possibly serious consequences may silently affect the athlete. *Prolonged QT syndrome* is a familial condition that involves an abnormal repolarization of the cardiac conduction system and may lead to syncope or fatal arrhythmia. Typically asymptomatic, prolonged QT syndrome may be diagnosed by a QT interval of more than 480 milliseconds on electrocardiography. *Congenital coronary artery abnormalities* may be asymptomatic or present as exertional chest pain from kinking of an anomalous vessel. "Pistol" Pete Maravich, a well-known collegiate and professional basketball player, collapsed after a recreational basketball game and died at an age of 40 years from a heart attack caused by a congenitally missing left coronary artery. *Valvular disease* also may afflict athletes without any symptoms. Abnormal heart murmurs on physical examination merit further evaluation.

Coronary artery disease is the most common cause of death in older athletes. Risk factors should be minimized to prevent complications, and athletes who report

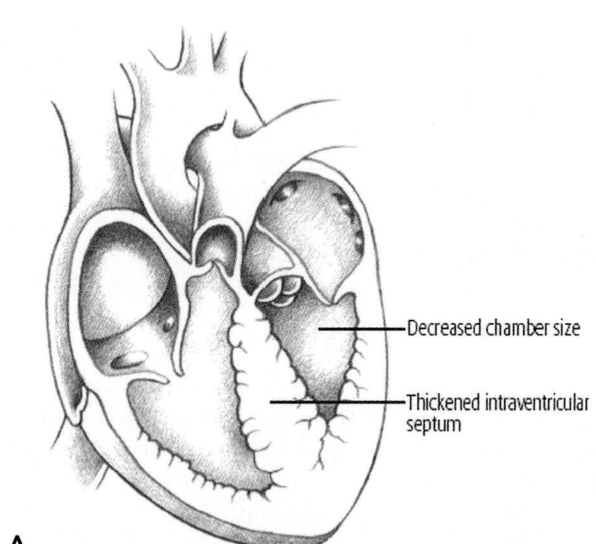

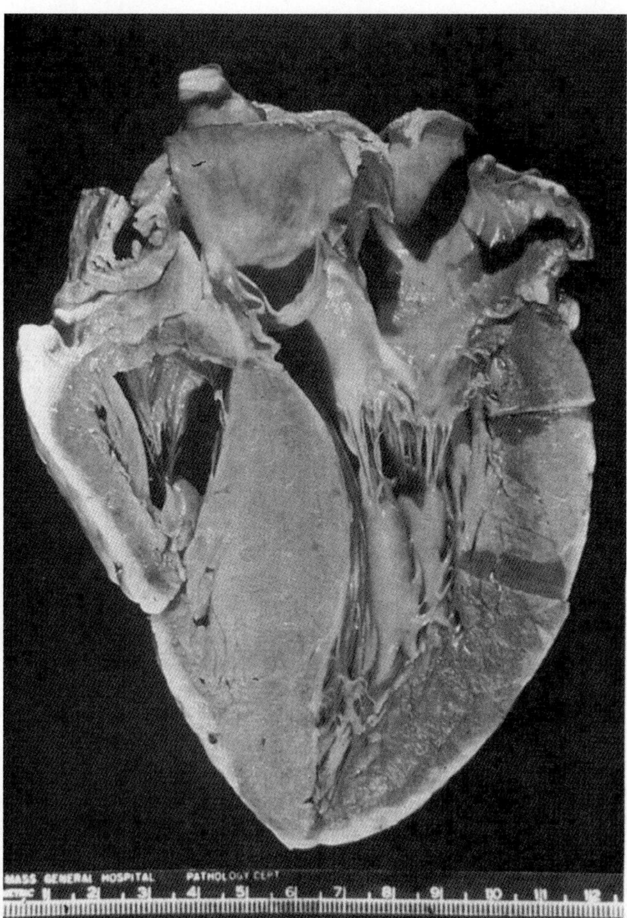

Figure 9.17 **(A)** Hypertrophic cardiomyopathy diagram. **(B)** Postmortem heart specimen from patient with hypertrophic cardiomyopathy. (**A:** *Reprinted with permission from* Springhouse, ed. *Just the Facts: Pathophysiology*. Philadelphia, PA: Lippincott Williams & Wilkins, 2004. **B:** *Reprinted with permission from* Lilly LS, ed. *Pathophysiology of Heart Disease*. 2nd ed. Baltimore: Williams & Wilkins, 1998.)

exercise-induced chest pain or palpitations should undergo stress testing. The American Heart Association recommends exercise testing in men older than 40 years and women older than 50 years who have at least one cardiac risk factor. All athletes older than 65 years should have exercise testing to screen for potentially serious coronary artery disease.

Asthma/Exercise-Induced Bronchospasm

Asthma, a condition marked by airway hypersensitivity with a range of severity, commonly affects athletes and deserves special consideration due to respiratory stress of athletics. Characterized by intermittent airway inflammation resulting in bronchoconstriction and increased mucus production, asthma causes potentially severe symptoms of wheezing, shortness of breath, chest tightness, and coughing. Asthma attacks, if untreated, may result in severe chest pain, hypoxia, and loss of consciousness. Triggers include allergens, exercise, physical or emotional stress, or viral illness. After addressing and eradicating environmental causes, medical management focuses on reversal of bronchospasm and reduction of inflammation. Inhaled β-agonists such as albuterol are a mainstay of treatment of acute asthma attack and act on β-adrenergic receptors in the smooth muscle of the airways to promote bronchodilation. Anticholinergics such as ipratropium also reduce bronchospasm. Preventive agents generally suppress chronic inflammation and hypersensitivity and include glucocorticoids, leukotriene blockers, and antihistamines.

Athletes with normal lungs may experience asthma-like symptoms during or after periods of exercise. Affecting up to 50% of cold weather athletes, *exercise-induced bronchospasm* presents screening challenges as athletes may have no medical history or family history of asthma and may be asymptomatic at rest. Challenge testing in which a 10% to 15% decrease in peak expiratory flow rate or 1-second forced expiratory volume after 6 to 8 minutes of strenuous exercise confirms the diagnosis. A greater than 50% decrease indicates severe disease. Athletes may also develop a cough with challenge testing, which is also indicative of exercise-induced bronchospasm. Treatment generally involves modification of exercise routine to minimize triggers and prophylactic bronchodilator therapy.

Asthma does not preclude athletic participation, and prevention of symptoms should be the goal of management. The athlete should be educated about early warning signs of attack, and appropriate pharmacological treatment should be readily available. A severe attack may warrant supplemental oxygenation and transfer to a hospital.

Infectious Disease

The nature of the sports lifestyle puts athletes at risk of acquiring and transmitting infection. The stress on the immune system of the training athlete combined with close quarters in locker rooms and on team buses and the sharing of equipment, towels, and water bottles create an environment conducive to spread of infection. While most infectious agents cause mild, self-limited disease, athletes may be exposed to potentially deadly organisms. The key to management of infectious diseases among athletes is prevention. Sanitary practices such as hand-washing and using clean towels must be emphasized and players showing signs or symptoms of infection should be evaluated and treated. Universal body fluid precautions should be maintained when treating all athletes, and all equipment should be cleaned thoroughly with an antimicrobial solution after use.

Staphylococcus Infection

Staphylococcus aureus, an organism that commonly colonizes the nares and skin of athletes, may cause serious infection if the body's natural defenses are breached. Even small cuts in the skin provide a portal for a virulent strain of this organism to establish an infection that may range from mild local cellulitis or inflamed boil to potentially fatal systemic bacteremia. Recently, outbreaks among athletes of community-acquired methicillin-resistant *Staphylococcus aureus*, an organism that previously existed only in health care facilities, have instigated national concern due to the virulence and tenacity of this infection. To prevent spread, athletes should practice good hygiene, avoid sharing of towels and equipment, and cover skin lesions. Antibiotics may be required to eradicate the organism.

Meningitis

Meningitis is most commonly caused by enteroviruses and is characterized by fever, headache, neck stiffness, and signs of meningeal irritation such as pain with passive neck flexion. Broad-spectrum antibiotics should be initiated after obtaining a cerebral spinal fluid specimen for analysis due to risk of bacterial etiology. Viral meningitis is typically a self-limited condition that needs only supportive care, but bacterial meningitis is associated with severe complications including death and requires emergent medical intervention. The most common organisms in the athletic population are *Streptococcus pneumoniae* and *Neisseria meningitidis*, and once speciated, an appropriate antibiotic regimen should be tailored specific to the organism. *N. meningitides* is of particular concern in the athletic population due to an increased prevalence found among college students living in close quarters.

Mononucleosis

Infectious mononucleosis is caused by the Epstein–Barr virus or cytomegalovirus and eventually affects 90% of adults at some point in their lives. Spread by oral secretions, sharing water bottles, or close contact, mononucleosis is characterized by a triad of fever, pharyngitis, and lymphadenopathy. Splenomegaly is also associated with this condition, and thus contact sports should be avoided during acute infection to prevent splenic injury. Symptomatic treatment and prevention of possible complications comprise standard treatment, and symptoms usually resolve in 4 to 8 months.

ENVIRONMENTAL ILLNESS

Heat Illness

The intensity inherent to athletics puts players at risk of heat illness even during moderate playing conditions since during maximal exercise, the muscles can produce 15 to 20 times more energy than at rest. This energy is converted to heat and is a major contributor to the development of heat illness. Involving a spectrum of conditions from minor dehydration to heatstroke, heat illness results when the heat-dissipating mechanisms of the body are overwhelmed.

The hypothalamus is the regulator of core temperature in the body and is responsible for orchestrating heat loss. Heat exchange requires a temperature gradient and occurs by conduction via direct contact between objects, convection by transfer to circulating air, radiation via direct release into atmosphere, and evaporation of perspiration. The body's most potent heat dispersion mechanism, perspiration, may transfer up to 1,000 kcal of heat per hour into the atmosphere as the exercising athlete produces 1 to 2 liters of sweat per hour. Other heat-dissipating mechanisms include peripheral vasodilation, increased cardiac output and minute ventilation, and elevation of core body temperature. If the thermoregulatory mechanisms of the body are overcome by inadequate hydration, poor conditioning and acclimatization, extreme heat, or inappropriate clothing, the thermoregulatory capacity of the body will fail and heat illness will ensue.

Minor Heat Illness

A number of minor heat-related conditions constitute early warning signs that an athlete is overheating. *Miliaria rubra*, or heat rash, is a pruritic papular rash that may erupt with overexposure to high heat and humidity, especially with clothing that impedes evaporation of sweat. Caused by occluded sweat glands, heat rash is treated with cooling and drying of the skin and may take 7 to 10 days to resolve. *Heat cramps* strike large muscle groups, such as the gastrocnemius, quadriceps, or hamstrings, and are caused by sodium deficiency from inadequate hydration and electrolyte intake coupled with profuse sweating. Athletes who lose excessive sodium in their sweat are at greater risk for heat cramps and may benefit from additional salt in their diet and fluids. Treatment involves rehydration with electrolyte or salt solution as well as cooling the athlete and stretching the cramping muscle group. Heat illness may also manifest as *heat syncope* from orthostasis caused by peripheral vasodilation, venous pooling, and dehydration. Mental status quickly improves once the athlete is supine, and management of heat syncope involves moving the athlete into a shaded area, elevating the legs, and rehydration.

Heatstroke

As the thermoregulatory system of the body fails and the core temperature rises, more serious heat-related illnesses may occur. *Heat exhaustion* presents with fatigue, malaise, nausea, and headache in an athlete with normal mentation and no neurological symptoms. The athlete may appear flushed, with profuse sweating and cold clammy skin, and core body temperature may approach 104°F (40°C). The athlete with symptoms of heat exhaustion should be removed from play immediately and rapidly cooled to prevent progression to heatstroke. *Heatstroke* represents an emergency as the thermoregulatory system has been overwhelmed beyond the point of spontaneous recovery. The athlete suffering from heatstroke experiences heat exhaustion symptoms coupled with severe mental status impairment and core body temperature of more than 104°F (40°C). With mortality rates in excess of 10%, heatstroke warrants immediate activation of emergency protocol while removing clothing and moving the athlete to a cool or shaded location. A direct correlation has been demonstrated between the duration of elevated core temperature and outcome with increased morbidity and mortality associated with hyperthermia lasting more than 60 minutes. Aggressive cooling should be initiated immediately with ice immersion, cooling blankets, fans, or internal cooling measures and should continue until core body temperature is less than 101.8°F (38.8°C). Intravenous hydration may be necessary, and vital signs and body temperature should be closely monitored to prevent overcorrection.

Prevention of Heat Illness

The key to management of heat illness is prevention. Encouraging copious hydration and recognition of the signs and symptoms of heat illness should be emphasized during extremely hot playing conditions. Athletes should have access to plenty of water and relief from the environment, and equipment and clothing should be lightweight and allow free evaporation of sweat. Those with a history of heat illness require evaluation prior to participation and should return to play in a graduated manner under supervision of the trainer. Any event in which heat illness is a risk should have ice immersion immediately available.

Hydration

Adequate hydration is critical to protecting athletes from untoward effects of heat, and optimal hydration entails matching fluid and electrolyte loss (Table 9.8). Hydration status may be assessed by weight monitoring before, during, and after exertion. Mild dehydration is represented by 2% to 3% body weight loss and signals need for hydration. Athletes with more than 5% weight loss are severely dehydrated and should be prohibited from playing. Sports drinks have evolved to address electrolyte depletion from exertion and should be used in conjunction with free water. Athletes who consume too much free water without adequate sodium intake may be at risk for developing *exertional hyponatremia*.

Acclimatization

Acclimatization is necessary prior to full participation in extreme playing conditions such as the summer preseason for most fall sports. Achieving an adequate level of fitness first is important before initiating acclimatization as getting fit in extreme environments is counterproductive. Involving a gradual increase in environmental exposure time and

TABLE 9.8
FLUID REPLACEMENT GUIDELINES

National Collegiate Athletic Association Sports Medicine Handbook

- 8–16 oz water 1 h prior to exertion
- Continue drinking every 15–20 min during activity
- After exercise, replace fluid lost (1 qt per 2 lb)

National Athletic Trainers Association

- 16 to 20 oz of fluid 2–3 h before exertion
- Immediately prior to exercise, consume 6–10 oz
- Take 6–10 oz every 15–20 min during exercise
- After exercise, consume fluid in excess of what was lost

(*Adapted from* Howe AS, Boden BP. Heat-related illness in athletes. *Am J Sports Med.* 2007;35(8):1384–1395.)

the degree and duration of exertion, proper acclimatization generally takes 10 to 14 days. During this time, physiological changes including enhanced cardiac output, heat exchange mechanisms, and renal function improve the athlete's ability to withstand hot playing conditions. Hydration requirements increase with acclimatization.

Cold Illness

Athletes participating in sports at cold temperatures are at risk for developing illness or injury from exposure. Normally, temperature homeostasis is maintained by hypothalamus-mediated mechanisms to conserve and produce heat such as peripheral vasoconstriction and shivering. Similar to heat illness, management of cold illness should focus on prevention. Weather forecasts should be monitored, and athletes should be alerted in the event of cold or inclement weather so that they may dress appropriately. Insulation is improved by layering of clothing. Hydration should be encouraged regardless of the level of thirst. Shelter and rewarming equipment should be available on site, and any athlete who shows early signs or symptoms of cold illness should be evaluated.

Hypothermia

Hypothermia occurs when these mechanisms are overcome by extreme cold and is defined as the cooling of core body temperature to less than 95°F (35°C). Athletes exposed to the elements without proper clothing, equipment, training, or shelter are at risk for developing hypothermia and may present with uncontrollable shivering, tachycardia, dysarthria, and altered mental status. Athletes with severe hypothermia, in which the core body temperature drops to less than 88°F (31°C), exhibit global physiological impairment that include hypotension, bradycardia, apnea, and reduced level of consciousness. The shivering response and level of alertness wane with increasing severity. Treatment of hypothermia varies with severity. Mild hypothermia may be managed with removal from cold environment, insulation, and rewarming with blankets, heaters, and warm fluids. Severe hypothermia warrants activation of the emergency response plan and requires aggressive yet cautious rewarming with external and internal methods. These patients should be monitored in an intensive care setting and rewarming should not exceed 2°C per hour to prevent ventricular arrhythmia and hypovolemic shock.

Frostbite

Athletes exposed to freezing temperatures are at risk for *frostbite*. Characterized by ice crystal formation in the extracellular spaces, frostbite generally affects bare skin and distal extremities as exposure combined with peripheral vasoconstriction and dehydration leave theses regions vulnerable to freezing. The lower extremities, in particular the great toe, are most commonly affected. Increasing pain and a gradual loss of both sensation and pliability indicate the development of a cold injury, and the affected area should be protected from the cold and gently rewarmed to prevent the irreversible damage of frostbite. Frostbitten tissue is hard, mottled, and insensate and may be superficial or involve the deep tissues including muscle, neurovascular structures, and bone. Often occurring in hypothermic patients, frostbite treatment should initially address core body temperature. The area of frostbite should be rewarmed in a water bath at 40°C to 42°C. Rubbing the tissue should be avoided to prevent further damage, and rewarming should not be initiated if there is any chance of refreezing. Demarcation of affected tissue may take several weeks, and debridement and amputation should be delayed for 90 days.

Altitude Illness

The reduced barometric pressure and low oxygen of high altitude introduce unique environmental factors to the athlete. Hypobaric hypoxia may result in high-altitude syndromes such as acute mountain sickness, high-altitude cerebral edema, or high-altitude pulmonary edema. Headache is generally the first symptom of altitude sickness. A headache along with one or more additional symptoms to include nausea, dizziness, fatigue, or sleep disturbance represents *acute mountain sickness*, a condition that usually occurs within 12 hours of arrival to an altitude. Cessation of ascent and adaptation to the current altitude may alleviate symptoms, and prophylactic acetazolamide or dexamethasone may prevent development of altitude sickness. Neurological or pulmonary symptoms may signify onset of potentially fatal cerebral or pulmonary edema and necessitate supplemental oxygenation and immediate descent.

THE FEMALE ATHLETE

Women represent a rapidly growing segment of the athletic population. The inaugural modern summer Olympic Games in Athens in 1896 featured no female athletes. Women represented 42% of the more than 10,500 athletes who competed in the 2008 summer Olympics in Beijing, and in the 2012 Olympics in London, the number of female athletes is expected to equal the number of male athletes. The female athlete has also experienced a substantial improvement in performance. The winner of the women's 2008 Boston Marathon would have defeated the 1968 winner by more than 1 hour.

With this rise in participation and performance, a number of conditions and injuries specific to this population have become apparent. Most of the differences between genders that influence athletic participation are clearly evident. Women are smaller, less muscular, and reach maturity at an age younger than their male counterparts. Osteoporosis, iron deficiency anemia, disordered eating, and pregnancy are conditions to consider in the female athlete.

Several musculoskeletal manifestations of the difference between the architecture of the male and female body have been identified, including a greater incidence of stress fractures, ACL injuries, patellofemoral dysfunction, shoulder instability, foot problems, and scoliosis among female athletes.

The Female Athlete Triad

The *female athletic triad* of disordered eating, amenorrhea, and osteoporosis is a condition that has garnered considerable attention since the term was conceived by the American College of Sports Medicine Task Force on Women's Issues in 1993. Most commonly affecting women in endurance sports (running, swimming), sports with weight categories (rowing), and sports that emphasize lean body type (gymnastics, dance, cheerleading), the female athletic triad is a preventable condition that may lead to severe short-term and chronic consequences. The training female athlete is prone to a potentially detrimental behavioral pattern of disordered eating and excessive exercise. Deliberately or unconsciously motivated by a desire to maintain weight or body type or by a fear of gaining weight, affected athletes may restrict calories (anorexia nervosa), binge and purge (bulimia nervosa), or engage in other patterns of disordered eating. Disordered eating may be coupled with inappropriate use of medications or excessive exercise and results in inadequate nutrition and poor energy. Amenorrhea, or at least 3 months of missed menstrual periods, may also be a consequence of this pathological behavior. Caused by reduced estrogen production from poor nutrition, lack of energy, and low body fat, amenorrhea constitutes an important sign that normal physiologic processes are impaired. The hypoestrogenemic and poor nutritional state signified by amenorrhea is associated with increased cardiovascular risk, poor immunological function, and loss of normal bone density. The resultant osteopenia from deficient estrogen and calcium leaves the bones brittle and susceptible to fracture, and severe postmenopausal osteoporosis may develop.

A high level of suspicion must be maintained when evaluating the female athlete. Warning signs including weight loss, alopecia, hypertrichosis, dry skin, oral caries, stress fracture, and depression should alert the physician that a serious condition may be developing. Prevention through multidisciplinary education is clearly the best approach for the female athlete triad, and any athlete who exhibits warning signs should promptly be referred to an appropriate health care professional who should collaborate with dieticians, psychiatrists, and psychologists. Coaches and family members should also be involved in the treatment. Pharmacological therapy may be indicated in severe cases including oral contraceptive pills to regulate hormone levels, vitamin D supplementation to aid in calcium absorption, bisphosphonates and calcitonin to slow bone resorption, and antidepressants to ameliorate depressive symptoms. To prevent complications, athletes exhibiting signs of the female triad who are less than 85% of ideal body weight should not be allowed to participate in regular physical activity.

REHABILITATION

The goal of rehabilitation is to restore the lost range of motion, strength, and function that resulted from an injury, allowing the athlete to return to their previous level of performance. Taking into account the nature and severity of athletes' injury, the physician in collaboration with a trainer or physical therapist is responsible for establishing an appropriate rehabilitation program that allows athletes to safely and quickly recover so that they may return to play. An understanding of the physiology of the injury is required for appropriate rehabilitation, and proper precautions should be maintained to minimize pain and prevent reinjury.

Rehabilitation is divided into an acute phase focused on controlling the inflammatory response, a subacute phase emphasizing range of motion and reconditioning, and a chronic phase of strengthening and gradual return to sports-specific activity. The initial objective of rehabilitation is the reduction of pain, swelling, and inflammation through the use of PRICE along with anti-inflammatory medications. Immobilization, while essential for proper healing, quickly results in loss of range of motion and muscle mass and early range of motion is important to limit stiffness and weakness. Several strategies may be implemented to restore mobility including active and passive range of motion, stretching, and joint mobilization and manipulation (Fig. 9.18). With the advancement of range of

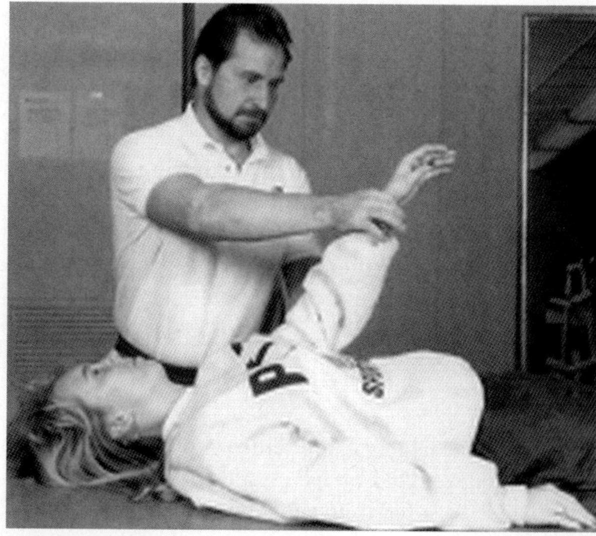

Figure 9.18 Range-of-motion exercises help to restore joint mobility. (*Reprinted with permission from* Fu FH, Stone DA, eds. *Sports Injuries: Mechanisms, Prevention, Treatment*. 2nd ed. Philadelphia, PA: Lippincott Williams & Wilkins, 2001.)

motion, a gradual muscular strengthening plan may be initiated through a combination of open and closed kinetic chain functional exercise techniques. During open chain exercises, in which the distal extremity is not fixed, contraction of the agonist muscle produces movement. Conversely, closed chain exercises, in which the distal extremity is fixed, rely on reciprocal co-contraction of agonist and antagonist muscles and more closely reproduces natural functional demands. Endurance training should be performed as an adjunct to strength exercises to limit fatigue, and proprioception and neuromuscular training promote dynamic stability and prevent reinjury. With the increase in strength and endurance, the focus of rehabilitation shifts to sports-specific exercise to prepare the athlete for return to play.

Athletes, especially high-performance athletes, may push the extremes of rehabilitation. Aggressive therapy may be counterproductive to recovery, and reinjury may occur. The team physician should be in communication with the athletic trainer and the physical therapists about reasonable rehabilitation goals and return to play.

PHARMACOLOGY OF SPORTS

Anti-Inflammatories and Analgesics

Medications have an important role in the management of sports injuries. Often used as an adjunct to rest or therapy, pharmacological treatment of sports injuries focuses on suppressing the inflammatory response and reducing the pain associated with the injury. In the acute response to tissue injury, high levels of inflammatory mediators such as prostaglandins, thromboxanes, and leukotrienes accumulate in the area of injury. These substances promote vasodilation, increased vascular permeability, and recruitment of leukocytes to breakdown and remove necrotic tissue and debris. This tissue process manifests clinically as swelling, local heat, and pain. Chronic inflammation is characterized by persistent symptoms of acute inflammation.

NSAIDs such as ibuprofen and naproxen have anti-inflammatory effects and analgesic and antipyretic properties. This class of drugs is used universally for athletic injuries and functions primarily by inhibition of the cyclooxygenase enzyme complex. Composed of two isoenzymes, COX-1 and COX-2, cyclooxygenase converts arachidonic acid to prostaglandins. COX-1 is involved in normal prostaglandin synthesis in the gastric mucosa, renal tissue, platelets, and endothelial cells, and inhibition of this isoenzyme is responsible for the majority of side effects from NSAIDs. The therapeutic effect of NSAIDs is exerted upon the COX-2 isoenzyme. In the acute response to injury, local COX-2 expression increases up to 80-fold, producing high levels of prostaglandins, which in turn lead to inflammation and pain. Selective COX-2 inhibitors such as celecoxib are effective at suppressing inflammation with fewer side effects. Ultimately, the goal of NSAID therapy is reduction of injury-associated pain and inflammation so that rehabilitation may occur. Untoward effects including dyspepsia, gastric ulceration, and renal failure should be considered when using NSAIDs.

Corticosteroids possess potent anti-inflammatory properties and function by inhibition of the vasoactive response to injury, suppression of leukocyte recruitment, and reduction of cytokine expression. A wide spectrum of activity and side effects exists among different corticosteroids, and the primary means of delivery in athletes is oral administration and local injection. Oral corticosteroids have excellent anti-inflammatory properties, but systemic side effects such as glucose intolerance, hypertension, osteoporosis, and impaired wound healing preclude routine use. Local injections are associated with fewer systemic complications and may be used to decrease local inflammation in bursitis, tendinitis, and arthritis. Corticosteroids should not be injected into tendons or ligaments due to increased risk of rupture.

Acetaminophen is an effective analgesic with limited anti-inflammatory properties. Possessing a more benign side effect profile than NSAIDs, acetaminophen may be used as a single agent for mild to moderate inflammation or as an adjunct to NSAID therapy. Hepatotoxicity constitutes the major danger of acetaminophen therapy and may be prevented by limiting acetaminophen intake to less than 4 g per day in adults.

Narcotics such as hydrocodone and oxycodone bind opiate receptors to inhibit conduction within central pain pathways. Powerful analgesics, narcotics, should be reserved for pain from severe injury or postoperative pain. Tolerance develops over 1 to 3 weeks from upregulation of opiate receptor expression, and physical dependence may result from prolonged use. Because of risk of addiction, narcotics should be used sparingly.

Commonly Used Supplements, Vitamins, and Drugs

Athletes use a variety of dietary and pharmacological substances to enhance performance, control weight, improve nutrition, and recover from injury. Most substances used by athletes are dietary supplements that are available over the counter and generally pose minimal risk to the athlete when taken as directed.

Creatine is among the most common supplements used by high school and college athletes and enhances short-term training stamina through augmentation of adenosine triphosphate regeneration. A 2001 survey of high school athletes found that 44% of high school senior athletes used creatine. Triggering a shift of fluid into the cells, creatine causes a theoretical risk of dehydration, and reports of cramps, muscle injury, and renal dysfunction have been associated with use.

Stimulants such as *pseudoephedrine* and *caffeine* may be used by athletes to increase energy and endurance. While caffeine is generally perceived to be benign, athletes should be aware of increased short-term risk of heart attack, arrhythmias, and sudden cardiac death with heavy use. Recognizing the ubiquity of use among the general public, caffeine is legal in most sports although the International Olympic Committee (IOC) has instituted a daily threshold of 9 mg/kg (approximately 5 cups of coffee). *Ephedrine* is a sympathomimetic initially developed as a weight loss aid. Abused by athletes who sought to take advantage of its "energizing" qualities, ephedrine has been banned by the IOC due to increased risks of cardiac dysfunction. Ephedrine is frequently combined with caffeine and aspirin ("ECA stack") and has been linked to numerous deaths among athletes.

Athletes who abuse *anabolic steroids* aim to augment the potent effects of endogenous androgenic hormones on muscle mass, strength, and recovery from injury. While *testosterone* and synthetic analogues have been shown to improve strength and performance when taken in supraphysiologic doses, they possess a substantial side effect profile. Increased rates of heart disease, increased aggression, hypercoagulability, testicular atrophy, gynecomastia, and hirsutism among athletes who abuse anabolic androgenic steroids reflect the dangers of use. *Dehydroepiandrosterone* and *androstenedione* are precursors in the gonadal steroid pathway and are converted by the body into testosterone. While the ergogenic benefits of these testosterone precursors have yet to be clearly demonstrated, the adverse effects of elevated testosterone has led to the banning of these substances by the IOC and many other sports organizations.

Human growth hormone (HGH) is also an endogenous occurring substance abused for its ergogenic effect. Developed to treat patients with endogenous growth hormone deficiency, HGH exerts an anabolic effect on muscle growth and increases fat metabolism. Abuse is associated with hypertension and acromegaly among other detrimental physiologic effects.

Athletes may boost aerobic capacity by blood doping. Homologous or autologous transfusion prior to a sporting event confers the advantage of increased circulating red blood cells for enhanced oxygen delivery. Athletes may also use synthetic *erythropoietin (EPO)* to improve aerobic capacity. Naturally produced by the kidneys to stimulate red blood cell formation, EPO abuse may result in consequences of hyperviscosity from polycythemia including heart attack, stroke, and pulmonary embolus.

NUTRITION

Athletes in training and competition have complex nutritional requirements to build and maintain muscle, maximize oxygenation delivery, optimize metabolism, and recover from injury. Insufficient caloric intake may result in loss of muscle mass, loss of bone density, menstrual dysfunction, and increased risk of fatigue, injury, or illness. A balanced diet that meets caloric needs with proper proportions of carbohydrates, fats, proteins, and vitamins is essential to maintaining physical well-being. Current recommendations outline a diet consisting of approximately 55% to 60% of calories from carbohydrates, 10% to 15% from protein, and 25% to 30% from fats.

Blood glucose and glycogen stores provide the substrate for energy production and are maintained by dietary carbohydrates found in sugars. Daily intake recommendations range from 6 to 10 g of carbohydrate per kilogram of body weight per day. Dietary carbohydrate that is not converted to energy or glycogen may contribute to adipose stores. Dietary proteins from meats and nuts supply amino acids for building and repair of muscle tissue. Daily intake recommendations for athletes range from 1.2 to 1.4 g per kilogram per day, although athletes who participate in sports that emphasize muscle bulk and strength may consume 1.6 to 1.7 g of protein per kilogram per day. Fat provides an energy substrate and fat-soluble vitamins and essential fatty acids. Ubiquitous in the American diet, excess intake builds adipose stores and elevates blood cholesterol levels. Polyunsaturated and monounsaturated fatty acids found in fish, nuts, and vegetable oils should compose the majority of fat intake, and saturated and *trans*-fatty acids as well as cholesterol should be avoided because of detrimental effects on the blood lipid profile.

Athletes must regulate their diets to ensure that they consume the appropriate amount and proportions of calories to optimize performance. The composition of the diet should be tailored to the individual sport as endurance athletes may benefit from increased carbohydrate intake to maximize energy storage and production while strength athletes may supplement their protein intake to promote muscle growth. Carbohydrate loading by maximizing intake while tapering training intensity in the days leading up to a competition may boost glycogen stores and increase endurance. Before exercise, a carbohydrate-rich snack or sports drink elevates blood glucose levels and provides energy. Fat should be avoided before exercise as high-fat foods delay gastric emptying and may cause abdominal discomfort. During and after exercise, the dietary objective is to adequately replace utilized calories. A well-balanced meal shortly after exercise serves to replace glycogen to restore energy and provide amino acids to repair muscle tissue.

Although disordered eating is more common in female athletes, all athletes are susceptible to maladaptive eating and training behavior. Certain sports such as gymnastics, wrestling, and crew are associated with higher risks of low body weight. Early recognition of disordered eating patterns is vital to preventing serious complications, and athletes who seek a certain weight or body type should be referred to a dietician who can assist in constructing a healthy diet that will safely allow achievement of these objectives. Basic weight loss guidelines include eating smaller and more frequent meals, limiting empty calories, and eating foods that promote satiety. Weight loss of 1 to 2 lb per week represents a healthy and reasonable goal. Basic weight gain guidelines consist of consuming an additional 500 to 1,000 cal per day and choosing higher calorie items. A reasonable and healthy goal is 1 lb of weight gain every 2 weeks.

CONCLUSION

Regardless of sport, level of participation, and degree of performance, athletes continuously challenges the knowledge and skills of sports physicians. The diversity within the athletic population requires sports physicians to play a number of roles. They must play the role of pediatrician to recognize conditions specific to childhood and adolescence, the role of internist to manage medical conditions, and the role of orthopaedist to treat musculoskeletal injuries. In addition, sports physicians must coordinate the multidisciplinary care for athletes. They must understand nutrition to encourage a balanced diet, identify maladaptive eating behavior, and counsel athletes on the use of dietary supplementation. Sports physicians should be familiar with the principles of exercise and rehabilitation from injury. Outside the realm of medicine, sports physicians should appreciate the politics and ethics of athletics and understand the rules and requirements specific to the sport in which athletes participate. They must ensure that appropriate health care policies and emergency plans are established. Successful sports physicians are able to integrate all of these principles into their practice while demonstrating the availability, affability, and ability required for optimal care of athletes.

RECOMMENDED READINGS

Botrè F, Pavan A. Enhancement drugs and the athlete. *Neurol Clin.* 2008;26(1):149–167.

Guskiewicz KM, Bruce SL, Cantu RC, et al. National Athletic Trainers' Association Position Statement: Management of Sport-Related Concussion. *J Athl Train.* 2004;39(3):280–297.

Rice SG. American Academy of Pediatrics Council on Sports Medicine and Fitness: Medical Conditions Affecting Sports Participation. *Pediatrics.* 2008;121(4):841–848.

Seto CK, Way D, O'Connor N. Environmental illness in athletes. *Clin Sports Med.* 2005;24(3):695–718.

The American Academy of Family Physicians, American Academy of Orthopedic Surgeons, American College of Sports Medicine, American Medical Society for Sports Medicine, American Orthopaedic Society for Sports Medicine, American Osteopathic Society for Sports Medicine. Consensus statements. http://www.aafp.org/online/en/home/clinical/publichealth/sportsmed.html.

Principles of Orthopaedic Trauma

10

Samir Mehta

INTRODUCTION

The diagnosis, management, and understanding of patients sustaining traumatic orthopaedic injuries covers a wide array of mechanisms of injury, fractures, soft tissue injuries, and urgency. At its heart, orthopaedic trauma care is based on the fundamental principles governing musculoskeletal injury, and its medical and surgical treatment. As with all surgical subspecialties, proper diagnosis of the orthopaedic patient requires a thorough history and physical examination. Radiographic analysis using plain radiographs and, in certain situations, computed tomography (CT) and magnetic resonance imaging (MRI) are essential in providing additional information as it correlates to the clinical examination.

This chapter is dedicated to highlighting principles utilized to evaluate the orthopaedic trauma patient and detailing a set of surgical emergencies that all orthopaedic surgeons should be familiar with and comfortable identifying and managing. A working knowledge of this list of diagnoses and treatment regimens is critical in avoiding significant morbidity and mortality in the patient with orthopaedic injuries.

EVALUATION OF THE ORTHOPAEDIC TRAUMA PATIENT

Nearly 60% of all trauma patients have an orthopaedic injury or musculoskeletal complaint. It is imperative to adhere to the Advanced Trauma Life Support (ATLS) guidelines in evaluating any trauma patient. It is the obligation of an orthopaedic surgeon called to the resuscitation bay to evaluate a patient to begin his/her examination with the ATLS protocol. Despite orthopaedic interests being predominantly musculoskeletal, the orthopaedic surgeon should assess the airway, check for breathing, and determine circulatory volume and hemodynamic stability. Typically, orthopedic injuries are diagnosed during the secondary survey once the patient is deemed hemodynamically stable. However, patients with severe musculoskeletal injuries that compromise circulation can be diagnosed during the primary survey.

The proper evaluation of the trauma patient requires a thorough understanding of the mechanism of injury as this allows for a high index of suspicion for specific injury patterns as well as associated injuries. In the unstable trauma patient with an unknown cause of hypotension, a high-energy blunt injury mechanism (e.g., motor vehicle or motorcycle collisions and falls from a height) may increase the likelihood of a pelvic ring injury, long bone fracture, or spinal cord injury. Unexplained hypotension in a patient, especially without a known thoracic or abdominal injury, should prompt consideration of a pelvic injury or long bone fracture as the source of exsanguination or significant blood loss (Table 10.1).

Physical Examination

As mentioned above, orthopaedic injures are typically diagnosed during the secondary survey. Injuries associated with a gross deformity of the involved extremity or large soft tissue defect with the underlying bone or joint exposed may be obvious on examination and require prompt treatment during the secondary survey. More subtle soft tissue injuries (i.e., lacerations, abrasions, and ecchymosis) should increase the suspicion for an underlying fracture or joint injury (Fig. 10.1). Deformity and soft tissue injury are

TABLE 10.1
OCCULT BLOOD LOSS IN ACUTE FRACTURES

Location of Fracture	Blood Loss (Units)
Ankle	0.5–1.5
Elbow	0.5–1.5
Femur	1.0–2.0
Forearm	0.5–1.0
Hip	1.5–2.5
Humerus	1.0–2.0
Knee	1.0–1.5
Pelvis	1.5–4.5
Tibia	0.5–1.5

essential in diagnosing orthopaedic injuries in the unconscious patient. All patients who are awake should be examined in a systematic fashion so as to minimize the likelihood of missing an injury. Unconscious patients are thoroughly examined once awake (tertiary survey) for injuries not obvious at the time of presentation to the resuscitation bay.

The musculoskeletal portion of the secondary survey starts with the proximal upper extremity and is conducted bilaterally while observing the patient's facial expression during the examination, which can provide additional information regarding subtle injuries. The patient's shoulders, elbows, and wrists are taken through range of motion. The upper arm and forearm are palpated for tenderness. The hand is assessed for soft tissue injury, which can be easily missed on the initial examination. Evaluation of "anatomical snuffbox" (space between the extensor pollicis brevis and extensor pollicis longus tendons at the level of the dorsolateral wrist) tenderness aids in the diagnosis of an underlying scaphoid fracture. The vascular supply of each upper extremity is then evaluated on the basis of the radial and ulnar artery pulses, as well as the degree of capillary refill. In the adequately resuscitated trauma patient, capillary refill should be less than two seconds.

The upper extremity examination terminates in a detailed neurologic examination with documentation of axillary, musculocutaneous, radial, ulnar, and median nerve function (Fig. 10.2). The radial nerve is assessed by testing for active wrist or thumb extension as well as sensation in the first dorsal webspace. Fractures about the distal humerus may result in injury of the radial nerve and may manifest as motor weakness or sensory loss. The ulnar nerve is evaluated with demonstration of good hand intrinsic muscle activity by way of grip strength or spreading the

A
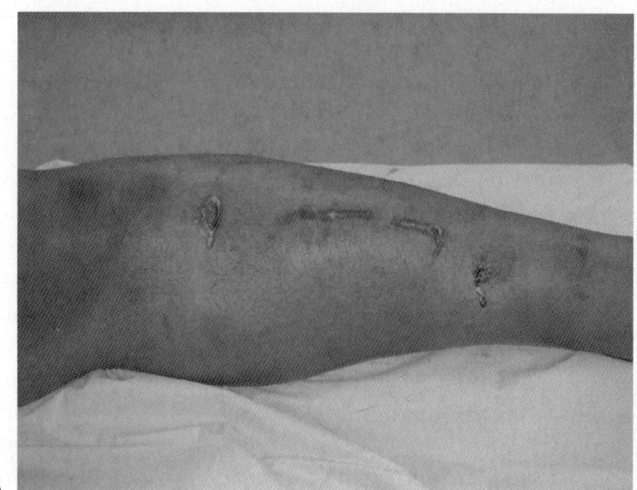

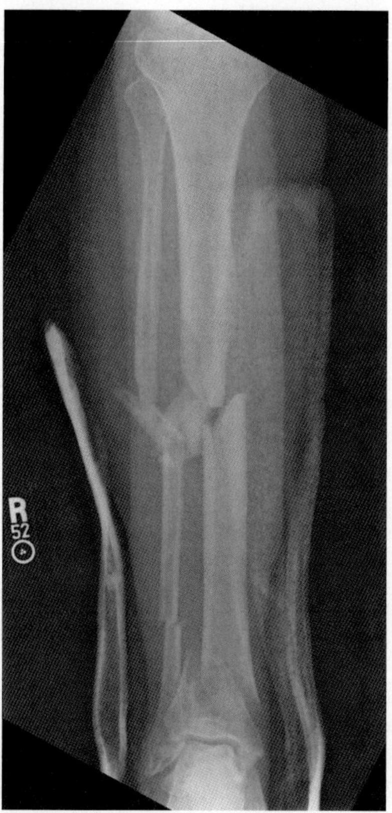

B

Figure 10.1 **(A)** A 37-year-old male patient with a blunt force trauma to the leg resulting in two small lacerations over the anteromedial tibia. A high index of suspicion should be maintained with this type of presentation. **(B)** Radiographs reveal a comminuted open tibia fracture.

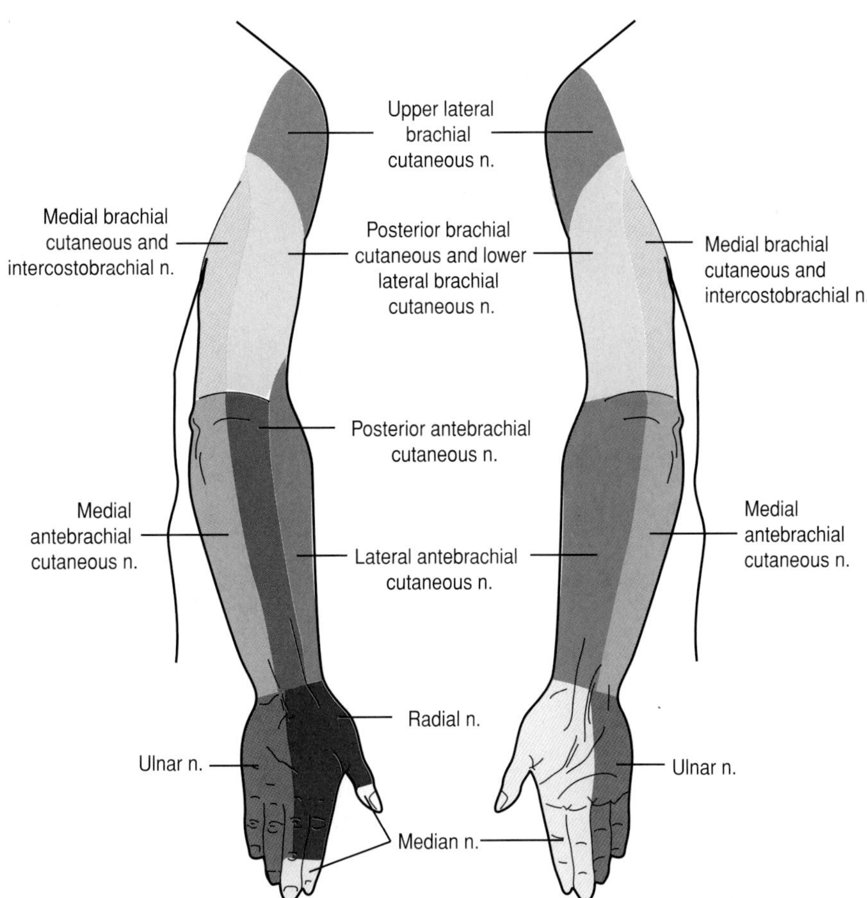

Figure 10.2 Sensory distribution of the upper extremity.

fingers to resistance as well as light touch sensation to the small and ulnar half of the ring finger. The median nerve is tested by asking the patient to give an "okay" sign with the thumb and index finger as well as by assessing sensation of the palmar aspect of the thumb, index, long, and radial half of the ring finger. Soft tissue injuries such as lacerations about the wrist may cause a disruption of the ulnar or median nerves. In addition, fractures such as distal radius fractures may result in significant volar wrist swelling and patients may develop an acute carpal tunnel syndrome requiring immediate decompression of the median nerve at the wrist.

Attention is then turned to the thorax. Each clavicle, as well as the sternum, is palpated for tenderness. The rib cage is gently squeezed toward the midline to assess for tenderness secondary to rib fractures. The thoracic examination extends distally to the pelvic ring. For the hemodynamically stable patient that was not noted to have findings consistent with a pelvic fracture during the primary survey, the pelvis is examined at this point during the examination. The pelvis is examined by applying gentle pressure on the anterior superior iliac spines in an anterior to posterior direction with the palm of both hands. In addition, gentle medial pressure is applied from the lateral aspect of each iliac wing with both hands. These maneuvers are often uncomfortable for patients with an underlying fracture. Patients with minimal pelvic bleeding associated with a pelvic fracture should not have this examination performed repeatedly by multiple examiners or with significant force in an effort to minimize the risk of fracture displacement and disruption of vessel tamponade. Patients with pelvic ring injuries should also undergo a thorough genitourinary examination to assess for open fractures within the pelvic vault (e.g., open fracture through the vaginal wall) or neurologic injury.

Examination of the lower extremities follows a similar progression as seen with the upper extremities. Each hip, knee, and ankle is taken through a range of motion. The thigh, lower leg, and foot are all palpated for tenderness. Particular focus should be given to the proximal tibia to avoid missing a subtle proximal tibia (tibial plateau) fracture. Tibial plateau fractures that are not obvious are notorious for appearing innocuous on plain radiographs and often require advanced imaging with a CT scan. The vascular examination includes palpation of the posterior tibial artery behind the medial malleolus and the dorsalis pedis artery between the first and second metatarsals on the dorsum of the foot.

The neurologic examination includes testing the terminal branches of the sciatic, tibial, and peroneal nerves (Fig. 10.3). The peroneal nerve is further subdivided into a superficial and deep branch. Foot eversion strength and sensation over the dorsum of the foot demonstrates adequate

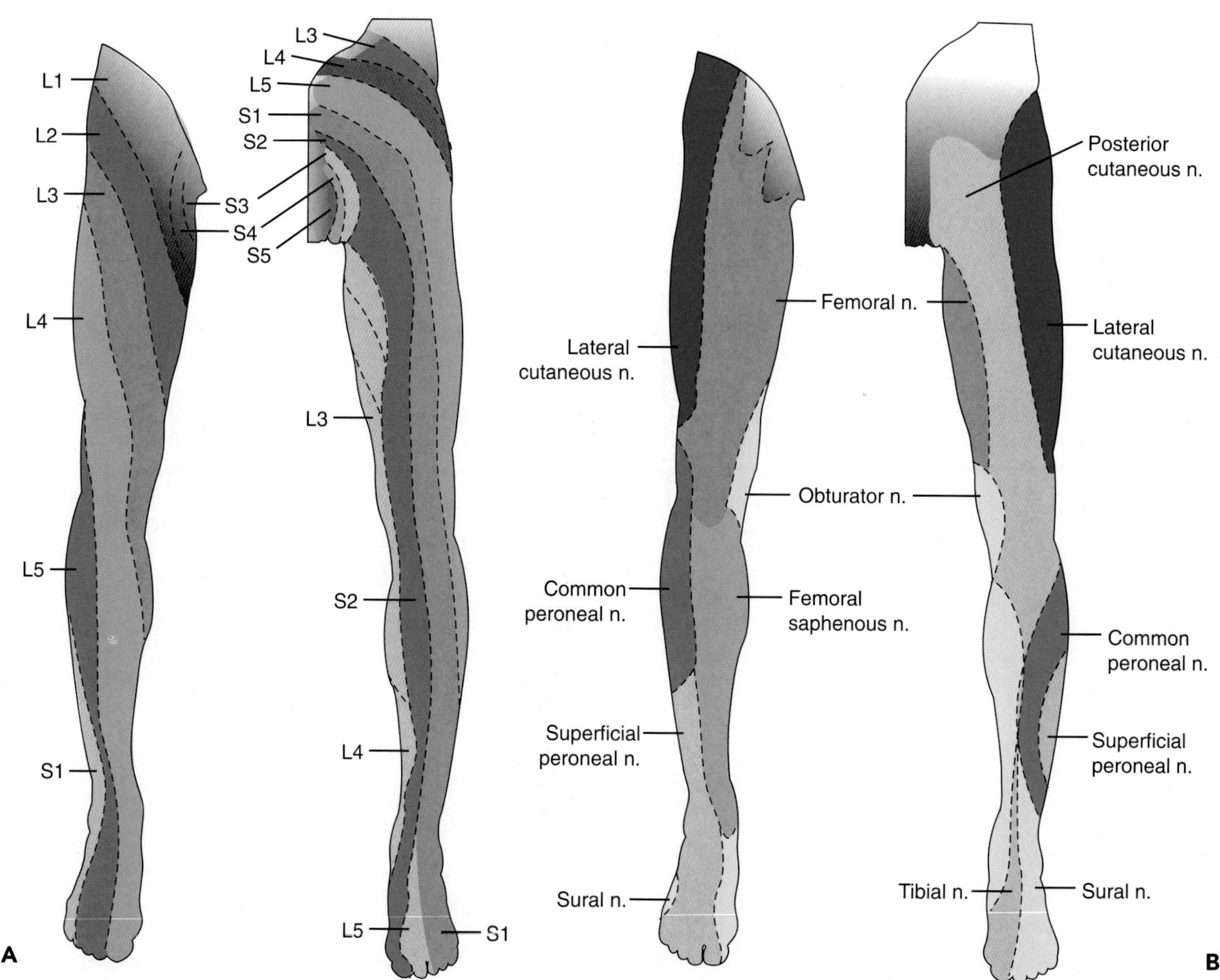

Figure 10.3 Sensory distribution of the lower extremity. **(A)** Dermatonal distribution and **(B)** peripheral nerve distribution.

motor and sensory function of the superficial peroneal nerve. The deep peroneal nerve motor function can be evaluated by testing ankle dorsiflexion or great toe extension while sensation should be intact to the first dorsal webspace. Injuries to the proximal fibula can result in injury to the peroneal nerve prior to its division and may manifest as loss of motor function, sensory function, or both. The typical presentation is a patient with a "foot drop" on the affected side—the foot is resting in a plantar flexed position and the patient is unable to dorsiflex the foot. The tibial nerve innervates the superficial and deep posterior compartments of the lower leg as well as several muscles in the foot via its terminal branches, the medial, and lateral plantar nerves. Motor function of the tibial nerve is tested by demonstration of ankle plantar flexion strength through the gastrocnemius-soleus muscle complex, while sensation should be intact on the plantar aspect of the foot. Any injury to the sciatic nerve proximally, either at the level of the lumbar spine or hip, may result in motor and sensory functional loss of the lower extremity distal to the knee.

Spinal Cord Injury

Every trauma patient must have a detailed cervical, thoracic, and lumbar spine examination documented. In addition, patients suspected of having a spinal cord injury require a thorough neurologic examination documenting motor distribution and sensory dermatomal distribution of each cervical and lumbar nerve root level. The upper and lower extremity examination is sufficient for patients not suspected of having a spinal cord injury. The clinical outcome of a patient with a spinal cord injury is based upon the initial functional level (lowest functioning motor and sensory nerve root).

A detailed motor and sensory examination of bilateral upper and lower extremities needs to be conducted to completely document spinal cord function. The examination commences at the level of the shoulder. Shoulder abduction denotes motor strength in the C5 nerve distribution. Flexion at the elbow tests C5 and C6 whereas elbow extension tests the C7 nerve root. Isolated C6 function can be evaluated with wrist extension. Both C8 and T1 motor functions are assessed by examining the intrinsic hand muscles. The associated dermatomal sensory pattern also should be documented. Sensation over the lateral shoulder is in the distribution of C5. Examination of the skin over the thumb, middle finger, and little finger constitutes intact sensation to light touch in the C6, C7, and C8 distributions, respectively. The T1 dermatomal distribution is located along the medial aspect of the upper arm.

Across the thorax and abdomen, there are no motor function tests to be conducted. Certain anatomic landmarks represent the dermatomal distribution of the thoracic spinal nerve roots. The T4 level is at the nipple. The T8 dermatome can be tested at the level of the xiphoid process, whereas the T10 level is at the umbilicus.

Physical examination of the lower extremity begins with motor testing of the major lumbosacral nerve roots. Hip flexion is associated with L2 and L3 motor function, whereas knee extension is associated with L3 and L4 nerve root function. Isolated L4 and L5 nerve root function can be tested with ankle and great toe dorsiflexion, respectively. Ankle plantar flexion assesses isolated S1 nerve root motor function. Dermatomal patterns for sensation to light touch are as follows: (1) the medial proximal thigh is L2; (2) the medial distal thigh is L3; (3) the medial lower leg is L4; (4) the lateral lower leg is L5; and (5) the plantar aspect of the foot is S1.

There are a series of reflexes that should also be tested and documented to complete the spinal cord evaluation. The biceps, brachioradialis, and triceps reflexes of the upper extremity demonstrate an intact spinal cord reflex at the level of C5, C6, and C7, respectively. The patellar and Achilles reflexes of the lower extremity demonstrate an intact spinal cord reflex at the level of L4 and S1, respectively. The presence of a Hoffman sign (involuntary flexion of the thumb with pressure on the distal long finger) or a Babinski sign (upward curling of the toes with posterior to anterior, lateral to medial irritation of the plantar foot) signify upper motor neuron signs. In the face of a suspected spinal cord injury, a rectal examination must also be documented. The bulbocavernosus reflex is tested by pulling of the Foley catheter with a finger in the rectum. The absence of this reflex classifies the patient to be in a state of spinal shock and may last up to 48 hours following the injury. A repeat examination at 48 hours with a similar finding signifies that the state of the spinal cord injury at that time is irreversible.

Although acute pharmacologic treatment of spinal cord injuries remains controversial, the current treatment regimen involves administration of intravenous high-dose steroids within eight hours of injury.

Fractures Associated with Vascular Injury

External sources of hemorrhagic shock (e.g., femoral artery laceration) may also be addressed during the primary survey as they are encountered after stabilization of the airway and breathing. Obvious vascular injuries with continued bleeding, regardless of whether they are associated with an underlying fracture, are initially treated with pressure application over the wound. Prompt diagnosis and stabilization of other life- and limb-threatening injuries are paramount while simultaneously addressing the external bleeding source. The patient is typically taken to the operating room with as minimal delay as possible, and the appropriate consult service(s) (i.e., vascular surgery) should be notified.

An injury to a major vessel such as the femoral artery that is associated with an underlying femur fracture requires the simultaneous consultation and intervention of orthopaedic surgery and vascular surgery. A multidisciplinary approach to this patient in the operating room is critical to optimize clinical outcomes with sequencing of care being essential. One scenario would involve urgent orthopaedic stabilization of the long bone injury with external fixation followed by definitive vascular repair (Fig. 10.4). By repairing the bone first, the subsequent vascular repair will not be jeopardized by the necessary manipulation of the fracture. Although blood loss from the vessel injury is time dependent as is reperfusion of the injured limb, repair of the vascular injury could be compromised while stabilizing the underlying fracture. Another potential option in the management of this patient would be temporizing vascular fixation with a commercially available shunt with care taken to have excess shunt material present. Once the limb is reperfused and bleeding controlled, the orthopaedic procedure can follow.

Tertiary Survey

All trauma patients admitted to the hospital with an orthopaedic component to their injury pattern should receive a thorough tertiary physical examination once stable. A tertiary survey should also be conducted on all patients who were examined in the resuscitation bay. Patients who sustain major injuries such as long bone fractures or cervical spine injuries are at risk for being distracted by their injuries and not recognizing pain elsewhere from a more minor injury (e.g., wrist/snuffbox tenderness from a scaphoid fracture or metatarsal fractures of the feet). The tertiary examination is specifically geared toward identifying more subtle musculoskeletal injuries that require treatment either as an inpatient or at a later date as an outpatient.

OPEN FRACTURES

An open fracture is defined as any fracture that communicates with the external environment via a soft tissue defect. Typically, open fractures are the result of high-energy trauma and may yield a spectrum of soft tissue injury—from a "poke" hole to complete soft tissue devitalization, periosteal stripping, and exposed bone. When a patient

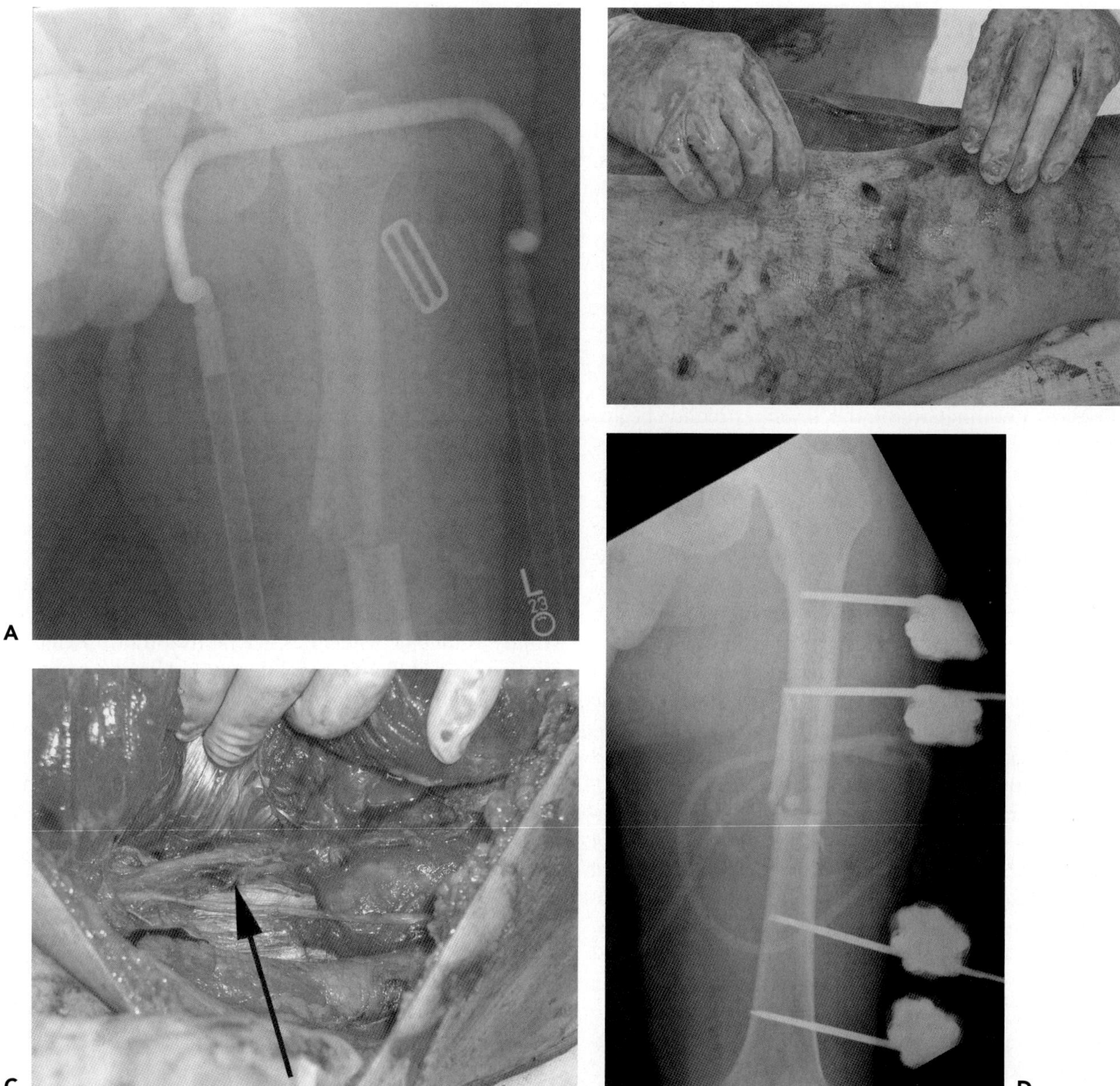

Figure 10.4 **(A)** Anteroposterior view of the left femur after a motor vehicle collision with a comminuted femoral shaft fracture. The patient also had decreased pulses in the limb and an abnormal ankle-brachial index (less than 0.9). **(B)** The patient had a small open wound on the medial side of the thigh. **(C)** Exploration of the thigh revealed the deep profundus artery (*arrow*) at the level of Hunters canal intact, but with direct compression by a fragment of bone. **(D)** The patient was temporized with an external fixator.

arrives in the trauma bay with an obvious extremity deformity and a large soft tissue injury, the diagnosis of an open fracture is self-evident. However, in the patient who presents with a deformed extremity and a small abrasion or laceration, an open fracture may be easily missed.

Open fractures are considered surgical emergencies and require prompt attention following hemodynamic stabilization of the trauma patient. Initially, tetanus prophylaxis should be administered if a tetanus booster has not been given in the previous 5 years (Table 10.2). In addition, intravenous antibiotics should be administered immediately upon recognition of the injury. Following diagnosis of an open fracture and documentation of a detailed neurovascular examination, the fracture site should be covered with a povidone-iodine soaked gauze. Although somewhat controversial, open fractures are generally considered a surgical emergency and should be taken to the operating room within 6 hours from the time of injury for thorough debridement and irrigation. The involved extremity should be splinted appropriately prior to subjecting the patient

TABLE 10.2
INDICATIONS FOR TETANUS PROPHYLAXIS

Tetanus Immunization (Prior Doses of Tetanus Toxoid)	Clean, Minor Wounds		Contaminated Wounds	
	Tetanus Toxoid	Tetanus Immune Globulin	Tetanus Toxoid	Tetanus Immune Globulin
Uncertain or <2	Yes	No	Yes	Yes
2	Yes	No	Yes	No*
≥3	No†	No	No‡	No

*Yes, if wound greater than 24 h old.
†Yes, if more than 10 yr since last dose.
‡Yes, if greater than 5 yr since last dose.

to further imaging studies (e.g., additional radiographs or CT scans for peri-articular fractures) as well for transport to the operating room. Splinting minimizes further injury to the injured extremity, particularly neurovascular structures that traverse the fracture site and the soft tissue envelope.

Open fractures are classified on the basis of the Gustilo and Anderson classification. This classification system is based on the degree of energy imparted to the limb at the time of the injury. Type I injures are low-energy open fractures and are typically associated with soft tissue defects of less than 1 cm (Fig. 10.1A). Type II injuries are considered to be medium-energy open fractures with an associated soft tissue defect that is usually between 1 and 10 cm (Fig. 10.5A). Type III injuries (Fig. 10.5B) are high-energy open fractures and are subcategorized on the basis of the degree of soft tissue injury: (A) large soft tissue defect with intact periosteum and minimal contamination; (B) large soft tissue defect with periosteal stripping, a greater degree of wound contamination, and needing additional soft tissue coverage (e.g., rotational flap, free flap); and (C) large soft tissue defect with an associated vascular injury requiring repair. Type I and II open fractures require prompt administration of a third generation cephalosporin such as cefazolin. All Type III fractures require the administration of cefazolin plus the addition of an aminoglycoside such as gentamicin. Patients who have sustained open fractures with severe contamination (e.g., "barnyard" injuries) require the addition of penicillin to cover gas-forming bacteria such as *Clostridium perfringens*. The major concern with open fractures is the increased incidence of infection associated with these injuries due to the degree of wound contamination as well as the degree of soft tissue loss.

Initial treatment in the operating room entails thorough debridement and irrigation of the wound with delivery of the bony edges of the fracture into the wound for debridement. The laceration is typically extended in a proximal and distal fashion to gain adequate access to the fracture site. Depending on the fracture type, the associated soft tissue defect, and extent of wound contamination, the treatment may include definitive plate fixation, intramedullary (IM) rod fixation, or temporary stabilization with external

A 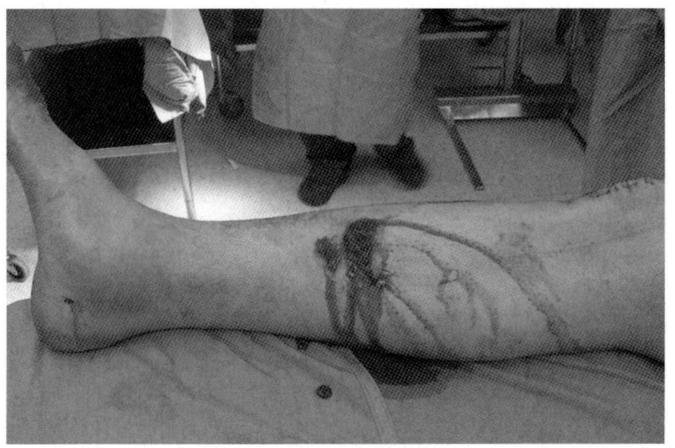

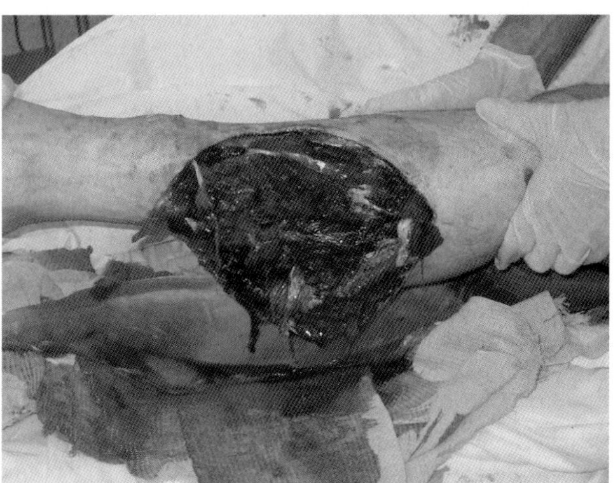 B

Figure 10.5 **(A)** Open type II tibia fracture with transverse tibial shaft fracture and a wound that is primarily closeable. **(B)** Open type III tibia fracture after significant high-energy soft tissue injury with muscle and skin loss.

fixation. As mentioned above, open fractures associated with a vessel injury (i.e., type IIIC injuries) may require external fixation of the fracture prior to definitive vascular repair to avoid undue tension on the repair.

FRACTURES WITH NEUROVASCULAR COMPROMISE

Gross deformities of an extremity identified in a trauma patient mandate the documentation of a detailed neurovascular examination, especially distal to the site of the deformity. A patient who presents with a neurovascular deficit distal to an extremity injury should undergo fracture reduction and/or gentle traction to pull the extremity out to length. It is imperative that a repeat neurovascular examination of the extremity be performed after any manipulation of the injured limb. If the neurovascular examination returns to normal following manipulation, the initial deficit noted on physical examination was likely due to traction or tension on the neurovascular structures resulting from the deformity. The extremity should at this point be splinted appropriately to avoid any additional undue stress on the neurovascular structures traversing the injury site. Ideally, patients should have radiographs obtained prior to manipulation of any deformed extremity. However, there should be no delay in waiting for radiographs if there is a neurovascular deficit in which case manipulation should be attempted without formal x-rays. Following manipulation, radiographs of the deformity site, as well as a joint proximal and distal to the injury should be obtained and reviewed thoroughly for associated bony injuries.

Patients with persistent neurovascular deficit following manipulation of a deformed extremity require additional evaluation. Nerve deficits sustained at the time of injury are often neurapraxic in nature as a result of the nerve stretching. These type of injuries typically are self-limited and may take anywhere from 3 to 6 months to completely resolve. Electromyography is the gold standard to monitor improvement of nerve function and may show activity or improvement as early as 6 weeks following the inciting event.

Fractures that result from high-energy injuries may result in nerve laceration (Fig. 10.6) and complete disruption of the neuronal axons. In this situation, the decision may be made to explore the nerve at the time of definitive treatment and perform a primary repair.

Vascular deficits that do not return after limb manipulation are considered vessel injuries until proven otherwise and require additional formal studies and imaging to confirm the diagnosis. The initial step is to determine the ankle-brachial index. This noninvasive measure of distal blood flow is done by measuring the systolic blood pressure at the level of the elbow and at the ankle. A Doppler signaling device is typically used to hear the pulsatile nature of arterial flow around each joint. A ratio (index) of the ankle to brachial pressure of less than 0.9 is considered positive

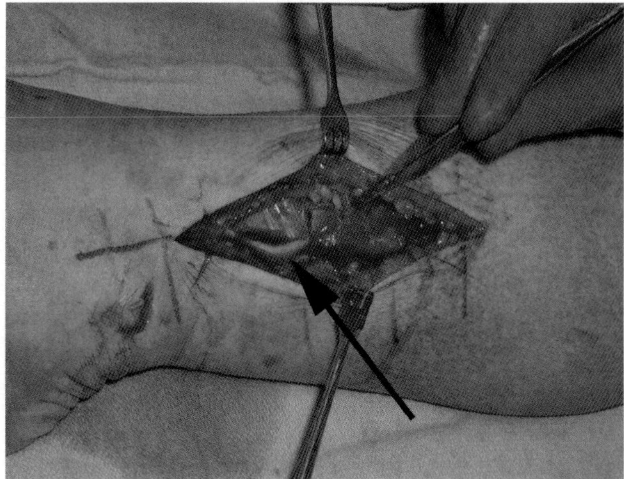

Figure 10.6 Unstable ankle fracture after a skateboarding accident resulting in a traumatic laceration of the superficial peroneal nerve (*arrow*) seen during fixation of the fibula fracture.

and points in the direction of a vessel injury. In these patients, a more formal study is required to identify intimal injures to the arterial wall versus a complete disruption of the vessel. The finding of an abnormal ankle-brachial index mandates an arteriogram that can be conducted in an interventional radiology suite or in the operating room at the time of surgical treatment of the injury.

SPINAL CORD INJURY

A complete physical examination must be conducted on all patients with a suspected spinal cord injury as was discussed previously in the evaluation of the trauma patient. There are several spinal cord injury patterns that are associated with predictable motor and sensory deficits. Brown-Sequard syndrome (Fig. 10.7A) is a hemicord transection, often by a penetrating injury (e.g., knife wound). An injury pattern of this nature results in ipsilateral motor, proprioception, and light touch loss with a contralateral loss of pain and temperature sensation distal to the injury level.

Central cord syndrome (Fig. 10.7B) is typically seen in middle-aged to elderly patients who have preinjury cervical spine degenerative joint disease. The classic scenario is that of a patient involved in a motor vehicle collision who sustains a hyperextension (e.g., whiplash) injury to the cervical spine. This injury pattern results in bilateral upper extremity motor weakness more so than bilateral lower extremity weakness. Central cord syndrome has the greatest potential for compete functional recovery when compared with the other injury patterns.

Anterior cord syndrome (Fig. 10.7C) is usually the result of a vascular insult to the anterior spinal cord (anterior spinal artery distribution). The deficit pattern is a loss of bilateral motor function, pain, and temperature sensation

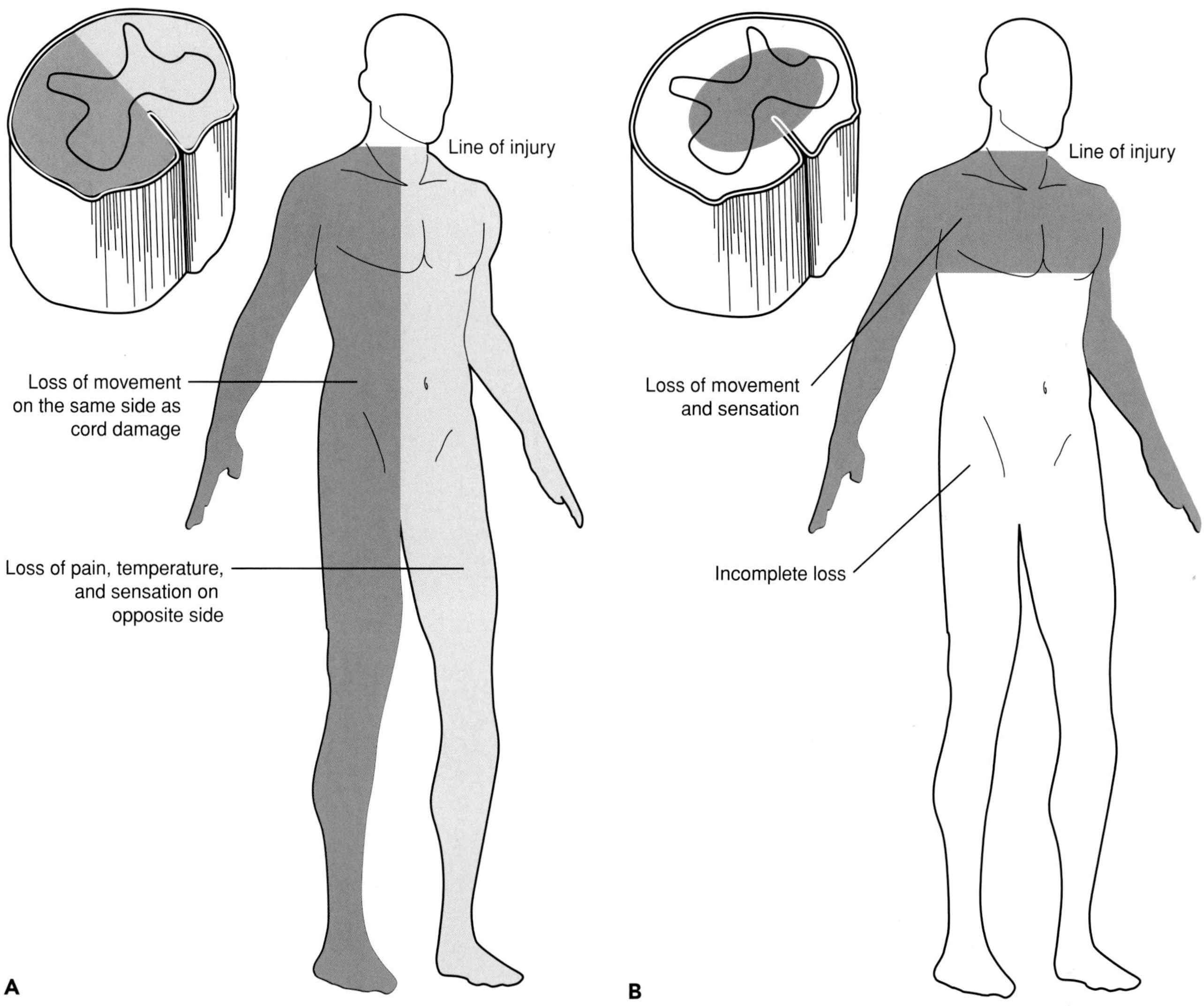

Figure 10.7 **(A)** Brown-Sequard syndrome, **(B)** central cord syndrome, and **(C)** anterior cord syndrome with affected anatomical locations. *(continued)*

distal to the level of injury. This injury pattern is associated with the lowest likelihood of functional recovery.

FRACTURE-DISLOCATIONS

Fracture-dislocations are fractures that occur around a joint and result in a fracture of the bone with an associated dislocation of the joint. This type of injury has several variations based on the fracture pattern, the bone that is involved, and the joint that is involved. Dislocations in general require prompt reduction due to the stress imparted on the traversing neurovascular structures and soft tissue (Fig. 10.8). In addition, joints that are left dislocated for a prolonged period of time, typically more than 6 hours, are at risk of irreversible cartilage damage and posttraumatic arthritis of the involved joint. Following reduction of a fracture-dislocation, the limb is splinted to prevent any further damage or loss of reduction during patient transport. These injuries often requires definitive operative fixation of the fracture as well as repair/reconstruction of any associated soft tissue disruption (e.g., ligaments).

Fractures surrounding a joint (periarticular fractures), whether associated with a dislocation or not, often require advanced imaging to fully delineate the injury pattern. CT scans are helpful in identifying the bony pattern of injury, whereas MRI is used to determine soft tissue (i.e., ligament or tendon) injuries. MRI is more useful when delayed treatment of the injury is undertaken since obtaining an MRI in the acute setting usually demonstrates a great deal of edema that can obscure soft tissue detail. Advanced imaging and diagnostic tools may be necessary in patients with abnormal vascular examination results after dislocation and reduction given that many joints lie in close proximity to vasculature.

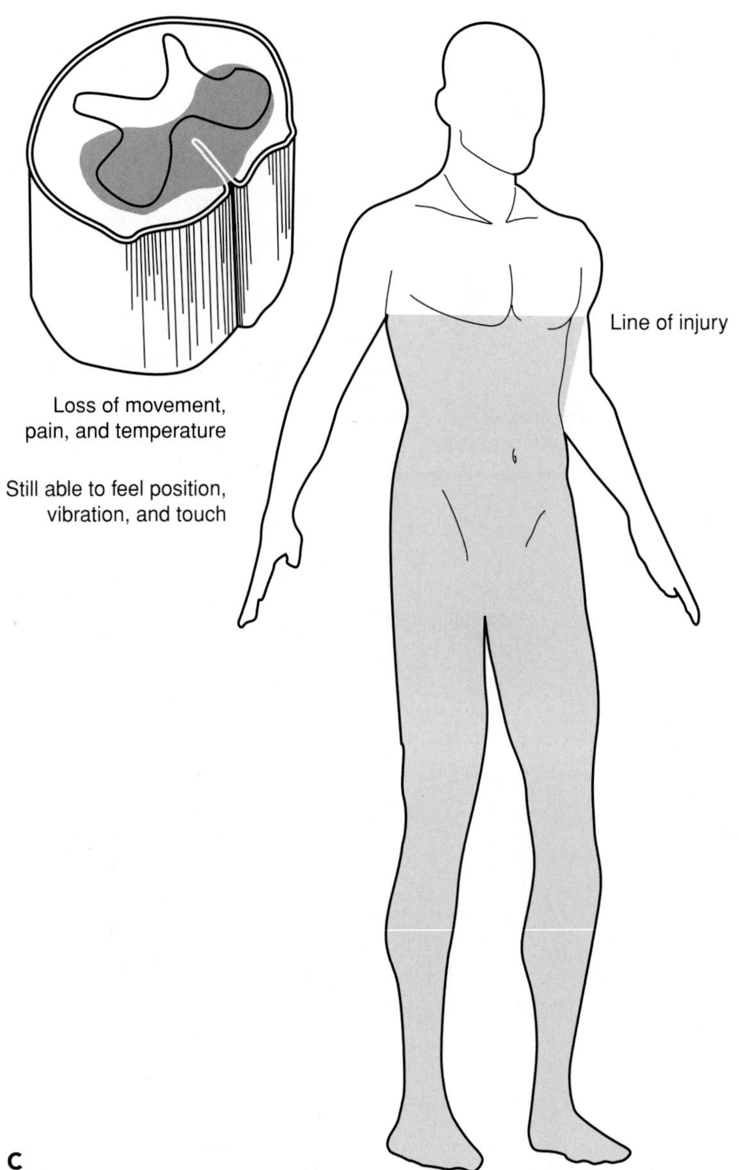

Figure 10.7 *(continued)*

COMPARTMENT SYNDROME

The phenomenon of compartment syndrome is a surgical emergency and requires a high index of suspicion. Each extremity contains several muscles that are separated by fascial compartments. When the pressure within any single or several compartments reaches a level beyond a threshold value, the venous return from the extremity is initially compromised. As the pressure continues to increase, the forward arterial flow of oxygenated blood is compromised resulting in intracompartmental muscle ischemia. Identification of an "impending" compartment syndrome is critical in minimizing the morbidity associated with irreversible muscle ischemia and eventual muscle cell death. The most common sites of compartment syndrome include the forearm and the lower leg (Fig. 10.9A). This phenomenon also can occur within the fascial compartments of the thigh, foot, and the gluteal muscles, although much less common.

Compartment syndrome is a clinical diagnosis. In the patient who is awake and alert and is able to comply with the physical examination, the diagnosis can be made clinically and usually is linked to a high index of suspicion. The following patient scenarios should increase the likelihood of the possible diagnosis of compartment syndrome: (1) high-energy closed fractures; (2) prolonged external pressure on the compartment (e.g., patients found down for a prolonged period of time); (3) intravenous ionic dye extravasation (e.g., patients receiving contrast dye for a CT scan that extravasates out of the intravascular system into a fascial compartment); (4) crush injuries; (5) reperfusion injuries (e.g., repair of arterial injuries resulting in reconstitution of blood flow and thus increased inflammation); (6) concomitant arterial and

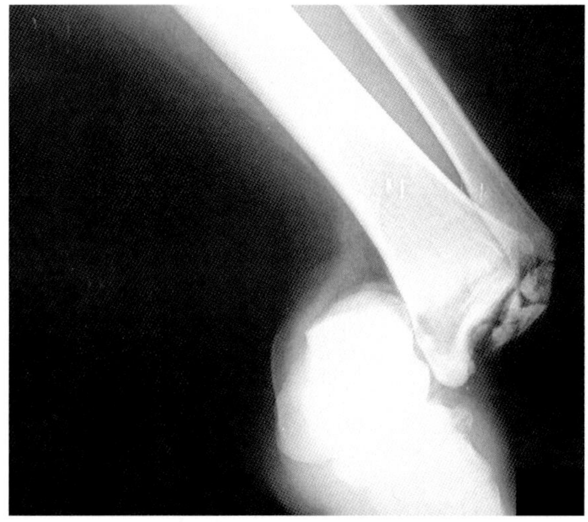

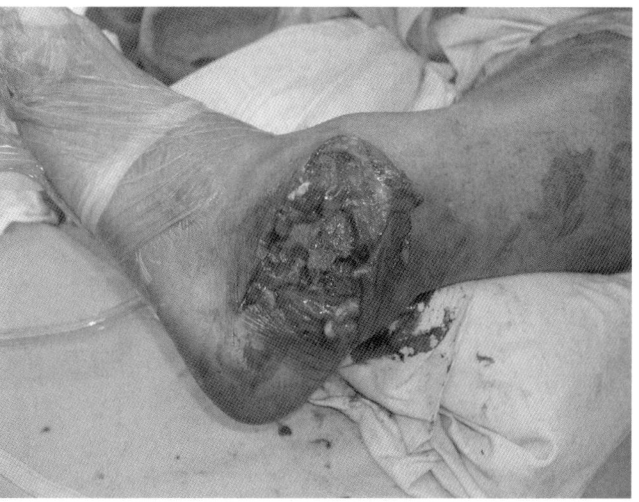

Figure 10.8 **(A)** Medial ankle dislocation with fibular fracture and **(B)** tension-type soft tissue defect requiring prompt reduction followed by irrigation and debridement with temporizing fixation in the operating room.

venous injuries to an extremity; and (7) limb ischemia more than 6 hours.

The physical examination in a conscious patient should begin with evaluating for pain with passive stretch of the distal extremity digits. This is the most sensitive test in making the clinical diagnosis of compartment syndrome. For example, a patient with an impending lower leg compartment syndrome following a closed proximal tibia fracture will present with pain out of proportion to what would be expected with dorsiflexion of the toes. In conjunction with this examination finding, patients typically exhibit very tense compartments on palpation and significant pain with compression of the involved area. Other pertinent physical findings could include pulselessness, poikilothermia (cool extremity), and paraesthesias. However, when these examination findings are present, the diagnosis has often been missed and it may be too late to administer effective surgical treatment.

The diagnosis of compartment syndrome is more difficult to make in the unconscious patient or in the pediatric population. Again, the most important concept in making the diagnosis, even in the unconscious patient, is a high index of suspicion. Specifically in the pediatric population, even though the child may be awake, compliance with the physical examination and ability to answer questions may be the limiting factor. In addition, the administration of

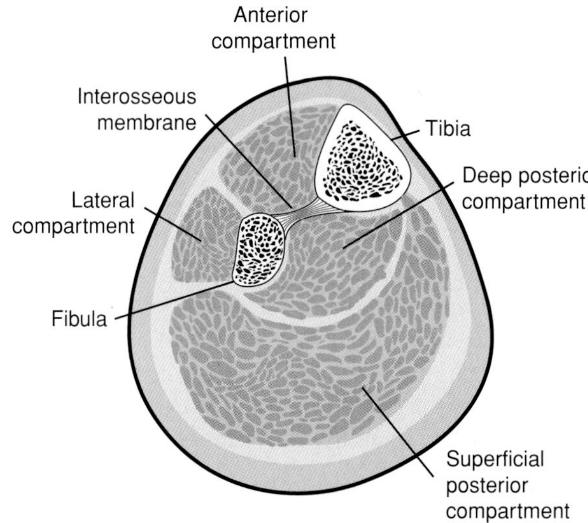

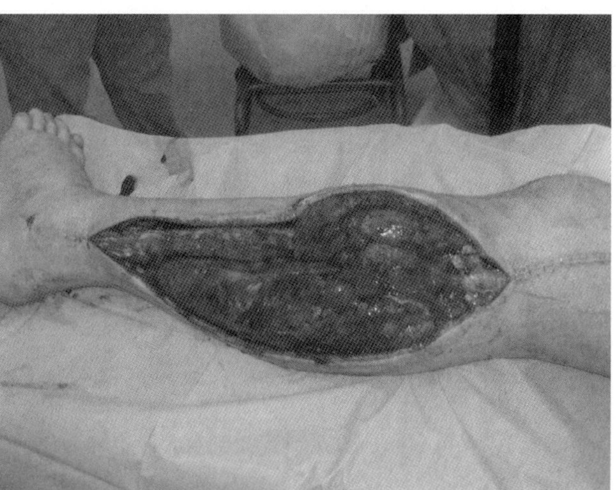

Figure 10.9 **(A)** The four compartments of the tibia include the anterior, lateral, superficial posterior, and deep posterior. **(B)** The anterior and lateral compartments are released through a lateral exposure. The superficial and deep posterior compartments can be released through a medial incision. The incisions should be extensile and should include both skin and fascia.

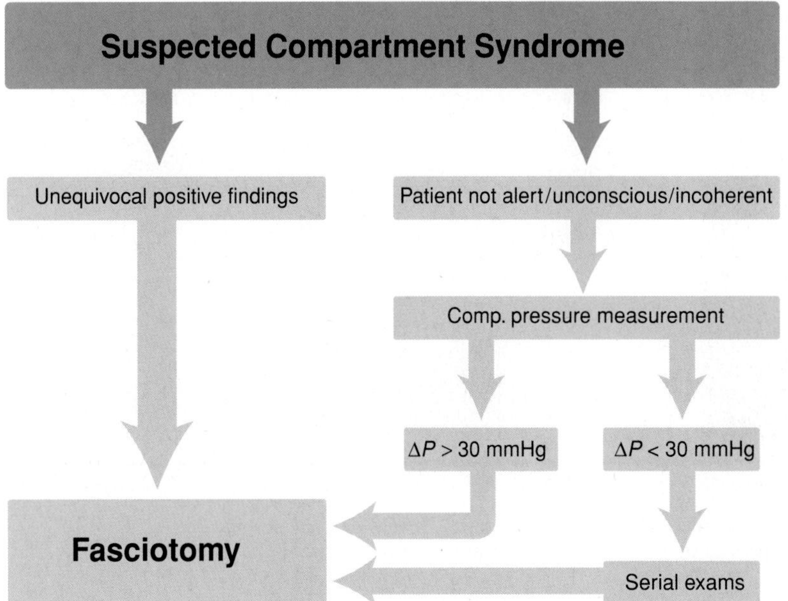

Figure 10.10 Management scheme for a patient with suspected compartment syndrome.

intravenous narcotic medications for pain control may also obscure the physical examination findings. In those patients, where the index of suspicion is high but the physical examination is equivocal, a more invasive diagnostic measure, intracompartmental pressure assessment, should be performed.

Several commercially available needle devices can be used to measure intracompartmental pressures. In general, a small amount of saline is introduced into the compartment under interrogation that then equilibrates within the compartment. The pressure measurement reading is then taken as the pressure within the fascial compartment. Typically, the forearm requires pressure measurement in three separate compartments: the flexor compartment, the extensor compartment, and the mobile wad (fascial compartment containing the brachioradialis, extensor carpi radialis longus, and extensor carpi brevis muscles). For the lower leg, the anterior, lateral, superficial, and deep posterior fascial compartments should be measured. Each compartment measurement should be documented as well as the patient's diastolic and mean arterial pressure (MAP) at the time of the measurement.

There are several measurement thresholds that can be used to determine whether an intracompartmental pressure is high and requires treatment. Some authors recommend an absolute value greater than 30 mmHg as the threshold value. The intracapillary pressure required for the forward flow of blood into a fascial compartment is 25 mmHg. Therefore, an intracompartmental pressure of 30 mmHg or more most likely impedes the forward flow of arterial blood into the compartment. However, other authors have demonstrated that each compartmental measurement should take into account the hemodynamics of the patient at the time of the measurement. With this in mind, an intracompartmental pressure that is within 40 mmHg of the diastolic or MAP of the patient should be considered a high pressure. Regardless of the technique used to define a high compartmental pressure, the method should be clearly recorded in the patient record and the decision making should reflect the documented pressure measurements or pressure differentials (Fig. 10.10). Measurement of elevated compartment pressures mandates immediate treatment, which consists of fasciotomy and complete release of the involved fascial compartments.

Surgical release of fascial compartments is not a cosmetic procedure (Fig. 10.9B). Extensile incisions are used to release the fascia under direct visualization to obtain adequate release and avoid inadvertent injury to the neurovascular structures traversing the compartment. All three forearm compartments are typically released through a single volar incision whereas the four compartments of the lower leg can be released through a single or dual extensile incision. Following fascial release, the wound is copiously irrigated and packed open with a wet to dry dressing. In addition, vessel loops stapled to the skin in an interwoven pattern or a negative pressure wound therapy dressing (vacuum assisted closure dressing) are commonly used in this setting. Patients are typically taken back to the operating room every 48 to 72 hours for repeat irrigation and debridement until the wound can be primarily closed, all necrotic muscle has been thoroughly debrided, and/or the decision is made for additional soft tissue (split thickness skin grafting) coverage.

If compartment syndrome is a possibility given a certain injury pattern (e.g., closed midshaft tibia fracture), then regional anesthesia, continuous epidurals, and patient controlled intravenous opiate analgesia should be avoided since they may mask the symptoms of compartment syndrome. Missed compartment syndrome in tibia fractures and other surgical patients managed postoperatively with these techniques have been reported and therefore they are generally avoided.

POLYTRAUMA

The management of the patient with polytrauma is a complex interplay of injuries, treatment options, and an appreciation for the complexity of the variability in presentation. A polytrauma patient is one who has an Injury Severity Score greater than 18 with multiple system injuries. There is a systemic inflammatory response after trauma, which may lead to sequelae such as acute respiratory distress syndrome (ARDS), sepsis, and/or multiorgan failure. This has given rise to the "two-hit" theory. The "first hit" is from the initial stimulus resulting in a systemic inflammatory response. The "second hit" comes from a subsequent proinflammatory event such as incomplete resuscitation, excessive blood loss, sepsis, or a surgical procedure. Two interleukins have been implicated in the polytrauma patient—IL-6 as a proinflammatory cytokine increasing likelihood of ARDS and IL-10 as an anti-inflammatory cytokine. Patients at risk include those who are clinically unstable, a difficult resuscitation, coagulopathic (platelet count less than 90,000), hypothermic (less than 32°C), in shock, require greater than 25 units packed red blood cells, or those with bilateral lung injury, and multiple long bone fractures and thoracic or abdominal injury.

A polytrauma patient who is adequately resuscitated has a normal or normalizing lactate, base deficit, or mixed venous oxygen saturation. The patient is adequately rewarmed with an international normalized ratio less than 1.25, platelet count greater than 90,000, and a cerebral perfusion pressure greater than 70 mmHg. However, it should be noted that there is a secondary period, where despite appropriate resuscitation, patients operated on 2 to 4 days after their initial trauma may have a worsening of their condition ("second hit"). Therefore, significant surgical intervention may need to be delayed 5 to 8 days after injury to the limit the impact of the "second hit" (Fig. 10.11). This has lead to two schools of thought in the management of the polytraumatized patient—early total care and damage control orthopaedics. Early total care involves immediate definitive management of orthopaedic injuries allowing for early mobilization and decreased pulmonary complications. However, increased mortality and morbidity has been associated with early total care in patients with chest trauma. Damage control orthopaedics temporizes fractures with external fixation avoiding the "second hit." When the patient is stable, definitive care is undertaken.

In the multiply injured patient, fat embolism is an important cause of ARDS and a major source of morbidity and mortality. It may be potentiated by fracture stabilization with IM nailing of long bones. Fat embolism syndrome is clinically apparent in 10% of polytrauma patients, although the actual incidence rate is probably much higher. It may not appear until 2 to 3 days after the injury and may present as respiratory distress (shortness of breath and tachypnea), arterial hypoxemia, tachycardia, fevers, and a deterioration of neurological status (restlessness, confusion, or coma). In addition, petechiae (which may be short

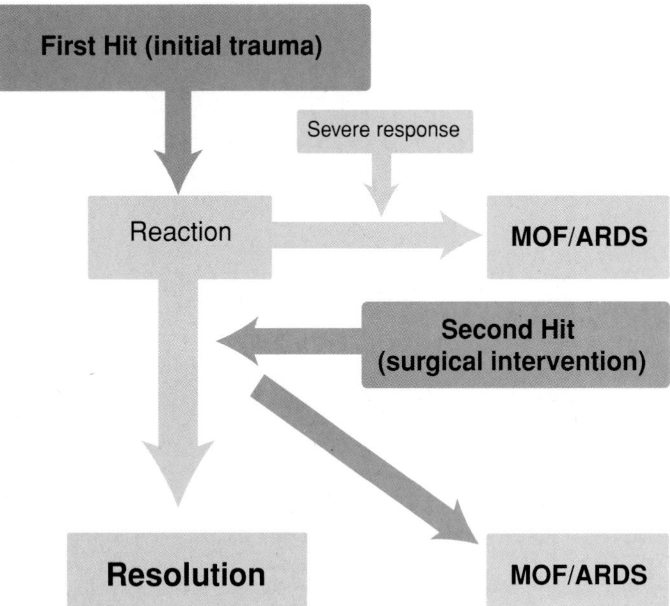

Figure 10.11 Damage control orthopaedics is often utilized in patients with thoracic trauma resulting in a proinflammatory state. The "second hit" results in further aggravation of an already heightened inflammatory response and may lead to multiorgan failure.

lived) can appear across the chest and axilla. Treatment consists of pulmonary support and early orthopedic care.

FRACTURE CLASSIFICATION

Once a fracture has been identified on radiographs, it is important to be able to convey this information to others who may not have access to the images. Fracture classification systems serve multiple functions including communication to other medical professionals about the severity, location, or complexity of the fracture. For example, the Schatzker classification for tibial plateau fractures indicates the severity of articular surface involvement and whether the diaphysis is associated with the metaphysis. The classification system may also guide treatment as is the case with the Garden classification for femoral neck fractures. Garden type I and type II fractures are considered stable and may be addressed with open reduction and internal fixation whereas Garden type III and type IV fractures are displaced requiring arthroplasty. Certain classification systems may portend prognosis of the fracture, such as the Hawkins classification system for talus fractures. The Hawkins classification ranges from one to four, where a type 1 fracture has a 5% to 10% chance of resulting in avascular necrosis, whereas a type IV has a 90% chance of avascular necrosis. Lastly, classification systems can aid in research for study design, describing results, and examining applicability of treatment interventions. Ultimately, the utility of a classification system is based on high inter- and intraobserver reliability.

A myriad of classification systems exist within orthopaedics and it is not realistic to memorize all of these systems. The most widely accepted fracture classification system is the AO/OTA system, which uses numbers and letters to describe fractures. Each bone has a number (1-humerus, 2-forearm, 3-femur, 4-tibia), which is first in the code. The second number is the segment of the bone that is involved (1-proximal, 2-diaphysis, 3-distal). The "type" of fracture is then described for diaphyseal injuries (A-simple, B-wedge, C-complex) (Fig. 10.12A). If the fracture is proximal or distal, then the letters represent extra-articular (A), partial articular (B), or complete articular (C) injuries (Fig. 10.12B).

However, not all physicians or residents may be familiar with the classification system being used to describe a

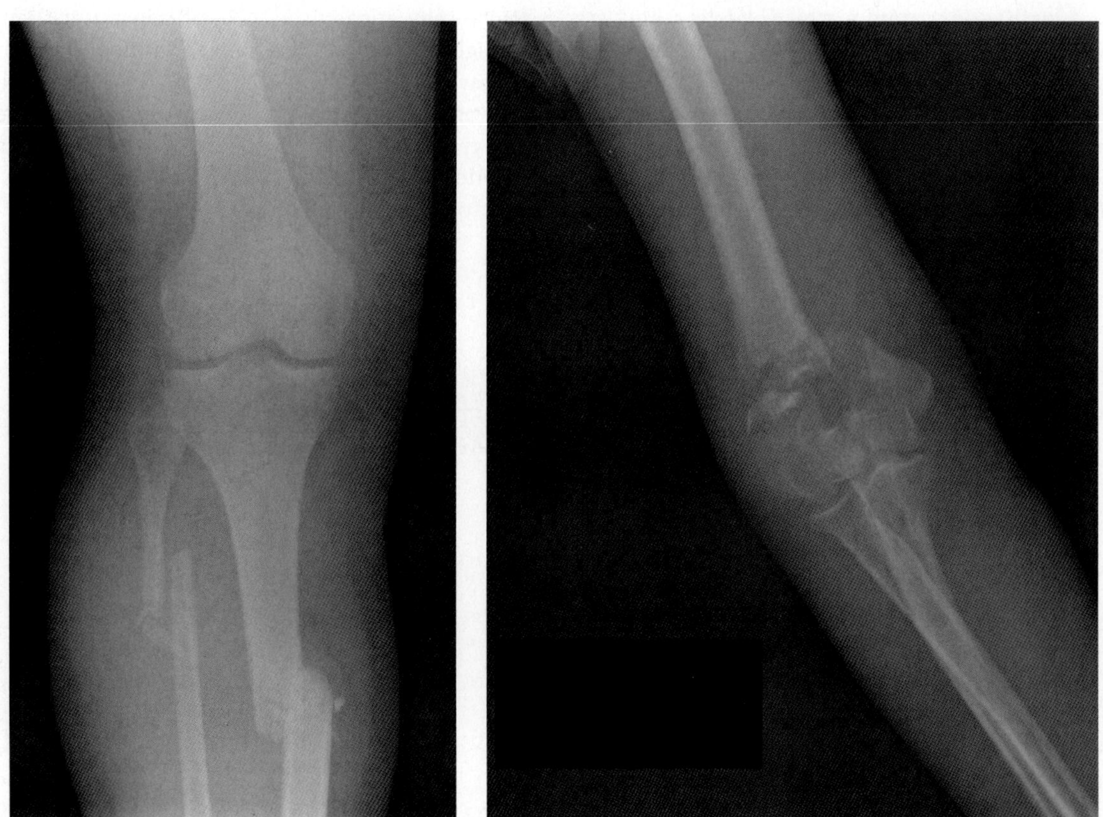

Figure 10.12 **(A)** The tibia fracture would be classified as an AO/OTA type 42A. The classification would indicate that the fractured bone is a tibia (4), it is midshaft/diaphyseal (2) in location, and is simple **(A)**. **(B)** The radiograph reveals an AO/OTA type 13C fracture that would indicate humerus (1), distal (3), and complete articular (C) since there is no articular surface attached the shaft and there is a split through the articular surface. Ultimately, using descriptive words is the best way to describe a fracture pattern.

fracture. The best method in communicating a fracture pattern is using descriptive words about the location of the fracture, the angulation, the displacement, the direction of the fracture line, and the degree of comminution.

FRACTURE MANAGEMENT

Bone Biology and Physiology

Bone has two major functions. The mechanical function involves supporting load, allowing muscle action, protecting vital organs, and enabling locomotion. The biologic function includes hematopoiesis and the important role of calcium homeostasis. Almost 99% of the body's calcium is contained within bone and it is essential in Vitamin D metabolism. In addition, bone is an end organ for parathyroid hormone, calcitonin, growth hormone, and corticosteroids—all of which are involved in bone (and calcium) regulation. Bone is a composite of two materials. The organic extracellular matrix (35% dry weight) is composed of collagen and provides flexibility and resilience. The mineral phase is composed of hydroxyapatite (calcium and phosphate) and provides for the hardness and rigidity of bone.

Cortical bone is peripheral and remodels slowly due to a poor porosity but is extremely strong. On the other hand, cancellous bone (medullary or central) has 10% of the strength of cortical bone, is spongy, and has porosity between 30% and 90%. Bone responds to stress by altering its mechanical characteristics (Wolff's law). With increased stress, bone will hypertrophy. The contrary is true—decreased stress can lead to increased bone resorption. Unlike articular cartilage, tendon, or ligament injury, bone regenerates tissue and repairs without scar. The blood supply to the cortical bone has two main contributions—the inner two-third of the cortical bone receives its blood supply from the nutrient vessel, whereas the outer one-third of cortical bone receives its blood supply from the periosteum (Fig. 10.13).

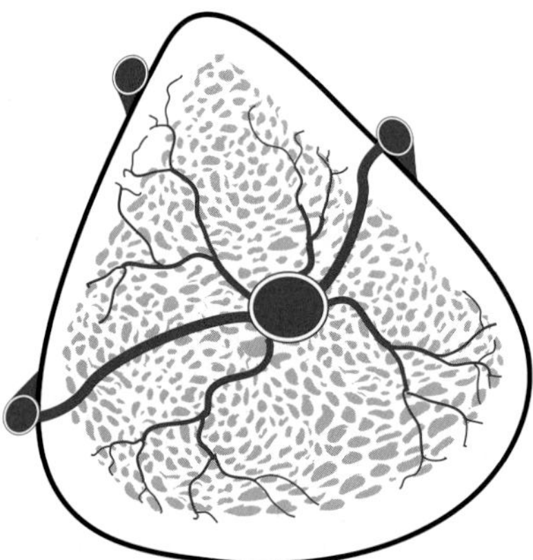

Figure 10.13 Contributions to the blood supply of cortical bone.

Fracture Healing

Fractures occur when the energy of the injury is sufficient to overload the bone resulting in loss of continuity, loss of support, soft tissue damage, and damage to the blood supply. Fracture healing requires an adequate biologic environment (soft tissue, pluripotential cells, and patient factors) and an appropriate mechanical environment (e.g., fracture stabilization technique). Within the appropriate biological and mechanical environment, fractures heal via primary or secondary modes. The biomechanics of fracture healing involve the amount of motion at the fracture site and the gap size between the fractured ends of the bone. Strain in bone is mechanical force producing elongation. Bone forms with low strain across a fracture gap. Low strain and no gap result in primary bone healing without callus. Low strain and a large gap will result in secondary bone healing with callus formation. Primary bone healing is direct remodeling of the fracture through rigid fixation. It is also known as a haversian remodeling or osteon remodeling and does not result in callus formation. There is direct contact between bone ends with no motion (Fig. 10.14). On the other hand, secondary bone healing (indirect bone healing) results from nonrigid fixation with callus formation through intramembranous and endochondral healing. It should be noted that in secondary bone healing, fragment motion stimulates callus formation (Fig. 10.15). However, excessive motion (or instability), at critical times during healing may lead to nonunion (Fig. 10.16).

Fracture healing occurs in three distinct phases—inflammatory (days), reparative (weeks), and remodeling (months) (Fig. 10.17). The inflammatory phase results from the torn periosteum, fracture hematoma, necrotic marrow and cortex, and inflammatory mediators. The pluripotential stem cells are locally derived and result in osteoblast and osteoclast differentiation and proliferation through cellular mediators. The repair phase organizes the hematoma with early subperiosteal woven bone and the start of cartilage formation. Finally, woven or fiber bone bridging the fracture gap is replaced by lamellar bone that revascularizes over time.

Preoperative Planning

Prior to an operation, the time which a surgeon devotes to a careful preoperative plan is of critical importance and often determines the success or failure of the procedure. Planning is essential as it allows for communication with the anesthesiologist, nursing, critical care, and imaging technicians. In addition, it allows for anticipation of problems, necessary supplies, instruments, and implants; shortens operating room time; and may improve outcomes. The basic steps to fracture fixation include the surgical incision, preparation of the bone ends, reduction, temporizing fixation, definitive fixation, closure, and aftercare. The components of a preoperative plan include operating room logistics

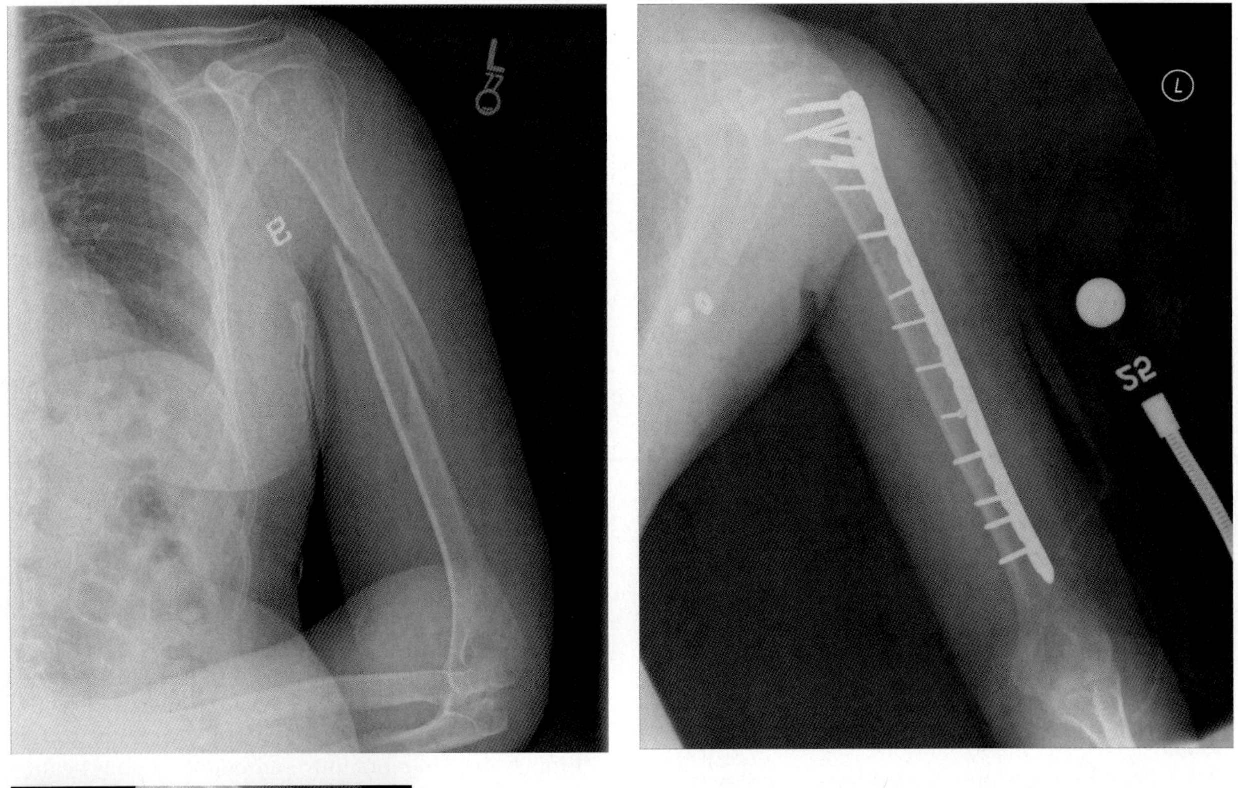

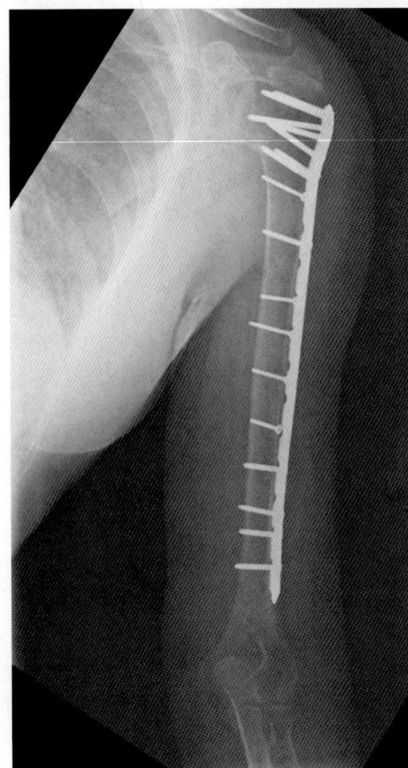

Figure 10.14 **(A)** A 42-year-old female with a left spiral fracture of the humeral shaft after fall while on a boat. **(B)** The oblique fracture was directly stabilized with three lag screws and a neutralization plate. **(C)** Three months later, the fracture lines are no longer visible and the fracture has healed primarily without callus formation.

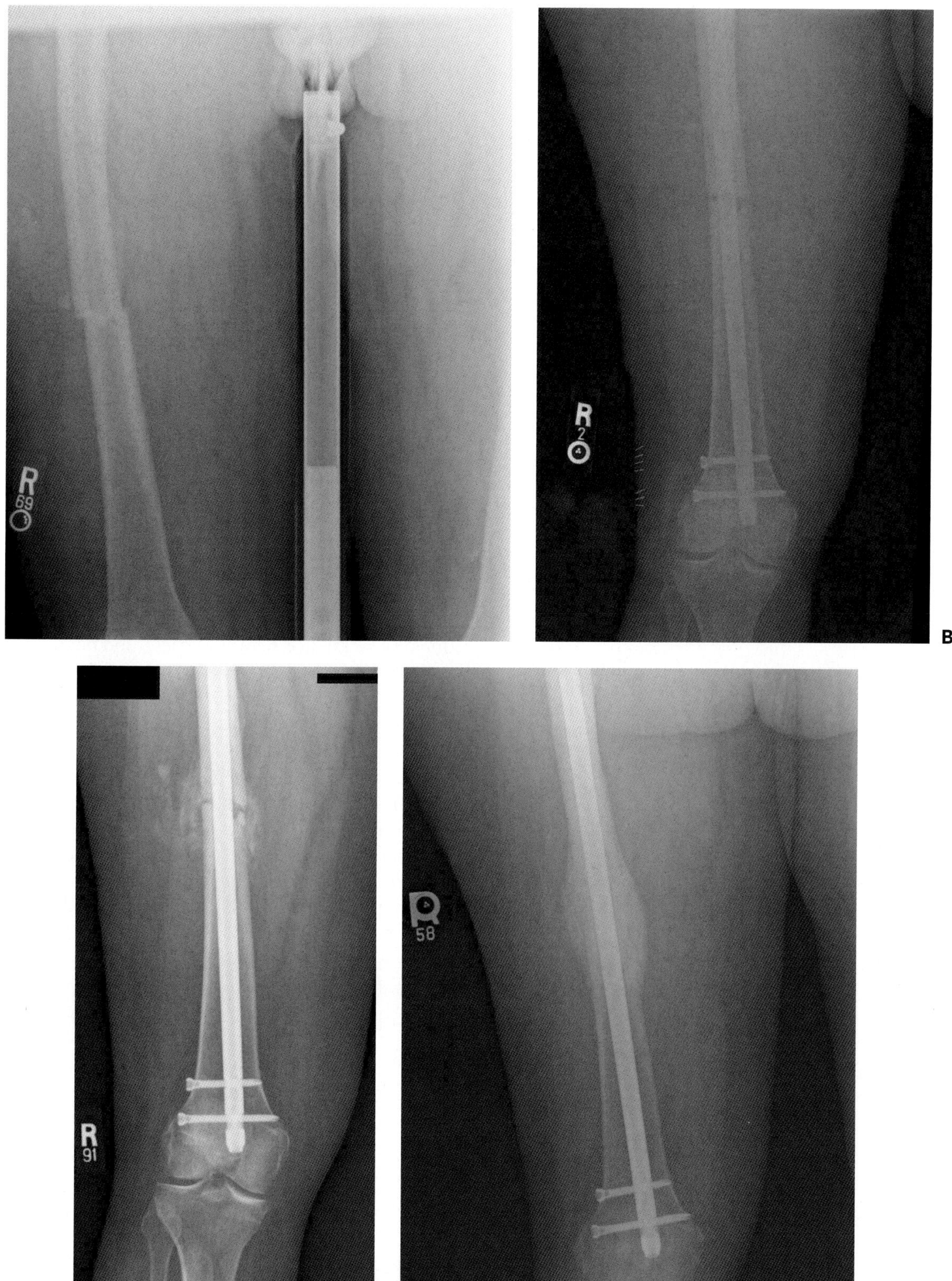

Figure 10.15 **(A)** Anteroposterior radiograph revealing a transverse mid-shaft right femoral shaft fracture after a motor vehicle collision. **(B)** The fracture has been stabilized with an intramedullary nail—a relative stability construct. **(C)** Two months after surgical fixation, the fracture shows brisk callus formation, but the fracture line is still evident. **(D)** By 6 months, the fracture has completely healed through secondary bone healing.

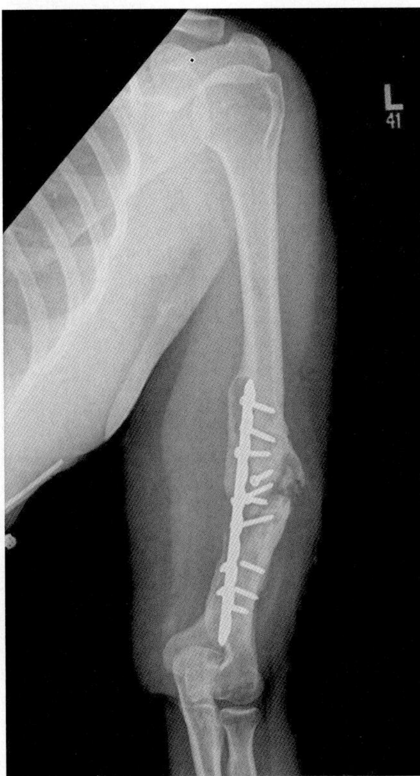

Figure 10.16 A 29 year-old female 2 years status post open reduction and internal fixation of her left distal humerus fracture. She has a nonunion due to significant motion at the fracture site due to lack of adequate stabilization. The presence of the broken hardware is likely due to the repetitive loading seen by the screws because of the excessive motion and lack of stability.

(room setup), anesthetic type, imaging, instruments, implants, and surgical tactic including multiple options for reduction and fixation strategy (Fig. 10.18).

Fracture Stabilization

Indications for fracture fixation include open fractures, articular fractures, polytrauma, encouraging patient mobilization, early joint mobilization, and correction of alignment. There are four broad categories of fixation methods to hold a fracture: (1) splinting and casting, (2) traction, (3) external fixation, and (4) internal fixation. The choice of treatment depends on many factors, including the inherent stability of the fracture. For the most part, the initial injury, particularly the amount of displacement and comminution, will determine the maximal degree of fracture instability. There are many fractures in which splinting or casting is the treatment of choice (e.g., clavicle, humerus, distal radius, and foot). In addition, most pediatric fractures can be treated successfully in a cast because of the rapid healing and remodeling potential in that patient population.

When splinting or casting a fracture, immobilization of the joints above and below the fracture site is critical. The main disadvantages of this form of stabilization are the inability to rigidly hold a reduction, joint stiffness from prolonged immobilization, and the danger of skin ulcerations at bony prominences. Traction is currently used mostly in the lower extremity, via longitudinal traction that is applied through a pin inserted either through the distal femur or through the proximal tibia. It is generally used as a temporizing measure in patients with unstable fractures who cannot tolerate an operation. The main drawbacks are suboptimal fracture fixation (with tendency for shortening and rotational malunion) and the need for prolonged immobilization (more than 6 weeks), which can lead to development of sacral ulcers, joint stiffness, and pneumonia. External fixation is indicated in fractures with segmental bone loss, associated vascular injuries, and massive soft tissue injuries with a high risk of infection (Fig. 10.19). In addition, because of the speed with which it can be applied, external fixation is also indicated in the multiply injured patient with extremity injuries and in the hemodynamically unstable patient (damage control orthopaedics). The main complications of external fixators are the risk of pin tract infection and less rigid fixation when compared with internal fixation.

The five main types of internal fixation devices are pins (such as Kirschner wires), screws (such as lag screws), plates, IM rods, and prosthetic replacements. Pins, which can be inserted percutaneously, are often used to stabilize fractures in the hand and foot and to supplement fixation elsewhere (Fig. 10.20). Lag screws, which provide compression across a fracture site, are used to fix simple transverse

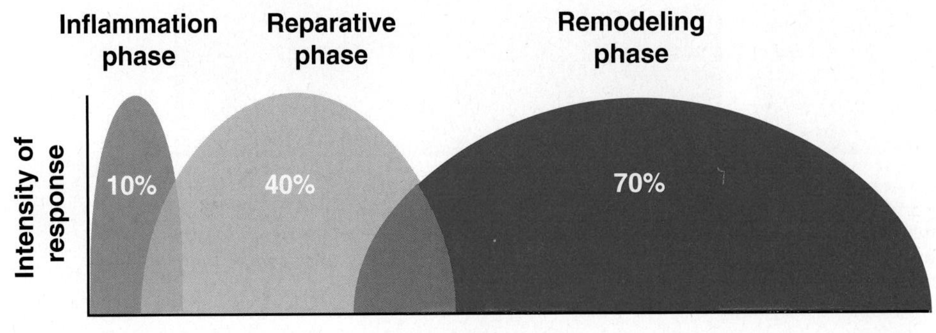

Figure 10.17 The bone healing timeline can be altered by patient factors, severity of soft tissue injury around the fracture bone, infection, and method of stabilization.

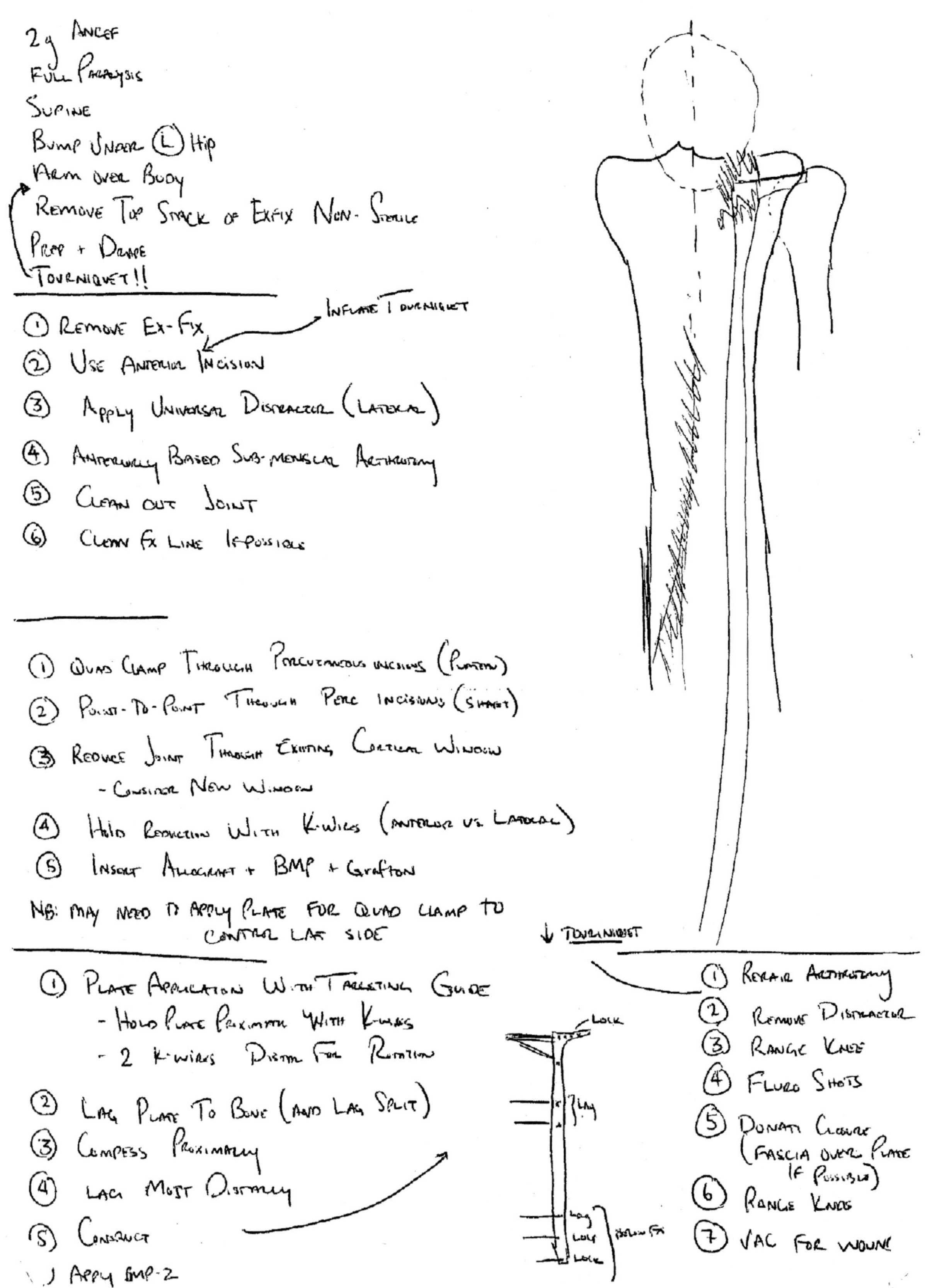

A

Figure 10.18 **(A)** Preoperative plan for a complex reconstruction of a **(B)** mal-united tibial plateau fracture. The preoperative plan is reviewed with the surgical team and posted in the operating room. (*continued*)

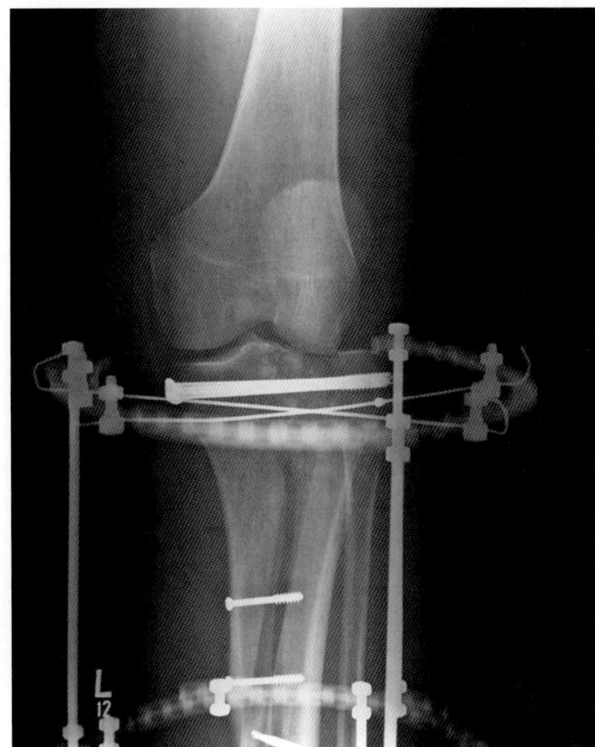

B

Figure 10.18 *(continued)*

or oblique fractures such as many femoral neck fractures (Fig. 10.21). Plates such as the dynamic compression plate and fixed-angle plates are useful in long-bone fractures and provide rigid fixation and compression across the fracture site. The IM rod is inserted from one end of a long bone down the IM canal, thus transfixing the fracture site and providing translational and angular stability. The smaller incision used to insert the IM rod avoids extensive soft tissue dissection and allows rapid healing and early return to function. Sometimes the IM canal is reamed to allow for insertion of a larger (and hence, stiffer) rod, and it is important to note that there have been reports of embolization of fat and marrow elements during IM reaming and rodding. Lastly, prosthetic replacement such as the hemiarthroplasty of the humeral and femoral head is used in situations in which comminution of the bone and cartilage is so severe that anatomic reduction cannot be restored (Fig. 10.22).

Absolute stability results in primary bone healing as there is no motion between the fracture ends and no callus formation. The prime example of an absolute stability construct is lag screw between fractured bone ends, neutralized with a plate. One the other hand, relative stability allows for callus formation with motion at the fracture site (e.g., IM nail, external fixation, bridge plating, or casting).

DIAPHYSEAL FRACTURES

The fracture pattern, the degree of soft tissue injury, and associated injuries determine the treatment of diaphyseal

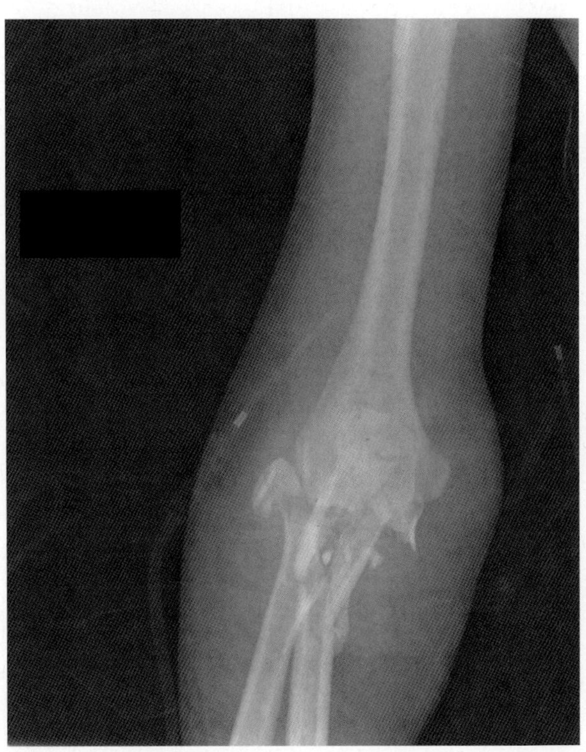
A

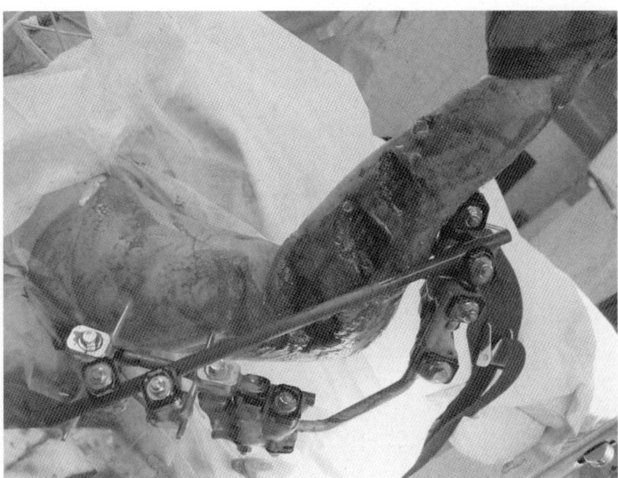
B

Figure 10.19 **(A)** An anteroposterior radiograph of an open elbow fracture in 18-year-old patient after a fall from two stories. The patient had a dislocation of the other elbow, an open femur fracture, and bilateral lung injury. He was placed into an external fixator **(B)** to stabilize his arm and prevent further injury to his soft tissue.

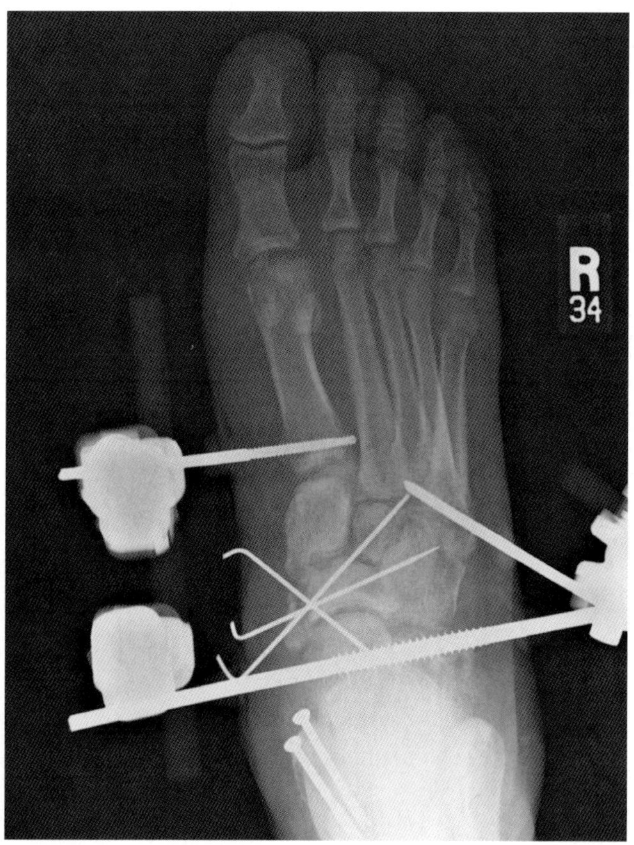

Figure 10.20 Navicular dislocation after a motor vehicle collision stabilized with multiple Kirschner wires. The entire foot was protected with an external fixator.

(long bone) fractures. The fracture location is generally described as diaphyseal, metaphyseal, or intra-articular, whereas the fracture pattern is described as transverse, oblique or spiral, simple, or comminuted. Diaphyseal fractures occur when energy imparted to the extremities cannot be dissipated in the soft tissues. Comminuted fractures are more likely with open fractures due to the higher energy required to create these injuries. The type and rate of stress loading determine the fracture pattern. Slow torque causes a spiral fracture, whereas a high-energy, direct blow causes a comminuted transverse fracture.

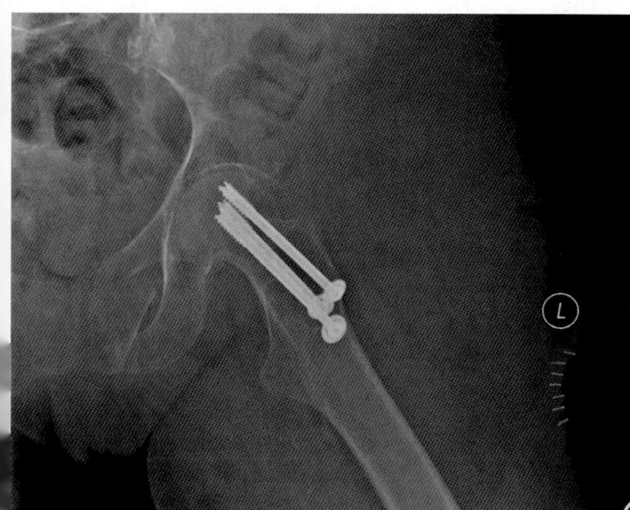

Figure 10.21 Lateral hip radiograph revealing lag screw fixation of a valgus-impacted femoral neck fracture in an elderly patient.

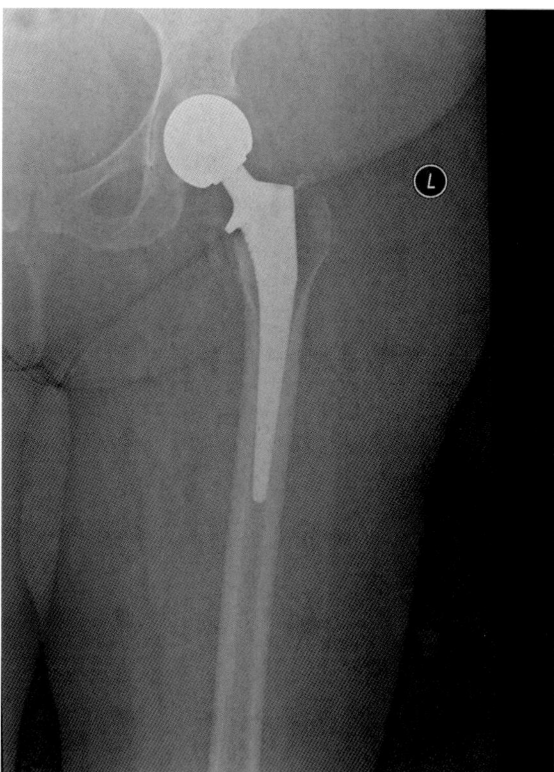

Figure 10.22 Anteroposterior radiograph of a left hip revealing a hemiarthroplasty for a displaced femoral neck fracture in an elderly patient.

Splints are used for initial immobilization because of their ease of application and ability to readily reassess the injury. Immobilization, traction, external fixation, and a variety of techniques of internal fixation are used for definitive stabilization. If casts are applied for definitive treatment, they must immobilize the joint above and below the fracture. Complications from casting include cast burns and compartment syndromes. Both complications are more likely to occur in the unconscious or insensate patient who cannot complain of pain.

Skeletal traction involves the application of longitudinal stabilization forces using a pin or wire through bone distal to the fracture site. Currently, the trend is to use skeletal traction only in the preliminary treatment of some fractures in adults until definitive stabilization may be completed. One reason for this is that prolonged skeletal traction is not conducive to early mobilization. In contrast, external fixation of diaphyseal fractures is a definitive, percutaneous stabilization technique that allows rapid stabilization of a fracture without further soft tissue injury resulting from open

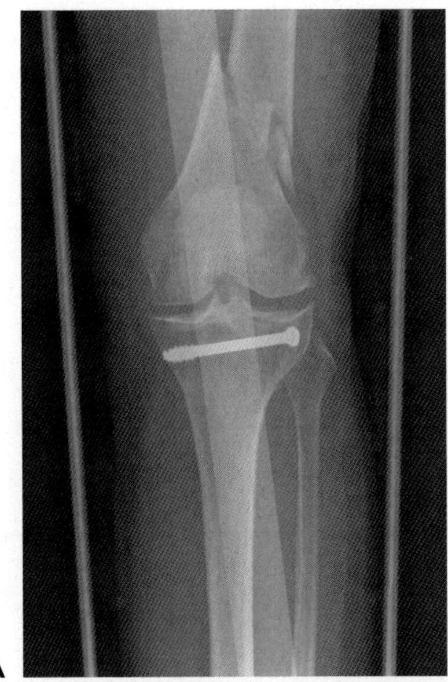

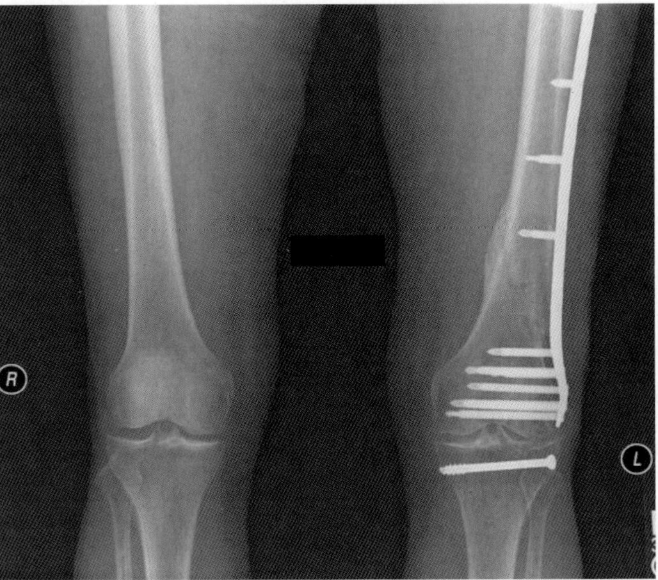

Figure 10.23 Anteroposterior view of the left femur **(A)** with an oblique distal femoral shaft fracture treated with bridge plating **(B).** Callus forms secondary to the relative stability fixation construct. If a lag screw had been placed across the fracture site to create absolute stability, the fracture would have healed without callus.

surgery. This technique also avoids the implantation of hardware at a site that is at risk for bacterial colonization and infection. Finally, external fixation facilitates wound care and patient mobilization. However, external fixation has been shown to be associated with pin tract infections and increased rates of malunion, nonunion, and delayed union.

Internal fixation has been advocated in the orthopaedically injured patient because it permits indirect reduction of the fracture, early motion of joints, and patient mobilization. The latter improves pulmonary toilet, decreasing the risk of infection, and reduces the risk of deep venous thrombosis. A disadvantage of internal fixation is the requirement for surgery, with additional tissue trauma and blood loss. Internal fixation with IM rodding may disrupt the endosteal blood supply to the bone.

Relative stability constructs are encouraged for diaphyseal fractures, which limit disruption of the periosteal blood supply. The goal of fracture fixation in diaphyseal fractures is restoration of length, alignment, and rotation. Fracture healing occurs through callus formation as a result of relative motion at the fracture site. Fracture fixation techniques promoting a relative stability construct include bridge plating (Fig. 10.23) and IM nailing.

ARTICULAR FRACTURES

Articular cartilage is composed of water (65% to 80%), proteoglycans, type II collagen, and chondrocytes, which are responsible for the resilience, elasticity, and compressive resistance of the joint surface. Articular cartilage is avascular, aneural, and sensitive to injury with limited healing potential as nutrition occurs through diffusion during motion and gentle loading.

Intra-articular fractures result in chondrocyte injury or death where collagen is broken, proteoglycan is lost, and subchondral bone is fractured. Studies have shown that there is lower proteoglycan synthesis and higher water content in areas of direct impact with possible irreversible cartilage damage occurring even after a single high-energy impact load. Cartilage and bone disruption (osteochondral fracture) results in the formation of a fibrin clot, inflammation, invasion of new cells, and production of new chondral and osseous tissue. Depending on the location and size of the lesion and the structural integrity, stability and alignment of the joint, the repair tissue may remodel and serve as a functional joint surface, or it may degenerate.

The treatment principles associated with articular fractures include anatomic reduction, absolute stability, restoration of axial alignment, and early joint range of motion (Fig. 10.24). Research has shown that nonanatomically reduced or noncompressed fractures heal with fibrocartilage only, as opposed to hyaline cartilage. In addition, improper alignment of the mechanical axis alters load transmission and accelerates joint degeneration. Early join motion increases cartilage nutrition through imbibition, improves range of motion, and maintains muscle tone. The foundation of absolute stability, which is the dictum in obtaining primary bone healing in articular fractures, is the placement of a lag screw.

PELVIC RING INJURIES

The pelvis is the supporting structure for the peritoneal contents and retroperitoneal structures. It connects the appendicular skeleton to the axial skeleton. Because the pelvis lies

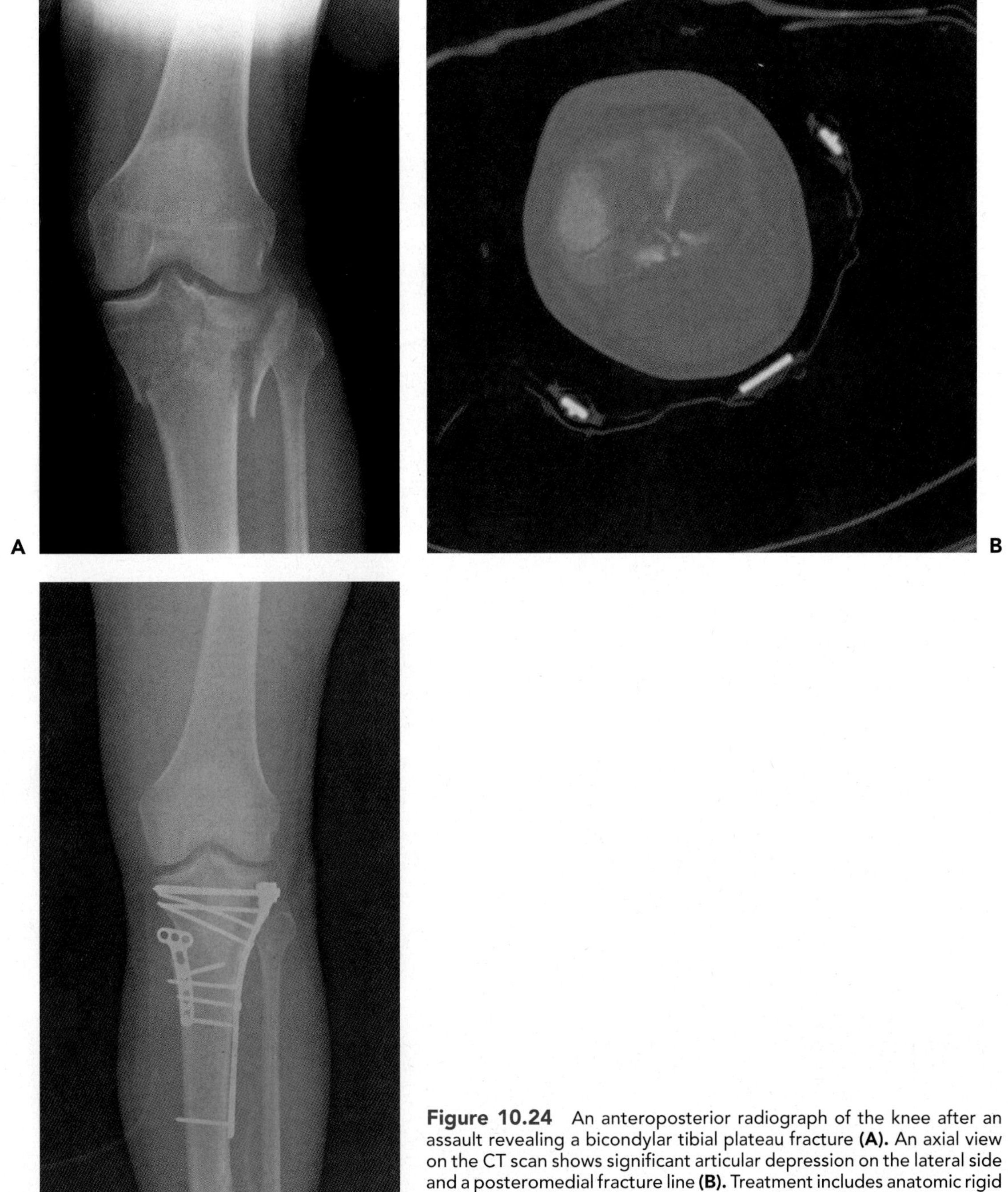

Figure 10.24 An anteroposterior radiograph of the knee after an assault revealing a bicondylar tibial plateau fracture **(A).** An axial view on the CT scan shows significant articular depression on the lateral side and a posteromedial fracture line **(B).** Treatment includes anatomic rigid surgical stabilization when the soft tissue is amenable with early range of motion and no weightbearing for 12 weeks **(C).**

in close proximity to vessels, the colon, and genitourinary structures, pelvic injuries can be associated with retroperitoneal bleeding and neurologic, bowel, and bladder injuries. The pelvis is made of three bones—two innominate bones and the sacrum—connected by a number of ligaments including the symphyseal ligament anteriorly and the posterior and anterior sacroiliac ligaments posteriorly. The sacrum and posterior ring are critical to the overall stability of the pelvic ring as the sacrum is the "keystone" to maintaining the biomechanics of ring congruity through force transmission.

Pelvic fractures may be defined as stable, rotationally unstable, or rotationally and vertically unstable. All unstable injuries involve disruption of the posterior portion of the pelvic ring. Unstable pelvic fractures result from high-energy injuries in the setting of multiple trauma and are associated with 50% mortality in the multiple trauma patient. They require rapid assessment for stabilization and triage. Mechanism of injury and history are essential, if they can be obtained from the patient. Physical examination should include a full trauma survey, including a through neurologic examination. The anterior and posterior pelvis should be inspected for open wounds. In males, the scrotal contents are palpated for testicular displacement and the penile meatus is examined for blood, which would suggest urethral injury. Rectal examination is completed for assessment of possible laceration and prostate displacement. Female patients should undergo both bimanual and speculum examinations to rule out vaginal, urethral, and bladder injury. Vaginal or rectal laceration requires specific treatment.

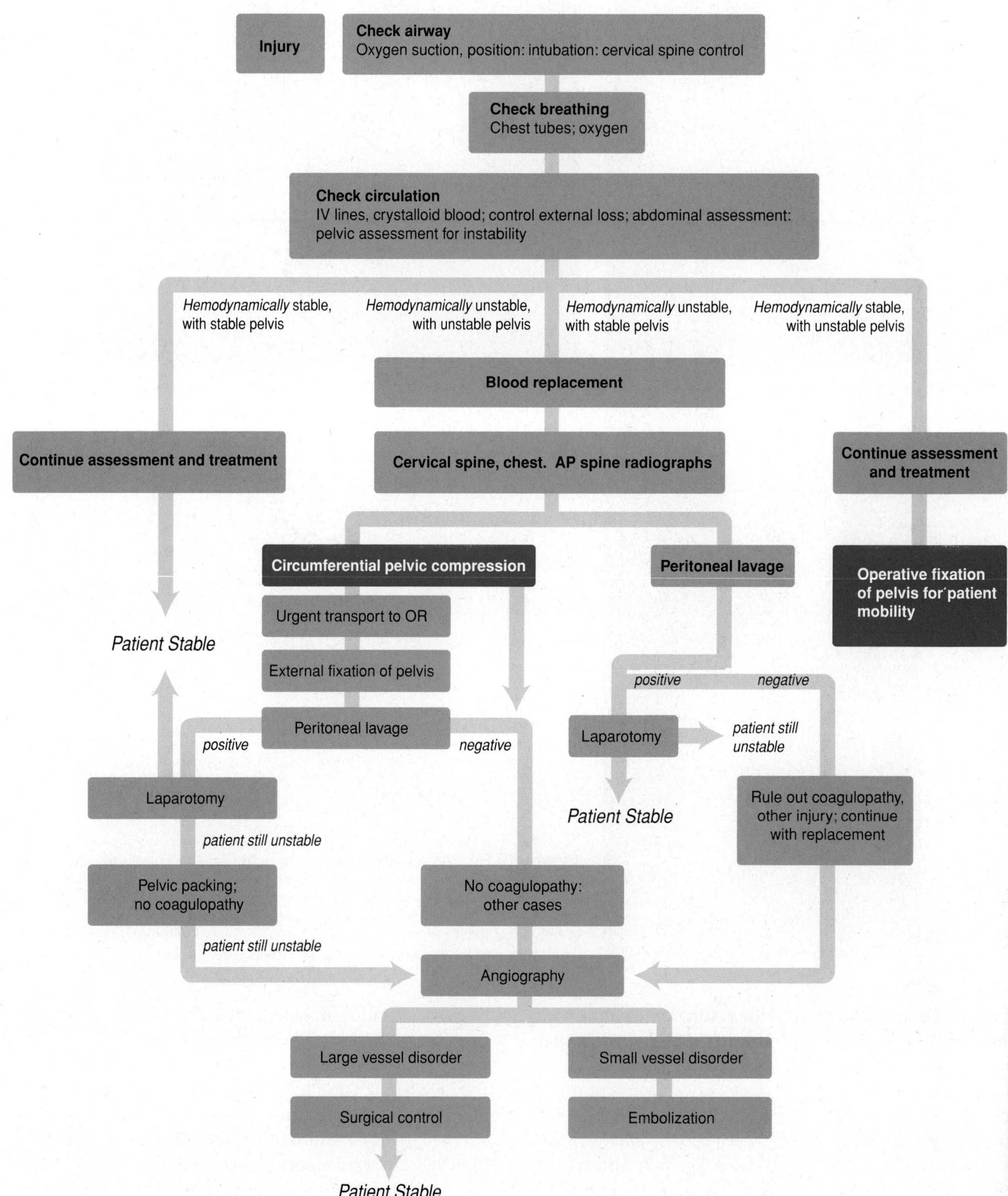

Figure 10.25 Pathway for management of pelvic ring injuries based on varying hemodynamics. AP, anteroposterior IV, intravenous; OR, operating room.

Pelvic ring injuries as a cause of hypotension (resulting in acidosis and hypothermia) in the hemodynamically unstable trauma patient require prompt diagnosis and treatment. Reducing the volume of the pelvis is often effective in tamponading pelvic bleeding, which most commonly is from a venous source (i.e., large pelvic veins). Posterior pelvic disruption can result in 3 to 4 L of blood loss and hemodynamic instability. Concomitantly, aggressive intravenous resuscitation is necessary and may require blood product administration to achieve adequate hemodynamic stability. Patients who respond to resuscitation should be optimized with respect to their hemodynamic status. Patients who do not respond to resuscitative efforts should be continually re-evaluated to avoid a missed diagnosis for the underlying hypotension. If the working diagnosis remains hypotension secondary to pelvic ring disruption, then the algorithmic approach for these patients calls for angiography of the pelvic vasculature after adequate reduction in pelvic volume. In this scenario, a "blush" or active arterial bleeding source may be identified via angiogram and embolized at the time of the study (Fig. 10.25). The most common source of arterial bleeding in the pelvis is injury to the superior gluteal artery.

Based on the fracture pattern, the acute treatment in the resuscitation bay may differ, but typically, a circumferential binder (bed sheet, commercially available wrap [e.g., T-pod]) is placed around the pelvis and greater trochanters to reduce the intrapelvic volume (Fig. 10.26). It is imperative that the commercially available binders be assessed for soft tissue pressure necrosis after 24 to 28 hours of application. Pneumatic antishock garments have been used in cases of shock with pelvic fractures, but their use remains controversial because of complications and the difficulties they present in examination and treatment of the patient.

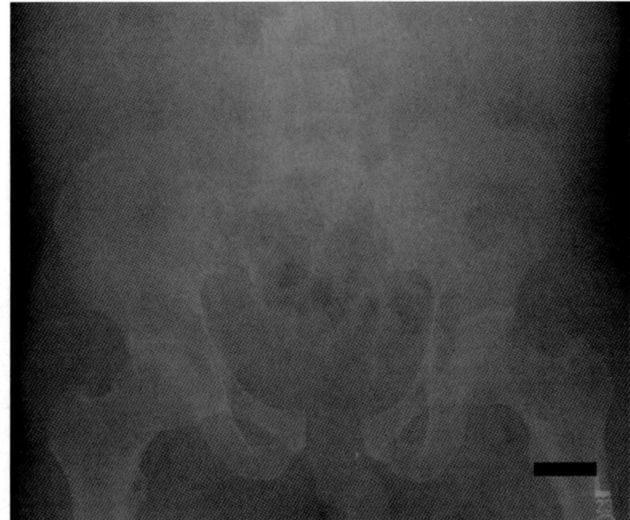

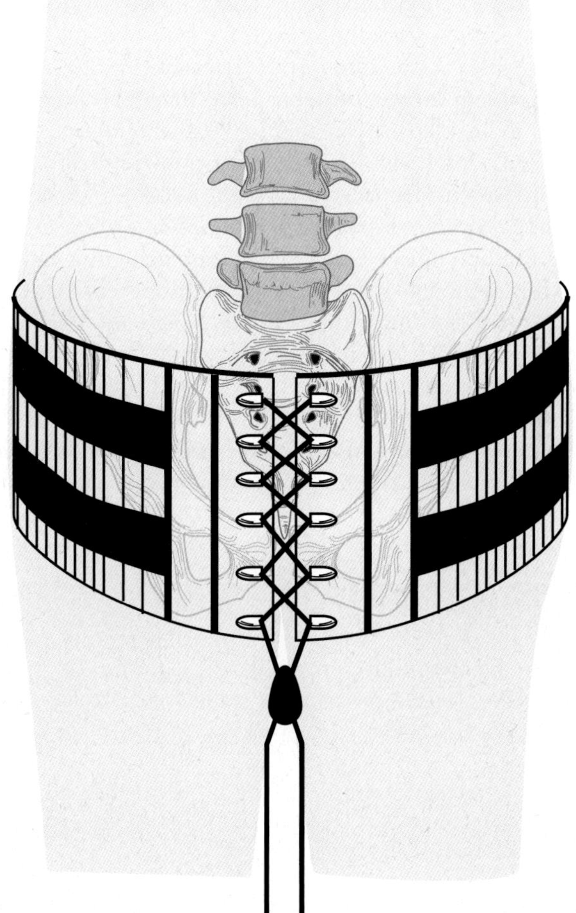

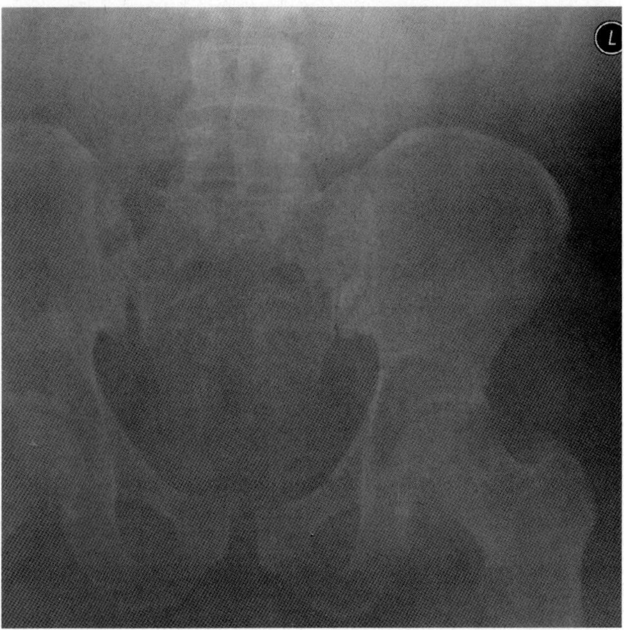

Figure 10.26 **(A)** Pelvis radiograph showing disruption of the pelvic ring including fractures of the sacrum, injury to both sacroiliac joints, and separation of the pubic symphysis. **(B)** Clinical picture of a commercially available circumferential binder stabilizing the pelvis and **(C)** reducing the intra-pelvic volume by restoring the anatomic relationship of the bones.

Complications of pneumatic antishock garments include lactic acidosis, cardiac collapse after deflation, diaphragmatic herniation, and lower extremity compartment syndrome. Another option for the extremity management of bleeding associated with pelvic fractures is percutaneous external fixation. External fixation is a temporary measure before definitive open reduction and internal fixation. If pelvic stabilization is not possible or bleeding continues despite application of external fixation, angiography and embolization are therapeutic alternatives.

Radiographic assessment includes an anteroposterior (AP) view of the pelvis, along with inlet and outlet views. Radiographic understanding the pelvic ring can be difficult as the pelvis normally sits obliquely when a person is in supine position. Further evaluation of identified fractures is obtained with pelvic CT, and a cystogram and retrograde urethrogram may also be indicated. If a bilateral posterior ring injury is identified (i.e., sacral fracture on the left and sacroiliac joint disruption on the right, bilateral sacral fractures, etc.), it is imperative that a lateral image of the pelvis be obtained to assess the sacrum for kyphotic deformity and possible cauda equina type symptoms (Fig. 10.27).

The patient with an unstable pelvic fracture is often admitted to the intensive care unit (ICU) after temporary stabilization of the pelvis. The use of a circumferential binder, although often adequate to reduce the fracture and control bleeding, does not provide extraordinary mechanical stability. Caution must be exercised in mobilizing the patient with this as the sole stabilization given the potential for resumption of bleeding with disruption of any clot. Vigilance in assessment of associated injuries should be maintained until the patient has stabilized.

Two major classification systems have been used for describing pelvic ring injuries. The tile classification is based on stability with a type A being considered stable, a type B partially stable, and type C being unstable. Young and Burgess suggested a classification system that used mechanism of injury as the basis for description of the fracture. In their schema, specific fracture patterns were present on the basis of the direction of force applied to the pelvis and included AP, lateral compression, and vertical sheer. AP injuries resulted from direct force against the anterior or posterior aspect of the pelvis and were associated with significant blood loss (Fig. 10.28A). Lateral compression injuries commonly occurred with a directed lateral blow to the pelvis as would be expected in a "T-bone" type motor vehicle collision. Lateral compression injuries have the highest associated rate of coup-countercoup head injuries due to the mechanism of injury (Fig. 10.28B). Vertical sheer fractures are an internal fracture-dislocation of the hemipelvis with the highest rates of associated neurologic injury as well as visceral injury (Fig. 10.28C).

In addition to the pelvic ring, Denis developed a classification for the sacrum to predict neurologic injury. The classification is based on the location of the fracture line relative to the sacral foramina (Fig. 10.29). Zone 1 fractures are across sacral ala and can cause L5 nerve root impingement, but only about 6% of these patients will have neurological injuries. Zone 2 fractures occur through the neuroforamina and can cause unilateral sacral anesthesia. If fracture fragments are present within the neural canal, this injury pattern requires operative debridement of the fracture fragments (usually through a posterior exposure) prior to reduction and fixation. Fractures through the sacral body are in zone 3 and are associated with the highest incidence of injury to cauda equina with the potential for neurogenic bladder. More than 50% of these patients will show neurological injuries.

Once patients are stabilized hemodynamically, they should return to the operating room for definitive care of unstable pelvic fractures. Stabilization of these fractures leads to earlier patient mobilization, minimizes the risk of pulmonary complications, decreases ventilator time, and improves morbidity and mortality. Stabilization of the anterior aspect of the pelvis includes definitive external fixation, plating of the symphysis pubis, or fixation of the rami. Posterior stabilization can be achieved through a variety of means including open reduction and internal fixation, percutaneous iliosacral screw fixation, tension band plating, transiliac compression rods, and in the case of spondylopelvic dissociation (bilateral sacral fractures) with lumbo-pelvic fixation (Fig. 10.30).

After stabilization of fractures, one should aggressively mobilize the patient as much as possible given the stability of the pelvic reconstruction. Large forces occur across the pelvis because it serves as a platform for transmitting the lower extremity forces to the torso. Often patients with pelvic fracture are unable to ambulate immediately. This is not only because of the severe nature of these injuries, but also because of the associated injuries. Mobilization starts with range of motion exercise to the extremities as soon as possible after injury. This is followed with upright sitting

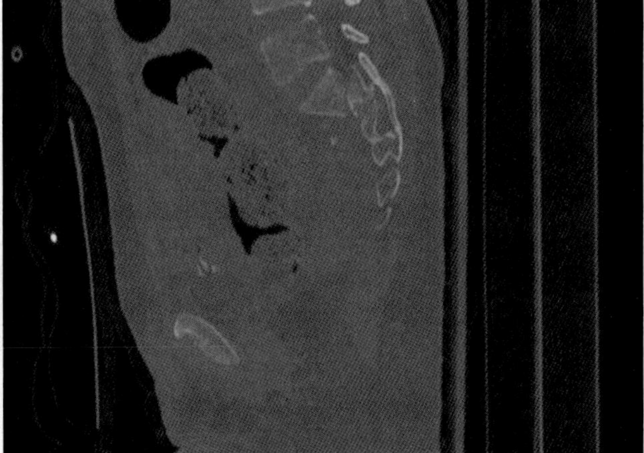

Figure 10.27 Sagittal reconstruction view of the posterior pelvic ring revealing severe kyphotic deformity of the sacrum after a three-story fall. The patient had fracture through the left and right sides of the sacrum connected in the middle—spondylopelvic dissociation. The physical examination findings included bilateral lower extremity numbness with no bowel or bladder function.

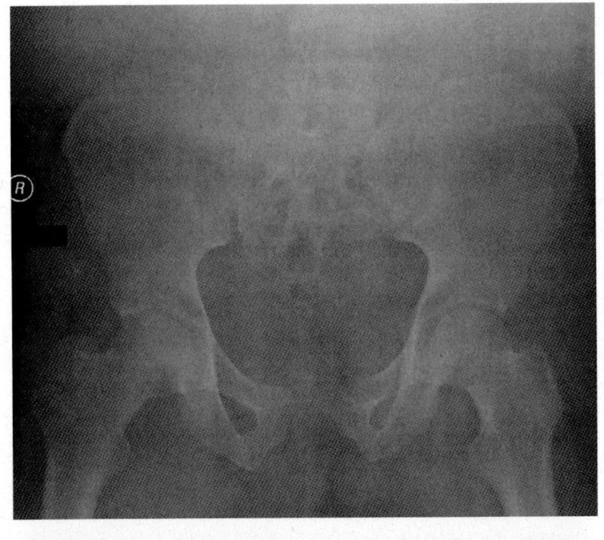

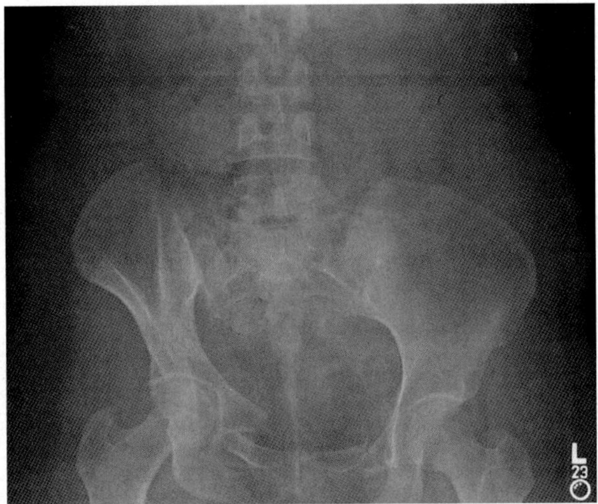

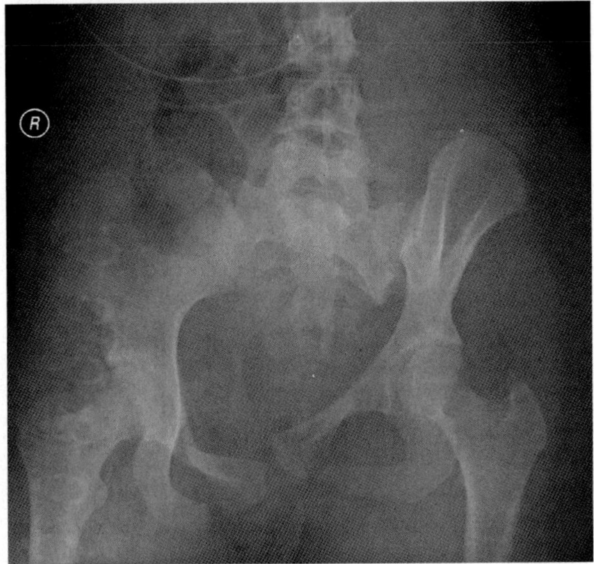

Figure 10.28 **(A)** Anteroposterior (AP) pelvis of a 32-year-old male involved in a head-on motor vehicle collision resulting in an AP compression type pelvic ring injury with symphyseal disruption and bilateral sacroiliac joint injury. **(B)** Lateral compression pelvic ring injury in a 41-year-old female struck by a motor vehicle. The entire right hemipelvis is internally rotated. **(C)** Vertical sheer pelvic ring injury on the left secondary to being thrown by a horse in a 17-year-old female.

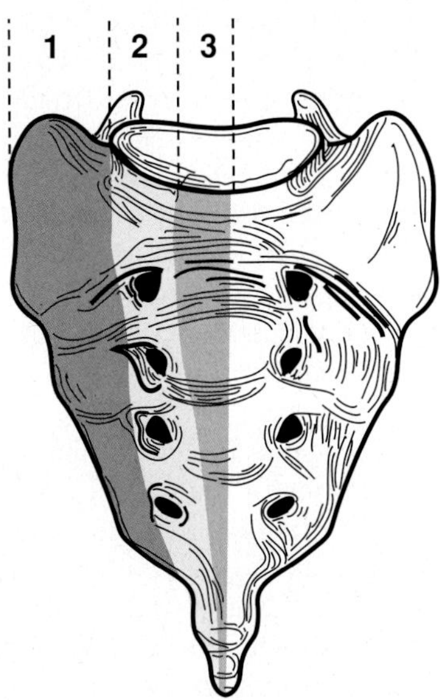

Figure 10.29 Denis classification of sacral fractures based on the position of the fracture line relative to the sacral tunnels.

and transfer to a chair. Ambulation is advanced depending on the pelvic stability and other injuries.

After pelvic stabilization, the patient is subject to normal orthopedic postoperative complications directly related to treatment, such as infection (5% to 50% based on operative procedure), loss of fixation, malunion, and nonunion (10% to 15%). In addition, there are more severe complications specific to these injuries, which include neurologic impairment, pulmonary embolism, and sepsis. Neurologic deterioration occurs in 2% to 5% of pelvic fractures. It is most frequently due to nerve root traction or avulsion. Therapeutically, the patients are initially treated with observation. Electrodiagnostic studies (electromyography and nerve conduction testing) are typically considered at approximately 4 weeks after injury to help determine the long-term treatment plan. Residual pain despite fixation can be as high as 30%. Pelvic trauma predisposes the patient to deep venous thrombosis, and prophylaxis for pulmonary embolism must be administered. However, because anticoagulants must be used with caution in the

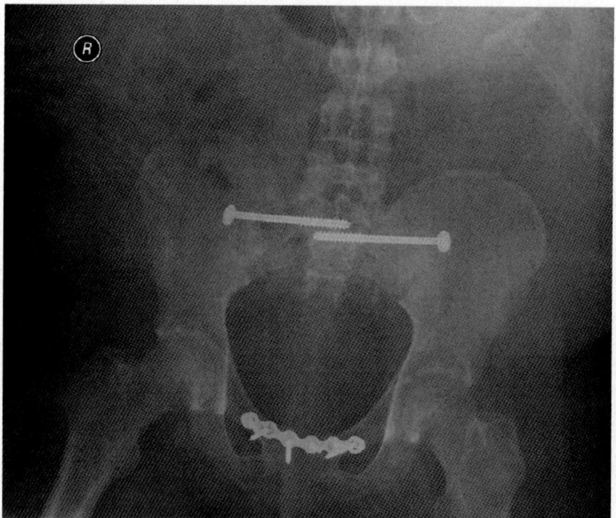

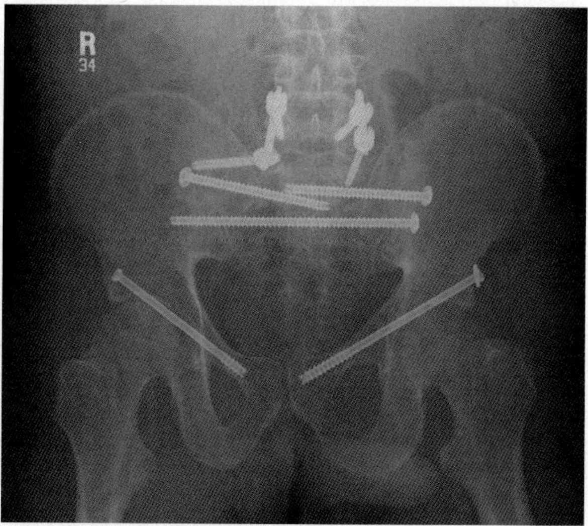

Figure 10.30 **(A)** Anteroposterior (AP) pelvis radiograph after fixation of a type C or AP compression type pelvic ring injury with open reduction and internal fixation of the pubic symphysis and percutaneous iliosacral screw lag fixation of the posterior ring. **(B)** Percutaneous fixation of the pelvic ring anteriorly and posteriorly after a fall from 50 feet. In addition, the patient had lumbopelvic stabilization due to multiple fractures through the sacrum.

setting of severe retroperitoneal bleeding, a vena cava filter is often placed angiographically to prevent pulmonary embolism.

Open Pelvic Fractures

Open pelvic injuries are associated with high-energy trauma and have higher morality rates than do closed injuries. Initially, these open injuries are life threatening because of bleeding, but later they become potential sources of deep-seated infection. Greater risk for infection is associated with disruption of the bladder and urethra as well as rectal and vaginal lacerations. Urologic injuries are generally treated with urinary diversion and rectal lacerations with a diverting colostomy, whereas vaginal injuries are treated in an open procedure. These measures, along with antibiotic therapy and surgical debridement, can decrease the risk of deep abscess, osteomyelitis, and sepsis.

ACETABULAR FRACTURES

After emergent resuscitation of the trauma patient who potentially has an acetabular fracture, assessment includes a careful physical examination and review of relevant radiographs. A physical examination focusing on the acetabular injury should include a well-documented, complete neurologic assessment of the pelvis and lower extremity, evaluation of the soft tissues in the trochanteric and gluteal regions, and the resting position of the leg. Because the sciatic nerve is damaged in as many as 20% of acetabular fractures that involve the posterior wall or column, the motor and sensory function of the extremity must be carefully documented. In particular, because the peroneal division is most at risk, foot dorsiflexion and eversion must be tested.

Closed soft tissue injuries may occur about the hip region, especially over the trochanter. A closed degloving injury is referred to as a "Morel-Lavallee lesion." The serosanguineous fluid collections that develop in these cavities are culture-positive in as many as 31% of cases. If this injury pattern is discovered, irrigation and debridement of these areas should be performed, and internal fixation should be delayed until the area is clean.

Plain-radiographic assessment of a patient with an acetabular injury begins with the five standard views of the pelvis: AP, iliac oblique, obturator oblique, inlet, and outlet (Fig. 10.31). These views will delineate associated pelvic fractures, femoral head injury, and hip dislocations. The standard AP radiograph is usually sufficient for recognition and classification of an acetabular fracture. However, the 45-degree oblique (Judet) views are needed to fully characterize the fracture and to determine whether there is subluxation of the hip joint, which may not be visible on the AP view. The obturator oblique view is taken with the affected side of the patient rotated 45 degrees forward. This allows clear visualization of the anterior column in the region of the hip, the posterior wall, and any posterior subluxation of the hip. The iliac oblique view is taken with the unaffected side of the patient rolled 45 degrees forward. This view profiles the posterior column from the notch to the ischium and the anterior wall, which is curvilinear and shallower than the posterior wall. The inlet and outlet pelvic radiographs may depict pelvic injuries that would affect the management of the acetabular fracture. Occasionally, anterior sacroiliac joint widening is present

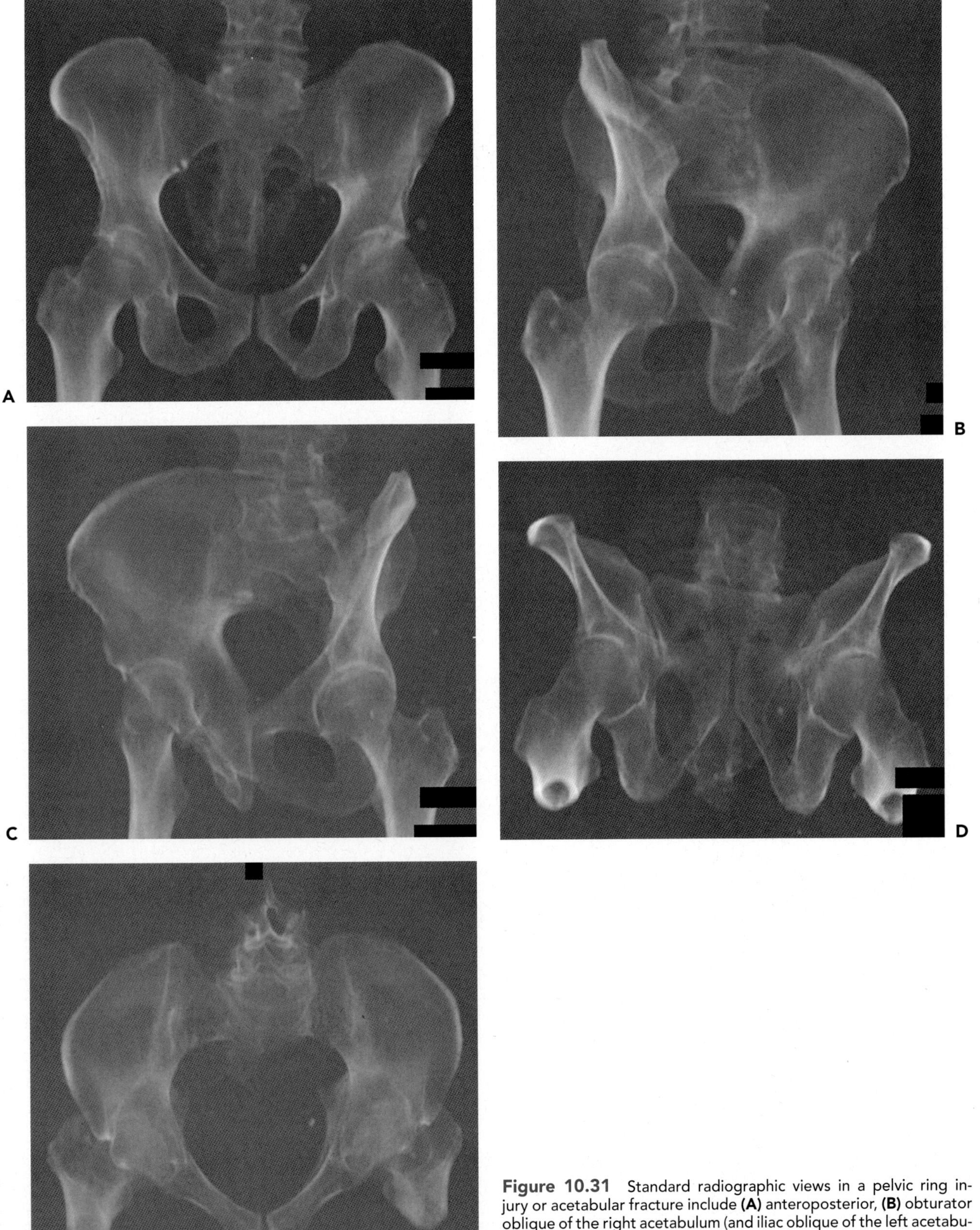

Figure 10.31 Standard radiographic views in a pelvic ring injury or acetabular fracture include **(A)** anteroposterior, **(B)** obturator oblique of the right acetabulum (and iliac oblique of the left acetabulum), **(C)** iliac oblique of the right acetabulum (and obturator oblique of the left acetabulum), **(D)** inlet, and **(E)** outlet.

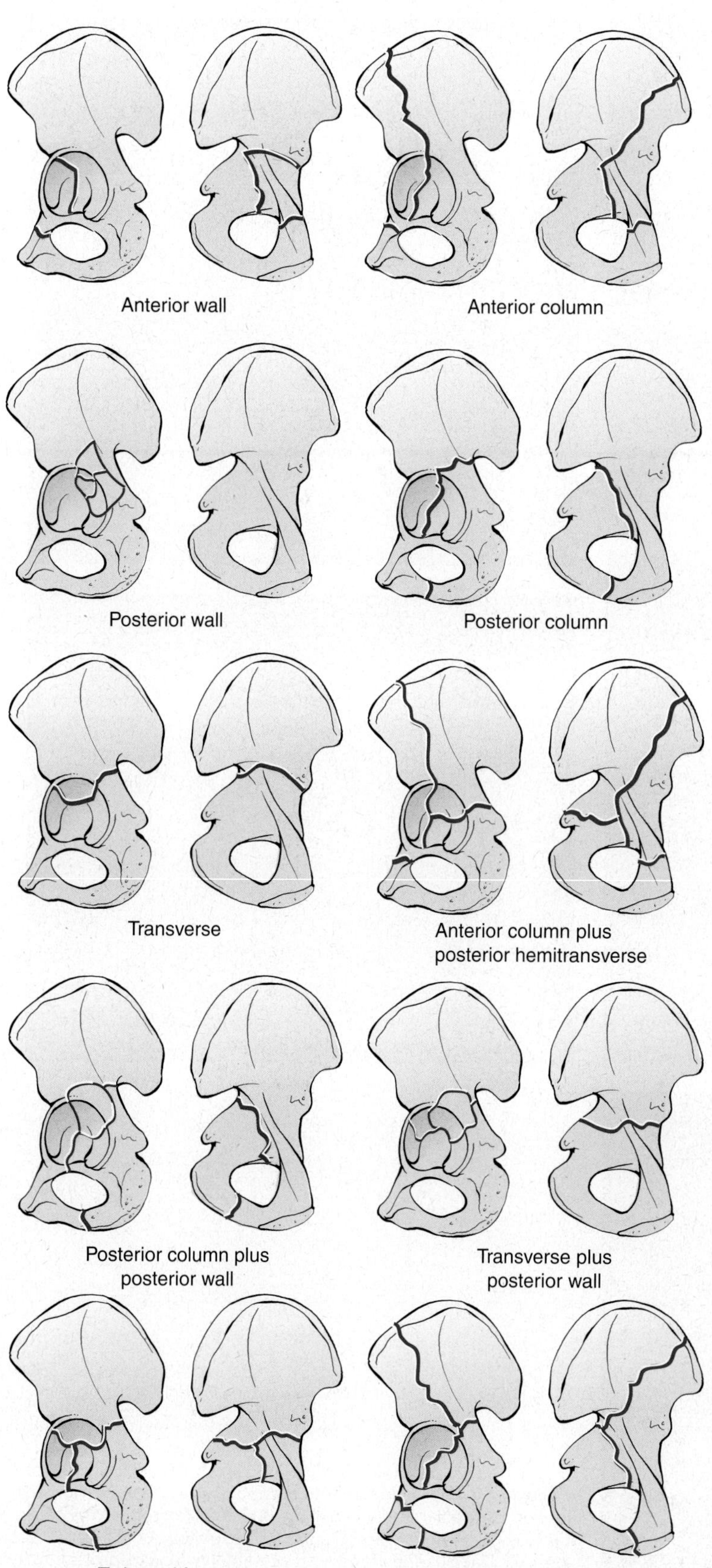

Figure 10.32 Letournel acetabular fracture classification. (*Reprinted with permission from* Bucholz RW, Heckman JD, Court-Brown C, et al. *Rockwood and Green's Fractures in Adults.* 7th ed. Philadelphia, PA: Lippincott Williams & Wilkins, 2010.)

with transverse and both-column acetabular fractures and this may be difficult to appreciate on the standard AP view.

A computed tomographic study with fine cuts (1.5 or 2 mm) through the affected area of the acetabulum allows more precise definition of the fracture than is possible with plain radiography. Two-dimensional and three-dimensional reconstructions of the fracture often help in understanding the rotational deformities of displaced fractures but are not necessary for decision making or operative planning. The information commonly available from the standard radiographic series allows classification of the fracture and definition of many associated variables affecting outcome.

The classification of acetabular fractures was standardized by Letournel (Fig. 10.32). He described five elementary and five associated fracture patterns. The five elementary fractures have a single fracture line through the acetabulum: posterior wall, posterior column, anterior wall, anterior column, and transverse (through both the posterior and anterior columns). The five associated patterns involve multiple fracture lines: posterior wall + posterior column, transverse + posterior wall, anterior column + posterior hemitransverse, T-type, and associated both column. The associated both column is a unique fracture pattern, which is different than the others within the Letournel classification system because the associated both column has no single piece of articular surface attached to the pelvis; that is, the entire acetabulum is dissociated from the stable pelvis (Fig. 10.33). The various fracture patterns have relevance to treatment alternatives and prognosis.

Indications for nonoperative management of acetabular fractures includes an intact superior acetabular dome, based on the three standard roof arc measurements (which should be greater than 45 degrees), or fractures, which show congruency. Location of the fracture lines will also portend nonoperative treatment if the fracture line does not involve the weight bearing done or only the pubic portion of the anterior column. Surgeons advocate early touch

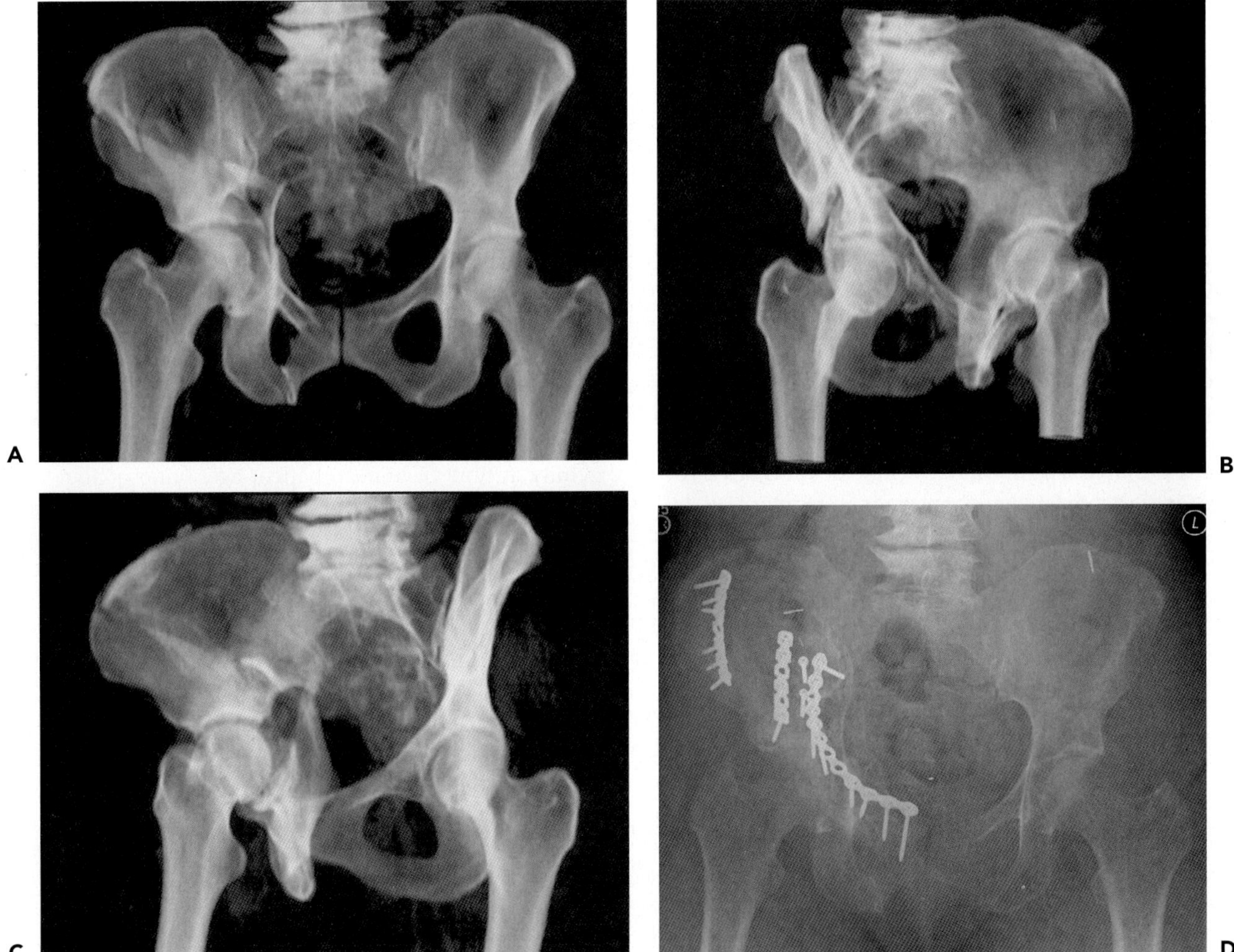

Figure 10.33 **(A)** Anteroposterior (AP), **(B)** obturator oblique, and **(C)** iliac oblique of a both column acetabular fracture showing no portion of the articular surface attached to the stable pelvis. The patient was initially placed into skeletal traction and then had an open reduction and internal fixation **(D)** performed through a Stoppa exposure with a lateral window.

TABLE 10.3
SURGICAL EXPOSURES FOR ACETABULAR FIXATION

Surgical Exposure	General Indications	Fracture Patterns	Complications
Kocher Langenbeck	Posterior column and posterior articular surface	Posterior wall Posterior column Transverse Transverse with posterior wall Some T-shaped fractures	HO: 8%–25% Sciatic nerve palsy: 3%–5% Infection: 2%–5%
Ilioinguinal	Anterior column and anterior articular surface	Anterior wall Anterior column Transverse with Anterior displacement Anterior column/posterior hemitransverse Associated both column	Lateral femoral cutaneous nerve dysesthesia (80%–90% returns by 1 year) HO: 2%–10% Femoral nerve palsy: 2% Infection: 2%–5%
Extended iliofemoral	Maximal simultaneous access to both columns	Transtectal transverse/posterior wall T-shaped fractures Greater than 21 days following injury Inability to reduce posterior column through ilioinguinal Associated SI joint disruption	Infection: 2%–5% Sciatic nerve palsy: 3%–5% HO: 20%–50%

down mobilization for a minimally displaced acetabular fracture, as long as there is close radiographic follow up.

Surgical management of acetabular fractures is technically demanding and has many potential complications. The goal of surgery is to accurately restore the anatomic configuration of the joint surface, as well as congruence and stability of the hip joint, while avoiding complications. The results after surgery correlate most closely with the quality of the reduction. Indications for open reduction and internal fixation of acetabular fractures include articular displacement of more than 2 mm or persistent displacement following closed reduction, a nonconcentric reduction after dislocation of the hip out of traction (on any radiographic view), any intra-articular loose bodies associated, an unstable fracture of posterior acetabular wall, lack of parallelism between the femoral head and acetabular roof, medial femoral head subluxation, or instability out of traction after closed reduction. After surgical stabilization, early postoperative mobilization with range of motion and touch-down weight bearing is encouraged.

Factors that are predictive of outcome include injury to cartilage or bone of femoral head, anatomic reduction, and age of patient. In treating acetabular fractures, a singe surgical exposure is preferred (see Table 10.3). Of note, the surgical windows in the ilioinguinal exposure are lateral, middle, and medial. The lateral window allows access to the internal iliac fossa, the sacroiliac joint, and the upper one-third of the pelvic brim. The middle window accesses the quadrilateral surface, the anterior rim, and the pelvic brim from the sacroiliac joint to the pectineal eminence. The medial window accesses the superior pubic ramus and the symphysis pubis. More recently, authors have advocated the use of the modified Stoppa exposure (Pfannenstiel incision allowing intrapelvic access to the sacroiliac joints posteriorly) in conjunction with the lateral window of an ilioinguinal exposure in lieu of the ilioinguinal approach.

Posterior Wall Fractures

Posterior wall fractures are the most common type of acetabular fractures and comprise approximately 50% of all acetabular fractures (associated and elementary patterns) in most published series. The amount of injury to the posterior wall will typically be dictated by such factors as mechanism of injury, position of the femoral head within the acetabulum at the time of injury, position of the lower extremity at time of impact, patient age, bone quality, and energy imparted. Posterior wall fractures are sometimes colloquially referred to as "dashboard injuries." Posterior wall fractures are associated with posterior dislocations of the hip joint between 40% and 70% of the time in various series (Fig. 10.34). An isolated posterior wall fracture can be classified as an "elementary" fracture pattern in the Judet-Letournel classification of acetabular fractures. Posterior wall fractures can also occur as a part of more complex fracture patterns, so when a posterior wall fracture is detected, the entire pelvic ring should be assessed. The posterior wall can be best visualized on an obturator oblique radiograph of the pelvis (Fig. 10.35). An isolated femoral head dislocation without an associated fracture of the posterior wall is a rare occurrence (10% in the highest series). More often, dislocation of the femoral head results in a fracture of the posterior wall (tension-type failure). If radiographs reveal a fracture-dislocation of the femoral head with an associated posterior wall fracture, then an immediate attempt at a closed reduction is warranted (Fig. 10.36). Posttraumatic

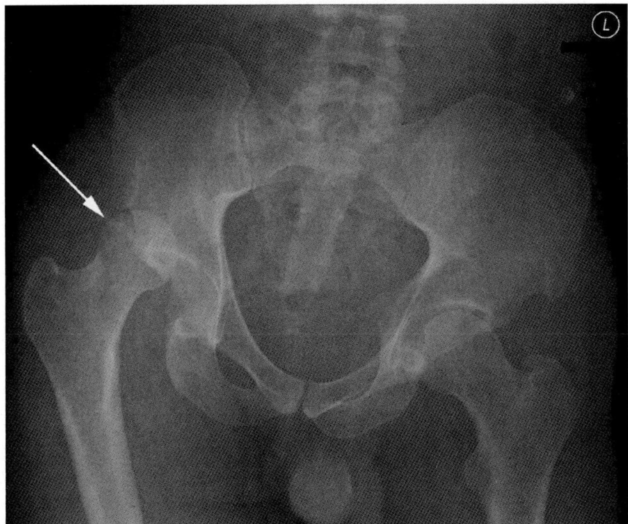

Figure 10.34 Anteroposterior (AP) pelvis of a 19 year-old male involved in a motor vehicle collision while riding his bicycle. The right hip is posteriorly dislocated and the posterior wall fragment is displaced (*arrow*).

injury to the sciatic nerve can occur up to 30% of the time with a posterior wall fracture-dislocation. Treatment involves open reduction and internal fixation of the unstable posterior wall component (Fig. 10.37).

TRAUMATIC AMPUTATION

Traumatic amputation is defined as a loss of a digit(s) or limb due to a traumatic injury. Technical advances in microvascular surgery have made replantation a common treatment of upper extremity traumatic amputations, and

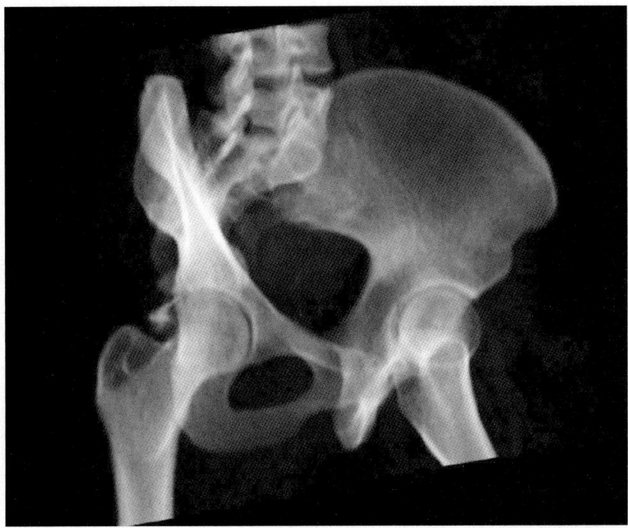

Figure 10.35 Obturator oblique of the right acetabulum in a 32-year-old female after a motor vehicle collision postreduction revealing a posterior wall fracture.

surgical success of these procedures continues to be enhanced with modern techniques. Similar injury patterns for the lower extremity often do not result in replantation due to the excellent outcomes with prosthetic use following below the knee amputation.

The most important factor determining whether a digit or limb can be replanted is the ischemia time, warm or cold. Warm ischemia time is the time the extremity distal to the injury site has been without blood flow with a normal temperature and metabolic rate. Cold ischemia time is defined as the time the extremity distal to the injury site has been without blood flow with a reduced metabolic rate due to lowering the temperature of the tissues. A patient with a traumatic amputation should have the amputated limb wrapped in moist gauze and placed in a bag, which is subsequently placed on ice to reduce the metabolic rate. If the amputated limb is placed directly on ice, there is an increased risk for frost bite as well as severe skin maceration, potentially rendering the limb useless for replantation. In general, warm ischemia time should be less than 6 hours and cold ischemia time should be less than 12 hours. Smaller limbs, such as a digit, may still be viable at 12 and 24 hours of warm and cold ischemia time, respectively.

The general sequence of replantation commences with bony fixation, extensor tendon and flexor tendon repair, arterial repair, nerve repair, and lastly venous repair. Immediate postoperative care requires elevating the replanted limb, elevating the temperature of the room environment, and avoidance of nicotine and caffeine, which may cause arterial constriction. In the event of significant venous congestion, leeches may be placed on the limb to relieve congestion via the secretion of the anticoagulant hirudin. Compromise of the arterial inflow to the limb warrants re-exploration within 48 hours following replantation. The use of aspirin, dipyridamole (Persantine), low-molecular-weight dextran, heparin, and sympathetic blockade may also minimize the risk for arterial thrombosis and spasm.

Determining the viability of a limb for salvage is an extremely daunting task. The decision to acutely amputate a limb should be grounded on as much clinical data as possible, should be life saving, and should only happen with documentation from two services (e.g., orthopaedic surgery and general surgery, or orthopaedic surgery and vascular surgery, etc.) detailing the need for the acute amputation. In addition, photographs of the limb should be recorded in the medical record (Fig. 10.38).

Scoring systems have been developed to help assist with determining the viability of limb salvage versus limb amputation. The most common scoring system used is the Mangled Extremity Severity Score (MESS) (Table 10.4). Earlier studies showed that an MESS score of greater than or equal to 7 had a 100% predictable value for amputation. This relatively simple, readily available scoring system of objective criteria was highly accurate in discriminating between limbs that were salvageable and those that were unsalvageable

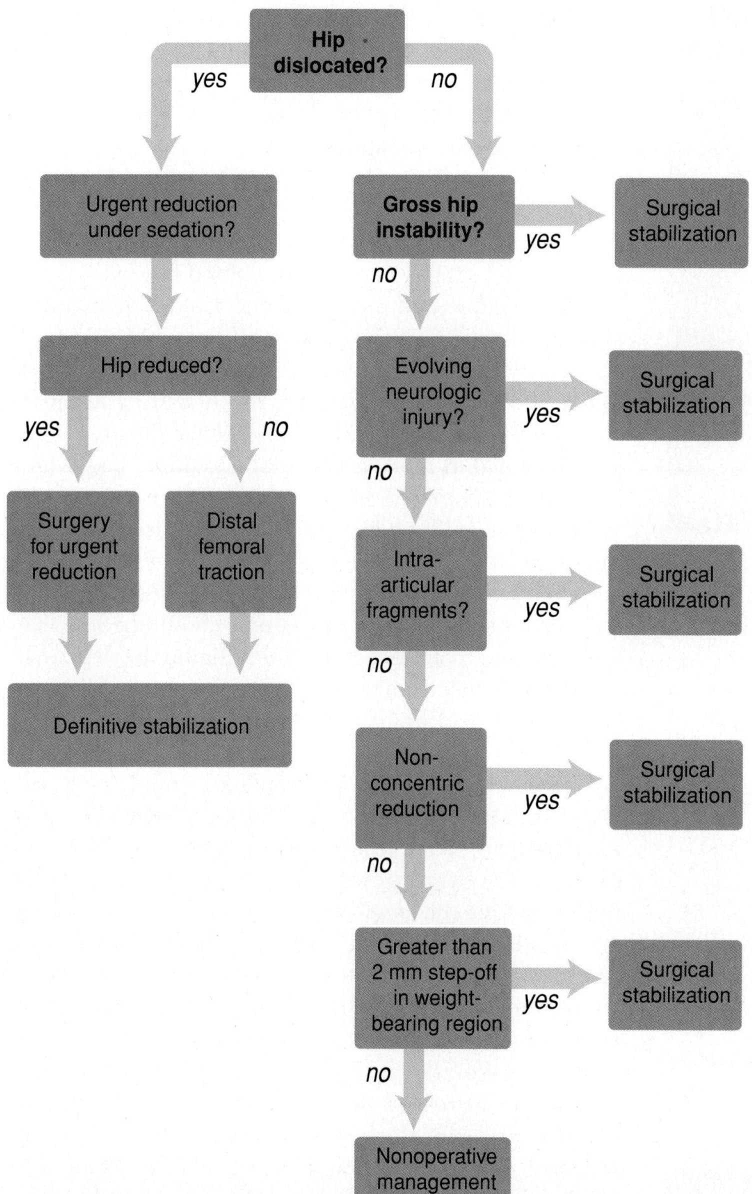

Figure 10.36 Management of posterior wall fracture-dislocations.

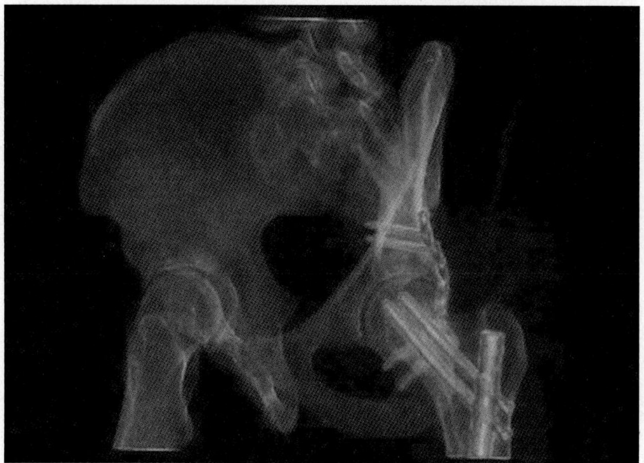

Figure 10.37 Obturator oblique of the left acetabulum after posterior wall fixation using a buttress plating technique to provide absolute stability and direct compression at the fracture site.

and better managed by primary amputation in these underpowered studies. More recent data from the multicenter, prospective Lower Extremity Assessment Program (LEAP) study have shown limited utility of scoring systems in outcomes of either limb salvage or limb amputation. The clinical utility of five lower extremity injury-severity scoring systems was also assessed in the LEAP study. Scoring systems for lower-extremity traumatic injuries designed to assist in the decision-making process were used to evaluate 546 patients—407 limbs remained in the salvage pathway 6 months after the injury. The analysis did not validate the clinical utility of any of the lower-extremity injury-severity scores. However, a high specificity of the scores in all of the patient subgroups did confirm that low scores could be used to predict limb-salvage potential. Yet, the converse was not true—low sensitivity of the indices failed to support the validity of the scores as predictors of

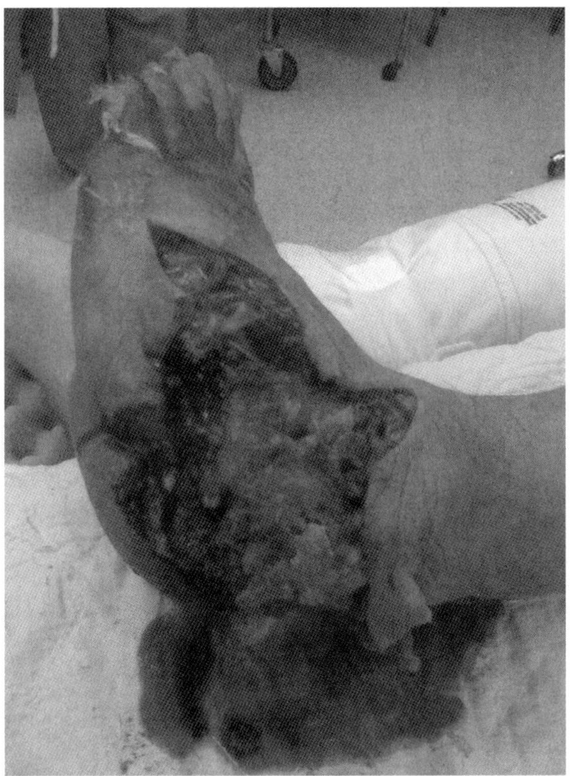

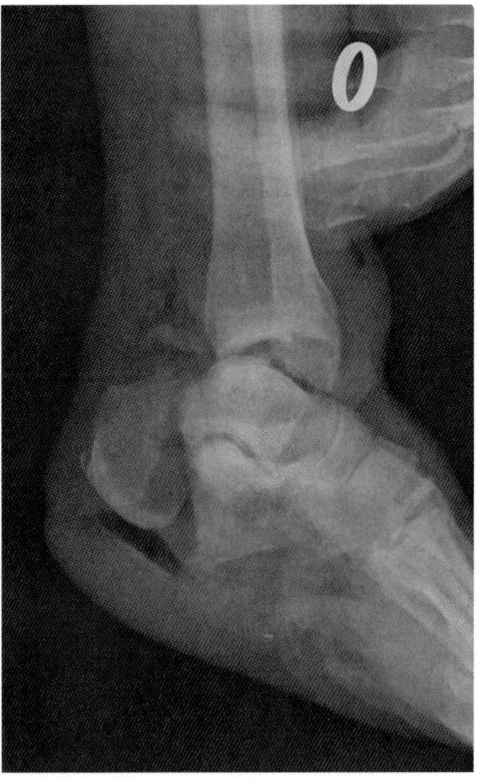

Figure 10.38 **(A)** A 48-year-old male with a crush injury to the left foot with significant soft tissue defect, contamination, and calcaneal bone loss **(B)**. Reconstruction options for this limb from a soft tissue and bone standpoint were limited and the patient elected to have a transtibial amputation. He returned to work 8 weeks after his surgery.

amputation. In addition, the data from this study revealed that lack of initial plantar sensation on presentation after lower extremity trauma is not predictive of ultimate return of nerve function or clinical outcome. More than one-half of the patients who presented with an insensate foot that was treated with limb reconstruction ultimately regained sensation at 2 years. Initial plantar sensation was not prognostic of long-term plantar sensory status or functional outcomes and should not be a component of a limb-salvage decision algorithm.

TABLE 10.4
MANGLED EXTREMITY SEVERITY SCORE

Criteria	Description	Points
Skeletal/soft tissue injury	Low energy (stab; simple fracture; pistol gunshot wound)	1
	Medium energy (open or multiple fractures, dislocation)	2
	High energy (high speed MVC or rifle GSI):	3
	Very high energy (high speed trauma + gross contamination):	4
Limb ischemia*	Pulse reduced or absent but perfusion normal	1
	Pulseless; paresthesias, diminished capillary refill	2
	Cool, paralyzed, insensate, numb	3
Shock	Systolic BP always >90 mmHg	0
	Hypotensive transiently	1
	Persistent hypotension	2
Age (years)	<30	0
	30–50	1
	>50	2

*Score doubled for ischemia >6 hours.
MVC, motor vehicle collision; GSI, gunshot injury.

COMPLICATIONS ASSOCIATED WITH ORTHOPAEDIC TRAUMA

Malunions

Although the majority of fractures go on to union, they may heal in an unacceptable position that causes significant impairment. There is no generic definition of a malunion. Historically, each bone has been labeled "healed" within certain parameters. For example, acceptable healing after a tibia fracture is more than 50% of cortical overlap, less than 10 degrees of angulation in any plane, less than 5 degrees of varus or valgus deformity, less than 10 degrees of anterior or posterior angulation, less than 10 degrees of rotation, and less than 1 cm of shortening. These parameters are not the same for humeral shaft fractures. Thus, simply because a bone has healed in a nonanatomic position does not necessarily mean the fracture is malunited.

In malunion, the bone may be angulated, may be rotated on itself, or the fractured ends may be overlapped causing shortening. Malunion may be caused by inadequate immobilization of the fracture, misalignment at the time of immobilization, premature removal of the cast or other immobilizer, or incomplete or limited surgical fixation. A malunited fracture can lead to impairment, disability, degenerative joint disease due to altered biomechanics, and referred pain (Fig. 10.39).

Clinically, malunions are fractures that have healed in a manner that leads to either functional and/or cosmetic deformity. Management of malunions, particularly with deformity correction, should result in functional improvement. A malunited articular injury (i.e., an articular fracture with step-off) can lead to early posttraumatic arthritis particularly with weightbearing and range of motion.

Nonunions

Despite meticulous care and the best of intentions, fractures may not heal. A nonunion is defined by the Food and Drug Administration as a fracture that has not healed 9 months after occurring, or a fracture that does not show progression of healing in three consecutive radiographs 1 month apart. Fractures typically do not heal for four reasons: infection, lack of blood supply, poor host factors, and biomechanical instability. In most clinical scenarios, it is combination of these factors at play. One of the most important aspects of nonunion care is diagnosing the etiology of the nonunion as this will directly impact the management of the patient.

The initial management of a nonunion starts with the patient's index procedure. Optimizing fracture care at the time of initial injury—through meticulous soft tissue management, limiting infection, and maximizing stabilization—can go a long way in preventing the development of a nonunion.

Diagnosis of a nonunion occurs through obtaining an adequate history and physical examination and reviewing imaging studies. Critical elements of the history include time of injury, types of surgery, development of infection, whether the fracture was open, and functional capacity.

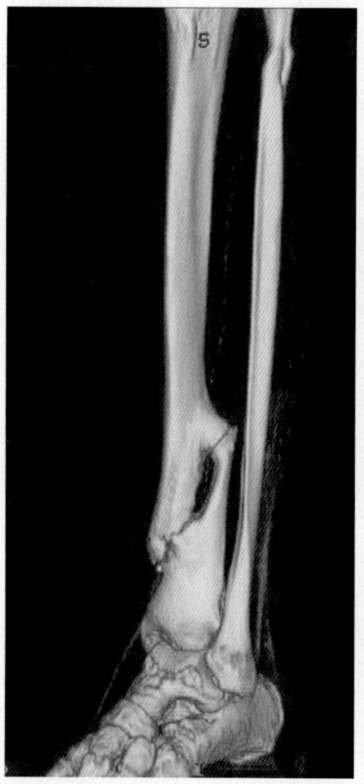

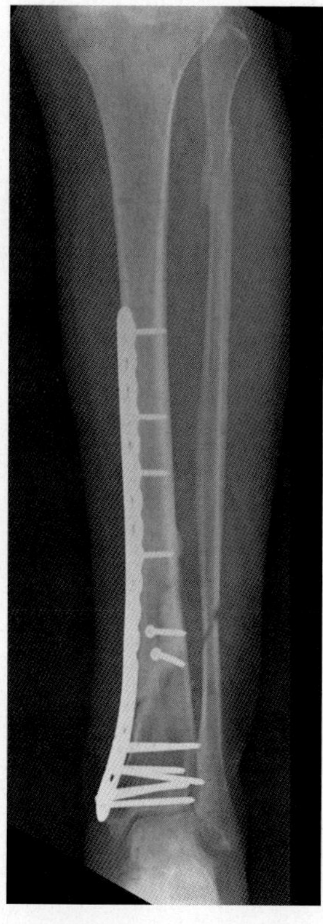

Figure 10.39 **(A)** A 35-year-old firefighter who fell from a ladder resulting in a distal third tibia fracture initially treated nonoperatively in a cast. Nine months later the patient was complaining of increasing difficulty walking, pain in the ankle, and a leg length discrepancy. **(B)** He underwent an osteotomy of his fibula and a take-down of his malunion with plate fixation to restore his length, alignment, and rotation.

Physical examination should focus on evaluation of the skin and soft tissue for surgical incisions and traumatic wounds, pain at the fracture site with direct palpation, sinus tracts, and instability.

In addition to the history and physical examination, imaging is essential in the diagnosis of a nonunion. Plain orthogonal radiographs are a critical first step in the imaging of a potential nonunion. Obtaining additional oblique radiographs has been shown to improve the sensitivity and specificity of detecting nonunions in long bones. Radiographic findings supporting nonunion include an absence of bone crossing the fracture site (bridging trabeculae), sclerotic fracture edges, persistent fracture lines, and lack of evidence of progressive change toward union on serial radiographs. Lack of callus is not a reliable radiologic parameter to use as callus would not be expected to be seen in patients undergoing primary bone healing (e.g., lag screw fixation with application of a neutralization plate) but would be expected in patients with secondary bone healing (e.g., IM nail). Advanced imaging modalities such as CT, MRI, and tagged white blood cell scans may be used to provide additional information regarding the configuration of the nonunion or potential sites of infection. Existing hardware may preclude the ability to obtain quality images.

Nonunions can be classified by their appearance on radiographs. The type of nonunion, as depicted by the plain x-rays, can often help the physician identify the etiology of the nonunion. Hypertrophic (or hyper-vascular) nonunions typically have a "horse hoof" or "elephant foot" appearance, which represents abundant callus as a result of a robust blood supply and inadequate biomechanical stability (Fig. 10.40). A hypertrophic nonunion has the biologic building blocks to heal, but lacks the stability to complete the process. Aside from exuberant callus on radiographs, patients may also exhibit increased uptake on radionucleotide scans, and this should not be confused with infection. Management of hypertrophic nonunions typically involves stabilization of the nonunion site through immobilization or, more commonly, surgical stabilization with a nail or compression plate.

At the opposite end of the spectrum, nonunions may be atrophic or avascular (Fig. 10.41). Radiographs show eburnated, osteopenic, and/or sclerotic bone ends. The nonunion is biologically devoid of healing and, as such, the ends of the bone have become atrophic and osteoporotic. Because of the lack of blood supply, a bone scan will typically be cold representing the lack of biologic activity. Surgical management involves stabilization and addition of biologically active material (e.g., autograft, bone morphogenic protein) to augment the healing response along with fixation.

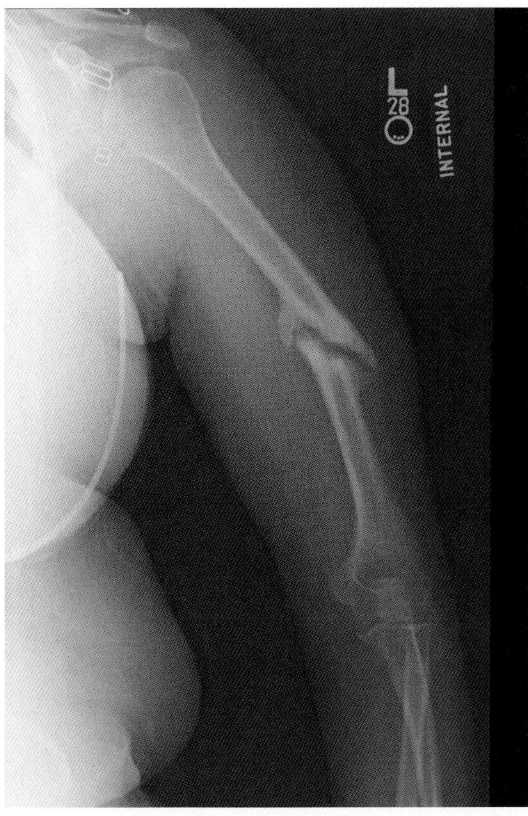

Figure 10.40 Hypertrophic nonunion of the humeral shaft. Despite callus formation, the humerus has not healed because of inadequate stabilization.

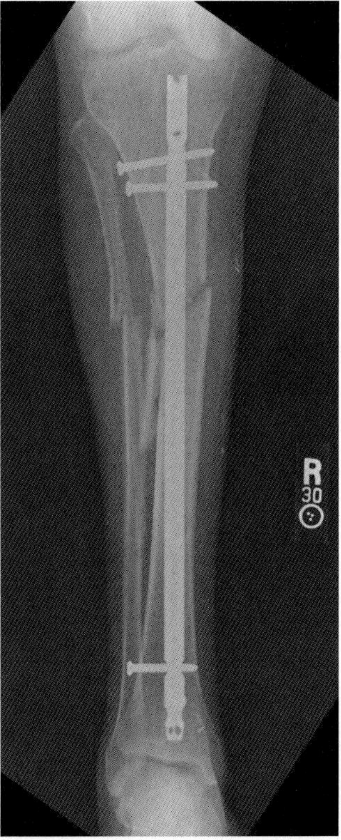

Figure 10.41 Atrophic nonunion of the tibial shaft in an elderly patient with diabetes, peripheral vascular disease, and poor nutrition. Despite surgical stabilization, there is no callus formation and the bone ends are sclerotic with little signs of vascularity.

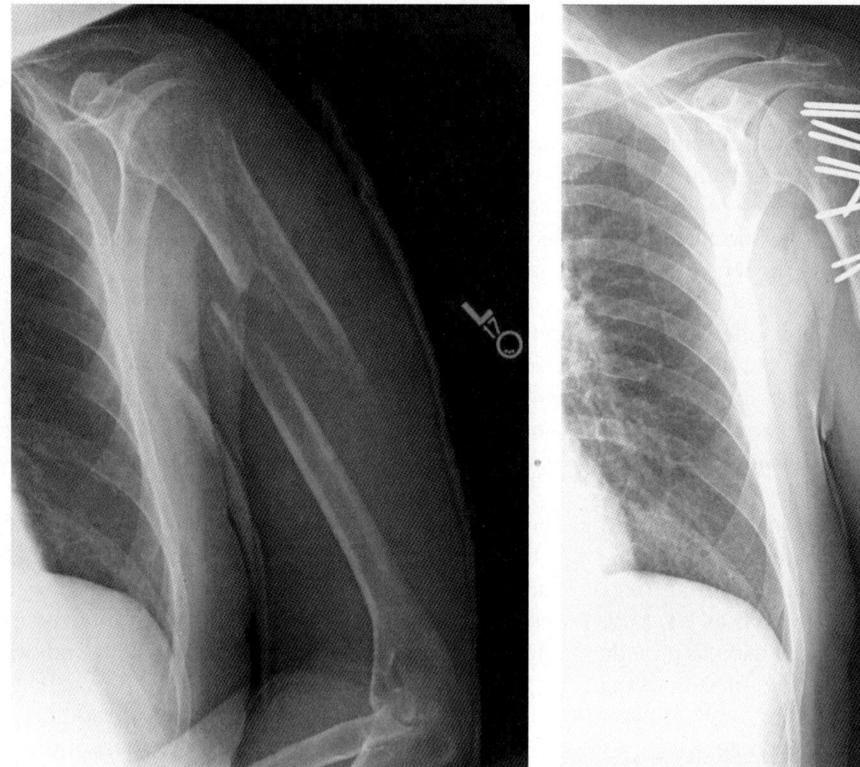

Figure 10.42 **(A)** Oligotrophic nonunion of the humeral shaft in a 42-year-old male who fell down the stairs. Despite several months of nonoperative management, the fracture showed no callus formation and no signs of healing. With surgical stabilization **(B)**, the fracture healed 8 weeks later. No orthobiologic agents were necessary as the fracture ends were not necrotic.

Oligotrophic nonunions do not show callus on radiographs but do not have signs of sclerosis or bone loss either (Fig. 10.42). Unlike atrophic nonunions, the blood supply is typically intact and a bone scan shows uptake. The healing response is inadequate, and this may be due to excessively rigid fixation, distraction at the fracture site, comminution, or host factors such as poor systemic levels of vitamin D and calcium.

Recent studies have examined the role of the host in fracture healing revealing the importance of the endocrine system. In the management of nonunions, some surgeons will obtain vitamin D, calcium, thyroid stimulating hormone, protein, albumin, magnesium, and phosphorus levels in conjunction with routine blood work. Pharmacologic correction of these important markers of healing in conjunction with appropriate musculoskeletal intervention has been shown to dramatically increase nonunion fracture healing rates.

Lastly, infection has been shown to delay or impede fracture healing. Infection typically occurs in the setting of an open fracture but may also be a risk in patients with prolonged surgical exposures, revision surgery, or medical comorbidities. All patients who present with a nonunion, hardware failure, or delayed healing, particularly with a history that is concerning, should undergo a work-up for infection as part of their nonunion evaluation. This work-up includes a complete blood cell count, erythrocyte sedimentation rate (ESR), C-reactive protein (CRP). Imaging may also be considered such as a tagged white blood cell scan or a triple-phase bone scan, as well as positron emission tomography. Lastly, some surgeons have advocated direct biopsy of the nonunion site with delayed management until formal biopsy results are available. None of these tests has been shown to have very high sensitivity or specificity, and, as such, the diagnosis of infection continues to be a combination of clinical suspicion, imaging, history, and physical examination.

Management of an infected nonunion is based upon the whether the infection needs to be eradicated or suppressed to obtain healing. In the presence of orthopaedic implants, it is extremely difficult to eradicate infection. Identification of the microorganism is critical to appropriate antibiotic selection for eradication or suppression until healing in conjunction with debridement and removal of hardware if necessary.

Osteomyelitis

Postoperative wound infections and osteomyelitis are usually related to high-energy injuries, which are associated with significant wound contamination and osseous devascularization. Other risk factors include prolonged open wound time, inadequate fixation, and extensive surgical dissection and periosteal stripping, which compromise blood flow to the wound. Patients can present with a myriad of signs and symptoms including pain, tenderness, fever, headache, nausea, vomiting, erythema, swelling, sinus tracts, drainage, and fluctuance.

Laboratory data can aid in the diagnosis of osteomyelitis. In acute osteomyelitis, the white blood cell count is elevated only 25% of the time and shows an abnormal differential only 65% of the time. Blood cultures in acute osteomyelitis are positive only 50% of the time. Chronic osteomyelitis often shows a mild anemia with elevations of ESR and CRP. There may be a leukocytosis with a left shit, but this is neither specific nor sensitive. Blood cultures are almost always negative.

Various imaging modalities can be utilized to help determine the presence and breadth of infection. Radiographs are positive in 90% of cases by 3 to 4 weeks after inoculation. The earliest bone changes are those of destruction or resorption, usually seen as mottled areas of decreased density in metaphyseal areas. Over time, a thin line of newly formed bone parallel to the shaft may be detected in the periosteal regions of the metaphysis as new bone results from infection progressing into the subperiosteal region and gradually extending along the shaft. If the infection is not controlled, the new periosteal bone thickens over succeeding few weeks becomes an involucrum. After several weeks have passed and the disease is in chronic phase, sequestra may appear as opaque areas of bone, usually surrounded by radiolucent zone consisting of exudate and granulation tissue. Occasionally, an acute metaphyseal osteomyelitis is contained locally by the host defenses. In such instances, the infection becomes surrounded by scar tissue and a rim of reactive bone, resulting cavity or cyst is filled with pus, which may ultimately become sterile. A bone abscess resulting from this localized form of the disease is called a Brodie's abscess. An MRI may help identify associated abscesses, sequestra, and sinus tracts and may also reveal specific changes in bone marrow. In bone marrow, inflammatory exudate has decreased signal on T1 as compared with normal marrow. Infected marrow will have higher signal on T2. A triple phase bone scan, often performed with either technetium 99m or indium 111, is positive 3 to 4 days after infection. The three phases of the bone scan involve a radionucleotide angiogram, immediate postinjection blood pooling, and ultimately decreased soft tissue presence with increased urinary excretion. Osteomyelitis shows increases in phases one and two, and focal increases in the third phase at the 3-hour time point.

An anatomic classification system for osteomyelitis has been provided by Drs Cierny and Mader (Fig. 10.43). The location of the osteomyelitis can be completely medullary (type I), superficial with a sinus tract from the skin extending down to the cortex (type II), localized where the cortex is violated, but the infection is contained (type III), and diffuse where the infection has eroded through each cortex (type IV). In addition to classifying the location of the osteomyelitis and its impact on the bone, Drs Cierny and

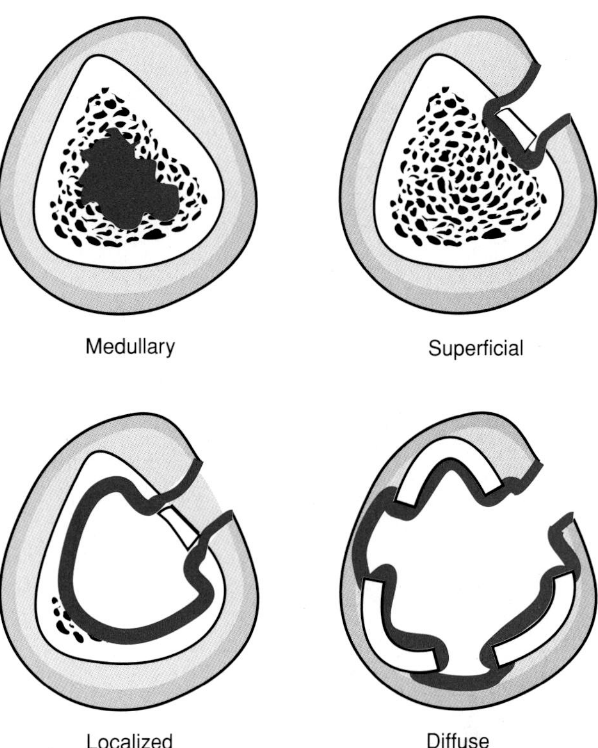

Figure 10.43 Anatomic classification of osteomyelitis based on the involvement of the soft tissue and location in the bone.

Mader also classified the host (patient). Type A hosts have a good immune system and delivery of antibiotics and nutrition to the infection site. Type B hosts are compromised either locally (type B^L), systemically (type B^S), or both (B^C). Type C hosts are patients who require suppressive therapy only or who have minimal disability where the treatment would result in greater morbidity than the infection itself. These patients are often not surgical candidates.

The primary treatment for osteomyelitis is prevention. Once a patient has osteomyelitis, the primary goal is identifying the correct organism and eradicating the infection. *Staphylococcus aureus* is the most common offending organism (90% of cases). Treatment for osteomyelitis consists of incisional drainage, debridement and irrigation, followed by intravenous antibiotics. Temporary implantation of antibiotic-impregnated cement beads and hyperbaric oxygen can help with more resistant cases. Osseous and soft tissue stability is essential with appropriate soft tissue coverage (Fig. 10.44).

Septic Arthritis

Patients with a distant focus of infection can present with new onset joint pain because of hematogenous spread of a bacterial organism within the confines of a joint capsule (i.e., synovial joint). The classic clinical scenario is a patient with pneumonia or bacterial endocarditis that presents with new onset hip pain. In the immunocompetent patient, the body's reaction to intra-articular infection is to mount a significant inflammatory response with the

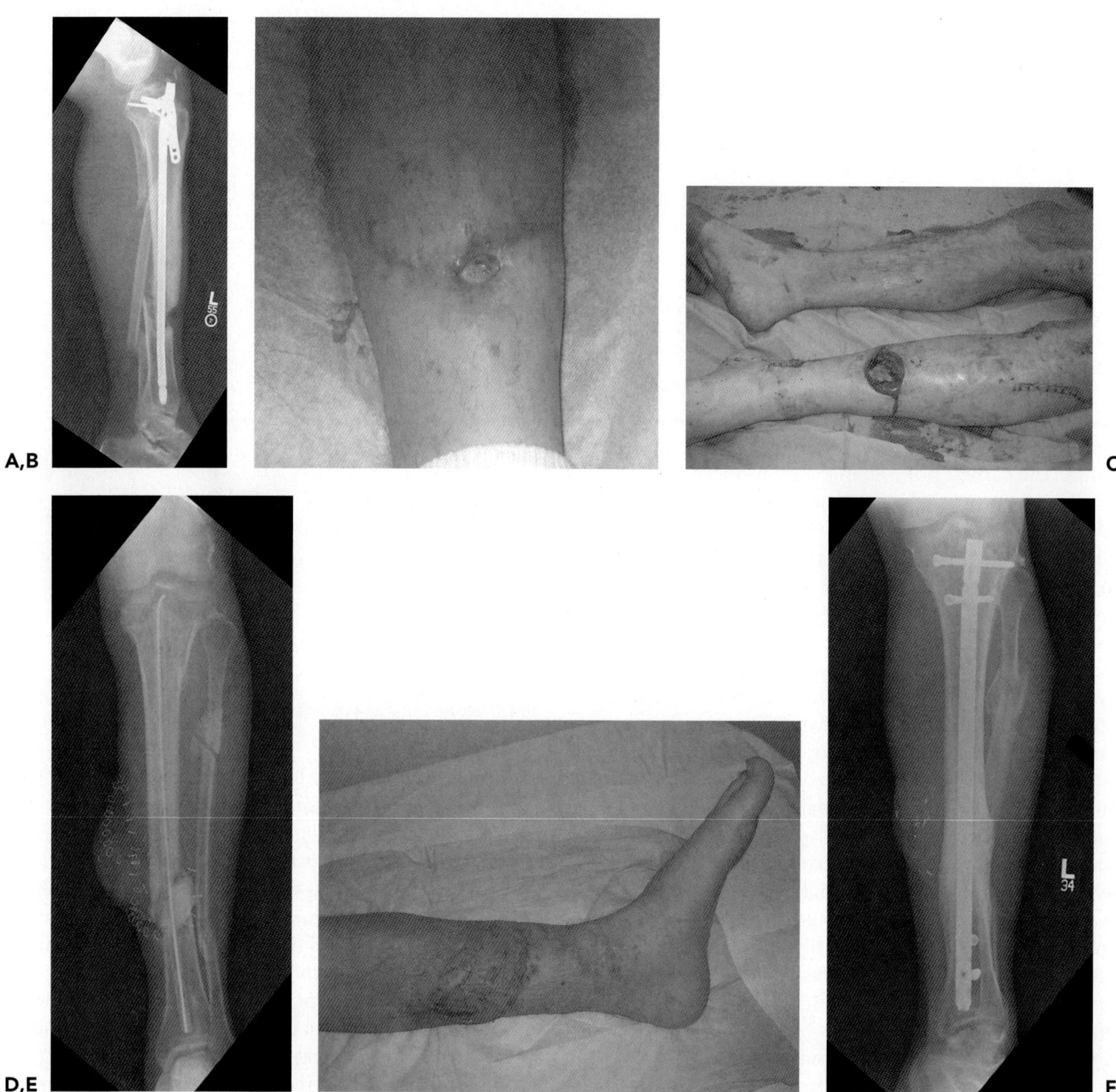

Figure 10.44 **(A)** Lateral radiograph of a 39-year-old male 18 months after operative stabilization of an open tibia fracture showing an atrophic nonunion. **(B)** Physical examination revealed a draining sinus tract directly over the nonunion site near the open fracture. The patient was taken to the operating room for debridement of his sinus tract and osteomyelitis **(C)** and placement of an antibiotic spacer and antibiotic nail **(D).** He also had a free flap performed to cover the defect **(E).** After 6 weeks of intravenous antibiotics, he was taken to the operating room for repair of his nonunion with bone grafting and intramedullary nailing. Six months later, he united his fracture **(F)** with no signs of recurrence of infection and intact soft tissue.

deposition of several cytokines, elastases, proteases, and other enzymes, which will lead to the eventual destruction of articular cartilage. Septic arthritis is a surgical emergency and involved joints should be irrigated and debrided as soon as possible.

The clinical examination may be equivocal in immunocompromised patients (e.g., diabetics, posttransplant, patients on chemotherapy, HIV positive, and intravenous drug abusers). The pathognomonic physical examination finding is micromotion pain with attempted joint range of motion. Patients with a septic joint often sit in a position to maximize the intracapsular volume so as to minimize the degree of stretch on the joint capsule and thus reduce pain. Immunocompromised patients as well as diabetics with peripheral neuropathy may present with a septic joint without much pain. One of the few clinical clues to aid in the diagnosis may be overlying cellulitis in conjunction with a history that raises the index of suspicion.

Diagnosis of a septic joint is based on a sterile aspirate of the intra-articular fluid, which is sent to the laboratory for white blood cell count, gram stain, and culture and sensitivity. In addition, the aspirate fluid should also be assessed for gouty crystals, which could result in a similar clinical picture. In aspirating a joint, it is imperative not to make the portal of entry through overlying cellulitic skin in an effort to avoid seeding the joint with bacteria from the skin infection. In addition, the systemic white blood cell count as well as the ESR and CRP may provide further information. The ESR and CRP may be elevated in the acute phase. Even if convincing evidence is present to make the diagnosis, it is important to not administer intravenous antibiotics until after sterile cultures are taken in the operating room at the time of definitive treatment.

When evaluating the cell count, a septic joint is defined as any joint with more than 50,000 white blood cells with greater than 85% to 90% polymorphonuclear cells. Cell counts of less than 50,000 may signify inflammatory disorders or crystalline disease and may warrant sending the fluid to the laboratory for crystal analysis (i.e., gout or calcium pyrophosphate disease—pseudogout).

The surgical treatment of septic arthritis is thorough irrigation and debridement. The involved joint can be irrigated using either an open technique or an arthroscopic technique, based on equipment availability. In the operating room, it is imperative to obtain sterile cultures before the administration of antibiotics. After cultures have been sent to the laboratory, a third-generation cephalosporin such as cefazolin is given to cover the most common offending organism, *S. aureus*. A large drain may be left in the joint to allow for egress of any additional purulent collections within the joint. Patients may require repeat irrigation and debridement within 48 to 72 hours to decrease the burden of inflammatory intra-articular mediators. The postoperative regimen warrants the placement of a peripheral intravenous central catheter for 6 weeks of organism-specific antibiotic therapy. Following successful treatment of septic arthritis, the goal is to regain range of motion and function of the joint/extremity.

Necrotizing Fasciitis

Necrotizing fasciitis is defined as an infection of the subcutaneous tissue overlying the fascia of an extremity. The most common organism involved in this type of infection is group A streptococcus. Patients typically present with a superficial skin infection that looks innocuous. However, the inciting physical examination finding is pain out of proportion to the clinical examination.

Cellulitis is a superficial infection of the epidermis and may present in similar fashion to necrotizing fasciitis. However, necrotizing fasciitis is often associated with an elevated body temperature and hemodynamic instability (hypotension). In the early stages, hemodynamic instability may be absent and by the time hypotension is present, the infection may have become more extensive. A missed diagnosis of necrotizing fasciitis is fatal.

Any patient with the diagnosis of necrotizing fasciitis requires emergent surgical debridement of the affected region. An extensile exposure is utilized to expose from the level of the skin to the underlying deep fascia. The infection has been described as "dishwater" pus and requires thorough irrigation and debridement. Hypotensive patients require close ICU care in the immediate postoperative period to optimize their hemodynamic status. Repeat irrigation and debridement is the standard of care and allows for exploration of the wound for evaluation of infection spread. Intravenous antibiotics are the mainstay of treatment and duration is typically 6 weeks.

SUMMARY

The management of the orthopaedic trauma patient is a multidisciplinary effort. The orthopaedic surgeon is critical in this evaluation, which includes an adequate history, thorough physical examination, and directed imaging techniques. A thorough understanding of common musculoskeletal conditions is necessary. Once the injuries have been defined, a plan is designed to manage the patient's injuries addressing life-threatening fractures initially with control of bleeding and temporizing stabilization. Great care is taken to prevent the "second hit." Preoperative planning is essential in the management of diaphyseal and articular injuries. Particular attention needs to be paid to the prevention of complications in this often challenging patient population.

RECOMMENDED READINGS

Bhandari M, Guyatt G, Tornetta P III, et al. Randomized trial of reamed and unreamed intramedullary nailing of tibial shaft fractures. *J Bone Joint Surg Am.* 2008;90(12):2567–2578.

Bosse MJ, MacKenzie EJ, Kellam JF, et al. An analysis of outcomes of reconstruction or amputation after leg-threatening injuries. *N Engl J Med.* 2002;347(24):1924–1931.

Garden RS. Stability and union in subcapital fractures of the femur. *J Bone Joint Surg.* 1964;46B(4):630–647.

Gustilo RB, Anderson JT. Prevention of infection in the treatment of one thousand and twenty-five open fractures of long bones: retrospective and prospective analyses. *J Bone Joint Surg Am.* 1976;58: 453–458.

Letournel E. Acetabulum fractures: classification and management. *Clin Orthop Rel Res.* 1980;151:81–106.

Routt ML, Nork SE, Mills WJ. High energy pelvic ring disruptions. *Ortho Clin North Am.* 2002;33(1):59–72.

Siebel R, LaDuca J, Hassett JM, et al. Blunt multiple trauma (ISS 36), femur traction, and the pulmonary failure-septic state. *Ann Surg.* 1985;202(3):283–293.

Winquist RA, Hansen ST, Clawson DK. Closed intramedullary nailing of femoral fractures. A report of five hundred and twenty cases. *J Bone Joint Surg Am.* 1984;66:529–539.

Pediatric Orthopaedics 11

Section 1 General and Regional Problems in Children

Wudbhav N. Sankar Karen Myung Robert M. Kay

Children are very different from adults. Youth is a time of rapid growth, musculoskeletal development, and emotional maturation. The unique physiology of children makes them susceptible to very different orthopaedic conditions compared with adults. In addition, most metabolic and congenital disorders present at an early age. Proper care of pediatric patients rests upon a proper understanding of normal growth and development; global neuromuscular, metabolic, and hereditary conditions; and several specific regional issues.

TORSIONAL AND ANGULAR VARIATIONS

Before one can diagnose and effectively treat diseases of the pediatric musculoskeletal system, one must understand what constitutes normal growth and development. Torsional and angular changes in the lower extremity are among the most common reasons for referral of a child. The complaint of in-toeing or out-toeing as well as knock-knees and bow-legs are a major preoccupation of parents and grandparents alike. In spite of these concerns, the vast majority of these children are normal children who are simply reflecting modest variations in growth and development. The physician evaluating a child with a torsional or angular variation should carefully assess the patient to be sure that there is no underlying pathologic condition before reassuring the family that the findings are indeed normal variations.

Physiology

Variations in axial rotational alignment are usually due to mechanical forces applied in utero. Inside the womb, the fetus can assume a position in which the feet are tucked inward, the tibiae are internally twisted, and the hips are medially rotated. These forces result in variable amounts of metatarsus adductus, internal tibial torsion, and femoral anteversion at birth. With normal growth, however, each of these three conditions will, to a large extent, remodel. For example, femoral anteversion is typically 30 to 40 degrees at birth but eventually decreases to an adult angle of 10 to 15 degrees. Frontal plane angulations such as knock-knees and bow-legs also follow a predictable course. Most neonates will demonstrate some amount of genu varum at birth due to intrauterine positioning and external rotation contractures of the hip. Before the walking age, genu varum may actually help a child cling to a parent's hip. This varus pattern persists through the first year of life with normalization to a neutral axis around 18 months of age. Most children actually develop increased genu valgum beginning at age 2. Maximum knock-knee is usually present in the 2- to 4-year-old age group with rapid spontaneous correction thereafter, with essentially adult alignment achieved by 6 to 7 years of age (Fig. 11.1).

Presentation

Parents of in-toeing children typically complain of the cosmetic appearance, frequent tripping, or an awkward "egg-beater" running style. The cause of in-toeing can often be deduced simply by the age at which the child presents. Children who are just beginning to walk typically have residual metatarsus adductus from intrauterine positioning. Between ages 1 and 3, internal tibial torsion is the most likely culprit (Fig. 11.2). After age 3, the most likely cause of in-toeing is persistent femoral anteversion that has yet to remodel. Out-toeing is a less common presentation and is also of no functional consequence.

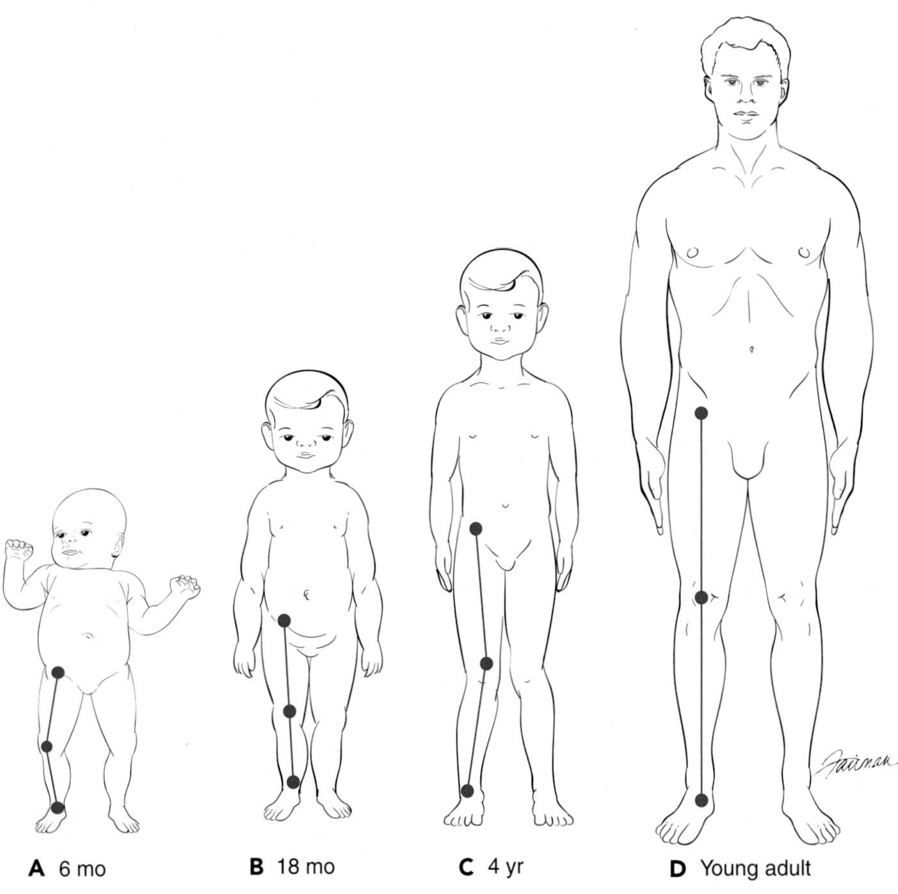

Figure 11.1 **(A)** A 6-month-old child with genu varum. **(B)** An 18-month-old child with straight legs. At some point in most children, usually around 18 months of age, the legs are perfectly straight as their developmental stage passes from genu varum to genu valgum. **(C)** A 4-year-old child with genu valgum. **(D)** Adults normally have a mild amount of genu valgum. (*Reproduced with permission from* Skaggs DL, Flynn JM. *Staying Out of Trouble in Pediatric Orthopaedics.* Philadelphia, PA: Lippincott Williams & Wilkins, 2006.)

Children with angular variations present according to their normal developmental sequence. Parents of toddlers typically complain of a "bow-legged" appearance while preschool children usually present with "knock-knees" (Fig. 11.3). These physiologic variations are not symptomatic but may cause anxiety for the parents due to the cosmetic appearance. The most common angular complaint in adolescents is persistent genu valgum, which may cause their knees to rub together when they run or play sports.

History and Physical Examination

Although most torsional and angular variations are physiologic, it is important to take an accurate history to screen for an underlying abnormality. A birth history should be taken

A

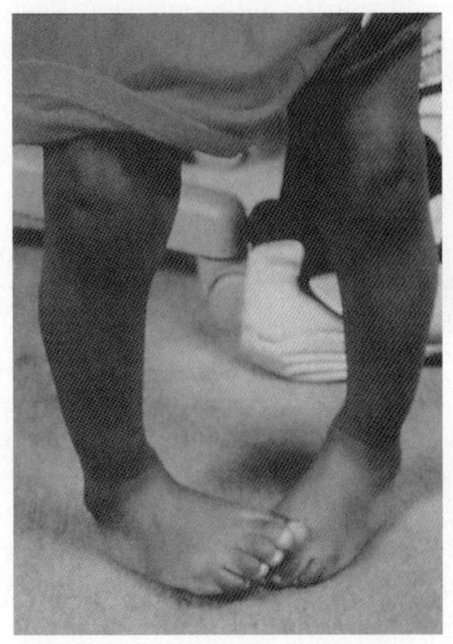

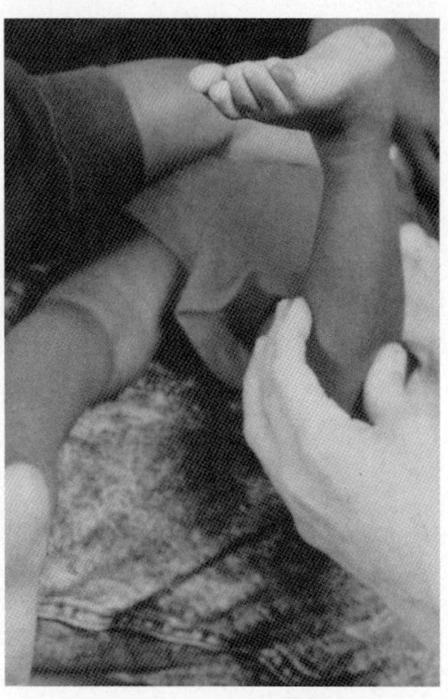

B

Figure 11.2 Internal tibial torsion is often seen in toddlers with an in-toed gait. (*Reprinted with permission from* Morrissy RT, Weinstein SL. *Lovell and Winter's Pediatric Orthopaedics.* Philadelphia, PA: Lippincott Williams & Wilkins, 2006.)

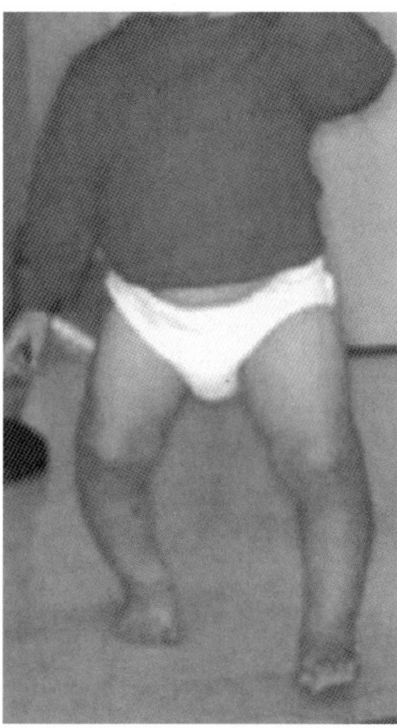

Figure 11.3 Genu varum in a toddler. (*Reproduced with permission from* Skaggs DL, Flynn JM. *Staying Out of Trouble in Pediatric Orthopaedics.* Philadelphia, PA: Lippincott Williams & Wilkins, 2006.)

and gross motor milestones should be assessed, including the age at which the child first walked. Patients who are not growing appropriately may have a skeletal dysplasia or an underlying syndrome.

The overall effect of torsional variations on a child's walking can be assessed by measuring the foot-progression angle. Normally, when a child walks, the foot should be slightly externally rotated from the line of progression by approximately 10 to 15 degrees. In-toeing is diagnosed if the foot progression angle is negative, and out-toeing refers to external rotation of the foot beyond 25 degrees (Fig. 11.4). The physical examination of a child with an abnormal foot progression angle focuses on each level of the

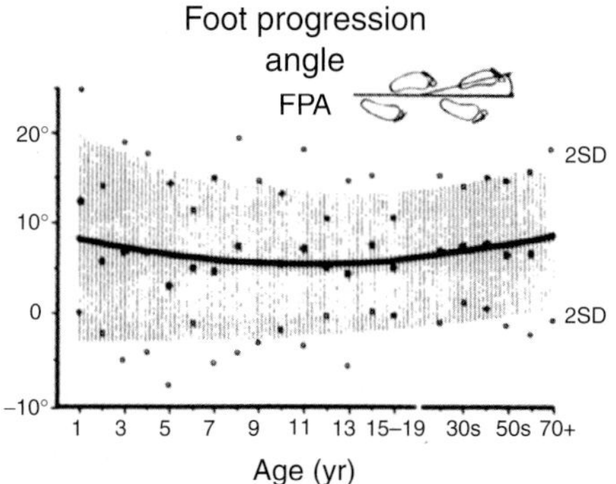

Figure 11.4 Normative values for foot progression angle. The solid line demonstrates mean values and the shaded area represents ±2 standard deviations. (*Reprinted with permission from* Morrissy RT, Weinstein SL. *Lovell and Winter's Pediatric Orthopaedics.* Philadelphia, PA: Lippincott Williams & Wilkins, 2006.)

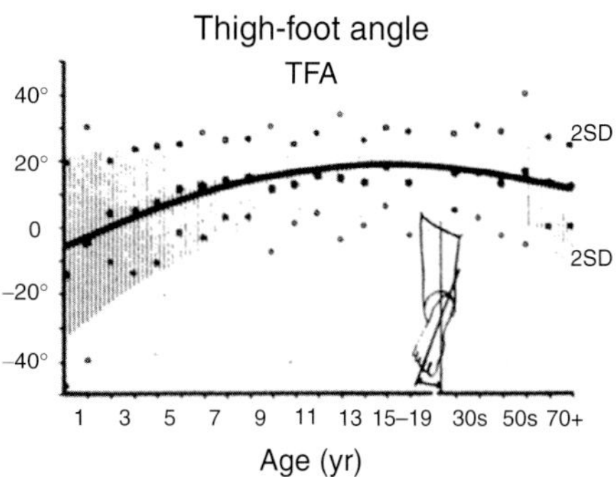

Figure 11.5 Normative values for thigh–foot angle. The solid line demonstrates mean values and the shaded area represents ±2 standard deviations. (*Reprinted with permission from* Morrissy RT, Weinstein SL. *Lovell and Winter's Pediatric Orthopaedics.* Philadelphia, PA: Lippincott Williams & Wilkins, 2006.)

lower extremity to develop a torsional profile. The feet are evaluated first to look for abnormalities such as metatarsus adductus. Tibial rotation can be quantified by measuring the thigh–foot angle (Fig. 11.5). With the child is lying prone and the knee is flexed at 90 degrees, the angle between the thigh and the long axis of the foot can be assessed. After age 8, the thigh–foot angle averages 10 degrees external (range 0–20 degrees). Measurements below this range indicate internal tibial torsion and values greater than 20 degrees indicate external tibial torsion. Drawbacks of this measurement are its sensitivity to the position of the foot and lack of reliability in cases of coexisting foot deformity. Alternatively, the transmalleolar axis can be measured. This is the angle formed between an imaginary line drawn through the femoral condyles and an imaginary line drawn through the medial and lateral malleoli. Values less than 10 degrees imply internal tibial torsion and measurements greater than 30 degrees indicate external tibial torsion. Femoral version is best evaluated by measuring hip rotation in the prone position with the hips extended and the knees flexed 90 degrees (Fig. 11.6). By age 10, internal hip rotation averages 50 degrees (range 25–65 degrees) and external rotation 45 degrees (range 25–65 degrees). Internal hip rotation greater than 70 degrees implies increased femoral anteversion. Likewise, diminished internal rotation is seen in children with femoral retroversion.

Angular variations can be quantified by measuring the intermalleolar distance (for genu valgum or knock-knees) or the intercondylar distance (for genu varum or bow-legs). These measurements provide an objective measure that parents and physicians can follow as the child grows. Up to 12 degrees of genu valgum and an intermalleolar distance of 8 cm is within the normal range (Fig. 11.7). Intercondylar distance should decrease by age 2. Examiners should be careful not to confuse apparent genu varum due to tibial torsion with a true bow-legged appearance. To remove the optical illusion caused by the knees pointing laterally, the legs should be rotated until the patellas point anteriorly (Fig. 11.8).

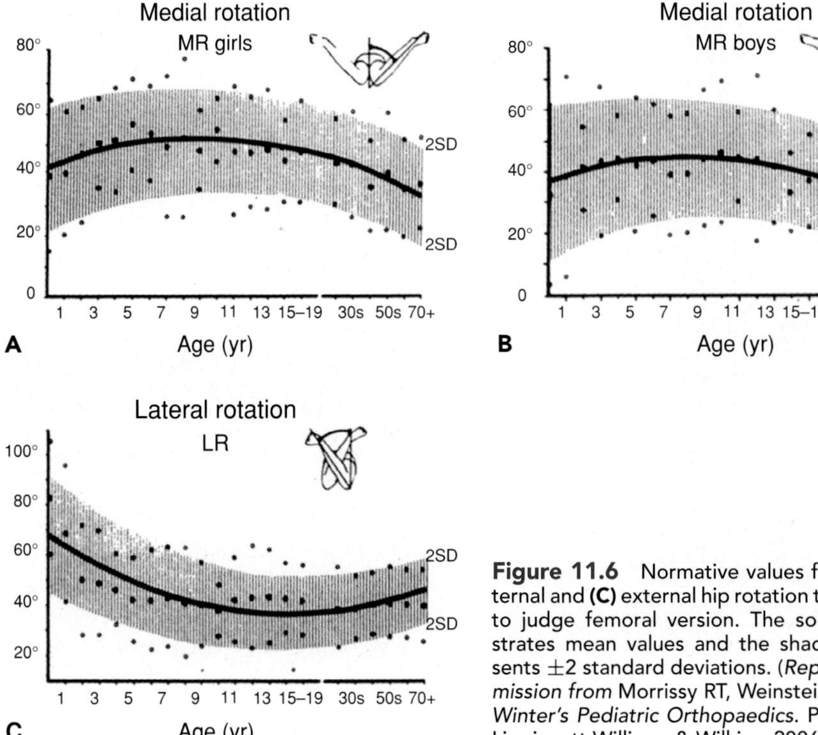

Figure 11.6 Normative values for **(A** and **B)** internal and **(C)** external hip rotation that can be used to judge femoral version. The solid line demonstrates mean values and the shaded area represents ±2 standard deviations. (*Reprinted with permission from* Morrissy RT, Weinstein SL. *Lovell and Winter's Pediatric Orthopaedics*. Philadelphia, PA: Lippincott Williams & Wilkins, 2006.)

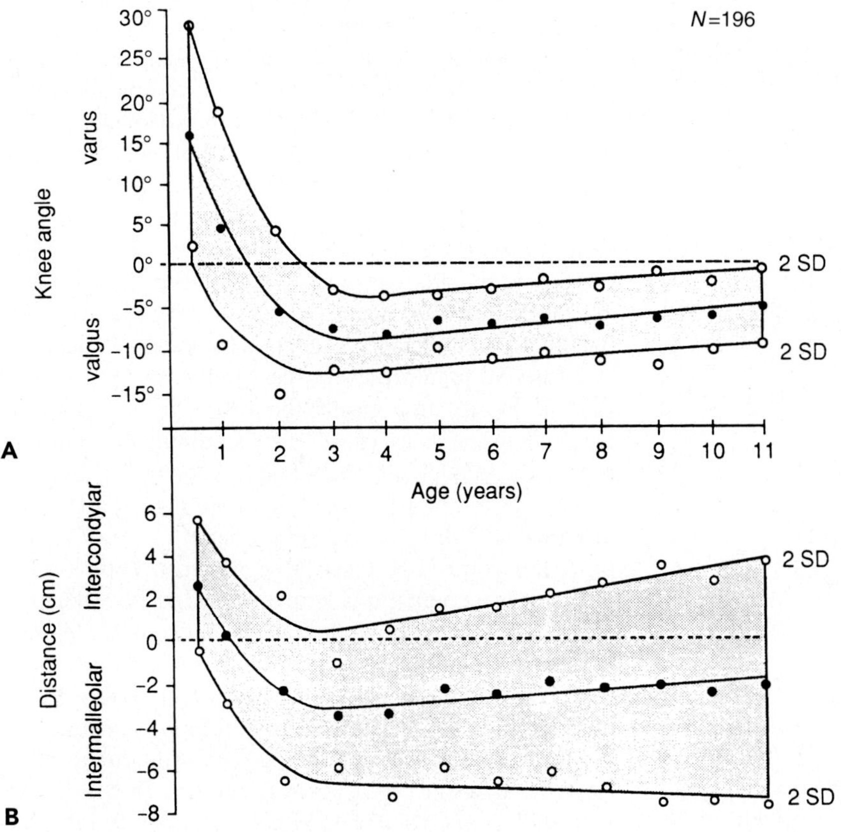

Figure 11.7 Mean values and standard deviations for **(A)** knee angle and **(B)** intercondylar or intermalleolar distance. (*Reproduced with permission from* Skaggs DL, Flynn JM. *Staying Out of Trouble in Pediatric Orthopaedics*. Philadelphia, PA: Lippincott Williams & Wilkins, 2006.)

Figure 11.8 **(A)** Child demonstrating the apparent genu varum of tibial torsion. The chief complaint of this child's parents was bowed legs. With the feet pointing forward, the legs have the appearance of genu varum when the child is supine or walking. The apparent "bowing" is a product of the knees pointing laterally, so knee flexion gives the appearance of bowing. **(B)** When the child's patellas point anteriorly, it is clear that there is not significant genu varum present. (*Reproduced with permission from* Skaggs DL, Flynn JM. *Staying Out of Trouble in Pediatric Orthopaedics.* Philadelphia, PA: Lippincott Williams & Wilkins, 2006.)

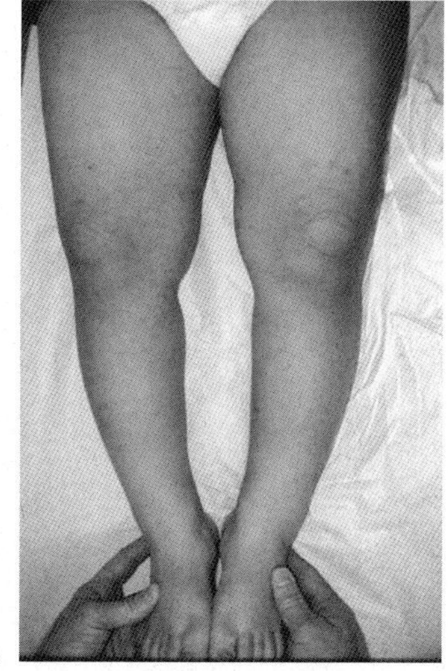

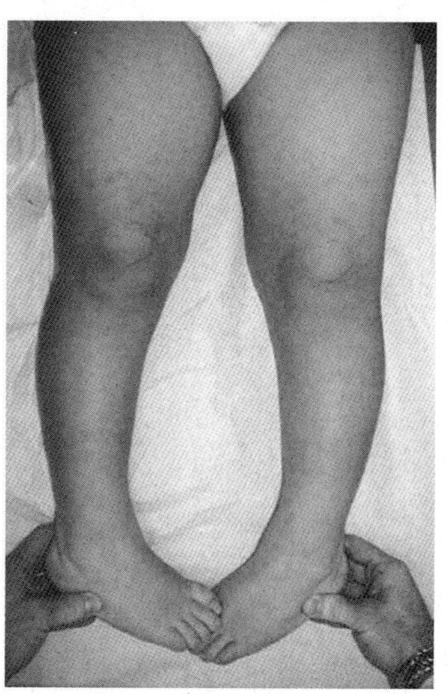

Radiographs

Although plain radiographs have limited utility in the evaluation of torsional variations, standing full-length radiographs can be very useful for working up moderate to severe angular variations (Fig. 11.9). Using this radiograph, the anatomic axis between the femur and the tibia can be measured to quantify the degree of knock-knees or bow-legs.

Figure 11.9 Physiologic genu varum in a toddler. Note that the weight-bearing axis falls medial to the knee joint.

In addition, one can evaluate the child's weight-bearing axis, which is the line intersecting the center of the femoral head and the center of the ankle. Normally, this axis runs through approximately the center of the knee joint. With increasing genu varum, the weight-bearing axis falls more medially. Similarly, increased genu valgum causes the axis to fall lateral to the center of the knee.

Special Studies

Advanced imaging is rarely necessary in the evaluation of torsional or angular variations. Occasionally, severe cases of femoral anteversion or retroversion may warrant a computed tomography (CT) to quantify the exact degree of rotational deformity.

Differential Diagnosis

Although the vast majority of torsional and angular variations are physiologic and will improve with age, it is important to rule out an underlying pathologic condition before reassuring the family that their child is normal. Torsional variations may cause tripping but should not cause a limp nor should it be painful. Existence of either of these two symptoms should prompt a workup for other causes. Unilateral in-toeing can be due to hemiplegic cerebral palsy (CP) or other neuromuscular condition. Out-toeing in an older child can be caused by a slipped capital femoral epiphysis (SCFE) or coxa vara.

Angular variations outside the range of normal can be caused by a number of different conditions, most of which are described in detail elsewhere in this chapter. In evaluating a toddler with bowed legs, the most important diagnosis to consider is Blount disease (tibia vara). In particular, Blount disease should be suspected when the child is older than 2 years, the varus deformity is sharply angular, a lateral knee thrust is present with ambulation, the bowing

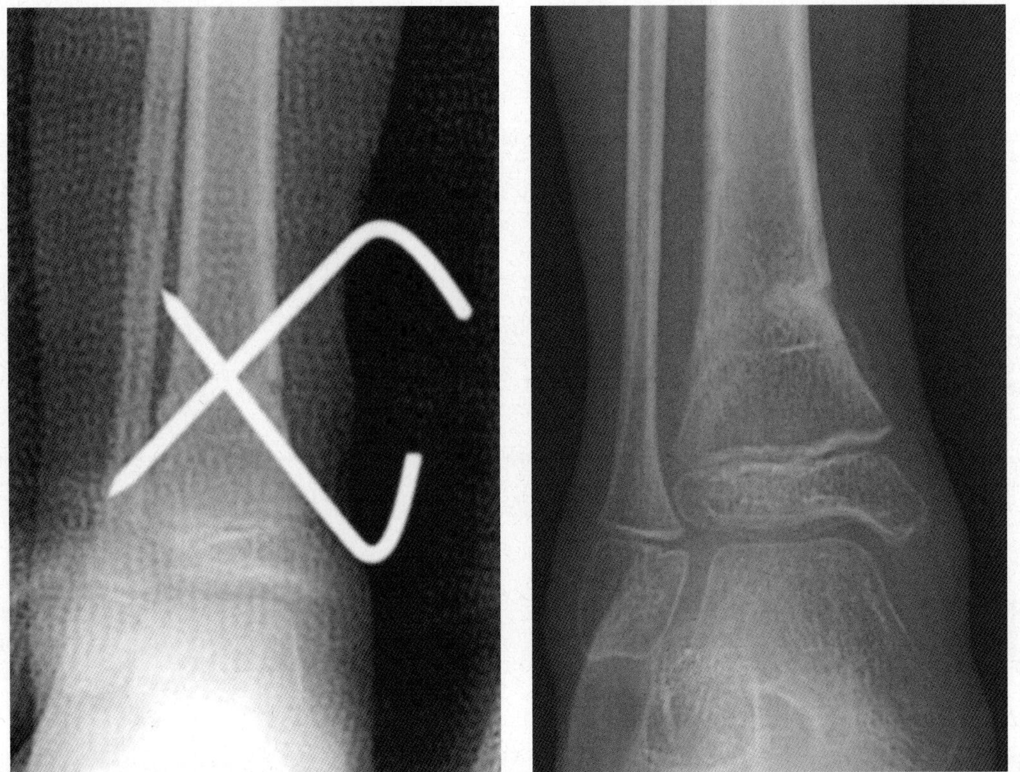

Figure 11.10 Anteroposterior radiographs **(A)** 4 weeks after and **(B)** 8 weeks after tibial rotational osteotomy. In this case, pins and a cast were used to achieve fixation at the osteotomy site. (*Reproduced with permission from* Skaggs DL, Tolo VT. *Master Techniques in Orthopaedic Surgery: Pediatrics.* Philadelphia, PA: Lippincott Williams & Wilkins, 2008.)

is particularly severe, and characteristic radiographic changes are seen in the proximal tibia. Rickets and skeletal dysplasias can present with either genu varum or genu valgum. Usually, these children have small stature and typical radiographic findings. Other potential causes of angular deformity include renal osteodystrophy, congenital pseudarthrosis of the tibia (CPT), trauma to the physis, and infection.

Treatment

Torsional variations rarely require formal treatment. Although the presence of in-toeing or out-toeing may frustrate parents, the vast majority of these conditions improve spontaneously with age. There is no evidence that bracing or special shoes help accelerate the natural history. On rare occasions, children with torsional deformities that persist into adolescence *and* cause functional problems can be treated with corrective osteotomy of the tibia or femur (Fig. 11.10).

Physiologic angular variations should also be observed for spontaneous improvement. Of course, all children with an underlying etiology should be treated for their diagnosis. Occasionally, children will present with persistent moderate to severe genu valgum in their early teenage years. Operative treatment can be considered for those adolescents who are symptomatic from pain or gait disturbance and for those with a weight-bearing axis that passes lateral to the knee. Prior to skeletal maturity, treatment usually consists of temporary hemiepiphysiodesis of the distal femur and/or proximal tibia, using staples or "8" plates (Fig. 11.11). After skeletal maturity, corrective osteotomy may be necessary.

NEUROMUSCULAR DISEASE

Children afflicted with neuromuscular diseases frequently manifest severe musculoskeletal abnormalities. Not only do they suffer from the intrinsic effects of the neuropathic or myopathic abnormalities but they are usually profoundly affected by the secondary bone and joint deformities that result from these diseases. For management to be effective, it is important that the physician recognize the basic differences between the neuromuscular disorders. Certain neurologic diseases are central, whereas others are peripheral; some affect only the motor system, whereas others affect both sensory and motor components. CP, for example, is a central neurologic condition with resulting spasticity in the periphery. Children with CP typically have reasonable sensation. In contrast, myelodysplasia affects the spinal cord and adjacent nerve roots, leaving little motor

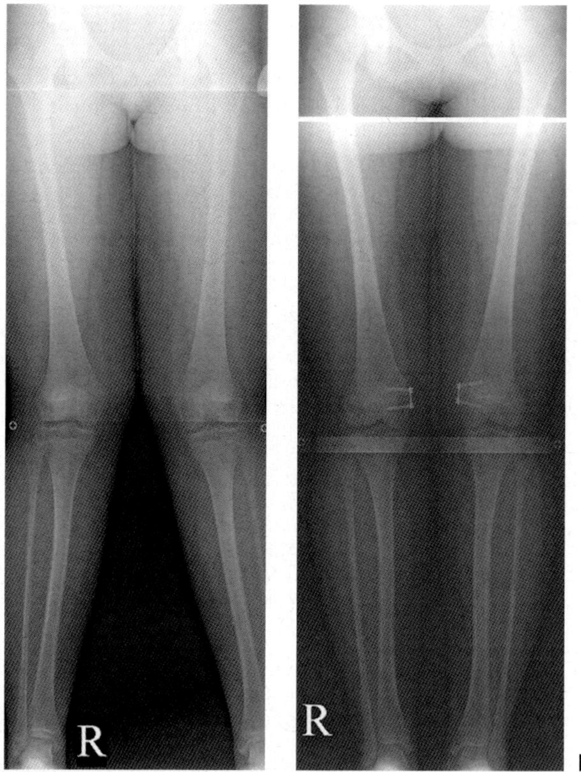

Figure 11.11 **(A)** This teenaged girl did not like the appearance of her genu valgum and complained that her knees rubbed together when she played sports. **(B)** Repeat standing radiograph after temporary hemiepiphysiodesis of the distal femur using "8" plates. (*Reproduced with permission from* Children's Orthopaedic Center, Los Angeles, CA.)

or sensory function below the lesion. Muscular dystrophies (Duchenne and others) affect the end organ, causing significant myopathic changes. Nerves, however, are typically unaffected. Arthrogryposis is a neuromuscular disease of unknown etiology. Typically, muscles are poorly developed but nerve function exists.

Cerebral Palsy

Pathophysiology

CP is really not one disease but rather a syndrome of motor disorders that result from an insult to the immature brain. The size and scope of the brain injury affects not only the severity of motor involvement but also the child's speech, cognition, and overall functional ability. CP is the most common neuromuscular disorder in children and is characterized by a static, nonprogressive central injury. As a consequence, the usual inhibitory role of the central nervous system (CNS) is suppressed, resulting in increased peripheral spasticity. Over time, this spasticity results in contractures and joint deformities. Prenatal causes include infections such as toxoplasmosis, rubella, cytomegalovirus, herpes, and syphilis, as well as maternal drug and alcohol use. Perinatal causes include birth trauma and anoxia. In fact, prematurity is the most common risk factor for CP. Infants less than 1,500 g have a 25 times increased risk of developing CP. Finally, head trauma, intraventricular hemorrhage, and meningitis are examples of postnatal causes of CP.

Classification

CP can be classified physiologically, geographically, or functionally. Physiologic grouping is based on the location of the brain lesion and the movement disorder that results. Spastic CP, the most common form of CP, occurs when the pyramidal tracts of the brain are affected. Dyskinesia, characterized by athetosis, chorea, and other involuntary motor movements, occurs when the extrapyramidal regions become injured. Some children may have a mixed picture, with both pyramidal and extrapyramidal features. Geographic classification is based on the distribution of limbs that are affected. *Hemiplegia* refers to arm and leg involvement on one side of the body, *diplegia* describes primarily bilateral lower extremity involvement, and *quadriplegia* affects all four extremities. Significant overlap can occur between the geographic classifications; for example, severe diplegia can often be confused with mild quadriplegia depending on the extent of upper extremity involvement. As a result, many physicians prefer a Gross Motor Function Classification System (GMFCS), which is based on the child's level of ambulation and use of assistive devices (Fig. 11.12).

Presentation

CP can present in many different ways. Common reasons for referral include limping, leg-length discrepancies, foot problems, toe-walking, tight muscles, and/or poor upper extremity function. Typically, gross motor development is delayed; however, this depends on the severity of central injury. In addition, intelligence and communication skills vary depending on the degree of involvement. Hemiplegic children often have normal intelligence, whereas some quadriplegic children demonstrate significant mental deficits and an inability to communicate in a meaningful manner.

History and Physical Examination

Most children with CP have a history of prematurity, prolonged delivery, and/or anoxic injury about the time of birth. A detailed birth history should also include problems during pregnancy and the duration of hospitalization after birth. A careful developmental history may reveal evidence of developmental delay. On average, children should sit by 6 months, stand by 8 months, and walk by 12 months. If a child does not reach these milestones by 1.5 times these ages (i.e., sit by 9 months, stand by 12 months, or walk by 18 months), an investigation into the developmental delay is warranted. Another useful historical detail is early handedness. A preference for a certain hand prior to 1 year of age may be a sign of hemiplegia.

Physical examination should include range of motion of all joints along with an assessment of muscle tone, selective motor control, and upper and lower extremity reflexes.

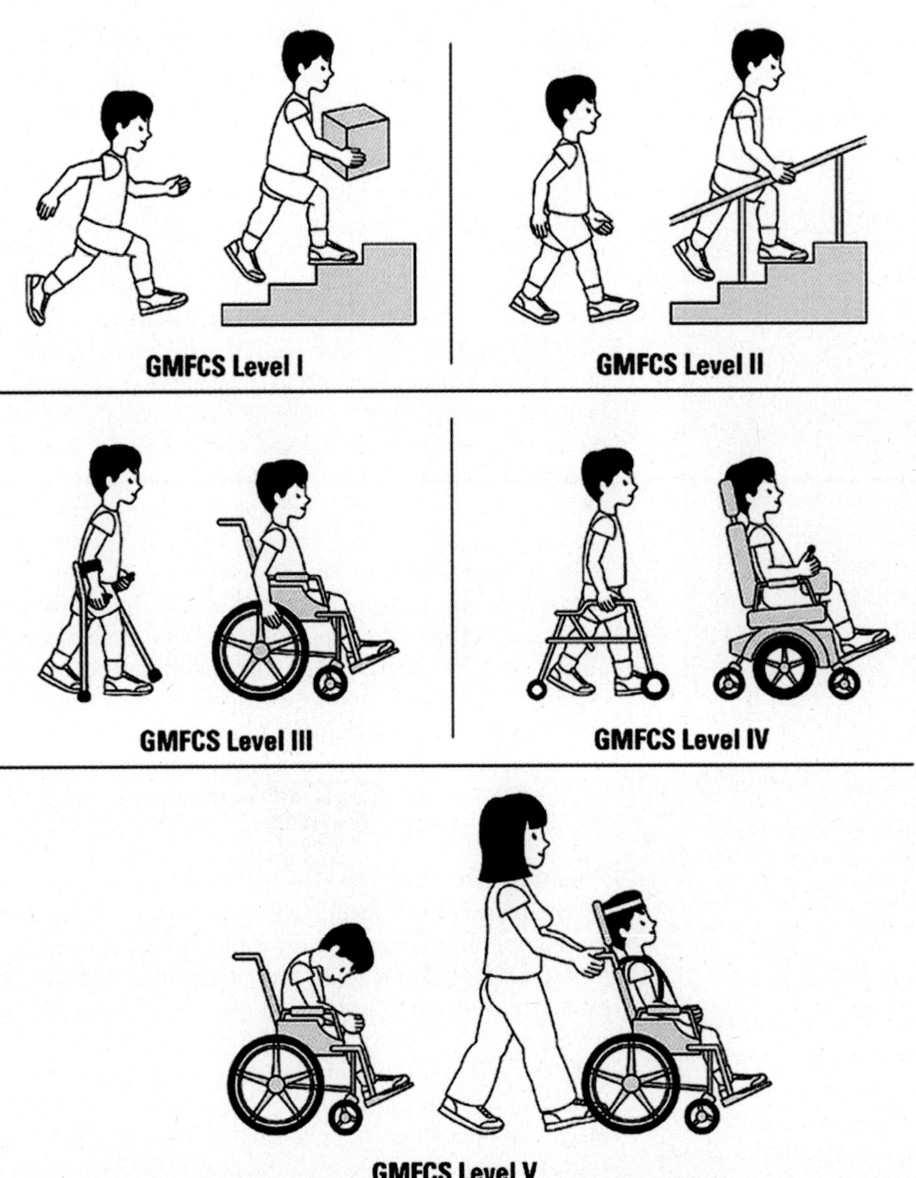

Figure 11.12 The Gross Motor Function Classification system (GMFCS). GMFCS level 1: Children walk indoors and outdoors and climb stairs without limitation. Children perform gross motor skills including running and jumping, but speed, balance, and coordination are impaired. GMFCS level II: Children walk indoors and outdoors and climb stairs holding onto a railing but experience limitations walking on uneven surfaces and inclines and walking in crowds or confined spaces. Children have, at best, only minimal ability to perform gross motor skills such as running and jumping. GMFCS level III: Children walk indoors or outdoors on a level surface with an assistive mobility device. Children may climb stairs holding onto a railing. Children may propel a wheelchair manually or are transported when traveling for long distances or outdoors on uneven terrain. GMFCS level IV: Children may continue to walk for short distances on a walker or rely more on wheeled mobility at home and school and in the community. Children may achieve self-mobility by using a power wheelchair. GMFCS level V: Physical impairments restrict voluntary control of movement and the ability to maintain antigravity head and trunk postures. All areas of motor function are limited. Children have no means of independent mobility and are transported. (*Redrawn with permission from* Graham HK. On the other hand: classifying cerebral palsy. *J Pediatr Orthop.* 2005;25(1):127.)

Typically, tone and reflexes are increased, whereas selective motor control is decreased. In particular, function at the ankle, knee, and hip should be carefully evaluated. Ankle dorsiflexion should be measured carefully with the hindfoot inverted to lock the subtalar joint and with the knee both flexed and extended to differentiate the contribution of the gastrocnemius (which crosses both joints) to the overall tightness of the Achilles tendon (Fig. 11.13). Hamstring tightness can be assessed by measuring the popliteal angle (the angle formed between the vertical and the leg) with the hip flexed 90 degrees and the contralateral hip and knee extended (Fig. 11.14). Adductor tightness is measured by the degree of abduction of the leg, with the hip and knee extended. Fixed joint contractures should also be evaluated as both hip and knee flexion contractures are common. To accurately measure a hip flexion contracture, the contralateral hip should be flexed to flatten the lumbar and stabilize the pelvis (Fig. 11.15). When both hips are flexed and brought together in the midline, a knee height difference is a "positive" Galleazi test and is suggestive of hip subluxation or dislocation on the shorter side. In quadriplegic children, the spine should be evaluated for scoliosis and the child's overall sitting balance and pelvic obliquity should be assessed. Perhaps the most important component of the physical examination in ambulatory children is watching the child walk. Evaluation of gait is the best functional assessment of the child. During gait, torsional abnormalities and dynamic issues can be diagnosed, and one can assess the overall effect of the static contractures and muscle tightness on function.

Radiographs

The most important radiograph in a child with CP is an anteroposterior (AP) view of the pelvis. Persistent

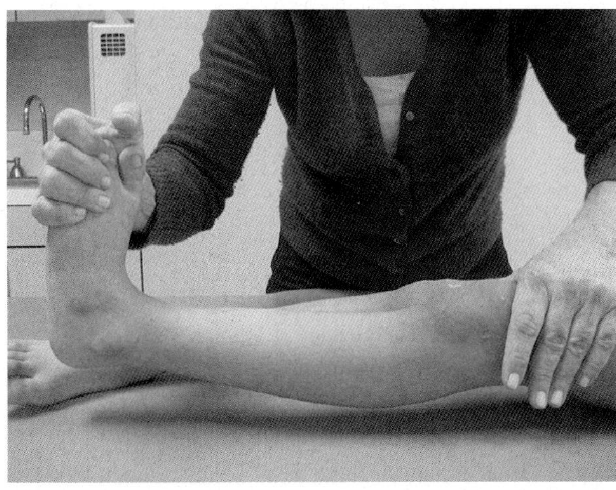
A

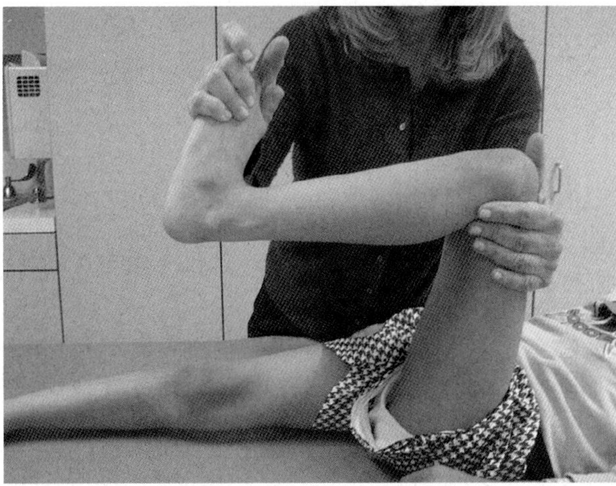
B

Figure 11.13 **(A)** Dorsiflexion should be measured in both with the knee extended **(A)** and the knee flexed 90 degrees **(B)**. The latter technique relaxes the gastrocnemius muscle. By comparing the range of motion in both positions, one can assess the contribution of the gastrocnemius to the overall tightness of the Achilles tendon. (*Reproduced with permission from* Children's Orthopaedic Center, Los Angeles, CA.)

hypertonicity around the hips can lead to "spastic hip disease" or progressive subluxation and dislocation of the hip due to overpull of the adductor and iliopsoas muscles. These hips are initially normal at birth, so it is important to monitor them radiographically over time to identify those hips that are "at risk" for subluxation. The most commonly used radiographic index for quantifying the severity of spastic hip disease is the Reimer migration percentage (or migration index). The migration percentage is calculated by dividing the width of the uncovered femoral head (A) by the total width of the femoral head (B) (Fig. 11.16). Indices greater than 25% may indicate the need for soft tissue surgery, whereas percentages greater than 50% probably require bony reconstruction.

Special Studies

In recent years, quantitative gait evaluation using three-dimensional computerized motion analysis has become increasingly popular to help plan appropriate surgical intervention. These studies are performed at specific gait laboratories and can be extremely useful for systematically evaluating the complex walking patterns of patients with CP.

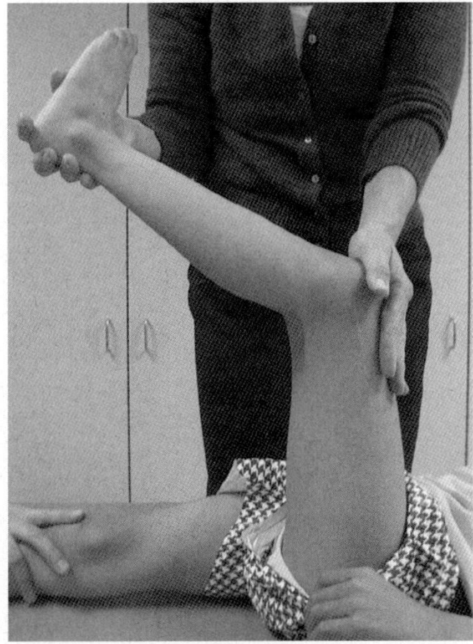

Figure 11.14 Hamstring tightness can be assessed by measuring the popliteal angle. This is the angle formed between the vertical and the child's leg when the hip is flexed to 90 degrees. (*Reproduced with permission from* Children's Orthopaedic Center, Los Angeles, CA.)

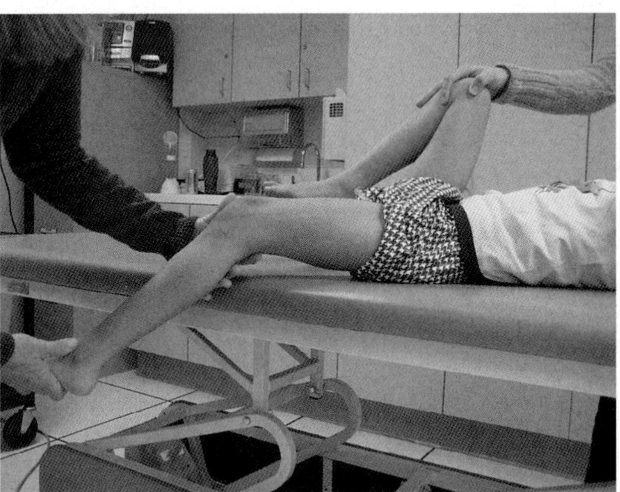

Figure 11.15 Hip flexion contracture is best assessed by using the Thomas test. The contralateral hip is flexed to flatten the lumbar spine and stabilize the pelvis. The residual flexion of the hip compared to the horizontal is the amount of hip flexion contracture that is present. (*Reproduced with permission from* Children's Orthopaedic Center, Los Angeles, CA.)

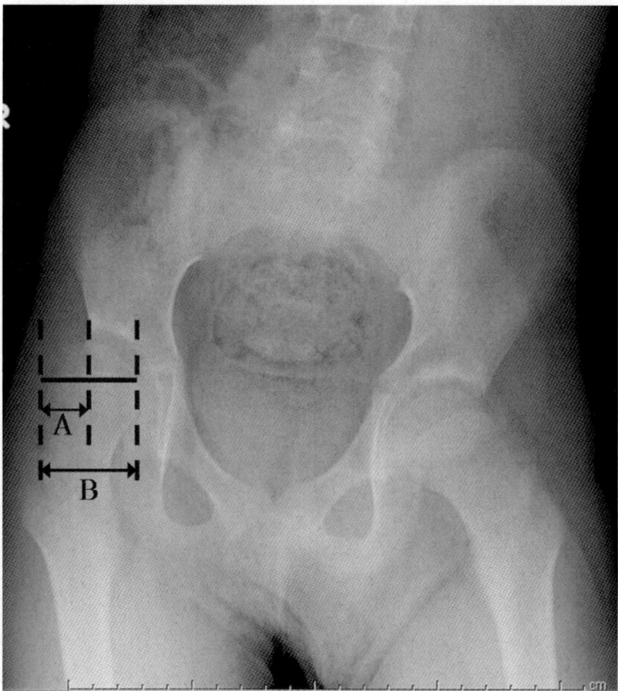

Figure 11.16 The migration index is calculated by dividing the width of the uncovered femoral head **(A)** by the total width of the femoral head **(B).** (*Reproduced with permission from* Children's Orthopaedic Center, Los Angeles, CA.)

General Treatment Principles

The management of CP is complex and is best accomplished as a team effort. Developmental pediatricians, neurologists, physical therapists, and orthotists all must participate in the overall decision-making process. Medical spasticity management may include oral muscle relaxants such as diazepam and baclofen. In severely involved patients, baclofen can be given intrathecally, where it has the advantage of more direct targeting, which allows for lower doses and less systemic CNS depression. Appropriate physical therapy and bracing can be extremely useful to maintain flexibility and delay the need for surgery. Botulinum toxin, a neurotoxin from *Clostridium botulinum,* prevents acetylcholine release at the neuromuscular junction. Although the effects last only for 3 to 6 months, the injections can be a useful adjunct to therapy and casting as a means to control peripheral spasticity. Selective dorsal rhizotomy, the cutting of certain dorsal spinal rootlets, is a neurosurgical procedure that can help in spasticity management. The ideal candidate is a young diplegic child with good selective motor control and ambulatory potential.

From a musculoskeletal standpoint, the spasticity associated with CP can affect multiple joints and may cause deformities at several levels. In the past, individual surgical problems were dealt with in isolation. This led to the "birthday syndrome," in which a child would come back nearly every year to have surgery on another part of the lower extremity. In reality, contractures or deformities at any level in the lower extremity affect the alignment and function at other levels. Failure to address the various problems simultaneously results in suboptimal treatment outcomes. Currently, single-event multilevel surgery (SEMLS) is the preferred treatment because it allows for simultaneous correction of multiple deformities, thus providing for optimal correction of the deformities while limiting the child to a single recuperative period.

Treatment of Regional Deformities

Hip

Surgery on the spastic hip accounts for the largest number of procedures performed on the pediatric hip. These children have significant hip disease initiated by muscle imbalance, the development of soft tissue contractures, subsequent bony deformity, and ultimately hip subluxation and dislocation. The contractures involve the hip flexors (psoas and rectus femoris) and the hip adductors. With progressive contracture, the axis of hip rotation is altered and secondary osseous changes develop. Femoral anteversion is present at birth, remains persistent in these children, and accentuates the rate at which hip subluxation and dislocation occur (Fig. 11.17). Radiographs of the spastic hip frequently are misinterpreted as demonstrating significant valgus, when in fact they are demonstrating anteversion. It is important to realize that children with CP are born with normal hips and that subsequent changes are the result of neuromuscular imbalance. Untreated, these hips may progress to severe subluxation or dislocation. Although it is somewhat controversial, there seems to be general agreement that a dislocated hip has a 50% chance of becoming painful. It is this observation, and the improved seating position, that makes the best argument for operative reconstruction of a subluxed or dislocated hip. Of course, the

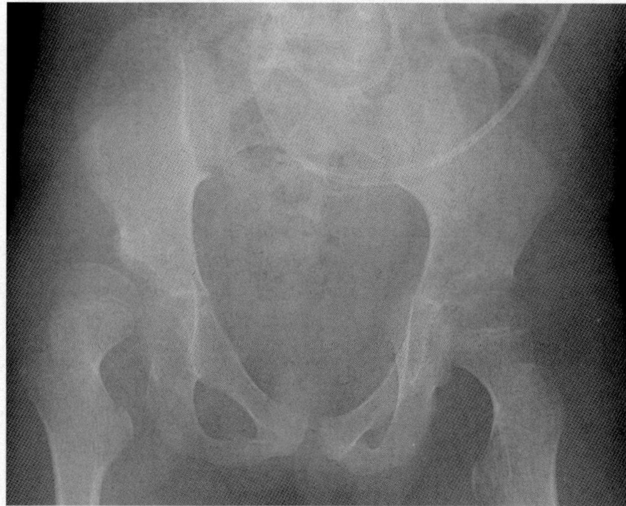

Figure 11.17 Anteroposterior radiograph of the pelvis in a child with spastic quadriplegic cerebral palsy. The right hip demonstrates severe subluxation and uncovering. (*Reproduced with permission from* Children's Orthopaedic Center, Los Angeles, CA.)

best way to manage these children is to prevent hip subluxation through early screening, spasticity management, and appropriate surgery.

Physical therapy, botulinum toxin injections, and abduction splinting can be effective to maintain hip range of motion and delay the need for surgery. In general, children who have less than 30 degrees of abduction and/or a migration index greater than 25% are at risk for progressive subluxation and should be treated with adductor tenotomy. If a coexisting hip flexion contracture exists, an iliopsoas recession should also be performed. For hips with more severe migration indices (>50%–60%), a varus derotational femoral osteotomy is warranted. The varus portion of the osteotomy helps redirect the femoral head so that it points more directly at the acetabulum, whereas the derotation is useful for correcting femoral anteversion. In severe cases, a formal open reduction may be required, and, if acetabular dysplasia exists, a reshaping acetabuloplasty such as the Dega or San Diego pelvic osteotomy should be included (Fig. 11.18). The management of the older child with a fixed, painful, spastic hip dislocation is problematic. Total hip replacement has been reportedly successful, but in many patients, arthroplasty is not considered appropriate. Resectional type arthroplasties, such as proximal femoral resection with soft tissue interposition, can be effective but are clearly a salvage option.

Knee

Hamstring contractures and the subsequent development of knee flexion deformities are common problems in the spastic child. Walking with flexed knees greatly increases the energy expenditure required for ambulation and can severely limit the functional abilities of children with CP (Fig. 11.19). Over time, excessive knee flexion can lead to patella alta, lengthening of the patella tendon, and patellofemoral pain. It is important to remember that crouched posture is not solely the result of knee flexion deformities: hip flexion contractures and calcaneus deformities of the foot both contribute to the overall positioning.

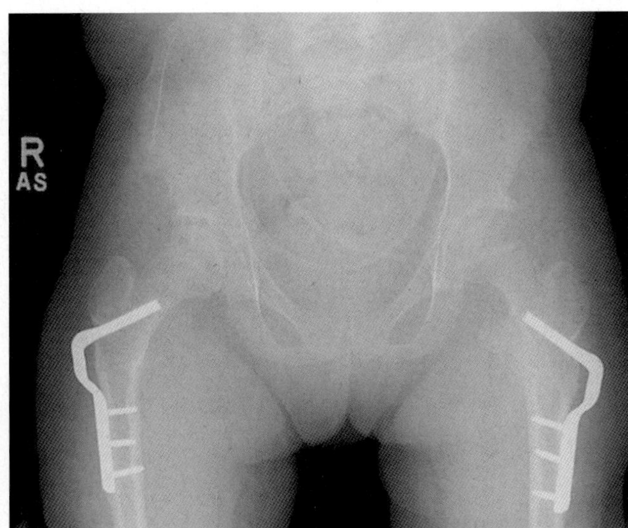

Figure 11.18 Postoperative anteroposterior radiograph after bilateral varus derotational femoral osteotomies and Dega pelvic osteotomies. (*Reproduced with permission from* Children's Orthopaedic Center, Los Angeles, CA.)

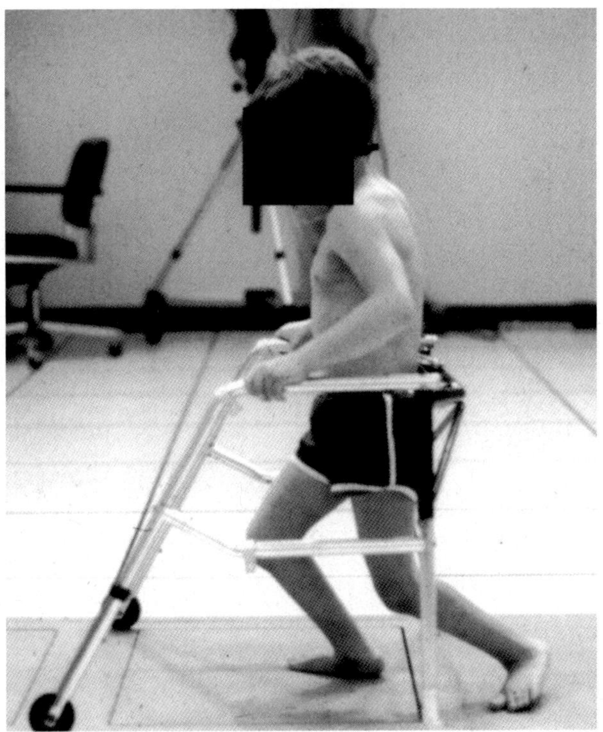

Figure 11.19 Crouched gait in a child with cerebral palsy. (*Reprinted with permission from* Morrissy RT, Weinstein SL. *Lovell and Winter's Pediatric Orthopaedics*. Philadelphia, PA: Lippincott Williams & Wilkins, 2006.)

Similar to the hip, conservative measures such as physical therapy, botulinum toxin injections, and nighttime extension splinting can be helpful to maintain flexibility and delay the need for surgery. Generally, hamstring lengthening is indicated for children with popliteal angles greater than 40 degrees. This procedure involves a tenotomy of the semitendinosus tendon and a fractional lengthening of the semimembranosus at the musculotendinous junction. Some surgeons also add a gracilis lengthening; in severe cases, a lengthening of the lateral hamstrings (i.e., biceps femoris) may also be necessary. If children have a stiff knee during the swing phase of gait along with overactivity of the rectus femoris in swing phase (based on gait analysis), the rectus femoris can be transferred to the distal hamstrings to help improve dynamic knee flexion.

In cases of fixed knee flexion contractures, a posterior capsulectomy or distal femoral extension osteotomy is occasionally necessary. Recently, some authors have advocated distal advancement of the patella tendon along with the extension osteotomy for those patients who have flexion contractures, patella alta, and patellofemoral pain (Fig. 11.20).

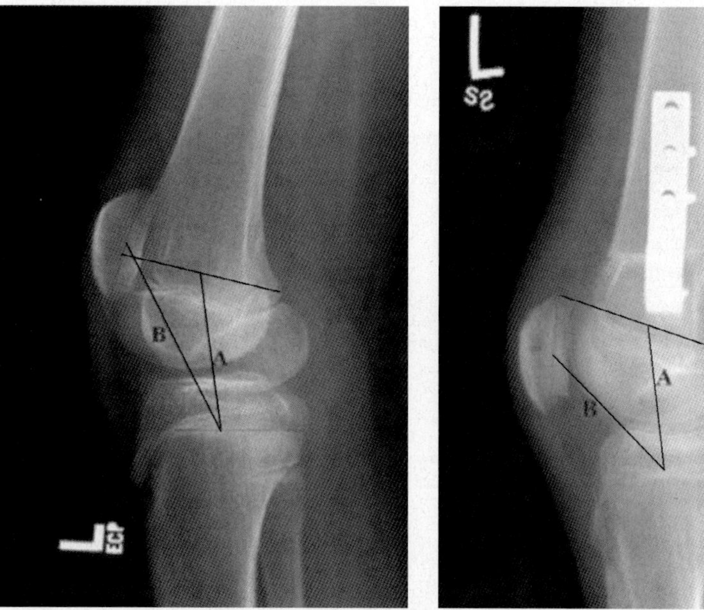

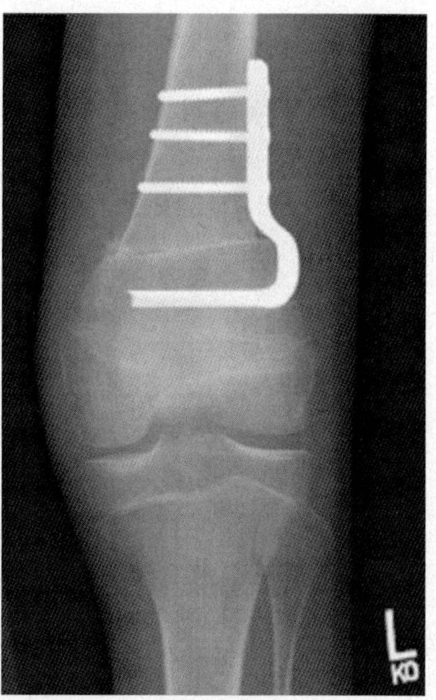

Figure 11.20 Preoperative **(A)** and postoperative **(B)** lateral radiographs and **(C)** postoperative anteroposterior radiograph of a left knee in maximum extension after treatment with distal femoralextension osteotomy with patellar advancement. The change in the patellar height can be quantified by relating the femur–tibia distance, (A), to the patella–tibia distance, (B). (*Reproduced with permission from* Stout JL, Gage JR, Schwartz MH, et al. Distal femoral extension osteotomy and patellar tendon advancement to treat persistent crouch gait in cerebral palsy. *J Bone Joint Surg.* 2008;90:2470–2484.)

Foot and Ankle

Equinus deformities of the ankle are probably the most common deformities seen in CP. Such positioning can lead to toe-walking and decreased functional ability. In hemiplegic children, equinovarus deformities are common, with the foot pointing down and in (Fig. 11.21). A recent study demonstrated that in one-third of these patients, the equinovarus deformity was due to overactivity of the posterior tibialis muscle; in another one-third, the cause was an overactive anterior tibialis muscle; and in the remaining one-third, the deformity was due to both muscles. Equinovarus at the ankle can lead to decreased toe clearance during swing, in-toeing, and tripping. Planovalgus is a common foot deformity seen in diplegic and quadriplegic children. At first, there is ligamentous laxity and a contracture of the heel cord. Over time, the forefoot begins to pronate and abduct and the hindfoot develops valgus (Fig. 11.22). As the deformity progresses, the posterior tibialis

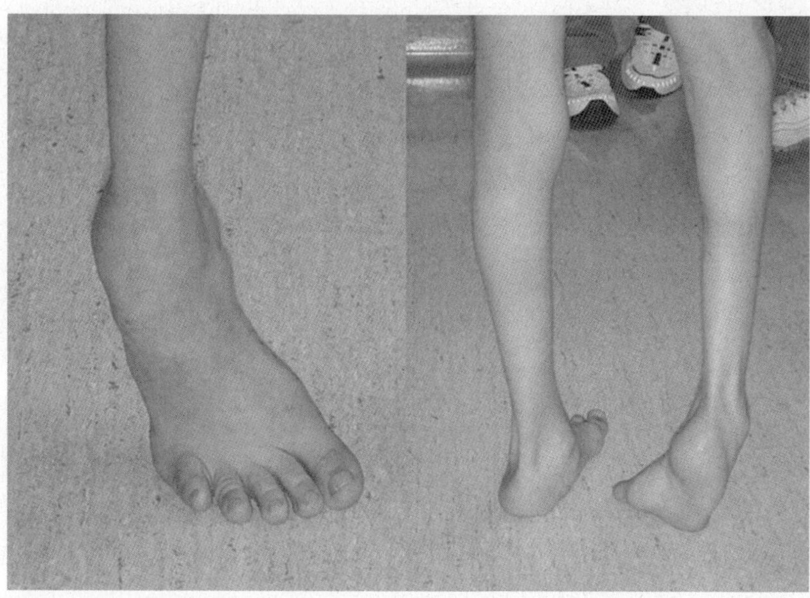

Figure 11.21 Typical appearance of an equinovarus foot in a patient with right-sided hemiplegic cerebral palsy. (*Reproduced with permission from* Children's Orthopaedic Center, Los Angeles, CA.)

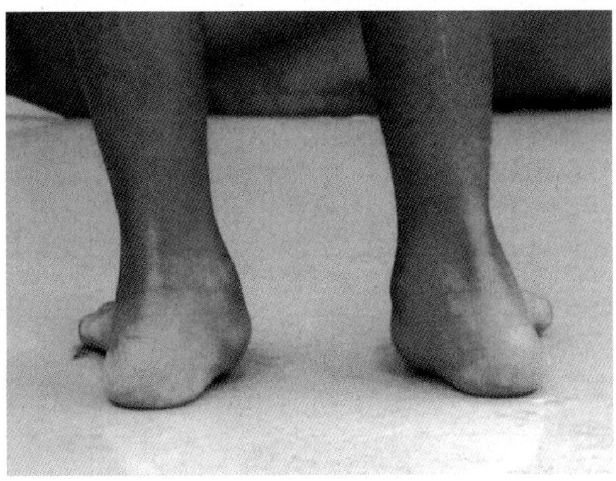

Figure 11.22 Bilateral posterior view of pes planovalgus. (*Reprinted with permission from* Morrissy RT and Weinstein SL. *Lovell and Winter's Pediatric Orthopaedics*. Philadelphia, PA: Lippincott Williams & Wilkins, 2006.)

stretches and becomes nonfunctional. These factors allow the foot to collapse through the arch. Spastic bunion deformity commonly complicates the planovalgus foot as the equinovalgus foot position often forces the medial border of the great toe into abduction.

For both equinus and equinovarus deformities, conservative measures should be exhausted before considering surgery. Botulinum toxin injections, physical therapy, stretching casts, and ankle–foot orthoses (AFOs) can be used to improve dorsiflexion or to maintain existing gains. It is important to remember that although the calf muscles are tight, they are also weak. Overzealous surgery can lead to overlengthening of the Achilles tendon, excessive weakness, and a calcaneus gait. Most children who require surgery for an equinus contracture can be treated with a gastrocnemius recession. This is performed at the musculotendinous junction and helps preserve more push off strength compared with open lengthening of the Achilles tendon (Fig. 11.23). For children who have dorsiflexion greater than 20 degrees short of neutral, an open sliding or Z-lengthening is probably warranted (Fig. 11.24). For children with equinovarus deformities, quantitative gait analysis is extremely useful to determine which muscle group is primarily responsible. For flexible deformities, a split

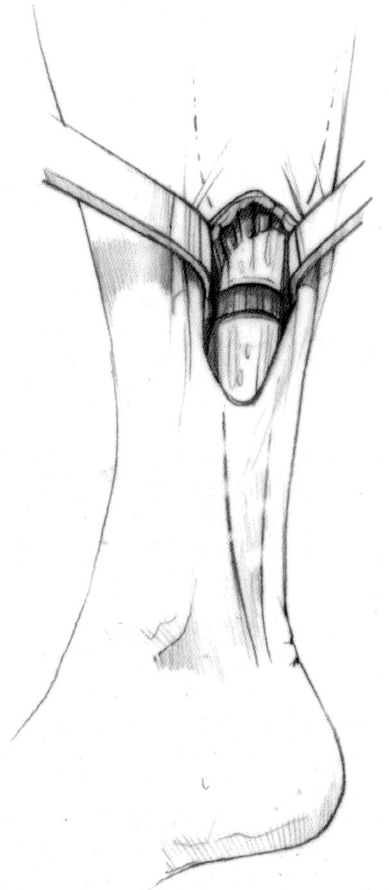

Figure 11.23 A gastrocnemius recession is performed by cutting the fascia (but not the muscle) at the musculotendinous junction. This technique helps preserve push-off strength. (*Reproduced with permission from* Skaggs DL, Tolo VT. *Master Techniques in Orthopaedic Surgery: Pediatrics*. Philadelphia, PA: Lippincott Williams & Wilkins, 2008.)

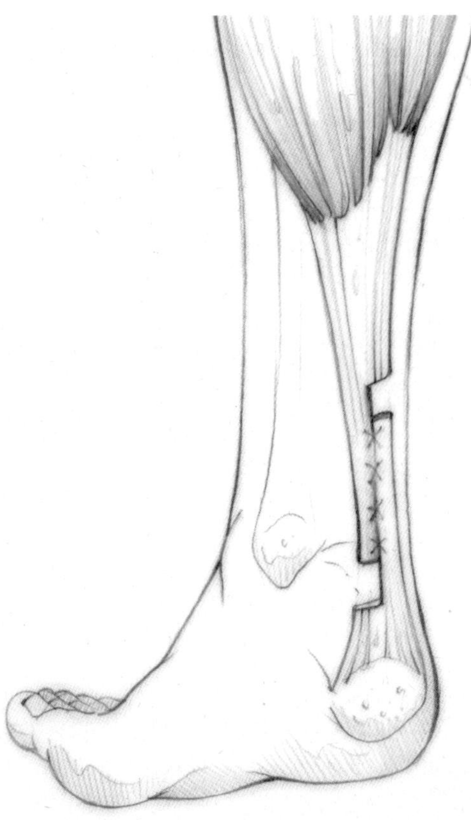

Figure 11.24 Z-lengthening of the Achilles tendon is indicated for more severe contractures. (*Reproduced with permission from* Skaggs DL, Tolo VT. *Master Techniques in Orthopaedic Surgery: Pediatrics*. Philadelphia, PA: Lippincott Williams & Wilkins, 2008.)

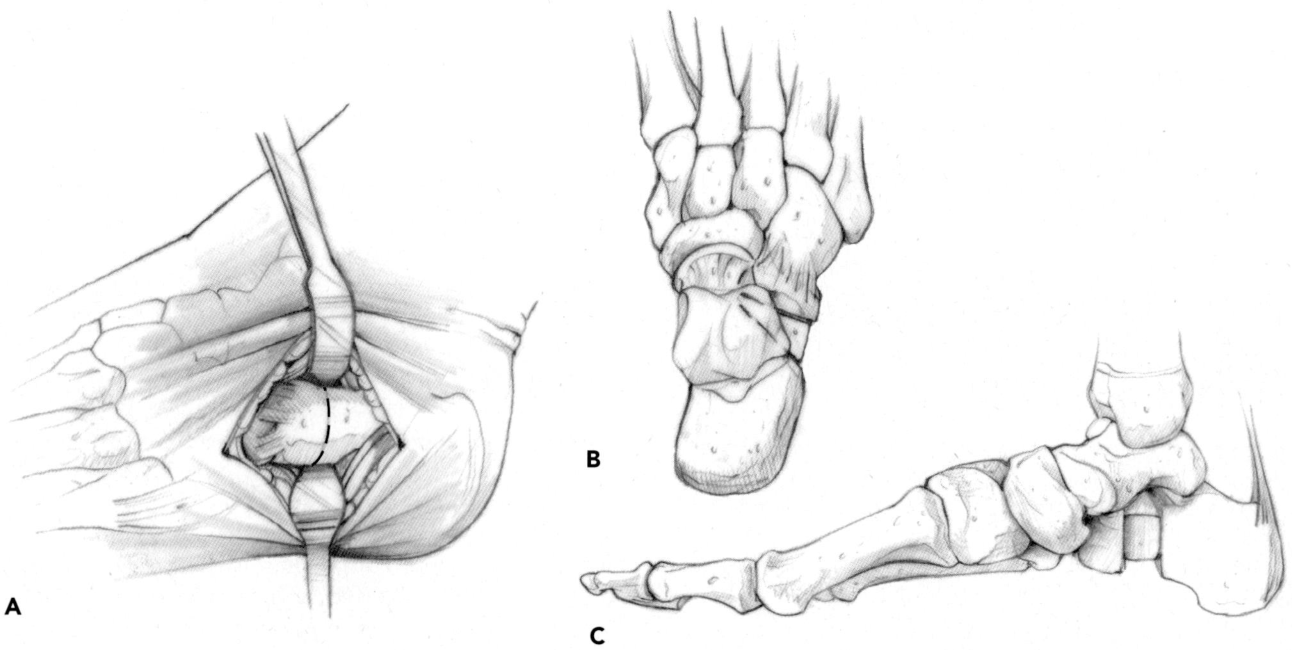

Figure 11.25 Calcaneal lengthening osteotomy. **(A)** The calcaneus is cut 2–2.5 cm proximal to the calcaneocuboid joint. **(B–C)** A trapezoidal bone graft is inserted to enhance talar coverage by the navicular. (*Reproduced with permission from* Skaggs DL, Tolo VT. *Master Techniques in Orthopaedic Surgery: Pediatrics.* Philadelphia, PA: Lippincott Williams & Wilkins, 2008.)

anterior tibial tendon transfer or split posterior tibial tendon transfer can help balance the foot. In more rigid deformities, a hindfoot osteotomy may also be necessary. Planovalgus feet that have failed bracing may be amenable to a lateral column lengthening. This procedure takes advantage of the windlass mechanism to develop an arch and correct the hindfoot. By placing a wedge of bone graft in the calcaneal neck, the previously short lateral column of the foot becomes elongated; this helps swing the foot into a more anatomic position (Fig. 11.25). For the spastic bunions, most authors feel that standard bunion procedures have an unacceptable rate of recurrence; and therefore, most prefer an arthrodesis of the first metatarsophalangeal (MTP) joint as a definitive procedure.

Upper Extremity

The upper extremity is also involved in patients with hemiplegic or quadriplegic CP. In mild cases, the extremity may lack some degree of coordination and selective muscle control; in severe cases, the extremity may be extremely spastic with the typical appearance of thumb-in-palm, wrist flexion, forearm pronation, and elbow flexion (Fig. 11.26). Although deformities may initially be dynamic, by the time children are 6 to 9 years of age, fixed contractures usually develop. The goals in treating the upper extremity are to improve its function as a helping hand; to improve its gross function in grasping, pinching, and releasing; and to improve its appearance. Occupational therapy is helpful for younger children to encourage the child to use the hand. Botulinum toxin and occasional splinting can help manage forearm and elbow contractures. Surgical techniques are available to correct the thumb-in-palm deformity, the instability of the first metacarpophalangeal joint, and the instability of the carpometacarpal joint of the thumb. Wrist flexion deformity has been managed by tendon transfers, tenodesis, and wrist fusion. In severe cases where improved

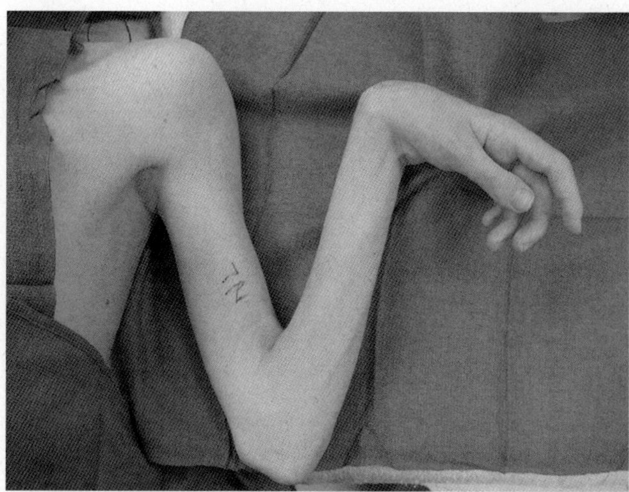

Figure 11.26 Clinical photograph demonstrating the characteristic appearance of a spastic upper extremity due to cerebral palsy. Note the elbow flexion, wrist flexion, and forearm pronation. (*Reproduced with permission from* Children's Orthopaedic Center, Los Angeles, CA.)

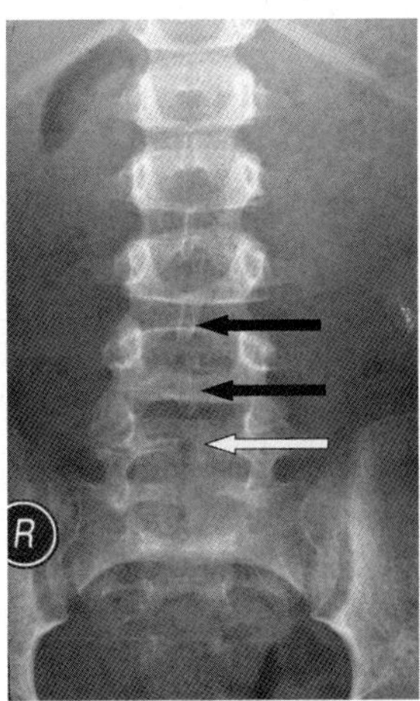

Figure 11.27 Spina bifida occulta. Spinous processes of L2 and L4 are visible (*black arrows*). An absent spinous process at L5 (*white arrow*) is consistent with spina bifida occulta in an otherwise normal child. (*Reproduced with permission from* Skaggs DL, Flynn JM. *Staying Out of Trouble in Pediatric Orthopaedics*. Philadelphia, PA: Lippincott Williams & Wilkins, 2006.)

hygiene and appearance are the primary goals, selective tenotomies may be appropriate.

Myelodysplasia (Spina Bifida)

Pathophysiology

Myelodysplasia, or spina bifida, can be divided into two main categories: spina bifida occulta and spina bifida cystica. Spina bifida occulta is present in 10% to 15% of the normal population and typically consists of a benign defect in one or more of the posterior elements of L4–S1 (Fig. 11.27). Although rarely associated with lower spinal cord malformations (e.g., lipomeningocele and tethered cord), spina bifida occulta usually does not cause any problems. Spina bifida cystica occurs when some portion of the spinal canal herniates through the defect in the posterior elements (Fig. 11.28). Depending on the contents of the herniated cyst, the lesion may be termed a meningocele (meninges only), myelocele (spinal cord and/or nerves), or a myelomeningocele (both). The underlying etiology for myelodysplasia is the failure of the neural tube to close during early embryogenesis. This results in a flaccid paralysis below the level of the lesion. Unlike CP, both motor and sensory functions are impaired. Although the areas of involvement are initially flaccid, it is not unusual for some children to develop spasticity in the lower extremities later in life.

Classification

Myelodysplasia is generally classified by the level of neurologic function. The functional motor level is the best means of determining prognosis, predicting deformities, and planning treatment. Thoracic level patients have almost no ambulatory potential because they lack active hip

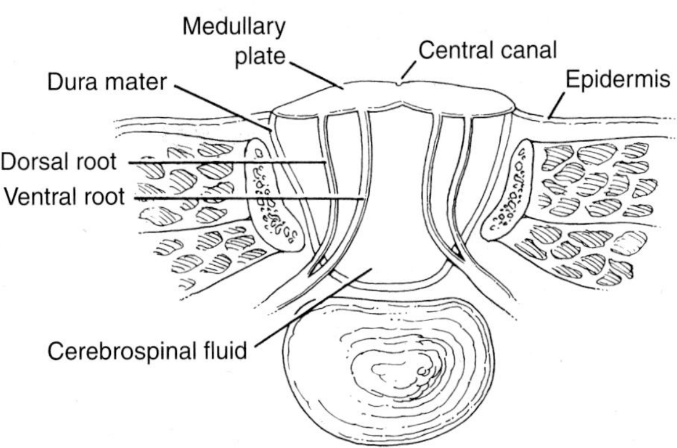

Figure 11.28 Cross section of myelomeningocele. The abnormal cord is part of the sac that has herniated out of the canal. (*Reprinted with permission from* Morrissy RT, Weinstein SL. *Lovell and Winter's Pediatric Orthopaedics*. Philadelphia, PA: Lippincott Williams & Wilkins, 2006.)

flexion and knee extension (Fig. 11.29). Major issues in these children include the development of scoliosis and/or kyphosis. Prolonged wheelchair use can lead to knee flexion contractures, and feet may develop equinus deformities, which inhibits the ability to fit shoes. High lumbar level children (L1–L2) have variable amounts of hip flexion and adduction (Fig. 11.30). These patients have similar issues as the thoracic level children but may be at increased risk for hip dislocation if there is unopposed force of the iliopsoas and adductor muscles.

Midlumbar myelodysplasia (L3–L4) patients have good quadriceps function, which is the most important determinant of ambulatory ability (Fig. 11.31). As a result, they generally are able to walk with the use of lower extremity orthoses and crutches. These patients are at high risk for hip dislocation. The implication of this is unclear since dislocated hips have not been proven to limit the ambulatory potential of these children. Because of significant abductor weakness, midlumbar myelodysplasia patients usually walk with a Trendelenburg gait and may develop valgus at the knee from the lateral sway. Although the quadriceps are functional, knee flexion contractures can develop, which lead to crouched gait and increased energy requirements

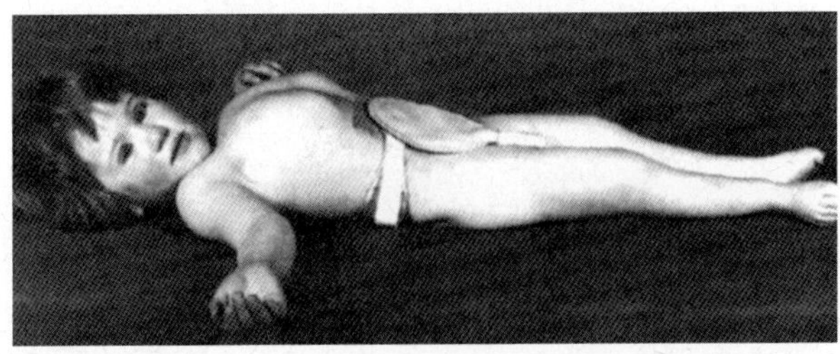

Figure 11.29 Patients with thoracic-level myelodysplasia lack motor function in the lower extremities and the legs lie, as they did in birth, in a position dictated by the effect of gravity. (*Reproduced with permission from* Broughton NS. *Textbook of Paediatric Orthopaedics*. London, England: WB Saunders, 1997.)

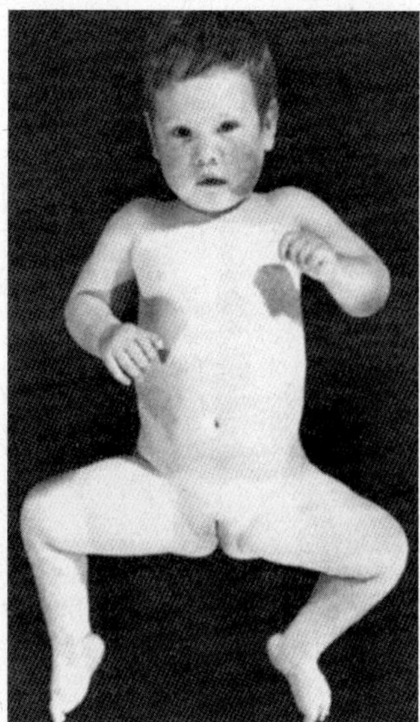

Figure 11.30 L1-level myelodysplasia. Flexion and external rotation of the hips leads to an abducted posture from weak hip adductors. (*Reproduced with permission from* Broughton NS. *Textbook of Paediatric Orthopaedics.* London, England: WB Saunders, 1997.)

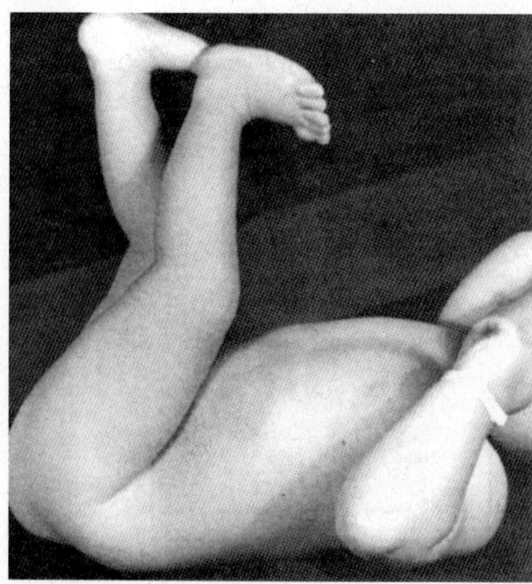

Figure 11.32 L5-level myelodysplasia. There is flexion at the hip and some flexion at the knee. Unopposed action of ankle dorsiflexors (due to weakness of the gastroc-soleus complex) leads calcaneus position of the feet. (*Reproduced with permission from* Broughton NS. *Textbook of Paediatric Orthopaedics.* London, England: WB Saunders, 1997.)

for ambulation. Patients with L4 function will often develop a calcaneal foot deformity due to the unopposed action of the anterior tibialis.

Low lumbar level (L5) myelodysplasia have adequate hip abductor strength in addition to strong quadriceps function (Fig. 11.32). Most of these patients walk with a minimal Trendelenburg gait using only AFOs. The incidence of hip problems is low as is the incidence of scoliosis. Foot deformities, however, occur quite frequently; the most common deformity is a calcaneal foot due to poor gastroc-

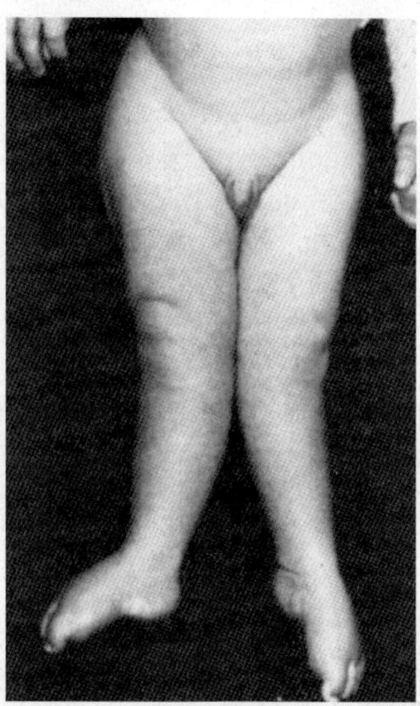

Figure 11.31 L3-level myelodysplasia: the hips lie in flexion and adduction and the knees in extension or hyperextension from functioning quadriceps. There is no muscle power in the feet. (*Reproduced with permission from* Broughton NS. *Textbook of Paediatric Orthopaedics.* London, England: WB Saunders, 1997.)

soleus function. The final type of myelodysplasia is sacral level involvement. These children are generally free of spine and hip problems and ambulate well with AFOs. Foot abnormalities are seen in 50% and may be cavus, equinus, or valgus deformities. One of the major issues in these children is skin breakdown since they are quite functional but have decreased sensation on the plantar aspect of their feet.

Presentation

Myelodysplasia is generally diagnosed in utero. The identification of elevated α-fetoprotein in the maternal blood (sampled at 15–16 weeks) will trigger an amniocentesis. This study is quite definitive for the diagnosis of open neural tube defects. Ultrasound has also been shown to be reasonably sensitive in the diagnosis of myelodysplasia. Either way, most cases are identified prior to birth. After delivery (usually by cesarean section to avoid trauma to the herniated sac), closure of the myelomeningocele is performed by a neurosurgeon within 48 hours of birth. Approximately 80% of these children will survive their first year, and 60% to 70% of patients will survive to adulthood. Patients are generally referred for orthopaedic care at an early age to determine ambulatory potential and manage lower extremity deformities.

History and Physical Examination

A careful history may elicit one or more of the major risk factors for spina bifida, including history of myelodysplasia in a previous pregnancy, inadequate folic acid intake, maternal diabetes, and maternal use of valproic acid during the pregnancy. Folic acid supplementation, in particular, is the best means of preventing neural tube defects and is a standard component of all prenatal vitamins.

The most important goal of the physical examination is to classify the neurologic level. This can be a far more challenging task than it first appears. In newborns, spontaneous motion can be the result of reflex rather than voluntary movement. Even in older children, there may be gaps in the neurosegmentation levels and side-to-side differences, which can make classification difficult. Periodic manual muscle testing of the entire lower extremity (preferably by the same examiner) is the most accurate method to determine the functional neurologic level. In addition, skin (particularly around the feet) should be carefully examined for signs of redness and potential breakdown. Much like a diabetic patient, children with myelodysplasia lack protective sensation and can easily develop severe pressure ulcers.

General Treatment Principles

Much like children with CP, patients with myelodysplasia are best treated by a multidisciplinary team of pediatricians, urologists, physical therapists, orthotists, neurosurgeons, and orthopaedic surgeons. Neurosurgical consultation, in particular, is extremely important. Many children with myelodysplasia have shunts placed to control hydrocephalus; proper follow-up is necessary to prevent shunt blockages and the resulting hydrocephalus. In addition, children should be monitored for signs of a tethered cord. These signs include changes in bladder function, increased lower extremity spasticity, sudden change in motor strength and function, or rapidly progressive scoliosis (Fig. 11.33). It is important to remember that almost all children with spina bifida will show signs of spinal cord tethering on magnetic resonance imaging (MRI) due to scar tissue created at the time of myelomeningocele closure. However, if clinical findings support the MRI, then patients should be referred for neurosurgical detethering. This is generally successful in stabilizing the neurologic status and preventing further deterioration.

Any surgery on patients with myelodysplasia should be performed in a latex-free environment. Because of early exposure to latex during infancy, the incidence of latex allergy is increased in these children and has been reported to be as high as 3% to 7%. Performing surgery in a normal latex environment can risk an anaphylactic reaction with a precipitous drop in blood pressure.

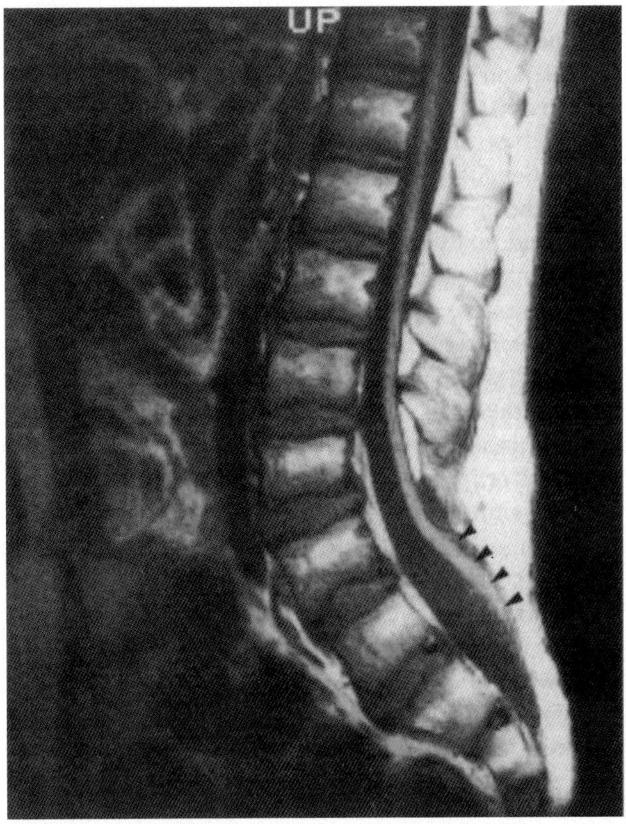

Figure 11.33 Magnetic resonance image of a child with myelomeningocele shows radiographic evidence of a tethered cord. The conus medullaris is low-lying. The placed is displaced posteriorly and is adherent to the dorsal dura (*arrowheads*). (*Reproduced with permission from* Weinstein SL. *The Pediatric Spine.* Philadelphia, PA: Lippincott Williams & Wilkins, 2001.)

Another issue that commonly arises in the care of children with myelodysplasia is pathologic fracture due to severely osteoporotic bone. These fractures often present with warmth, redness, and swelling but minimal pain due to impaired sensation (Fig. 11.34). As a result, they can

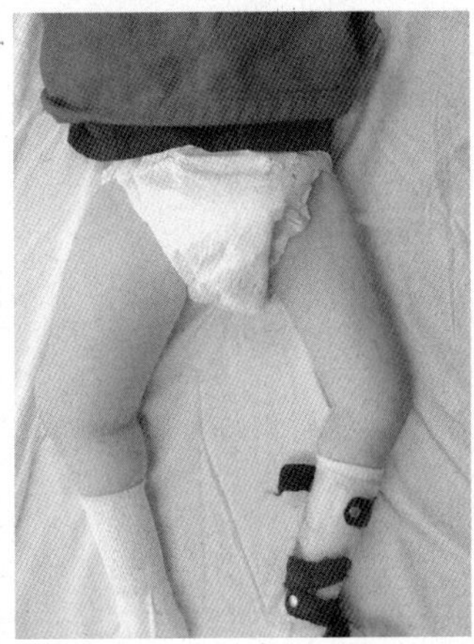

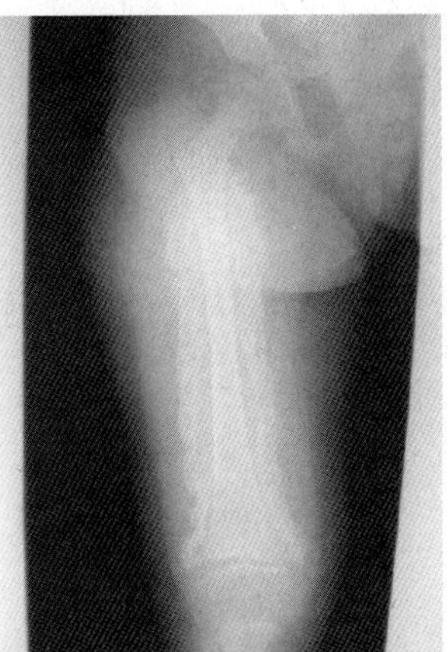

Figure 11.34 **(A)** This boy with thoracic level spina bifida presented with a chief complaint of painless leg swelling. The leg was warm to touch. **(B)** Radiographs demonstrate copious new bone formation. (*Reproduced with permission from* Skaggs DL, Flynn JM. *Staying Out of Trouble in Pediatric Orthopaedics.* Philadelphia, PA: Lippincott Williams & Wilkins, 2006.)

often be confused with osteomyelitis or other infection. Generally, careful palpation will reveal some crepitus and inflammatory markers such as erythrocyte sedimentation rate (ESR) or C-reactive protein (CRP) level will be normal. These fractures are best managed by short-term immobilization, often with soft bulky dressings or soft braces. Prolonged immobilization in hard casts may lead to worsened osteopenia and skin breakdown.

Treatment of Regional Deformities

Spine

The incidence of scoliosis or kyphosis in children with spina bifida is approximately 60%. The vast majority of these patients have thoracic or high lumbar neurologic levels. Since these patients are usually nonambulatory, the goal of treatment is to preserve adequate sitting balance and limit progression of the deformity. In general, curves less than 20 degrees should be observed. Curves between 20 and 40 degrees can be treated with a brace to improve upright posture and sitting balance; however, there is no evidence that the use of a spinal orthosis will prevent curve progression. Curves greater than 50 degrees and pelvic obliquity that adversely affects sitting balance may require spinal fusion and instrumentation (Fig. 11.35). Surgery is generally performed from both an anterior and posterior approach because the lack of posterior bony elements can increase the risk of pseudarthrosis if bone graft is applied only posteriorly. Even with this dual approach, complications are common: 10% to 30% of patients will have loss of neurologic or bladder function, pseudarthrosis, or wound breakdown after surgery.

Kyphosis can occur in 10% to 15% of children with myelodysplasia. Untreated, progressive kyphosis can lead to loss of truncal height, decreased pulmonary function, and skin breakdown over the apex of the deformity. Kyphectomy, which involves vertebral resection at the apex of the kyphotic segment followed by instrumentation usually to the pelvis, is the most accepted form of surgical treatment. Prior to any surgery in which the thecal sac may be ligated, it is important to verify proper function of the shunt to prevent acute hydrocephalus.

Hips

Management of hip dislocation and hip dysplasia in children with myelodysplasia is somewhat controversial but should be guided by the level of neurologic function. Thoracic level patients rarely dislocate their hips because they lack any muscle activity about the hip. Children with upper lumbar level spina bifida usually should not undergo procedures to reconstruct dislocated hips since the status of the hip will not affect the child's ability to walk. If hip flexion contractures are greater than 20 to 30 degrees and

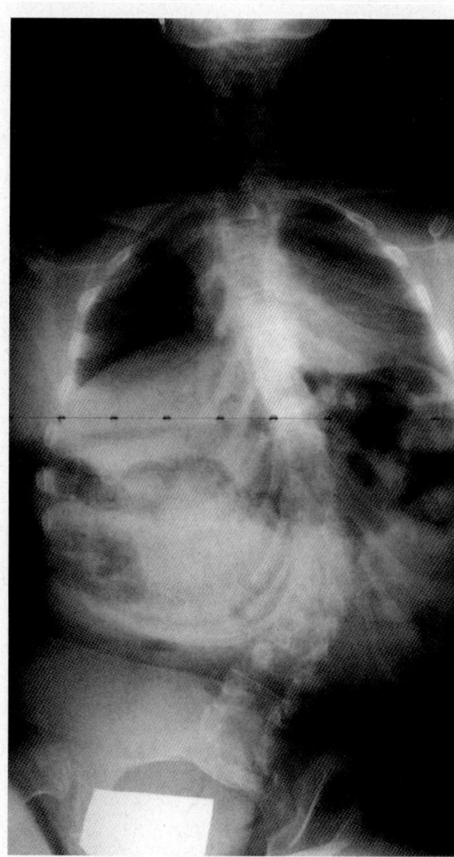
A

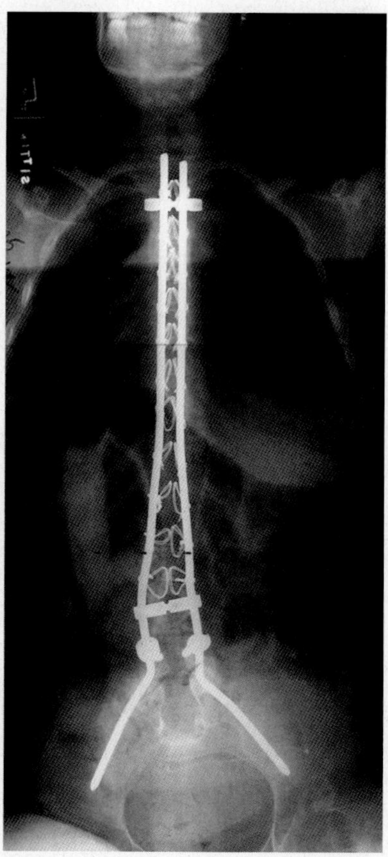
B

Figure 11.35 Thirteen-year-old boy with thoracic-level myelomeningocele and progressive curve and with pelvic obliquity. Posterior spine fusion to the pelvis stabilizes the curve and provides a level-sitting platform. (*Reprinted with permission from* Morrissy RT, Weinstein SL. *Lovell and Winter's Pediatric Orthopaedics*. Philadelphia, PA: Lippincott Williams & Wilkins, 2006.)

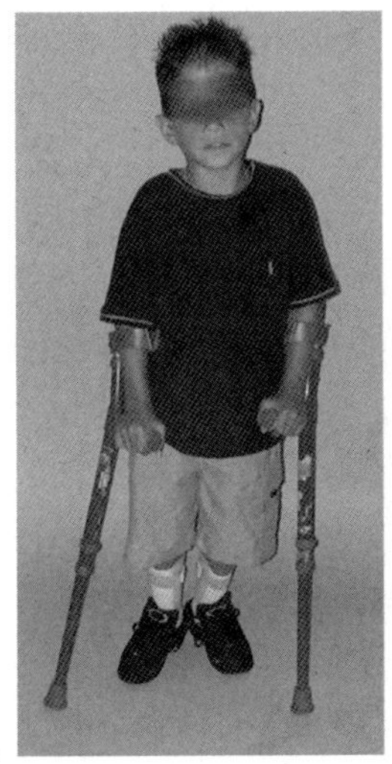

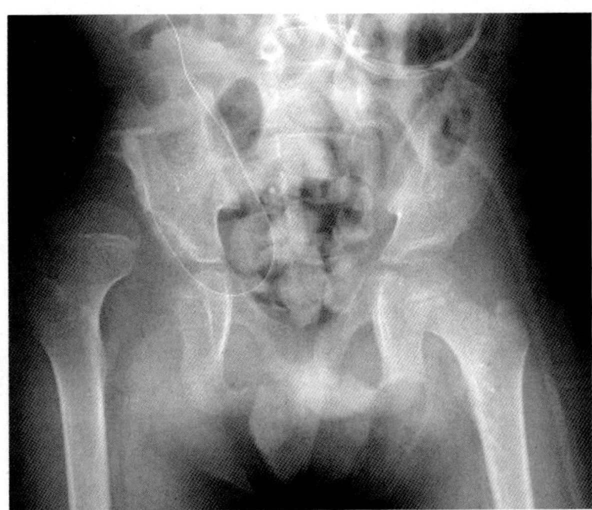

Figure 11.36 Community ambulatory child with L3 functional level. He uses Lofstrand crutches and bilateral ankle–foot orthoses. He is able to ambulate with a swing-through gait despite a unilaterally dislocated hip. (*Reprinted with permission from* Morrissy RT, Weinstein SL. *Lovell and Winter's Pediatric Orthopaedics*. Philadelphia, PA: Lippincott Williams & Wilkins, 2006.)

interfere with bracing, hip flexor release or anterior capsulotomy may be indicated. In children with midlumbar myelodysplasia, most authors prefer to leave bilateral dislocations untreated. Select unilateral dislocations may warrant reduction; however, this is controversial because of the high incidence of recurrent dislocation (Fig. 11.36). Again, any hip contracture that interferes with bracing or walking should be released. Low lumbar and sacral level spina bifida are at low risk for hip dislocation since muscle forces around the hip are well balanced. For those dislocations that do develop, anterior releases and bony surgery should be performed as needed to achieve a stable, concentric hip reduction.

Knee

Several different knee deformities may develop in spina bifida. Extension contracture, flexion contracture, and valgus deformity have all been reported depending on the specific pattern of muscle function. Knee flexion contractures are common, particularly in patients with thoracic or upper lumbar spina bifida. If a child predominantly uses a wheelchair, treatment may not be necessary; however, if the deformity interferes with bracing or ambulation, then posterior soft tissue release and/or distal femoral extension osteotomy is indicated. Patients with midlumbar myelodysplasia are at high risk for severe knee valgus due to their Trendelenburg gait. Crutches along with knee–ankle–foot orthoses (KAFOs) can help protect the knees in these patients.

Foot and Ankle

Foot deformities are extremely common in spina bifida, occurring in up to 75% of patients. In patients with higher levels of involvement, equinus contractures, vertical talus, and rigid clubfoot deformities predominate. The goal of treatment is a supple, plantigrade foot that easily accommodates shoewear. Since most children will require braces, tenotomies (with excision of a tendon segment) are preferred over tendon lengthenings since flail extremities are easier to deal with than recurrent deformities. Simple equinus contractures are best treated with an open Achilles tenotomy. A vertical talus will require open reconstruction with release of the tight anterior structures. Open reduction of the talonavicular joint with pin fixation is the norm. Clubfoot deformities can be initially treated with early manipulation and casting; however, a higher percentage of patients will require open release compared with idiopathic clubfeet. In certain severe cases, a talectomy may be required as a salvage option. In children with mid to low lumbar myelodysplasia, calcaneal foot deformities are more common due to unopposed pull of the anterior tibialis muscle. These children are best treated with tenotomy and bracing since transfers of the anterior tibialis tendon have not been shown to provide added benefit. Equinovarus and equinovalgus deformities may also be seen. Equinovarus deformity is best treated by release of the posterior tibialis tendon; a calcaneal osteotomy can be added for cases of residual hindfoot varus. Equinovalgus feet that fail bracing can be treated by peroneal and calcaneal lengthening. Sacral level patients can also have equinus or valgus but may also develop cavus deformities. If this latter deformity is supple, release of the peroneus longus and plantar fascia may control the deformity. In more severe cases, a dorsiflexion osteotomy of the first ray or even a calcaneal osteotomy may be necessary.

Charcot–Marie–Tooth Disease

Charcot–Marie–Tooth (CMT) disease is the most common form of hereditary motor sensory neuropathy. Other neuropathies are primarily adult diseases without orthopaedic implications; thus, they are not included in this section. CMT disease itself is actually a group of different diseases with different genotypes but similar phenotypes.

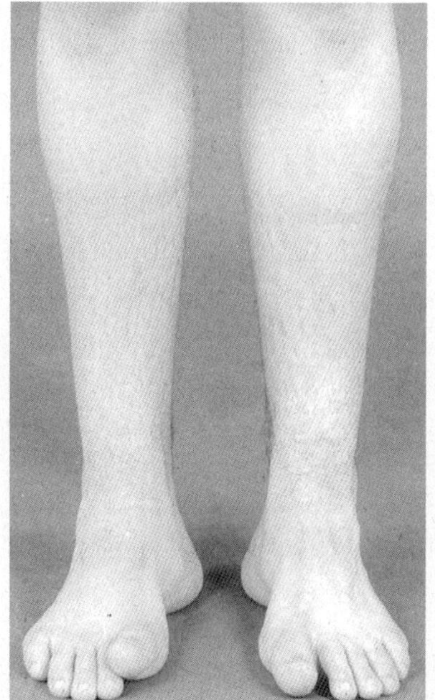
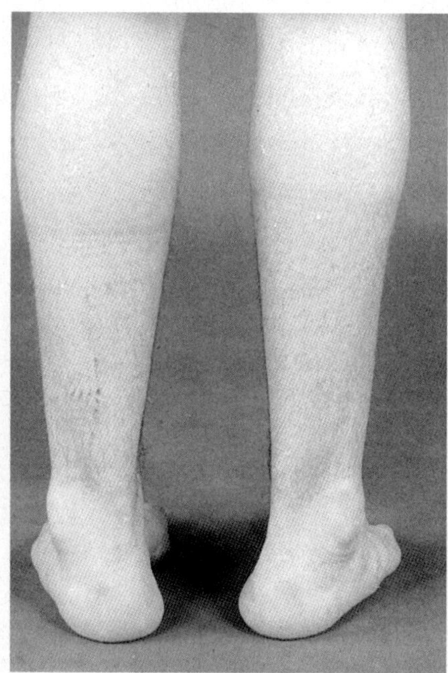
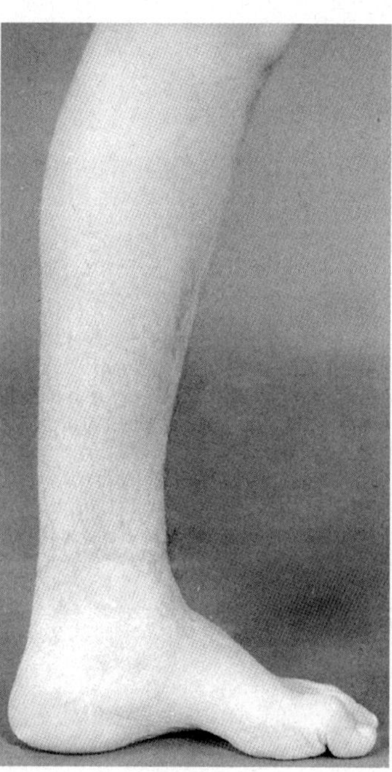

A,B C

Figure 11.37 **(A)** Front view of the lower legs and feet of a 16-year-old boy with Charcot–Marie–Tooth disease. His calves are thin, and he has symptomatic cavus feet. Clawing of the toes is minimal. **(B)** Posterior view demonstrates moderate heel varus. **(C)** The cavus foot deformity is most apparent when viewed from the medial side. A mild flexion deformity of the great toe interphalangeal joint is present. (*Reprinted with permission from* Morrissy RT, Weinstein SL. *Lovell and Winter's Pediatric Orthopaedics*. Philadelphia, PA: Lippincott Williams & Wilkins, 2006.)

Pathophysiology and Classification

CMT disease is a progressive demyelinating peripheral neuropathy. Two major forms of CMT disease exist. The type I form is usually inherited in an autosomal dominant fashion and accounts for 60% to 80% of all patients with CMT disease. The genetic defect in 70% of type I patients is a duplication in the peripheral myelin protein (PMP) gene on chromosome 17. This mutation causes an overproduction of the protein, which causes demyelination of the peripheral nerves. The type II form of CMT disease is inherited in an X-linked fashion and is responsible for 20% to 40% of all cases. Type II CMT disease is caused by a deficiency in the connexin gene, which codes for a gap junction protein that enhances conduction between peripheral nerves. Deficiency in this protein results in an axonal neuropathy.

Presentation

Patients with CMT disease typically present during early adolescence with progressive cavovarus deformities of the feet, although some children present during preschool years (Fig. 11.37). This characteristic foot deformity is caused by the pattern of peripheral demyelination in CMT disease, which affects distal muscle groups first. This results in weakness of the tibialis anterior, peroneus brevis, and foot intrinsics with relative preservation of peroneus longus, posterior tibialis, and toe extensor strength. The discrepancy in strength allows the peroneus longus to overpower its antagonist, the tibialis anterior, leading to plantarflexion of the first ray. In an effort to balance the tripod of the foot, the hindfoot compensates by swinging into a varus position. As a result, patients tend to overload the lateral border of the foot and often present with calluses in this location. Atrophy and contracture of the intrinsic musculature of the foot lead to clawing of the toes, contracture of the plantar fascia, and elevation of the arch. Plantar flexion of the metatarsal heads can lead to increased pressure in these areas and metatarsalgia.

The innervation of the hand is also affected in CMT disease, which leads to intrinsic atrophy. Hand involvement, however, usually does not develop until late in the disease course. Hip dysplasia can also occur, perhaps because of subtle weakness of the proximal musculature about the hip. Scoliosis is seen in up to 37% of adolescents with CMT disease. Deformities are similar to idiopathic curves but tend to have more kyphosis than lordosis.

Physical Examination

Observation of gait in patients with CMT disease usually reveals a drop foot during swing. A steppage gait can develop, which is characterized by hyperflexion of the knee and hip in an attempt to help clear the foot. Toe extension during swing can also be seen as this helps compensate for the weakness of the primary ankle dorsiflexors. Lower extremity examination will reveal diminished deep tendon

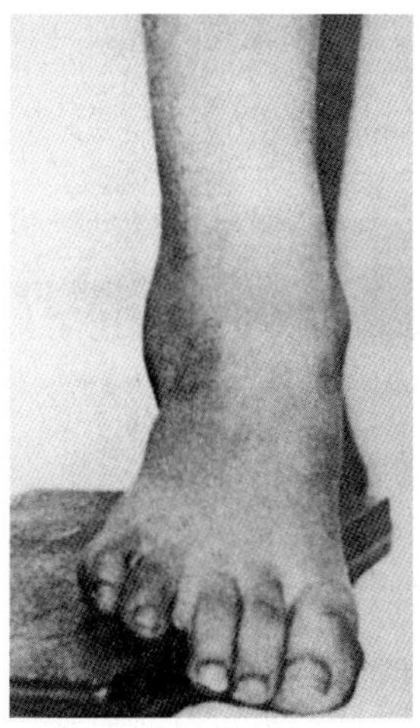
A

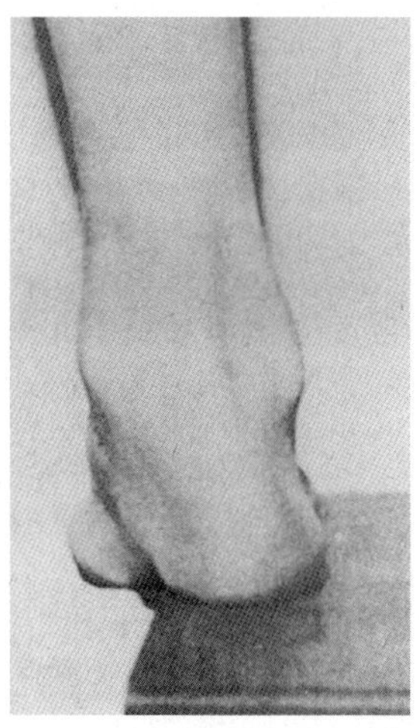
B

Figure 11.38 The Coleman block test for determination of hindfoot flexibility. The flexible varus deformity of the hindfoot will correct to valgus when the plantar flexed first metatarsal is allowed to drop down off the edge of the block of wood. Failure to correct to valgus indicates the need for surgical correction of the hindfoot, in addition to the procedures on the forefoot. (*Reproduced with permission from* Coleman SS, Chestnut WJ. A simple test for hindfoot flexibility in the cavovarus foot. *Clin Orthop.* 1977;123:60–62.)

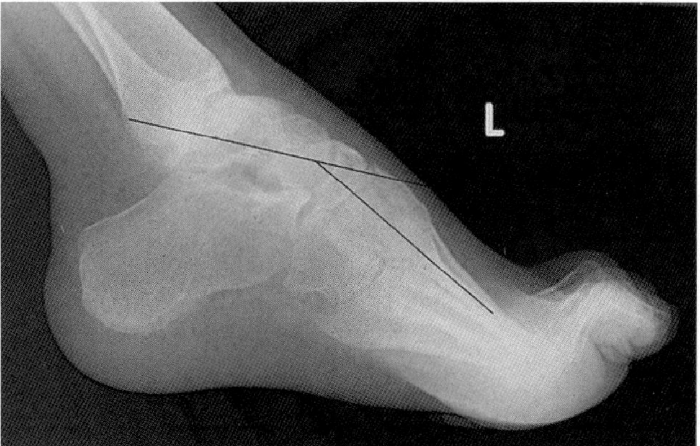

Figure 11.39 Lateral radiograph of a typical cavovarus foot due to Charcot–Marie–Tooth disease. Note the increase in Meary angle from plantar flexion of the forefoot relative to the hindfoot. (*Reproduced with permission from* Children's Orthopaedic Center, Los Angeles, CA.)

reflexes and decreased calf circumference from global atrophy. Distal sensation is usually decreased to all modalities.

Evaluation of the cavovarus foot in patients with CMT disease begins with a careful assessment of the skin. Lateral overloading may cause large calluses along the lateral border of the foot. As patients may be partially insensate, it is important to identify areas at risk for breakdown to prevent the formation of deep ulcers. To develop an appropriate treatment plan for the cavovarus foot, it is essential to assess the flexibility of hindfoot. This is best done by using the Coleman block test (Fig. 11.38). This test is performed by having the patient stand on a block with the head of the first metatarsal hanging free over the medial edge. If the hindfoot varus is a compensatory response to plantar flexion of the first ray (i.e., flexible), the heel will correct to neutral on the block. If the varus deformity has become rigid over time, it will not correct.

Hands should be examined by manual muscle testing to monitor atrophy of the intrinsic musculature. In certain cases, hand dynamometers may be useful to provide quantitative data about the change in muscle strength over time. Hips should be ranged and examined for subtle instability. A standard scoliosis examination should be performed (see pediatric spine section) to screen for spinal deformity.

Radiographs

Standing lateral radiographs of the foot will demonstrate the characteristic findings of the cavovarus deformity. Usually, the angle of the inferior border of the calcaneus and the tibia exceeds 30 degrees, indicating that the ankle is actually dorsiflexed not plantarflexed. The apparent equinus of the deformity is usually due to plantar flexion of the forefoot rather than plantar flexion of the ankle (Fig. 11.39). This can be quantified by measuring Meary angle, the angle between the long axis of the talus and the first metatarsal shaft. In the normal foot, these two axes line up and the angle is 0 degrees. With progressive plantar flexion of the first ray, Meary angle increases. Hibb angle is defined as the angle between the long axis of the calcaneus and the first metatarsal shaft. Normally, this angle is greater than 150 degrees; increased cavus results in a smaller Hibb angle.

Special Studies

Genetic testing is helpful to diagnose many patients with CMT disease. However, since many different genotypes cause a similar disorder, a negative test does not rule out the disease. In general, patients suspected of having CMT disease should be referred to a neurologist for electromyography and nerve conduction testing. Patients with type I CMT disease tend to have decreased nerve conduction velocity on electrodiagnostic studies. In patients with type II CMT disease, electrodiagnostic studies typically demonstrate normal or minimally decreased conduction velocity but decreased amplitude of action potentials. In rare cases, the combination of genetic testing and electrophysiologic testing is still insufficient to make the diagnosis. In these situations, a sural nerve biopsy should be performed.

Differential Diagnosis

Many different diseases can produce a similar cavovarus foot deformity as does CMT disease, including spinal cord tumors, Friedreich ataxia, diastematomyelia, and syringomyelia. A unilateral cavovarus deformity, in particular, should raise suspicion of spinal cord pathology. It is important to remember that a cavovarus foot is never normal; if a patient does not have electrodiagnostic or genetic

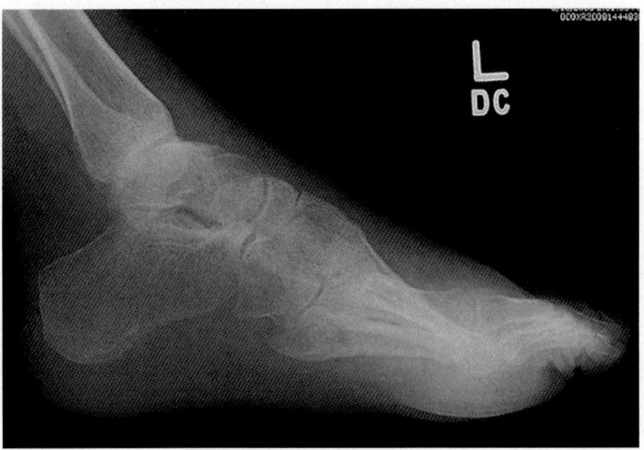

Figure 11.40 Postoperative lateral radiograph of the same foot from Figure 11.39 after dorsiflexion osteotomy of the first metatarsal, plantar fascia release, and transfer of the extensor hallucis longus from the toe to metatarsal head (Jones transfer). Note the improvement in the Meary angle and the clawing of the great toe. (*Reproduced with permission from* Children's Orthopaedic Center, Los Angeles, CA.)

evidence to support the diagnosis of CMT disease, a spinal MRI should be ordered.

Treatment

There is no clinically proven medical treatment that halts or slows progression of CMT disease. Treatment, therefore, is directed at correcting deformities and maximizing function. Conservative measures are largely unsuccessful for treating cavovarus feet. Occasionally, shoe inserts can be useful to elevate the metatarsal heads and reduce the symptoms of metatarsalgia. In patients with significant drop foot gait, an AFO can improve toe clearance by preventing excessive plantar flexion during swing phase. Early in the disease process, transfer of the peroneus longus to the peroneus brevis and plantar fascia release can remove the deforming forces and limit progression of the deformity. Once the first ray becomes plantar flexed, a dorsiflexion osteotomy of the first metatarsal along with tendon transfers is necessary to balance the foot. If the hindfoot is rigid, as assessed by the Coleman block test, a calcaneal osteotomy should be added to correct the varus deformity (Fig. 11.40). Claw deformities of the great and lesser toes can be managed by Jones transfers of the extensor tendons to the metatarsal necks. A triple arthrodesis should be avoided if at all possible, although in severe, rigid deformities, it may be the only means of obtaining a plantigrade foot.

Muscular Dystrophy

Muscular dystrophies are a group of genetic diseases, characterized by progressive deterioration of skeletal muscle. By definition, the pathologic changes are confined to the muscle itself with no abnormalities seen in the peripheral nerves. This section will focus on the most common and representative muscular dystrophy seen in children, Duchenne muscular dystrophy.

Pathophysiology

The underlying etiology of Duchenne muscular dystrophy is the absence of the muscle protein dystrophin. The gene responsible for producing dystrophin resides on the X chromosome, which explains why Duchenne muscular dystrophy is inherited in an X-linked manner. In most cases, the genetic defect is a frameshift mutation that results in no protein being produced. Normally, dystrophin acts to stabilize the cell membrane cytoskeleton in muscle. Absence of dystrophin leads to increased fragility of the myofiber membrane and leakage of cellular contents into the extracellular space. This creates an inflammatory response that results in loss of muscle fibers and fibrosis of the muscle.

Presentation and Natural History

Boys with Duchenne muscular dystrophy typically present between ages 3 and 8. The presenting complaint is often a waddling gait, difficulty with stairs, clumsiness, or progressive lower extremity weakness. The muscle weakness that develops is symmetric, and proximal muscles are affected before distal muscles. Lower extremity involvement tends to precede upper extremity involvement by 3 to 5 years. Weakness of hip extensors leads to anterior pelvic tilt and compensatory lumbar lordosis. In addition, weak abductors can result in a Trendelenburg gait. Children may also present with ankle equinus due to fibrosis and contracture of the gastroc-soleus complex. As the disease progresses, walking becomes more difficult. By age 12, most patients with Duchenne muscular dystrophy become full-time wheelchair users. Once patients lose the ability to ambulate, scoliosis develops in the vast majority of patients. Spinal deformity tends to progress relentlessly and can complicate worsening pulmonary function due to a weakened diaphragm and chest wall. Death usually occurs in the second or third decade of life due to respiratory failure.

History and Physical Examination

Since Duchenne muscular dystrophy demonstrates X-linked inheritance, any family history of the disease should prompt an early workup. One-third of all cases, however, are due to spontaneous mutations, so lack of family history is by no means conclusive. Any young boy who has a history of progressive clumsiness or weakness should be evaluated for muscular dystrophy. While tripping and falling are common parental complaints in the orthopaedic clinic, a boy who is falling more frequently than he did in the past should be taken seriously.

Observation of the child walking may reveal a waddling gait due to lumbar lordosis and abductor weakness.

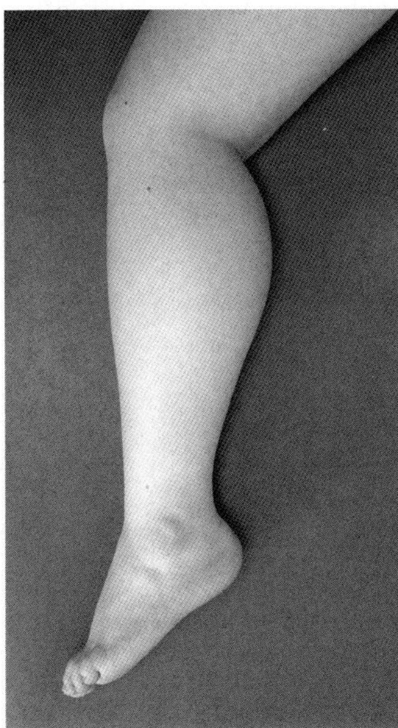

Figure 11.41 Pseudohypertrophy of the calf in the setting of weakness suggests Duchenne muscular dystrophy. (*Reproduced with permission from* Skaggs DL, Flynn JM. *Staying Out of Trouble in Pediatric Orthopaedics.* Philadelphia, PA: Lippincott Williams & Wilkins, 2006.)

Toe-walking can also be seen from fibrosis and contracture of the triceps surae. Although the gastroc-soleus muscle is weaker than normal, the muscle belly often appears enlarged. This finding is termed "pseudohypertrophy," is present in approximately 85% of children with Duchenne muscular dystrophy, and results from fibro-fatty replacement of the muscle fibers (Fig. 11.41). In these cases, range-of-motion testing of the ankle will reveal decreased ankle dorsiflexion, although a true equinus contracture does not typically develop for several years.

Careful manual muscle testing of children with Duchenne muscular dystrophy will reveal weakness in the proximal muscle groups. The most classic and useful screening test for Duchenne muscular dystrophy is the Gowers sign. This test is performed by asking the child to sit on the floor of the examining room and to stand up quickly without assistance. Patients with muscular dystrophy and proximal muscle weakness will have difficulty completing this task and will often use their upper extremities to help extend their knees and hips. Children who appear to "walk" their hands up their legs to help raise the trunk into an upright position have a positive Gowers sign (Fig. 11.42).

As the disease progresses, children often develop knee and hip flexion contractures. As the child becomes more dependent on a wheelchair, the spine should be carefully monitored for signs and symptoms of scoliosis.

Diagnostic Studies

If a diagnosis of muscular dystrophy is suspected, the first step is to measure the creatine kinase level in the blood. In normal patients, the creatine kinase level is less than 300 U/L; patients with muscular dystrophy can have values greater than 10,000 U/L. Children with elevated blood creatine kinase levels should be referred for genetic testing, which can yield a definitive diagnosis in up to 95% of patients. For those few patients in whom the diagnosis is still uncertain after genetic testing, a muscle biopsy may be necessary. By performing a Western blot test on the biopsy specimen, one can determine conclusively whether or not dystrophin is present.

Differential Diagnosis

The differential diagnosis of Duchenne muscular dystrophy includes other forms of muscular dystrophy and myotonic dystrophy. Becker muscular dystrophy is a more benign disease that also results from a mutation in the dystrophin gene. In contrast to Duchenne disease, the deletion in Becker muscular dystrophy results in either a truncated dystrophin molecule or lower amounts of normal dystrophin. Becker muscular dystrophy is characterized by similar pathology but a milder disease course than Duchenne muscular dystrophy.

Limb girdle muscular dystrophy actually refers to a large group of muscle diseases that are characterized by progressive muscle deterioration, predominantly in the muscles of the pelvic and shoulder girdle. Most cases are inherited in an autosomal recessive manner; onset of symptoms is often in late adolescence or early adulthood. In general, the clinical course is more benign than in Duchenne muscular dystrophy. Genetic tests for dystrophin abnormalities will

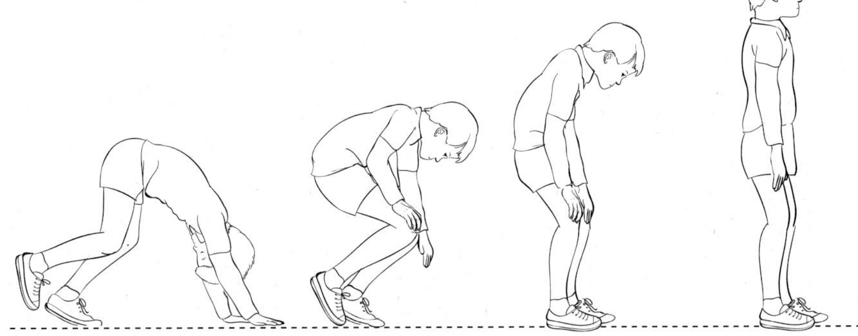

Figure 11.42 Weakness of proximal muscles from muscular dystrophy causes children to use their upper extremities to manually assist in knee extension and to achieve an upright stance. (*Reproduced with permission from* Skaggs DL, Flynn JM. *Staying Out of Trouble in Pediatric Orthopaedics.* Philadelphia, PA: Lippincott Williams & Wilkins, 2006.)

be negative, but muscle biopsy will yield a definitive diagnosis.

Facioscapulohumeral dystrophy is inherited as an autosomal dominant trait. It has a highly variable age of onset and severity. Weakness typically involves the shoulder girdle and facies. Classically, patients demonstrate an inability to whistle.

The most common form of myotonic dystrophy in children is congenital myotonic dystrophy. The disease is caused by a trinucleotide repeat on a noncoding region of chromosome 9. This results in deficient amounts of myotin protein kinase, which is important in ribonucleic acid metabolism. These children have profound hypotonia at birth and often require ventilator assistance to breath in the newborn period. Those who survive become progressively stronger and can usually walk independently by age 5. In this period, equinus contracture is common similar to patients with Duchenne muscular dystrophy. The two diagnoses, however, are easily distinguished on the basis of the history of hypotonia and developmental delay and the location of the weakness. Patients with myotonic dystrophy typically demonstrate distal weakness rather than the proximal weakness that characterizes Duchenne disease. Two other distinguishing features of myotonic dystrophy are the presence of myotonia (maintenance of muscle contraction even after the patient tries to relax) and the characteristic drooping face.

Treatment

The most promising medical treatment for Duchenne muscular dystrophy is the use of corticosteroids. Steroids are thought to alter the disease process by stabilizing the myofiber membrane and reducing the inflammatory response caused by leaking cell contents. Several recent studies have proven the efficacy of corticosteroids in prolonging ambulatory ability, preserving pulmonary function, and delaying the onset of scoliosis. In one study, one-third of patients receiving treatment were still walking at 18 years of age. Subjects in the treatment group were also found to have 40% greater forced vital capacity and a 50% lower rate of scoliosis than controls. The benefits of prolonged steroid therapy need to be balanced with the risks, which include weight gain, osteopenia, and cataracts.

Orthopaedic treatment generally focuses on maximizing ambulatory potential and treating spinal deformity. Early in the disease process, physical therapy and appropriate use of lower extremity orthoses can delay or limit the development of contractures. As muscle weakness worsens and contractures do develop, surgical release of hip and knee flexion deformities may help preserve walking ability, although such surgery is rarely performed currently. Equinus and equinovarus contractures resistant to conservative modalities can be treated with Achilles tendon lengthening and/or transfer of the posterior tibial tendon (Fig. 11.43). As children lose the ability to ambulate, adaptive equipment such as power wheelchairs are essential to allow independent function. One of the major responsibilities of an orthopaedic surgeon who cares for the child with Duchenne muscular dystrophy is the management of spinal deformity. Scoliosis tends to progress rapidly once the children become wheelchair bound. Unfortunately, this occurs at the same time that cardiac and pulmonary function decline sharply. As a result, the general recommendation is to operate on curves once they reach 20 degrees, before cardiopulmonary function decreases to a point that surgery is dangerous. Surgery usually consists of posterior spinal fusion and instrumentation to the pelvis.

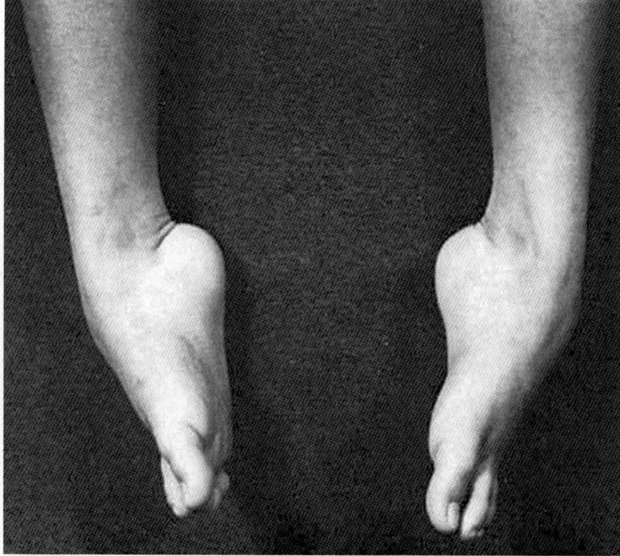

Figure 11.43 A boy with Duchenne muscular dystrophy and a severe equinovarus foot deformity. (*Reproduced with permission from* Chapman MW. *Chapman's Operative Orthopaedics.* 2nd ed. Philadelphia, PA: Lippincott Williams & Wilkins, 1993.)

Arthrogryposis

The term *arthrogryposis* actually applies to a variety of conditions that are characterized by decreased fetal movement and congenital joint contractures. Collectively, the incidence of arthrogryposis is approximately 1 per 3,000 live births. The incidence of amyoplasia, the most common type of arthrogryposis, is 1 in 10,000.

Pathophysiology

The final common pathway that causes arthrogryposis is decreased fetal movement, which leads to multiple joint contractures in utero. This lack of motion is most often due to failure of skeletal muscle development due to an underlying neuropathic or myopathic abnormality. Occasionally, space limitations in utero or maternal disease can limit fetal mobility. Although major joints initially develop normally from an embryological standpoint, lack of movement in utero leads to fibrosis of the joint capsules, atrophy and fibrosis of tendons, and an absence of skin creases. Several inheritance patterns have been described, but most cases of arthrogryposis are sporadic.

Classification

Arthrogryposis can be classified into three general categories based on the degree of nonmusculoskeletal organ involvement. Group 1 affects only the limbs and includes the most typical form of arthrogryposis, amyoplasia. Group 2 disorders affect the abdominal viscera and other organs in addition to the limbs. Examples include multiple pterygium syndrome and Larsen syndrome. Group 3 conditions involve the CNS in addition to the joint contractures.

Presentation

Children with classic arthrogryposis typically present soon after birth with multiple rigid joint contractures, absent skin creases, and atrophy of the limbs. The most common appearance is the waiter's tip posture caused by shoulder internal rotation and adduction, elbow extension, and wrist flexion (Fig. 11.44). Lower extremities usually demonstrate knees that are stiff in either flexion or extension and equinovarus deformities of the foot. One form of arthrogryposis, called *distal arthrogryposis,* presents with primarily hand and foot involvement (Fig. 11.45). These children have typical overlapping fingers and thumb in palm deformities in addition to clubfoot or vertical talus deformities. Unlike many syndromes, children with arthrogryposis have normal intelligence and actually perform better than average in school.

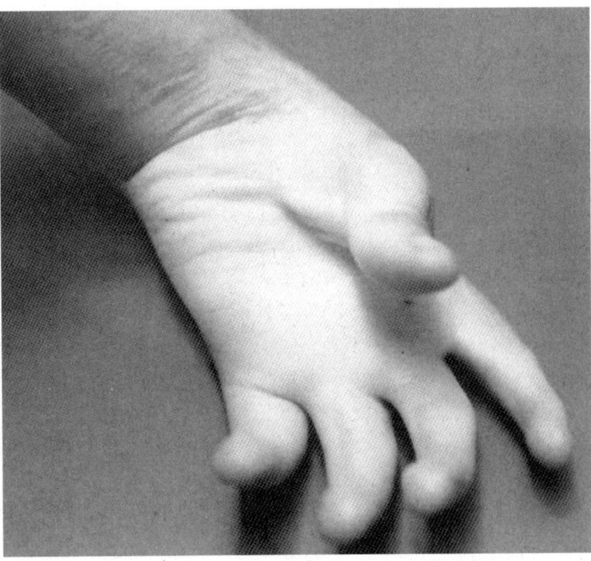

Figure 11.45 Distal arthrogryposis. Characteristic hand is the result of ulnar deviation at the metacarpophalangeal (MCP) joints. Notice the deeply cupped palm and webbing of the MCP joint of the thumb. (*Reproduced with permission from* Morrissy RT, Weinstein SL. *Lovell and Winter's Pediatric Orthopaedics.* Philadelphia, PA: Lippincott Williams & Wilkins, 2006.)

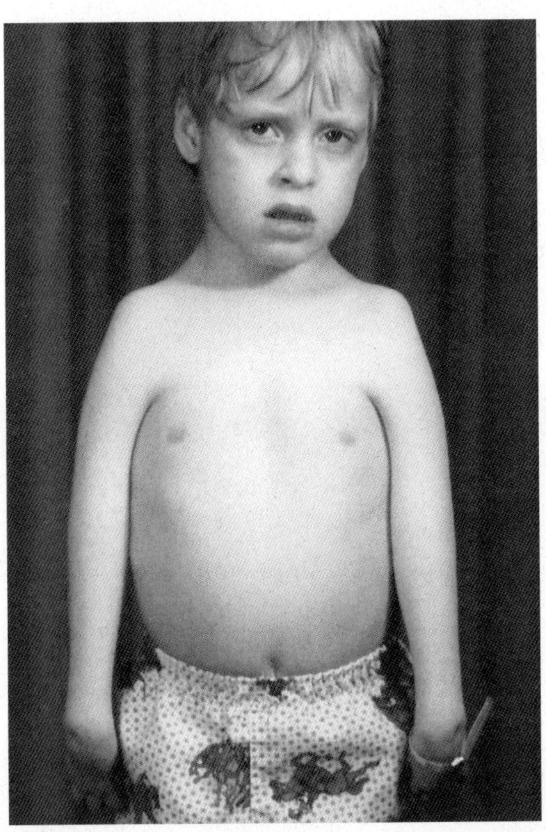

Figure 11.44 Arthrogryposis multiplex congenital. The picture shows the classic limb position and fusiform limbs lacking flexion creases. (*Reproduced with permission from* Morrissy RT, Weinstein SL. *Lovell and Winter's Pediatric Orthopaedics.* Philadelphia, PA: Lippincott Williams & Wilkins, 2006.)

History and Physical Examination

A thorough history should be performed to screen for other potential diagnoses including a number of genetic syndromes. Mothers often report decreased fetal movement in utero. Physical examination should determine which limbs are involved and what part of each limb is primarily affected. Cutaneous examination reveals absent skin creases and spindle-shaped extremities; sensory examinations are usually normal. The range of motion of each joint should be carefully measured. Affected joints usually demonstrate marked limitation of both active and passive motion although most retain at least a small degree of motion. Hip motion, in particular, is relatively spared especially in flexion and extension. Foot examinations typically reveal an equinovarus deformity from a rigid clubfoot or a rocker bottom deformity from a vertical talus. The spine should also be examined for evidence of scoliosis, which can occur in 2% to 70% of patients.

Differential Diagnosis

Since as many as 150 different syndromes can exhibit features of arthrogryposis; the most important step in making the diagnosis of amyoplasia or classic arthrogryposis is ruling out another known genetic syndrome. Multiple pterygium syndrome resembles amyoplasia in terms of the multiple joint contractures. However, dense, fibrotic webbing will be seen across the flexor surfaces of the knee in particular (Fig. 11.46). These children will also have genitourinary and craniofacial involvement. Larsen syndrome is officially considered a group 2 disorder but has many distinguishing features compared with amyoplasia. Children with Larsen syndrome have a characteristic facial appearance (flattened face, depressed nasal bridge, and widely set eyes) and joint dislocations due to ligamentous laxity. There is also a high incidence of spinal deformity in this condition, particularly cervical kyphosis. Occasionally, some skeletal dysplasias that exhibit restricted joint motion (e.g., diastrophic dysplasia) can be confused with amyoplasia. Usually, the findings of short stature and limb shortening are sufficient to differentiate these diagnoses.

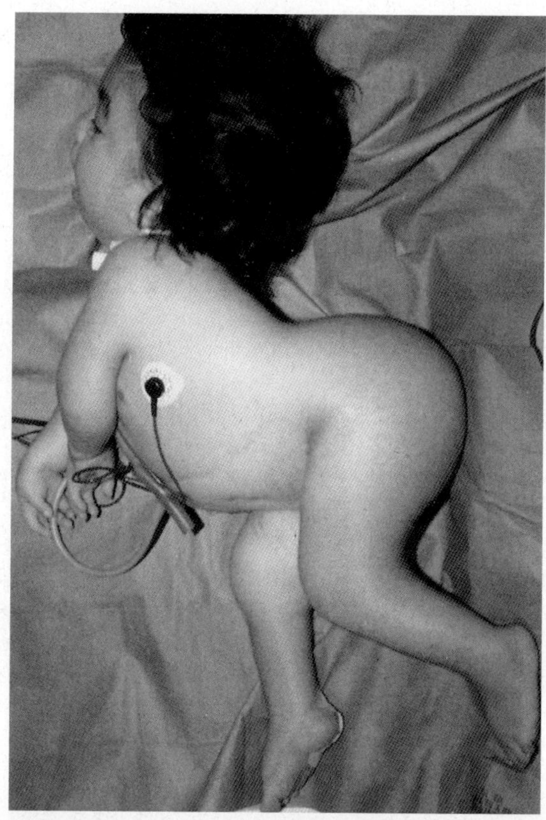

Figure 11.46 Multiple pterygium syndrome. Note the popliteal webbing. Severe limitation of trunk growth was caused by vertebral fusions and lordoscoliosis. (*Reproduced with permission from* Morrissy RT, Weinstein SL. *Lovell and Winter's Pediatric Orthopaedics.* Philadelphia, PA: Lippincott Williams & Wilkins, 2006.)

Treatment

The two major goals of treatment are maximizing ambulatory ability and upper extremity function to allow independent functioning for activities of daily living. It is important to remember that arthrogrypotic joints function poorly for a number of different reasons, including a thickened joint capsule, fibrotic tendons, atrophied muscles, tight skin, and poorly developed bursa. Therefore, even the best surgical options cannot be expected to recreate normal anatomy nor yield freely mobile joints.

Depending on the severity of the condition, early stretching and cast correction is useful to minimize deformity. Hip deformities are common in arthrogryposis and usually consist of dislocation and contracture (Fig. 11.47).

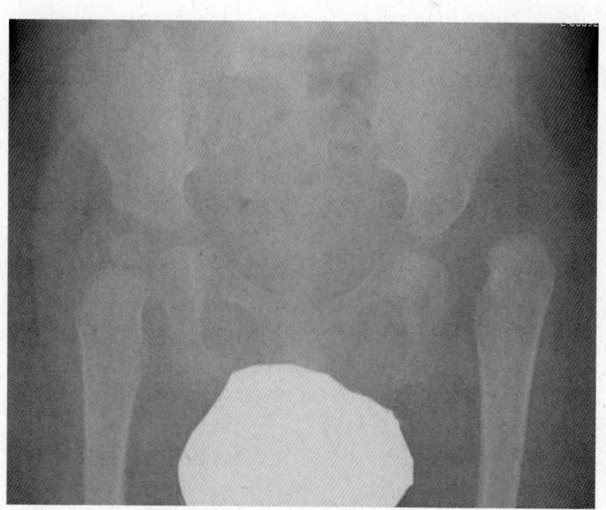

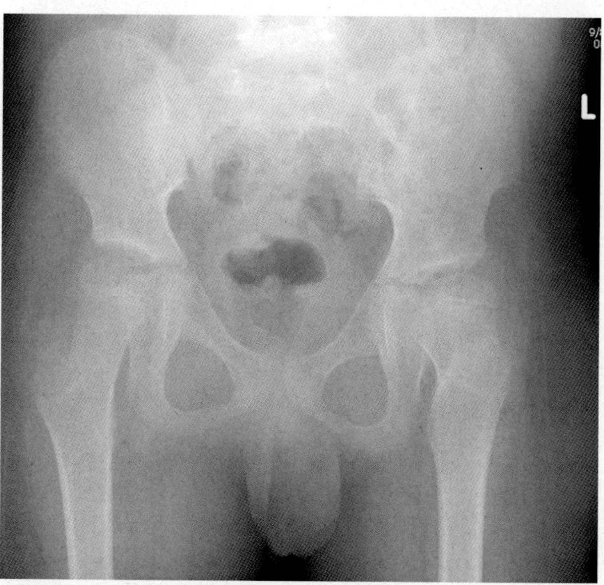

Figure 11.47 **(A)** Left teratologic hip dislocation in a child with arthrogryposis. **(B)** Seven years after open reduction, the left hip remains well reduced. (*Reproduced with permission from* Children's Orthopaedic Center, Los Angeles, CA.)

Unless they are severely contracted, most children should have open reductions performed for unilateral dislocations. The management of bilateral dislocations, however, is controversial; some authors prefer not to do surgery because of the risks of stiffness and osteonecrosis, whereas others routinely perform bilateral open reductions. Hip flexion contractures greater than 30 to 40 degrees warrant soft tissue release; abduction contractures can be treated by release of the iliotibial band with or without varus producing femoral osteotomy.

Knee flexion contractures greater than 20 degrees adversely impact a child's ambulatory ability. Most can be managed with some combination of posterior soft tissue release, femoral shortening, and/or distal femoral extension osteotomy. This latter procedure is extremely effective initially but carries a high recurrence risk as the distal femur tends to remodel back into flexion. Certain authors prefer gradual correction of knee deformities by using circular external fixators.

Several foot deformities can be seen in arthrogryposis, including calcaneovalgus feet or, more commonly, talipes equinovarus (clubfoot). Arthrogrypotic clubfeet are often extremely rigid. Serial manipulation and casting is occasionally successful, but most patients require radical posteromedial release around the age that the child begins to walk. Similarly, the treatment of the arthrogrypotic vertical talus is more often surgical, consisting of open release, reduction of the talonavicular joint, and pin fixation. In salvage cases of both clubfoot and vertical talus, a talectomy may be necessary.

Upper extremity surgery should be performed to improve self-care, improve self-feeding, and allow computer use. In the past, it was thought that one arm in full extension and one in flexion was best for function. Since grip strength is limited in both hands, most authors now prefer positioning both limbs to allow bimanual function. Shoulder contractures are best treated by derotation osteotomies of the humerus. Passive elbow motion can be improved by posterior elbow release and triceps lengthening. Active elbow flexion can sometimes be improved by pectoralis, latissimus, or triceps transfer. Wrist flexion deformities are typically treated by proximal row carpectomy, dorsal wedge osteotomies of the midcarpus, or wrist fusion. Thenar release and hand orthoses are used to treat thumb-in-palm deformities.

METABOLIC AND ENDOCRINE DISORDERS

Rickets

Pathophysiology

Rickets is a syndrome rather than a specific disease entity. Regardless of the specific etiology, the underlying cause of the disorder is the lack of available calcium, phosphorus, or both, ultimately resulting in the failure of bone and cartilage to mineralize appropriately. The effect of this impaired mineralization is most characteristically seen in the physis. Calcium is typically incorporated at the level of the zone of provisional calcification. Because of the lack of calcium, this zone is all but absent but the preceding zone of hypertrophy becomes enlarged and grossly distorted from "back-up" of the unmineralized physis. Along the trabeculae, osteoblastic activity is normal, so osteoid continues to be produced at a normal rate. The lack of normal mineralization, however, prevents osteoclastic mediated reorganization of this osteoid. As a result, the amount of osteoid builds up and remains disorganized, causing widening of the osteoid seams.

Normally, calcium metabolism is regulated primarily by vitamin D and parathyroid hormone (PTH) (Fig. 11.48). PTH is produced in the parathyroid glands in response to a drop in serum calcium or phosphate. Increasing PTH levels cause a release of calcium and phosphate from bone (where the vast majority of calcium is stored in the body) and increased calcium reabsorption in the kidney. Vitamin D production is stimulated by exposure to sunlight and the inactive form, 25-hydroxyvitamin D, is stored in the liver. Increasing PTH level also stimulates the activation of 25-hydroxyvitamin D to 1,25-dihydroxyvitamin D in the kidney. Activated vitamin D, in turn, stimulates increased absorption of calcium in the gastrointestinal tract and the proximal tubule of the kidney. Any abnormality in this complex system that decreases serum calcium or phosphate levels can lead to rickets.

Classification

Rickets is classified on the basis of the specific etiology. Nutritional rickets (vitamin D–deficient rickets) is the most classic form of the disease. Although rare in the developed world due to the fortification of milk products, nutritional rickets can still occur in those who are exclusively breast-fed and are sheltered from sun exposure. Vitamin D–dependent rickets has two forms: type I and type II. Type I disease is caused by a deficiency in α-hydroxylase, the enzyme that converts the inactive form of vitamin D to the active form in the kidney. Type II disease results from a defect in the intracellular receptor for active vitamin D. The most common form of rickets is vitamin D–resistant rickets, also known as *familial hypophosphatemic rickets*. This X-linked disorder causes impaired renal tubular reabsorption of phosphate. Other causes of rickets or rickets-type conditions include renal osteodystrophy (osteomalacia from renal disease), hypoparathyroidism (low production of PTH), and pseudohypoparathyroidism (lack of effect of PTH at the target cells).

Presentation and Physical Examination

Children with rickets have generalized muscular weakness, lethargy, and irritability. Motor developmental milestones such as sitting and walking may be delayed. The child

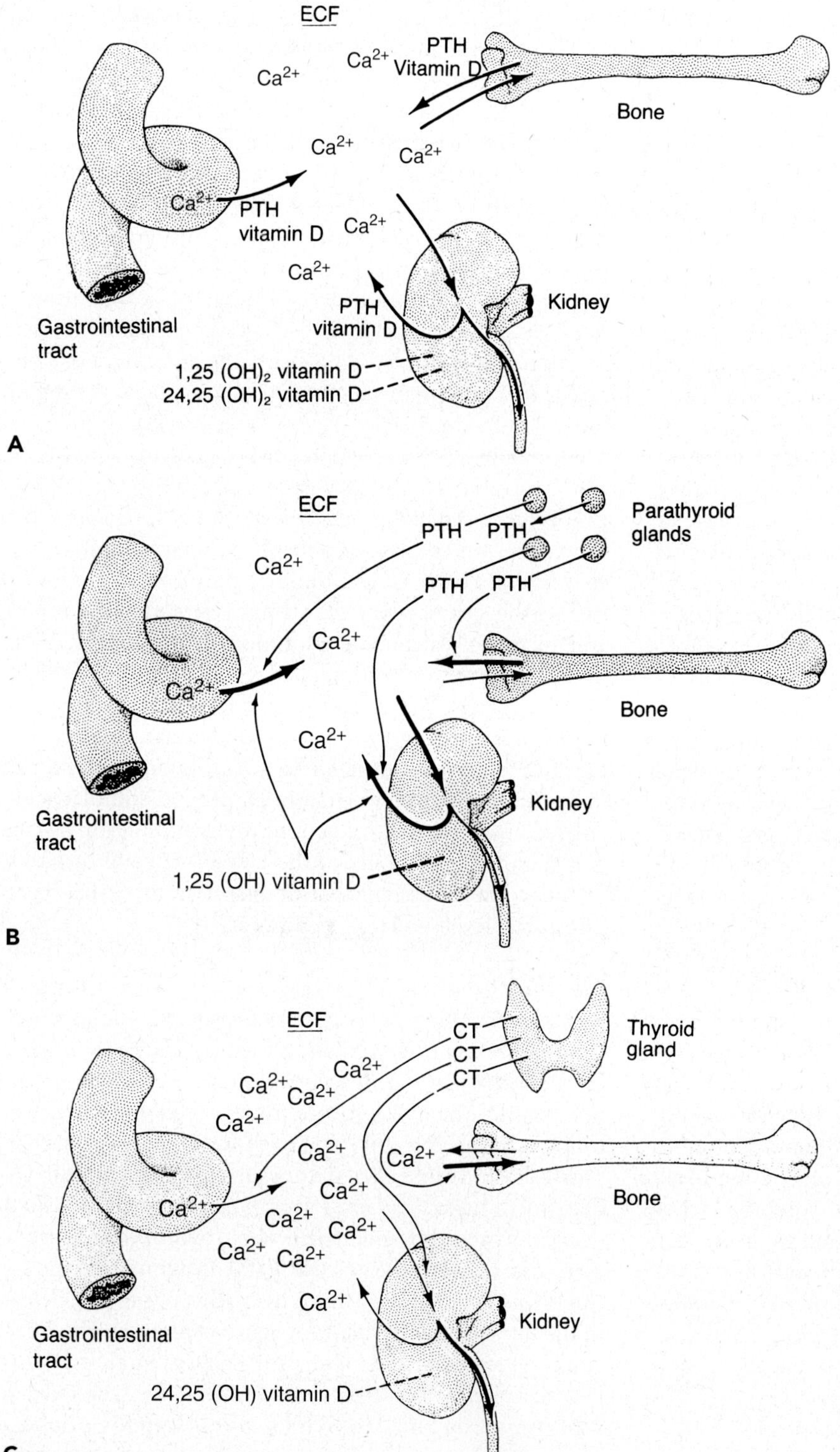

Figure 11.48 The roles of the bone, kidneys, gastrointestinal tract, parathyroid gland, and thyroid gland in calcium kinetics. These organs act to maintain calcium in the extracellular fluid (*ECF*) at the appropriate levels for normal cellular function. Vitamin D and parathyroid hormone (*PTH*) act to transport calcium ions across the gut wall and regulate renal excretion, and thereby, bone calcium content. Depending on the need for increased transport, 25-hydroxyvitamin D is converted to 24,25- or 1,25-dihydroxyvitamin D. **(A)** In the normocalcemic state, an equilibrium between calcium intake and excretion is maintained by the various organs. **(B)** In the hypocalcemic state, a reduced concentration of calcium signals the parathyroid glands to release more PTH, which acts at the levels of the gut cell, renal tubule, and bone to increase transport of calcium and rapidly replenish body fluids with it. An increase in PTH also favors the synthesis of 1,25-dihydroxyvitamin D in the kidney and acts to promote renal phosphate excretion by markedly diminishing the tubular reabsorption of phosphate. **(C)** In the hypercalcemic state, low concentrations of calcium and PTH act independently to diminish the synthesis of 1,25-dihydroxyvitamin D and decrease transport of calcium in the gut cell, tubule, and bone. Increased concentrations of calcium also cause the release of calcitonin (*CT*) from the C-cells of the thyroid gland, thereby diminishing calcium concentration. This mechanism principally involves stabilizing the osteoclast and decreasing its action on the bone, but it is not very effective in humans. (*Reproduced with permission from* Morrissy RT, Weinstein SL. *Lovell and Winter's Pediatric Orthopaedics*. Philadelphia, PA: Lippincott Williams & Wilkins, 2006.)

usually has short stature. Cranial features include frontal bossing and dental caries. Truncal abnormalities include enlargement of the costal cartilages (rachitic rosary), indentation of the lower ribs where the diaphragm inserts (Harrison groove), pectus carinatum, and long thoracic kyphosis. The lower extremity long bones are deformed, shortened, and often bowed. Knee deformity is very common and can manifest as either genu varum or genu valgum. If rickets is active during the normal age of physiologic genu varum (ages 1–2 years), then pathologic genu varum deformity prevails. On the other hand, if rickets is active during the normal age of physiologic genu valgum (ages 2–4 years),

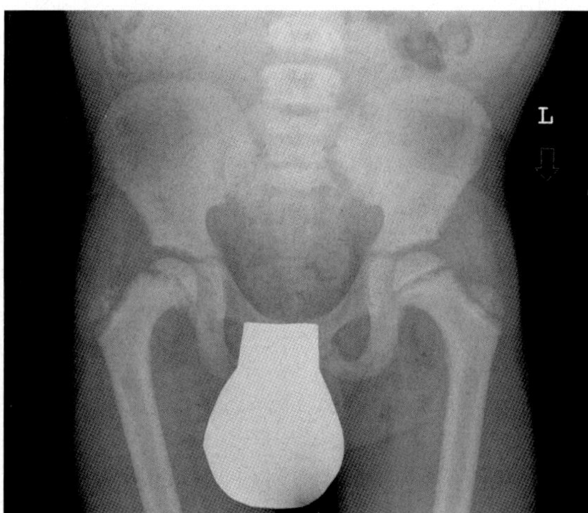

Figure 11.49 Renal osteodystrophy in a 12-year-old boy. An anteroposterior pelvis radiograph reveals an early slipped capital femoral epiphysis (SCFE) on the right. SCFE is common in renal osteodystrophy but rare in rickets. For more information on this condition, refer to the section on slipped capital femoral epiphysis. (*Reproduced with permission from* Morrissy RT, Weinstein SL. *Lovell and Winter's Pediatric Orthopaedics*. Philadelphia, PA: Lippincott Williams & Wilkins, 2006.)

then genu valgum deformity prevails. Ligamentous laxity and fractures are common findings. The upper extremities demonstrate apparent enlargements of the joints, as in the lower extremity, but are otherwise generally spared. In renal osteodystrophy, the additional findings of painful periarticular calcifications and slipped epiphyses, especially SCFE, may occur (Fig. 11.49).

Radiographs

The radiographic findings in rickets mirror the histologic changes (Fig. 11.50). The cortices of long bones are thin, and the trabeculae are indistinct. Osteopenia is the hallmark of rickets in the child. Since there is no zone of provisional calcification with the resultant "pile up" of hypertrophic zone cells, the width of the physis is increased. Similarly, the classic cupping of the metaphysis is noted from stunting of the growth plate centrally while normal peripheral appositional growth of the perichondral ring continues. Renal osteodystrophy has some unique radiographic features, including a "salt and pepper" skull; the absence of a cortical outline at the distal end of clavicles; and subperiosteal resorption of the ulnas, terminal tufts of the distal phalanges, and medial proximal tibia. In long-standing renal osteodystrophy, brown tumors, seen as expanded destructive bone lesions, may appear.

Special Tests

The main diagnostic tests include serum calcium, phosphate, alkaline phosphatase, and PTH levels. Other laboratory tests include vitamin D, urine calcium, and urine phosphate levels. Based on the salient laboratory findings, the underlying etiology of rickets can be identified (Table 11.1).

Differential Diagnosis

Osteomalacia is the adult counterpart to rickets and occurs only after the physes have closed. Physiologic genu varum, Blount disease, and idiopathic genu valgum should be considered in the differential diagnosis of genu varum and

TABLE 11.1
RICKETS

Etiology	Primary Effects	Secondary Effects
Nutritional rickets		
▪ Vitamin D deficiency	↓ 25-Hydroxyvitamin D	↓ 1,25-Dihydroxyvitamin D, ↑ PTH
▪ Calcium deficiency	↓ Calcium in diet	↑ Vitamin D, ↑ PTH
▪ Phosphate deficiency	↓ Phosphate	↑↑↑ 1,25-Dihydroxyvitamin D, normal PTH
Vitamin D–dependent rickets		
▪ Type I (α-hydroxylase deficiency)	↓↓↓ 1,25-Dihydroxyvitamin D	Normal or ↑ 25-hydroxyvitamin D
▪ Type II (vitamin D receptor defect)	↑↑↑↑ 1,25-Dihydroxyvitamin D	Normal or ↑ 25-hydroxyvitamin D
Hypophosphatemic rickets	↓↓↓ Phosphate	Other laboratory tests are normal except ↑ alkaline phosphatase
Renal osteodystrophy		
▪ High turnover	Chronically ↑↑↑ PTH	↑↑↑ Phosphate, ↓ calcium
▪ Low turnover	Aluminum results in ↓ PTH	
Parathyroid disorders		
▪ Hypoparathyroidism	↓↓↓ PTH	↓ 1,25-Dihydroxyvitamin D
▪ Pseudohypoparathyroidism	Normal to ↑ PTH	↓ 1,25-Dihydroxyvitamin D

PTH, parathyroid hormone.

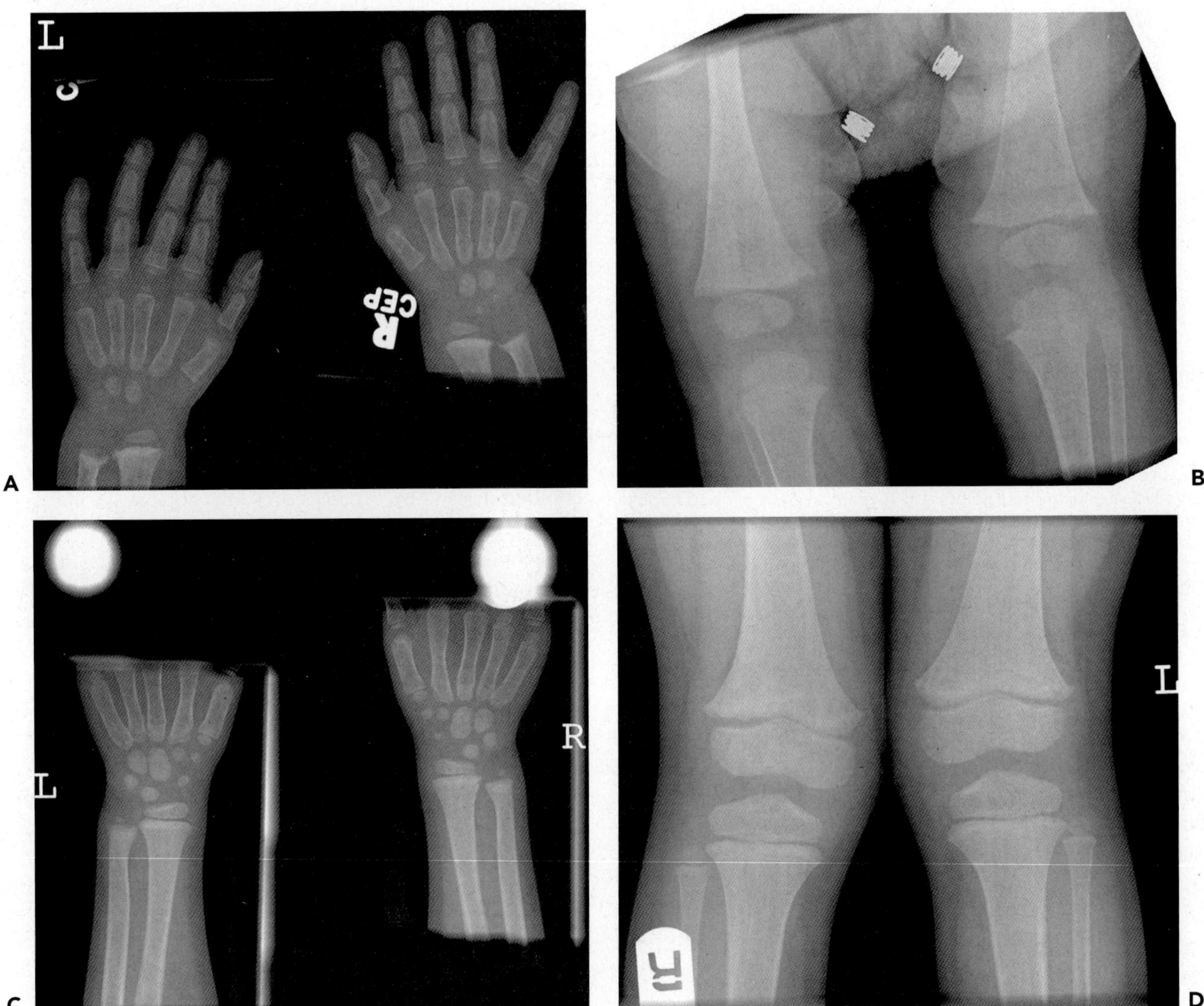

Figure 11.50 Rickets. Change caused by rickets can be seen **(A)** at the wrist and **(B)** at the knees of this 1-year-old child with familial hypophosphatemic rickets. The growth plates are widened and the metaphyses are cupped, particularly at the ulna and femur. At 4 years of age **(C** and **D)** the changes have resolved with medical treatment. (*Reproduced with permission from* Morrissy RT, Weinstein SL. *Lovell and Winter's Pediatric Orthopaedics*. Philadelphia, PA: Lippincott Williams & Wilkins, 2006.)

genu valgum, respectively. Other causes of short stature, such as skeletal dysplasias, should also be considered in the differential diagnosis of rickets.

Treatment

Medical management of the underlying metabolic disturbance, usually coordinated by a pediatric endocrinologist, is the mainstay of treatment. Depending on the specific cause of the rickets, treatment may include administration of supplemental vitamin D, calcium, and/or phosphate. The extent of remodeling likely to occur depends on the amount of growth remaining after correction of the underlying metabolic disturbance. Renal osteodystrophy involves complex management of the kidney, usually by a pediatric nephrologist. In some patients, aggressive management of renal function may abrogate the need for surgical intervention for deformity correction and even proximal femoral physeal abnormalities.

Orthopaedic intervention is required for fracture management and deformity control. Fractures are treated with standard methods of closed treatment and open reduction/internal fixation. Initial management of lower limb deformities includes brace management. Patients with renal osteodystrophy, however, are often recalcitrant to brace management. Patients with lower limb deformities that adversely affect function may be candidates for surgical intervention. Guided growth techniques or realignment osteotomies with internal or external fixation methods can be utilized to correct alignment and restore an adequate mechanical axis. Healing time may be prolonged and recurrence is common, especially in patients with persistent metabolic derangement. Displaced or symptomatic slipped

TABLE 11.2
CLASSIFICATION OF OSTEOGENESIS IMPERFECTA

Type	Skeletal Manifestation	Sclerae	Teeth	Collagen Defect
I	Mild	Blue	Normal (IA) or dentinogenesis imperfecta (IB)	Quantitative deficiency but normal collagen
II	Lethal			Abnormal collagen or severe quantitative deficiency
III	Severe	White	Dentinogenesis imperfecta	Abnormal collagen
IV	Moderate	White	Normal (IVA) or dentinogenesis imperfecta (IVB)	Abnormal collagen

From Morrissy RT, Weinstein SL. *Lovell and Winter's Pediatric Orthopaedics*. Philadelphia, PA: Lippincott Williams & Wilkins, 2006.

capital femoral epiphyses should be fixed with partially threaded screws.

Osteogenesis Imperfecta

Pathophysiology

Osteogenesis imperfecta (OI), or brittle bone disease, is a rare condition, with an estimated prevalence of 1 in 20,000 children. OI is not a single disorder but is rather a spectrum of clinical conditions that have increased bone fragility in common. In almost all cases, OI results from a quantitative or qualitative defect in type I collagen formation. Type I collagen is the major structural protein found in bone, skin, tendon, ligament, cornea, sclera, and dentin, and deficiency in this type of collagen results in fragility of the entire skeleton. The most common mutations responsible for OI involve one of two genes that encode the chains of type I collagen, the *COL1A1* gene or the *COL1A2* gene.

Classification

The most commonly used classification system for categorizing OI is the Sillence classification (Table 11.2). Although the Sillence system accounts for the majority of patients, recent genetic and biochemical research has led to the discovery of four additional types of OI. Type V disease is characterized by excessive callus formation, which can occasionally be confused with osteosarcoma. Type VI is similar to types III and IV but have normal collagen formation. Type VII is a rhizomelic variant with a predisposition to the proximal appendicular bones.

Presentation and Physical Examination

The clinical picture varies according to the severity and type of OI. Multiple pathologic fractures are the hallmark of the disease. In general, the earlier the fractures occur, the more severe the disease. The lower limbs are more frequently involved as they are more prone to trauma. Repetitive fractures in the epiphysis or physis may limit growth and contribute to the short stature that is commonly seen in these patients. Bowing of the long bones often develops due to microfractures occurring over time (Fig. 11.51). The frequency of fracture declines sharply after adolescence. In addition to the increased fracture risk, children may exhibit increased ligamentous laxity, joint hypermobility, and spinal deformity (including marked kyphoscoliosis). Abnormal collagen in the eyes may cause the classic blue or gray sclerae associated with some forms of OI. Craniofacial

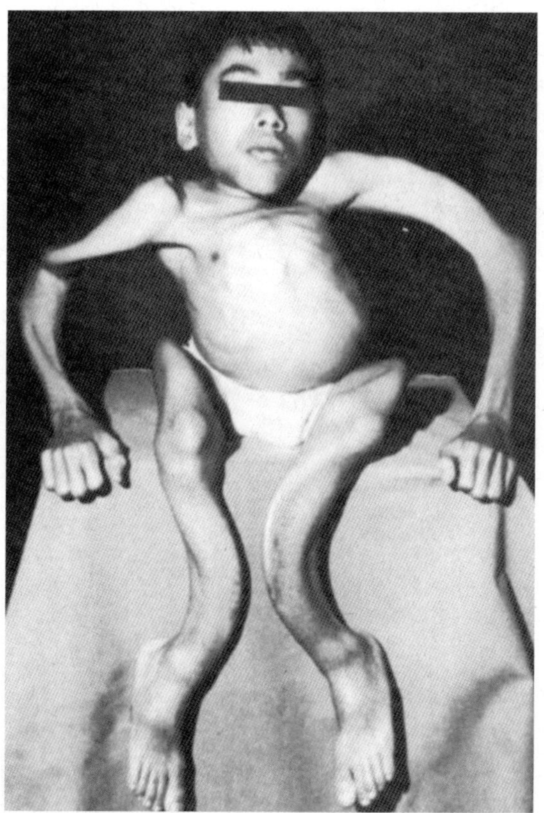

Figure 11.51 Osteogenesis imperfecta type III. Multiple fractures have created significant bowing in all four extremities. (*Reproduced with permission from* Broughton NS. *Textbook of Paediatric Orthopaedics*. London, England: WB Saunders, 1997.)

findings include small, triangular faces; defective dentinogenesis (small, fragile teeth); and defective hearing from otosclerosis. Cranial nerve palsies, headaches, apneic episodes, spasticity, nystagmus, or weakness should alert the physician to the potential for basilar invagination in patients with OI.

Radiographs

Generalized osteopenia is detected on plain radiographs in patients with OI. Since intramembranous bone growth is aberrant, the normal cylinderization of long bones does not occur, leaving behind thin, stenotic diaphyses as the hallmark of OI. The long bones appear bowed with thin cortices (Fig. 11.52). Deformities are present from multiple fractures (Fig. 11.53). The pelvis may show acetabular protrusion. The spine demonstrates osteopenic vertebrae that fracture easily, resulting in flattened or biconcave shape. Thoracic or thoracolumbar scoliosis is not uncommon. In addition, the skull manifests wormian bones, isolated lakes of bone typically found in and around the cranial sutures.

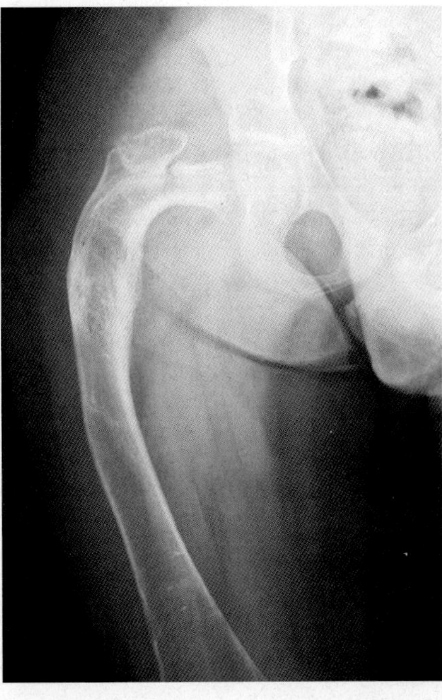

Figure 11.52 Multiple microfractures over time have led to bowing and coxa vara of the right femur in this child with osteogenesis imperfecta. This patient presented with hip pain and a femoral neck fracture, caused, in part, by the proximal femoral deformity.

Special Tests

In spite of genetic advances, there is no single test that is sufficient to make the diagnosis of OI. This is in part due to the wide variety of genetic and biochemical conditions that can present with a similar phenotype. The diagnosis of OI, therefore, remains a clinical one based on the entire clinical picture including the appearance of the patient, a history of fractures, the presence of abnormal sclerae or teeth, and characteristic radiographic findings.

In certain cases, prenatal diagnosis of OI can be accomplished by ultrasound when long bone deformity, severely reduced femoral length, and decreased echogenicity of the skull are recognized. Quantitative abnormalities in collagen production can be detected in 87% of patients with collagen analysis of skin biopsies and fibroblast cultures.

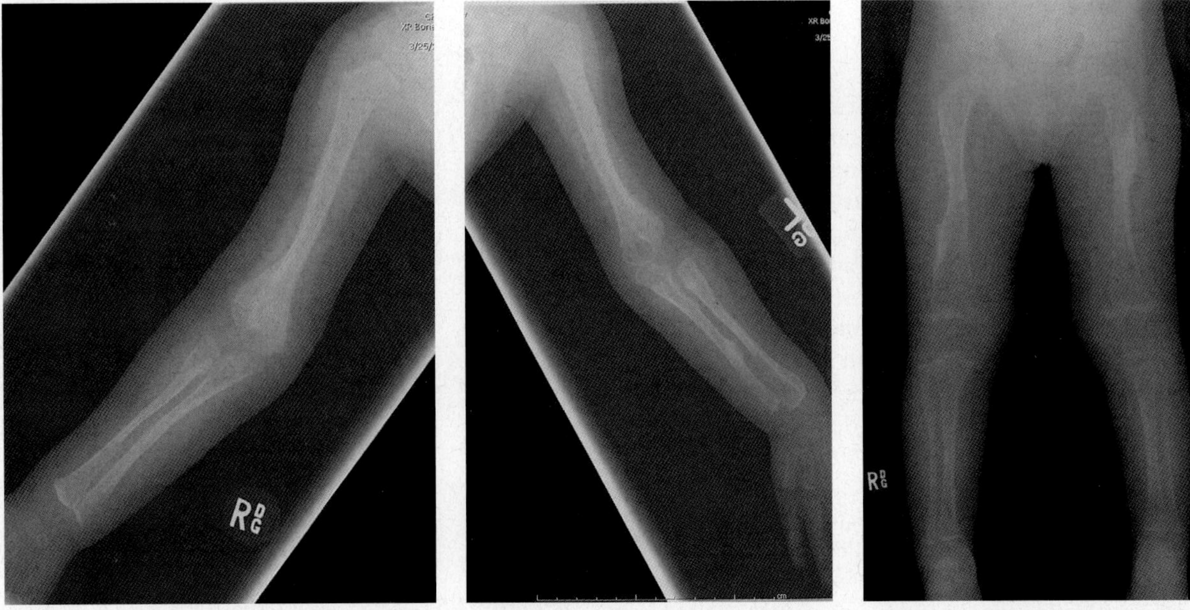

Figure 11.53 **(A** and **B)** Anteroposterior views of the upper extremities and **(C)** the lower extremities in a child with osteogenesis imperfecta. Note the deformity and callus formation from multiple previous fractures. (*Reproduced with permission from* Children's Orthopaedic Center, Los Angeles, CA.)

Bone densitometry (dual-energy x-ray absorptiometry) measurements show a decrease in mineralization. In children, the *z* score is utilized to evaluate the effect of treatment.

Differential Diagnosis

The differential diagnosis of OI includes child abuse, idiopathic juvenile osteoporosis, and rarely fibrous dysplasia. The presence of osteopenia, blue sclerae, family history of OI, and hearing difficulties helps to distinguish OI from child abuse. Mild cases of OI, however, are often extremely difficult to distinguish from nonaccidental trauma. The diagnosis idiopathic juvenile osteoporosis, unlike OI, is usually a transient, self-limiting phenomenon. Fibrous dysplasia is not characterized by the presence of thin, stenotic diaphyses on radiographs and has more localized involvement than OI.

Treatment

Recent advances in medical therapy have greatly improved the management of children with OI. By decreasing osteoclastic resorption of bone, bisphosphonates have been shown to increase cortical bone thickness, decrease the incidence of fractures, relieve chronic bone pain, and increase the height of collapsed vertebrae in patients with OI. The best choice of bisphosphonates remains unknown as does the optimal dosing regimen. Downsides of bisphosphonate therapy include a risk of delayed healing after osteotomy and the potential for osteonecrosis of the jaw. The administration of calcium, vitamin D, and calcitonin have been less successful than bisphosphonate treatment. Bone marrow transplant can be considered in the most severe cases in young infants.

The goals of orthopaedic treatment are to maximize function, to prevent disability from multiple fractures, and to correct deformity. Protective bracing (e.g., KAFOs) to prevent fractures and aid ambulation is an important component of the management of patients with OI. When fractures do occur, they heal at the normal rate. Although nonunions are relatively rare, the callus that forms is also weak, which increases the risk of refracture. Thus, closed management of fractures is initially employed with thoughtful avoidance of excessive immobilization that can result in disuse osteopenia. When open management is indicated, load-sharing devices, such as intramedullary nails, are preferred over plates and screws, which tend to lose purchase in weak bone and cause a stress riser at the edge of the implant. For significant deformity, realignment osteotomies with intramedullary fixation can improve mechanical alignment and prevent recurrent fractures (Fig. 11.54).

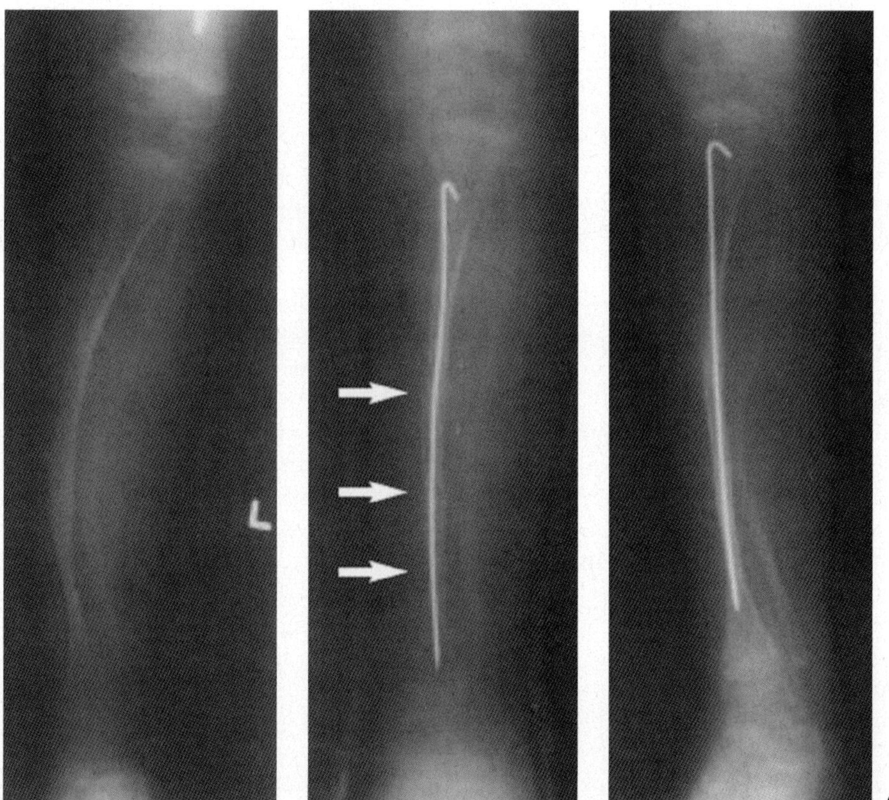

Figure 11.54 Leg deformity in a patient with type III osteogenesis imperfecta. **(A)** Preoperative anteroposterior radiograph obtained at age 6 years demonstrates left tibial deformity. **(B)** Postoperative radiograph with leg in a cast shows multiple osteotomies (*arrows*) with intramedullary fixation. **(C)** Films obtained after healing of osteotomies. (*Reproduced with permission from* Kocher MS, Shapiro F. Osteogenesis imperfecta. *J Am Acad Orthop*. 1998;6:225–236.)

Scoliosis tends to progress relentlessly in patients with OI, regardless of brace management, and often requires posterior spinal fusion with instrumentation before the curve gets too severe. The surgeon must be prepared to achieve fixation in osteopenic elements by using a combination of wires, hooks, and screws. Pseudarthrosis may occur in this mechanically disadvantageous environment. Finally, symptomatic basilar invagination may require formal decompression and stabilization.

Osteopetrosis

Pathophysiology

Osteopetrosis is a sclerosing bone dysplasia characterized by a diffuse increase in skeletal density and obliteration of marrow spaces. The primary defect is osteoclastic dysfunction that impairs the body's ability to resorb and remodel bone. Histologically, the skeleton shows cores of calcified cartilage surrounded by areas of normal new bone formation. Although this bone contains normal to increased numbers of osteoclasts, the cells are abnormal in function, as demonstrated by the absence of ruffled borders and clear zones. As a result, bone and cartilage cannot be resorbed and a dense pile of primitive trabeculae and calcified chondroid accumulates over time. Despite its density, osteopetrotic bone is brittle and more likely to fail under stress compared with normal bone. The inability to remodel bone also leads to narrowed medullary spaces and impaired hematopoietic function.

Classification

There are three forms of osteopetrosis: infantile malignant, intermediate, and adult tarda. Infantile and intermediate osteopetrosis are transmitted as an autosomal recessive trait. Adult form is inherited in an autosomal dominant pattern.

Presentation and Physical Examination

Children with osteopetrosis often present with pathologic fractures due to the fragility and brittleness of their bones. Bony overgrowth of the cranial foramina may manifest as cranial nerve palsies, blindness, or deafness. Osteomyelitis and dental caries are not uncommon because of diminished vascularity of the bone and a defective immune response. The lack of sufficient medullary space can cause depressed bone marrow function and pancytopenia; affected patients typically present with signs and symptoms of anemia, recurrent infections, abnormal bleeding, easy bruising, fatigability, and failure to thrive in severe cases. In addition, this marked diminution of bone marrow results in hepatosplenomegaly as extramedullary sites of hematopoiesis are stimulated. For malignant infantile osteopetrosis, the clinical course is rapidly progressive, and death may occur at a young age from sepsis or anemia. On the other hand, patients with the adult form have a normal life expectancy.

Radiographs

The hallmark of osteopetrosis is increased density of the bones (Fig. 11.55). The marble-like osseous structures appear densely white without medullary cavities. Bone within bone, known as *endobone,* is an area of radiodense tissue that exists inside the cortices of other bones; the presence of this radiographic finding is pathognomonic of osteopetrosis. Sclerosis at the vertebral end plates with normal density of the central body leads to a "rugger jersey" appearance of the spine (Fig. 11.56). In the appendicular skeleton, the metaphyses are abnormally dilated (Erlenmeyer flask appearance) because of impaired remodeling and tubularization of the long bones. On skull films, the basilar portions of the skull are sclerotic, and the supraorbital ridge is dense and quite prominent. Frequently, alternating bands of sclerosis and lucency are seen subjacent to the growth plate, which correlates with periods of high and low disease activity.

Special Tests

Routine blood tests are indicated in most patients to screen for pancytopenia or anemia.

Prenatal diagnosis of osteopetrosis has been accomplished in the 25th week of pregnancy with the use of fetal radiography, which reveals sclerosis of osteopetrotic bone. Ultrasound has also been used to identify affected fetuses.

Treatment

Treatment for infantile osteopetrosis is bone marrow transplantation at a young age. A successful transplant can resolve both the skeletal and hematologic abnormalities. High dose 1,25-dihydroxyvitamin D therapy with a low calcium diet has been employed because of its ability to stimulate osteoclasts and bone resorption.

Orthopaedic treatment tends to focus on fracture care and deformity management. Most fractures respond well to closed treatment, although healing may be delayed. When open treatment is necessary, the extremely hard bone can make fixation difficult: broken screws, drill bits, and even drivers are a common experience. Severe deformity may require corrective osteotomies, especially coxa vara of the hip. Similar to the treatment of fractures, surgery is technically challenging due to the difficulty in making the osteotomy and achieving adequate fixation.

Scurvy

This nutritional defect is a classic bone dystrophy that largely affects the metaphyseal region. The extrinsic defect is a deficiency in vitamin C, which is a cofactor in the normal pathway of bone collagen synthesis. In its absence, the resulting collagen is poorly cross-linked and

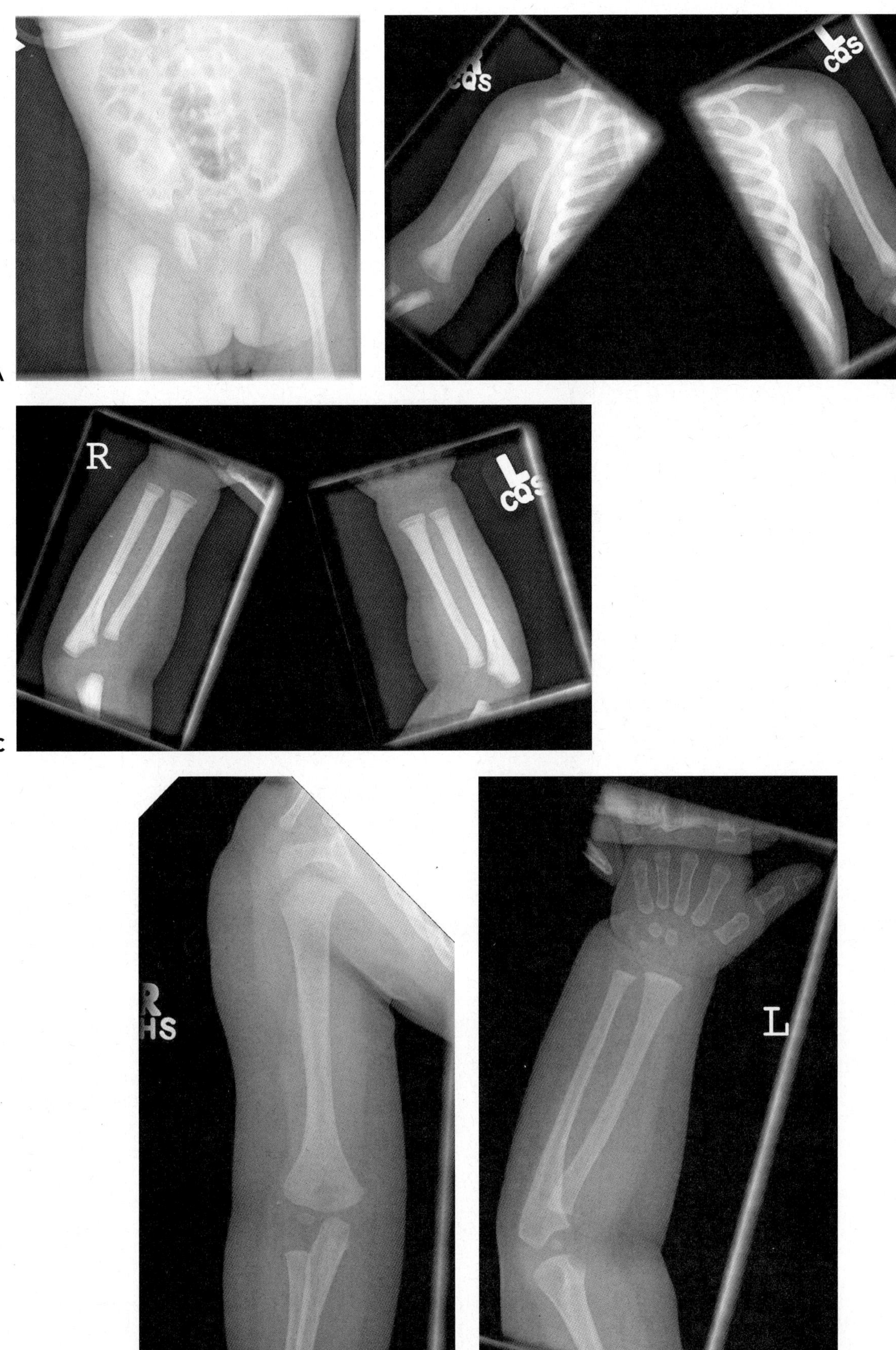

Figure 11.55 Six-month-old male infant with severe osteopetrosis and pancytopenia. **(A–E)** Dense sclerotic bones at the pelvis **(A)**, humerus **(B)**, and forearm **(C)**, without evident medullary cavities. **(D** and **E)** After successful bone marrow transplantation, the bony architecture in the humerus **(D)** and the forearm **(E)** were normalized. (*Reproduced with permission from* Morrissy RT, Weinstein SL. *Lovell and Winter's Pediatric Orthopaedics*. Philadelphia, PA: Lippincott Williams & Wilkins, 2006.)

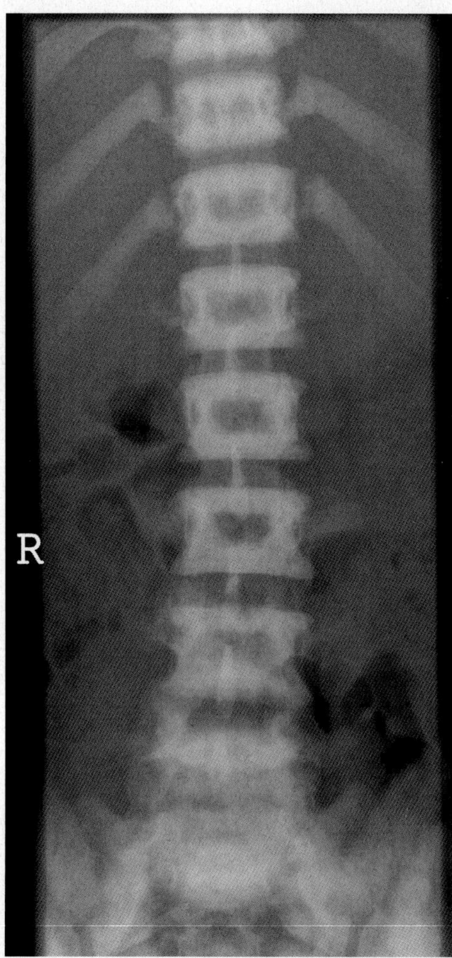

Figure 11.56 The classic rugger jersey appearance of the spine is seen in this 15-year-old girl with osteopetrosis. (*Reproduced with permission from* Morrissy RT, Weinstein SL. *Lovell and Winter's Pediatric Orthopaedics.* Philadelphia, PA: Lippincott Williams & Wilkins, 2006.)

mechanically deficient. Not surprisingly, the clinical state mirrors this deficiency in collagen. "Slipping" of the epiphyseal plates with minimal, if any, trauma is a hallmark of the disease. With physeal displacement, hemorrhage occurs under the periosteum. This results in stripping of the adjacent metaphyseal periosteum and subsequent subperiosteal bone formation. The petechial hemorrhages seen in these children are due to the defect in collagen located in the basement membrane of skin. Vitamin C supplementation is generally sufficient to cure this condition.

SHORT STATURE AND SKELETAL DYSPLASIAS

Not infrequently, children are referred to an orthopaedic surgeon for an evaluation of short stature. It is initially important to determine whether the short stature is physiologic or pathologic. In general, growth is considered aberrant when it falls two standard deviations below the mean height for age. Arguably, this will include some normal individuals; however, it should stimulate the examiner to more carefully pursue a diagnosis before assuming that the child is "physiologically short." The pathologic causes of short stature are many but include both skeletal dysplasias and mucopolysaccharidoses (MPSs). An accurate diagnosis must be established to provide appropriate medical care for these patients and to provide genetic counseling to the patient and family.

Achondroplasia

Pathophysiology

Achondroplasia is the most common type of skeletal dysplasia, with an estimated worldwide prevalence of 1 in 15,000 to 40,000 live births. It can be inherited in an autosomal dominant fashion, although as many as two-thirds of cases arise from spontaneous mutations. The defect in achondroplasia is an activating missense mutation in the gene encoding fibroblast growth factor receptor-3 (FGFR-3), mapped to chromosome 4. The mutated gene product ultimately results in retardation of cell division in the proliferative zone of the physis, thereby limiting enchondral bone growth. Intramembranous bone growth is not affected.

History and Physical Examination

In the workup of achondroplasia, as with all skeletal dysplasias, a family history of short stature or skeletal dysplasia should be sought. A history of mental retardation tends to move the diagnostic emphasis toward chromosomal defects rather than true skeletal dysplasias since dysplasias are rarely associated with cognitive deficits. Physical examination can yield a great deal of information and is extremely helpful for distinguishing achondroplasia from physiologic short stature and other skeletal dysplasias. Standing and sitting height should be measured over time and percentiles should be determined from standard charts. Head circumference should also be noted but is often preserved in achondroplasia since the skull enlarges by intramembranous ossification. The proportionality of trunk length to limb length should be assessed; achondroplasia, like most skeletal dysplasias, exhibits disproportionate short stature. The pattern of limb shortening should also be evaluated. Certain skeletal dysplasias including achondroplasia have shortening primarily of the proximal segment of the limbs (arms and thighs). This is termed *rhizomelic shortening*. When the middle segment of the limb (forearm and leg) is short, this is called *mesomelic shortening*. If the distal segments (hand and feet) demonstrate the shortening, this is referred to as *acromelic shortening*.

In addition to the overall examination of height and proportionality, specific regions of the body should be examined in patients with achondroplasia. Bowing at the knees or tibia is common and an accurate assessment of lower limb alignment should be performed at each office visit. A careful neurologic examination is warranted in all patients with achondroplasia because of the high incidence of spinal stenosis.

Presentation

Infants present soon after birth with a characteristic appearance (Fig. 11.57). The skull is normal in size but appears large relative to the shortened skeleton; frontal bossing and midface hypoplasia are typical. Trunk length is within the lower range of normal, but the limbs are significantly shortened in a rhizomelic pattern. Likewise, the ribs are also short, causing the chest wall to be small and constricted. This results in the appearance of a protuberant abdomen. Thoracolumbar kyphosis is common but can improve with age. Compensatory hyperlordosis in the lumbar region frequently occurs. Scoliosis is seen in one-third of these patients but is usually mild.

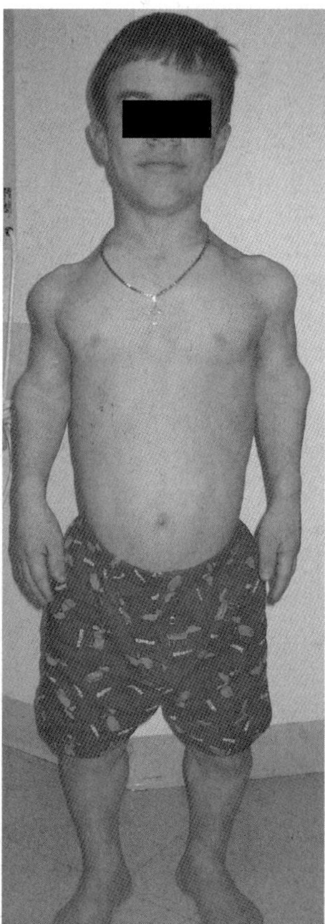

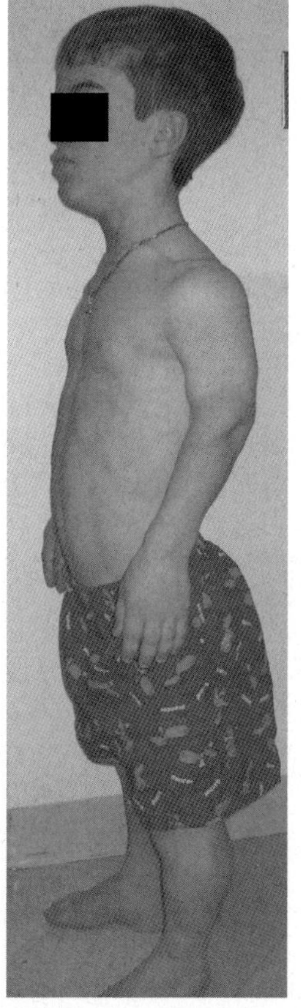

Figure 11.57 A 16-year-old boy with achondroplasia. **(A)** Pronounced shortening of the proximal limb segments (rhizomelic pattern). There is mild genu varum. The humeri are most affected. **(B)** The elbows have a mild flexion contractures. He has had previous osteotomies of the tibias and fibulas for genu varum. (*Reproduced with permission from* Morrissy RT, Weinstein SL. *Lovell and Winter's Pediatric Orthopaedics*. Philadelphia, PA: Lippincott Williams & Wilkins, 2006.)

Most patients with achondroplasia have some degree of spinal stenosis from shortened pedicles and a decreased interpedicular distance. Some patients may present with exercise intolerance and early fatigability; in severe cases, frank myelopathy or radiculopathy can occur. The upper extremities typically demonstrate extra space between the third and fourth rays of the hands, causing a "trident hand" appearance. The lower extremities often exhibit increased ligamentous laxity, genu varum, and internal tibial torsion.

Developmental milestones may be initially delayed, but normal motor coordination eventually develops. Independent ambulation is typically achieved by 18 to 24 months of age. Achondroplasia, like other skeletal dysplasias, is typically associated with normal intelligence. Life expectancy is somewhat diminished, but quality-of-life studies have shown similar scores compared with the general population.

Radiographs

All patients who are suspected of having achondroplasia or any other type of skeletal dysplasia should receive a skeletal survey. This includes a lateral radiograph of the skull and neck and AP views of the entire spine, pelvis, arms, hands, and legs. The radiographic changes seen in achondroplasia reflect those regions that are most dependent on enchondral ossification. In the long bones, the metaphyses are flared and the diaphyses are thick from appositional growth. Unlike other types of skeletal dysplasia, the epiphyses are spared. Lower extremity radiographs may demonstrate genu varum from abnormalities of the distal femur, proximal tibia, or relative overgrowth of the fibula. The radiographic appearance of the pelvis is classic in achondroplasia. Since the height of the pelvis is a function of enchondral bone growth, the achondroplastic pelvis is underdeveloped and flattened with a "champagne glass" outlet, small sciatic notches and squared iliac wings. At the hip, the proximal femoral metaphyses are widened and the femoral necks are short.

Spine radiographs are necessary to screen for scoliosis and kyphosis. In the latter condition, the apical vertebrae may become progressively wedge-shaped in the sagittal plane. The AP view should also be evaluated for decreasing interpedicular distance, which indicates the presence of spinal stenosis (Fig. 11.58).

Special Tests

Direct deoxyribonucleic acid analysis to identify mutations in the *FGFR3* gene can be performed postnatally or prenatally to screen families at risk. In addition, prenatal ultrasonography can identify characteristic skeletal anomalies and hydrocephalus. Advanced imaging studies, either CT

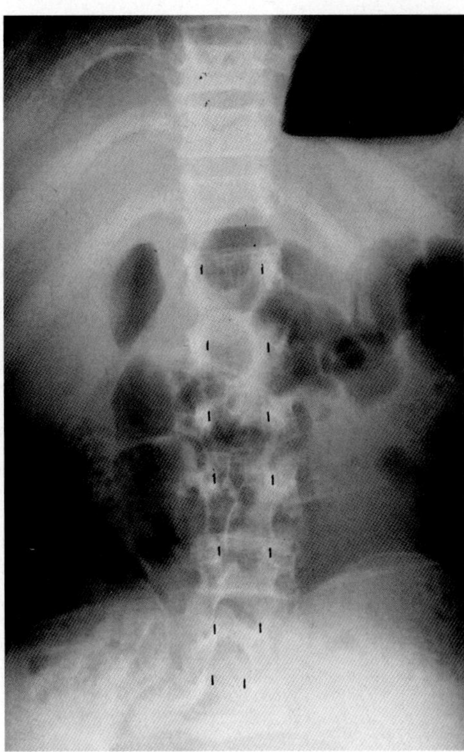

Figure 11.58 This anteroposterior view of the entire spine shows the progressive narrowing of the interpedicular distance at more caudal levels of the lumbar spine; this is the opposite of the normal pattern and suggests spinal stenosis. (*Reproduced with permission from* Morrissy RT, Weinstein SL. *Lovell and Winter's Pediatric Orthopaedics*. Philadelphia, PA: Lippincott Williams & Wilkins, 2006.)

or MRI, may be necessary to evaluate for foramen magnum stenosis, which is common due to the disproportionate growth of the calvarium relative to the basilar skull and neck. MRI is also useful in the workup of spinal stenosis to localize areas of central or foraminal compression.

Differential Diagnosis

The differential diagnosis of achondroplasia includes other causes of short stature such as rickets and other types of skeletal dysplasia. Many different skeletal dysplasias have been described, and a complete discussion of all of these conditions is beyond the scope of this text. Some brief differences will be mentioned and select conditions (diastrophic dysplasia, spondyloepiphyseal dysplasia [SED], and multiple epiphyseal dysplasia) will be discussed in the following section. Short-limbed dysplasias include hypochondroplasia, metatropic dysplasia, chondroectodermal dysplasia (also known as Ellis–van Creveld syndrome), diastrophic dysplasia, chondrodysplasia punctata, and pseudoachondroplasia. Hypochondroplasia resembles achondroplasia but is less severe. In metatropic dysplasia, the infant child has short limbs and a relatively long trunk, but as the child grows, severe kyphoscoliosis develops, resulting in an apparent short trunk. The head and face are usually normal, and there is often a small, tail-like appendage overlying the lower sacrum. Chondroectodermal dysplasia is a short-limbed dwarfism but is also characterized by postaxial polydactyly; abnormalities of the nail, hair, and teeth; and congenital heart failure. Patients with chondrodysplasia punctata present with multiple punctate epiphyseal calcifications at birth, but these resolve over the first year of life. Children later have joint contractures, coxa vara, atlantoaxial instability, and congenital kyphoscoliosis, in addition to proximal limb shortening. Pseudoachondroplasia involves both the epiphyses and metaphyses of long bones. The head and face are normal, and hip dysplasia and premature osteoarthritis are common.

Treatment

From a medical standpoint, infants with achondroplasia should be carefully monitored during the first few years of life for sleep apnea, spasticity, or hypertonia, which may be the result of foramen magnum stenosis. Although this generally improves with growth, severe cases may warrant decompression of the brain stem. Ear, nose, and throat problems are frequent because of midface hypoplasia, and early referral to an otorhinolaryngologist may be indicated.

From an orthopaedic standpoint, treatment is generally aimed at controlling deformity, maximizing function, and preventing neurologic deterioration. Genu varum is typically managed by corrective osteotomy since there is no evidence that bracing is effective in children with achondroplasia (Fig. 11.59). Hip deformities should be corrected surgically to preserve a neutral mechanical axis and maximize function. The thoracolumbar kyphosis seen in infants with achondroplasia should initially be observed. In most cases, the deformity resolves as the child begins to ambulate and muscle tone improves (Fig. 11.60). In the 10% to 15% of cases that do not resolve, bracing may be used for flexible curves. Occasionally, posterior fusion and instrumentation may be necessary to correct persistent deformity. Spinal stenosis should be treated with wide decompression (several levels above the stenotic segment to several levels below) followed by posterior stabilization. The use of pedicle screws is preferred over wires or hooks, which occupy space in the already narrowed spinal canal.

The topic of limb lengthening is a source of significant controversy in the orthopaedic community. Quality-of-life studies in patients with achondroplasia have demonstrated excellent function, and critics complain that limb lengthening is a long and difficult process to undertake for primarily a cosmetic result. Proponents of lengthening cite the ability to improve self-image and enhance function in an otherwise adult-sized world. Unlike most other types of skeletal dysplasia, achondroplasia is amenable to lengthening because the joints are normal and the tendons, vessels, and nerves have a capacity to stretch. The decision to

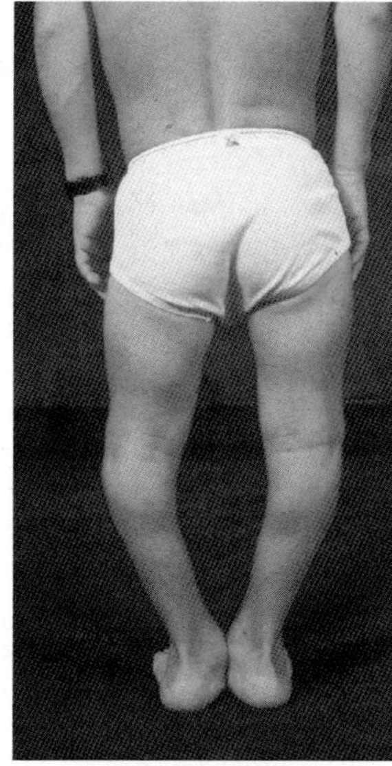
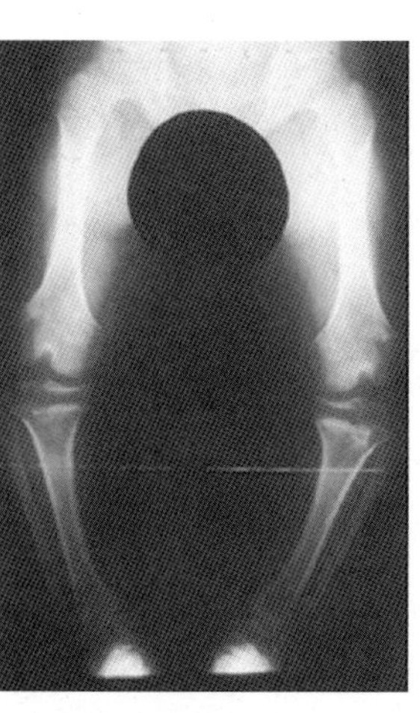
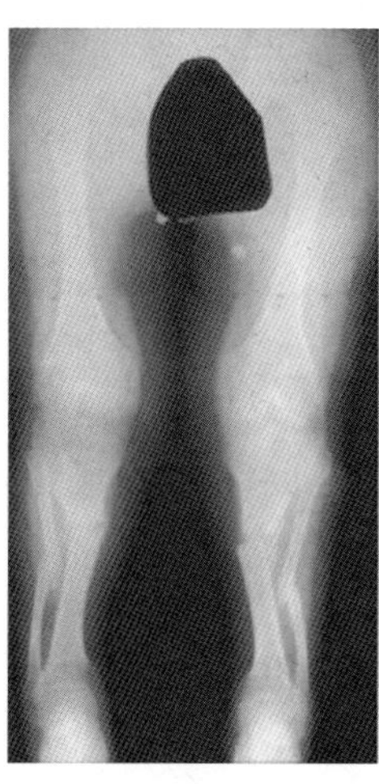
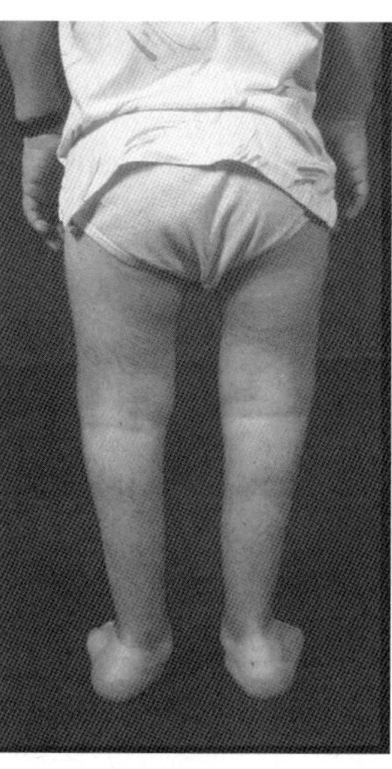

A,B C,D

Figure 11.59 **(A)** This 9-year-old boy with achondroplasia has genu varum frequently seen in this condition. **(B)** Standing anteroposterior (AP) radiograph of the lower extremities confirms genu varum due to fibulae being longer than the tibiae. **(C)** Standing AP radiograph of the lower extremities following corrective tibial and fibular osteotomies demonstrates reestablishment of a normal mechanical axis. **(D)** Postoperative clinical photograph confirms improvement in genu varum. (*Reproduced with permission from* Skaggs DL, Flynn JM: *Staying Out of Trouble in Pediatric Orthopaedics*. Philadelphia, PA: Lippincott Williams & Wilkins, 2006.)

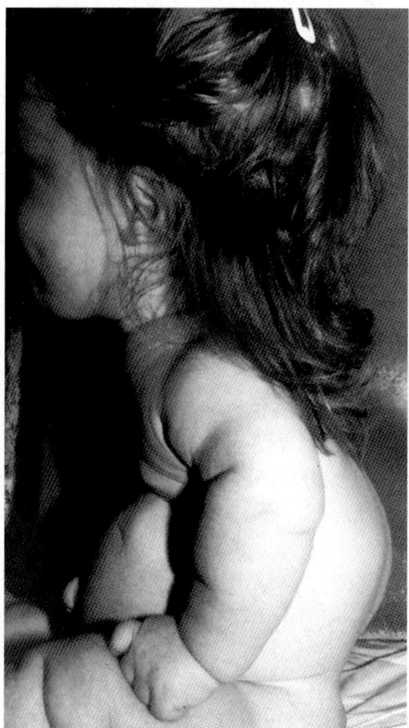
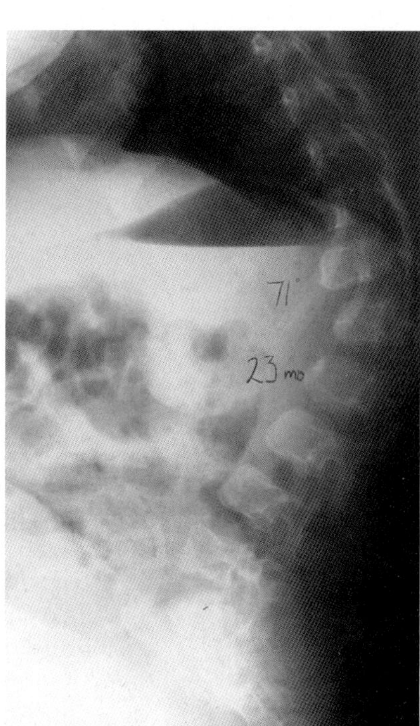

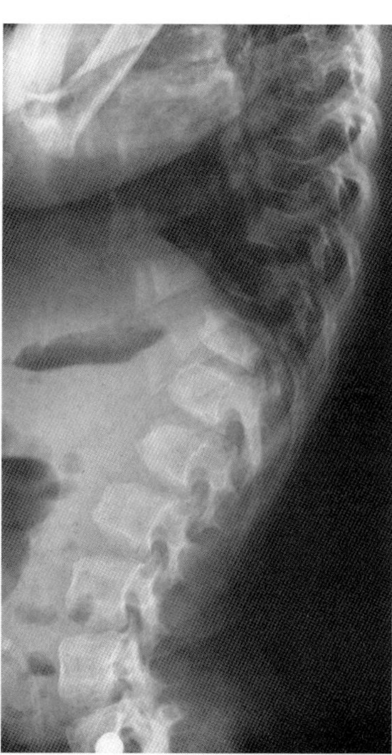

A,B C

Figure 11.60 Thoracolumbar kyphosis in a 23-month-old achondroplastic child who has not walked yet. **(A)** It is most pronounced in the sitting position. **(B)** Radiograph shows hypoplasia of L1, with rounding-off of the anterior vertebral body corners. **(C)** At 5 years of age, after a period of brace treatment, the shape of L1, as well as the overall kyphosis has improved. (*Reproduced with permission from* Morrissy RT, Weinstein SL. *Lovell and Winter's Pediatric Orthopaedics*. Philadelphia, PA: Lippincott Williams & Wilkins, 2006.)

undergo limb lengthening, however, should be made only after frank and open discussions have been held regarding the length of treatment (often 2 years), the potential complications, and the personal motivation of the patient. If undertaken, gradual correction with distraction osteogenesis and external fixation is the method of choice. Often, several courses of lengthening in both the upper and lower extremities are necessary to improve proportionality of the skeleton. Angular deformity, joint stiffness, and neurovascular injury are possible complications from limb-lengthening procedures.

MISCELLANEOUS SKELETAL DYSPLASIAS

As mentioned, many different skeletal dysplasias exist, and a complete discussion of all of these conditions is beyond the scope of this text. A few select conditions including diastrophic dysplasia, SED, and multiple epiphyseal dysplasia will be discussed.

Diastrophic Dysplasia

Diastrophic dysplasia is a severe short-limbed dwarfism that is extremely rare, affecting approximately 1 in 100,000 live births. Diastrophic dysplasia is inherited in an autosomal recessive fashion and involves the gene *DTDST,* which encodes a sulfate transporter protein that is involved in proteoglycan metabolism in cartilage. As a result, cells in affected cartilage have an impaired growth response to fibroblast growth factor. Ultimately, enchondral growth is impaired.

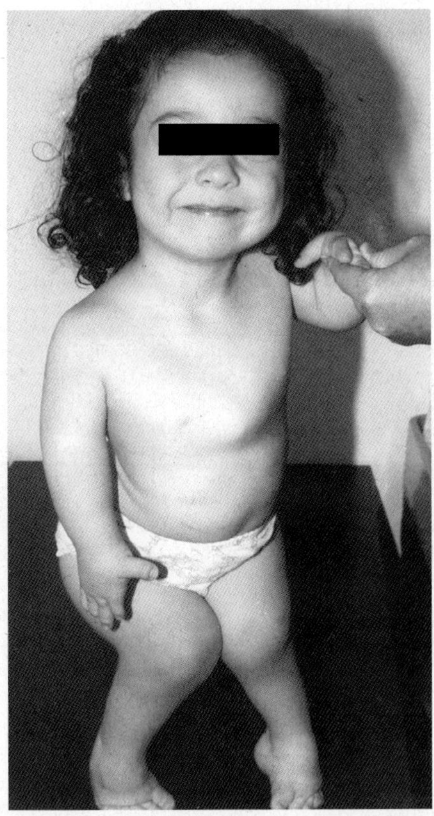

Figure 11.61 A 5-year-old girl with diastrophic dysplasia. Note the prominent cheeks, circumoral fullness, equinovarus feet, valgus knees with flexion contractures, and abducted or "hitchhiker" thumbs. (*Reproduced with permission from* Morrissy RT, Weinstein SL. *Lovell and Winter's Pediatric Orthopaedics.* Philadelphia, PA: Lippincott Williams & Wilkins, 2006.)

Diastrophic dysplasia is quite apparent at birth, noted by extremely short stature, rhizomelic shortening of the limbs, and rigid foot deformities (Fig. 11.61). The head is normal-sized but the face is dysmorphic with a narrow nasal bridge, flared nostrils, and a broad midnose. Prominent cheeks and fullness around the mouth have sometimes led to the term "cherub dwarf." At approximately 3 to 6 weeks of age, the external part of the ear develops cystic swelling that later calcifies in florets, resulting in the characteristic "cauliflower ear." The hands are typically short and broad with ulnar deviation. Abduction and shortening of the first metacarpal leads to the characteristic appearance of a "hitchhiker thumb." Flexion contractures often develop at the elbow, hip, and knee joints, resulting in severe functional limitation and gait disturbance. Hip dysplasia or frank dislocation is a common finding; bilateral dislocations are seen in up to 25% of cases. Unlike achondroplasia, the epiphyses in diastrophic dysplasia are affected and may become flattened and arthritic over time. At the knees, genu valgum frequently occurs and may be associated with patellar dislocation. A wide spectrum of foot deformities is seen in patients with diastrophic dysplasia. The most common findings include adduction and valgus or clubfoot. There may be a wider space between the great toe and the second toe, resulting in a "hitchhiker toe" appearance. These deformities are often rigid and recalcitrant to stretching casts. The cervical spine is kyphotic in 30% to 50% of patients. Some of these deformities resolve spontaneously, whereas others progress. Scoliosis of the thoracolumbar spine can be seen in up to a third of patients. Curves may be idiopathic-like or sharply angulated with concomitant kyphosis. Unlike achondroplasia, spinal stenosis occurs infrequently.

Prenatal diagnosis may be suggested on the basis of the ultrasonographic identification of classic findings such as short limbs, "hitchhiker thumbs," and foot deformities. Prenatal diagnosis is also available during the first trimester by mutation analysis of chorionic villous DNA. Postnatally, radiographic evaluation should include a complete skeletal series (as in all skeletal dysplasias). In particular, patients with diastrophic dysplasia should have serial lateral radiographs of the cervical spine to diagnose and monitor any existing cervical kyphosis or instability.

The management of children with diastrophic dysplasia focuses on each of the affected regions. Cervical kyphosis often improves with growth; therefore, close observation is initially indicated for all children except those with

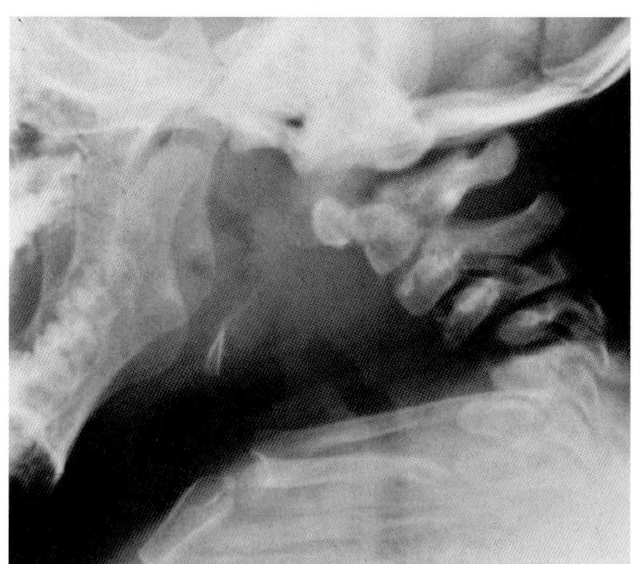
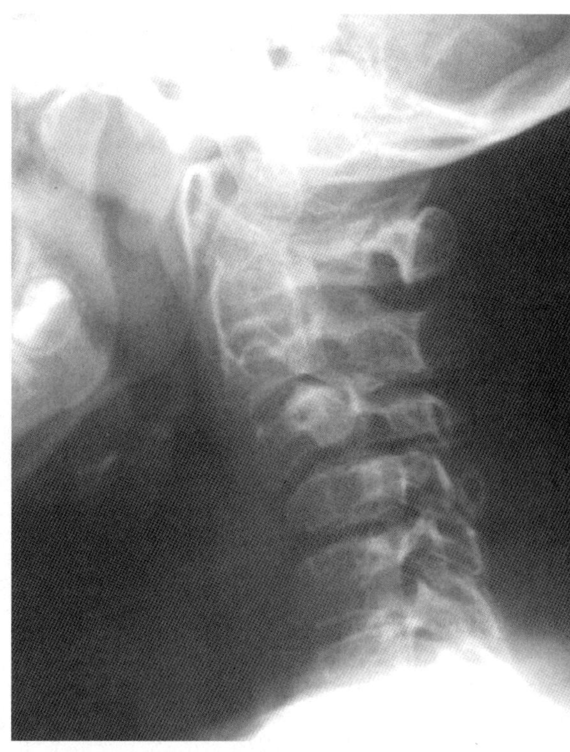

Figure 11.62 **(A)** Cervical kyphosis in a 1-year-old child with diastrophic dysplasia and marked deformity of C4. The patient was neurologically normal. **(B)** Seven years later, the vertebral bodies have been restored to a nearly normal shape without any intervention. (*Reproduced with permission from* Morrissy RT, Weinstein SL. *Lovell and Winter's Pediatric Orthopaedics.* Philadelphia, PA: Lippincott Williams & Wilkins, 2006.)

neurologic impairment (Fig. 11.62). Progressive, symptomatic, or unstable deformities require cervical decompression and fusion usually followed by halo immobilization. Scoliosis rarely responds to bracing, and posterior fusion is recommended for progressive curves greater than 50 degrees.

Deformed hips may require corrective osteotomy. In dislocated hips, closed reduction is seldom successful and open reduction with pelvic and/or femoral osteotomies and soft tissue releases is usually necessary to achieve adequate reduction. Despite one's best efforts, hips in diastrophic dysplasia often develop early osteoarthritis and may require joint arthroplasty in adulthood. Foot deformities are often rigid in diastrophic dysplasia, and thus are resistance to stretching casts. Surgical correction to achieve a plantigrade foot is often necessary once the child's foot has reached an operable size. Surgical reconstruction includes appropriate osteotomies and soft tissue releases catered to the individual foot. Postoperative bracing is recommended. Recurrence is common, often necessitating repeat surgery. Severe deformities may warrant salvage procedures such as talectomy or fusion.

Multiple Epiphyseal Dysplasia

As the name implies, multiple epiphyseal dysplasia (MED) is a skeletal dysplasia that affects multiple epiphyses in the skeleton with relative sparing of the physes and metaphyses. MED is a heterogeneous disorder, but in most cases, a mutation in the gene on chromosome 19 that codes for cartilage oligomeric matrix protein is responsible for the disorder.

Patients with MED typically present later in childhood and occasionally as late as adulthood. Short stature is moderate: most patients achieve an average adult height of between 54 and 60 in. Presenting complaints include joint pain, decreased range of motion, difficulty walking, and angular deformities of the lower extremity. MED affects multiple joints in both lower and upper extremities, but the spine and face are normal. The most severe site of involvement is usually the hips. Coxa vara and joint subluxation are common, and coexisting avascular necrosis can develop in up to 50% of patients; early degenerative changes result from the flattened and misshapen epiphysis. Knees generally demonstrate genu valgus from hypoplastic femoral condyles and sloping of the proximal tibia. The ankles are also in valgus, usually from squaring of the talus. In the upper extremities, common findings include flexion contractures, finger deformities, and dislocation of the radial head with compensatory capitellar enlargement.

Radiographs, including a complete skeletal series, are an essential part of the diagnostic workup. Involvement of multiple joints is characteristic, and secondary ossification centers are generally delayed in appearance. The epiphyses

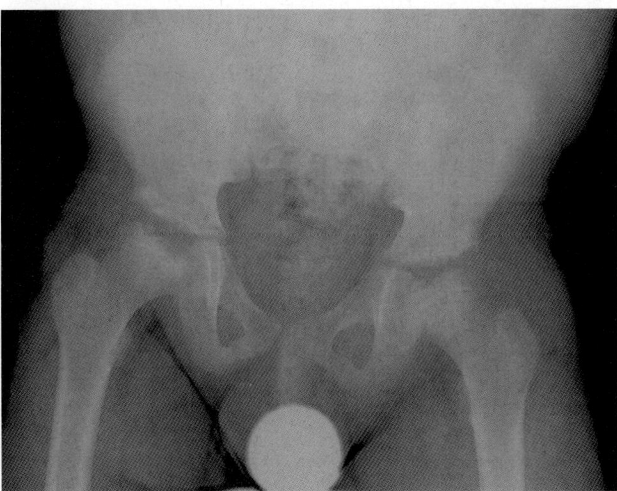

Figure 11.63 Multiple epiphyseal dysplasia. Note the deformity in the femoral epiphyses. Such changes can occasionally be confused with those seen in Legg–Calvé–Perthes disease (see hip section).

eventually appear but are small and fragmented. During skeletal maturation, these fragmented regions coalesce, but the final shape of the epiphysis is flattened, enlarged, and dysmorphic. Often, an arthrogram or MRI is necessary to assess the true shape of the epiphysis. Abnormal joint morphology predisposes patients with MED to early degenerative arthritis. The radiographic appearance of hips in MED can often be confused with bilateral Perthes disease (Fig. 11.63). Unlike Perthes disease, the radiographic findings in MED are usually symmetric and the acetabular changes more pronounced. Skeletal surveys will generally reveal involvement of other joints in MED.

Treatment is aimed at managing deformity and preserving function. During childhood, realignment procedures of the lower extremity through guided growth or corrective osteotomy can improve pain and mechanical loading of the knees and ankles. Hips that exhibit progressive subluxation or pain should be reconstructed with femoral osteotomies and/or acetabular procedures. Degenerative arthritis later in life often requires total joint arthroplasty.

Spondyloepiphyseal Dysplasia

SED is an extremely rare skeletal dysplasia occurring in approximately 1 in 4 million people. The condition comes in two major forms: congenita and tarda. SED congenita is typically inherited in an autosomal dominant fashion, whereas SED tarda is usually X-linked. In both cases, however, the condition can arise from spontaneous mutation or different patterns of genetic transmission. Both forms of the disorder result from a genetic defect in the production of type II collagen.

SED tarda presents at a later age with milder clinical features than SED congenita. In the latter form, patients present with a characteristic appearance of short stature (involving both trunk and extremities), small mouth, pectus carinatum, small rib cage, and protuberant abdomen (Fig. 11.64). Hips usually have varus deformities and flexion contractures that lead to a compensatory lumbar lordosis and a waddling gait. Knees typically are in varus, and the most common foot deformity is equinovarus. As the name implies, SED congenita affects the spine in addition to the extremities (unlike MED). Neck instability is common from odontoid hypoplasia, and a careful neurologic assessment is necessary in all patients to screen for myelopathy. Scoliosis is present in approximately 50% of patients.

In contrast, SED tarda results in a mildly shortened stature, mostly due to shortening of the trunk rather than the extremities. Spine involvement is equally mild and usually consists of mild platyspondyly. Angular deformities of the lower extremity are relatively rare, but degenerative changes can occur in the hips and knees by early adulthood.

A skeletal survey including appropriate views of the spine are necessary as part of the diagnostic workup. Varus deformities of the proximal femur are typical of SED congenita, and ossification of the femoral epiphysis may be delayed. In both forms of SED, radiographs of the hip may reveal flattening, enlargement, and progressive extrusion of the epiphysis (Fig. 11.65). In the lower extremities, genu valgum is more common than genu varum. Spine radiographs will demonstrate flattening of the vertebral bodies (platyspondyly), posterior wedging of the vertebra, and disc space narrowing. The pattern of scoliosis, when present, is sharply angulated over a few vertebral segments. As mentioned, cervical views should be obtained periodically to look for os odontoideum, odontoid hypoplasia, or atlantoaxial instability.

Like other skeletal dysplasias, the orthopaedic treatment of SED focuses on deformity management. Valgus producing osteotomies of the proximal femur are indicated for progressive varus deformities of the hips. Slight overcorrection should be the goal because of the high risk for recurrence, and coexisting flexion contractures should be released under the same anesthetic. Subluxation or extrusion should be reconstructed with femoral and/or pelvic osteotomy. Angular deformities of the lower extremities are best managed with corrective osteotomy. Clubfeet in SED are usually less stiff than in diastrophic dysplasia; as a result, conventional principles of serial manipulation and casting should be attempted before resorting to open release and osteotomy. Cervical instability that exceeds 8 mm or that is symptomatic should be treated by cervical fusion along with decompression for cases with coexisting stenosis. Because the cervical bones are usually quite small, segmental fixation is difficult and halo immobilization is usually necessary.

Mucopolysaccharidoses

Although they are not primary bone dysplasias, MPSs are frequently included in discussions of skeletal dysplasias because they lead to short stature.

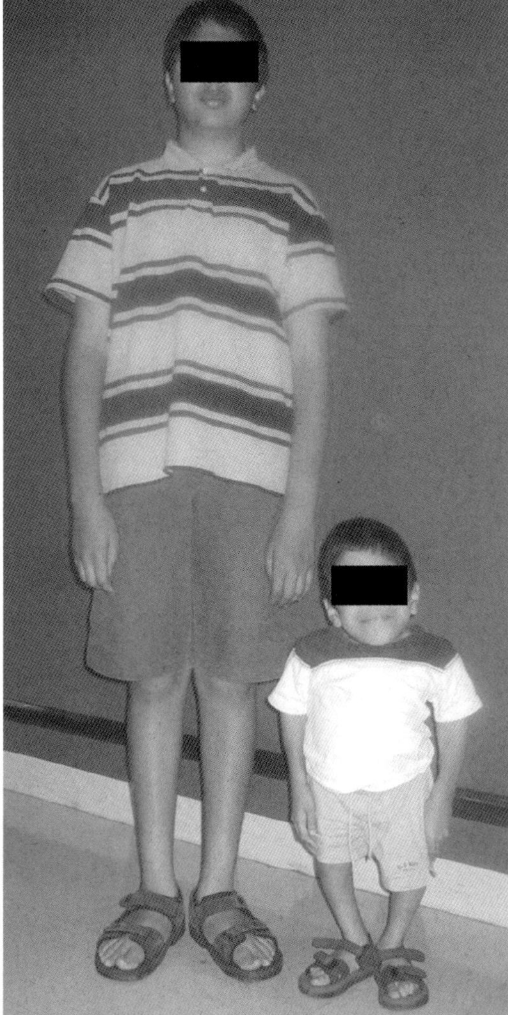

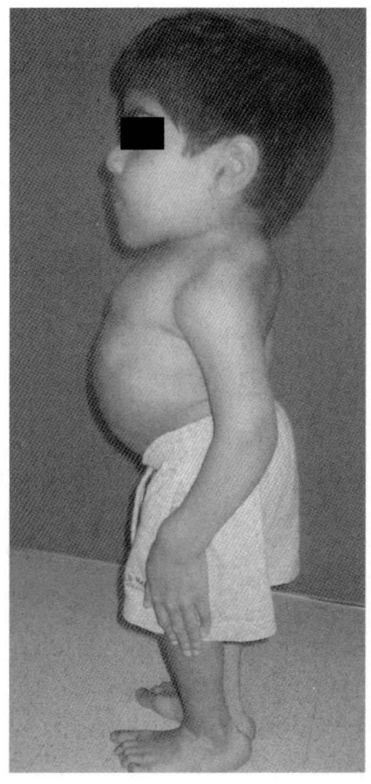

Figure 11.64 Spondyloepiphyseal dysplasia congenita produces extreme short stature. **(A)** This 12-year-old boy is with his 14-year-old brother. **(B)** Note the extreme trunk shortening, increased lumbar lordosis, and hip flexion contracture. (*Reproduced with permission from* Morrissy RT, Weinstein SL. *Lovell and Winter's Pediatric Orthopaedics.* Philadelphia, PA: Lippincott Williams & Wilkins, 2006.)

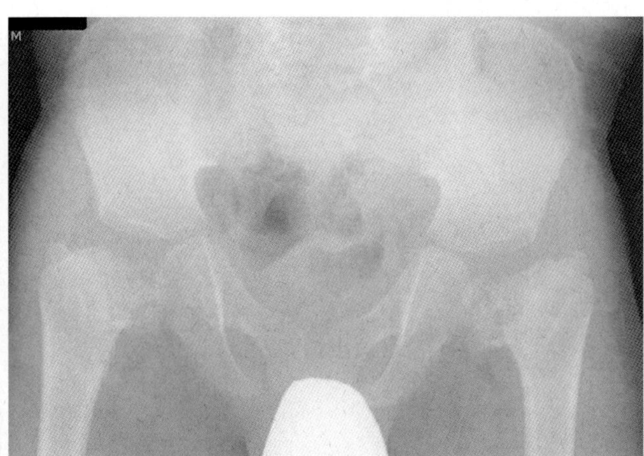

Figure 11.65 Anteroposterior radiograph of the pelvis in a 6-year-old boy with spondyloepiphyseal dysplasia congenita demonstrates marked coxa vara and delayed epiphyseal ossification typical of this condition. Proximal femoral valgus–extension–internal rotation osteotomy is often required for these patients. (*Reproduced with permission from* Skaggs DL, Flynn JM. *Staying Out of Trouble in Pediatric Orthopaedics.* Philadelphia, PA: Lippincott Williams & Wilkins, 2006.)

Pathophysiology

MPSs are a group of inherited metabolic disorders caused by a deficiency of various lysosomal enzymes. Normally, lysosomal enzymes are involved in glycosaminoglycan processing and degradation. Deficiency of these enzymes results in the accumulation of metabolic end products in the brain, viscera, and musculoskeletal tissues. Excess sugars spill over and are detectable in the urine. Normal physeal growth becomes disrupted when these end products accumulate at the growth plate and characteristic histologic changes in the proliferative and hypertrophic zones of the physis can be seen.

The overall incidence of MPSs is 1 in 25,000 live births. The more prevalent MPSs are transmitted by an autosomal recessive mode of inheritance, with the exception of Hunter syndrome, which is transmitted in an X-linked recessive fashion. Morquio and Hurler syndromes are the most common types of MPSs.

TABLE 11.3
MUCOPOLYSACCHARIDOSES

Syndrome	Enzyme Deficiency	Accumulated End Products	Mental Status
Hurler	α-L-iduronidase	Dermatan sulfate Heparan sulfate	Rapid deterioration
Hunter	Sulfo-iduronate sulfatase	Dermatan sulfate Heparan sulfate	Variable deterioration
Sanfilippo	Multiple enzymes	Heparan sulfate	Severe deterioration
Morquio	Galactosamine-6-sulfatase β-galactosidase	Keratan sulfate	Normal
Maroteaux–Lamy	β-glucuronidase	Dermatan sulfate	Variable

Classification
MPSs are classified by the deficient lysosomal enzyme and the type of accumulated end product (Table 11.3).

Presentation and Physical Examination
The diagnosis usually becomes clinically apparent between 6 months and 10 years of life, depending on the type of MPS and the speed at which the mucopolysaccharide accumulates. While there is clinical variability within this group of syndromes, these disorders share some common clinical features (Fig. 11.66). These include facial dysmorphism, short stature, hepatosplenomegaly, neurologic deficits, cardiac problems, and joint contractures. Mental retardation is associated with most types, as is deafness. Morquio syndrome, however, is characterized by normal intelligence. All patients with MPS have thick and inelastic skin with varying degrees of severity.

The facial dysmorphic features include a flat nasal bridge, hypertelorism, a prominent forehead and corneal clouding. Patients typically demonstrate short trunk dwarfism. An abnormal gait often results from angular deformities of the lower extremities (usually genu valgum) or joint contractures due to deposition of mucopolysaccharides in the joint capsule and periarticular tissues. One exception is Morquio syndrome in which patients usually develop generalized joint laxity instead of contracture. Hips may develop progressive dysplasia and coxa valga.

A careful neurologic examination is warranted in children with MPS because of the high incidence of odontoid hypoplasia and atlantoaxial instability, especially in patients with Morquio syndrome. Patients with tonal changes are usually flaccid, not spastic; myelopathy can develop early, and sudden death has been reported. The remainder of the spine may demonstrate platyspondyly and kyphoscoliosis.

Radiographs
Just like the clinical features, the radiographic findings in MPS are not present at birth but develop over time as the metabolic products accumulate. A skeletal survey, standing hip to ankle radiographs, and dynamic views of the cervical spine are generally indicated in the diagnostic workup of any MPS. Pelvic radiographs will often demonstrate enlarged and dysplastic acetabuli and coxa valga of the proximal femur. The femoral epiphysis may appear underdeveloped because of a small ossific nucleus, but MRI or arthrogram will demonstrate a large, dysmorphic cartilaginous femoral

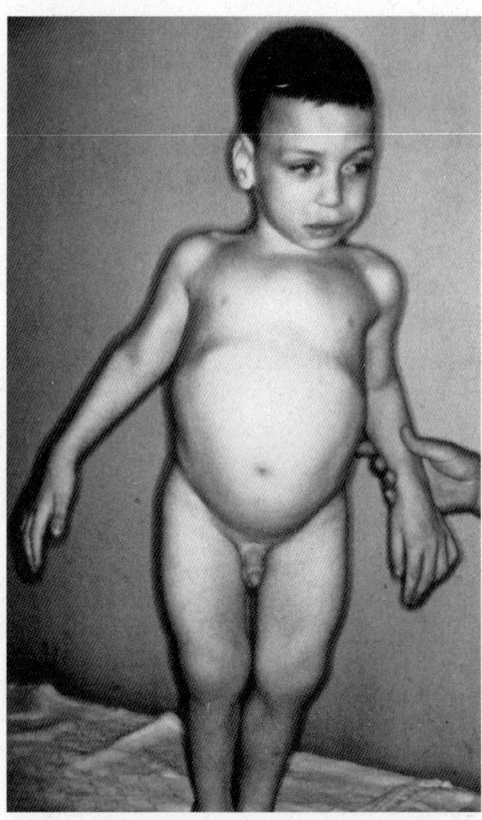

Figure 11.66 The classic appearance of a mucopolysaccharidosis in a 3-year-old patient includes facial features that are mildly coarsened, an abdominal protuberance from an enlarged spleen and liver, a short trunk, and stiff interphalangeal joints of the fingers. (*Reproduced with permission from* Morrissy RT, Weinstein SL. *Lovell and Winter's Pediatric Orthopaedics*. Philadelphia, PA: Lippincott Williams & Wilkins, 2006.)

head. Skull radiographs show a thick and enlarged calvarium. The clavicles are broad, especially medially and anteriorly. On spine radiographs, the vertebrae are somewhat flattened and "flame-shaped" with anterior-inferior beaking. Lateral cervical views will usually reveal odontoid hypoplasia; flexion and extension views are necessary to screen for atlantoaxial instability (Fig. 11.67).

Special Tests

MPS are generally diagnosed by urine screening for elevated sugar levels by using a toluidine blue-spot test. Positive tests are followed by more sophisticated biochemical analyses of both urine and serum to determine the specific mucopolysaccharide that has accumulated. Identification of the metabolic end product alone is not sufficient to

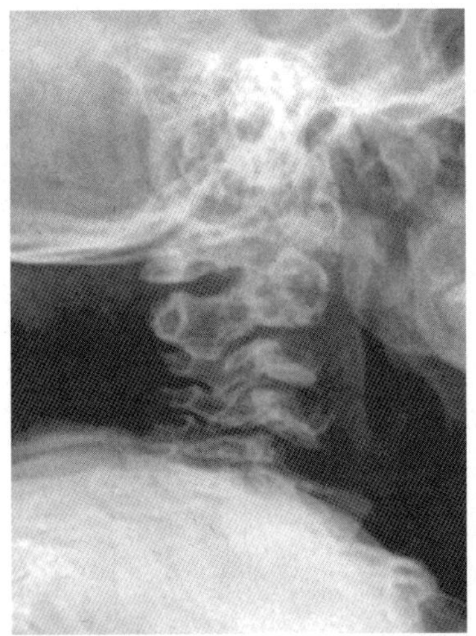

A

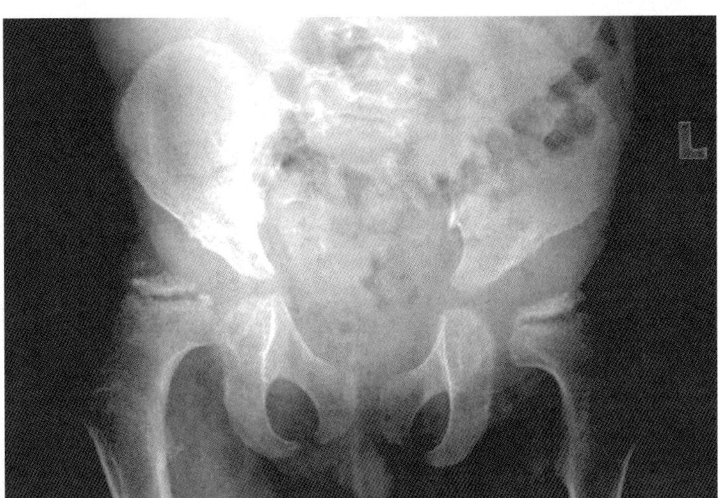

B

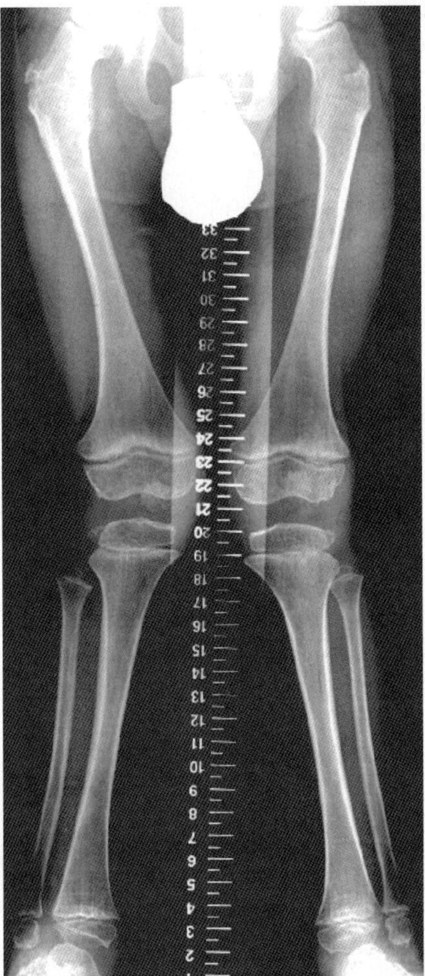

C

Figure 11.67 Characteristic radiographic features in a child with Morquio syndrome including an absent odontoid **(A),** a pelvis with capacious acetabuli and coxa valga **(B),** and marked genu valgum **(C).** (*Reproduced with permission from* Morrissy RT, Weinstein SL. *Lovell and Winter's Pediatric Orthopaedics*. Philadelphia, PA: Lippincott Williams & Wilkins, 2006.)

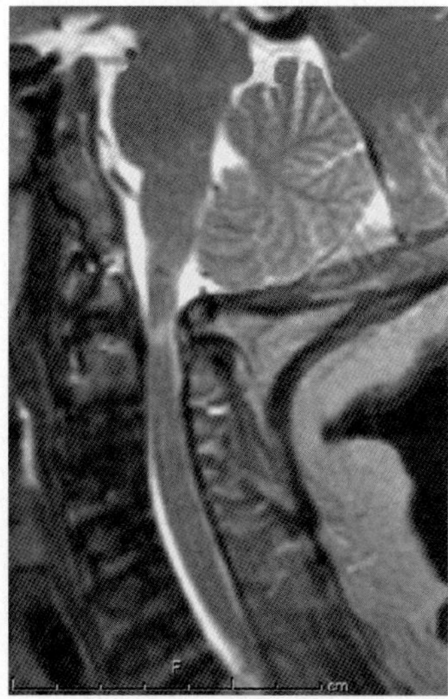

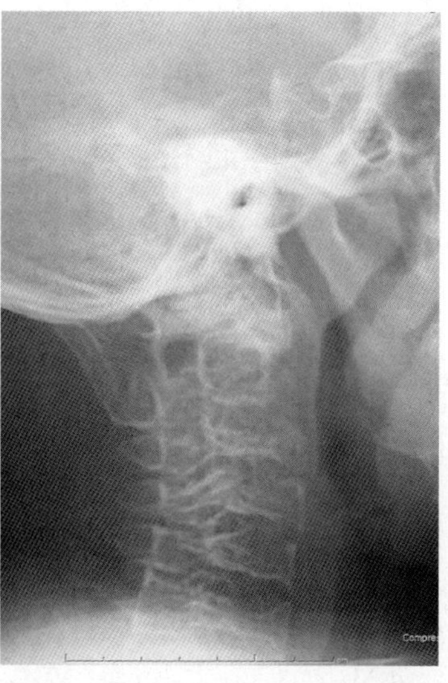

Figure 11.68 **(A)** Sagittal cut of magnetic resonance image in a 12-year-old boy with Morquio syndrome and declining ability to walk shows spinal cord compression and signal change associated with upper cervical instability resulting from his odontoid hypoplasia. **(B)** Postoperative lateral radiograph of the upper cervical spine illustrates solid occipital–C2 posterior fusion 6 months following the surgery. (*Reproduced with permission from* Skaggs DL, Flynn JM. *Staying Out of Trouble in Pediatric Orthopaedics.* Philadelphia, PA: Lippincott Williams & Wilkins, 2006.)

diagnose MPS but should be coupled with qualitative analysis and enzyme estimations for more definitive diagnosis.

Prenatal diagnosis for most of the MPS types is available to high-risk mothers, such as those with another affected offspring. Carrier status can be determined by enzymatic assays in high-risk individuals.

Differential Diagnosis

It is difficult to distinguish the various types of MPSs on the basis of radiographic and clinical findings alone. One exception is Morquio syndrome, which can sometimes be distinguished from the others on the basis of normal intelligence and generalized joint laxity rather than contracture. Generally, enzymatic assays and biochemical tests of both urine and serum are necessary to make the specific diagnosis. True skeletal dysplasias can be differentiated from MPS by the presence of characteristic clinical features, genetic testing, and the lack of abnormal urinary metabolites.

Treatment

No cure exists for patients with MPS. Treatment, for the most part, is supportive and directed at symptoms. In patients with Hurler syndrome, enzymatic replacement with recombinant α-L-iduronidase may improve some of the clinical manifestations of the disorder. Unfortunately, patients usually present after the onset of symptoms, and treatment cannot reverse the permanent tissue damage has already occurred. Allogeneic bone marrow transplantation may improve the facial features and the hepatosplenomegaly but does not seem to alleviate the musculoskeletal abnormalities. Patients with MPS have multiple medical problems due to the involvement of several organ systems. Consultation with the appropriate medial specialists is necessary to manage the cardiac, respiratory, and neurologic issues that can arise.

Orthopaedic treatment involves correction and/or stabilization of the musculoskeletal manifestations of the disorder. Joint contractures that are recalcitrant to stretching may require surgical release if they adversely affect function. Angular deformities of the lower extremities that impair ambulation should be treated by guided growth techniques or corrective osteotomy. Cervical instability, especially in Morquio syndrome, warrants atlantoaxial fusion and occasionally occipitocervical fusion (Fig. 11.68). Progressive kyphoscoliosis should be stabilized by spinal fusion and instrumentation.

CHROMOSOMAL AND INHERITED SYNDROMES

Down Syndrome (Trisomy 21)

Pathophysiology

Down syndrome occurs in patients who have a third copy of chromosome 21. In more than 95% of patients, this consists of a complete duplication of the entire chromosome. A very small percentage of children (3%) actually have a translocation of part of chromosome 21 with a normal total number of chromosomes. Either way, it is the duplication of several genes (all of which reside on the long arm of chromosome 21) that is responsible for producing the syndrome. The male:female incidence is equal, and the overall incidence is approximately 1.5 children per 1,000 live births. The major risk factor for having a child with Down syndrome is advanced maternal age.

Presentation and Physical Examination

Down syndrome is one of the most common and recognizable syndromes in humans. Patients with Down syndrome have a characteristic facial appearance, which includes upward-slanting eyes, epicanthal folds, arched palate, and flat face (Fig. 11.69). Short stature is typical, although patients are not nearly as short as in most skeletal dysplasias. Mental retardation is common but most children are able to function at a low-normal level, perform activities of daily living, and work as adults in certain capacities. Gross motor

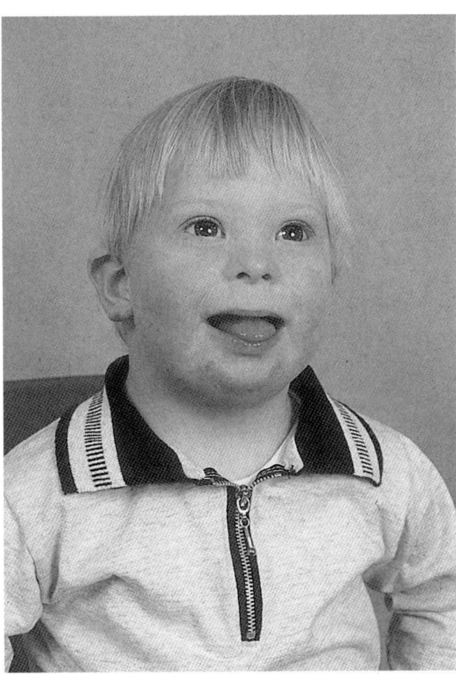

Figure 11.69 Clinical photograph of a child with Down syndrome (trisomy 21). Note the characteristic features including a small, rounded head; a flattened nasal bridge; oblique palpebral fissures; prominent epicanthal folds; small, low-set, shell-like ears; and a relatively large tongue. (*Reproduced with permission from* Pillitteri A. *Maternal and Child Health Nursing*. 4th ed. Philadelphia, PA: Lippincott Williams & Wilkins, 2003.)

development is somewhat delayed—children generally do not walk until 2 to 3 years of age. Congenital heart disease is present in up to 50% of patients and usually consists of a septal defect. Life expectancy in Down syndrome is somewhat shorter than normal, and a major cause of early mortality is cardiac disease. Other associated conditions include duodenal atresia, leukemia, and endocrinopathies such as hypothyroidism.

The orthopaedic manifestations in Down syndrome have a common thread of pathology, namely increased ligamentous laxity and joint hypermobility. Laxity at the C1–C2 articulation or the occipitocervical joint can result in cervical instability in up to 30% of patients. Most patients are asymptomatic, but others may present with subtle neurologic findings such as easy fatigability, abnormal gait, and clumsiness. Any concern should prompt a careful neurologic examination including an assessment of tone, reflexes, motor strength, and sensory deficits. Spinal deformity, which behaves like idiopathic scoliosis, is seen in approximately 50% of patients. Hip subluxation and dislocation is a major problem in Down syndrome, occurring in up to 10% of children. Unlike developmental dysplasia of the hip (DDH), hip dysplasia in Down syndrome is not present at birth but develops between the ages of 2 and 10 as a result of ligamentous laxity and joint hypermobility. Other common hip disorders include SCFE and avascular necrosis.

At the knee, patellar instability and subluxation is a direct result of ligamentous laxity. Because the medial patellofemoral ligament and the retinaculum are believed to be the major restraints in keeping the patella in the intercondylar groove, insufficiency of both of these structures allows subluxation. In addition, many children with Down syndrome have genu valgum, which increases the likelihood of patellar instability. Foot abnormalities are typical. Because of severe ligamentous laxity, the arch of the foot collapses and develops a planovalgus deformity. Many children also have a prominent metatarsus primus varus and a coincident bunion deformity.

Radiographs

Because of the high incidence of upper cervical instability, flexion–extension lateral views of the cervical spine should be obtained to measure the atlantodens interval. Values greater than 5 mm are considered diagnostic of instability. Screening radiographs of the cervical spine are generally required by the Special Olympics before a child with Down syndrome can be cleared for participation. In cases of suspected hip pathology, an AP and frog lateral view of the pelvis is warranted. Radiographs typically demonstrate flat, dysplastic acetabuli, and flared iliac wings. In certain children who complain of hip instability, the femoral heads may be well covered with a normal femoral neck–shaft angle and moderately increased femoral anteversion. In these cases, the source instability is laxity of the hip capsule and supporting ligaments.

Special Studies

Prenatal screening for Down syndrome includes measures of serum α-fetoprotein, estriol, and human chorionic gonadotropin. These levels are decreased, decreased, and increased, respectively, in the presence of a Down fetus. If these screening tests demonstrate an increased risk of trisomy 21, amniocentesis and chromosomal analysis can be performed to yield a definitive diagnosis.

CT scans may be useful prior to hip reconstruction to evaluate the version of the acetabulum and to identify areas of acetabular deficiency. MRI of the cervical spine is indicated in cases of severe atlantoaxial instability or neurologic compromise.

Treatment

The surgical treatment of children with Down syndrome can be frustrating since the same ligamentous laxity that causes the initial deformity also increases the chance of recurrence. As a result, conservative treatment is preferred whenever possible.

The management of upper cervical spine instability is somewhat controversial. Since most patients with moderate degrees of atlantoaxial instability will remain asymptomatic, and the complications of surgery can be significant, the role of prophylactic surgical stabilization remains unclear. In general, asymptomatic children with an atlantodens interval between 5 and 10 mm should be counseled to avoid high-risk sports such as diving and gymnastics.

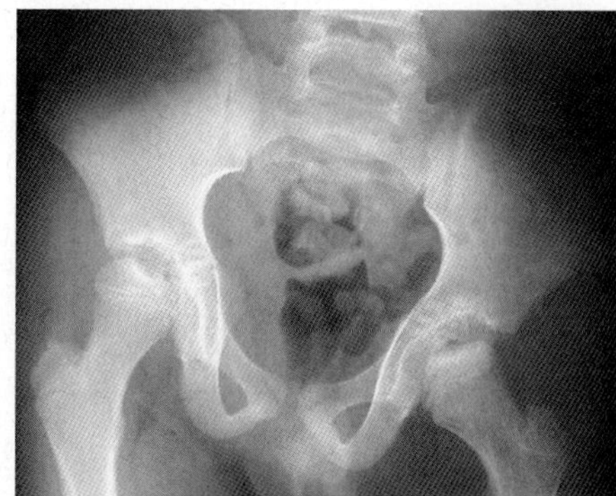

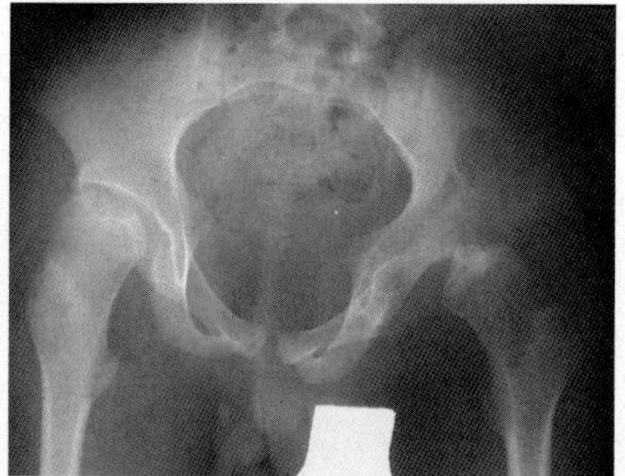

Figure 11.70 The management of hip instability from Down syndrome can be challenging. This boy presented after a few episodes of acute pain, but radiographs demonstrate a reduced, irregularly shaped femoral heads, and irregularly shaped acetabuli that seem to provide good "coverage." **(B)** He returns 3 years later with a painful, fixed dislocation of the left hip, subluxation of the right hip, and shallow, dysplastic acetabuli. (*Reproduced with permission from* Skaggs DL, Flynn JM. *Staying Out of Trouble in Pediatric Orthopaedics*. Philadelphia, PA: Lippincott Williams & Wilkins, 2006.)

Patients with instability that exceeds 10 mm should be considered for upper cervical fusion. Of course, any child with a neurologic deficit should undergo realignment and fusion. In cases of deficient posterior elements or occipitocervical instability, the arthrodesis should be extended to the occiput.

The management of hip disorders is equally challenging. Hip instability and recurrent dislocations are generally painless but may hasten the development of degenerative arthritis (Fig. 11.70). Spica casting and abduction bracing can help stabilize a hip in younger patients. In older patients, especially those that are symptomatic, reconstruction can be performed via a varus femoral osteotomy and/or redirectional acetabular osteotomy. Complications after surgery are common, most notably redislocation and infection.

Patellar instability should be initially treated by quadriceps strengthening and stabilizing braces. For those that fail conservative management, both soft tissue and bony surgery should be performed to minimize the risk of recurrence. Usually this involves a medial patellofemoral plication or reconstruction in addition to a tibial tubercle transfer for skeletally mature patients or a medial transfer of the lateral half of the patellar tendon (Roux–Goldthwaite procedure) for skeletally immature patients. In certain cases, treatment of coexisting genu valgum with hemiepiphysiodesis or corrective osteotomy will improve the success rate following surgery.

Pes planovalgus is generally painless and treatment is unnecessary unless symptoms develop. In these cases, shoewear modifications and orthotics should be the first line of treatment. For recalcitrant cases, calcaneal osteotomy to correct the hindfoot valgus can be considered. Similar to the flatfoot deformity, hallux valgus should be treated conservatively whenever possible. If surgery is necessary, the first MTP joint should be fused to minimize the risk of recurrence.

Marfan Syndrome

Pathophysiology

Marfan syndrome results from a defect in the gene that codes for fibrillin, located on the long arm of chromosome 15. Fibrillin is a glycoprotein that is closely associated with elastin and is an important component of several types of tissues, including skin, ligament, tendon, and blood vessels. A defect in this gene changes the mechanical properties of all of these tissues, leading to increased laxity. Fibrillin mutations also are thought to increase the availability of certain extracellular growth factors to cell receptors, leading to an increase in longitudinal growth. Marfan syndrome is generally inherited in an autosomal dominant fashion, although up to 30% of patients may have a spontaneous mutation. The prevalence of the disease is approximately 1 per 10,000 people in the United States.

Presentation and Physical Examination

Like many syndromes of orthopaedic importance, Marfan syndrome presents with a characteristic appearance (Fig. 11.71). Patients are generally tall and lanky with long, thin limbs. The digits are long and spider-like (arachnodactyly). Two characteristic examination findings in the hands and digits, while not diagnostic, are highly suggestive of the disease. The first is the Steinberg sign, in which the thumb extends past the ulnar border of the hand when the fist is clenched (Fig. 11.72). The second is overlap of the thumb and index finger when the patient's hand is wrapped around the contralateral wrist. Facial deformities include a high-arched palate, narrow face, and prognathism. Chest wall deformities such as pectus excavatum or pectus carinatum are typical. Joint laxity can lead to pes planovalgus, genu recurvatum, or joint dislocation. Scoliosis occurs in more than 30% of patients. Kyphosis and spondylolisthesis can also be seen.

Children with Marfan syndrome have many nonorthopaedic issues that warrant evaluation by a specialist.

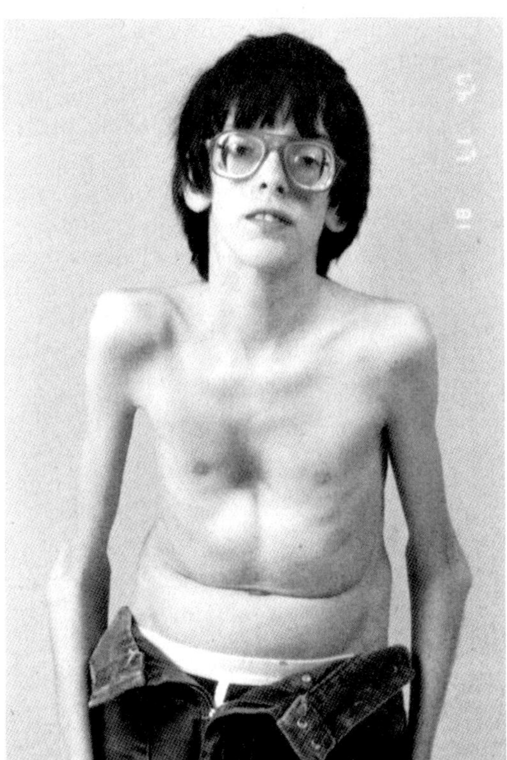

Figure 11.71 Clinical appearance of a patient with Marfan syndrome. Note extreme myopia (represented by thick corrective lens), severe pectus excavatum, long limbs, and arachnodactyly. The patient also has scoliosis and severe planovalgus feet. This appearance is typical of patients with florid manifestations of this syndrome. (*Reproduced with permission from* Herring JA. *Tachdjian's Pediatric Orthopaedics*. 3rd ed. St. Louis, MO: Saunders, 2002.)

Ophthalmologic consultation is necessary to screen for ectopia lentis (dislocated lens) that is caused by lax suspensory ligaments that allow superior migration of the lens. Testing of visual acuity may reveal myopia that results from the abnormal shape of the globe. Referral to a cardiologist is essential as patients with Marfan syndrome can develop dilation of the ascending aorta and mitral valve insufficiency. Altered elasticity in the vessel walls can lead to aortic aneurysm or dissection. Murmurs from aortic or mitral valve insufficiency are often audible.

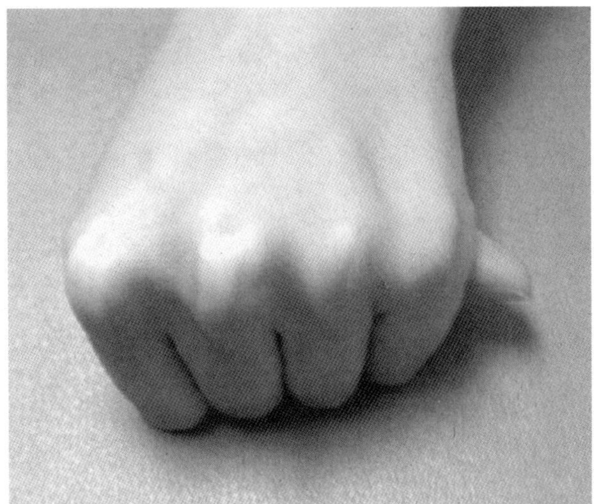

Figure 11.72 Steinberg thumb sign is useful in the diagnosis of Marfan syndrome. (*Reproduced with permission from* Skaggs DL, Flynn JM. *Staying Out of Trouble in Pediatric Orthopaedics*. Philadelphia, PA: Lippincott Williams & Wilkins, 2006.)

Radiographs

The diagnosis of Marfan syndrome is a clinical one; however, radiographs can be helpful to support the diagnosis and to evaluate anatomical areas of concern. Spinal radiographs may show scoliosis, kyphosis, or spondylolisthesis. In particular, signs of dural ectasia and pedicle dysplasia can be seen (increased interpedicular distance and increased sagittal diameter of L5). Radiographically, arachnodactyly can be quantified by measuring the length to width ratios of the second through fifth metacarpals on a posteroanterior view of the hand (Fig. 11.73). An AP view of the pelvis may show signs of protrusio acetabuli; this is defined as intrapelvic intrusion of the acetabulum such that the medial edge of the femoral head lies medial to the ilioischial line (Fig. 11.74).

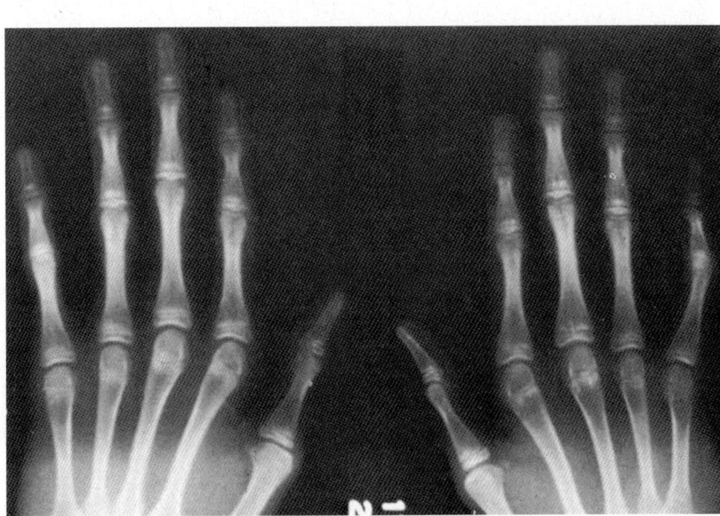

Figure 11.73 Hands showing arachnodactyly. Notice the long, thin metacarpals and phalanges. (*Reproduced with permission from* Morrissy RT, Weinstein SL. *Lovell and Winter's Pediatric Orthopaedics*. Philadelphia, PA: Lippincott Williams & Wilkins, 2006.)

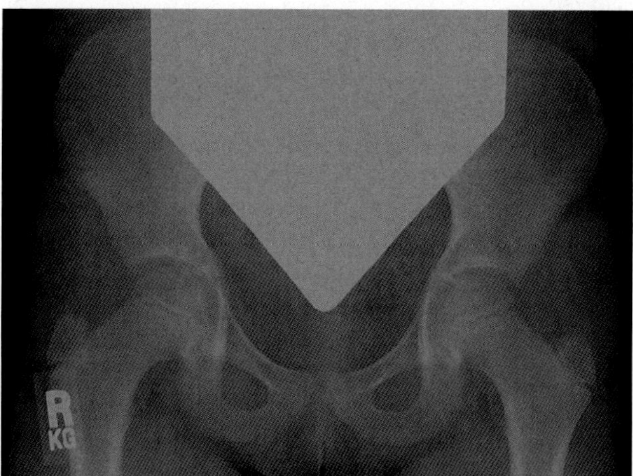

Figure 11.74 Anteroposterior radiograph of the pelvis in an 8-year-old girl with Marfan syndrome. Note the bilateral acetabular protrusio with intrusion of the medial wall of the acetabulum to the ilioischial line.

Special Studies

In spite of the knowledge of which gene causes Marfan syndrome, no specific laboratory test exists to make a definitive diagnosis. CT scans can be useful to define the bony anatomy of complex hip or spine deformities. Dural ectasia is best demonstrated on a lumbosacral MRI. Slit lamp examination and echocardiography are essential studies for ophthalmologic and cardiac evaluations respectively.

Differential Diagnosis

Marfan syndrome is a clinical diagnosis that is based on defined major and minor criteria involving several organ systems (Table 11.4). The differential diagnosis for Marfan syndrome includes several other conditions that can exhibit similar features. Homocystinuria is caused by a defect in the enzyme that converts cysteine to methionine. The condition resembles Marfan syndrome except that it is often associated with mental retardation and a coagulopathy. In addition, the direction of lens dislocation is classically inferior as compared with the superior direction that occurs in Marfan syndrome. The diagnosis can be confirmed by testing the urine for homocystine. Stickler syndrome (hereditary progressive arthro-opthalmopathy) presents with long, thin limbs such as in Marfan syndrome. However, radiographs will demonstrate features similar to mild spondyloepiphyseal dysplasia. Ocular manifestations more commonly include myopia and retinal detachment rather than ectopia lentis. Ehlers–Danlos syndrome is a collection of disorders characterized by excessive joint laxity and skin hyperelasticity. Joint dislocations, easy bruisability, and "cigarette paper" skin are the major manifestations, but height is generally normal and arachnodactyly is rare.

TABLE 11.4

BERLIN CRITERIA FOR DIAGNOSIS OF MARFAN SYNDROME[a]

Major Involvement	Minor Involvement
Ocular system	Skeletal system
Cardiovascular system	Ocular system
Dural ectasia	Cardiovascular system
	Pulmonary system
	Skin
	Central nervous system

[a]If a patient has an affected first-degree relative, at least two systems of any class must be involved. In the absence of an affected first-degree relative, involvement of the skeleton and one major system and two minor systems are required.

(*Adapted from* Morrissy RT, Weinstein SL. *Lovell and Winter's Pediatric Orthopaedics.* Philadelphia, PA: Lippincott Williams & Wilkins, 2006.)

Treatment

Currently, there is no specific treatment for the genetic defect responsible for Marfan syndrome. Therefore, treatment is aimed at managing the conditions associated with the syndrome. As mentioned, early referral to an ophthalmologist and cardiologist is important to prevent or treat ocular and cardiac problems. The use of β-blockers can reduce the risk of aortic dilation. For incompetent aortic roots, aortic valves, or mitral valves, replacement should be considered.

The treatment of scoliosis in Marfan syndrome is similar to that of idiopathic scoliosis. Bracing is recommended for curves greater than 25 degrees, although some authors have suggested that bracing may be less effective in this patient population. Surgery (usually posterior spinal fusion and instrumentation) is indicated for progressive curves that exceed 45 to 50 degrees. Complications are more common than with idiopathic scoliosis and include pseudarthrosis, infection, dural tear, residual curve decompensation, and loss of fixation in dysplastic posterior elements. Protrusio acetabuli is generally observed. In skeletally immature patients, Steel has described closure of the triradiate cartilage to minimize further acetabular deepening. In older, symptomatic patients, hip arthroplasty can be considered. The flatfeet and occasional joint dislocations that result from generalized laxity are best managed conservatively with bracing and physical therapy. For severe cases, surgical correction may be warranted.

LIMB DEFICIENCIES

Proximal Femoral Focal Deficiency

Pathophysiology

Proximal femoral focal deficiency (PFFD) refers to a spectrum of disorders characterized by a variably shortened femur with or without an abnormality of the femoroacetabular articulation. The incidence of the deficiency ranges from 1 case per 50,000 to 1 case per 200,000. The etiology of PFFD is not well understood, but certain theories have been proposed. The sclerotome subtraction theory suggests

Type		Femoral Head	Acetabulum	Femoral segment	Relationship among components of femur and acetabulum at skeletal maturity
A	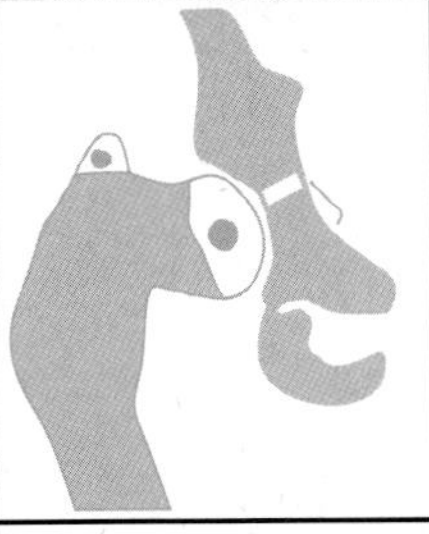	Present	Normal	Short	Bony connection between components of femur Femoral head in acetabulum Subtrochanteric varus angulation often with pseudarthritis
B	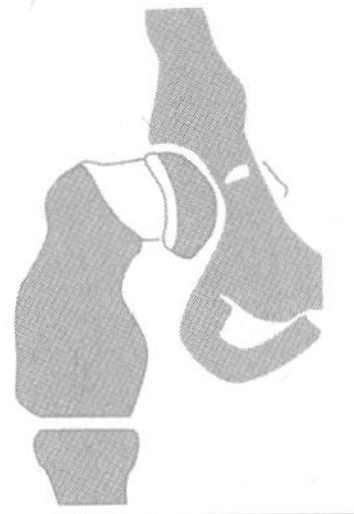	Present	Adequate or moderately displastic	Short, usually proximal bony tuft	No osseous connection between haed and shaft Femoral head in acetabulum
C	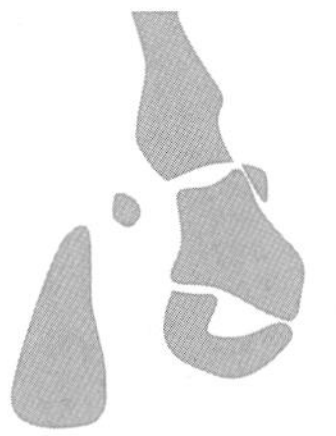	Absent or represented by ossicle	Severely displastic	Short, usually proximally tapered	May be osseous connection between shaft and proximal ossicle No articular relationship between femur and acetabulum
D	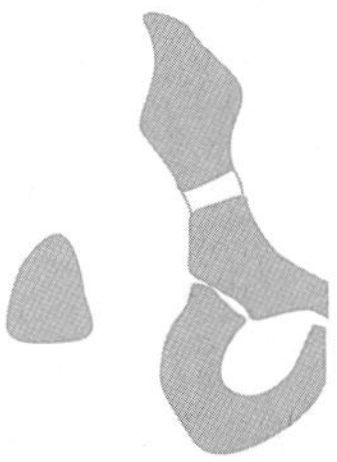	Absent	Absent Obturator fpramen enlarged Pelvis squared in bilateral cases	Short, deformed	(none)

Figure 11.75 Aitken classification for proximal femoral focal deficiency. (*Redrawn from* Herring JA. *Tachdjian's Pediatric Orthopaedics.* 3rd ed. St. Louis, MO: Saunders, 2002.)

that injury to the neural crest cells that form the precursors to the peripheral sensory nerves of L4 and L5 results PFFD. A second theory contends that PFFD may be the result of a defect in proliferation and maturation of chondrocytes in the proximal growth plate. Anoxia, ischemia, irradiation, bacterial and viral infections, toxins, hormones, mechanical energy, and thermal injury have all been suggested as possible causative factors. One well-known teratogen, thalidomide, has been implicated as a direct cause of PFFD when taken by the mother between the fourth and sixth weeks of gestation. Currently, no evidence exists for a genetic etiology.

Classification

The Aitken classification is the most widely used classification. It divides PFFD into four categories based on the radiographic appearance of the hip and the length of the femoral segment (Fig. 11.75). Gillespie proposed a more functional classification system in which he divided his patients into three groups based on treatment options. Group A consists of cases previously called congenitally short femurs; these children have normal hip joints and the length of the affected limb comes to the contralateral tibia or lower. Group B patients have hip involvement similar to Aitken A, B, or C but have larger leg length discrepancies than group A, with the length of the affected limb coming to the level of the contralateral knee or above. Gillespie group C patients are similar to Aitken D with near absence of the femur.

Presentation and Physical Examination

Children present soon after birth with obvious shortening and deformity of the affected limb. The bulbous proximal

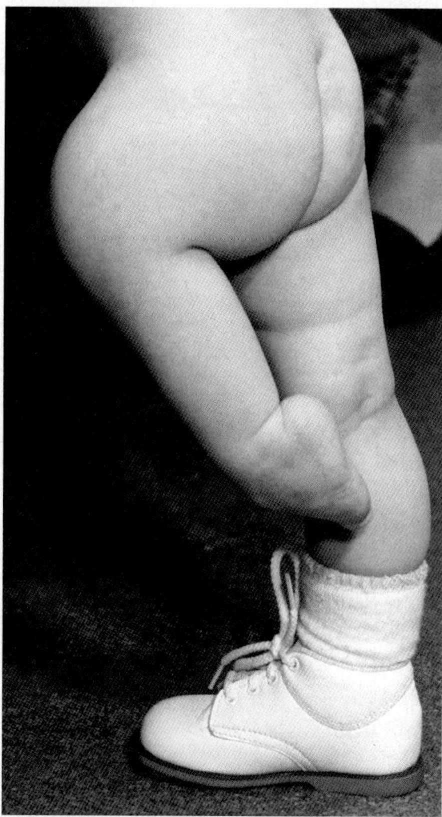

Figure 11.76 Photograph of a 12-month-old girl who demonstrates the clinical features of proximal femoral focal deficiency: a very short and bulbous femoral segment which is flexed, abducted, and externally rotated. (*Reproduced with permission from* Morrissy RT, Weinstein SL. *Lovell and Winter's Pediatric Orthopaedics*. Philadelphia, PA: Lippincott Williams & Wilkins, 2006.)

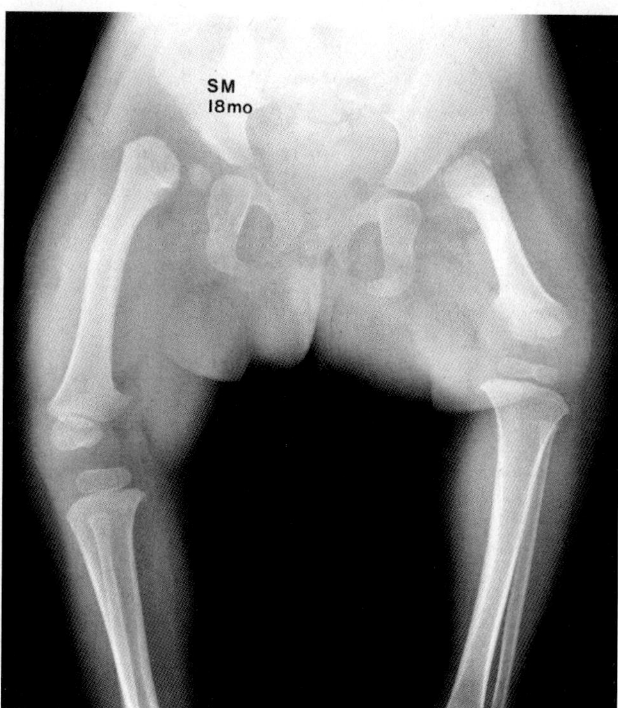

Figure 11.77 Anteroposterior view of the pelvis and lower extremities in an 18-month-old child with bilateral proximal femoral focal deficiency. The right hip is an Aitken class A and demonstrates the presence of an ossific nucleus and a good acetabulum. The opposite hip is an Aitken class C. (*Reproduced with permission from* Morrissy RT, Weinstein SL. *Lovell and Winter's Pediatric Orthopaedics*. Philadelphia, PA: Lippincott Williams & Wilkins, 2006.)

thigh quickly tapers to the knee, and the thigh is usually flexed, abducted, and externally rotated (Fig. 11.76). Physical findings may include proximal joint instability, knee instability (from absence of the anterior cruciate ligament), and variable deficiency of the proximal musculature. Flexion contractures of both the hip and the knee are common. In up to 50% of cases, the child will have an ipsilateral fibular deficiency with a equinovalgus foot deformity. Lateral rays of the foot may be missing. PFFD can be bilateral in up to 15% of cases.

Remarkably, children with PFFD compensate well for their deformity and do not have a delay in their gross motor development. Most children walk at the expected age either by toe-walking on the short side (for mild cases) or by bearing weight on the knee of the normal side and the foot of the shortened limb (for more severe cases).

Imaging

Radiographs are essential to determine the degree of femoral hypoplasia and to establish the status of the hip joint (Fig. 11.77). The percentage of the discrepancy can be estimated by comparing the short limb with the contralateral side. Often, ossification of the proximal femur will be delayed, making arthrography or MRI necessary to determine the presence or absence of a cartilaginous anlage.

Differential Diagnosis

The diagnosis of PFFD is generally straightforward. Occasionally, PFFD can be confused with congenital coxa vara with an associated short femur. The latter condition has a varus neck–shaft angle with deformation of all of the components of the head, neck, and trochanteric area and shortening of the femur. This is, however, an entirely different entity, and radiographs at approximately 1 year are generally sufficient to distinguish the two conditions.

Treatment

The management of PFFD requires a multidisciplinary team, which includes the pediatric orthopaedic surgeon, prosthetists, and physical therapists. No single treatment approach applies to all cases, and each patient with PFFD must be assessed individually.

In general, treatment is guided by the expected discrepancy at maturity and stability of the hip joint. Since the relative proportion of the shortened limb to the normal limb remains constant during growth, the expected discrepancy can be calculated by multiplying the percentage of the existing discrepancy (at the time of diagnosis) with the average length of an adult femur. Those children who have a predicted discrepancy less than 20 cm (Gillespie A) are good candidates for limb lengthening. To prevent iatrogenic hip dislocation, the hip joint should be stabilized before lengthening the femur.

Children with greater than 20 cm of expected discrepancy (Gillespie B) can be managed in several different ways. If the hip is stable, knee fusion followed by either Van Nes rotationplasty or Syme amputation preserves length of the limb and facilitates prosthetic fitting. The Van Nes rotationplasty rotates the limb 180 degrees such that the ankle becomes the new knee joint (Fig. 11.78). While highly functional, rotationplasties are sometimes difficult to accept from a cosmetic standpoint and can derotate somewhat

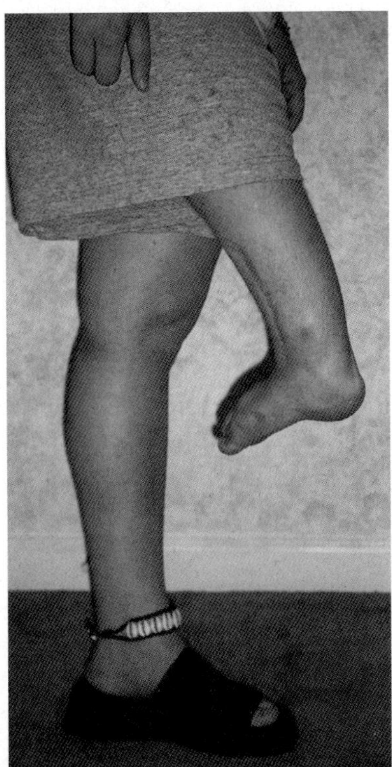
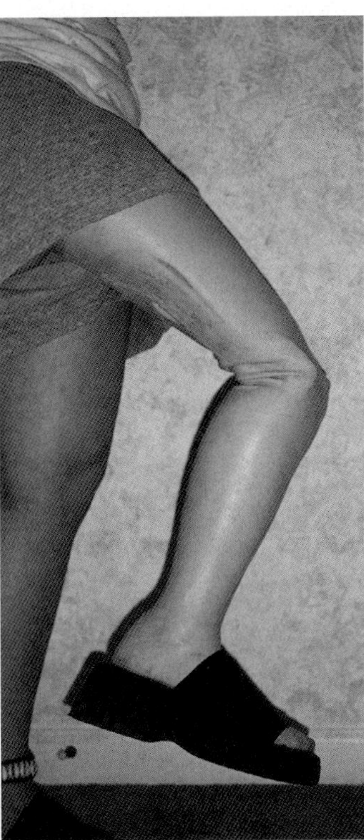
A,B

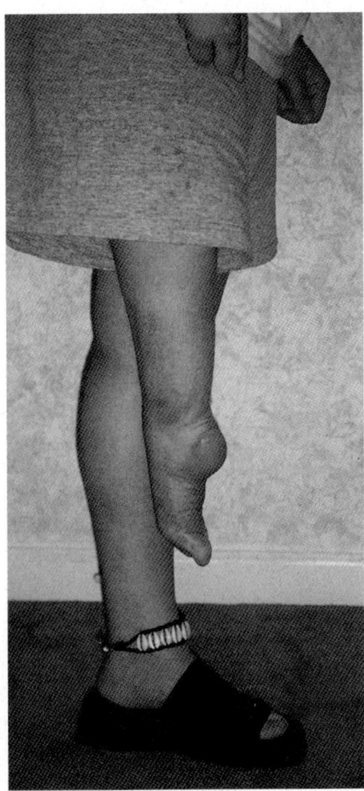
C

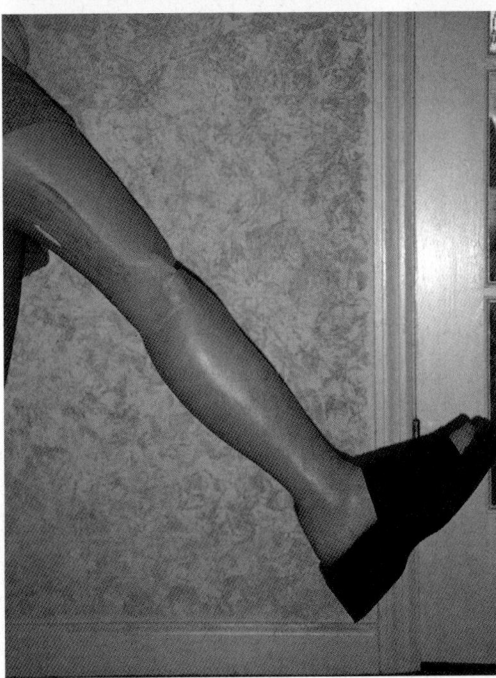
D

Figure 11.78 Results of a Van Nes rotationplasty in a 17-year-old girl with proximal femoral focal deficiency. With the ankle rotated 180 degrees, dorsiflexion of the ankle **(A)** results in flexion of the prosthetic knee **(B)**, and plantar flexion **(C)** results in extension of the prosthetic knee **(D)**. (*Reproduced with permission from* Morrissy RT, Weinstein SL. *Lovell and Winter's Pediatric Orthopaedics.* Philadelphia, PA: Lippincott Williams & Wilkins, 2006.)

with continued growth. Syme amputations are preferred if the foot and ankle do not function well or if the patient cannot tolerate the cosmetic appearance of the rotationplasty. For Gillespie B patients with an unstable hip, iliofemoral fusion may be necessary to stabilize the hip prior to a Syme amputation or rotationplasty. Most patients with near total absence of the femur (Gillespie C) should be managed with a prosthesis.

Fibular Hemimelia

Pathophysiology

Fibular hemimelia, or postaxial hypoplasia of the lower extremity, is the most common lower limb deficiency syndrome. By definition, fibular hemimelia is a longitudinal deficiency of the lateral portion of the lower limb in which part or all of the fibula may be missing. It can occur in isolation or as part of PFFD and varies in severity from mild to severe deformity. The etiology of fibular hemimelia remains unclear, but the most popular theory proposes that interference with the early development of the limb bud plays an essential role.

Classification

Several classification systems exist for fibular hemimelia. The Achterman–Kalamchi classification system is based on fibular morphology. In type IA, the proximal fibular epiphysis is distal to the level of the tibial growth plate with the distal fibular physis proximal to the talar dome. Type IB is characterized by a proximal fibula that is 30% to 50% shorter than normal (Fig. 11.79). The distal fibula is present but does not adequately support the ankle. Type II deformities refer to complete absence of the fibula.

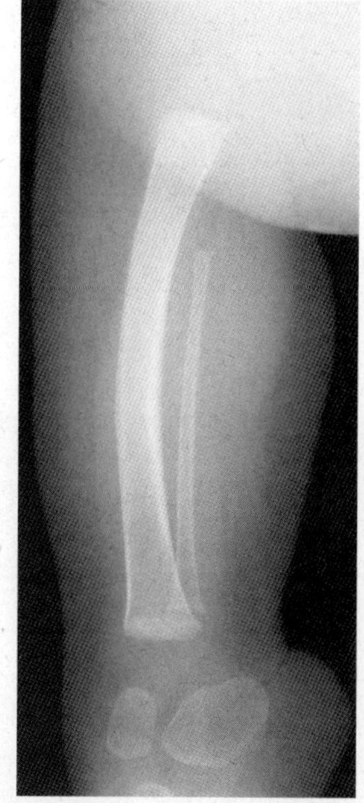

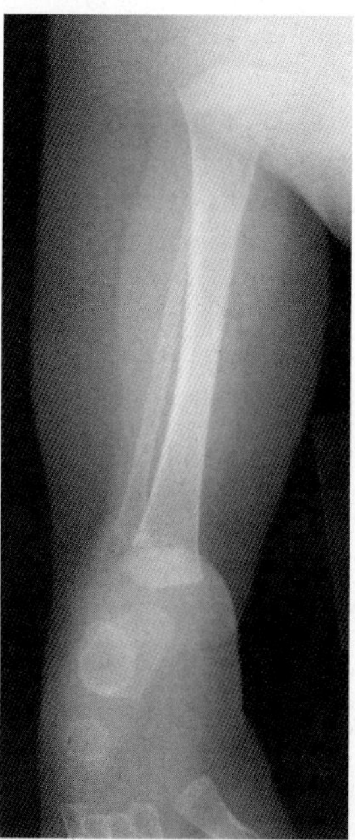

Figure 11.79 **(A** and **B)** Type IB fibular deficiency in which the proximal fibula is missing. (*Reproduced with permission from* Morrissy RT, Weinstein SL. *Lovell and Winter's Pediatric Orthopaedics.* Philadelphia, PA: Lippincott Williams & Wilkins, 2006.)

Presentation and Physical Examination

Children with fibular deficiency present early in life with shortening and deformity of the affected extremity (Fig. 11.80). Depending on the degree of fibular hypoplasia (or aplasia), a variable amount of femoral shortening can be seen. Other coexisting conditions can include genu valgum, a hypoplastic lateral femoral condyle, tarsal coalition, and

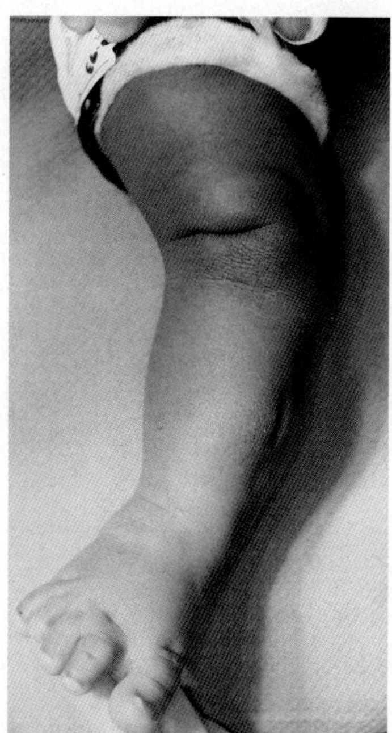

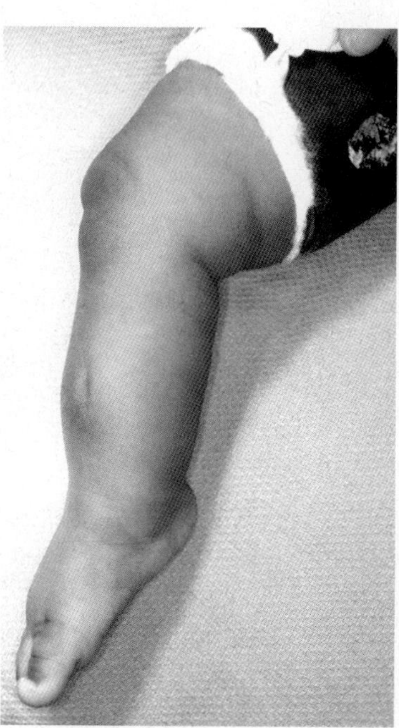

Figure 11.80 **(A** and **B)** Clinical appearance of a child with complete absence of the fibula (type II deformity). Note the short tibial segment, the valgus knee and foot, and the dimple over the tibia. (*Reproduced with permission from* Morrissy RT, Weinstein SL. *Lovell and Winter's Pediatric Orthopaedics.* Philadelphia, PA: Lippincott Williams & Wilkins, 2006.)

absence of the anterior cruciate ligament. Without a proper lateral malleolus as part of the ankle mortise, the foot tends to develop an equinovalgus deformity, and ankle instability is common. In cases of complete fibular absence, anteromedial bowing of the tibia can be seen. Depending on the severity of the fibular deficiency, the lateral rays of the foot can be missing.

Radiographs

A standing AP view of the hips to ankles shows the overall alignment of the affected lower extremity and permits use of the contralateral side as a control. Limb-length discrepancies are best measured by using scanograms (see section on leg length discrepancy). Abnormalities in specific parts of the lower extremity can be seen and, if necessary, imaged further with specific views. For example, if there is concern about coexisting PFFD and/or acetabular dysplasia, a pelvis and/or hip series should be ordered. Similarly, a knee series is useful for evaluating distal femur valgus, hypoplasia of the lateral femoral condyle, and flattening of the tibial eminence.

Differential Diagnosis

The characteristic clinical appearance and plain radiographs are generally sufficient to make the diagnosis. As mentioned, several other conditions are associated with fibular hemimelia and each should be evaluated individually.

Treatment

As with PFFD, the ultimate goal of surgery is to achieve symmetrical, stable, and well-aligned joints with the minimal number of surgical procedures. No single set of operations should always be performed; instead, individual procedures should be planned that address the specific abnormalities in each patient. Finally, realistic expectations of the timing, the duration of recovery, and the ultimate outcome must be communicated to patients and their families.

Treatment is generally guided by the degree of fibular shortening, the expected leg length discrepancy at skeletal maturity, and the quality of the foot. Patients with mild to moderate discrepancies (0%–10%) and a functional foot can be managed with shoe lifts, orthoses, and/or a well-timed contralateral epiphysiodesis. Patients with larger discrepancies and an adequate foot generally require one or more limb lengthening procedures. If the foot is nonfunctional either due to an unstable ankle or due to an insufficient number of rays (generally three or fewer), strong consideration should be given toward an early Syme amputation. Studies have shown improved function and normalized gait parameters in patients who underwent early amputation and prosthetic fitting compared with those who underwent (often several) limb salvage procedures. Amputation is certainly indicated for those patients with complete absence of the fibula.

Several of the associated conditions with fibular hemimelia may warrant treatment. Genu valgum is often progressive, and it can adversely affect alignment of the lower limb. This can be treated in several ways. Acute correction can be obtained by means of a distal femur corticotomy during a femoral lengthening procedure or by means of temporary medial epiphyseal stapling. As mentioned, ankle abnormalities can range from complete absence of the fibula to ankle valgus and/or a ball-and-socket ankle. In mild cases, a medial malleolar screw epiphysiodesis can improve alignment and provide good results. Procedures in the foot include resection of tarsal coalitions or fusions and addressing any problems with shoe fit that might arise for any deformity.

Tibial Hemimelia

Tibial hemimelia is a rare congenital anomaly characterized by deficiency of the tibia with a relatively intact fibula. The extent of the deficiency is variable: the type I form is characterized by total absence of the tibia; type II has a persistent proximal tibia; type III (rare) is characterized by the presence of a distal tibia only; and in type IV, there is a divergence of the distal tibia and fibula, with proximal displacement of the talus. The prevalence of tibial hemimelia is estimated at 1 in 1,000,000 live births. Although the majority of cases with tibial hemimelia are sporadic, affected families with possible autosomal dominant or autosomal recessive inheritance have been reported

Most children present early in life with the characteristic deformity of the lower limb (Fig. 11.81). If the entire tibia is absent, there is often a fixed proximal and lateral position of the fibula with severe flexion deformity. The affected limb is usually short, with the foot in an "apparent clubfoot" position of equinovarus. The most important component of the evaluation is to determine the amount of proximal tibial that exists and to determine whether there is a functional quadriceps. Radiographs are usually helpful to determine the degree of tibial hypoplasia, but ossification of the proximal tibia is often delayed so ultrasonography or MRI may be necessary to establish the presence or absence of a cartilaginous anlage.

If the entire tibia is absent, there is often a fixed proximal and lateral position of the fibula with severe flexion deformity. Knee disarticulation is generally preferred for this condition, although centralization of the fibula (Brown procedure) combined with Syme amputation has been described. If enough proximal tibia is present such that the quadriceps attachment is preserved, the end of the tibia can be fused to the fibula with a Syme amputation, and a very reasonable functional limb can be achieved.

Radial Clubhand

Axial deficiencies on the radial side of the forearm are the most common limb deficiencies in the upper extremity.

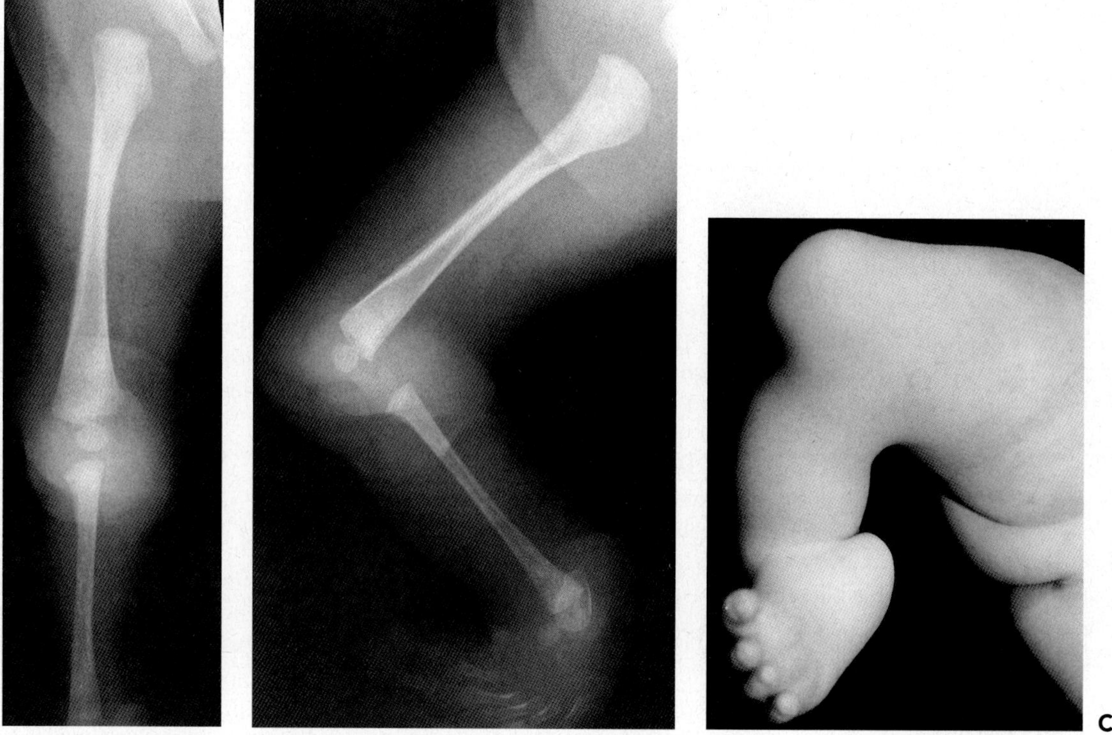

Figure 11.81 **(A** and **B)** Radiographs of an infant with complete absence of the tibia (type I deficiency). **(C)** The clinical appearance, with the medial deviation and severe equinus of the foot and the absence of any tibial structure below the distal femur. (*Reproduced with permission from* Morrissy RT, Weinstein SL. *Lovell and Winter's Pediatric Orthopaedics*. Philadelphia, PA: Lippincott Williams & Wilkins, 2006.)

This particular congenital longitudinal deficiency is reportedly transmitted as an autosomal dominant trait. Radial clubhand is characterized by partial or complete absence of the radius, with rare involvement of the ulnar ray. The hand is typically radially deviated and may be lacking a thumb (Fig. 11.82). The incidence is 1 in 100,000 live births, with approximately one-half of the cases being bilateral.

It is important for the treating physician to recognize that radial deficiencies may be associated with other syndromes in up to 50% of cases. TAR syndrome (thrombocytopenia and absent radius) is one of the more common of these conditions. VATER syndrome also has radial deficiencies along with vertebral, anal, tracheoesophageal, and renal abnormalities.

Despite the deformity, hand function is usually surprisingly good. As with many of these anomalies in young children, adaptive techniques develop rapidly. Therefore, it is important not to sacrifice a competent functioning hand in an effort to correct what the physician may feel is an unacceptable position. Stretching and splinting are largely ineffective for the definitive treatment of radial clubhand but can sometimes be helpful to stretch the soft tissues preoperatively. Surgically, several different centralization procedures have been described. All involve a soft tissue release and centralization of the carpus onto the distal ulna. Such procedures should be considered only in children with

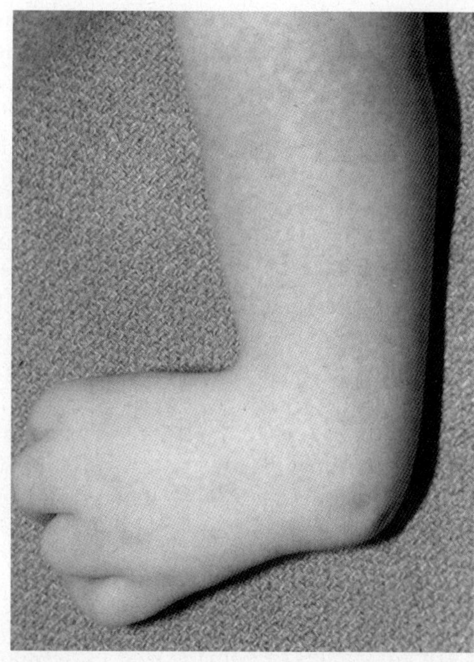

Figure 11.82 A patient with complete absence of the radius and thumb aplasia. Note the foreshortening of the forearm and the 90-degree radial deviation at the wrist. (*Reproduced with permission from* Morrissy RT, Weinstein SL. *Lovell and Winter's Pediatric Orthopaedics*. Philadelphia, PA: Lippincott Williams & Wilkins, 2006.)

sufficient elbow flexion so that they can still get the hand to the mouth after a centralization procedure. Internal fixation techniques and the use of external fixators have both been described.

ARTHRITIS

Inflammation or irritation of the joint can occur due to both infectious and noninfectious etiologies. The most important cause of acute arthritis in children is septic arthritis, which is discussed in Chapter 5. Other common causes of arthritis include transient synovitis, Lyme disease, and juvenile rheumatoid disease.

Transient Synovitis

Pathophysiology

Transient synovitis or toxic synovitis is a reactive arthritis that characteristically affects the hip. While the true cause is unknown, most authors believe that transient synovitis is a nonspecific inflammatory condition. Others have suggested that the condition is a postviral allergic synovitis since it tends to follow recent viral illnesses.

Presentation

Transient synovitis is one of the most common causes of hip pain and limp in young children. Children typically present between the ages of 3 and 9 with the acute onset of groin or thigh pain and limping. Most patients are afebrile or maintain a low-grade fever (temperature below 38°C).

History and Physical Examination

With a careful history, one can frequently uncover a history of upper respiratory tract infection or ear infection within several weeks of the onset of the limp. As a result, some authors have suggested that the condition is a postviral allergic synovitis. Physical examination will reveal restricted motion of the hip, particularly in internal rotation and extension. Most patients are ambulatory and systemic findings of infection are absent.

Diagnostic Studies

Laboratory studies are helpful in distinguishing transient synovitis from septic arthritis.

Inflammatory markers are relatively normal, but on occasion, a mild elevation in the ESR is observed. Radiographs are typically normal; in rare cases, MRI or CT may be necessary to rule out other diagnoses. Ultrasound will often demonstrate a mild to moderate joint effusion (Fig. 11.83). In cases in which septic arthritis is still a concern, aspiration of the joint will yield a definitive diagnosis as the cell counts in transient synovitis are within the range of normal.

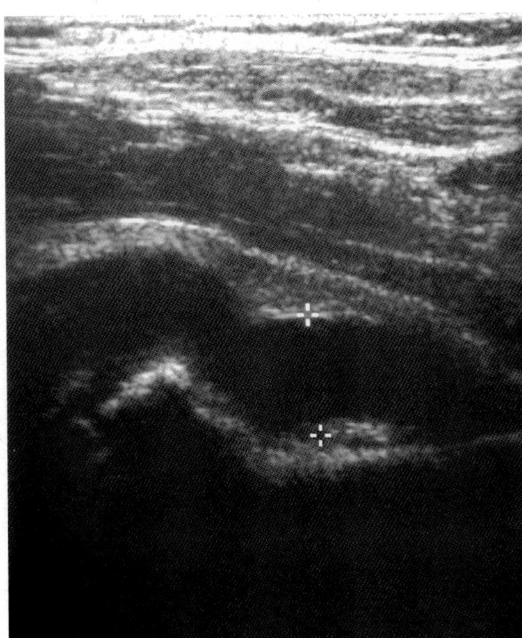

Figure 11.83 Longitudinal linear ultrasonographic view of the hips in a 6-year-old girl with transient synovitis. Ultrasonographic scan of the symptomatic hip demonstrates a large effusion in the joint as indicated between the cursor markings. Depending on the clinical presentation, aspiration may be necessary to differentiate an effusion from transient synovitis from a septic effusion. (*Reproduced with permission from* Morrissy RT, Weinstein SL. *Lovell and Winter's Pediatric Orthopaedics*. Philadelphia, PA: Lippincott Williams & Wilkins, 2006.)

Differential Diagnosis

Although the condition is common, transient synovitis is a diagnosis of exclusion; other cause of pain and limp must be ruled out before one settles on the diagnosis. The differential diagnosis includes lyme arthropathy, juvenile rheumatoid arthritis (JRA), and trauma. The most important diagnosis to rule out is septic arthritis. Usually, patients with septic arthritis will refuse to bear weight, have fevers with temperature higher than 38.5°C, and have elevated laboratory results, including white blood cell count, sedimentation rate, and C-reactive protein. If there is any doubt regarding the diagnosis, an arthrocentesis should be performed.

Treatment

The treatment of transient monoarticular synovitis of the hip is symptomatic as the condition is self-limited. Recommended therapies include activity limitation and relief of weight-bearing until the pain subsides. Anti-inflammatory agents and analgesics may shorten the duration of pain. Most children recover completely within 2 to 3 weeks.

Lyme Arthritis

Pathophysiology

Lyme disease is a tick-borne inflammatory disorder caused by the spirochete *Borrelia burgdorferi*. It is most commonly

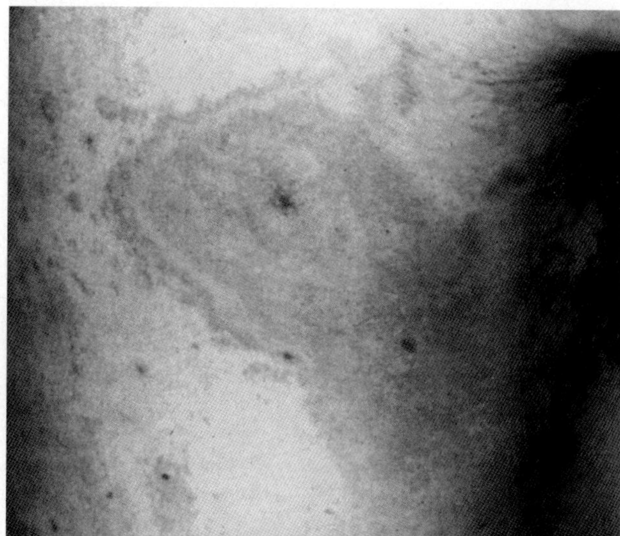

Figure 11.84 Primary erythema chronicum migrans lesion. (*Reproduced with permission from* Fleisher GR, Ludwig S, Henretig FM, et al. *Textbook of Pediatric Emergency Medicine.* 5th ed. Philadelphia, PA: Lippincott Williams & Wilkins, 2006.)

transmitted by the deer tick, *Ixodes dammini.* Named for the town in Connecticut where one of the original outbreaks occurred, Lyme disease is endemic to the northeast United States although it has been reported across the country. As one would expect, the highest rates of disease occur in the summer and fall and coincide with high deer activity and high outdoor activity by children.

Presentation

Typically, the disease presents in three stages. The first stage lasts days to weeks and is characterized by systemic symptoms (fever, malaise) and the classic erythema chronicum migrans (ECM) (Fig. 11.84). ECM is an expanding macular erythematous rash with a central clearing. This "bulls-eye" rash is seen only in 50% of children and usually occurs on the thigh, groin, or axilla. The second stage, which lasts weeks to months, is typified by cardiac and neurologic involvement. The cardiac sequelae can include varying degrees of heart block and myocarditis, and the neurologic findings can include meningitis, encephalitis, chorea, and Bell palsy. The third stage, which can persist for months to years, is characterized by frank arthritis. Intermittent attacks of asymmetrical joint swelling and pain, primarily in the large joints (e.g., knee), are typical. Children are, in general, more susceptible to the acute symptoms of Lyme disease than the chronic effects.

History and Physical Examination

Important elements of the history include living in, or recent travel to, the northeast United States, especially in regions that are heavily wooded, and other potential environmental exposures. Children and families will often not remember being bitten by a tick, although they may recall the presence of the ECM rash. Physical examination can reveal single or multiple joint involvement. These joints are usually hot, swollen, and painful and often resemble classic pyogenic septic arthritis. Ambulatory ability is variable as is the presence of a fever. Range of motion is normally restricted because of the effusion, but patients have less pain with micromotion compared with pyogenic infections.

Diagnostic Studies

Laboratory tests may show mild elevation in levels of inflammatory markers such as sedimentation rate or C-reactive protein but are usually not increased to the levels seen in pyogenic arthritis. Arthrocentesis will reveal white blood cell counts in the range of 25,000 to 50,000 cells/mL. Attempts at culture, when positive, are clearly diagnostic of the disease, but retrieval of organisms is very low. Blood tests for antibodies should be routinely performed as part of the diagnostic workup; however, there is a substantial false-negative rate early in the disease process. A two-tiered test including an enzyme-linked immunosorbent assay (ELISA) test (high sensitivity) and a Western blot (high specificity) is the diagnostic method of choice.

Differential Diagnosis

Depending on the severity of the presentation, Lyme disease can be difficult to separate from pyogenic septic arthritis or toxic synovitis. History and physical examination consistent with Lyme disease should prompt appropriate laboratory tests to confirm or rule out the diagnosis.

Treatment

Children with Lyme disease are usually treated with a prolonged course of amoxicillin. Advanced cases that have crossed the blood–brain barrier may require ceftriaxone. Most children who are diagnosed early and treated appropriately will make a rapid and full recovery.

Juvenile Rheumatoid Arthritis

JRA, also known as Still disease, currently affects nearly 400,000 children in the United States. There are two incidence peaks during childhood: one group younger than 6 years and another between 10 and 15 years of age.

Pathophysiology

The exact etiology of the disease remains unknown. Occasional references have been made to an association with an initiating traumatic event. The common thread that relates this entity to the adult form of rheumatoid arthritis is an exaggerated immunologic response in the synovium. This synovial proliferation and release of lysosomal enzymes cause the characteristic progressive joint destruction. In addition, the thickened pannus and resultant effusion cause ligamentous stretching and mechanical damage to the joint (Fig. 11.85). An additional risk in children is the effect of the hypervascular granulation tissue on the physis.

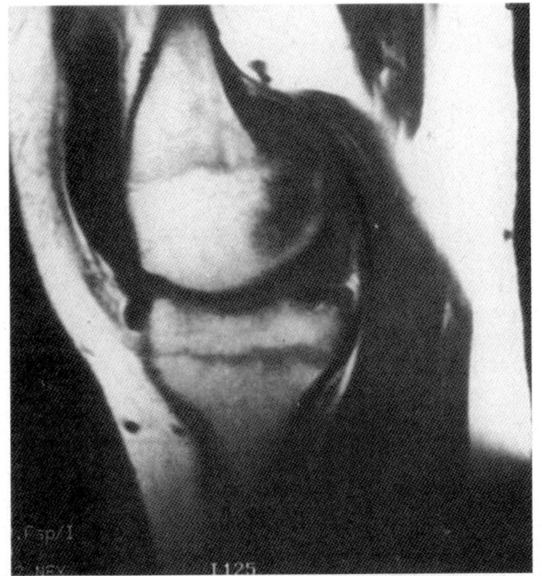

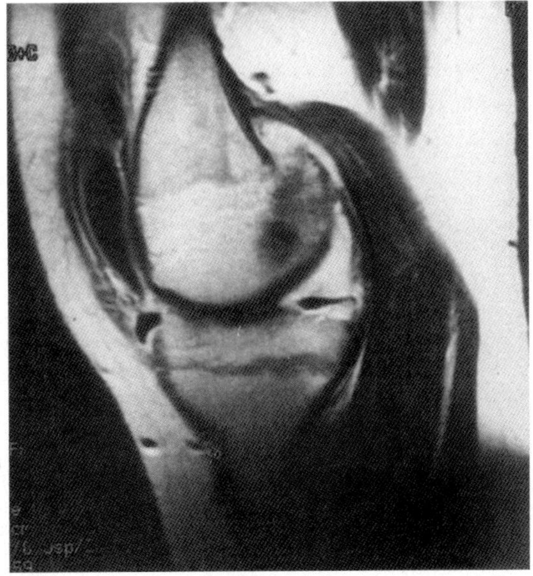

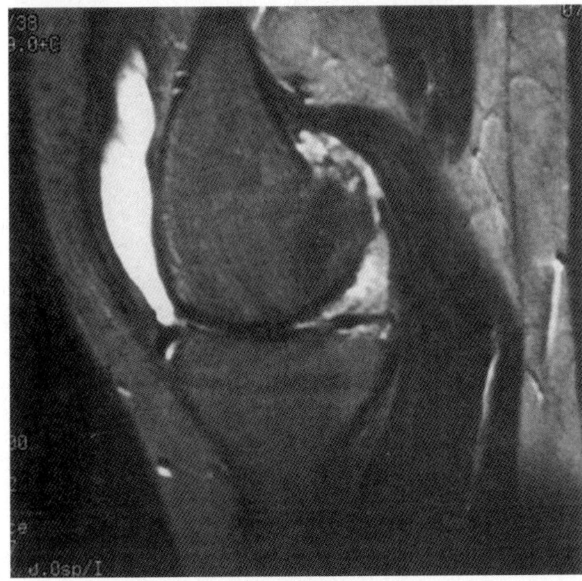

Figure 11.85 Synovitis and fluid in the knee of a 15-year-old girl with juvenile rheumatoid arthritis. **(A)** A sagittal T1-weighted magnetic resonance image (MRI). **(B)** T1-weighted MRI after gadolinium injection. **(C)** T2-weighted MRI showing high-signal areas (*white*) in the suprapatellar pouch and the posterior compartment. By comparing the pre **(A)** and post **(B)** contrast studies, the hypervascular inflamed synovium is enhanced (appears white). (*Reproduced with permission from* Koopman WJ. *Arthritis and Allied Conditions: A Textbook of Rheumatology.* 13th ed. Philadelphia, PA: Lippincott Williams & Wilkins, 1997.)

Stimulation of the growth plate frequently causes overgrowth of the limb.

Classification and Presentation

JRA can be classified into one of three forms: systemic, polyarticular, or monoarticular (pauciarticular) disease. The systemic form of JRA is an acute febrile illness representing approximately 20% of all patients. These children consistently present with a waxing and waning fever and a rash that is nonpruritic and evanescent (Fig. 11.86). Approximately 85% will also demonstrate hepatosplenomegaly. Polyarticular disease is seen in approximately 50% of involved children. Although chronically ill in appearance and stunted in their growth, these children do not manifest the generalized systemic symptoms seen in the previous group. Characteristically, multiple large joints (classically the knee) are involved (Fig. 11.87). However, small joints of the hand and feet are commonly affected as are facets of the cervical spine and temporomandibular joint. The monoarticular or pauciarticular form of the disease is seen in approximately 30% of cases. This is the most benign of the forms of JRA, but the type most likely to present for the first time to an orthopaedic surgeon. Onset of the disease is usually insidious and occurs in a seemingly otherwise-normal child. Effusions occur most commonly in the knee, followed in frequency by the elbow and the ankle. The small joints are usually spared, as is the cervical spine. The pain from the pauciarticular form of JRA is more manageable than other forms of the disease; over a period of 3 to 10 years, the disease usually resolves.

History and Physical Examination

A history of chronic symptoms often helps distinguish JRA from other forms of arthritis. In fact, to make a true

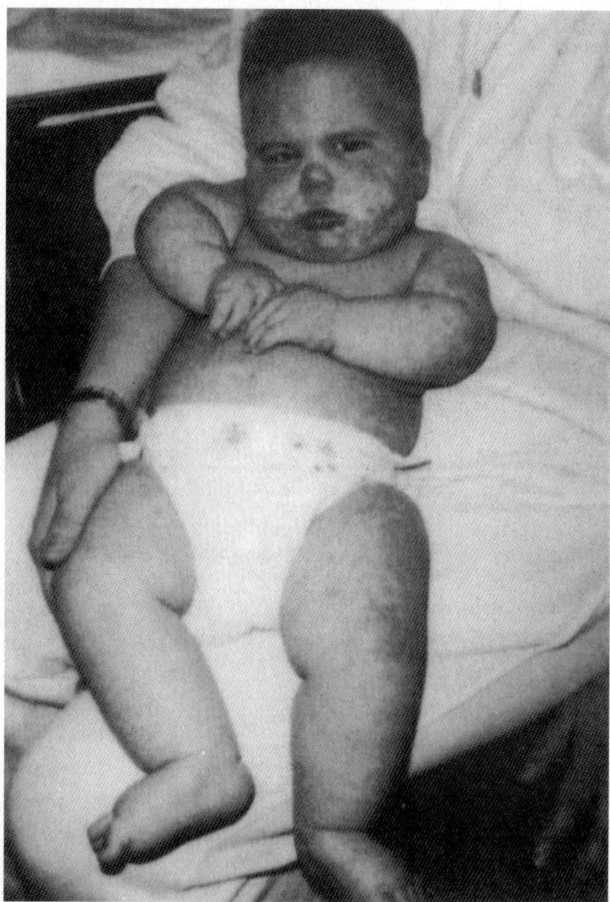

Figure 11.86 Erythematous maculopapular rash of a child with systemic juvenile rheumatoid arthritis. This rash appeared with a fever and then faded. (*Reproduced with permission from* Koopman WJ. *Arthritis and Allied Conditions: A Textbook of Rheumatology*. 13th ed. Philadelphia, PA: Lippincott Williams & Wilkins, 1997.)

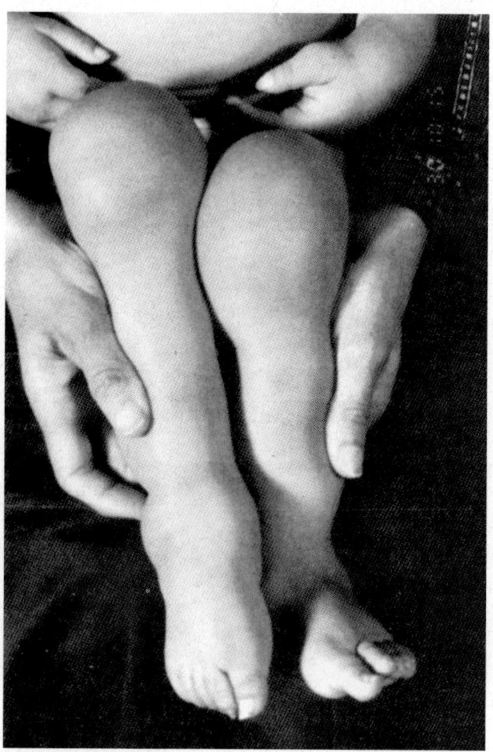

Figure 11.87 Arthritis of the knees and ankles in a child with seropositive polyarticular juvenile rheumatoid arthritis. (*Reproduced with permission from* Herring JA. *Tachdjian's Pediatric Orthopaedics*. 3rd ed. St. Louis, MO: Saunders, 2002.)

diagnosis of JRA, symptoms must be present for 6 weeks. Onset of symptoms is usually insidious without precipitating trauma. Patients often report morning stiffness with partial resolution of symptoms as the day goes on. Patients should also be asked about constitutional symptoms such as fever, malaise, and weight loss.

Patients suspected of having JRA can have many nonmusculoskeletal findings on physical examination; as a result, consultation with a pediatrician and/or rheumatologist is often warranted. Iridocyclitis is the most common cause of disability in these children (Fig. 11.88). The onset is insidious and vision becomes impaired as a result of adhesions and band keratopathy. Frequently, the ocular changes may occur before joint involvement or coincident with it. Since iridocyclitis is seen in 20% of children with the monoarticular form of the disease, routine slit lamp examination at 6-month intervals is critical. In the systemic form of the disease, the abdomen should be palpated to screen for hepatosplenomegaly, and patients should be assessed for lymphadenopathy. Enlarged mesenteric nodes can cause abdominal pain that mimics a surgical abdomen.

Children with JRA, particularly those with the polyarticular subtype, should have their necks examined for C1–C2 instability, including a careful neurologic assessment. The stretching of the transverse ligament of C1 results from

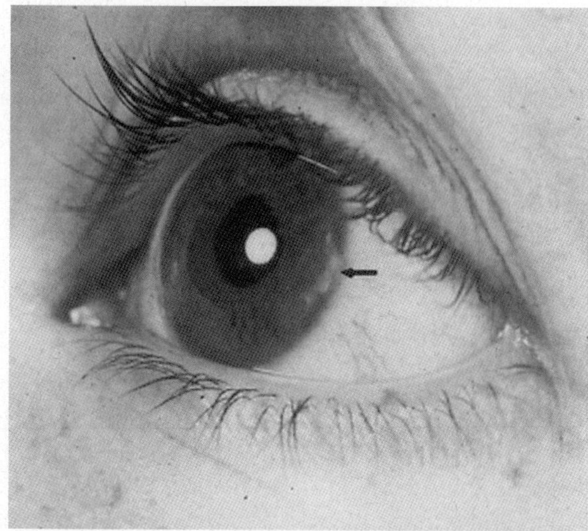

Figure 11.88 The *arrow* points to an area of band keratopathy just inside the corneal limbus in a girl who had anti-nuclear antibody (ANA)-positive juvenile rheumatoid arthritis. Her chronic uveitis was bilateral and had resulted in a decrease in vision to 20/400 in the right eye. (*Reproduced with permission from* McMillan JA, Feigin RD, DeAngelis C, et al. *Oski's Pediatrics: Principles and Practice*. Philadelphia, PA: Lippincott Williams & Wilkins, 2006.)

chronic synovial proliferation in the small bursa between the posterior aspect of the dens and the anterior surface of the transverse ligament. In addition, the temporomandibular joint can be symptomatic in one-third of patients. These children frequently complain of earaches and, because of alterations in mandibular growth, have a micrognathic appearance.

All joints in both the upper extremity and lower extremity should be systematically evaluated. Range of motion, warmth, and deformity should be assessed. In the upper extremity, the shoulder is usually spared. Elbow motion, however, can be markedly restricted and overgrowth of the radial head is frequently seen. Changes in the hand begin with early fusiform swelling of the interphalangeal joints, followed by joint subluxation and the development of flexion contractures. Radial deviation of the carpometacarpal joint and ulnar drift of the fingers are characteristic. In the lower extremity, loss of motion in the hip and knee are common. Alterations in growth with angular deformities and leg length inequality have also been reported. Foot examination often reveals involvement of the subtalar joint, which presents as a painful pes planovalgus.

Radiographs

Plain radiographs are the most important form of imaging, but MRI can be useful in early stages of the disease to evaluate synovial hypertrophy. Classic radiographic changes in JRA include symmetric joint space narrowing, subchondral erosions, periarticular osteopenia (Fig. 11.89). In addition, the epiphysis may be overgrown from hyperemia or undersized from growth retardation. Joint subluxation can occur in both large and small joints. Typical examples include ulnar subluxation of the metacarpophalangeal joints and volar subluxation of the wrist (Fig. 11.90). In late stages of the disease, fibrous or bony ankylosis can be seen. In the cervical spine, flexion–extension views should be obtained to look for atlantoaxial instability. An atlantodens interval greater than 4 to 4.5 mm is considered diagnostic for C1–C2 instability. Other radiographic findings include spontaneous fusions of the subaxial cervical spine and erosion of the odontoid process (Fig. 11.91).

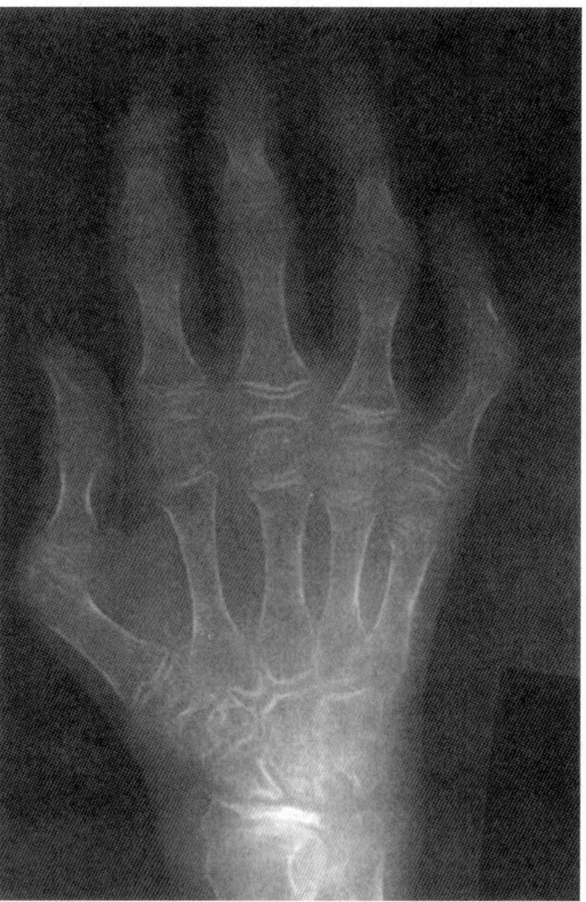

Figure 11.90 Hand radiograph in a 9-year-old girl with juvenile rheumatoid arthritis. Note the severe osteopenia, joint erosions, and subluxation of the first metacarpophalangeal joint. (*Reproduced with permission from* Koopman WJ. *Arthritis and Allied Conditions: A Textbook of Rheumatology.* 13th ed. Philadelphia, PA: Lippincott Williams & Wilkins, 1997.)

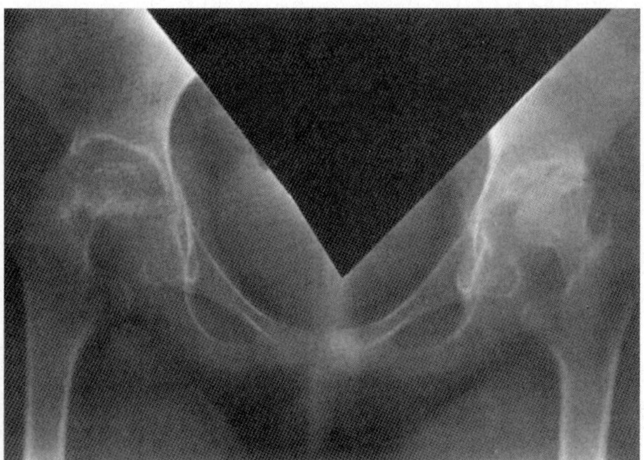

Figure 11.89 Anteroposterior radiograph of the pelvis of a 13-year-old girl with longstanding juvenile rheumatoid arthritis and severe joint damage. Note the osteopenia, subchondral erosions, and loss of joint space. (*Reproduced with permission from* Koopman WJ. *Arthritis and Allied Conditions: A Textbook of Rheumatology.* 13th ed. Philadelphia, PA: Lippincott Williams & Wilkins, 1997.)

Laboratory Studies

Complete blood cell counts often show low-grade anemia and/or leukocytosis. The platelet count, ESR, and CRP level are often elevated to a moderate degree. Rheumatoid factor is elevated only in 10% to 15% of patients. As there is no single diagnostic test for JRA, a constellation of physical findings, radiographic changes, and abnormal laboratory values is usually required to make the diagnosis.

Treatment

Medical treatment for JRA depends on the severity and type of disease. Mild, monoarticular disease can often

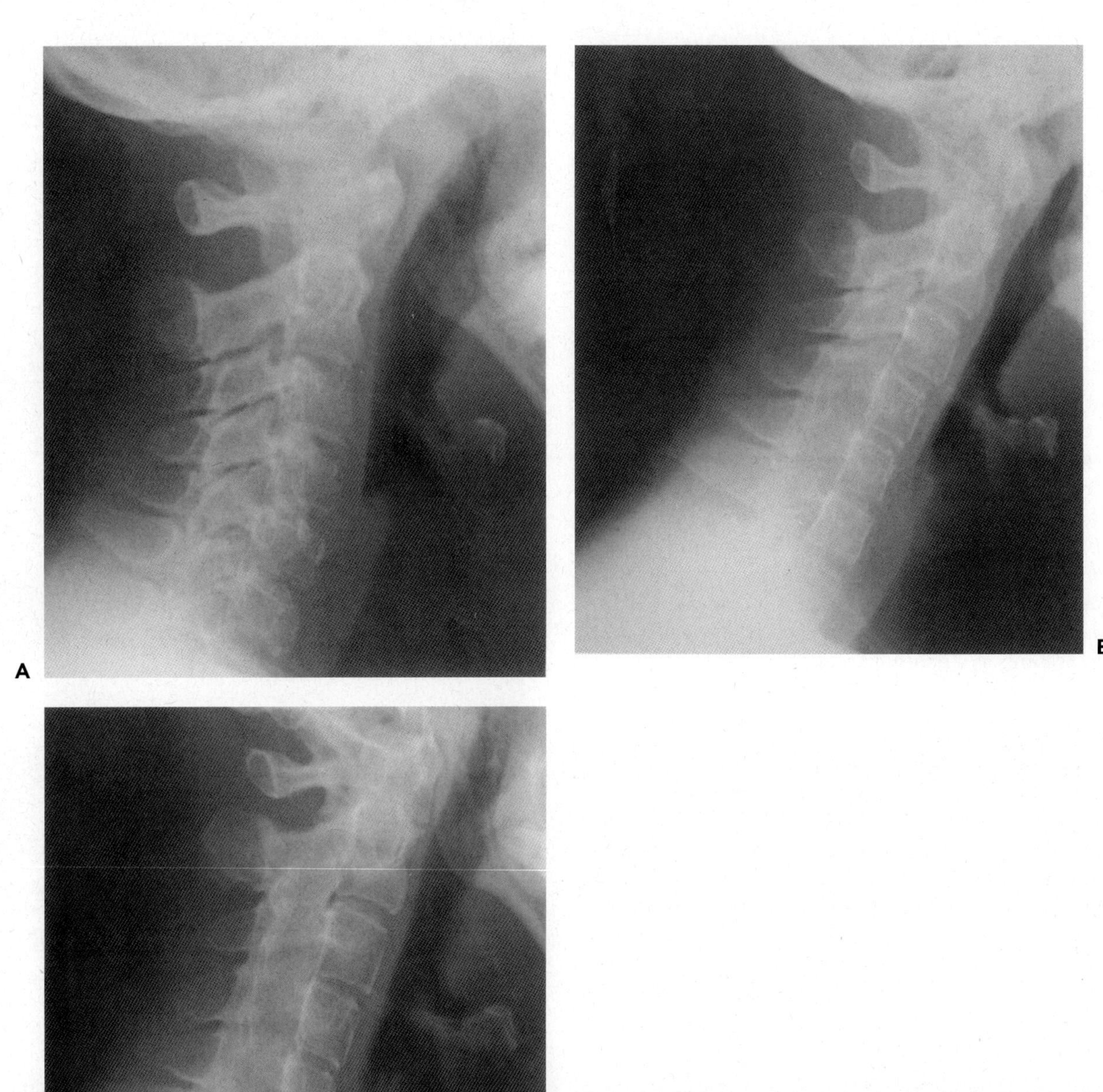

Figure 11.91 Cervical spine radiographs of a boy with systemic-onset juvenile rheumatoid arthritis. **(A)** Note the facet joint narrowing posteriorly from C2 to C6, observed at 10 years of age. **(B)** At 17 years of age, the facet joints from C3 to C6 have totally fused, with complete bony ankylosis. Also note the apple-core odontoid. **(C)** By 21 years of age, there has been complete bony ankylosis between C2 and C3. (*Reproduced with permission from* Morrissy RT, Weinstein SL. *Lovell and Winter's Pediatric Orthopaedics*. Philadelphia, PA: Lippincott Williams & Wilkins, 2006.)

be managed with nonsteroidal anti-inflammatory drugs (NSAIDs). For acute flares, intraarticular corticosteroid injections can be helpful. In more severe forms of JRA, several medications are available including cytotoxic drugs (e.g., methotrexate) and the newer anti-TNFα agents (e.g., infliximab). Although effective, these medications carry a risk for side effects and should be prescribed by a rheumatologist.

Physical therapy and bracing can be effective in reducing pain, increasing range of motion, and recovering function after surgery. Surgery can be considered for joint contractures, abnormal alignment, cervical spine instability, or joint deterioration. Synovectomy (either open or arthroscopic) can improve symptoms and prevent joint destruction. Knee and hip flexion contractures that impair function should be released. Growth disturbances or angular deformities may require epiphysiodesis or corrective osteotomies. Some severely affected joints may be amenable to fusion (e.g., subtalar joint). Larger joints may require total joint arthroplasty. Prior to any surgical procedure, patients should be screened for cervical instability or stiffness that may complicate intubation. When indicated, upper cervical fusion should be performed.

REGIONAL CONDITIONS

Hip

Perhaps no other joint in pediatric orthopaedics has attracted more attention than the hip. Several well-known pediatric diseases can affect the immature hip, including developmental hip dysplasia, SCFE, and Legg–Calvé–Perthes disease (LCPD). Knowledge of the normal growth and development of the hip joint and the vascular anatomy is essential for understanding the pathophysiology and treatment of these conditions.

Normal Development of the Hip

The hip joint begins to develop around the seventh week of gestation, when a cleft appears in the mesenchyme of the primitive limb bud. By the 11th week of gestation, precartilaginous cells differentiate into a fully formed cartilaginous femoral head and acetabulum (Fig. 11.92). At birth, the vast majority of both the femoral head and the acetabulum are cartilaginous.

The acetabulum is composed of four different cartilage types. The articular surface is covered by hyaline cartilage. Continuous with this hyaline cartilage is the Y-shaped triradiate cartilage, which is the acetabular physis. This structure connects the three pelvic bones (ilium, ischium, and pubis) and allows the acetabulum and to grow in height and increase in depth. The fibrocartilaginous labrum surrounds the acetabulum and increases the depth of the femoroacetabular articulation (Fig. 11.93). Finally, epiphyseal cartilage exists on the lateral edge of the acetabulum. This represents a secondary ossification center and is an important contributor to acetabular depth and lateral coverage. This lateral growth center and the triradiate cartilage generally fuse by the early teenage years.

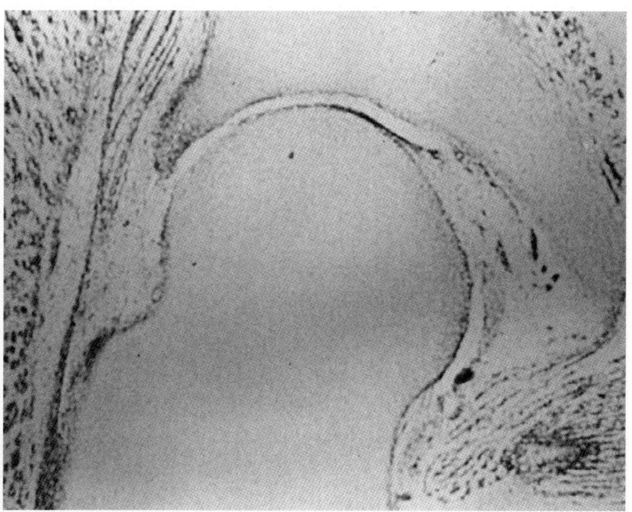

Figure 11.92 Embryonic hip. The components of the hip joint, the acetabulum, and the femoral head develop from the same primitive mesenchymal cells. A cleft develops in the precartilaginous cells at approximately the 7th week of gestation, defining the acetabulum and the femoral head. (*Reproduced with permission from* Morrissy RT, Weinstein SL. *Lovell and Winter's Pediatric Orthopaedics.* Philadelphia, PA: Lippincott Williams & Wilkins, 2006.)

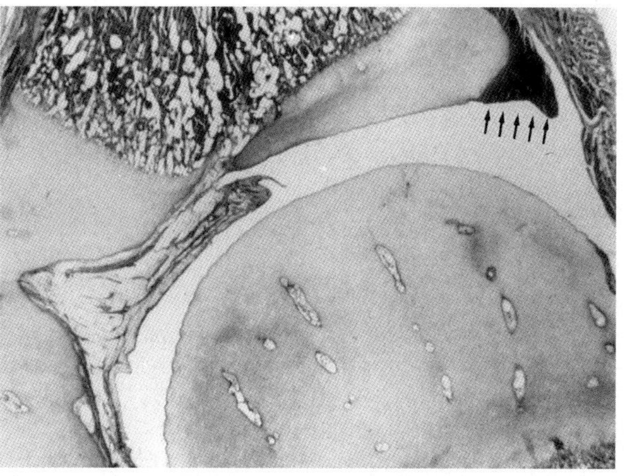

Figure 11.93 Coronal section through the center of the acetabulum in a full-term infant. Note the fibrocartilaginous edge of the acetabulum, the labrum (*arrows*), at the peripheral edge of the acetabular cartilage. The hip capsule inserts just above the labrum. (*Reproduced with permission from* Morrissy RT, Weinstein SL. *Lovell and Winter's Pediatric Orthopaedics.* Philadelphia, PA: Lippincott Williams & Wilkins, 2006.)

The ossification center of the femoral head typically appears between the fourth and sixth months of postnatal life. Initially, this center is spherical; subsequently, it expands into an ovoid shape. The femoral neck physis is initially continuous with a growth plate on the lateral surface of the femoral neck and the trochanteric growth plate (Fig. 11.94). The femoral neck physis and the trochanteric physis contribute primarily to the longitudinal growth of the proximal femur; however, the specific pattern of growth in all three physes is what determines the width of the femoral neck, the neck–shaft angle, and the relationship of the femoral head to the greater trochanter. With increasing age and mechanical loading, the trabeculae become more and more stress oriented. By the age of 6 years, the calcar of the proximal femur becomes prominent. The greater trochanter initially ossifies, as a secondary center, between 5 and 7 years of age. Fusion is generally complete by age 18.

An important concept is that the acetabulum and the femoral head develop in a concordant fashion. Proper acetabular development requires a well-reduced, spherical femoral head to provide the necessary template about which to form. The even distribution of contact forces supplied by a round femoral head allows the acetabulum to achieve an appropriate depth and coverage. Similarly, the contact pressures provided by a close-fitting acetabulum are necessary to shape the femoral head. Any abnormality of this articulation during early development can alter the biomechanics and result in a dysplastic acetabulum and/or proximal femur (Fig. 11.95).

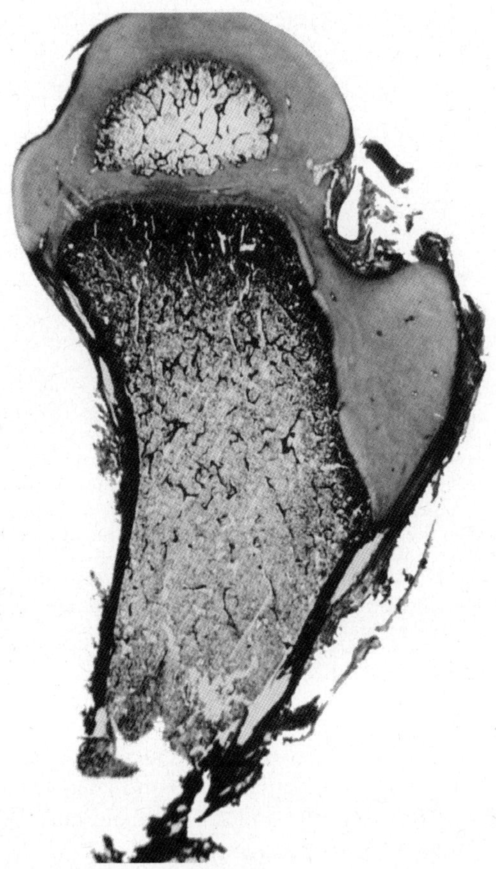

Figure 11.94 The proximal femur in an infant has three physeal plates: the growth plate of the greater trochanter, the growth plate of the proximal femoral physis, and the growth plate of the femoral neck isthmus connecting the other two. (*Reproduced with permission from* Morrissy RT, Weinstein SL. *Lovell and Winter's Pediatric Orthopaedics*. Philadelphia, PA: Lippincott Williams & Wilkins, 2006.)

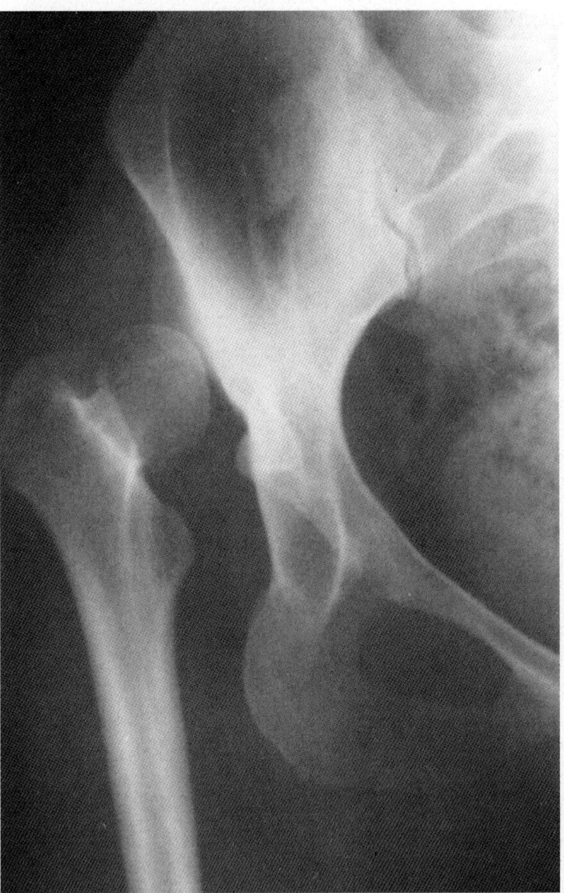

Figure 11.95 Untreated dislocation of the hip. Note the lack of concave shape and the shallowness of the acetabulum due to the lack of development with a concentrically reduced femoral head. (*Reproduced with permission from* Morrissy RT, Weinstein SL. *Lovell and Winter's Pediatric Orthopaedics*. Philadelphia, PA: Lippincott Williams & Wilkins, 2006.)

Vascular Anatomy

The blood supply of the hip joint is critical to its normal development. In general, the blood supply to the hip is divided into the extracapsular circulation and the intracapsular circulation. The extracapsular blood supply of the proximal femur is predominantly from the profunda femoris artery via its two major branches: the lateral circumflex artery (LCA) and the medial circumflex artery (MCA). These two arteries form an extracapsular ring around the trochanteric and basilar neck regions. The LCA supplies the anterior portion of the ring, whereas the MCA supplies the medial, posterior, and lateral portions of the ring. Both arteries give rise to ascending cervical branches, which provide the blood supply to the femoral neck and contribute to the intracapsular circulation (Fig. 11.96). The most important of these branches is the lateral ascending cervical artery, a terminal branch of the MCA that supplies the majority of the femoral epiphysis. This artery traverses the lateral capsule in the posterior trochanteric fossa via a narrow passage and is, therefore, vulnerable to constriction. The extracapsular ring is a constant finding, although its size and configuration are variable.

The intraarticular circulation is formed from the four ascending cervical arteries (medial, anterior, posterior, and lateral) that create a subsynovial anastomotic ring at the margin of the articular surface, although this ring is often incomplete. At birth, branches of both the lateral and medial circumflex arteries provide equal amounts of flow to the capital femoral epiphysis. The artery of the ligamentum teres, however, does not contribute significantly to the blood supply of the femoral head. By 3 to 4 years of age, the flow from the LCA diminishes and supplies predominantly the anterior neck and metaphysis. The physis establishes a firm barrier between the metaphysis and the epiphysis, which reduces the contributions of the metaphyseal branches. At this point, the MCA provides the majority of the blood flow to the capital femoral epiphysis through its lateral ascending cervical artery (lateral epiphyseal branches) (Fig. 11.97). After closure of the physis, the epiphyseal and metaphyseal vessels again are able to form an intraepiphyseal anastomotic network. Damage to one or both of the vascular systems of the proximal femur can

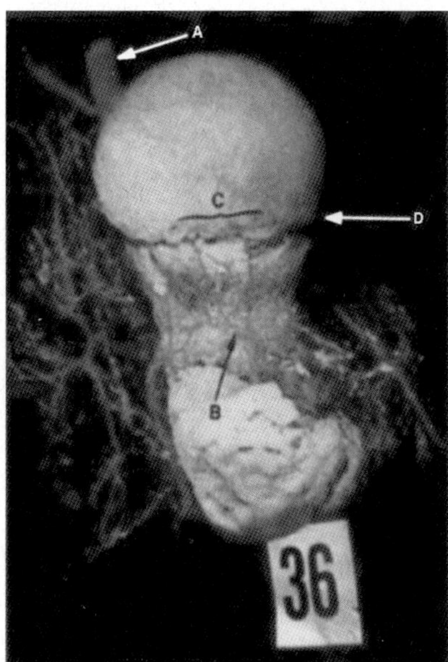

Figure 11.96 Extracapsular blood supply to the proximal femur. **(A)** Femoral artery. **(B)** Extracapsular ring from the medial circumflex artery and lateral circumflex artery. **(C)** Ascending lateral cervical artery. **(D)** Physis. (*Reproduced with permission from* Chung SM. The arterial supply of the developing proximal end of the human femur. *J Bone Joint Surg Am.* 1976;58:961–970.)

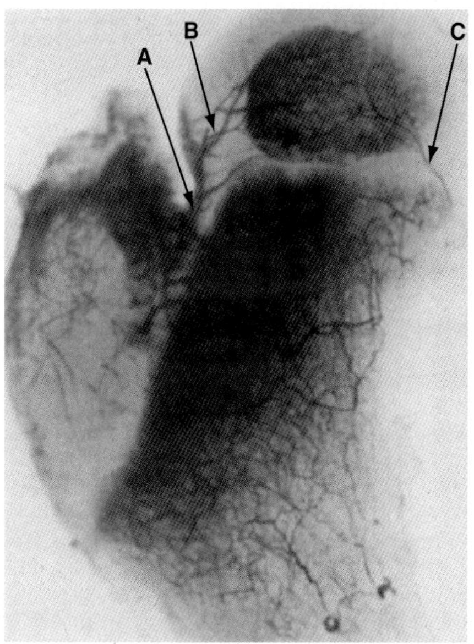

Figure 11.97 By age 3 to 4, most of the blood supply to the femoral epiphysis comes from the medial femoral circumflex artery, which gives rise to the lateral ascending cervical artery **(A)** and its lateral epiphyseal branches **(B).** A smaller contribution is provided by the medial ascending cervical artery **(C).** Note that by this age, the physis acts as a barrier that prevents metaphyseal vessels from supplying the epiphysis. (*Reproduced with permission from* Chung SM. The arterial supply of the developing proximal end of the human femur. *J Bone Joint Surg Am.* 1976;58:961–970.)

produce avascular necrosis of the femoral head and permanent deformity of the hip.

Developmental Dysplasia of the Hip

DDH refers to a spectrum of pathology in the development of the immature hip joint. The original term for the condition, *congenital dislocation of the hip,* was replaced by the current name to more accurately reflect the variable presentation of the disorder and to encompass mild dysplasias and frank dislocations. The incidence of this condition is approximately 1 per 1,000 live births for true dislocation and approximately 1 per 100 live births for dysplasia and mild subluxation. There is, however, marked geographic and racial variation in the incidence of DDH. The reported incidence based on geography ranges from 1.7 per 1,000 babies in Sweden to 188 per 1,000 in a district in Manitoba, Canada. The incidence of DDH in Chinese and African newborns is almost 0%, whereas it is 1% for hip dysplasia and 0.1% for hip dislocation in white newborns.

Pathophysiology

Although the exact etiology remains unknown, the final common pathway in the development of DDH is the increased laxity of the hip capsule, which fails to maintain a stable femoroacetabular articulation. This increased laxity is probably due a combination of hormonal, mechanical, and genetic factors. One major risk factor for DDH is female gender; the increased incidence of DDH in females is thought to result from increased susceptibility to maternal hormones such as relaxin, which increases ligamentous laxity. Breech positioning, especially when the infant's knees are extended, has been shown in animal models to increase the risk for dislocation. In humans, the incidence of DDH in breech infants is up to 20%. Any other condition that leads to a tighter intrauterine space and, consequently, less room for normal fetal motion may be associated with DDH. These conditions include oligohydramnios, large birth weight, and first pregnancy. The high rate of association of DDH with other intrauterine molding abnormalities, such as torticollis and metatarsus adductus, supports the theory that the "crowding phenomenon" has a role in the pathogenesis. Finally, genetic factors clearly play a role. A major risk factor for DDH is a positive family history, which is present in 12% to 33% of patients. Twin studies have shown a 34% incidence of DDH in both identical twins compared with 3% in fraternal twins. Genetic predispositions most likely reflect intrinsic differences in collagen and connective tissue laxity.

Depending on the severity of DDH, the neonatal hip may be completely dislocated, partially dislocated, or mildly displaced. Some of these hips probably spend some time dislocated and some time reduced. During the neonatal period, some of these unstable hips will gradually dock in the acetabulum and will end up normal from a radiographic and anatomic standpoint. Other hips will fail to reduce and will remain out of the acetabulum permanently. This latter group will develop several secondary

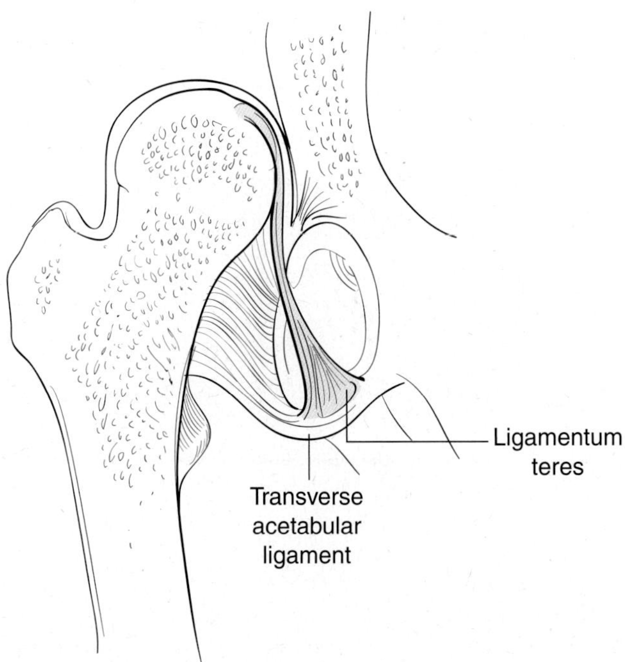

Figure 11.98 The hypertrophied ligamentum teres and the transverse acetabular ligament can block reduction. (*Reproduced with permission from* Skaggs DL, Flynn JM. *Staying Out of Trouble in Pediatric Orthopaedics.* Philadelphia, PA: Lippincott Williams & Wilkins, 2006.)

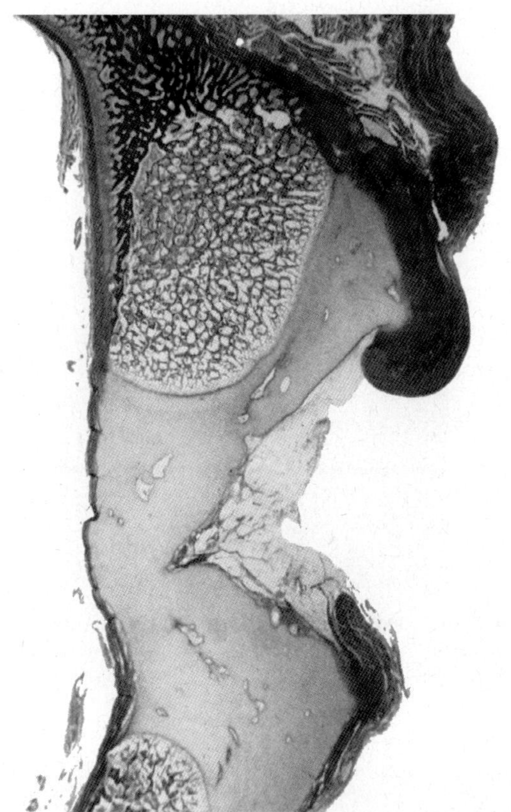

Figure 11.99 A coronal section of the acetabulum demonstrating the infolded hypertrophic labrum (limbus), which extends over the margin of the thickened acetabular cartilage. (*Reproduced with permission from* Morrissy RT, Weinstein SL. *Lovell and Winter's Pediatric Orthopaedics.* Philadelphia, PA: Lippincott Williams & Wilkins, 2006.)

anatomic changes that can prevent reduction. Both the fatty tissue in the depths of the socket, known as the *pulvinar,* and the ligamentum teres can hypertrophy, blocking reduction of the femoral head. The transverse acetabular ligament also usually thickens, which effectively narrows the opening of the acetabulum (Fig. 11.98). In addition, the shortened iliopsoas tendon becomes taut across the front of the hip, creating an hourglass shape to the hip capsule, which limits access to the acetabulum. Over time, the dislocated femoral head places pressure on the acetabular rim and labrum, causing the labrum to infold and become thick (Fig. 11.99).

As previously discussed, the shape of a normal femoral head and acetabulum depends on a concentric reduction between the two. The more time that a hip spends dislocated, the more likely that the acetabulum will develop abnormally. Without a femoral head to provide a template, the acetabulum will become progressively shallow with an oblique acetabular roof and a thickened medial wall. The point at which these changes become irreversible remains unknown; however, early treatment is preferred to maximize the chances for femoral and acetabular remodeling.

Classification

The spectrum of DDH can be divided into dislocated, subluxated, and dysplastic hips. Dislocated hips are those in which the femoral head no longer has any contact with the acetabulum. Subluxation occurs when the femoral epiphysis has partially lost contact with the acetabulum (Fig. 11.100). Radiographically, this is defined as a break in Shenton line (see later). Dysplasia refers to those hips that are still reduced but have shallow, saucer-shaped acetabuli. Although dislocations and subluxations are generally diagnosed early in childhood, acetabular dysplasia may be undetectable clinically until the patient becomes symptomatic during early adulthood.

Presentation

Girls present with DDH more often than do boys, by a 4:1 ratio. In 60% of cases, the left side is the affected side. In the newborn period, the majority of patients are referred because of instability found during routine clinical examinations by their pediatricians. After the walking age, children usually present with a limp and/or leg length discrepancy. For most children, pain is not a part of the presenting complaints. In contrast, those patients with mild acetabular dysplasia that escapes detection during childhood may present in early adulthood with groin pain and instability of their hip.

Physical Examination

In the newborn period, careful physical examination is essential for the diagnosis of DDH. The child should be

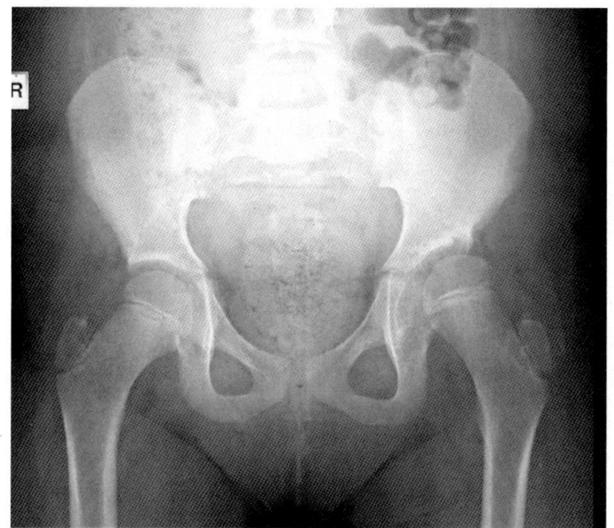

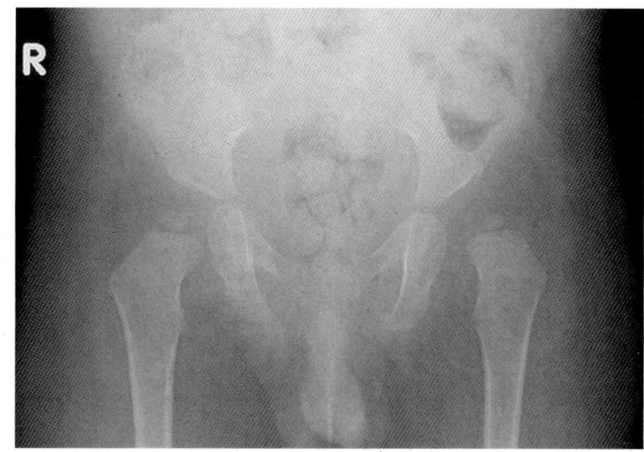

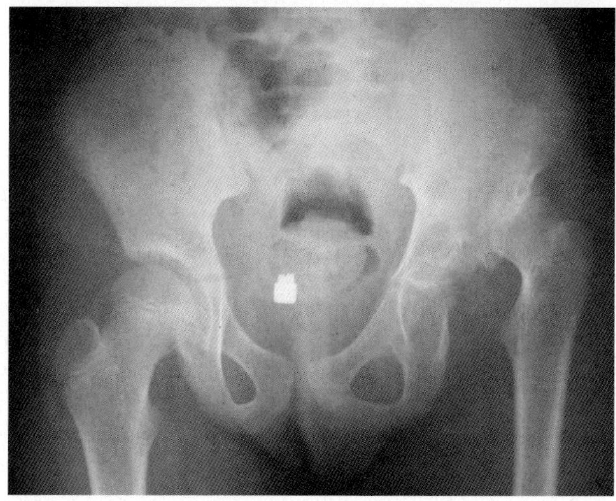

Figure 11.100 Anteroposterior radiographs of the pelvis showing three different left hips with **(A)** dysplasia alone, **(B)** hip subluxation, and **(C)** hip dislocation.

examined on a firm surface in the supine position. Obviously, the infant should be completely undressed to perform an adequate examination. An upset child will contract the proximal muscles and make the diagnosis of instability nearly impossible; it is, therefore, important to keep the child relaxed by warming the room, providing a blanket, or feeding with a bottle. The examiner should grasp the infant's thigh with the thumb over the lesser trochanter medially and the ring or middle finger around the greater trochanter laterally. The Ortolani test is performed by gently abducting the hip while exerting an upward force on the greater trochanter (Fig. 11.101). A palpable "clunk" represents the reduction of a dislocated (but reducible) hip. The Barlow test is performed in the same position with the hip in neutral or slight adduction and a gentle downward force applied to the hip joint. If the femoral head moves out of the acetabulum, the hip is considered dislocatable (Fig. 11.102). These findings can be subtle and often require a delicate touch. It is important to distinguish the "clunk" associated with a truly positive examination from a "click" that is frequently reported by pediatricians. Clicks

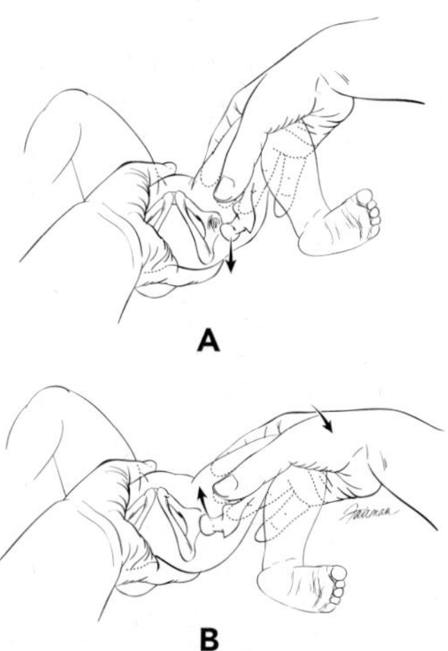

Figure 11.101 Ortolani maneuver: fingers up on the greater trochanter to lift the hip into place. (*Reproduced with permission from* Skaggs DL, Flynn JM. *Staying Out of Trouble in Pediatric Orthopaedics.* Philadelphia, PA: Lippincott Williams & Wilkins, 2006.)

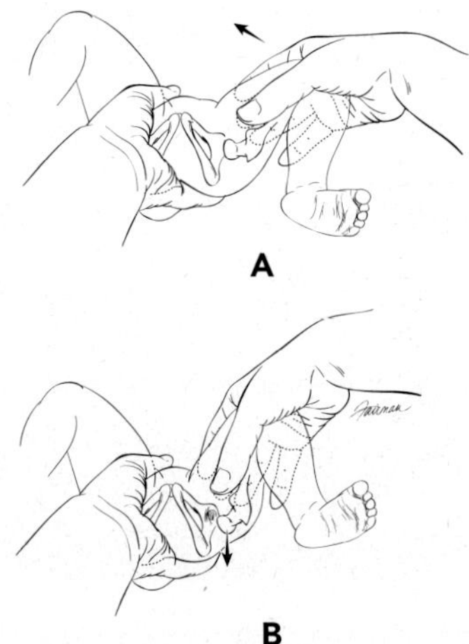

Figure 11.102 Barlow maneuver: palm pushes down on the knee to push the hip out the back. (*Reproduced with permission from* Skaggs DL, Flynn JM. *Staying Out of Trouble in Pediatric Orthopaedics*. Philadelphia, PA: Lippincott Williams & Wilkins, 2006.)

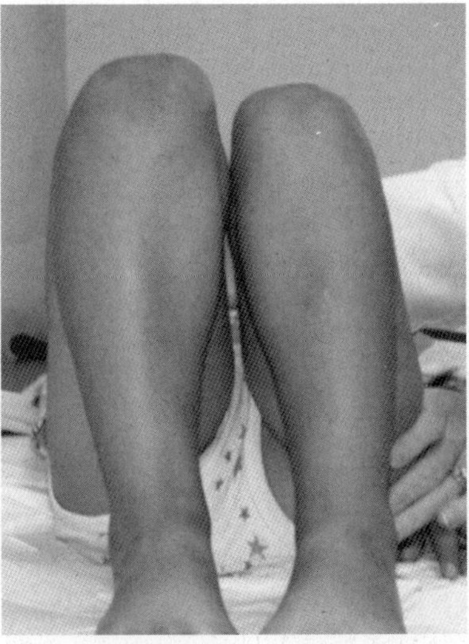

Figure 11.104 Galeazzi test is positive when knees are at different height. When positive, there may be a unilateral dislocated hip. (*Reproduced with permission from* Skaggs DL, Flynn JM. *Staying Out of Trouble in Pediatric Orthopaedics*. Philadelphia, PA: Lippincott Williams & Wilkins, 2006.)

are usually high-pitched snaps that occur at the extremes of abduction. These are usually caused by the ligamentum teres, fascia lata, or psoas tendon and do not represent a pathologic condition.

After approximately 6 weeks of age, the soft tissues around the hip tend to contract making the Ortolani and Barlow test less reliable. At this point, asymmetric and/or limited abduction is the most sensitive indicator for a unilateral hip dislocation (Fig. 11.103). Another useful test for diagnosing a hip dislocation is the Galeazzi test (Fig. 11.104). This test is performed on a flat surface with the hips flexed 90 degrees. Unequal knee heights suggest the presence of a dislocated hip on the shortened side. Historically, asymmetric thigh folds were considered another sign of DDH; however, this finding is a common variant and does not reliably predict the presence of a dislocation.

In the walking child, observation of gait will reveal a lurch from abductor dysfunction (Trendelenburg gait). In bilateral dislocations, excessive lordosis and hip flexion contractures can develop (Fig. 11.105). As in the younger child, unilateral dislocations will demonstrate limited abduction on the affected side and a positive Galeazzi test.

Regardless of age, care should be taken during the physical examination not to miss a bilateral hip dislocation. Bilateral dislocations may be present without asymmetry of leg length or hip abduction. One test that can help identify a bilateral dislocation is the Klisic test, in which the middle finger is placed over the greater trochanter with the index finger on the anterior superior iliac spine. An imaginary line between these two fingers should point to the umbilicus. In

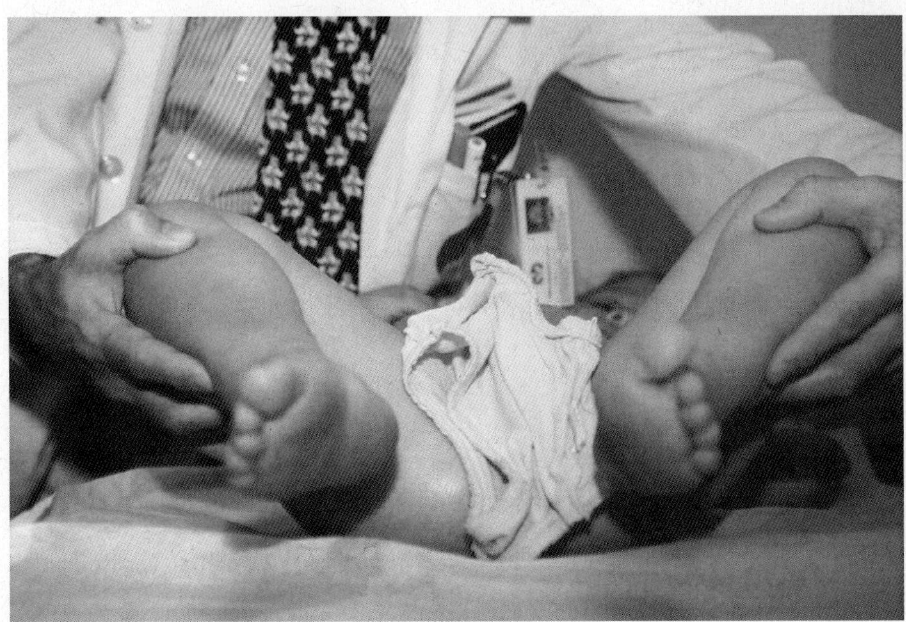

Figure 11.103 Asymmetry of hip abduction is associated with a unilateral dislocation in the hip that abducts less. A potential pitfall is not leveling the pelvis on the examination table; subtle asymmetry may be missed in that event. (*Reproduced with permission from* Skaggs DL, Flynn JM. *Staying Out of Trouble in Pediatric Orthopaedics*. Philadelphia, PA: Lippincott Williams & Wilkins, 2006.)

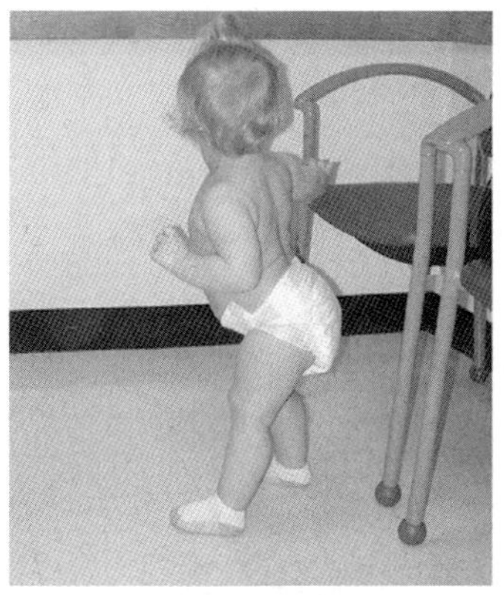
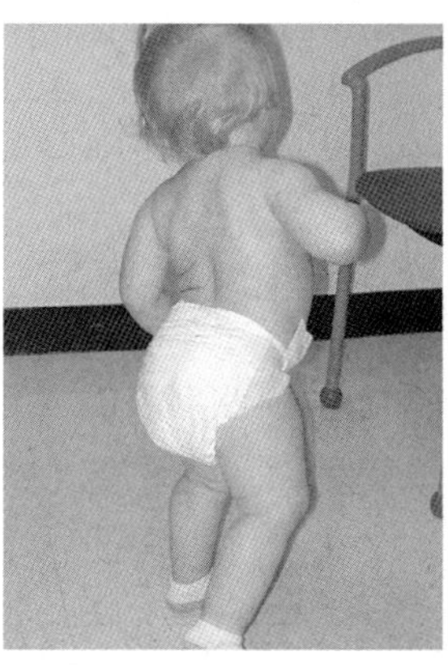
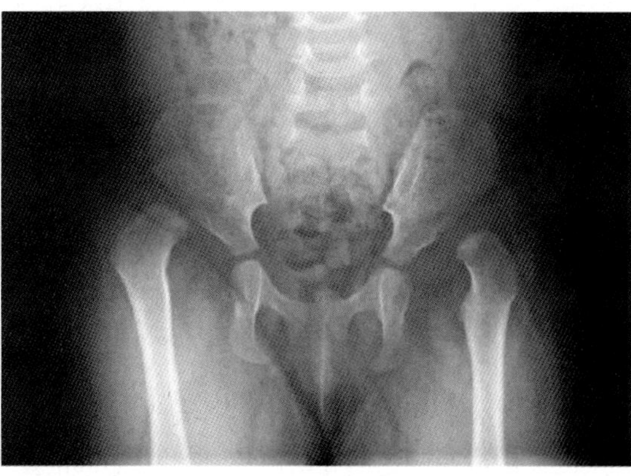

Figure 11.105 **(A** and **B)** Parents of this 16-month-old girl were concerned that she was not walking correctly. She has significant lordosis and a waddling gait. **(C)** An anteroposterior radiograph of the pelvis demonstrates bilateral dislocated hips. (*Reproduced with permission from* Skaggs DL, Flynn JM. *Staying Out of Trouble in Pediatric Orthopaedics.* Philadelphia, PA: Lippincott Williams & Wilkins, 2006.)

a hip dislocation, the greater trochanter moves proximally, causing this line to point somewhere between the umbilicus and the pubis. The results of this test are unaffected by the status of the contralateral side, making it an extremely useful test when bilateral dislocations are suspected.

Diagnostic Studies

Because it is superior to radiographs for evaluating cartilaginous structures, ultrasonography is the diagnostic modality of choice for DDH before the appearance of the femoral head ossific nucleus (4–6 months) (Fig. 11.106). During

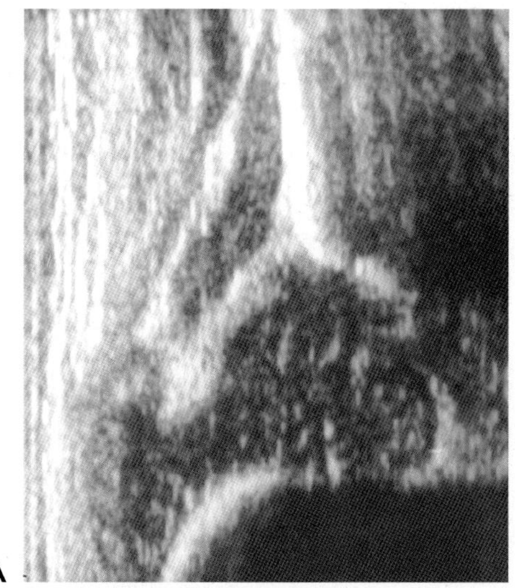
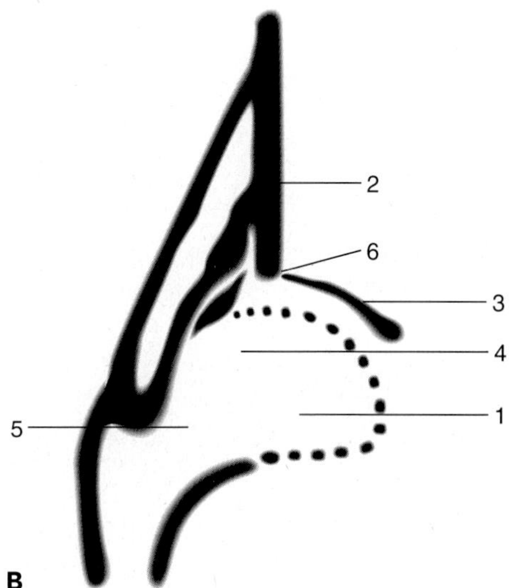

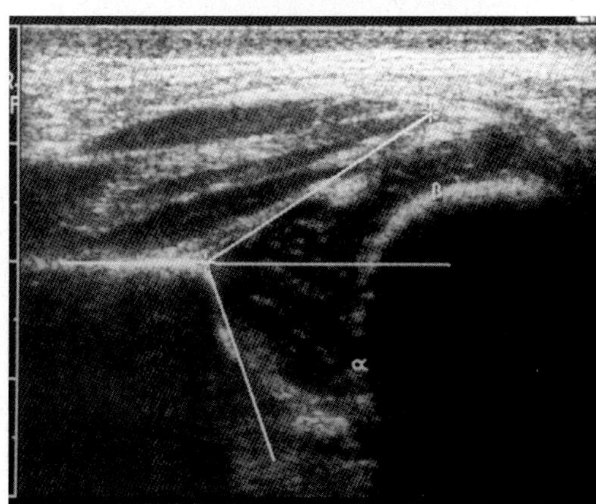

Figure 11.106 **(A)** Ultrasonography of a normal newborn. **(B)** Anatomic drawing of hip landmarks: 1, femoral head; 2, ilium; 3, bony acetabular floor; 4, acetabular labrum; 5, joint capsule; 6, osseous rim. **(C)** α and β angles are identified on this normal ultrasonograph of a newborn hip. (*Reproduced with permission from* Morrissy RT, Weinstein SL. *Lovell and Winter's Pediatric Orthopaedics.* Philadelphia, PA: Lippincott Williams & Wilkins, 2006.)

the early newborn period (0–4 weeks), however, physical examination is preferred over ultrasonography since there is a high incidence of falsely positive sonograms in this age group. Ultrasonography is extremely effective for evaluating the cartilaginous anatomy of the hip and the relationship of the femoral epiphysis to the acetabulum. Two different methods have been popularized, and often, both methods are used on the same child. The first method is the static technique described by Graf. The transducer is placed over the greater trochanter, which allows visualization of the ilium, the bony acetabulum, the labrum, and the femoral epiphysis. The angle formed by the line of the ilium and a line tangential to the bony roof of the acetabulum is termed the α angle and represents the depth of the acetabulum. Values greater than 60 degrees are considered normal, whereas those less than 60 degrees imply acetabular dysplasia. The β angle is formed by a line drawn tangential to the labrum and the line of the ilium; this represents the cartilaginous roof of the acetabulum. A normal β angle is less than 55 degrees; as the femoral head subluxates, the β angle increases. Another useful test is to evaluate the position of the center of the head compared with the vertical line of the ilium. If the line of the ilium falls lateral to the center of the head, the epiphysis is considered reduced. If the line falls medial to the center of the head, the epiphysis is undercovered and is either subluxated or dislocated (Fig. 11.107). The second ultrasonographic method used in DDH is the dynamic technique described by Harcke. This technique measures the degree of subluxation while the hip is being stressed. It is particularly useful in monitoring the response of a hip to brace treatment.

Screening for DDH with ultrasound remains controversial. Although routinely performed in Europe, ultrasonographic screening has not been shown to be cost-effective in the United States largely because of the cost associated with treating false-positive results. The current recommendations are that every newborn undergo a clinical examination for hip instability. Those children who have findings suspicious for DDH should be followed up with an ultrasound. Most authors agree that infants with risk factors for DDH (breech position, family history, torticollis, etc.) should probably be screened with an ultrasound regardless of the clinical findings.

After 4 to 6 months of age, the proximal femur has ossified to a sufficient degree that plain radiographs can be used to evaluate the position of the hip. Prior to this age, radiographs may document grossly dislocated teratologic hips but cannot declare a hip as being located or normal. Several classic radiographic lines have been used for many years to assist in the evaluation of the pediatric hip (Fig. 11.108). Hilgenreiner line is a horizontal line through the upper margin of the radiolucent triradiate cartilages. Perkins line is a vertical line drawn from the lateral margin of the ossified acetabulum and is perpendicular to Hilgenreiner line. The intersection of these two lines creates four quadrants around the hip. In the normal hip, the medial end of the ossified upper femoral metaphysis should lie medial to Perkin line and inferior to Hilgenreiner line (down and in). If the metaphyseal beak lies outside this

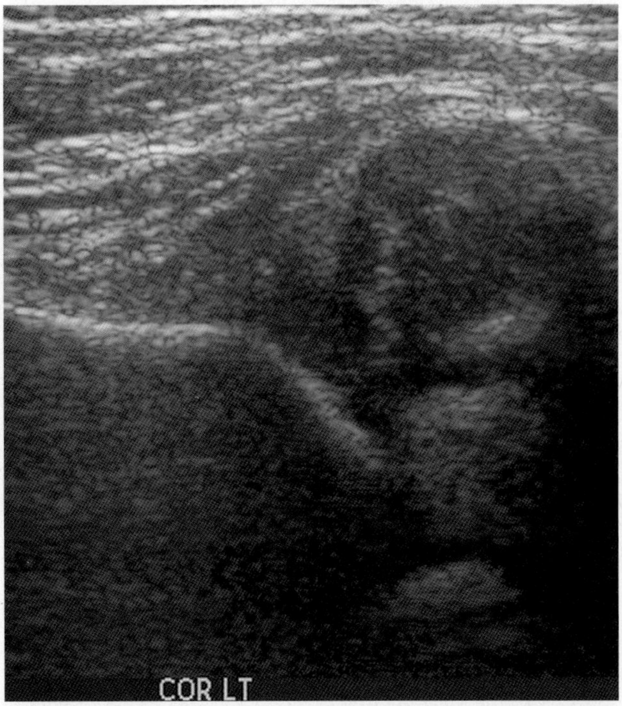

Figure 11.107 Coronal ultrasonographic image of a left hip that remains dislocated in spite of Pavlik harness treatment. Note that a line drawn tangential to the ilium falls medial to the center of the head.

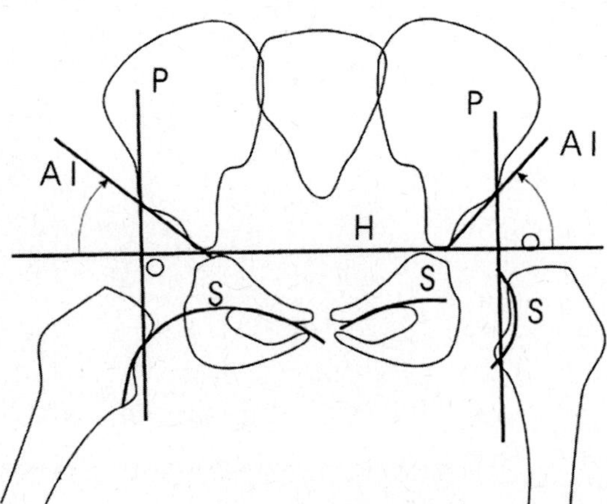

Figure 11.108 Radiographic lines in DDH. Hilgenreiner's line (H) is the horizontal line intersecting the left and right tri-radiate cartilages. Perkins' line (P) is drawn perpendicular to Hilgenreiner's line at the lateral corner of the acetabulum. The acetabular index (AI) is the angle between the acetabular roof and Hilgenreiner's line and is a measure of acetabular development. The intersection of Hilgenreiner's line and Perkins' line creates four quadrants around the hip. In a normal, reduced hip, the medial beak of the proximal femoral metaphysis shoudl be in the lower, inner quadrant. A disruption of Shenton's line (S) also indicates subluxation or dislocation of the hip. (*Reproduced with permission from* Morrissy RT, Weinstein SL. *Lovell and Winter's Pediatric Orthopaedics*. Philadelphia, PA: Lippincott Williams & Wilkins, 2006.)

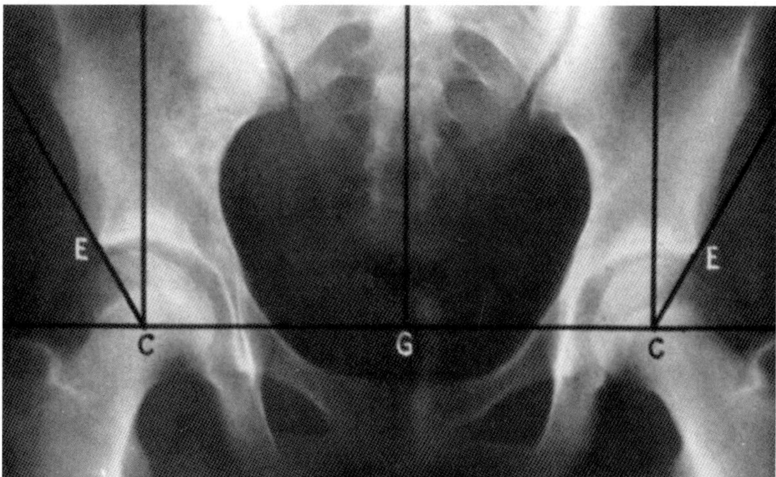

Figure 11.109 The center-edge angle is the angle formed between the perpendicular to a line connecting the center of both femoral heads and the line drawn between the center of the femoral head (C) and the lateral margin of the acetabulum (E). (*Reproduced with permission from* Morrissy RT, Weinstein SL. *Lovell and Winter's Pediatric Orthopaedics.* Philadelphia, PA: Lippincott Williams & Wilkins, 2006.)

quadrant, the hip is either subluxated or dislocated. Shenton line is formed by the medial border of the femoral neck and the superior border of the obturator foramen. Normally, this line should form a continuous arc. By definition, interruption of Shenton line implies subluxation at the least, if not, frank dislocation of the hip.

Two other radiographic measures are frequently used to evaluate acetabular dysplasia. The acetabular index is the angle formed between Hilgenreiner line and a line drawn tangential to the bony roof of the acetabulum. In the normal newborn period, the acetabular index averages 27.5 degrees. By 6 months of age, the mean index drops to 23.5 degrees, and by 2 years of age, the acetabular index is normally 20 degrees or less. For infants, 30 degrees is considered the upper limit of normal. After age 8 or so, the acetabular index becomes less reliable because the triradiate cartilage becomes harder to visualize. For older children (older than 6–8 years), the center–edge angle can be used to assess the degree of femoral head coverage. Prior to this age, the femoral epiphysis is not ossified sufficiently to judge an accurate center point. The center–edge angle is formed by the intersection of Perkins line and the line drawn between the center of the femoral head and the lateral margin of the acetabulum (Fig. 11.109). For children 6 to 13 years of age, a normal center–edge angle is greater than 19 degrees. After the age of 14, a normal center–edge angle is 25 degrees or greater. Values less than normal indicate undercoverage of the femoral head from acetabular dysplasia.

In general, advanced imaging (CT or MRI) is not necessary to make the diagnosis of DDH. CT scans, however, are the most widely used imaging modality for confirming hip reduction after open or closed treatment of a dislocated hip. In revision cases, CT scans can also be useful to define the bony anatomy of the hip. The downsides of CT include radiation exposure and the relatively poor visualization of soft tissue structures. Upsides include the rapid nature of the test, ease of scheduling, and widespread availability. Recently, some authors have advocated the use of MRI to confirm the adequacy of reduction following treatment of DDH. In addition to demonstrating the femoroacetabular relationship, MRI allows visualization of soft tissue structures (which can potentially block reduction) without the risk of ionizing radiation. Gadolinium-enhanced MRI can also be used to assess the perfusion of the femoral head inside the spica cast; this could potentially reduce the chance of avascular necrosis from immobilization in an at-risk position. In young adults with acetabular dysplasia, MRI is extremely useful for evaluating the health of the articular cartilage/labrum and for determining whether a patient is a suitable candidate for hip conserving surgery.

Arthrography is a useful intraoperative test for evaluating the depth and concentricity of a closed or open reduction. Pooling of dye in the medial joint implies that the femoral epiphysis is not deeply seated in the acetabulum (Fig. 11.110). Potential blocks to reduction include the ligamentum teres, transverse acetabular ligament, pulvinar, iliopsoas, or constricted capsule. In addition, the acetabular coverage can be estimated by looking for the "rose thorn" or

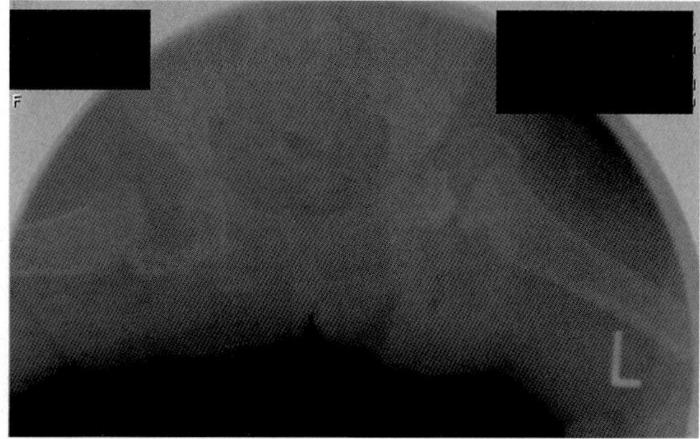

Figure 11.110 Arthrogram of the left hip showing medial dye pool after attempted closed reduction. (*Reproduced with permission from* Children's Orthopaedic Center, Los Angeles, CA.)

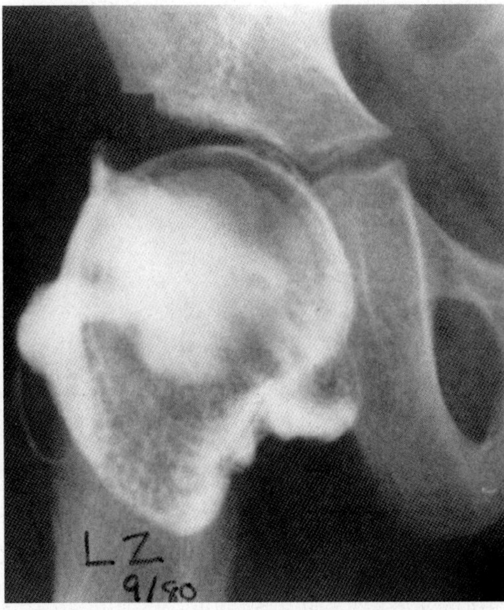

Figure 11.111 Arthrogram of a 5-year-old girl three years after open reduction. The sharp demarcation in the dye superior to the femoral head is the "rose-thorn" sign from the acetabular labrum. (*Reproduced with permission from* Morrissy RT, Weinstein SL. *Lovell and Winter's Pediatric Orthopaedics.* Philadelphia, PA: Lippincott Williams & Wilkins, 2006.)

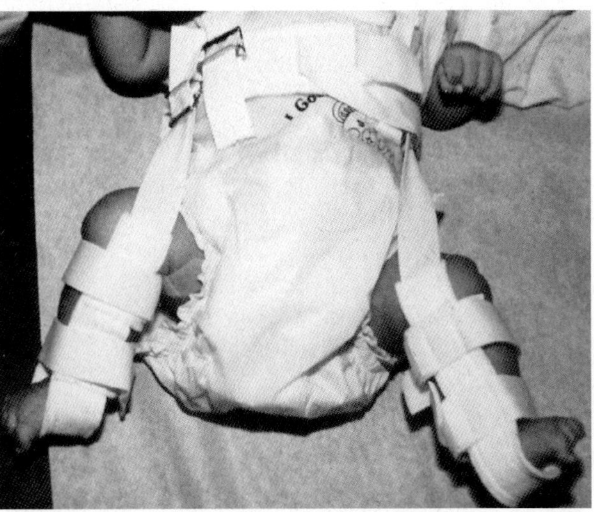

Figure 11.112 Newborn with bilateral hip dislocations in a Pavlik harness. Appropriately applied, the harness prevents hip extension and adduction, which can lead to redislocation, but allows flexion and abduction, which lead to reduction and stabilization. (*Reproduced with permission from* Morrissy RT, Weinstein SL. *Lovell and Winter's Pediatric Orthopaedics.* Philadelphia, PA: Lippincott Williams & Wilkins, 2006.)

sharp demarcation in the dye from the edge of the labrum (Fig. 11.111). A major advantage of arthrography is the dynamic nature of the test; the stability of reduction can be assessed in a wide variety of positions to determine the optimal position for immobilization.

Differential Diagnosis

Idiopathic DDH should be distinguished from teratologic hip dislocations, which occur in utero. Teratologic hips have extremely limited range of motion and are not reducible on examination. In general, teratologic dislocations are associated with other conditions including arthrogryposis, myelodysplasia, and a variety of genetic syndromes. Diagnosis is usually made on the basis of the clinical examination and the presence of other associated findings. The management of teratologic dislocations depends on the specific condition and the ambulatory potential of the child. In general, closed reduction is not successful for teratologic dislocations.

Treatment

The treatment of DDH varies depending on the age of the patient and the reducibility of the hip. Regardless of whether operative or nonoperative modalities are used, the goals of treatment are a concentric reduction of the femoral head into the acetabulum, maintenance of this reduction over time, and avoidance of complications, specifically avascular necrosis.

Birth to 12 Months

For infants younger than 6 months of age with a dislocated or dysplastic hip, a Pavlik harness is the preferred method of treatment (Fig. 11.112). This soft harness consists of Velcro straps around the chest that are connected to stirrups around both feet. The anterior straps of the harness can be adjusted to maintain the hips in flexion (usually approximately 100 degrees); excessive flexion is discouraged because of the risk of femoral nerve palsy. The posterior straps are designed to encourage abduction. These are generally set to allow adduction just to neutral, as forced abduction by the harness can lead to avascular necrosis of the femoral epiphysis. By positioning the hips in flexion and limiting the amount of adduction, the Pavlik harness points the femoral heads more directly at the acetabulum. For dysplastic hips, this allows for "deepening" of the socket by encouraging acetabular remodeling. For dislocated hips, the harness can guide the epiphysis into the acetabulum and maintain it in position while the soft tissues around the hip tighten.

Newborns hips that are Barlow positive (reduced but dislocatable) or Ortolani positive (dislocated but reducible) should generally be treated with a Pavlik harness as soon as the diagnosis is made. The management of newborns with dysplasia who are younger than 4 weeks is less clear. A significant proportion of these hips will normalize within 3 to 4 weeks; therefore, many physicians prefer to reexamine these newborns after a few weeks, before making treatment decisions. After applying a Pavlik harness, a follow-up ultrasound should be performed within 2 to 3 weeks to confirm hip reduction. Harness treatment should be abandoned at 4 weeks if the hip is not reduced by this

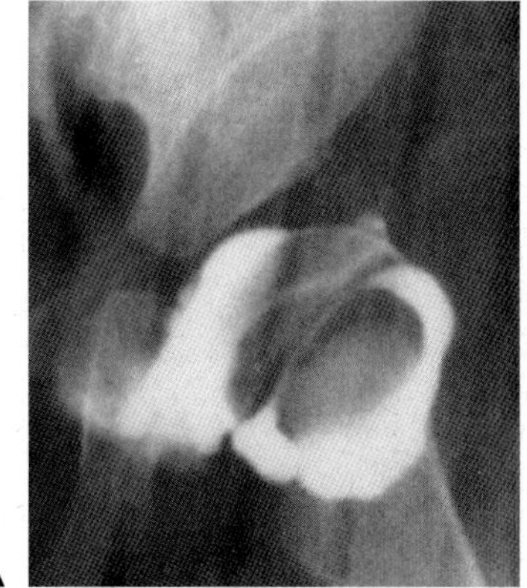

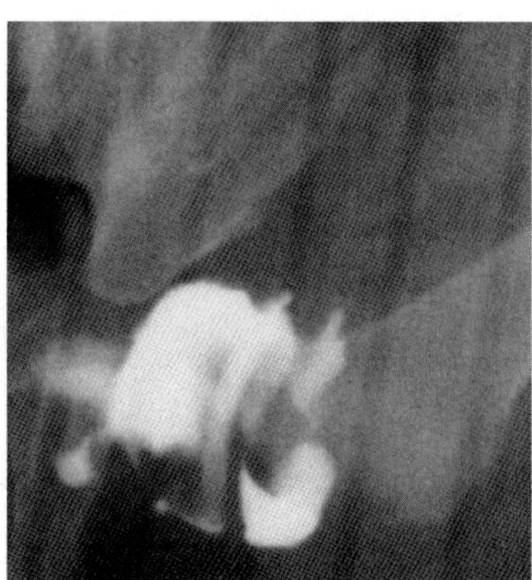

Figure 11.113 Arthrograms demonstrate closed reduction of the developmental dysplasia of the left hip in an 8-month-old girl. **(A)** Untreated. **(B)** Reduced. (*Reproduced with permission from* Morrissy RT, Weinstein SL. *Lovell and Winter's Pediatric Orthopaedics.* Philadelphia, PA: Lippincott Williams & Wilkins, 2006.)

time. Continued use of the harness beyond this period in a persistently dislocated hip can cause "Pavlik harness disease," or wearing away of the posterior aspect of the acetabulum, which can make the ultimate reduction less stable. For these hips that have "failed" Pavlik harness treatment, abduction bracing can occasionally be successful in achieving a stable reduction. If the Pavlik harness is successful in achieving a reduction, the harness is generally continued until both the clinical examination and the ultrasound parameters (α and β angles) normalize, followed by a 3- to 4-week weaning period. For the most part, Pavlik harness is extremely effective for treating DDH in the newborn period with reported success rates of more than 90% for acetabular dysplasia and 85% for reducible dislocations.

For those patients with persistent instability in spite of a Pavlik harness or those who present after 6 months of age, the next step in treatment is closed reduction and spica casting. Historically, traction was used prior to closed reduction because it was thought that this decreased the risk of avascular necrosis. Recent studies, however, have not supported this contention, and the use of traction has diminished in popularity. Closed reduction and casting is typically done under general anesthesia or heavy sedation. Arthrography is performed along with the procedure to confirm the adequacy of reduction (see earlier) (Fig. 11.113). The reduction maneuver usually consists of hip flexion and abduction with minimal force applied. If a reduction is felt, the hip should be evaluated under fluoroscopy to determine the most stable position. In particular, one should assess the amount of abduction/adduction before the hip redislocates. By comparing this to the maximum range of motion, a "safe zone" can be determined. If the safe zone is relatively wide (i.e., close to the maximum range of motion), the reduction is considered stable. If the safe zone is narrow, abduction can be improved by performing an adductor tenotomy. Once the safe and stable position for the hip has been determined, the child should be immobilized in a bilateral hip spica cast. The cast should be molded to maintain the child in the "human" position of Salter: roughly 90 degrees of flexion, 10 to 20 degrees of internal rotation, and 30 to 50 degrees of abduction (Fig. 11.114). Excessive abduction (>60 degrees) should be avoided as this increases the risk of avascular necrosis. Because plain radiographs are difficult to interpret, CT or MRI is typically used to confirm reduction after cast application (Fig. 11.115). Cast immobilization is usually continued for 3 to 4 months, with a cast change at 6 weeks, if necessary.

Walking Age

Before 18 months of age, the preferred method of treatment is still closed reduction and casting as long as excessive force is not necessary to achieve reduction. As children

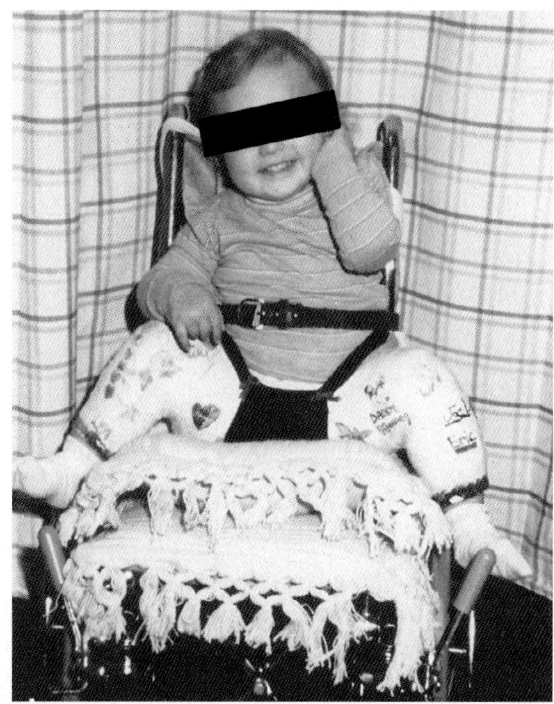

Figure 11.114 After closed reduction, the patient should be positioned in the "human position" of flexion and moderate abduction for the spica cast. (*Reproduced with permission from* Morrissy RT, Weinstein SL. *Lovell and Winter's Pediatric Orthopaedics.* Philadelphia, PA: Lippincott Williams & Wilkins, 2006.)

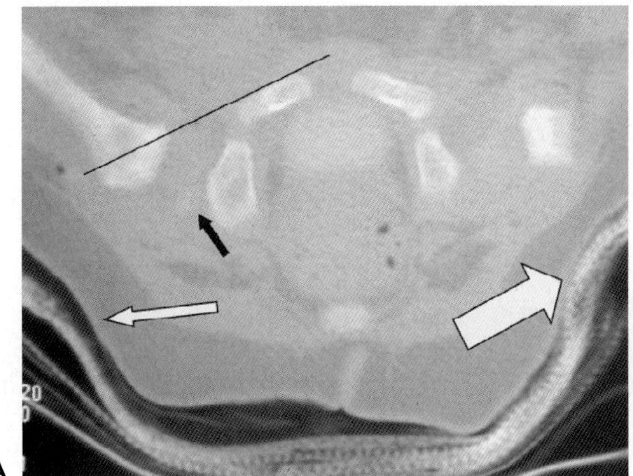

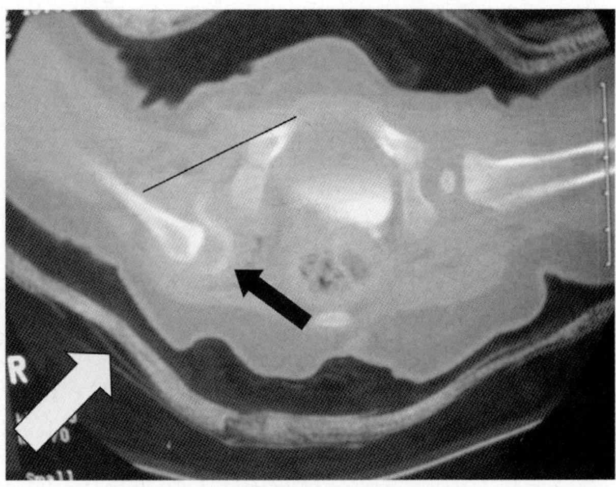

Figure 11.115 **(A)** Computed tomography (CT) scan following closed reduction of the right hip. The hip is located as judged by a line along the anterior cortex of the pubis which intersects the proximal femoral metaphysic, the so-called CT Shenton line (*thin black line*). The *small black arrow* demonstrates the characteristic apparent posterior subluxation of the femoral head within the acetabulum, which is present even when the hip is located. The *small white arrow* demonstrates mediocre molding of the cast under the greater trochanter to help keep the hip reduced. The trochanteric molding on the other hip (*large white arrow*) is actually better in this patient. **(B)** This CT scan demonstrates a dislocation following attempted closed reduction and spica casting. The line along the pubis does not intersect the proximal femoral metaphysic (*thin black line*). There is no molding under the greater trochanter (*large white arrow*). (*Reproduced with permission from* Skaggs DL, Flynn JM. *Staying Out of Trouble in Pediatric Orthopaedics.* Philadelphia, PA: Lippincott Williams & Wilkins, 2006.)

age, however, it becomes less likely that a stable reduction can be achieved via closed means. Indications for open reduction of the hip include failure to obtain a stable hip with closed reduction/casting, unacceptable widening of the joint space on arthrography, and older children. One of two different approaches can be used to perform the open reduction. For children between 6 and 18 months of age, some authors prefer the medial approach of Ludloff. The interval for this approach is either anterior or posterior to the pectineus. Advantages of this technique include minimal dissection and a direct approach to several of the obstructions to reduction (iliopsoas, transverse acetabular ligament). Disadvantages include risk to the medial femoral circumflex artery and the inability to perform a capsulorrhaphy or concomitant pelvic osteotomy. Most authors prefer an anterior approach for open reduction that is performed through the Smith–Peterson interval (tensor fascia lata/sartorius). This approach can be used in a child of any age and allows for a capsulorrhaphy and/or pelvic osteotomy to be performed through the same incision. Regardless of the approach, the principles of open reduction remain the same. All potential obstructions to reduction should be addressed in a systematic manner. These include a shortened iliopsoas tendon, constricted capsule, hypertrophic transverse acetabular ligament and ligamentum teres, infolded labrum, and pulvinar. Postoperatively, patients are immobilized in a one-and-a-half–legged spica cast with the hip more extended and less abducted than in closed reductions.

The addition of a pelvic osteotomy to the open reduction should be considered for all children older than 18 months. These procedures can improve the acetabular coverage and the stability of the hip following open reduction. Performing an early innominate osteotomy also maximizes the amount of acetabular remodeling following open treatment, thereby minimizing the risk for residual dysplasia in the future. The Salter, Pemberton, and Dega osteotomies are the most popular types of pelvic osteotomies for DDH in walking-aged children. The Salter osteotomy is a complete cut through the ilium at the level of the sciatic notch; the acetabulum is then rotated forward and outward, hinging on the pubic symphysis. A wedge of bone graft and internal fixation are used to maintain the acetabular position. The Pemberton osteotomy is a curved but incomplete cut in the ilium that hinges on the intact medial wall and the triradiate cartilage. The Dega osteotomy is another incomplete transiliac osteotomy that hinges on the intact posteromedial iliac cortex and sciatic notch. The correction from the Dega and the Pemberton osteotomies is maintained with a wedge of bone graft, but internal fixation is usually not necessary. All three procedures improve anterior and lateral coverage of the acetabulum, which is the area that is primarily deficient in DDH.

After 2 years of age, it is more likely that a femoral procedure will be necessary in addition to the open reduction $\pm$ pelvic osteotomy (Fig. 11.116). If excessive pressure is required to reduce the femoral head intraoperatively, a femoral shortening osteotomy should be performed. This

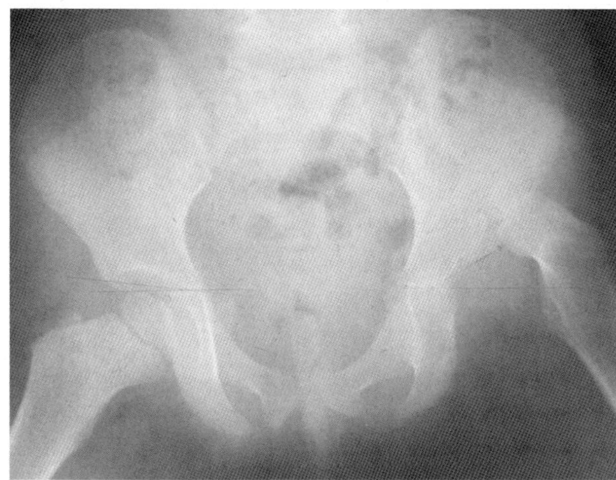

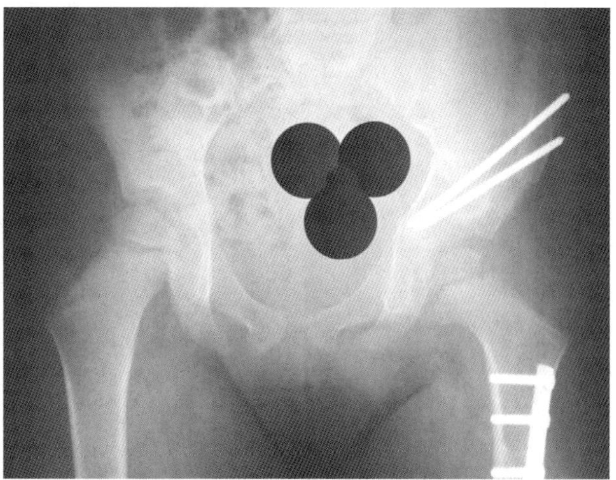

Figure 11.116 **A**: Preoperative radiograph demonstrating left hip dislocation. **(B)** Postoperative anteroposterior radiograph of the pelvis 1 year after open reduction, Salter osteotomy, and femoral shortening osteotomy. (*Reproduced with permission from* Skaggs DL, Tolo VT. *Master Techniques in Orthopaedic Surgery*: *Pediatrics*. Philadelphia, PA: Lippincott Williams & Wilkins, 2008.)

reduces the soft tissue tension around the hip, thereby decreasing the risk of osteonecrosis. The indications for concomitant derotation to correct femoral anteversion are somewhat controversial. Several cases have been reported of excessive derotation causing postoperative dislocation in a posterior direction. Other authors believe that femoral anteversion is an important part of the deformity in DDH and should be treated. Most authors agree, however, that varus osteotomy of the proximal femur (which was traditionally advocated) is not necessary in the management of DDH.

The upper age limit for open reduction is also controversial. Because the likelihood of successful treatment decreases with advancing age and because a dislocated hip is often painless until well into adulthood, most authors do not advocate open reduction for unilateral dislocations in children older than 8 years. In patients with bilateral dislocations, issues of leg length discrepancy are not applicable. In addition, the chances of two highly successful outcomes following open reduction are modest. For both of these reasons, the upper age limit for performing surgery on children with bilateral dislocations is often lowered to approximately 6 years of age.

Residual and Late-Presenting Dysplasia

Acetabular remodeling following treatment of DDH is most predictable up to 4 years of age. Some degree of remodeling does occur between the ages of 4 and 8; after this age, however, the acetabulum cannot be relied upon to remodel sufficiently. In addition, many patients with mild to moderate dysplasia may not present until their hips become symptomatic during early adulthood. Treatment of residual or late-presenting acetabular dysplasia is important because untreated dysplasia can increase the risk of osteoarthritis later in life. It is estimated that 20% to 50% of all patients requiring total hip arthroplasty for degenerative arthritis have underlying acetabular dysplasia (Fig. 11.117).

The treatment of choice for significant acetabular dysplasia is pelvic osteotomy. There are two general categories of osteotomies: reconstructive and salvage. Reconstructive osteotomies require the presence of a concentric and congruent reduction. These procedures can be further subdivided into redirectional and reshaping osteotomies. Redirectional osteotomies change the orientation of the acetabulum without changing the shape or volume of the

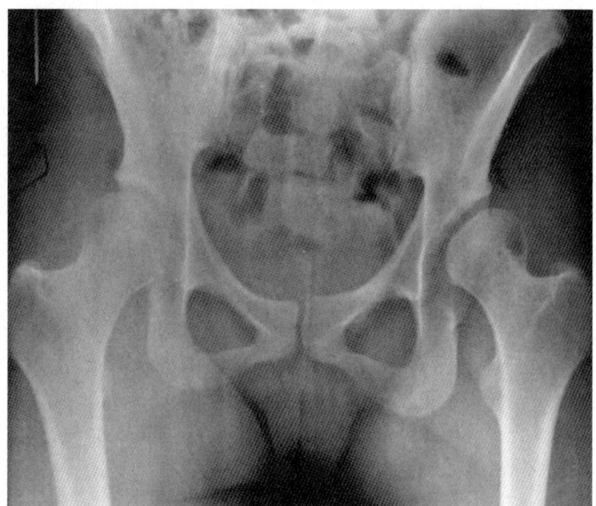

Figure 11.117 Anteroposterior view of the pelvis in a 15-year-old girl with of treated developmental dysplasia of the hip as an infant. Note the bilateral acetabular dysplasia as evidenced by a steep, shallow, acetabulum and a decreased center–edge angle bilaterally. The left hip is radiographically subluxated. (*Reproduced with permission from* Morrissy RT, Weinstein SL. *Lovell and Winter's Pediatric Orthopaedics*. Philadelphia, PA: Lippincott Williams & Wilkins, 2006.)

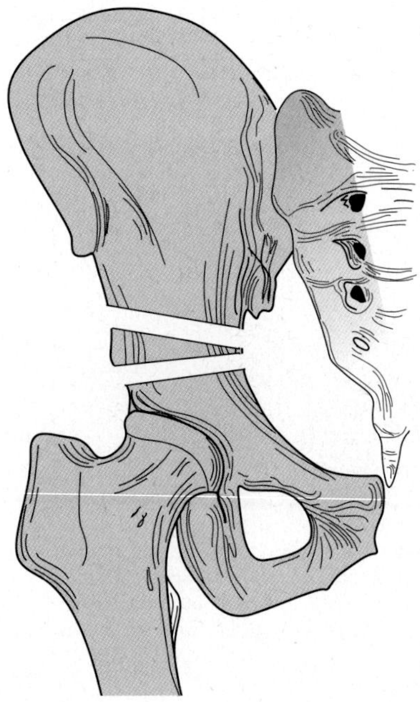

Figure 11.118 Salter single innominate osteotomy.

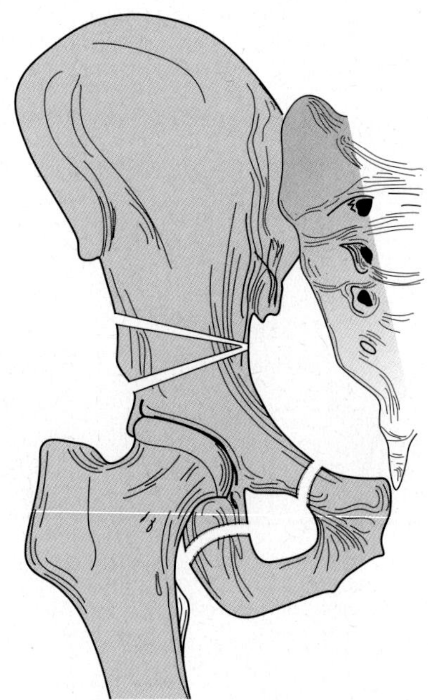

Figure 11.119 Triple innominate osteotomy.

socket. All involve a complete transection of the ilium plus additional cuts in the pelvis depending on the specific technique. The previously described Salter osteotomy is the simplest type of redirectional osteotomy and can be used in children up to 8 to 10 years of age to improve anterolateral coverage (Fig. 11.118). For older children who lack mobility of the pubic symphysis, a triple innominate osteotomy can be effective to achieve greater degrees of correction. This procedure involves transection of the ilium, the pubis, and the ischium but preserves the integrity of the triradiate cartilage; internal fixation is required to maintain the position of the acetabular fragment (Fig. 11.119). For older patients after closure of the triradiate cartilage, the preferred procedure is the Ganz periacetabular osteotomy. This technically demanding osteotomy involves a complete cut of the pubis, a partial cut of the ischium and ilium, and a posterior column osteotomy that connects the ischial and iliac cuts (Fig. 11.120). This osteotomy allows for significant degrees of correction but should not be performed in younger children because it violates the triradiate cartilage. Since the posterior column is preserved, the osteotomy is quite stable and requires only 3 to 4 screws to achieve adequate fixation (Fig. 11.121).

Reshaping osteotomies change the volume and shape of the socket and are, therefore, most useful for a capacious or shallow acetabulum. Both the Pemberton and the Dega osteotomy involve incomplete cuts in the ilium directed toward the triradiate cartilage. The acetabular fragment is then bent downward, hinging on the triradiate cartilage. A wedge of bone graft is placed in the osteotomy to maintain the acetabular position (Fig. 11.122). By varying the direction of the osteotomy and the position of the bone graft wedge, the increased acetabular coverage can be preferentially made more anterior, lateral, or posterior. Because the bone cuts are incomplete, the osteotomies are quite stable and internal fixation is not necessary.

For incongruent hip joints, reconstructive osteotomies cannot be performed and a salvage procedure may be necessary. The goal of these osteotomies is to increase the weight-bearing surface and reduce the amount of edge-loading. Because they do not redirect native hyaline cartilage, salvage osteotomies rely on capsular metaplasia to

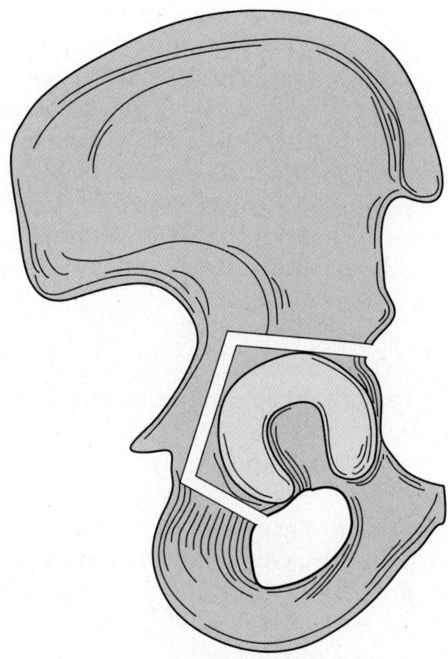

Figure 11.120 Bernese (Ganz) periacetabular osteotomy.

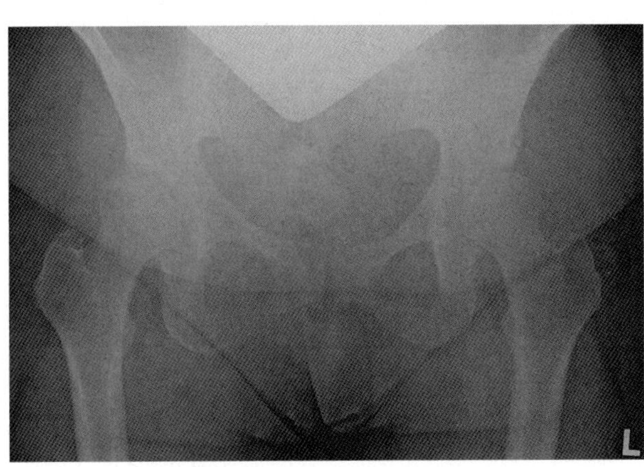

A

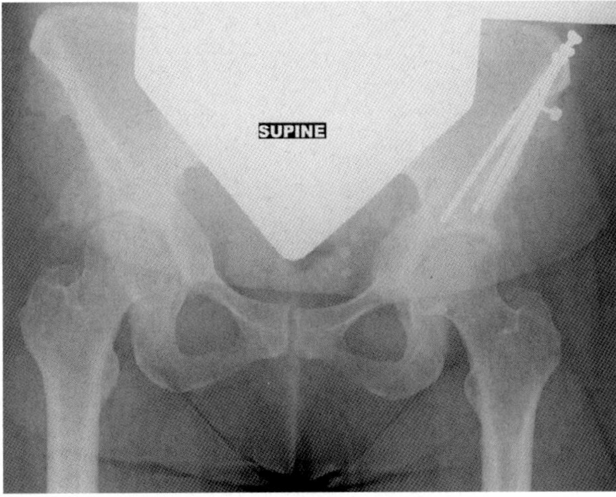

B

Figure 11.121 **(A)** Anteroposterior (AP) radiograph of the pelvis demonstrating bilateral acetabular dysplasia in a 45-year-old woman. **(B)** AP radiograph of the pelvis after bilateral periacetabular osteotomies to improve femoral head coverage. The hardware on the right side has already been removed.

provide an articulating surface. The Chiari osteotomy is performed by making a complete cut in the ilium just above the level of the hip joint. The proximal fragment is then translated laterally while the acetabulum is medialized, thereby providing increased lateral coverage (Fig. 11.123). Internal fixation holds the fragments in place and a spica cast is rarely necessary. The Staheli shelf procedure increases femoral head coverage by building a buttress on the anterior and lateral edge of the acetabulum. A slot is made along the rim of the acetabulum just above the level of the joint, and strips of corticocancellous bone are placed inside to create a "shelf" (Fig. 11.124). Over time, this shelf will remodel and hypertrophy from the pressure of the femoral head.

Figure 11.122 The cut for the Dega acetabuloplasty is oriented toward the sciatic notch above the level of the triradiate cartilage. The cut is incomplete and relies on hinging at the triradiate cartilage. Local bone graft wedges are used to hold the osteotomy open. (*Reproduced with permission from* Skaggs DL, Tolo VT. *Master Techniques in Orthopaedic Surgery*: *Pediatrics*. Philadelphia, PA: Lippincott Williams & Wilkins, 2008.)

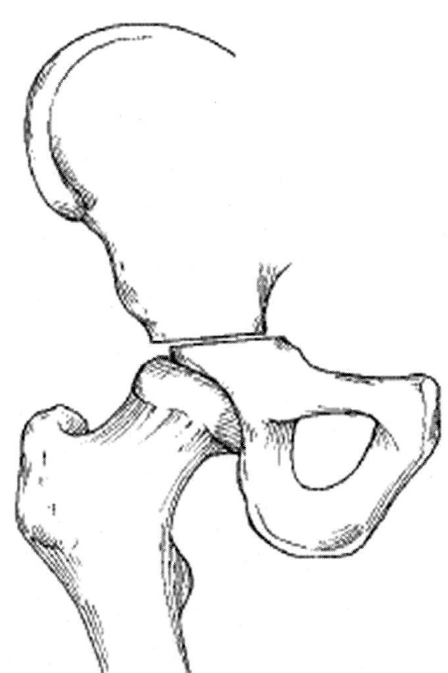

Figure 11.123 Chiari salvage osteotomy. (*Reproduced with permission from* Gillingham BL, Sanchez AA, Wenger DR: Pelvic Osteotomies for the Treatment of Hip Dysplasia in Children and Young Adults. *Am Acad Orthop Surg* 1999;7:325–337.)

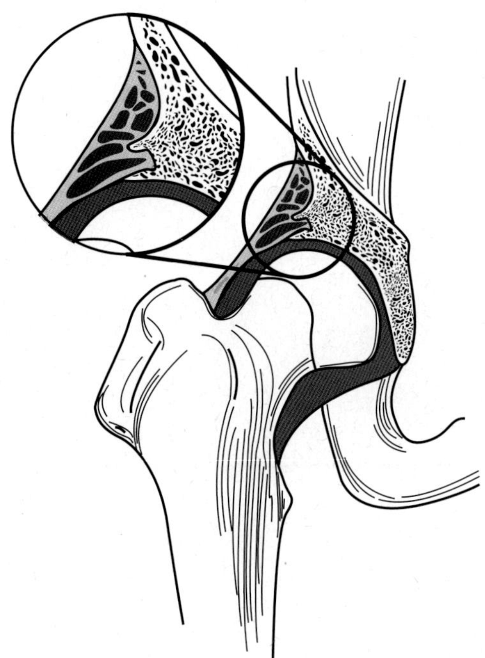

Figure 11.124 Slotted-shelf augmentation.

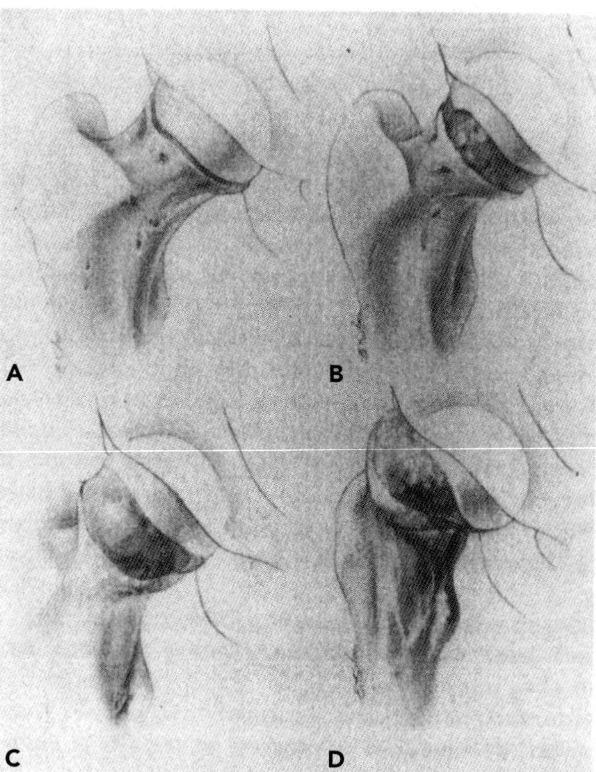

Figure 11.125 Pathoanatomy of the slipped capital femoral epiphysis is demonstrated. **(A)** No displacement is seen. **(B)** Rotation of the proximal femoral neck with the femoral head (which is anchored in the acetabulum) posterior relative to the femoral neck. **(C)** Progressive external rotation, with progressive posterior relation of the femoral head to the femoral neck. **(D)** Proximal migration of the femoral neck due to the markedly posterior relation of the femoral head to the femoral neck. (*Reproduced with permission from* Morrissy RT, Weinstein SL. *Lovell and Winter's Pediatric Orthopaedics*. Philadelphia, PA: Lippincott Williams & Wilkins, 2006.)

Slipped Capital Femoral Epiphysis

SCFE is the most common hip disorder in adolescents, with an approximate cumulative incidence of 50 per 100,000 persons. By definition, a SCFE is posterior and inferior displacement of the femoral epiphysis in relation to the femoral neck (Fig. 11.125). In reality, it is the femoral head that remains stationary in the acetabulum, whereas the neck displaces anteriorly and superolaterally. Early diagnosis is important because delayed or inadequate treatment can be a source of significant morbidity.

Pathophysiology

SCFEs are most likely caused by a combination of mechanical and endocrine factors. The plane of cleavage in most SCFEs occurs through the hypertrophic zone of the physis. During normal puberty, the physis becomes more vertically oriented, which converts mechanical forces from compression to shear. In addition, the hypertrophic zone becomes elongated in pubertal adolescents due to high levels of circulating hormones. This widening of the physis decreases the threshold for mechanical failure. Any other factor that causes a delay in metaphyseal ossification will also cause a relative increase in physeal height and mechanical weakening of the physis. Normal ossification depends on a number of different factors including thyroid hormone, vitamin D, and calcium. It is, therefore, not surprising that SCFEs occur with increased incidence in children with medical disorders such as hypothyroidism, hypopituitarism, and renal osteodystrophy. Obesity, one of the greatest risk factors for SCFE, affects both the mechanical load on the physis and the level of circulating hormones. The combination of mechanical and endocrine factors results in gradual failure of the physis that allows displacement of the femoral neck in relation to the head. If the displacement occurs acutely, the injury is analogous to a Salter–Harris type I fracture of the proximal femoral physis.

Classification

Historically, SCFEs have been classified on the basis of chronology. Acute SCFEs are defined by hip pain for less than 3 weeks. A chronic SCFE, on the other hand, is one in which the symptoms have lasted longer than 3 weeks, often for many months prior to presentation. Children with a history of prolonged hip pain who present with a sudden increase in their symptoms are said to have an acute-on-chronic SCFE. Although easy to use, the chronologic classification has two major limitations. First, it does not offer much information regarding prognosis, and second, it depends on recall of the patient and family, which may not be accurate. Currently, the preferred classification method for SCFEs is based on the stability of the slip. By definition, a stable SCFE is one in which the child is able to walk and bear weight on the affected leg with or without crutches. In contrast, an unstable SCFE is one in which the child is unable to bear weight regardless of walking aids. Unlike chronicity, the stability-based classification provides important prognostic information. Stable slips have a very low rate of avascular necrosis; the incidence of avascular necrosis (AVN) in unstable slips, however, has been reported to be as high as 50%.

Presentation

The classic patient presenting with a SCFE is an obese, African American boy between the ages of 11 and 16. Girls present earlier, usually between 10 to 14 years of age. Chronic and stable SCFEs tend to present after weeks to months of symptoms. Patients usually limp to some degree and have an externally rotated lower extremity. Most patients complain of groin symptoms, but isolated thigh pain or knee pain is a common presentation from referred pain along the course of the obturator nerve. In fact, missed or delayed diagnosis often occurs in children who present with knee pain and do not receive appropriate imaging of the hip (Fig. 11.126). Unstable SCFEs usually present in an urgent fashion. Children typically refuse to allow any range of motion of the hip; much like a hip fracture, the extremity is shortened, abducted, and externally rotated.

Physical Examination

Observation of gait in a child with a stable SCFE reveals several characteristic findings. Children typically limp and demonstrate out-toeing of the involved extremity. This latter finding is because as part of the displacement, the femoral neck externally rotates in relation to the epiphysis. Attempts to range the hip will reveal significant restrictions to flexion and internal rotation as the proximal metaphysis impinges on the rim of the acetabulum. In typical

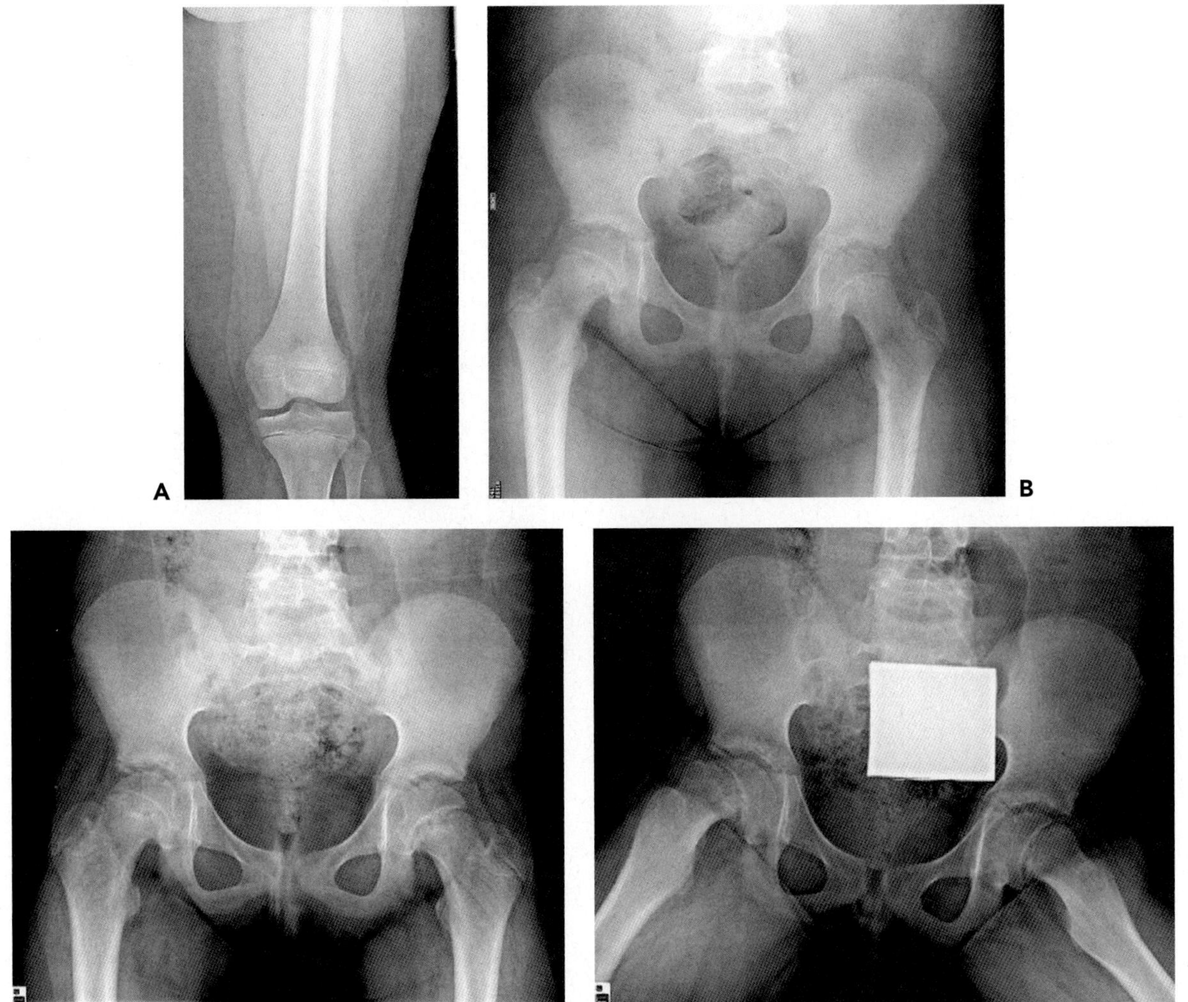

Figure 11.126 This 9-year-old girl presented to her primary care doctor with a 4-month history of knee and thigh pain. Knee **(A)** radiographs and an anteroposterior view of the pelvis **(B)** were obtained but no frog lateral views. The radiographs were interpreted as normal. Two months later, the child was referred to a pediatric orthopaedist who ordered appropriate radiographs. These radiographs revealed a now moderately displaced slipped capital femoral epiphysis bilaterally **(C** and **D)**. (*Reproduced with permission from* Skaggs DL, Flynn JM. *Staying Out of Trouble in Pediatric Orthopaedics.* Philadelphia, PA: Lippincott Williams & Wilkins, 2006.)

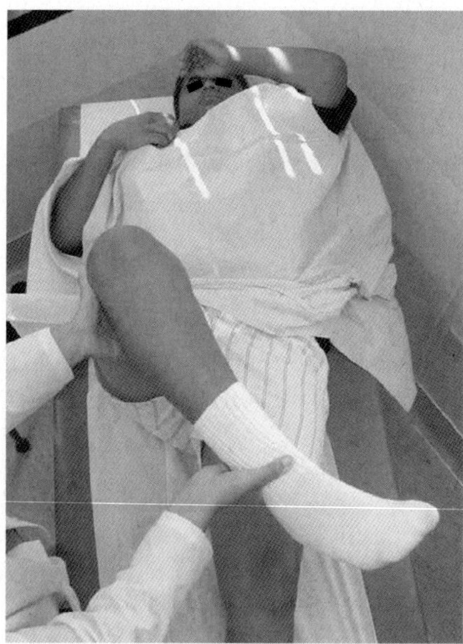
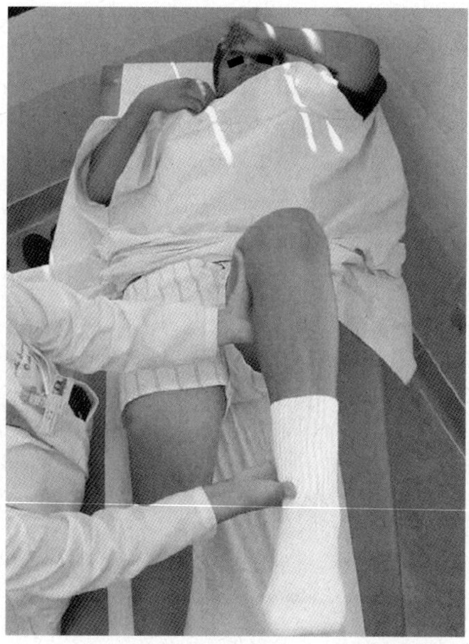

Figure 11.127 In this boy with right slipped capital femoral epiphysis, the examination demonstrates obligate external rotation as the hip is flexed **(A)**. No rotation with hip flexion is seen on the normal side **(B)**. (*Reproduced with permission from* Skaggs DL, Flynn JM. *Staying Out of Trouble in Pediatric Orthopaedics*. Philadelphia, PA: Lippincott Williams & Wilkins, 2006.)

cases, bringing the hip into flexion will cause obligate external rotation of the hip and extremity as the acetabulum forces the femoral neck laterally (Fig. 11.127). This range-of-motion limitation from femoroacetabular impingement can be painless at first. Over time, however, damage can occur to the labrum and the articular cartilage, which results in pain with flexion and internal rotation of the hip.

Radiographs

Most SCFEs can be diagnosed with an AP view of the pelvis and frog lateral views of both hips (Fig. 11.128). In patients with an unstable SCFE, a shoot-through lateral is preferred over the frog lateral to minimize unnecessary trauma to the epiphysis from moving the leg. One of the earliest radiographic findings is widening and blurring of the physis. On the AP view, Klein line can be drawn along the superior femoral neck. Normally, this line should intersect some portion of the lateral epiphysis. With the typical posteroinferior displacement of the epiphysis, this line will no longer touch the epiphysis. Another finding is the metaphyseal blanch sign, described by Howard Steel. This is a crescent-shaped area of increased density in the proximal metaphysis that results from overlap of the femoral neck and the posteriorly displaced femoral epiphysis. Although some of these radiographic findings can be subtle, most diagnoses can be readily made on the frog lateral view, which will reveal the characteristic posterior and inferior displacement of the epiphysis in relation to the femoral neck.

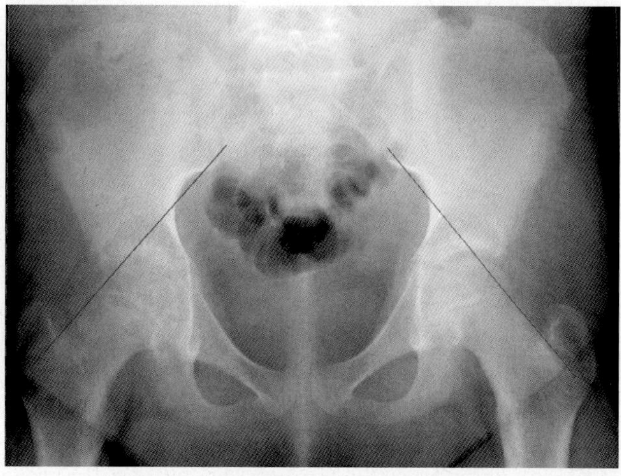
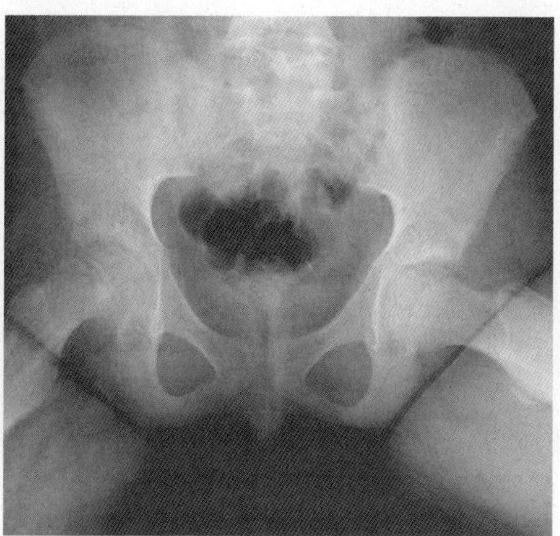

Figure 11.128 Radiographs of a 12 year-old-boy with 3 months of hip pain show typical findings of a slipped capital femoral epiphysis (SCFE). **(A)** Anteroposterior (AP) view demonstrates physeal widening, osteopenia, decreased epiphyseal height, increased metaphyseal-teardrop distance, and asymmetry of Klein line. **(B)** Although many of these features are seen on the AP view, the most striking feature is how much more easily the displacement is seen on the frog lateral view. The importance of obtaining lateral views when evaluating for SCFE cannot be overemphasized. (*Reproduced with permission from* Morrissy RT, Weinstein SL. *Lovell and Winter's Pediatric Orthopaedics*. Philadelphia, PA: Lippincott Williams & Wilkins, 2006.)

Plain radiographs are also useful for grading the severity of a SCFE. The slip angle is calculated by measuring the femoral head–shaft angle of the involved side and comparing this to the normal, contralateral side (if both sides are slipped, 10 degrees can be used as a normal value) (Fig. 11.129). Differences less than 30 degrees are considered mild. Slip angles between 30 and 60 degrees are moderate, and values greater than 60 degrees are severe.

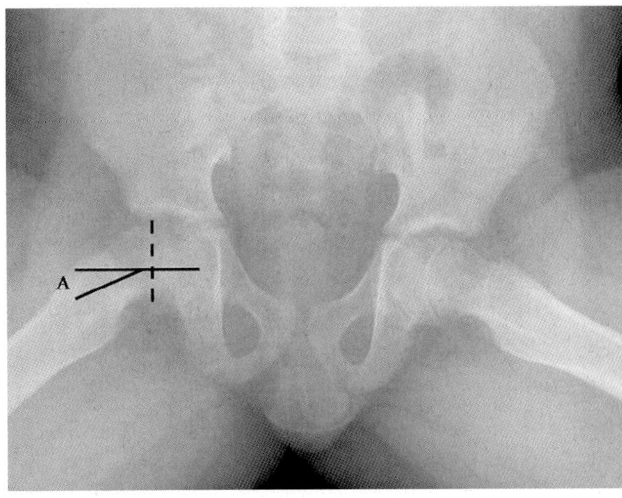

Figure 11.129 The slip angle is the angle between the axis of the femoral shaft and the perpendicular to the base of the epiphysis. This angle **(A)** is generally compared with the contralateral, normal side. In this case, the left side demonstrates a mild slip, so 10 degrees may be used as normative value for comparison.

Special Studies

Advanced imaging is rarely necessary during the initial diagnosis of most SCFEs. Bone scans or MRI can be useful for assessing femoral head perfusion in unstable slips and for monitoring patients postoperatively for AVN. In addition, MRI can aid in the diagnosis of "preslips," a condition characterized by inflammation of the physis that has yet to displace (Fig. 11.130). CT scans are useful for assessing the severity of deformity after initial treatment and for planning corrective osteotomies (Fig. 11.131).

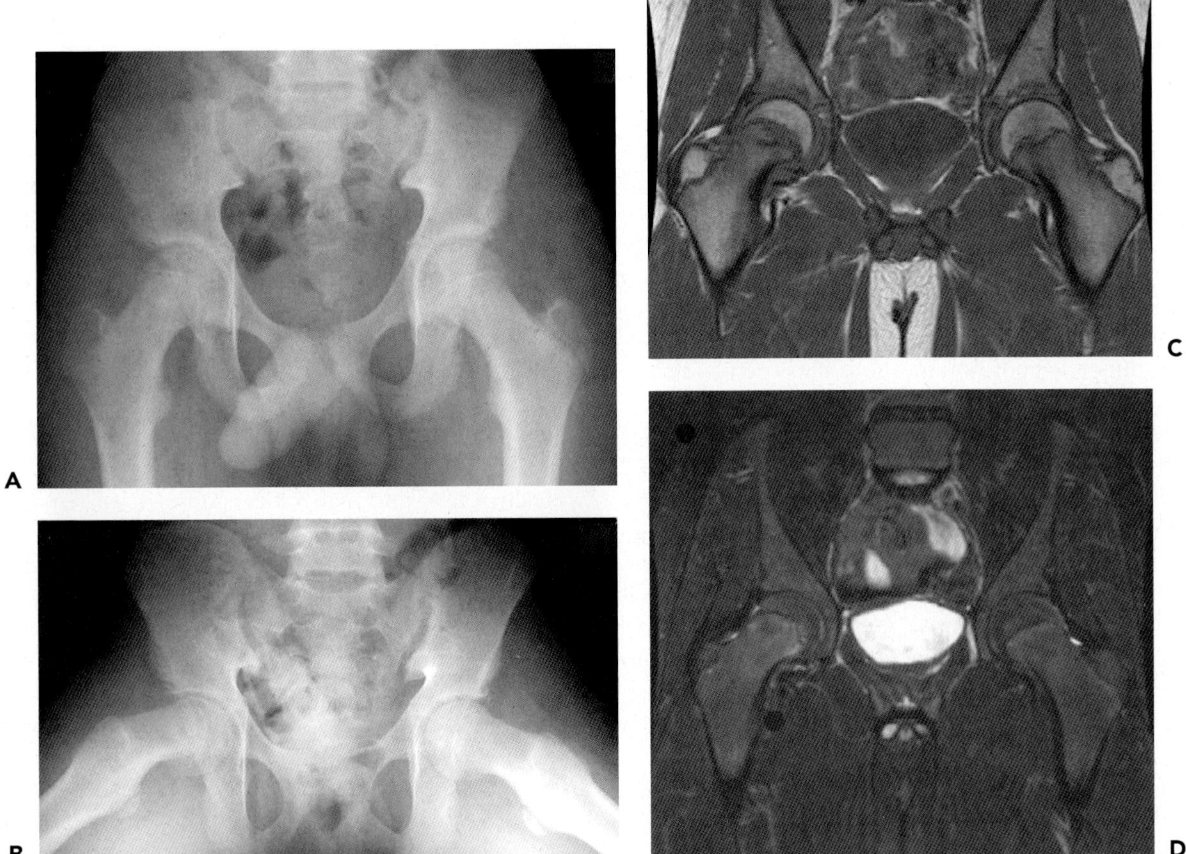

Figure 11.130 A 12-year-old boy presented with pain in the right hip for 2 months. On further questioning, he reported some vague, intermittent symptoms in the left hip. **(A** and **B)** Anteroposterior and frog lateral view of the pelvis show evidence of a right-sided slip, but no definitive signs of a left slipped capital femoral epiphysis. **(C)** T1- and **(D)** T2-weighted magnetic resonance image of the same patient demonstrate physeal widening and irregularity consistent with a "pre-slip." (*Reproduced with permission from* Morrissy RT, Weinstein SL. *Lovell and Winter's Pediatric Orthopaedics.* Philadelphia, PA: Lippincott Williams & Wilkins, 2006.)

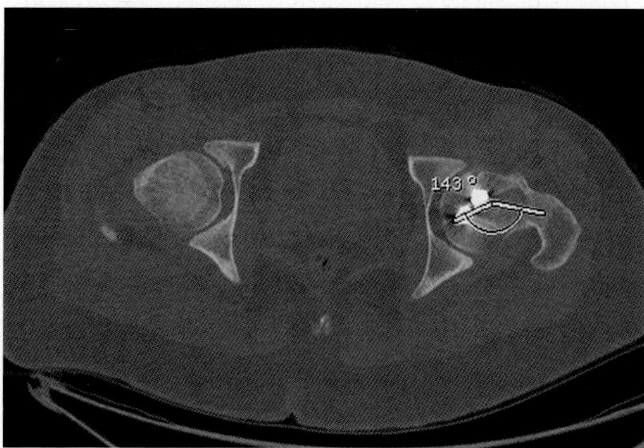

Figure 11.131 Computed tomography is useful to assess the severity of residual deformity after in situ pinning and allows for a more accurate measurement of the slip angle.

Treatment

Once the diagnosis is made, the patient should be admitted to the hospital immediately and placed on bed rest. Allowing the child to go home prior to definitive treatment increases the risk that a stable SCFE will become an unstable SCFE and that further displacement will occur. Children with atypical presentations (younger than 10 years, thin body habitus) should have screening laboratory tests performed to rule out an underlying endocrinopathy.

The goal of treatment is to prevent further progression of the slip and to stabilize (i.e., close) the physis. Although various forms of treatment have been used in the past, including casting and threaded pins, the current gold standard for the treatment of SCFE is in situ pinning with a single, large cannulated screw (Fig. 11.132). Screws are typically placed percutaneously under fluoroscopic guidance. The recommended position for the screw is perpendicular to the physis and in the center of the head on both the AP and lateral views. Generally, 3 to 5 threads across the physis are sufficient to achieve adequate fixation, but care should be taken to ensure that the screw has not entered the joint (Fig. 11.133). Because the epiphysis is posterior and inferior in relation to the neck, the initial entry point for the screw becomes progressively anterior on the femoral neck with increasing slip severity. Placing the screw too anterior, however, can increase the chances that the screw head will impinge on the acetabular rim. Postoperatively, most patients are allowed partial or complete weight-bearing with crutches for 4 to 6 weeks. Gradual return to normal activities ensues, with resumption of full activity by 4 to 6 months following hip pinning. Patients should be monitored with serial radiographs to be sure that the physis is closing and that the slip is stable. After healing from the initial stabilization, patients with severe deformity may be candidates for a flexion, valgus, and internal rotation proximal femoral osteotomy to reduce impingement and improve range of motion (Figs. 11.134 and 11.135).

The management of patients with an unstable SCFE presents additional challenges. Because of the high risk of osteonecrosis and the gross instability of the physis, unstable SCFEs should be treated in an urgent/emergent fashion. It remains unclear whether AVN is caused more by damage to the blood supply of the femoral epiphysis sustained at the time of injury or more by iatrogenic trauma from reduction during surgery. Regardless, most authors support the gentle reduction of an unstable SCFE that occurs during patient positioning. The unstable SCFE should then be pinned in situ, accepting whatever residual deformity that exists (Fig. 11.136). In general, two screws are advised to improve the rotational stability of the physis. A recent report has described increased intracapsular pressures in children with unstable SCFEs and has advocated decompressing the hematoma within the capsule to reduce the risk of AVN. Unlike stable SCFEs, most patients are kept non–weight-bearing postoperatively for 4 to 6 weeks, followed by a gradual return to weight-bearing.

The incidence of bilateral SCFEs is approximately 20% at the time of presentation. An additional 20% to 40% of children will develop a contralateral slip in the future. As a result, some surgeons recommend prophylactic pinning of the contralateral side in patients with a unilateral SCFE. The benefits of preventing a possible slip must be balanced with the risks of performing a potentially unnecessary surgery. A decision analysis, based on the risk of contralateral slip and incidence of complications reported in the literature, favored prophylactic pinning. A more recent analysis based on expected values found that prophylactic pinning of the contralateral side would be warranted if the probability of a contralateral slip exceeded 27%. The question as to whether or not to pin the contralateral side remains a source of constant debate.

Complications

Chondrolysis, the global loss of articular cartilage within the hip joint, is a major complication of SCFEs. With modern treatment, the incidence of chondrolysis is approximately 1.5%, although older studies have reported an incidence as high as 10%. Patients with chondrolysis typically present 1 to 4 months after treatment with extreme pain and loss of motion; radiographs demonstrate severe joint space narrowing (Fig. 11.137). The etiology of chondrolysis is poorly understood. Some authors have shown a correlation between transient penetration of the joint during surgery (by a guide pin or implant) and an increased risk of chondrolysis. Other reports describe the spontaneous development of chondrolysis in patients who have not been treated. The joint fluid of these patients demonstrates elevated levels of certain types of immunoglobulins, suggesting an autoimmune etiology. The pathologic findings include hypertrophy of the synovium, degeneration of the articular cartilage, and intraarticular adhesions. Although the joint space narrowing and range of motion may recover somewhat, most of these hips have unsatisfactory

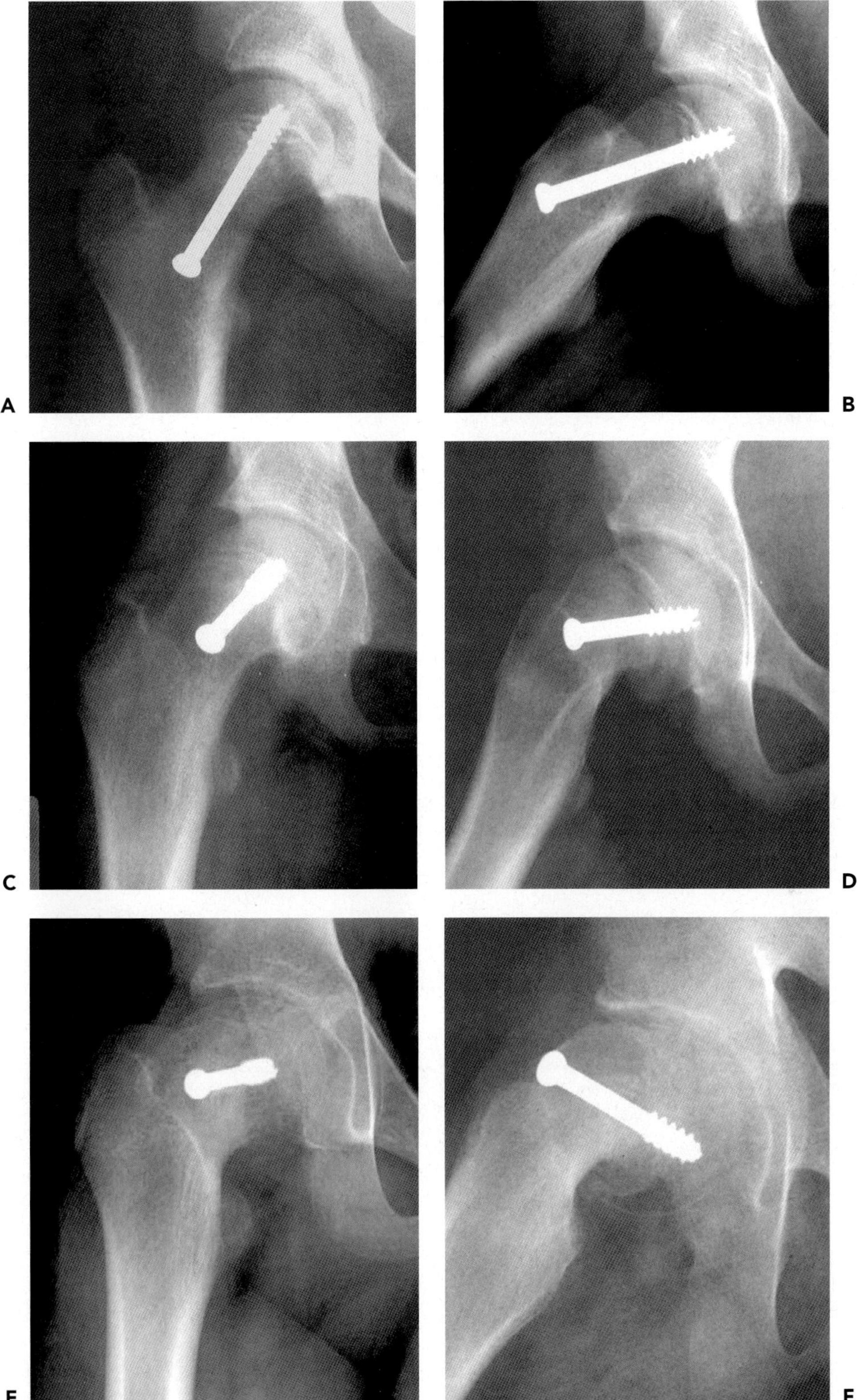

Figure 11.132 Proper screw locations in slips of varying severity **(A** and **B)**, **(C** and **D)**, and **(E** and **F)**. In all three cases, the screws enter the anterior femoral neck, are perpendicular to the physis, and are located in the center of the femoral head. The starting point is more proximal and the screw is angled progressively more posterior as the magnitude of slip progresses from least **(A** and **B)** to most **(E** and **F)** severe. (*Reproduced with permission from* Morrissy RT, Weinstein SL. *Lovell and Winter's Pediatric Orthopaedics*. Philadelphia, PA: Lippincott Williams & Wilkins, 2006.)

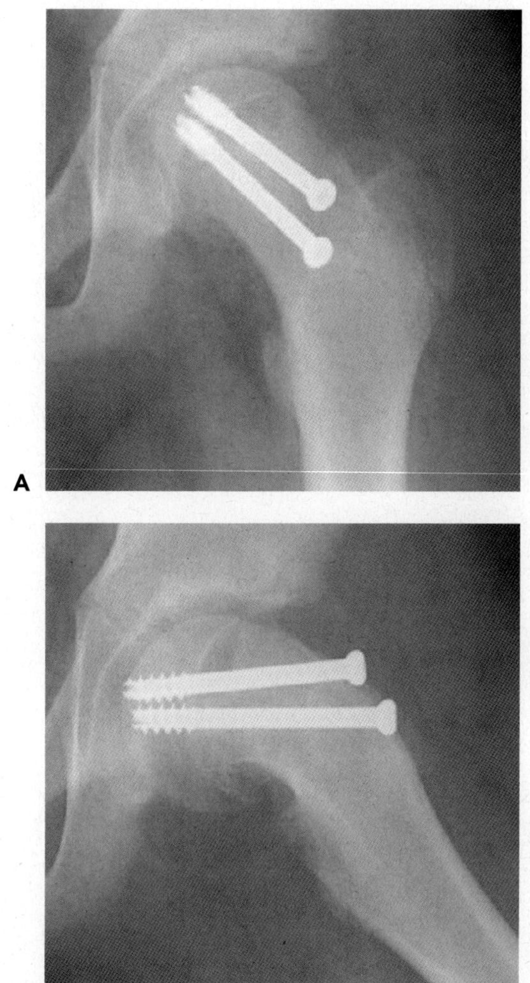

Figure 11.133 A $11\frac{1}{2}$-year-old boy with hip pain for 1 month after in situ screw fixation of a stable slipped capital femoral epiphysis. Anteroposterior radiograph **(A)** demonstrates what appears to be adequate alignment of the hardware. The frog lateral view **(B),** however, demonstrates penetration of the joint surface by one screw. This case highlights the importance of keeping the screw at least 5 mm from subchondral bone even if the hip is imaged through the full range of motion at the time of surgery. (*Reproduced with permission from* Morrissy RT, Weinstein SL. *Lovell and Winter's Pediatric Orthopaedics*. Philadelphia, PA: Lippincott Williams & Wilkins, 2006.)

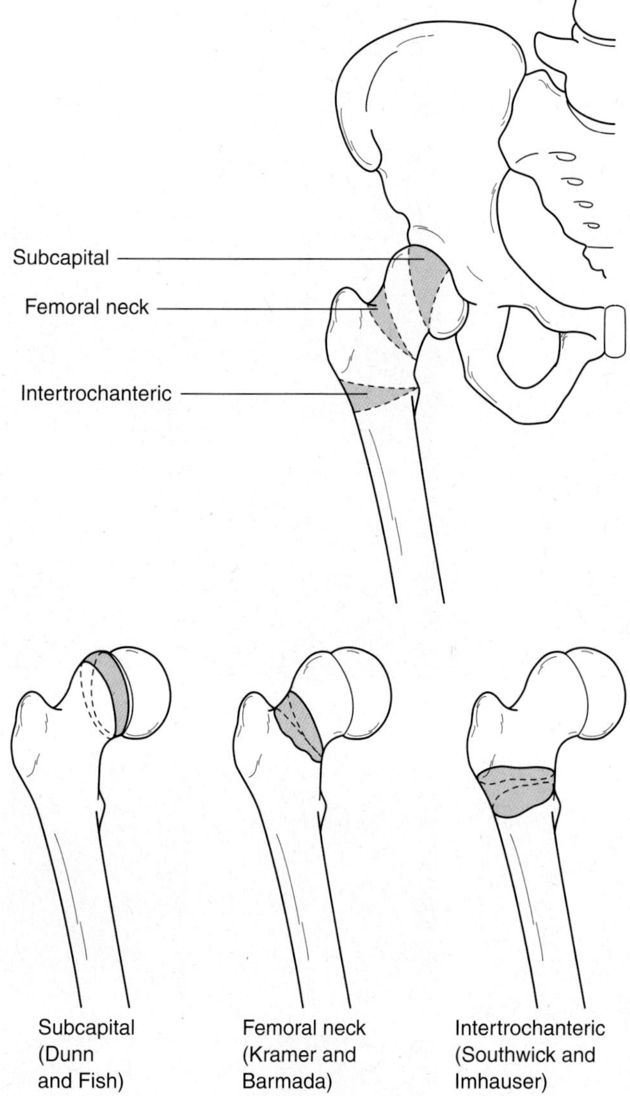

Figure 11.134 The three levels of osteotomy to correct the proximal deformity following slipped capital femoral epiphysis. The ability to correct the deformity is greatest with a subcapital osteotomy, least with a femoral neck osteotomy, and intermediate with an intertrochanteric osteotomy. The risk of osteonecrosis is inversely related to the distance from the physis to the osteotomy. Intertrochanteric osteotomies are the most commonly performed osteotomies because of the low rate of AVN and the ability to obtain good correction. (*Reproduced with permission from* Morrissy RT, Weinstein SL. *Lovell and Winter's Pediatric Orthopaedics*. Philadelphia, PA: Lippincott Williams & Wilkins, 2006.)

outcomes with severe degenerative arthritis and joint contractures. In the short term, symptoms can be managed with rest, gentle range-of-motion exercises, and NSAIDs.

The second important complication associated with SCFE treatment is avascular necrosis (AVN) of the femoral head. The underlying cause of AVN is a disruption in the blood supply to the epiphysis, leading to devascularization of the femoral head. It is, therefore, not surprising that the risk of osteonecrosis varies with the stability of the slip. In several large series, the risk of AVN after treatment of a stable slip approached zero. Unstable slips, however, have a 15% to 50% incidence of AVN. As mentioned, unstable slips should be treated in an urgent/emergent fashion with gentle reduction, secure fixation, and capsular decompression to minimize the chances of developing AVN. The first radiographic sign of osteonecrosis is increased sclerosis of the epiphysis because the lack of a normal blood supply prevents the normal resorption of bone from disuse. Eventually, the necrotic bone is absorbed, followed by collapse of the femoral head (Fig. 11.138). This results in severe joint pain and restricted range of motion. Often, the posterior portion of the epiphysis is relatively spared. In these cases, a flexion and valgus-producing proximal femoral

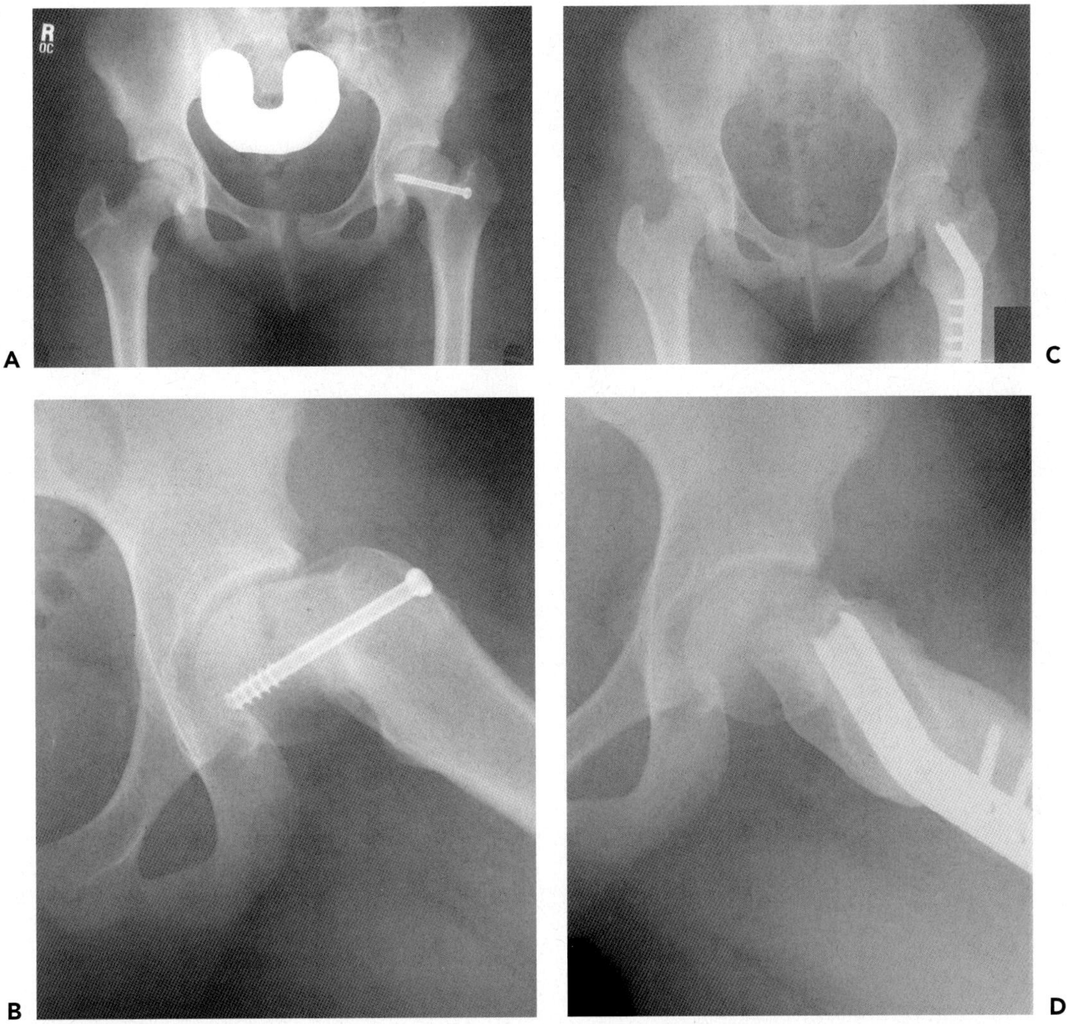

Figure 11.135 A 13-year-old girl with pain on sitting and difficulty riding a bike from impingement and external rotation of the left leg 16 months following in situ fixation of the left slipped capital femoral epiphysis. **(A)** Anteroposterior (AP) pelvis and **(B)** lateral radiographs showing the residual deformity after in situ fixation. **(C)** AP and **(D)** lateral views 1 year after flexion–valgus–internal rotation osteotomy of the proximal femur. The osteotomy increases the neck–shaft angle, increases the articulotrochanteric distance, and moves the metaphysis away from the joint. A downside of the surgery is that if total hip arthroplasty is necessary in the future, distortion of the proximal femoral anatomy will make such a replacement more difficult. (*Reproduced with permission from* Morrissy RT, Weinstein SL. *Lovell and Winter's Pediatric Orthopaedics*. Philadelphia, PA: Lippincott Williams & Wilkins, 2006.)

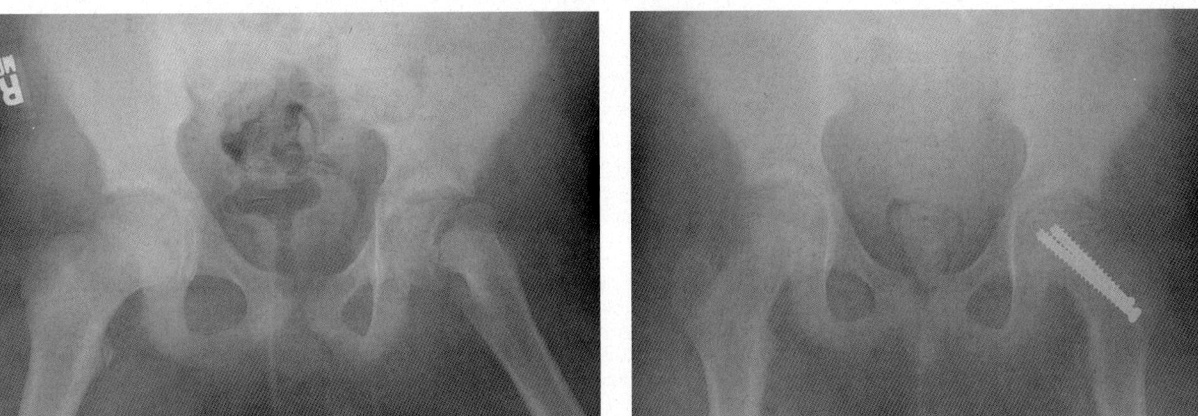

Figure 11.136 **(A)** Preoperative radiograph of a left acute, unstable slipped capital femoral epiphysis. **(B)** Radiographs after gentle closed reduction and screw fixation with two screws. (*Reproduced with permission from* Children's Orthopaedic Center, Los Angeles, CA.)

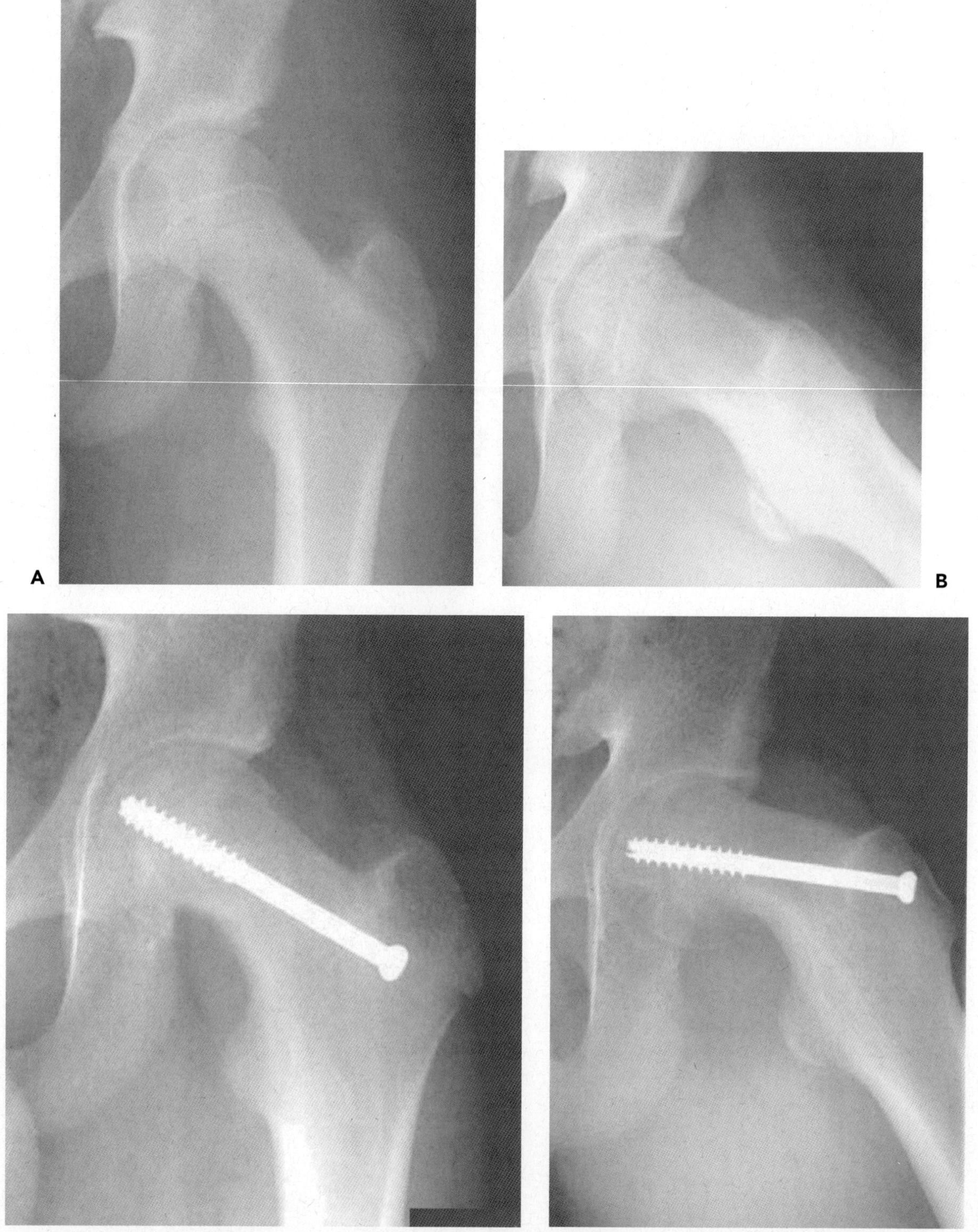

Figure 11.137 Left hip chondrolysis in a 13-year-old body. (**A** and **B**) Normal joint space of the left hip when the patient presented with a right slipped capital femoral epiphysis. Ten months later, the patient developed a left-sided slip and was pinned in situ with prompt resolution of symptoms. However, 2 months postoperatively, the patient began to have increased hip pain, difficulty walking, and decreased hip range of motion. (**C** and **D**) Radiographs at that time reveal joint space narrowing consistent with chondrolysis. (*Reproduced with permission from* Morrissy RT, Weinstein SL. *Lovell and Winter's Pediatric Orthopaedics*. Philadelphia, PA: Lippincott Williams & Wilkins, 2006.)

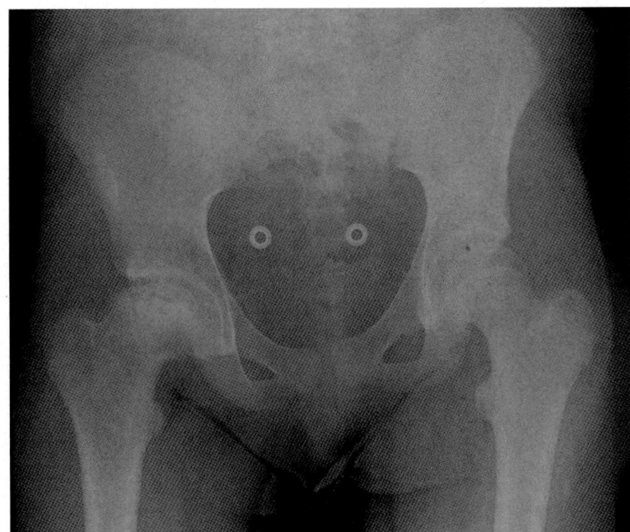

Figure 11.138 Avascular necrosis of the right hip following in situ screw fixation of an unstable slipped capital femoral epiphysis. The hardware has been removed to allow magnetic resonance imaging.

osteotomy can be useful to rotate the relatively preserved articular cartilage into the weight-bearing zone. In severe cases, however, arthrodesis or arthroplasty may be the only viable options.

Legg–Calvé–Perthes Disease

LCPD, or idiopathic osteonecrosis of the femoral head, was simultaneously described in the literature in 1910 by Arthur Legg in the United States, Jacques Calvé in France, and Georg Perthes in Germany. Henning Waldenström of Sweden actually published the first description of the condition in 1909, but since he attributed the cause to a mild form of tuberculosis, his name is not frequently associated with the disease. Since its initial description, LCPD continues to be one of the most vexing problems in pediatric orthopaedics, as both the etiology and the treatment of this condition remain poorly understood.

Pathophysiology

Although the underlying etiology remains obscure, most authors agree that the final common pathway in the pathogenesis of LCPD is disruption of the vascular supply to the femoral epiphysis, which results in ischemia and osteonecrosis. Several factors in the coagulation cascade have been suggested to play a role including protein C, protein S, and antithrombin III. Deficiencies in all three have been demonstrated in some patients with LCPD, which increases blood viscosity and the risk for venous thrombosis. Poor venous outflow leads to increased intraosseous pressure, which in turn impedes arterial inflow, causing ischemia and cell death. Although several studies support this theory of thrombophilia as the cause of vascular disruption, other recent studies have failed to show definitive abnormalities in the levels of fibrinolytic factors. Alternative theories for the cause of LCPD include trauma to the lateral epiphyseal vessels and a systemic abnormality in growth and development (based on the findings that children often have delayed skeletal growth).

Regardless of the underlying etiology, the early pathologic changes in the femoral head are consistent with ischemia and necrosis; subsequent changes result from the repair process. Waldenström originally separated the course of the disease into four stages, although several modifications of his system have been described (Fig. 11.139). The initial stage of the disease, which often lasts 6 months, is characterized by synovitis, joint irritability, and early necrosis of the femoral head. Revascularization then leads to osteoclastic-mediated resorption of the necrotic segment. The necrotic bone, however, is replaced by fibrovascular tissue and not new bone. This compromises the structural integrity of the femoral epiphysis. The second stage is the fragmentation state, which typically lasts 8 months. During this stage, the femoral epiphysis begins to collapse, usually laterally, and begins to extrude from the acetabulum. The healing stage, which lasts approximately 4 years, begins with new bone formation in the subchondral region. Reossification begins centrally and expands in all directions. The degree of femoral head deformity depends on the severity of collapse and the amount of remodeling that occurs. The final stage is the residual stage, which begins after the entire head has reossified. A mild amount of remodeling of the femoral head still occurs until the child reaches skeletal maturity. LCPD often damages the proximal femoral physis; during this stage, relative overgrowth of the greater trochanter can occur.

Classification

At the present time, three major classification systems exist for LCPD, all of which are based on radiographic assessment of the involved hip. The Catterall classification system, first described in 1971, separates the disease into four groups based on the percentage of the head involved and the degree of collapse (Fig. 11.140). Catterall group I includes patients with less than 25% head involvement, which is usually in the anterocentral region. Group II defines hips with 50% head involvement; more of the anterolateral region is affected and a central sequestrum may be present. Group III patients have up to 75% of the epiphysis affected with large areas "sequestrated." Group IV describes total head involvement. Widespread use of the Catterall classification has waned in recent years because the groupings can be difficult to define and because several studies have demonstrated a lower interobserver reliability compared with other classification systems.

The Salter–Thompson classification system is also based on the percentage of subchondral collapse. Two groups are defined: those in group A have less than 50% of the

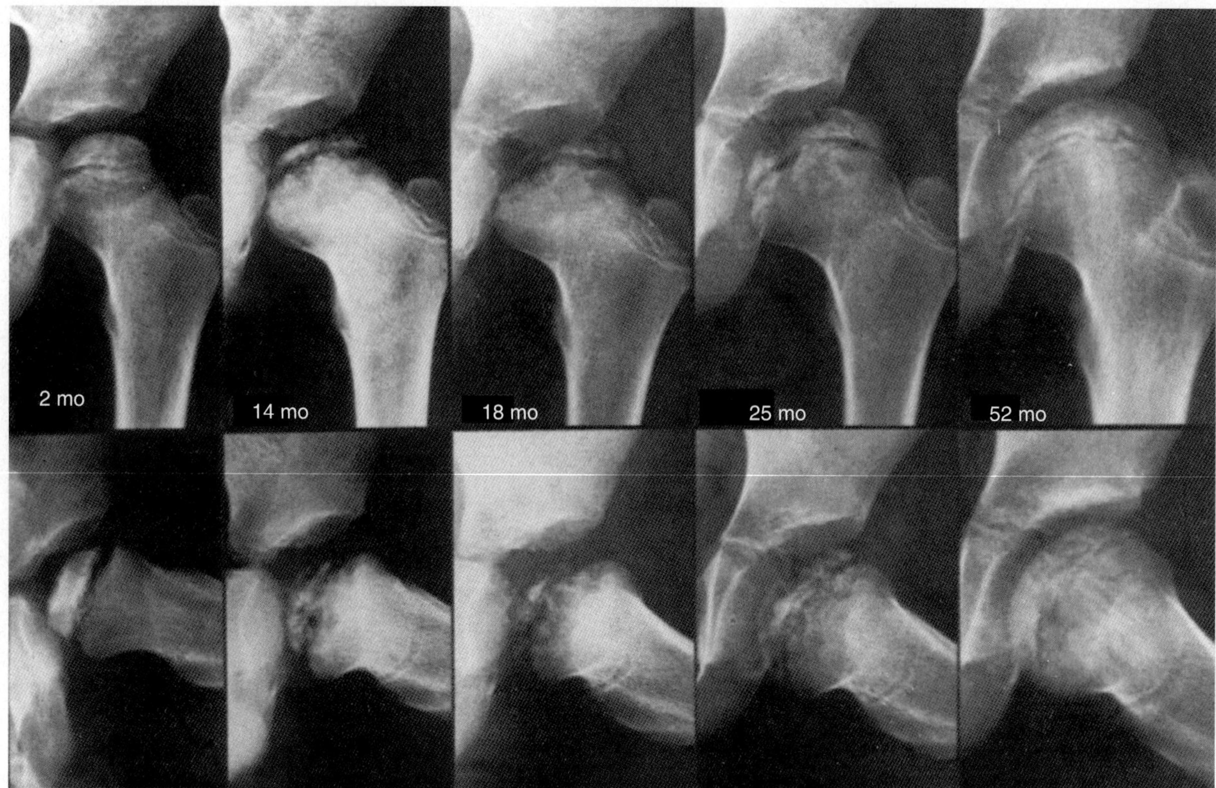

Figure 11.139 Legg–Calvé–Perthes disease with whole head involvement. Note the stages of disease progression by month after initial presentation. Two months, initial; 14 months, fragmentation; 18 months, early healing; 25 months, late healing; 52 months, residual stage. (*Reproduced with permission from* Morrissy RT, Weinstein SL. *Lovell and Winter's Pediatric Orthopaedics.* Philadelphia, PA: Lippincott Williams & Wilkins, 2006.)

head involved, and those in group B have more than 50% of the head involved. Typically, Catterall groups I and II represent hips in Salter group A and Catterall groups III and IV represent hips in Salter group B. A major drawback of the Salter–Thompson system is its reliance on the presence of a subchondral fracture, which in some series is present only in 30% of patients.

The lateral pillar classification, described by Anthony Herring, has gained popularity because of its improved interobserver reliability. Lateral pillar group A hips are those with minimal collapse of the lateral column of the epiphysis. In lateral pillar group B patients, up to 50% loss of height of the lateral epiphysis can be seen. Group C describes those patients with more than 50% collapse of the lateral pillar (Fig. 11.141). Recently, Herring has added a B/C border group to the classification, which describes patients with approximately 50% collapse of the lateral epiphysis. A major advantage of the lateral pillar system is that it offers some information for predicting the prognosis of a given hip. One difficulty with the system, however, is the timing of assessment. The original description classified radiographs during the first 6 months of fragmentation. Depending on when the child is evaluated during the fragmentation process, the final grouping can vary.

Presentation

The most common presenting complaint is pain or a limp. The onset of symptoms is often insidious, and pain may be referred to the thigh or knee. Parents may recall a history of trauma or viral illness preceding the onset of pain, and the severity of symptoms may wax and wane in the months prior to presentation. Children typically present between 4 and 9 years of age, although an adolescent onset pattern has been described. Boys are more commonly affected than girls, by a 3:1 ratio. Approximately 10% of patients may have bilateral involvement, although both hips rarely present at the same disease stage. Affected children are often small in stature and demonstrate a delay in their bone age.

Physical Examination

Observation of a child's gait is important, as a subtle limp is often the only sign of early disease. The limp seen in LCPD is a combination of an antalgic gait from hip irritability and a Trendelenburg gait from abductor dysfunction. Patients will generally have a positive Trendelenburg sign on the involved side. Depending on the duration of symptoms, atrophy of the proximal muscles can be seen. Careful assessment of hip range of motion is absolutely essential in the evaluation of any child with LCPD. Abduction is best

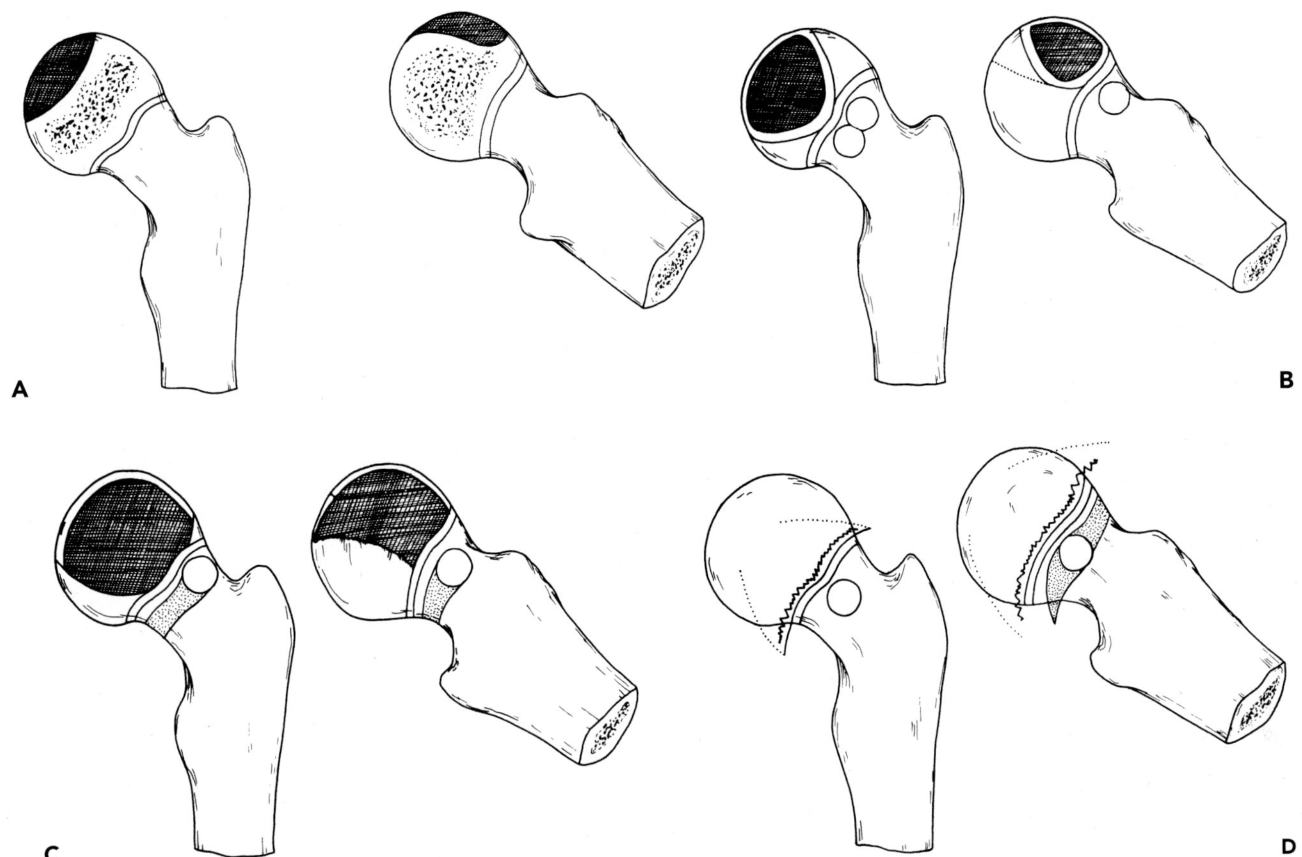

Figure 11.140 **(A)** Catterall group I disease shows anterior femoral head involvement with no evidence of sequestrum, subchondral fracture line, or metaphyseal abnormalities. **(B)** Catterall group II disease showing anterolateral involvement, sequestrum formation, and a clear junction between the involved and uninvolved areas. **(C)** Catterall group III disease shows large sequestrum involving three-fourths of the femoral head. The junction between the involved and the uninvolved portions is sclerotic. **(D)** Catterall group IV disease shows involvement of the whole head of the femur, with either diffuse or central metaphyseal lesions and with posterior remodeling of the epiphysis. (*Reproduced with permission from* Morrissy RT, Weinstein SL. *Lovell and Winter's Pediatric Orthopaedics*. Philadelphia, PA: Lippincott Williams & Wilkins, 2006.)

measured with the hip in extension and the pelvis well stabilized. Rotation can be assessed in either the supine or prone position. Early in the disease process, loss of motion may be minimal but pain may be elicited at terminal abduction and internal rotation of the hip. As the disease progresses through the fragmentation stage, loss of motion usually worsens, especially in abduction and internal rotation. Extension and flexion is generally spared. As the femoral epiphysis reconstitutes, children generally regain some degree of motion.

Radiographs

Standard radiographs for LCPD include an AP of the pelvis and frog lateral views of both hips. The radiographic findings in LCPD parallel the stage of the disease. During the initial stage, joint space widening and soft tissue swelling can be seen. The ossific nucleus is usually smaller and becomes more radiodense than the contralateral side (Fig. 11.142). Other findings include metaphyseal lucencies or cysts. During the fragmentation stage, the epiphysis becomes irregular with radiolucencies from resorption of the necrotic bone (Fig. 11.143). Often, a central region will become demarcated from the medial and lateral columns. The healing stage is marked by new bone formation in the subchondral region (Fig. 11.144). The lucent regions of the epiphysis gradually fill in until the entire head is reossified. During the final, residual stage, radiographs will usually demonstrate the sequelae of the disease process: an enlarged femoral head (coxa magna), a widened and shortened femoral neck (coxa breva), and trochanteric overgrowth (Fig. 11.145).

In addition to these radiographic changes, several classic radiographic signs have been reported that describe a "head at risk" for severe deformity. Lateral extrusion of the epiphysis, a horizontal physis, calcification lateral to the epiphysis, subluxation of the hip, and a radiolucent horizontal "V" in the lateral aspect of the physis (Gage sign) have all been associated with a poor prognosis (Fig. 11.146).

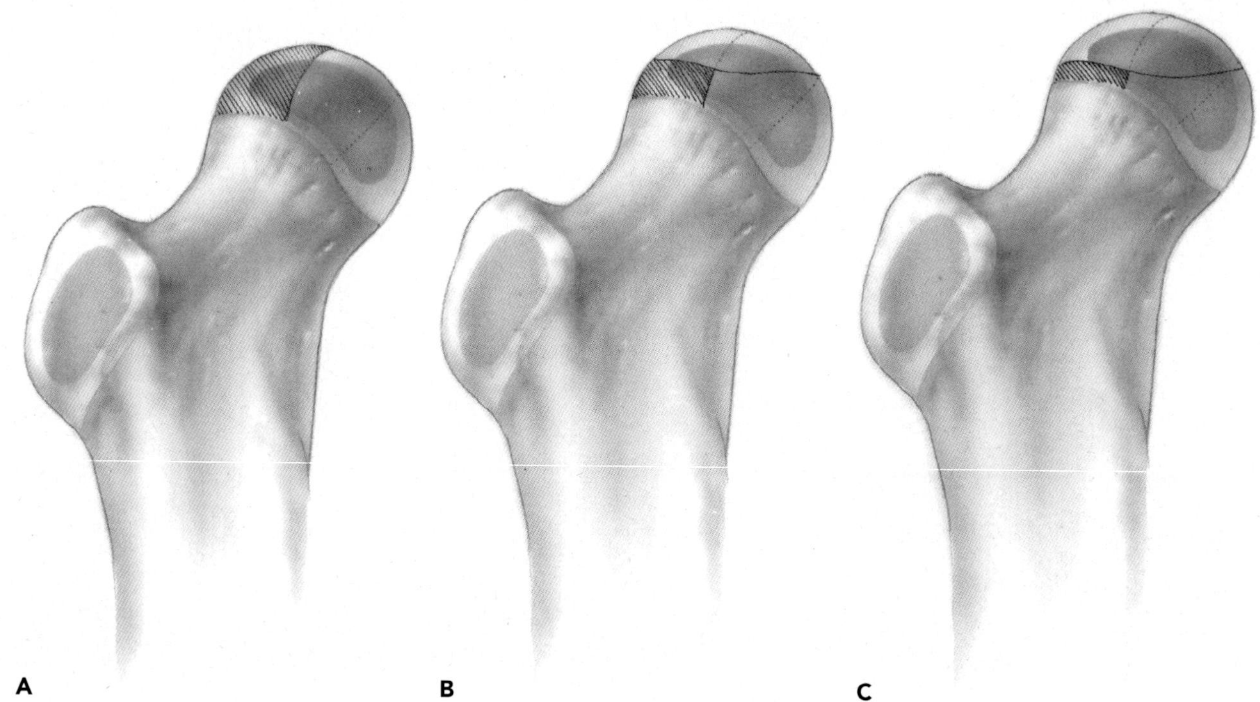

Figure 11.141 **(A)** Lateral pillar type A demonstrates preservation of the height of the lateral pillar. **(B)** Type B has more than 50% of the height of the lateral pillar maintained. **(C)** Type C has less than 50% of the lateral pillar height maintained. Recently, Herring has added a B/C subgroup to define those patients with approximately 50% collapse of the lateral pillar. (*Reproduced with permission from* Morrissy RT, Weinstein SL. *Lovell and Winter's Pediatric Orthopaedics*. Philadelphia, PA: Lippincott Williams & Wilkins, 2006.)

Special Studies

Although not routinely used in the evaluation of LCPD, MRI offers several theoretical advantages. Because if its ability to define soft tissue anatomy, MRI can offer information about the shape of the largely cartilaginous femoral epiphysis and the congruity with the acetabulum. In addition, MRI can provide early information on the extent of necrosis and the pattern of revascularization. One of the major drawbacks with the current radiographic classification

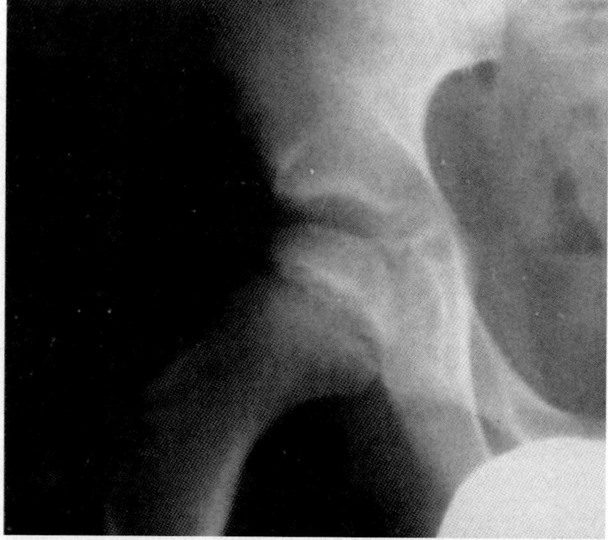

Figure 11.142 The initial stage of Legg–Calvé–Perthes disease demonstrates subtle widening of the joint space and increased sclerosis of the epiphysis. (*Reproduced with permission from* Morrissy RT, Weinstein SL. *Lovell and Winter's Pediatric Orthopaedics*. Philadelphia, PA: Lippincott Williams & Wilkins, 2006.)

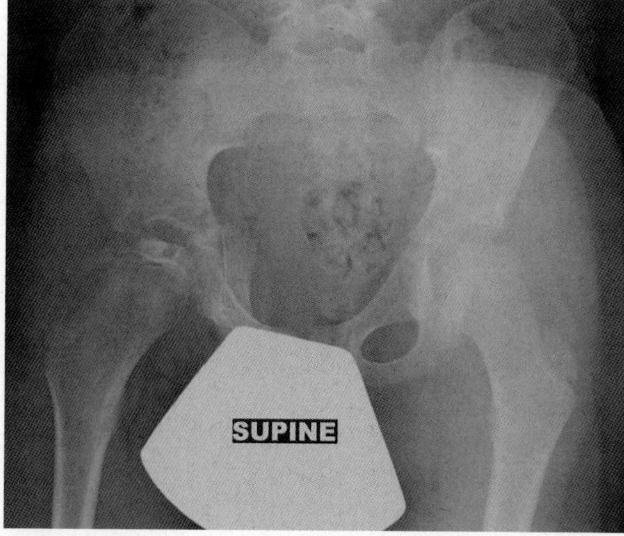

Figure 11.143 Anteroposterior radiograph of the pelvis demonstrates a right hip in the fragmentation stage of Legg–Calvé–Perthes disease. Note the irregular radiolucencies in the epiphysis.

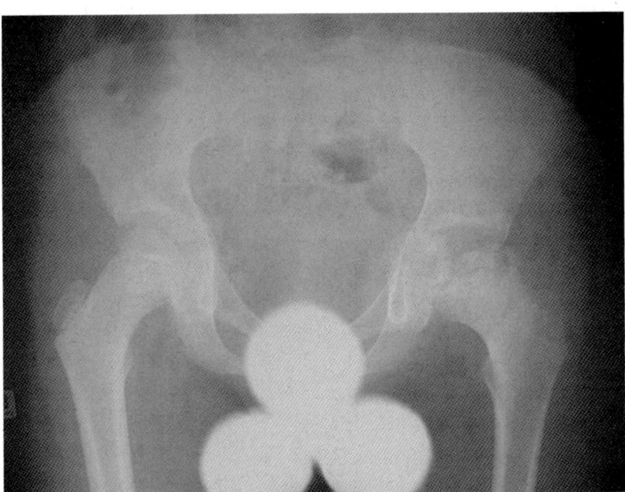

Figure 11.144 Anteroposterior radiograph of the pelvis shows a left hip in the healing stage of Legg–Calvé–Perthes disease. The overall contour of the femoral head is visible and the lucent areas of the epiphysis are filling in with new bone.

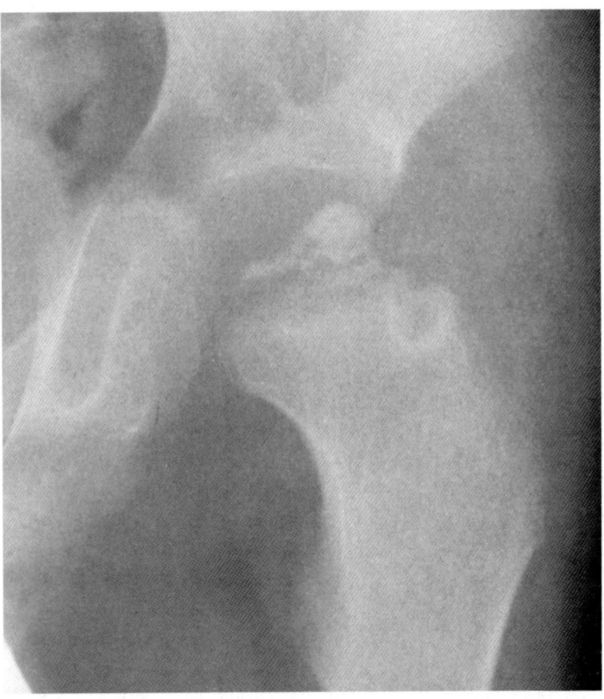

Figure 11.146 A 6-year-old boy with Legg–Calvé–Perthes disease of the left hip. Several Catterall "at-risk" signs are present, including a Gage sign, calcification lateral to the epiphysis, metaphyseal lesions, lateral joint subluxation, and a horizontal growth plate. (*Reproduced with permission from* Morrissy RT, Weinstein SL. *Lovell and Winter's Pediatric Orthopaedics*. Philadelphia, PA: Lippincott Williams & Wilkins, 2006.)

systems is that they rely on collapse of the epiphysis, the prevention of which is one of the major goals of treatment. In the future, MRI may be a better imaging option to provide early staging information that can guide treatment geared at preventing femoral collapse.

Arthrography is the other special study that is frequently used to guide treatment in LCPD. Although invasive, arthrograms can provide dynamic information about the shape of the femoral head, incongruities in the femoroacetabular articulation, and the position of optimal containment. Perhaps the best use of arthrography is to make the diagnosis of hinged abduction (Fig. 11.147). Hinged abduction occurs when the femoral head is too large or misshapen to rotate under the acetabulum during abduction. Instead, the head "hinges" on the lateral edge of the acetabulum; this leads to widening of the medial joint, which is marked by pooling of dye.

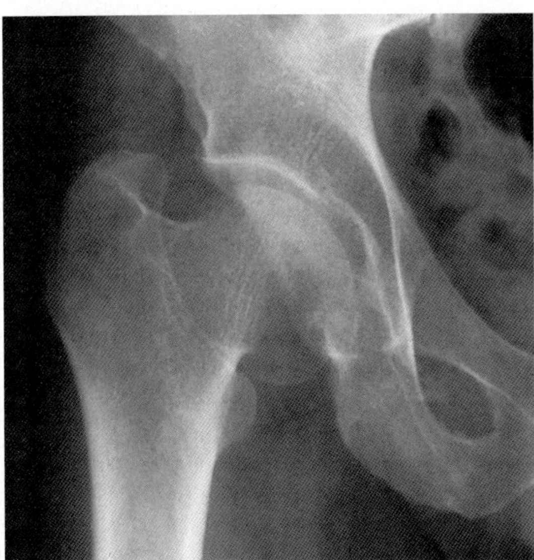

Figure 11.145 Adult patient with residual deformity from Legg–Calvé–Perthes disease. Note the enlarged head (coxa magna), shortened neck (coxa breva), and overgrowth of the greater trochanter. (*Reproduced with permission from* Morrissy RT, Weinstein SL. *Lovell and Winter's Pediatric Orthopaedics*. Philadelphia, PA: Lippincott Williams & Wilkins, 2006.)

Differential Diagnosis

The differential diagnosis for LCPD includes other causes of avascular necrosis, including trauma, leukemia, sickle cell disease, and hemophilia. An appropriate history and physical examination will generally rule out these other conditions. Hypothyroidism can cause similar radiographic findings as early LCPD; however, the findings are generally bilateral and symmetric. In contrast, bilateral involvement in LCPD occurs in a sequential rather than simultaneous fashion. In unclear cases, a thyroid function panel may be necessary. Although radiographically similar, children with MED are generally less symptomatic than those with LCPD. These patients are short in stature and almost always have abnormalities in other epiphyses. In addition, both hips are affected symmetrically. Older children with a history of DDH who developed iatrogenic osteonecrosis can resemble patients with LCPD. A history of treatment

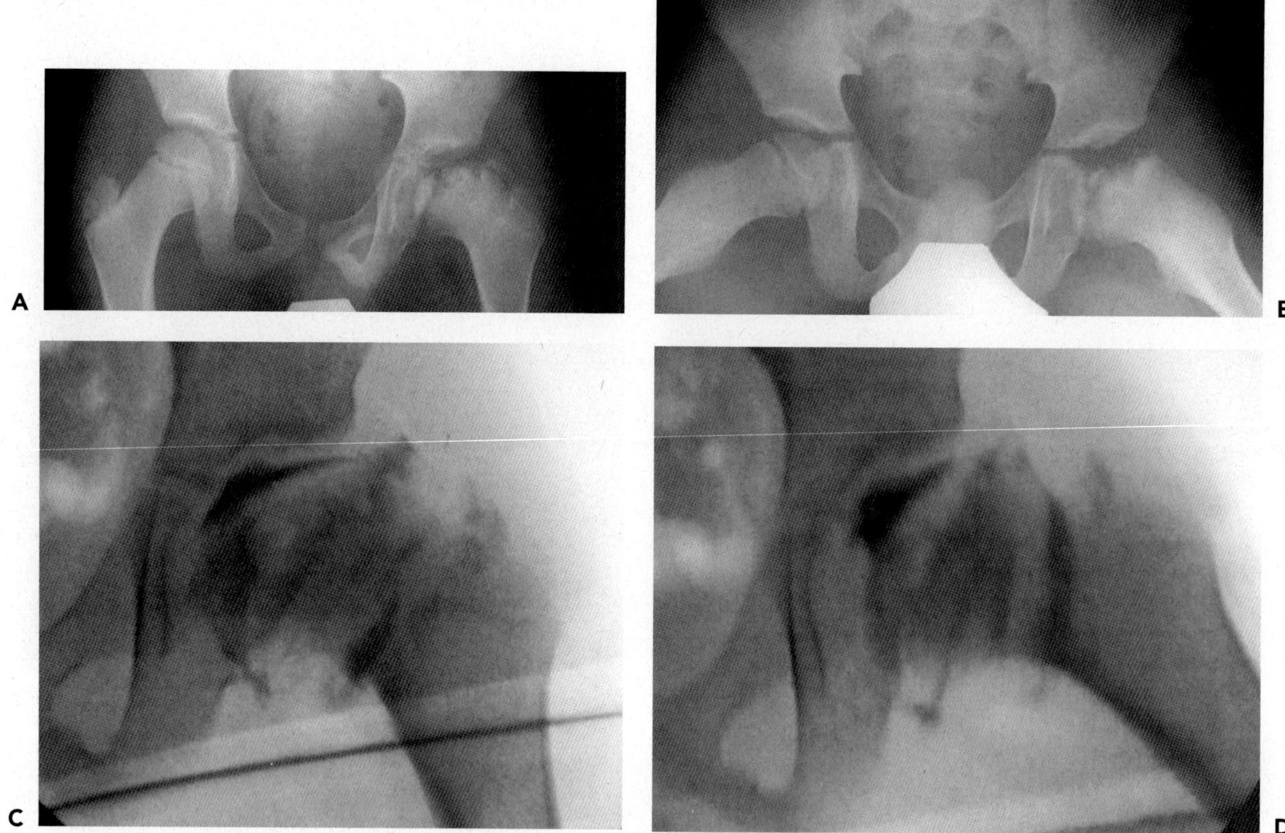

Figure 11.147 A 9-year-old boy with Legg–Calvé–Perthes disease. **(A** and **B)** Anteroposterior and lateral radiographs demonstrate total head involvement in the reossification stage of the disease. **(C)** Arthrogram in neutral position showing considerable flattening of the head. **(D)** Arthrogram in abduction demonstrating hinge abduction. Note the medial dye pool. (*Reproduced with permission from* Morrissy RT, Weinstein SL. *Lovell and Winter's Pediatric Orthopaedics*. Philadelphia, PA: Lippincott Williams & Wilkins, 2006.)

for hip dysplasia is generally sufficient to distinguish this diagnosis.

Treatment

Treatment of LCPD remains challenging because of the variability in disease severity. In general, the two most helpful prognostic factors are age at the time of disease onset and the lateral pillar classification. Children younger than 6 years at the time of disease onset, especially those with lateral pillar A and B hips, usually do well with nonoperative treatment. This is due to the greater remodeling potential of younger children and the higher percentage of cartilage in the femoral epiphysis, which helps resist collapse. On the other hand, children with delayed onset of disease (older than 8 years) and lateral pillar C hips tend to have poor long-term outcomes regardless of treatment. Those children that fall between these two extremes (i.e., 6–9 years of age, lateral pillar B or B/C hips) may be the best candidates for early surgical intervention.

For nearly half a century, the treatment of LCPD has been guided by the principle of containment. This principle is predicated on the fact that while the femoral head is fragmenting and, therefore, in a softened condition, it is best to contain it entirely within the acetabulum; by doing so, the femoral head will remodel, assuming the shape superimposed by the acetabulum. Conversely, failure to contain the head permits it to deform, with resulting extrusion and impingement on the lateral edge of the acetabulum (hinge abduction). Essentially, the implication of the containment theory is that the acetabulum will act as a mold for the regenerating femoral head. If containment is successful, the end result will be a spherical femoral head with a congruous hip joint.

During the early stages of the disease, the initial goal should be to alleviate discomfort and regain range of motion. Historically, this was accomplished by a period of bed rest with or without the application of longitudinal traction. Nowadays, most symptoms are managed with the appropriate use of NSAIDs, activity modification, and protected weight-bearing. Some authors advocate specific range-of-motion exercises, but vigorous physical therapy should be avoided as this can often exacerbate symptoms.

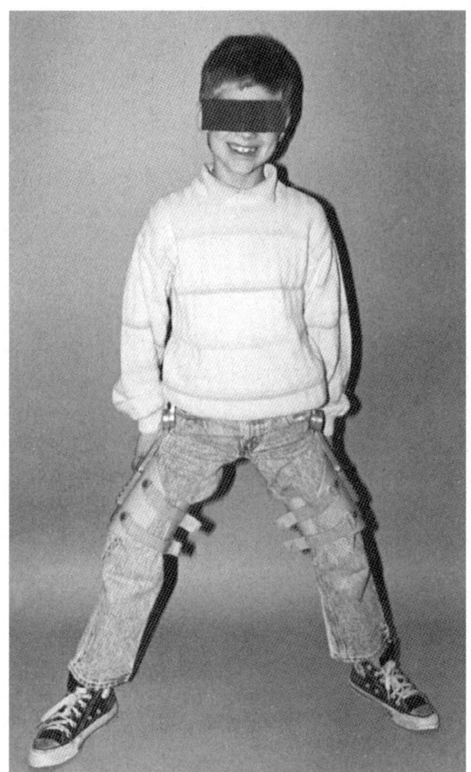
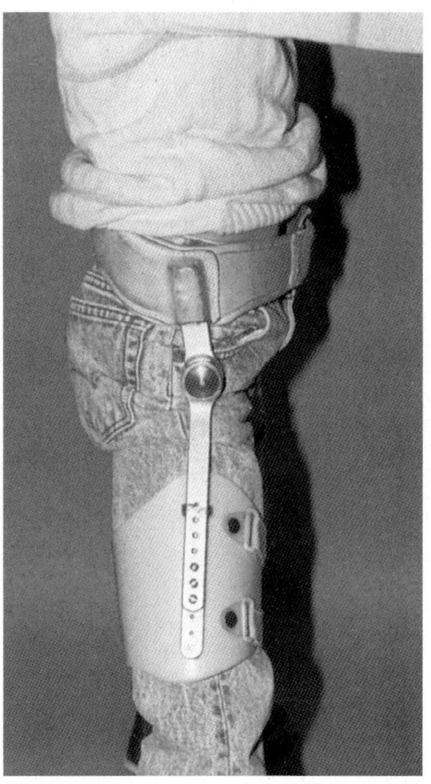

Figure 11.148 An abduction orthosis. (*Reproduced with permission from* Morrissy RT, Weinstein SL. *Lovell and Winter's Pediatric Orthopaedics*. Philadelphia, PA: Lippincott Williams & Wilkins, 2006.)

Once range of motion has improved, containment options should be discussed with the family. It is important to remember that to be successful, containment must be instituted early while the femoral head is still moldable; once the head has healed, repositioning the femoral epiphysis will not aid remodeling and may in fact worsen symptoms.

Nonoperative containment techniques employ devices, whether they be casts or orthoses, to position the hips in abduction and internal rotation (Fig. 11.148). In this position, the femoral head is solely contained within the acetabulum. In 1971, Gordon Petrie reported success using two long leg casts connected by a bar. The legs were placed in at least 45 degrees of abduction and 10 degrees of internal rotation. If necessary, an adductor tenotomy can be added to increase the amount of abduction. These Petrie casts were changed every 2 months or so until the femoral head was well into the healing stage. Orthoses such as the Toronto brace and the Atlanta Scottish Rite brace are based on these same principles of containment but allow some degree of hip motion and limited ambulation. Although bracing and casting can be helpful for maintaining motion, recent studies have not proven their efficacy for improving the long-term outcome of LCPD.

Surgical containment methods include both femoral and pelvic osteotomies. In the early stages of the disease, varus-producing intertrochanteric femoral osteotomy is the most popular means of achieving containment (Fig. 11.149). Correction should be limited to 10 to 15 degrees to minimize the risks of shortening the leg and causing abductor dysfunction (i.e., Trendelenburg gait). Results are best if surgery is performed before the epiphysis extrudes more than 20%. Alternatively, a pelvic osteotomy can be performed to enhance lateral coverage of the epiphysis. Most commonly, a shelf arthroplasty is the procedure of choice. Downsides include the risk of iatrogenic impingement from excessive coverage and stiffness from increased pressure on the femoral head. Regardless of whether a femoral or pelvic osteotomy is favored, arthrography should be performed before the procedure to confirm that containment is possible.

After healing of the epiphysis, surgical treatment shifts from containment to managing the residual deformity. Patients with hinge abduction or joint incongruity may benefit from a valgus-producing proximal femoral osteotomy (Fig. 11.150). Patients with coexisting subluxation or severe lateral uncovering may need a salvage pelvic osteotomy (e.g., shelf arthroplasty or Chiari) in addition to the femoral procedure. Coxa breva and overgrowth of the greater trochanter can be managed by performing an advancement of the trochanter. This helps restore the length–tension relationship of the abductor mechanism and can alleviate abductor fatigue. Patients with femoroacetabular impingement from irregularity of the femoral head can

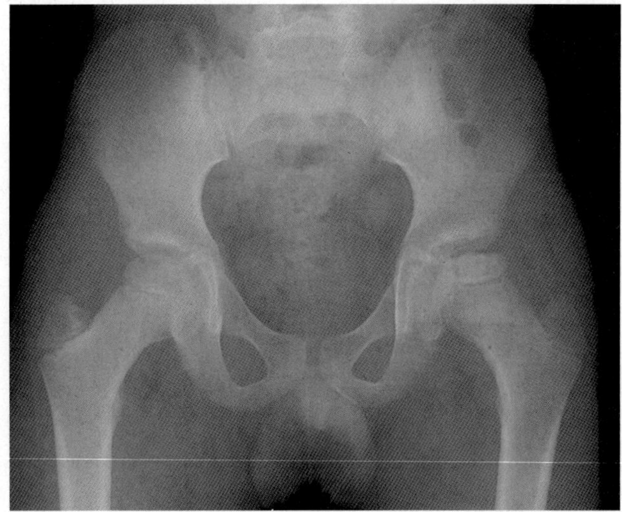
A

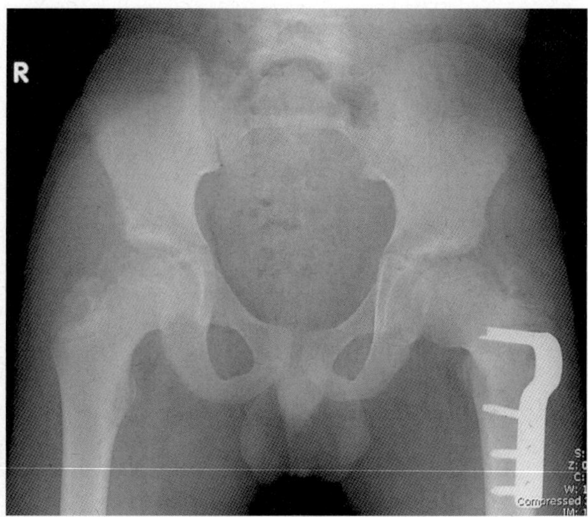

B

Figure 11.149 **(A)** Legg–Calvé–Perthes disease of the left hip. **(B)** Two years after varus proximal femoral osteotomy. (*Reproduced with permission from* Children's Orthopaedic Center, Los Angeles, CA.)

often be helped with an osteoplasty or cheilectomy of the offending prominence.

Long-Term Prognosis

As mentioned, the goal of containment is to preserve a spherical femoral head since the long-term outcome of LCPD depends on the shape of the femoral head. The Stulberg classification separates hips into five different categories based on the radiographic appearance of the hip after skeletal maturity. Stulberg group I hips are essentially normal, whereas group II hips are enlarged but spherical. Stulberg group III hips are oval or mushroom-shaped; these hips have an approximately 50% risk of developing osteoarthritis in adulthood but generally not until after the age of 40. Stulberg group IV hips have an area of flattening of the femoral head but are congruous with the acetabulum; patients with group IV deformities have a greater than 50% risk of developing significant osteoarthritis by the age of 40. Finally, Stulberg V hips are characterized by a flattened femoral head that is incongruous with the acetabulum. In one series, up to 86% of these patients had severe degenerative changes by the age of 40.

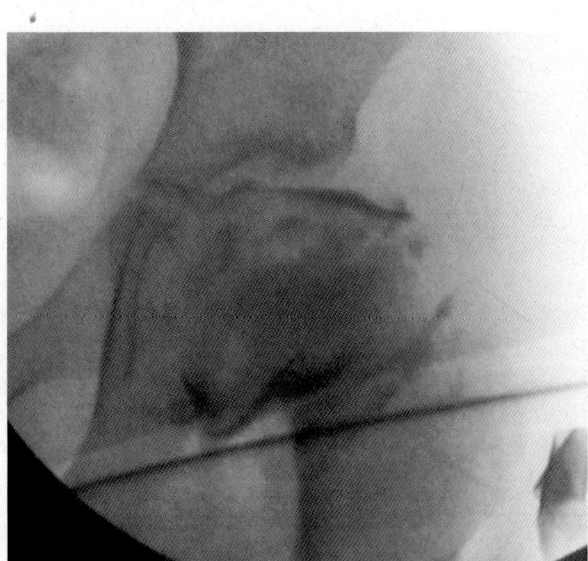
A

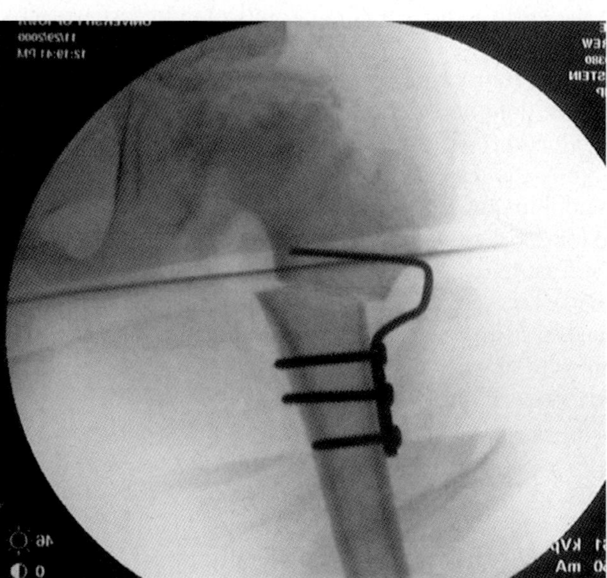
B

Figure 11.150 Same patient from Figure 11.148. **(A)** Arthrogram in adduction demonstrates improved congruity. **(B)** Valgus osteotomy was performed. (*Reproduced with permission from* Morrissy RT, Weinstein SL. *Lovell and Winter's Pediatric Orthopaedics*. Philadelphia, PA: Lippincott Williams & Wilkins, 2006.)

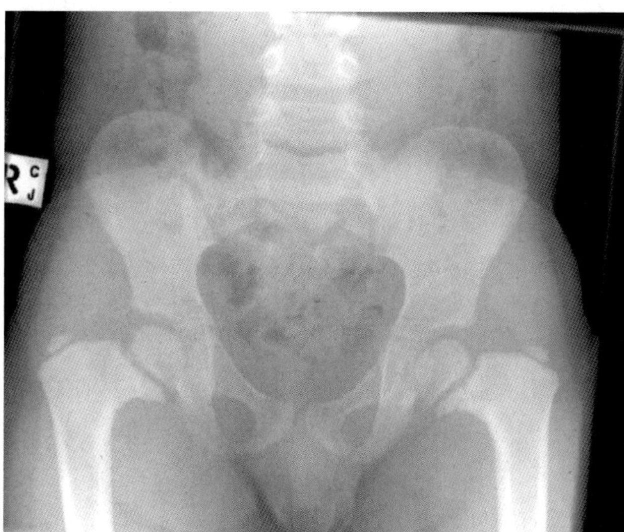

Figure 11.151 Bilateral congenital coxa vara in a 3-year-old child. Note the decreased neck–shaft angle and more vertical orientation of the physis. (*Reproduced with permission from* Morrissy RT, Weinstein SL. *Lovell and Winter's Pediatric Orthopaedics*. Philadelphia, PA: Lippincott Williams & Wilkins, 2006.)

Congenital Coxa Vara

Congenital coxa vara is an abnormality of the hip that results in a decreased neck–shaft angle and overgrowth of the greater trochanter. The incidence of coxa vara is much rarer than other pediatric hip conditions; 1 per 25,000 live births is generally affected, and the incidence does not seem to be affected by race.

Pathophysiology

Congenital coxa vara most likely results from a primary defect in the ossification of the medial femoral neck. The stress of weight-bearing causes fatigue failure of this weakened region, resulting in progressive varus deformity of the proximal femur (Fig. 11.151). As the neck–shaft angle decreases, the physis becomes more vertical, which converts the normal compressive forces to shear forces. The abnormal physeal orientation and mechanical loading pattern of a hip with coxa vara leads to relative shortening of the femoral neck and overgrowth of the greater trochanter.

Presentation

Congenital coxa vara is equally common in males and females. Approximately 25% to 33% of cases present with bilateral involvement. Patients with congenital coxa vara typically present after walking age with a painless limp. Families may also complain of an apparent leg length discrepancy. In older children, abductor fatigue from the abnormal mechanics of the hip may cause pain with physical activity.

Physical Examination

Observation of gait is extremely important in suspected cases of congenital coxa vara. Children with bilateral involvement will typically demonstrate a waddling gait; unilateral cases have an ipsilateral Trendelenburg gait. On range-of-motion assessment, abduction and internal rotation are generally restricted. Because of trochanteric overgrowth, abductor strength is often decreased and patients typically have a positive Trendelenburg sign. Leg lengths should be carefully assessed; modest discrepancies (<3 cm) are not uncommon with unilateral coxa vara.

Radiographs

Plain radiographs of the proximal femur are sufficient to make the diagnosis. In addition to the decreased neck–shaft angle (<120 degrees), radiographic findings include a widened and more vertically oriented physis, shortened femoral neck, and overgrowth of the greater trochanter. The most characteristic radiographic sign of congenital coxa vara is an inverted radiolucent "V" in the medial femoral neck that straddles a triangular piece of bone. The superior and more horizontal arm of the "V" represents the capital femoral physis. The inferior, more vertical line is the area of abnormal ossification. In addition to the neck–shaft angle, the severity of coxa vara can be graded by using the Hilgenreiner epiphyseal angle (HEA) (Fig. 11.152). This HEA is formed by the intersection of Hilgenreiner line and a line drawn through the capital femoral physis. Children with a HEA less than 45 degrees tend to have spontaneous resolution of their deformity. Values greater than 60 degrees have a high rate of progression. Angles between 45 degrees and 60 degrees represent a gray area; these children should be followed closely for signs of progression.

Differential Diagnosis

Several other conditions can cause varus deformity of the proximal femur, including PFFD, a variety of skeletal dysplasias, and rickets. Pathologic conditions of bone, including OI, fibrous dysplasia, and renal osteodystrophy, can also lead to progressive deterioration of the neck–shaft angle. In addition, coxa vara may be a long-term sequela of infection or trauma to the proximal femoral physis. A careful history and physical examination is usually sufficient to rule out these other diagnoses. Limb deficiency syndromes, metabolic disturbances, and conditions with pathologic bone generally affect more regions than just the hip. Skeletal dysplasias can generally be distinguished on the basis of family history and short stature. Skeletal surveys can be extremely helpful if the diagnosis remains uncertain.

Treatment

For progressive cases of congenital coxa vara, the goal of treatment is normalization of the biomechanics around the hip, which will help stimulate healing of the pathologic femoral neck. To do so, one must restore the normal neck–shaft angle, improve abductor function, and increase range of motion. As mentioned, surgery is recommended when the HEA is greater than 60 degrees and when progression

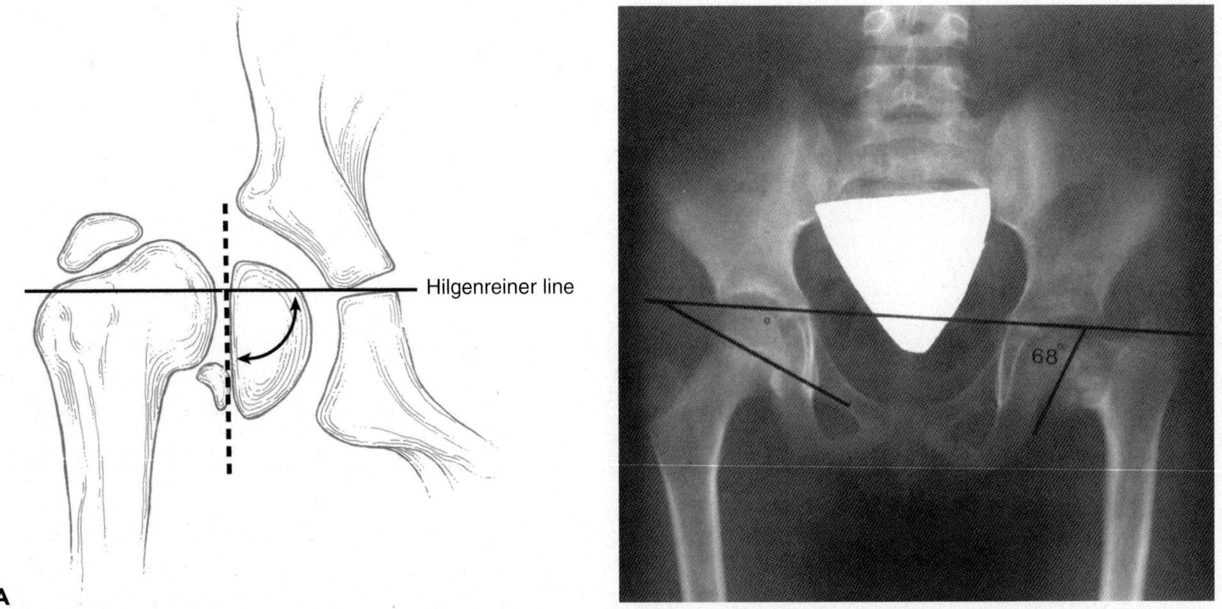

Figure 11.152 Hilgenreiner epiphyseal angle (HEA). **(A)** The HEA is the angle between Hilgenreiner line and a line drawn parallel to the capital femoral physis. **(B)** An HEA angle of 68 degrees in a patient with coxa vara; this value is associated with a progressive deformity. (*Reproduced with permission from* Morrissy RT, Weinstein SL. *Lovell and Winter's Pediatric Orthopaedics*. Philadelphia, PA: Lippincott Williams & Wilkins, 2006.)

is documented in children whose HEA is between 45 degrees and 60 degrees. Valgus osteotomy of the proximal femur is the most popular surgical technique for correcting congenital coxa vara. Performed at either the intertrochanteric region or the subtrochanteric region, valgus osteotomy corrects the neck–shaft angle, lowers the trochanter, improves abduction, and corrects the orientation of the physis (Fig. 11.153). Several osteotomy techniques have been described, but fixation usually consists of a blade plate or screw and side plate device. Correction of the HEA to less than 40 degrees has been associated with a decreased risk of recurrence.

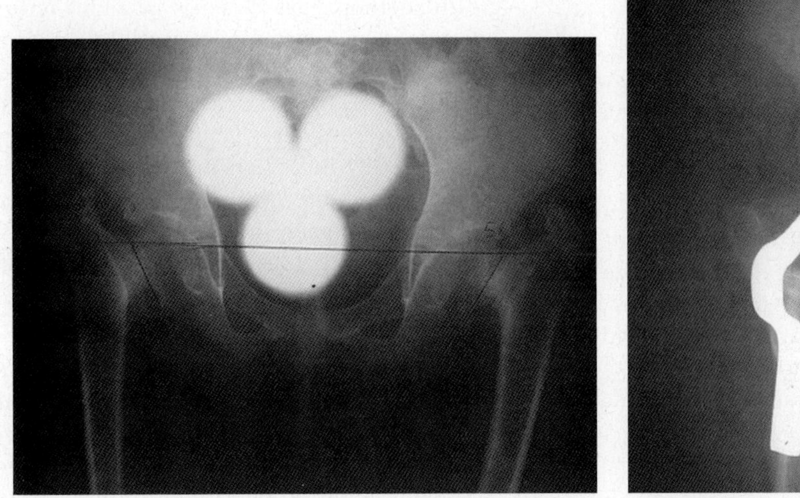

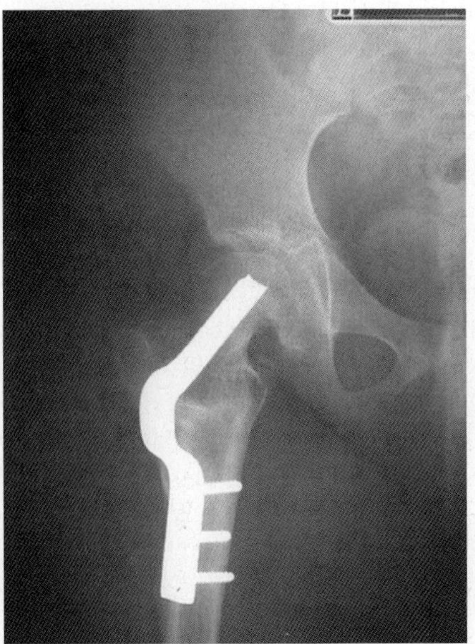

Figure 11.153 **(A)** Anteroposterior (AP) view of the pelvis showing bilateral congenital coxa vara. **(B)** AP view of the right hip 1 year after valgus-producing intertrochanteric femoral osteotomy.

KNEE AND LEG

Osgood–Schlatter Disease

Osgood–Schlatter disease is really more appropriately considered a condition rather than a disease. This condition is an osteochondrosis of the tibial tubercle. Unlike epiphyses, which are loaded in compression, apophyses are loaded in tension. In the case of Osgood–Schlatter disease, the pull of the strong quadriceps causes a traction apophysitis at the tibial tubercle. This low-grade inflammatory condition results from chronic mechanical overload and causes localized pain and swelling.

The typical child with Osgood–Schlatter disease presents in the preadolescent or adolescent years complaining of anterior knee pain. These children invariably localize their pain to the tibial tubercle. Characteristically, the pain is made worse by strenuous physical activity and stair climbing. Although the diagnosis is rarely in question based on the clinical evaluation alone, most physicians will obtain radiographs of the knee. Radiographic findings include irregular ossification of the tibial tubercle and traction osteophytes.

The treatment of Osgood–Schlatter disease focuses on activity modification since symptoms are primarily activity related. Moderation of activity and the selection of one sport versus many is usually the most help. Adjunctive therapy with icing after activity, lightweight knee straps or braces, and intermittent NSAID administration are all of value. In severe cases in which an ossicle is present, surgical excision can be considered.

Osteochondritis Dissecans

Osteochondritis dissecans is an osteochondral lesion that typically occurs in the distal femur. Although the exact etiology remains unknown, most authors believe that some sort of vascular insult causes osteonecrosis of the subchondral bone that leads to weakening of the overlying articular cartilage. The most common location is the lateral aspect of the medial femoral condyle, although lesions can also occur in the lateral femoral condyle, trochlea, or patella.

Children usually present in their preadolescent or adolescent years with either chronic knee pain or acute knee pain after a traumatic event. Depending on the stability of the lesion, children may complain of mechanical symptoms (locking, catching, popping, etc.). Physical examination will often reveal direct tenderness over the site of involvement, and range of motion may be restricted. Unless there is precipitating trauma, most knees do not demonstrate an effusion. Plain radiographs (including a tunnel view) are usually adequate to make the diagnosis (Fig. 11.154). However, MRI scans are helpful to determine the stability of the lesion and to monitor healing after treatment (Fig. 11.155).

Several classification systems exist for osteochondritis dissecans, but most differentiate lesions based on stability of the osteochondral fragment. Type I lesions are considered stable and have intact cartilage on the surface of the joint. Type II lesions may have some fissuring, but the osteochondral fragment is still attached to the base by an osseous bridge. Type III lesions are completely detached

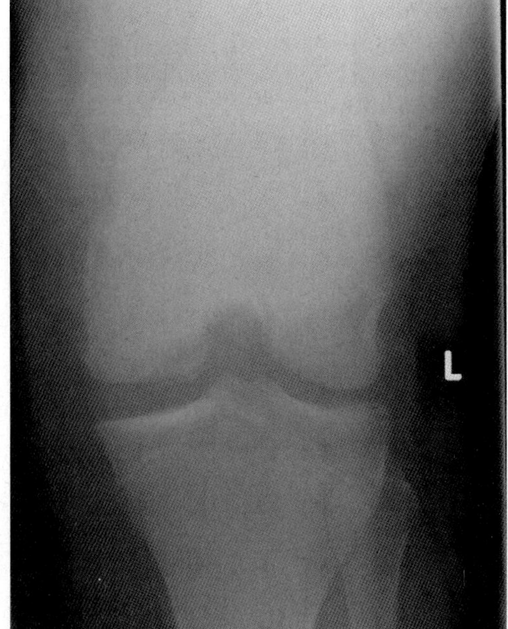

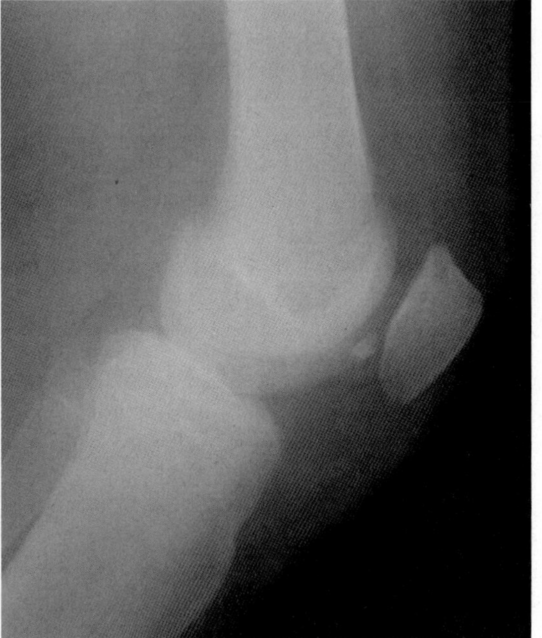

Figure 11.154 **(A)** Tunnel view of the left knee showing a loose body from a detached osteochondritis dissecans (OCD) lesion. **(B)** Lateral view confirms the loose body. (*Reproduced with permission from* Children's Orthopaedic Center, Los Angeles, CA.)

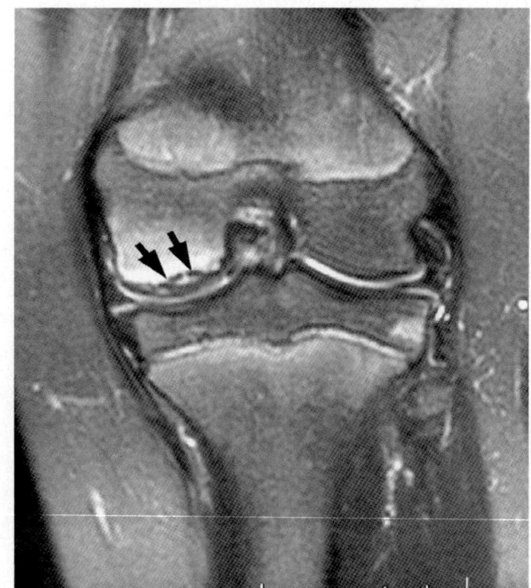
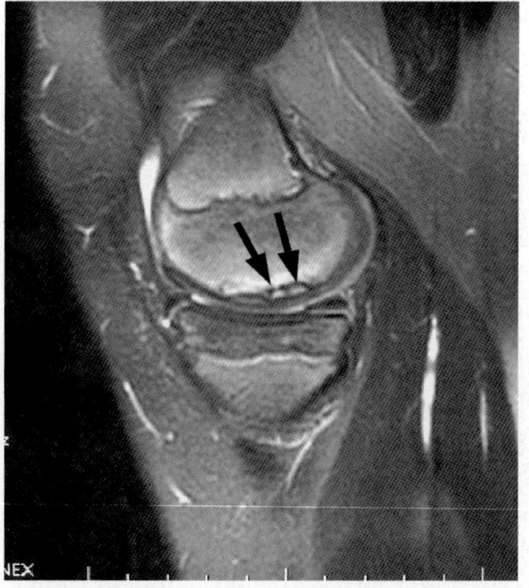

Figure 11.155 **(A)** Magnetic resonance image of a knee demonstrating an OCD lesion (*black arrow*) in the classical location (lateral aspect of the medial femoral condyle). The lesion appears to be stable, with an intact articular surface. **(B)** Lateral image of the same knee (*black arrows outline lesion*). (*Reproduced with permission from* Morrissy RT, Weinstein SL. *Lovell and Winter's Pediatric Orthopaedics*. Philadelphia, PA: Lippincott Williams & Wilkins, 2006.)

but are nondisplaced, and type IV lesions are completely displaced.

Treatment of osteochondritis dissecans depends on the stability of the lesion and the age of the patient. Children with an open distal femoral physis are considered to have juvenile osteochondritis dissecans; these younger patients tend to have higher healing rates with nonoperative treatment. As a result, conservative management in the form of activity restriction and/or cast immobilization should be tried for at least 6 months for all stable lesions. Those that fail nonoperative management can be treated with arthroscopic debridement and microfracture. After skeletal maturity, patients are more likely to fail conservative treatment and require surgery. For unstable lesions, regardless of age, arthroscopic fixation using headless screws or bioabsorbable implants is indicated.

Popliteal Cysts

Popliteal cysts are synovial cysts located behind the knee joint that are typically composed of gelatinous material. Primary cysts arise from the bursa under the medial head of the gastrocnemius or from the fascia of the semimembranosus muscle. Secondary cysts communicate directly with the knee joint and usually indicate an intraarticular process such as a meniscal tear or synovitis. Whereas the majority of popliteal cysts in adults are secondary to intraarticular disease, most cysts in children are a primary phenomenon.

Children typically present with a painless mass behind the knee. Parents may report that the mass waxes or wanes in size. Plain radiographs can be used to rule out other conditions, but clinical examination and transillumination of the cyst are generally sufficient to make the diagnosis. In certain cases, ultrasonography can be helpful to distinguish cysts from solid tumors. MRI is generally not necessary but may be indicated in ambiguous cases.

The vast majority of popliteal cysts will resolve within 6 months. Therefore, most cysts should be treated conservatively with warmth, compressive bandages, and NSAIDs (if necessary). Surgical excision should be avoided unless the mass fails to resolve, enlarges rapidly, or causes significant symptoms.

Discoid Meniscus

A discoid meniscus is an abnormally large and abnormally shaped meniscus that usually occurs in the lateral hemijoint. The etiology of the discoid meniscus remains controversial. The theory of embryologic delay has been popular for many years. Simply stated, this proposes that the normal "C" shaped meniscus is the result of differential changes that occur in an initial "hockey-puck" shaped structure. Current literature, however, has suggested that this may not be the cause since discoid menisci have never been reported in the autopsies of newborns or stillbirths.

A discoid meniscus can present anywhere between the age of 3 and early adulthood. Young children generally do not complain of pain but may present with a limp, intermittent effusions, or a loud clunk with flexion and rotational motions of the knee. As the child grows older, the meniscus can tear, resulting in pain, locking, and other mechanical symptoms. Physical examination may reveal pain along the lateral joint line and lack of terminal extension. Gait is notable for a persistent knee flexion through stance phase.

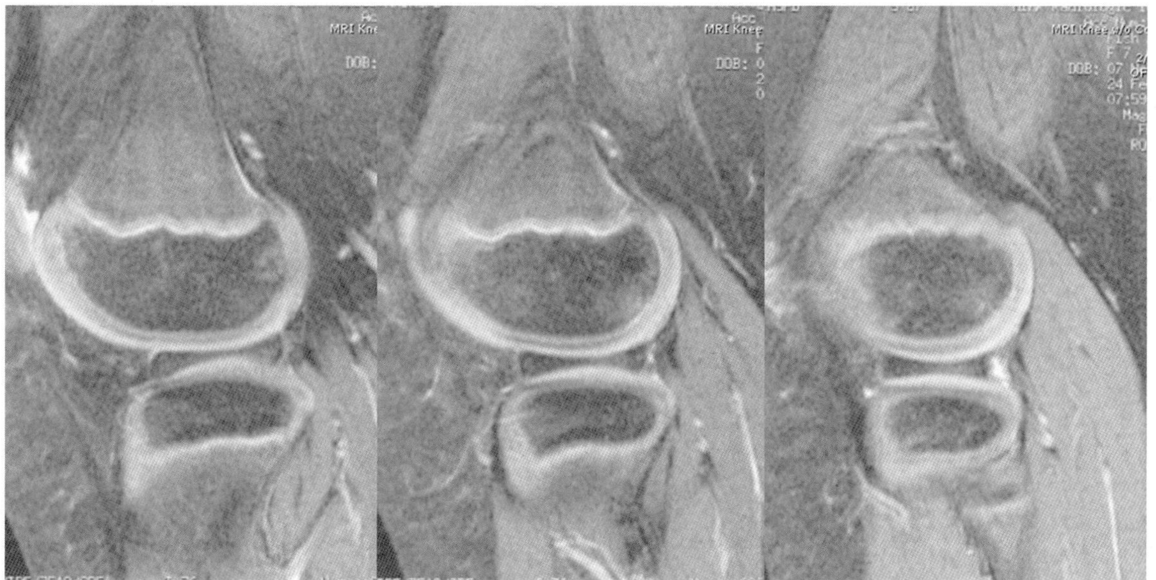

Figure 11.156 Three successive sagittal magnetic resonance image cuts demonstrating contiguous anterior and posterior horns of the lateral meniscus. This finding is diagnostic of a discoid meniscus. (*Reproduced with permission from* Children's Orthopaedic Center, Los Angeles, CA.)

Radiographs are of limited utility; occasionally, squaring of the lateral femoral condyle can be seen. MRI, however, is extremely useful in evaluating meniscal anatomy. Evidence of contiguous anterior and posterior horns of the lateral meniscus on three successive sagittal plane cuts is diagnostic (Fig. 11.156).

Discoid menisci can be classified into three types: complete, incomplete, and Wrisberg variant. This latter type is really not an abnormality in meniscal shape but rather an abnormality in the peripheral attachment of the meniscus. A complete absence of the meniscotibial ligaments makes the Wrisberg type hypermobile and prone to tearing.

Asymptomatic patients do not require treatment. Patients who complain of pain or mechanical symptoms should undergo arthroscopic treatment. If possible, only the central portion of the discoid meniscus should be removed (saucerized) to preserve some meniscal function (Fig. 11.157). Occasionally, the meniscus too is damaged

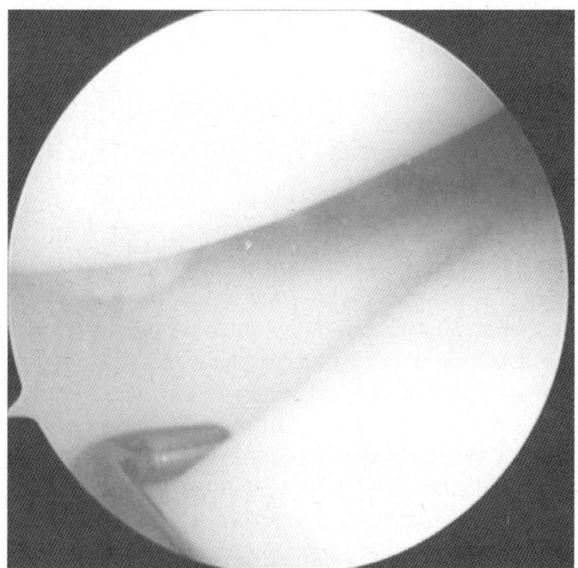

A

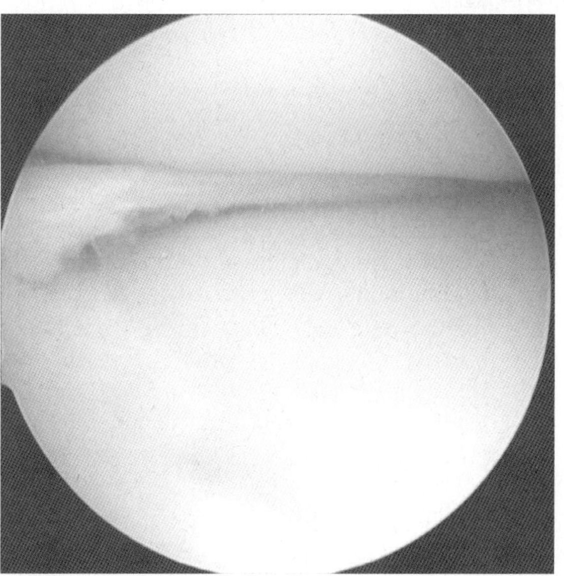

B

Figure 11.157 **(A)** Complete discoid meniscus viewed from the lateral compartment. **(B)** Appearance of the meniscus after arthroscopic saucerization. (*Reproduced with permission from* Skaggs DL, Tolo VT. *Master Techniques in Orthopaedic Surgery: Pediatrics*. Philadelphia, PA: Lippincott Williams & Wilkins, 2008.)

and the entire meniscus must be resected. Unstable discoid menisci, including the Wrisberg type, can be stabilized by suturing the edge to the capsule.

BLOUNT DISEASE (TIBIA VARA)

Pathophysiology

Blount disease, or tibia vara, is an abnormality in the medial aspect of the proximal tibial epiphysis and physis that results in progressive varus deformity of the tibia. The term *Blount disease* really applies to two distinct conditions: infantile tibia vara and adolescent tibia vara. The true etiology of both conditions remains poorly understood.

Infantile tibia vara has not been reported at birth and is, therefore, considered a true developmental condition. The etiology is considered multifactorial, but early ambulation and African American heritage both are risk factors for developing tibia vara. As part of the condition, damage occurs to the medial physis of the proximal tibia that results in progressive bowing of the tibia from relative overgrowth of the lateral side. Histologic studies have demonstrated disorganization of the physis and a disruption of the normal endochondral ossification process. In later stages, a true bony bridge can form across the medial physis that prevents any remaining growth on the medial side. Adolescent tibia vara occurs when the tibial physis is more mature. Repetitive microtrauma from compressive loads is thought to cause retardation of the growth of the medial physis. This theory is consistent with the high prevalence of obesity in children with adolescent tibia vara. Histopathologically, fissures and clefts can be seen in the physeal cartilage and are highly suggestive of repetitive microinjury. Unlike infantile tibia vara, bony bridges are rarely seen.

Classification

As mentioned, Blount disease is typically separated into infantile and adolescent forms on the basis of the age of onset. The severity of infantile tibia vara is described by the Langenskiöld classification (Fig. 11.158). The classification is based on the radiographic appearance of the proximal tibia. The condition of the growth plate, the extent of the medial beaking, changes in the medial tibial metaphysis, and evidence of premature fusion of the growth plate medially are all factors in differentiating the grades. The stages represent progressive medial physeal inclination of the proximal tibia with physeal bar presence in stage 6. The Langenskiöld grade and the age of the patient are factors in determining treatment.

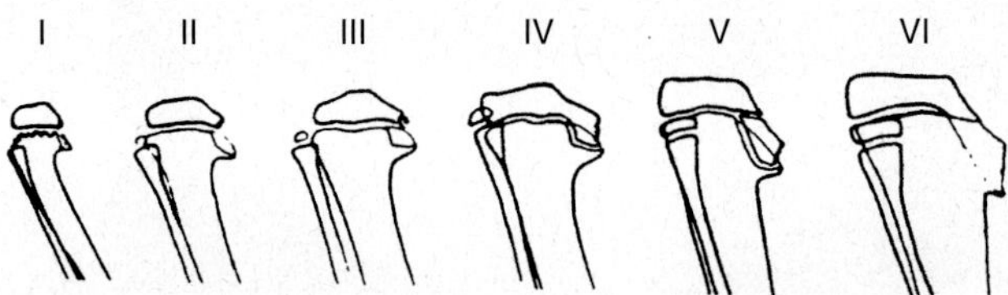

Figure 11.158 The six stages of radiographic changes seen in Langenskiöld classification of infantile tibia vara. (*Reproduced with permission from* Langenskiöld A. Tibia vara. *Clin Orthop Relat Res.* 1989;246:195.)

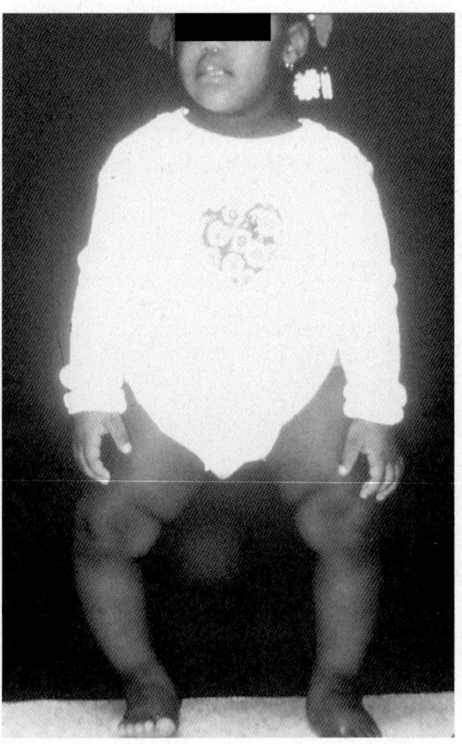

Figure 11.159 Clinical appearance of a 30-month-old girl with right-sided Blount disease. The left side, in contrast, demonstrates physiologic bowing. (*Reproduced with permission from* Morrissy RT, Weinstein SL. *Lovell and Winter's Pediatric Orthopaedics.* Philadelphia, PA: Lippincott Williams & Wilkins, 2006.)

Presentation and Physical Examination

Patients often present with the characteristic appearance of significant genu varum (Fig. 11.159). Patients with infantile-onset types typically have bilateral involvement, whereas adolescent-onset disease is usually unilateral. Most patients are asymptomatic, but some adolescents may report aching pain on the medial aspect of their knee. The majority of patients, regardless of the age of presentation, are significantly obese, with weights that are often greater than the 95th percentile for age (Fig. 11.160). During the physical examination, careful attention should be paid to the child's gait. Evidence of a "lateral thrust" (lateral translation of the tibia under the femur) with weight-bearing is usually indicative of Blount disease. Internal tibial torsion is often present in addition to the varus deformity. A concomitant leg length discrepancy can be seen in children with unilateral disease.

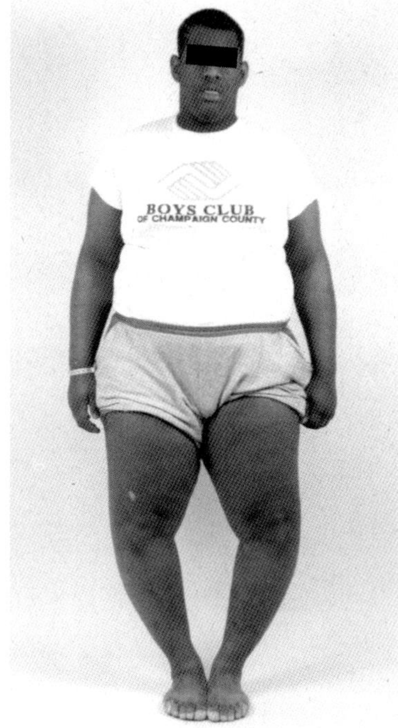

A

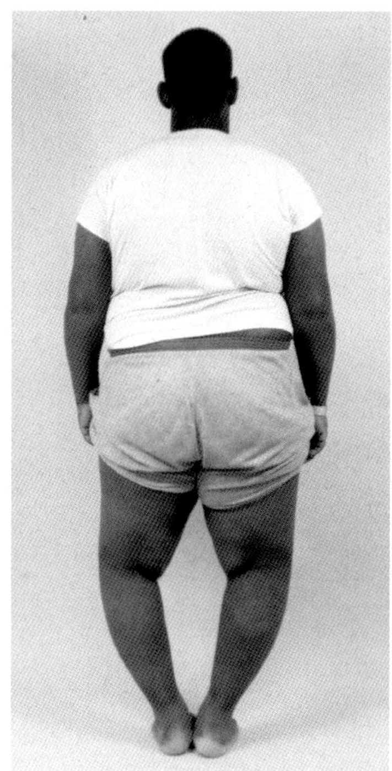

B

Figure 11.160 A 13-year-old boy with adolescent Blount disease. As is often seen in this group of patients, he is morbidly obese. The large thigh circumference in such patients contributes to the deformity and increased load across the medial distal femur and proximal tibia. (*Reproduced with permission from* Morrissy RT, Weinstein SL. *Lovell and Winter's Pediatric Orthopaedics*. Philadelphia, PA: Lippincott Williams & Wilkins, 2006.)

Imaging

Radiographic evaluation includes views of the proximal tibia and a standing AP view of both hips to ankles, with the patellas (not the feet) facing forward. The characteristic radiographic findings in infantile tibia vara include varus angulation of the proximal tibial epiphysis/metaphysis, widening and irregularity of the medial tibial physis, a medially sloped epiphysis, and prominent beaking of medial metaphysis. Prior to the appearance of these findings, it can be difficult to distinguish infantile Blount disease from severe physiologic bowing. For these cases, Levine and Drennan described the metaphyseal–diaphyseal angle (MDA) to help predict the likelihood of a given limb developing infantile Blount disease. A child with an MDA of less than 9 degrees is unlikely to progress to tibia vara, whereas the one with greater than 16 degrees is at high risk for progression (Fig. 11.161). Unlike the infantile form, the shape of the tibial physis is relatively normal in adolescent Blount disease. Sloping of the medial epiphysis and beaking of the metaphysis are not usually seen. The hallmark of adolescent tibia vara is widening of the medial physis. Occasionally, widening of the physis can also be seen in the lateral side of the distal femur. Advanced imaging, such as CT scan or MRI, is generally not needed to make the diagnosis of Blount disease. In certain cases, these studies may be useful to rule out the presence of a bony bar and to evaluate the health of the medial physis.

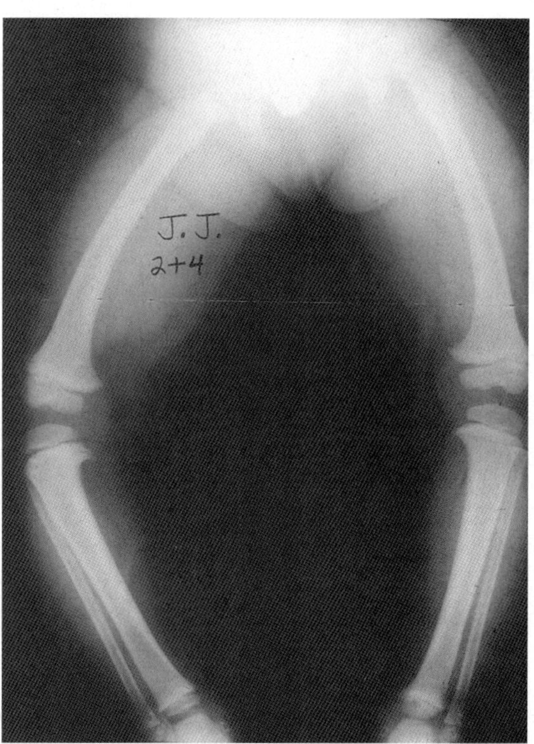

Figure 11.161 Standing radiograph of the same patient from Figure 11.159. The metaphyseal–diaphyseal angle on the right is 20 degrees, compared with 10 degrees on the left. This is consistent with stage II Blount disease on the right and physiologic bowing on the left. (*Reproduced with permission from* Morrissy RT, Weinstein SL. *Lovell and Winter's Pediatric Orthopaedics*. Philadelphia, PA: Lippincott Williams & Wilkins, 2006.)

Differential Diagnosis

The most important diagnosis to distinguish from Blount disease is physiologic genu varum, which can be a difficult

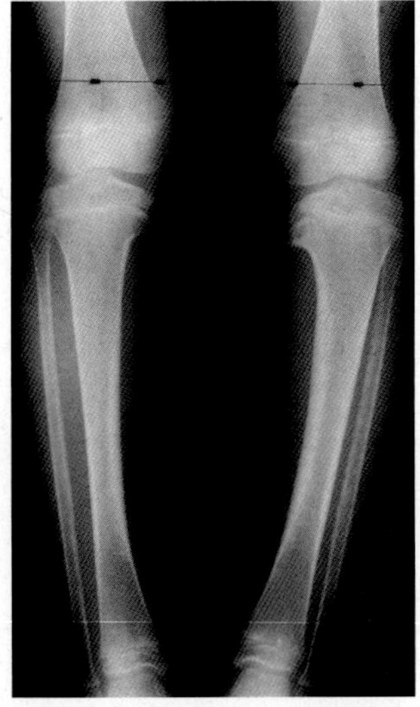

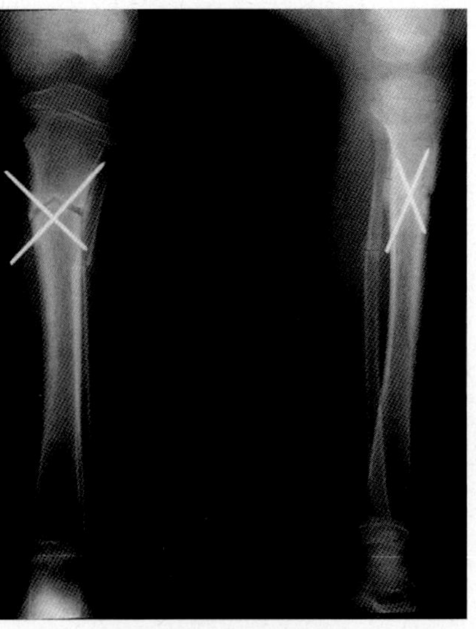

Figure 11.162 **(A)** Anteroposterior (AP) radiograph showing focal changes of Langenskiöld stage IV infantile Blount disease. The medial tibial physis is indistinct and concerning for a physeal bar. A follow-up computed tomography scan showed a bridge of bone across the medial physis. **(B)** AP and lateral radiographs after bar excision and proximal tibial osteotomy. (*Reproduced with permission from* Morrissy RT, Weinstein SL. *Lovell and Winter's Pediatric Orthopaedics.* Philadelphia, PA: Lippincott Williams & Wilkins, 2006.)

task in a child younger than 2 years. The lack of characteristic "Blount findings" on radiographs and a low MDA is indicative of physiologic genu varum. In addition, the deformity in physiologic genu varum is symmetric and global, often involving both the femur and the tibia. However, the presence of a focal deformity or a lateral thrust during gait is more suggestive of Blount disease. Other nonphysiologic causes of genu varum include skeletal dysplasias, rickets, trauma, and infection.

Treatment

Treatment is guided by both the age of the patient and the severity of the condition. Observation may be indicated when the diagnosis is still uncertain, but treatment should be initiated as soon as the radiographic diagnosis of infantile Blount disease is confirmed since early treatment has been associated with a better prognosis. A brace, such as a valgus-producing KAFO, can be effective in treating mild to moderate infantile tibia vara (Langenskiöld II or better) before 3 years of age. For older children, patients with more severe disease, and those who do not respond to bracing, surgery is recommended. The results of corrective osteotomy are best if surgery is performed by 4 years of age. Various techniques have been described, including transverse, domed, and angled osteotomies, but in all cases, the limb should be overcorrected into valgus to minimize the risk of recurrence. The internal tibial torsion should also be corrected. In more severe Langenskiöld stages, consideration should be given to resection of the medial bar and interposition of fat or other material to reduce the chances of recurrent deformity (Fig. 11.162).

For children with adolescent Blount disease and open physes, temporary hemiepiphysiodesis using a staple or plate or a more permanent lateral hemiepiphysiodesis can be used to gradually correct the deformity over time (Fig. 11.163). For severe deformities and for those patients with closed physes, a valgus producing proximal tibial osteotomy with internal fixation is the most commonly used approach. Alternatively, external fixation using a circular or multiaxial frame can be used to achieve gradual correction of the deformity and to minimize the risk of neurovascular complications from an acute correction.

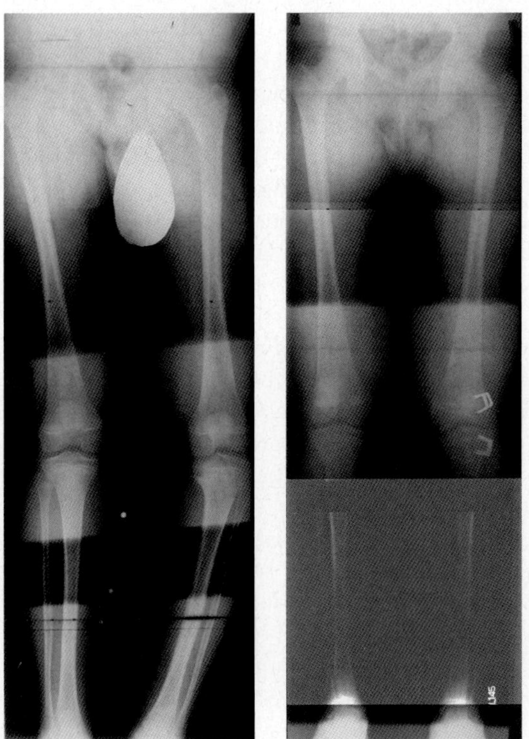

Figure 11.163 **(A)** Long-cassette radiographs of a teenager with unilateral adolescent Blount disease and open physes. **(B)** Hemiepiphyseal stapling was used. Correction is noted 1 year after staple insertion in the lateral distal femur and proximal tibia. This technique is optimal in mild to moderate deformities, in which 1 to 2 years of growth remain. (*Reproduced with permission from* Morrissy RT, Weinstein SL. *Lovell and Winter's Pediatric Orthopaedics.* Philadelphia, PA: Lippincott Williams & Wilkins, 2006.)

ANTEROLATERAL BOWING AND CONGENITAL PSEUDARTHROSIS OF THE TIBIA

Pathophysiology

Anterolateral bowing of the tibia is, as the name implies, an abnormal bow of the tibia with an apex that is anterior and lateral. This deformity renders the tibia susceptible to fracture and is closely associated with the development of a pseudarthrosis at the fracture site (Fig. 11.164). In reality, anterolateral bowing of the tibia and the subsequent CPT should be considered a continuum. It is a rare condition, occurring in 1 per 100,000 live births, and is unilateral in the vast majority of cases. Its etiology remains unclear. Several theories have been proposed, including intrauterine trauma, generalized metabolic disease, and vascular malformation. The fibula is affected in approximately one-third of patients. Histologically, there is a thickened periosteum and a cuff of abnormal, highly cellular fibrovascular tissue at the site of the pseudarthrosis.

Neurofibromatosis (NF) is the most commonly associated condition. Approximately 6% of patients with NF type I develop deformity of the tibia, whereas up to 55% of case of anterolateral bowing and pseudarthrosis are associated with NF. Other associated conditions include Ehler–Danlos syndrome, fibrous dysplasia, and amniotic band syndrome.

Classification

Numerous classification systems of CPT have been described, including those of Boyd, Anderson, and Crawford. Radiographic classification of CPT as described by Crawford is as follows: type I has anterolateral bowing with medullary sclerosis and cortical thickening at the apex; type II has constriction or narrowing of the cortical diameter with cortical sclerosis; type III has a cystic-appearing lesion; type IV has frank pseudarthrosis with tapered bone ends (Fig. 11.165). These systems generally describe the radiographic appearance of the untreated bone at the pseudarthrosis site, the presence of fracture at birth, and the appearance of the fibula. However, none of these classification systems provides specific guidance for management or is predictive of outcome. Also the type of CPT in these classification systems will change with growth. Consequently, the criteria that may be most relevant to treatment were suggested by Johnston and are based on the presence or

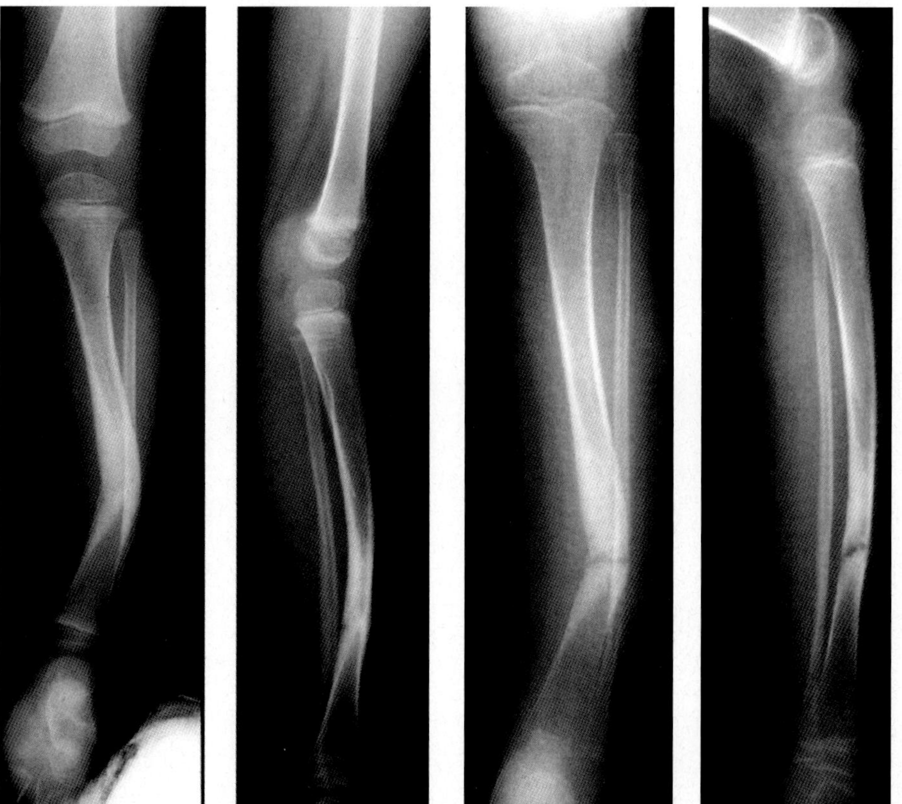

Figure 11.164 **(A)** Anterolateral bowing of the tibia may be apparent at birth or may progress with weight-bearing. Bowing usually occurs between the middle and distal third of the tibia. **(B)** Even though this deformity was protected in a total-contact orthosis, fracture and pseudarthrosis developed at the apex of the bow. (*Reproduced with permission from* Morrissy RT, Weinstein SL. *Lovell and Winter's Pediatric Orthopaedics.* Philadelphia, PA: Lippincott Williams & Wilkins, 2006.)

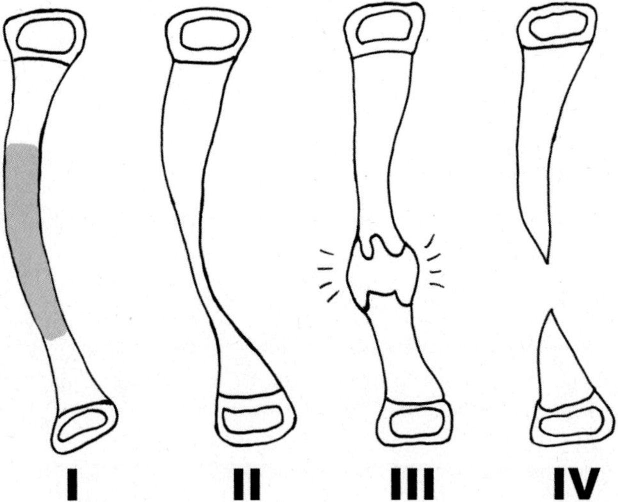

Figure 11.165 Crawford classification for congenital pseudarthrosis of the tibia. Type 1: anterolateral bowing with medullary sclerosis. Type II: "failure of tabulation with constriction or narrowing of the cortical diameter. Type III: cystic lesion. Type IV: frank pseudarthrosis with tapered bone ends. (*Reproduced with permission from* Johnston CE. Congenital pseudarthrosis of the tibia: results of technical variations in the Charnley-Williams procedure. *J Bone Joint Surg Am.* 2002;84:1799–1810.)

absence of fracture and the age at which the first fracture occurs (early onset before age 4 years and delayed onset after age 4 years).

Presentation and Physical Examination

CPT is characterized by anterolateral angulation of the tibia (Fig. 11.166). This bowing, combined with an overall de-

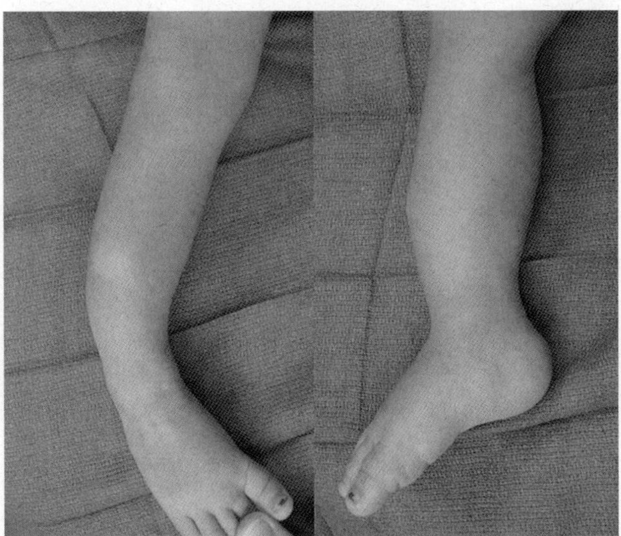

Figure 11.166 Clinical photographs of a child with anterolateral bowing and congenital pseudarthrosis of the tibia. The extremity is shortened, and the apex of the deformity is anterior and lateral. (*Reproduced with permission from* Children's Orthopaedic Center, Los Angeles, CA.)

crease in distal tibia growth, results in shortening of the limb. Usually, the disease becomes evident during the first year of life, but milder forms may manifest later, up to age 12 years. The deformity is an apical prominence in the leg laterally with the foot inverted or medially displaced relative to the lower leg. If fracture has already occurred, motion at the pseudarthrosis site is appreciated. Mild deformity may present as a limp because of shortening or impending fracture. The foot on the involved side may be normal or slight smaller than the contralateral foot.

Imaging

AP and lateral views of the tibia demonstrate anterolateral bowing of the tibia. The site of pseudarthrosis may appear dysplastic with diaphyseal narrowing, sclerosis and even obliteration of the intramedullary canal, or may appear cystic. Most of the lesions are localized to the middle or distal third of the tibia. However, the location may change during the course of the disease. MRI may define the extent of periosteal thickening and pathology. In Crawford types I, II, and IV, the pseudarthrosis appears hypointense on T1-weighted images. In Crawford type III patients, the pseudarthrosis appears slightly hyperintense. In all patients, the lesion appears hyperintense on T2-weighted and fat-suppressed imaging.

Differential Diagnosis

Bowing of the tibia can occur in various planes with the apex of the deformity defining the direction of bowing. Anterolateral bowing as seen in CPT should be distinguished from posteromedial and anteromedial bowing of the tibia. Posteromedial bowing is associated with calcaneovalgus feet and generally resolves with growth. Anteromedial bowing, on the other hand, is associated with fibular hemimelia.

Treatment

Treatment of anterolateral bowing and CPT is challenging. Prior to fracture, anterolateral bowing of the tibia is best managed with a brace such as a clamshell AFO or KAFO. This is the best means of protecting the bone, minimizing the risk of fracture, and controlling the deformity. Certain authors have suggested that surgery can be considered in patients with anterolateral bowing to prevent fracture; this usually consists of an allograft or autograft fibular strut, which is used to bypass the region of at-risk bone.

Unfortunately, most patients present after a fracture has already occurred and an established pseudarthrosis is already present. For these patients, surgical intervention attempts to repair the pseudarthrosis and prevent progressive deformity. The appropriate age for surgical intervention is not known. The basic tenets of the surgical treatment

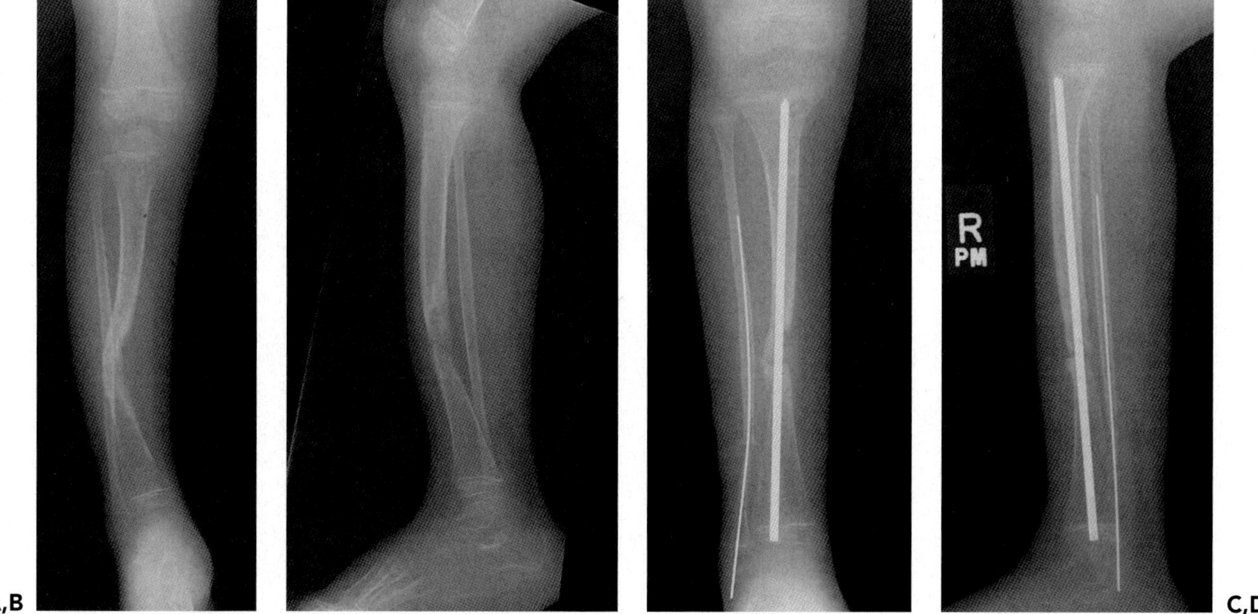

Figure 11.167 **(A** and **B)** Preoperative anteroposterior and lateral radiographs of the tibia demonstrating congenital pseudarthrosis and anterolateral bowing. **(C** and **D)** Postoperative radiographs 2 months after bone grafting and intramedullary fixation of the tibia and fibula. (*Reproduced with permission from* Children's Orthopaedic Center, Los Angeles, CA.)

of CPT include resection of the pseudarthrosis, biologic bone bridging of the defect, stable fixation, and correction of angular deformity. The highest rates of union have been reported after surgical intervention although no single method of surgery has proved to be superior.

Intramedullary stabilization is often recommended as the first line of surgical treatment. Several intramedullary nail designs, including telescoping nails, fixed-length nails, and the Williams nail, have been used to treat CPT (Fig. 11.167). All of these intramedullary devices provide load sharing and reinforcement of the bone long after the pseudarthrosis has been treated. Ring external fixators are sometimes used when a significant limb length discrepancy is also present: the pseudarthrosis is resected and the gap is compressed, whereas a corticotomy is performed at a separate proximal site for distraction osteogenesis. Other concomitant modalities include contralateral vascularized fibular graft and bone morphogenic protein. Complications of surgical treatment include refracture, persistent pseudarthrosis, residual deformity, ankle valgus deformity, and residual limb length discrepancy. The need for fibular surgery remains controversial. Some studies show that when the fibula is intact, fibular osteotomy is needed for optimal limb alignment and union. Finally, multiple unsuccessful attempts to maintain union or limb alignment, significant limb length discrepancy (>5 cm), a permanently deformed foot, or functional loss are relative indications for an amputation. The Symes amputation offers excellent function. In some cases, amputation at the pseudarthrosis is necessary.

IDIOPATHIC TOE-WALKING

Although it is not uncommon for toddlers to toe-walk, lack of normal heel strike after 3 years of age is abnormal. Typically, toe-walking starts as a habitual phenomenon, and when asked to most children, they are able to walk plantigrade. Over time, however, a contracture of the heel cord can develop, which makes the gait disturbance more difficult to control.

Patients typically present between 3 and 4 years of age. Most patients are asymptomatic, but some children may complain of fatigue or pain in the gastroc-soleus complex. Idiopathic toe-walking is more common in male children, and a family history of the condition can often be elicited. The toe-walking gait is best appreciated with the child barefoot. As mentioned, if the child concentrates, the degree of toe-walking can often be controlled. If distracted or asked to run, however, the true severity of the gait disturbance is revealed. Ankle plantar flexion is generally normal, but dorsiflexion should be carefully evaluated to determine the degree of heel cord tightness. Toe-walking is often a sign of more serious conditions such as CP, primary muscle disease, and disturbances of the CNS. As a result, the diagnosis of idiopathic toe-walking should be made only after these other conditions have been ruled out. Unlike these other diagnoses, children with idiopathic toe-walking have normal muscle tone and muscle strength; spasticity and clonus are absent.

Treatment generally consists of heel cord stretching to maintain range of motion and an articulated AFO with a plantar flexion stop to prevent the toe-walking and encourage normal heel strike gait. For patients with tight heel cords who lack significant motion, serial stretching casts may be necessary to regain sufficient ankle dorsiflexion. If toe-walking persists in spite of maximal conservative treatment, surgical lengthening of the gastrocnemius should be considered.

FOOT AND ANKLE

Metatarsus Adductus

Metatarsus adductus is a common foot deformity seen after birth, occurring in as many as 1 in 100 live births, and is thought to result from intrauterine positioning. The deformity consists of an adducted forefoot, curved lateral border, and a neutral heel, creating the characteristic "bean-shape" sole of the foot (Fig. 11.168). A deep medial crease is usually present. Most cases present during infancy as caregivers are often concerned about the appearance of the foot. After the walking age, an in-toeing gait may be the presenting complaint. Physical examination should focus on determining the flexibility of the deformity. In addition, one can quantify the severity of the deformity by determining the heel bisector line. Normally, a line drawn through the long axis of the heel should exit between the second and third toes. With increasing severity of the condition, the heel bisector line moves laterally.

Flexible deformities can be treated with observation or stretching; 90% to 95% will spontaneously resolve regardless of treatment. Rigid deformities should undergo serial manipulation and casting before 6 months of age. Surgery is rarely required and is indicated only for children older than 3 years with a rigid deformity that has not responded to serial casting.

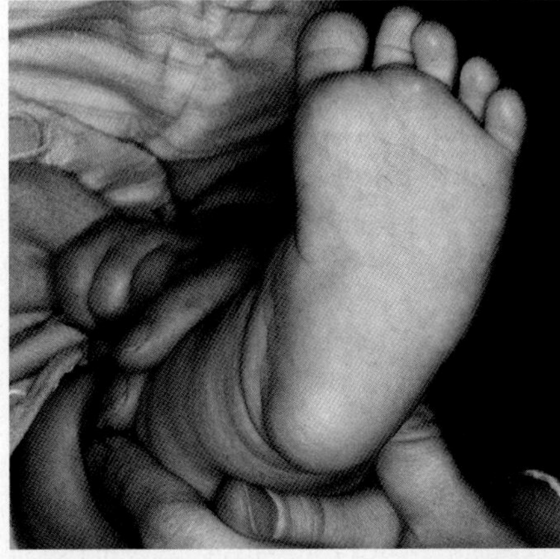

Figure 11.168 Metatarsus adductus in an infant. Note the convex lateral border of the foot and the neutral hindfoot alignment. (*Reproduced with permission from* Morrissy RT, Weinstein SL. *Lovell and Winter's Pediatric Orthopaedics*. Philadelphia, PA: Lippincott Williams & Wilkins, 2006.)

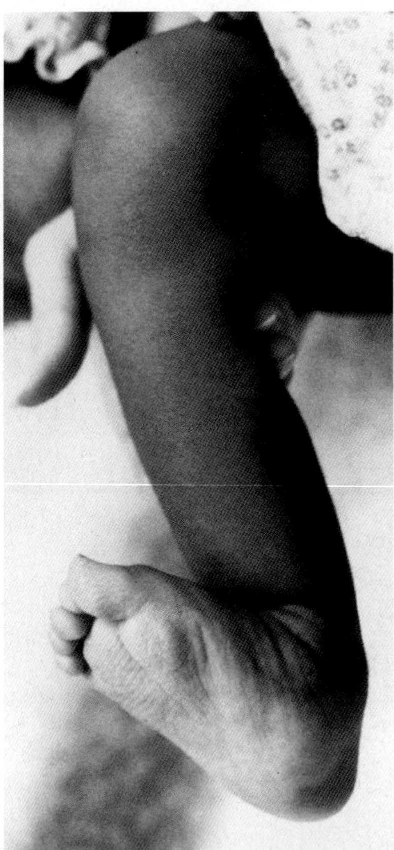

Figure 11.169 Positional calcaneovalgus foot deformity. Note that the dorsum of the foot is almost in contact with the anterior leg. (*Reproduced with permission from* Morrissy RT, Weinstein SL. *Lovell and Winter's Pediatric Orthopaedics*. Philadelphia, PA: Lippincott Williams & Wilkins, 2006.)

Calcaneovalgus Foot

In a calcaneovalgus foot deformity, the hindfoot externally rotates and hyperdorsiflexes. In some cases, this causes the dorsum of the foot to be in contact with the anterior tibia (Fig. 11.169). The deformity is primarily positional and is thought to occur from intrauterine positioning. The estimated incidence of calcaneovalgus foot deformity is 0.4 to 1 in 1,000 live births, although some believe that a mild form can be see in up to 30% to 40% of newborns.

Although a calcaneovalgus foot is generally considered a benign condition, it is important to rule out other, more pathologic conditions. Posteromedial bowing of the tibia is a condition in which the distal tibia is hypoplastic and bowed; this can result in an apparent calcaneovalgus deformity. Posteromedial bowing can generally be distinguished from a true calcaneovalgus foot by determining the location of the apex of the deformity: in posteromedial bowing, the apex is in the distal tibia, whereas in calcaneovalgus foot, the apex is in the joint (Fig. 11.170). Vertical talus can sometimes present with a similar, dorsiflexed appearance of the foot. In contrast to the calcaneovalgus foot, a vertical talus has far less flexibility.

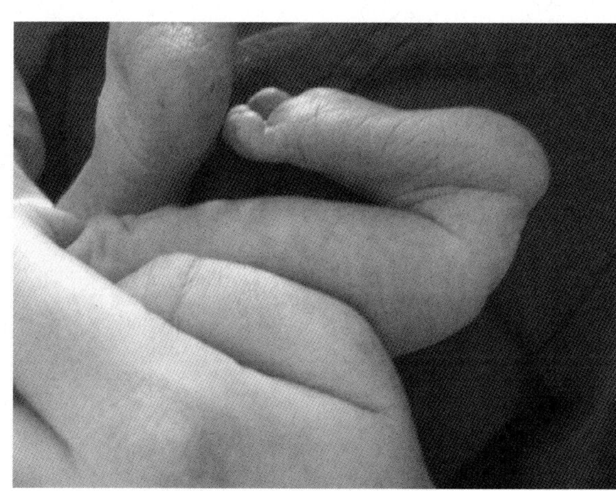
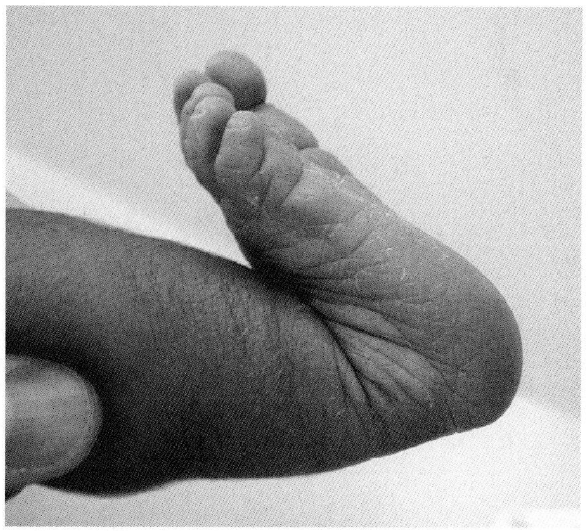

Figure 11.170 **(A)** In posteromedial bowing, the apex of the deformity is in the distal tibia. **(B)** In a calcaneovalgus foot, the apex of the deformity is in the joint. (*Reproduced with permission from* Skaggs DL, Flynn JM. *Staying Out of Trouble in Pediatric Orthopaedics.* Philadelphia, PA: Lippincott Williams & Wilkins, 2006.)

For calcaneovalgus feet, gentle stretching of the foot into plantar flexion and inversion can be helpful; however, most deformities will resolve spontaneously by 3 to 6 months regardless of treatment. In patients with posteromedial bowing of the tibia, parents should be counseled that a leg length discrepancy (usually 3–6 cm) will most likely result.

Congenital Vertical Talus

Congenital vertical talus (CVT) is a rare foot deformity that is characterized by a hindfoot that is in equinus and a forefoot that is dorsiflexed, resulting in a fixed midfoot dislocation through the talonavicular joint. Unlike calcaneovalgus feet, which are flexible, CVT is a rigid deformity with a convex plantar surface that forms a rocker bottom deformity (Fig. 11.171). Although CVT can occur in isolation, more than 50% of cases are associated with a neuromuscular or genetic disorder such as myelomeningocele, arthrogryposis, and trisomy 18.

Children typically present during infancy with the characteristic foot appearance. The head of the talus is usually palpable in the medial aspect of the midfoot. The anterior soft tissue structures are contracted, including the toe extensors, peroneals, and anterior tibial tendon. The Achilles tendon also is shortened, which fixes the hindfoot in an equinovalgus position. True CVT should be distinguished from an oblique talus, a condition in which the navicular is subluxated dorsally in relation to the talus but is still reducible. Plantar flexion lateral radiographs are useful to differentiate these two clinical entities: if the navicular reduces onto the talus when the foot is positioned in maximal plantar flexion, the diagnosis of an oblique vertical talus can be made (Fig. 11.172). If the navicular remains dislocated in this position, the child has a vertical talus.

Initially, serial manipulation and casting is useful to stretch the anterior skin as well as capsular and musculotendinous soft tissues. Historically, however, cast treatment alone has been insufficient to completely correct the deformity. Definitive surgical correction typically consists of a comprehensive open release, pin fixation of the talonavicular joint, and lengthening of the anterior tendons and triceps surae. Surgery is usually performed between 6 and 12 months of age, and results are better if surgery is performed before 2 years of age. Recently, Dobbs has described a new technique consisting of serial manipulation and cast immobilization followed by percutaneous talonavicular pin fixation and Achilles tenotomy. Early results have

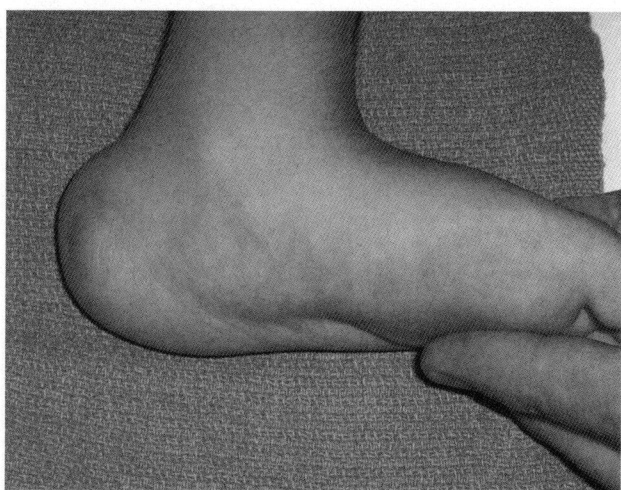

Figure 11.171 Clinical appearance of a foot with a congenital vertical talus. Note the rocker bottom deformity. (*Reproduced with permission from* Children's Orthopaedic Center, Los Angeles, CA.)

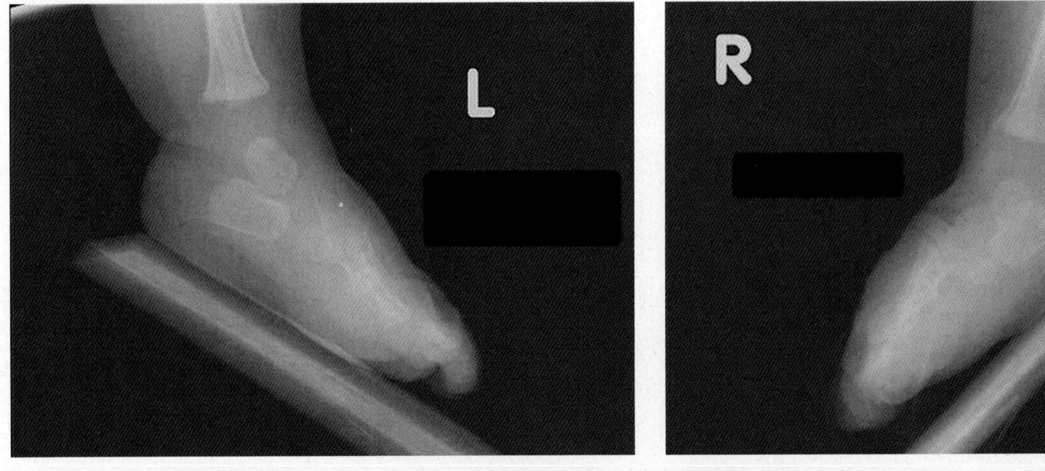

Figure 11.172 Plantar flexion lateral views of an oblique **(A)** and vertical talus **(B).** In the oblique talus, the navicular (unossified), and first metatarsal reduce on the talus. In a true congenital vertical talus, the talus remains plantar flexed in relation to the navicular (unossified) and metatarsal. (*Reproduced with permission from* Children's Orthopaedic Center, Los Angeles, CA.)

demonstrated excellent results in terms of clinical appearance, deformity correction, and foot function.

Flexible Flatfoot (Pes Planus)

A flexible flatfoot is characterized by a decrease in the longitudinal arch of the foot during stance along with valgus alignment of the hindfoot. The condition is considered flexible if subtalar mobility is preserved, as this helps distinguish it from other more pathologic processes (Fig. 11.173). Although a flexible flatfoot was thought to be pathologic for many years, at the present time, it is considered a variation of normal and not a true pathologic entity. All children are flatfooted at birth as the arch does not normally develop until after 2 years of age. Up to 25% of normal adults will retain some degree of flat feet; the vast majority does not cause any functional limitations.

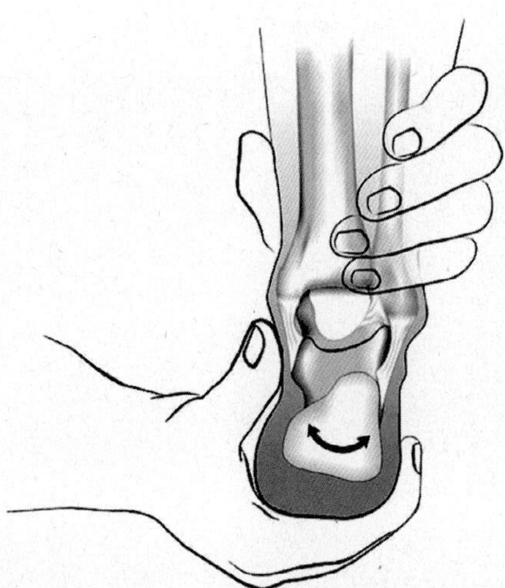

Figure 11.173 Hindfoot mobility can be assessed by cupping the heel and shifting it from side to side (inverting and everting). (*Reproduced with permission from* Skaggs DL, Flynn JM. *Staying Out of Trouble in Pediatric Orthopaedics.* Philadelphia, PA: Lippincott Williams & Wilkins, 2006.)

Most children present because their caregivers are concerned about the appearance of their feet. Pain is less often the cause for seeking care. The foot is characterized by a collapsed arch with weight-bearing. When weight-bearing is discontinued, the arch reconstitutes itself. The hindfoot is usually in valgus but should correct to varus when children stand on their toes (Fig. 11.174). Ankle range of motion and tightness of the heel cord should be assessed by checking dorsiflexion with the hindfoot inverted and the knee both extended and flexed (Silfverskiöld test). Radiographs are rarely necessary to make the diagnosis; however, lateral views of the foot will often demonstrate a sag at the talonavicular joint and an increase in Meary angle (the angle between the long axis of the talus and the long axis of the first metatarsal).

Most children are asymptomatic, but some may have activity-related pain. If the child does not complain of pain, it is best to reassure the caregivers, explain the benign natural history of the condition, and avoid expensive orthotics. If symptoms are present and the heel cords are tight, a stretching program is indicated. Arch supports can often be helpful to reduce symptoms, but if more control of the hindfoot is desired, a larger orthosis such as a UCBL (named for the University of California Biomechanics Laboratory, where it was developed) or supramalleolar orthosis may be necessary. Surgery should be reserved for patients with continued pain in spite of maximal conservative management. Generally, it is best to avoid foot arthrodeses as these procedures can increase the risk of arthritis in adjacent joints. The two most popular surgical procedures for correction are the medial sliding calcaneal osteotomy

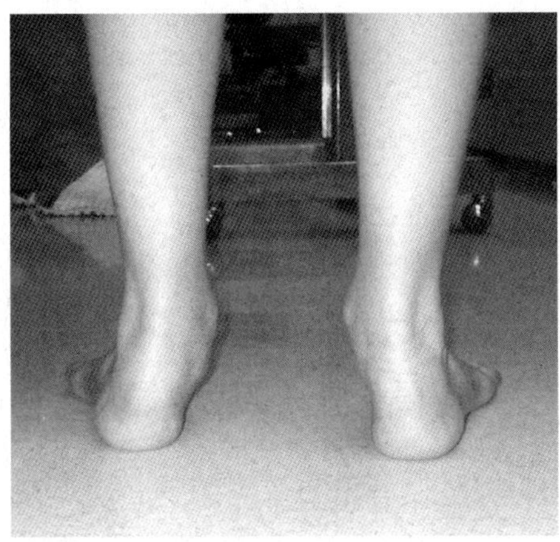
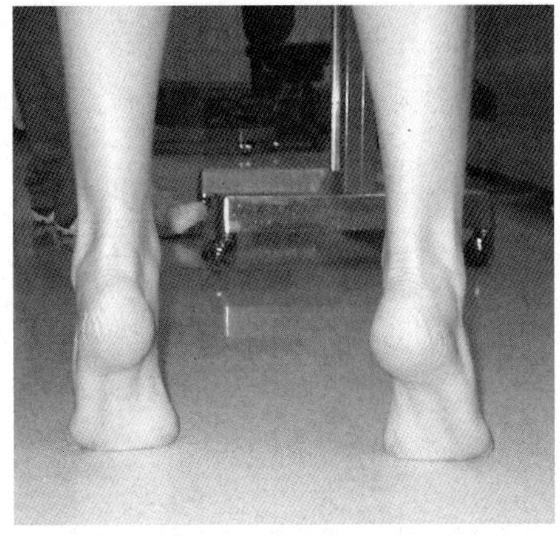

Figure 11.174 **(A)** Patient with flatfeet and hindfoot valgus. **(B)** When standing on the toes, the hindfoot goes into varus, proving that the hindfoot is mobile, and the arch elevates, thus confirming a flexible flatfoot. (*Reproduced with permission from* Skaggs DL, Flynn JM. *Staying Out of Trouble in Pediatric Orthopaedics*. Philadelphia, PA: Lippincott Williams & Wilkins, 2006.)

and the lateral column lengthening. The former procedure translates the calcaneus medially to reestablish the weight-bearing axis of the hindfoot. If the forefoot remains abducted after the hindfoot osteotomy, a closing wedge osteotomy of the medial cuneiform and an opening wedge osteotomy of the cuboid can restore forefoot and midfoot alignment. The lateral column lengthening takes advantage of the windlass mechanism to develop an arch and correct the hindfoot. By placing a wedge of bone graft in the calcaneal neck, the previously short lateral column of the foot becomes elongated; this helps swing the foot into a more anatomic position.

Tarsal Coalition

By definition, a tarsal coalition is an abnormal fibrous, cartilaginous, or bony connection between two bones of the hindfoot or midfoot. The overall prevalence of tarsal coalitions has been reported to be 2% to 6% in the general population. The true prevalence, however, is difficult to ascertain since many patients are asymptomatic and do not present for medical care. The most common sites of coalition occur between the anterior process of the calcaneus and the navicular and between the talus and the calcaneus (through the middle facet of the talocalcaneal joint). Approximately 50% of patients have bilateral coalitions. Although most cases occur in isolation, tarsal coalitions have been associated with other disorder such as clubfoot, fibular hemimelia, and Apert syndrome.

Most patients present during adolescence when the cartilaginous or fibrous connections begin to ossify. Frequent ankle sprains and aching pain over the medial aspect of the foot or the sinus tarsi are typical complaints. The most characteristic finding in a tarsal coalition is limited subtalar motion and a valgus hindfoot. This lack of mobility is thought to be the source of pain as the stress of weight-bearing gets transferred to adjacent joints. Unlike the flexible flatfoot, patients with tarsal coalitions have a rigid flatfoot deformity that does not correct when children rise on their toes. Weight-bearing radiographs are essential in the workup of a suspected coalition. Calcaneonavicular coalitions are best visualized on an oblique radiograph of the foot. On the lateral view, an elongated anterior process of the calcaneus, the so-called anteater nose sign may be seen (Fig. 11.175). Radiographic findings of a talocalcaneal coalition include the "C-sign," a line formed from the outline of the talar dome that extends around the inferior margin of the sustentaculum tali, and beaking of the dorsal talus (Fig. 11.176). Since these findings can be unreliable, CT scans are often necessary to diagnose talocalcaneal coalitions. Because of the significant incidence of multiple coalitions and bilateral involvement, the presence of one coalition should prompt further imaging of both feet.

Up to 75% of tarsal coalitions are asymptomatic; as a result, the mere presence of a coalition does not indicate the need for treatment. For patients who are symptomatic, initial management should consist of activity modification, NSAIDs, and a trial of cast immobilization and/or orthotics. In many cases, these measures will be sufficient to decrease inflammation and eliminate pain. For those who remain symptomatic in spite of conservative treatment, surgical options include resection of the coalition or arthrodesis. Most calcaneonavicular coalitions respond well to excision of the coalition and interposition of fat or the extensor digitorum brevis. The surgical treatment of talocalcaneal coalitions, however, is less clear. The classic teaching is that a resection should be performed if less than 50% of the middle facet is involved and an arthrodesis should be performed if the coalition is more extensive. In reality, outcomes have been somewhat unsatisfactory following isolated resection, and further studies are needed to determine which patients are best treated by this procedure. For patients with moderate to severe valgus, results

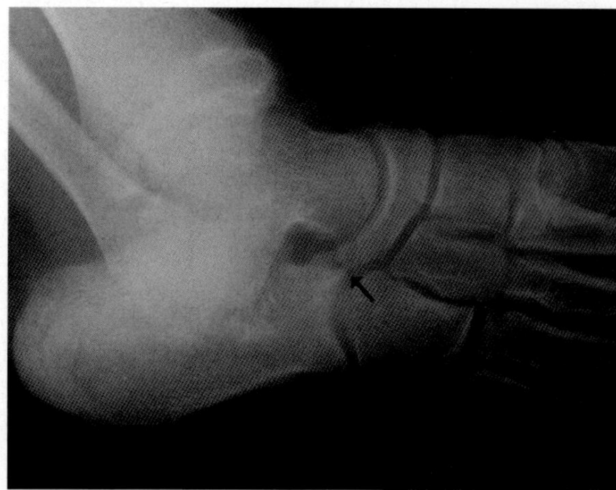

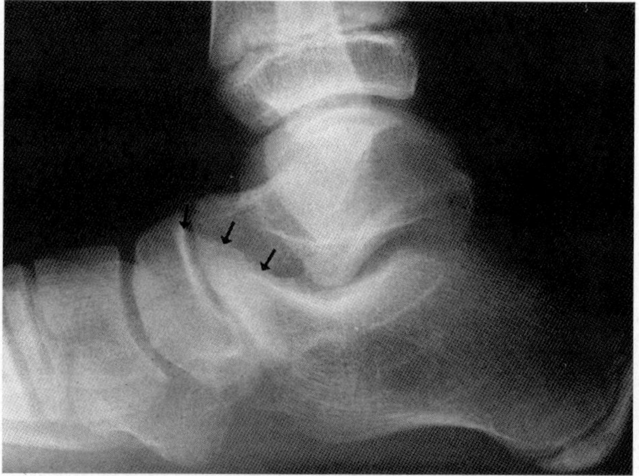

Figure 11.175 **(A)** A calcaneonavicular coalition (*arrow*) is best seen on an oblique radiograph of the foot. **(B)** Lateral radiograph demonstrating the anteater nose sign (*arrows*), indicating a calcaneonavicular coalition. (*Reproduced with permission from* Morrissy RT, Weinstein SL. *Lovell and Winter's Pediatric Orthopaedics*. Philadelphia, PA: Lippincott Williams & Wilkins, 2006.)

after talocalcaneal coalition excision are improved if a concomitant calcaneal osteotomy is performed.

Clubfoot

Clubfoot or talipes equinovarus is a congenital foot deformity that is characterized by the CAVE mnemonic (*c*avus, forefoot *a*dductus, hindfoot *v*arus, and *e*quinus). The incidence of this condition is approximately 1 to 2 per 1,000 births, and 30% to 40% of cases occur bilaterally. Clubfeet can have a wide spectrum of presentations from the mild, postural forms to the severe, rigid deformities. The latter are usually associated with arthrogryposis, myelomeningocele, Larsen syndrome, or another underlying syndrome. The etiology of talipes equinovarus remains unknown, but postulated theories include an in utero arrest in the fetal development of the foot, a retractile fibrotic response in the medial ligaments, and a primary genetic defect.

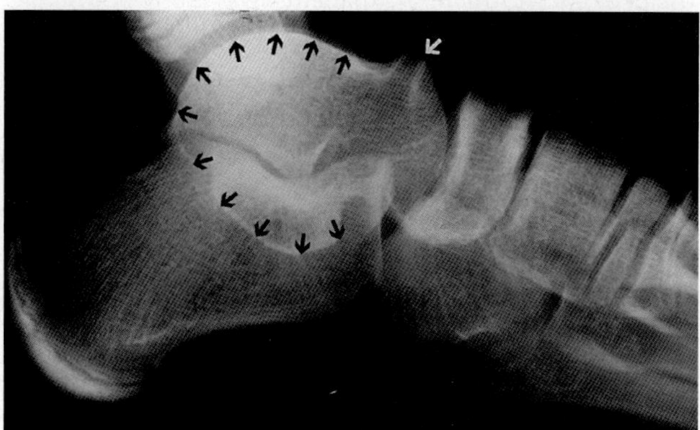

Figure 11.176 A dorsal talar beak (*white arrow*) in a foot with a talocalcaneal coalition. This represents a traction spur, not degenerative arthritis. The C-sign of Lafleur (*black arrows*) is a nonspecific indication of a talocalcaneal coalition. (*Reproduced with permission from* Morrissy RT, Weinstein SL. *Lovell and Winter's Pediatric Orthopaedics*. Philadelphia, PA: Lippincott Williams & Wilkins, 2006.)

The pathophysiology of clubfeet involves more than just the osseous components of the foot and should be considered a local dysplasia of all the tissues of the lower extremity from the knee down. The neck of the talus is shortened and deviated medially and plantarward, causing the subjacent calcaneus to rotate into varus. In turn, the calcaneus dislocates from the calcaneocuboid articulation, and as the forefoot medially subluxes, the navicular becomes displaced dorsally and medially onto the neck of the talus. This can be so extreme that the navicular will articulate with the medial malleolus. It is important to recognize that not only is the talus deviated in an abnormal direction but the shape of the talus itself is dysmorphic. Associated with these osseous deformities are contractures of the capsules and ligaments of the ankle and subtalar joints. The tendons of the tibialis posterior, flexor hallucis longus, and flexor digitorum longus are contracted. These muscles of the lower extremity are also smaller and weaker than normal. Histologic studies of muscle tissue have demonstrated increased intracellular connective tissue, muscle atrophy, and loss of myofibrils.

Patients typically present soon after birth with the characteristic clinical appearance of the foot (Fig. 11.177). With improvements in prenatal ultrasonography, the diagnosis can often be made in utero; as a result, expecting mothers may occasionally present for counseling prior to the birth of their child. Examination of the foot will reveal the typical supination of the forefoot and equinovarus positioning of the hindfoot. The flexibility of the foot should be assessed by direct manipulation. Radiographs are seldom necessary to make the diagnosis but can be useful for surgical planning. In normal feet, the talus should line up with the first metatarsal on both the AP and lateral views. With

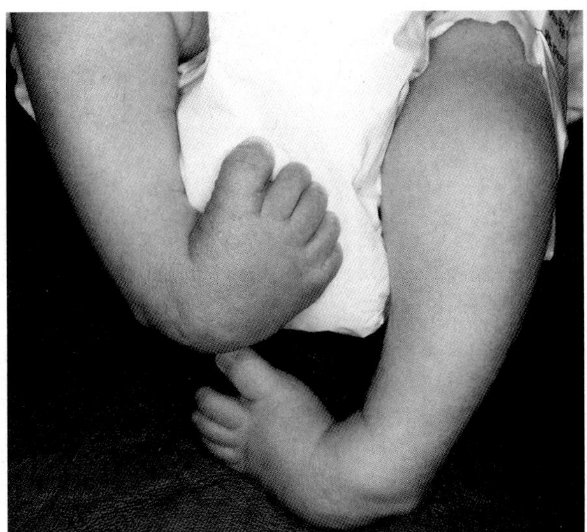

Figure 11.177 Clubfoot deformity is associated with forefoot supination, deep medial creases, and equinovarus of the hindfoot. (*Reproduced with permission from* Morrissy RT, Weinstein SL. *Lovell and Winter's Pediatric Orthopaedics.* Philadelphia, PA: Lippincott Williams & Wilkins, 2006.)

increasing deformity in clubfeet, the long axis of these two bones progressively diverges. In addition, the talocalcaneal angle can be measured on both views. On the AP radiograph, the long axis of the talus and the calcaneus normally diverge, creating a talocalcaneal angle between 20 and 30 degrees. With increasing hindfoot varus seen in clubfeet, the talocalcaneal angle falls below 20 degrees. On the lateral view, the angle between the talus and the calcaneus should be between 35 and 50 degrees. Increased parallelism of the two bones, such that the lateral talocalcaneal angle decreases below 35 degrees, is indicative of a clubfoot (Fig. 11.178).

Although surgical release has been historically favored as the treatment for clubfeet, the Ponseti method of serial manipulation and casting has gained widespread support and has revolutionized the management of talipes equinovarus. This protocol aims to first correct forefoot adduction, supination and hindfoot varus using stretching and a series of well-molded long-leg plaster casts. These casts are changed every 1 to 2 weeks to effect gradual correction. Equinus should be addressed only after the other deformities have been corrected; forced dorsiflexion in an incompletely corrected foot can result in a midfoot breach and a rocker bottom deformity. In the vast majority of cases, an Achilles tenotomy is necessary to completely correct the equinus contracture. Several studies have shown excellent mid- and long-term results and decreased stiffness by using the Ponseti method, compared with feet that have been treated surgically. In certain cases, especially those involving arthrogryposis, myelomeningocele, or other syndromes, surgery may still be necessary. Surgery is performed through a posterior (Cincinnati) incision or double-incision approach and typically consists of open reduction of the talonavicular joint, rebalancing the medial and lateral soft tissue structures, lengthening of the

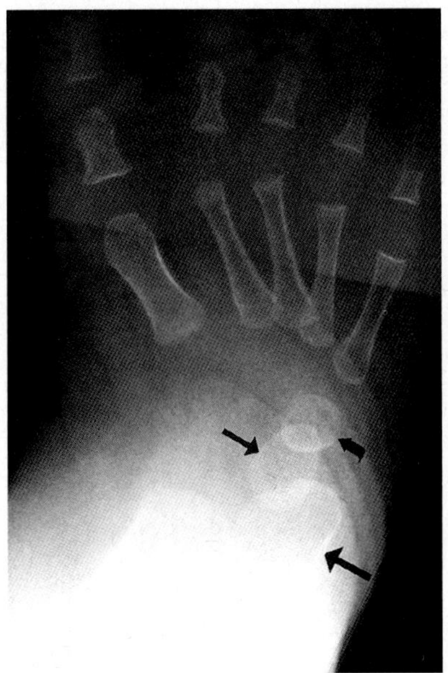

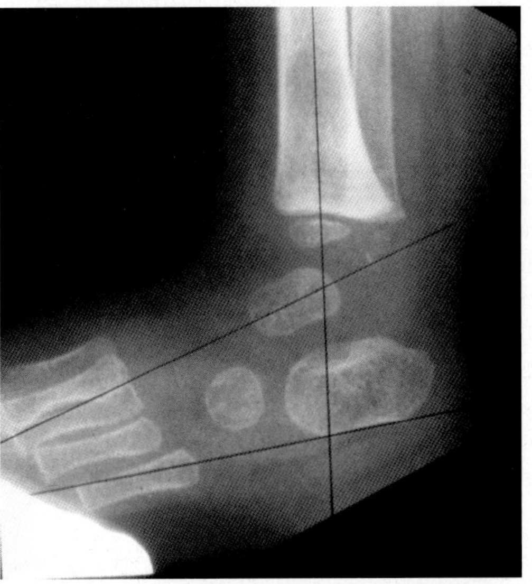

Figure 11.178 **(A)** Simulated weight-bearing anteroposterior radiograph of a clubfoot. The talus (*small straight arrow*) and calcaneus (*large straight arrow*) are parallel, rather than divergent. The cuboid ossification center (*curved arrow*) is medially aligned on the end of the calcaneus. **(B)** Maximum dorsiflexion lateral radiograph of a clubfoot. The talus and calcaneus are somewhat parallel to each other and plantar flexed in relation to the tibia. (*Reproduced with permission from* Morrissy RT, Weinstein SL. *Lovell and Winter's Pediatric Orthopaedics.* Philadelphia, PA: Lippincott Williams & Wilkins, 2006.)

Achilles tendon, and pin fixation to hold the correction. The advantage of open release is the ability to correct severe deformities; downsides include the risk of stiffness and overcorrection.

Osteochondroses

Osteochondroses (local disorders of enchondral growth) are a common cause of foot pain in growing children. Kohler disease is osteonecrosis of the tarsal navicular. Typically, this is seen in 4- to 6-year-old children who present with pain and swelling around the arch of the foot. The etiology of the condition is thought to be repetitive trauma. The radiograph will demonstrate increased density and sclerosis of the navicular. Occasionally, the bone will appear flattened on the lateral view. Treatment should be conservative. During the symptomatic phase, short leg casting followed by a longitudinal arch support is usually adequate to control symptoms. Within 1 year of onset, radiographs usually demonstrate normalization of the tarsal navicular.

Avascular necrosis of the second metatarsal head, known as *Freiberg infraction,* typically affects adolescents. The increased incidence in females suggests that the frequent discrepancy in length between the first and second metatarsal may be a factor. Again, repetitive microtrauma has been implicated as a causative factor. The radiographs usually demonstrate flattening of the involved metatarsal head. Conservative treatment is best, with short-term immobilization and appropriate orthotic use. Activity restriction particularly from jumping or contact sports may be necessary. For those cases that do not respond to conservative management, surgery may be indicated. Techniques include excision of the necrotic bone with grafting or simple shortening of the metatarsal to relieve the weight-bearing stress on the plantar surface.

Sever disease is the most common cause of heel pain in children. The condition is an osteochondrosis of the calcaneal apophysis. Typically, the patient is 5 to 10 years of age and presents with heel pain during or after activity. Physical findings generally consist of tenderness over the tuberosity of the os calcis; radiographs usually demonstrate fragmentation changes of the apophysis that can be misinterpreted as pathologic. These latter changes reflect the normal irregular ossification of this secondary ossification center. Treatment consists of activity modification, judicious use of NSAIDs, heel cups, and heel cord stretching. Injections with lidocaine or cortisone are generally avoided.

Juvenile Hallux Valgus

Similar to the adult bunion deformity, juvenile hallux valgus is characterized by lateral deviation of the great toe and prominence of the first metatarsal head. Both metatarsus primus varus and pes planus can be associated with hallux valgus. A strong family history of the disorder is usually present, with most patients inheriting the condition from their mother.

Most adolescents with hallux valgus are asymptomatic but may present because of concerns about the cosmetic appearance of their feet. When pain is present, it is generally located over the prominence of the metatarsal head and is exacerbated by wearing tight-fitting shoes. Weight-bearing radiographs are essential to accurately quantify the severity of the deformity. As in adults, the hallux valgus angle, the intermetatarsal angle, and the distal metatarsal articular angle can all be measured on the AP radiograph; these measures help identify the causes of the deformity and aid in planning surgical correction.

Treatment of the adolescent bunion should be largely conservative. Shoe modifications, toe spacers, and splints can all be useful to provide symptomatic relief. Most authors recommend waiting until skeletal maturity before pursuing surgical treatment for adolescent bunions. In younger patient, recurrence following surgical correction is common, and many series report only 50% to 60% good results. Depending on the preoperative radiographic assessment, surgical treatment after skeletal maturity generally consists of a double metatarsal osteotomy or proximal crescentic osteotomy of the first metatarsal along with distal soft tissue realignment.

Other Toe Deformities

Congenital deformities of the toes are relatively common. Syndactyly can occur and, as with fingers, can be partial or complete. Radiographs are useful to distinguish simple (soft tissue involvement only) from complex (soft tissue and bone involvement). Unlike in the hand, separation is not typically necessary, since syndactyly of toes does not cause a functional deficit. Congenital curly toe is another common finding. Frequently, this condition is bilateral and usually affects the second or third toe. Curly toe has a high familial incidence and causes a great deal of parental concern. Unfortunately, it does not correct spontaneously and tends to worsen with growth. Initially, taping and stretching can be used but when symptoms worsen, flexor tendon reconstruction may be necessary.

SHOULDER AND ELBOW

Sprengel Deformity

Sprengel deformity is characterized by a failure of the scapula to descend from its normal embryologic level at C4 to the thoracic region. Typically, the scapula develops adjacent to the cervical somites and completes its descent to the thoracic region by 3 months of fetal life. In Sprengel deformity, the scapula is retained in its cervical position by a fibrous, cartilaginous, or osteocartilaginous bar. The

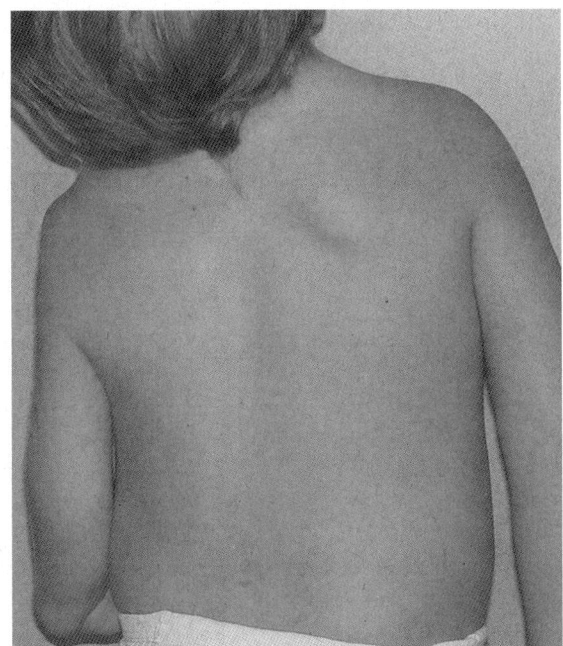

Figure 11.179 Three-year-old child with right-sided Sprengel deformity in addition to Klippel–Feil syndrome. Note the elevated and hypoplastic right scapula. (*Reproduced with permission from* Children's Orthopaedic Center, Los Angeles, CA.)

condition is more common in females than males and affects the left shoulder more often than the right.

The clinical features of Sprengel deformity include a hypoplastic, high-riding scapula with a variable degree of generalized muscular atrophy about the entire shoulder girdle (Fig. 11.179). In approximately one-third of cases, an omovertebral bone can be identified. Some patients will demonstrate decreased range of motion in the shoulder, particularly in abduction; however, in many cases, the complaints are primarily cosmetic in nature. It is essential for the treating physician to recognize that Sprengel deformity can be associated with other congenital anomalies, including congenital scoliosis, Klippel–Feil syndrome, congenital muscular torticollis, and renal and facial deformities.

The treatment of Sprengel deformity varies with the severity of the condition. For the vast majority of patients in whom the cosmetic deformity is mild and motion is adequate, only observation is required. For more severe cases, surgical correction usually consists of the Woodward procedure in which the omovertebral bone is resected and the trapezii, rhomboids, and levator musculature are released from their spinal attachments and advanced distally to lower the scapula. Resection of the superior border of the scapula improves the cosmetic outcomes. In children older than 7 years, the midportion of the clavicle should be resected and morselized to minimize the risk of traction palsy to the brachial plexus as the scapula is advanced distally.

Congenital Pseudarthrosis of Clavicle

Congenital pseudarthrosis of the clavicle is a rare condition in which the medial and lateral ossification centers of the clavicle fail to unite (Fig. 11.180). Typically, infants with this defect present with a palpable mass in the center of the clavicle. The condition almost always occurs on the right side, unless dextrocardia is present. The radiographic appearance is often confused with a clavicle fracture, but the condition is not painful. The diagnosis is confirmed by lack of callus on subsequent radiographs. The natural history of this condition is benign as virtually no functional deficits have been reported. As a result, most children do not require treatment. Open excision of the pseudarthrosis site, bone grafting, and fixation are generally successful for those children who report discomfort or are concerned about the cosmetic appearance of the bump.

Brachial Plexus Palsy

The incidence of brachial plexus palsy has been estimated between 0.13 and 3.6 cases per 1,000 live births. Risk factors

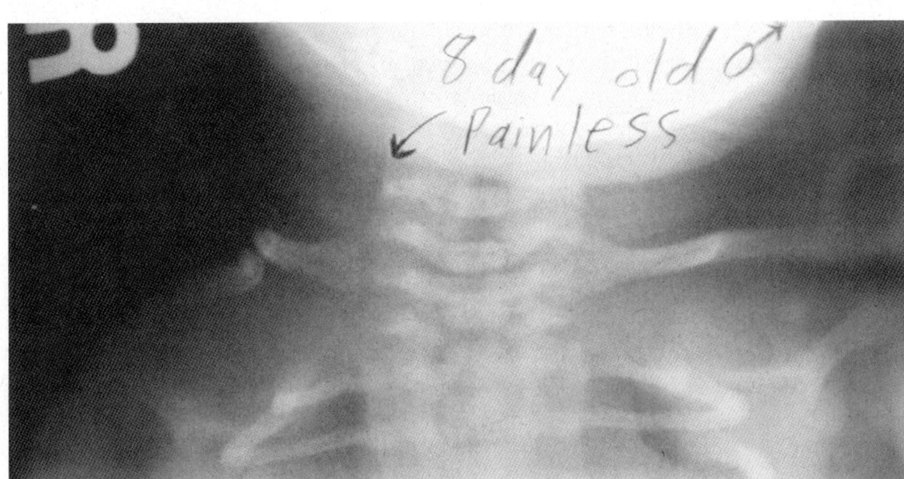

Figure 11.180 Pseudarthrosis of the right clavicle in an 8-day-old male infant. (*Reproduced with permission from* Skaggs DL, Flynn JM: *Staying Out of Trouble in Pediatric Orthopaedics.* Philadelphia, PA: Lippincott Williams & Wilkins, 2006.)

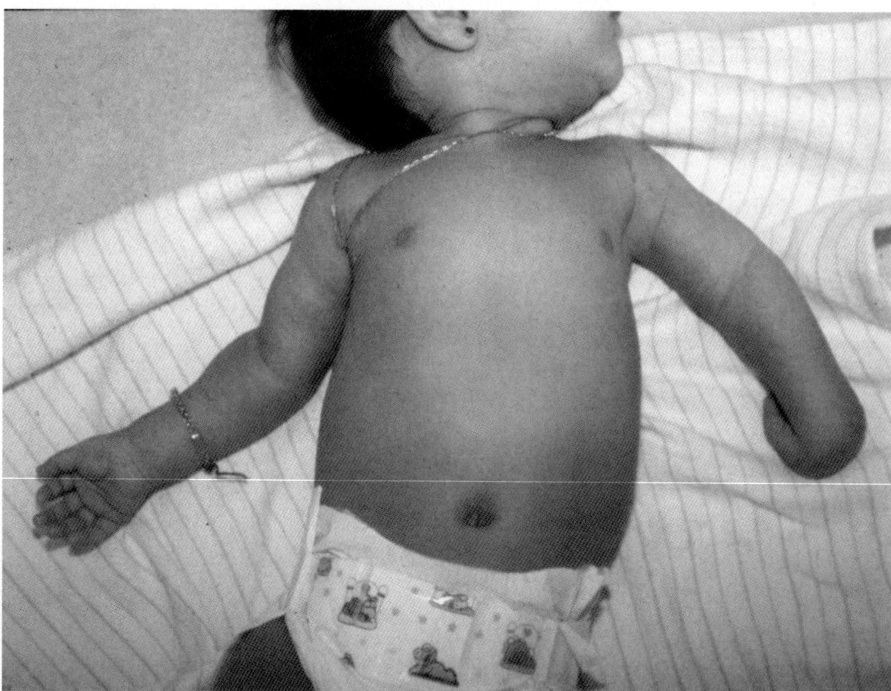

Figure 11.181 This patient with Erb palsy has the left arm in the characteristic "waiter's tip" position. (*Reproduced with permission from* Skaggs DL, Flynn JM. *Staying Out of Trouble in Pediatric Orthopaedics.* Philadelphia, PA: Lippincott Williams & Wilkins, 2006.)

include maternal diabetes, large birth weight, prolonged labor, forceps delivery, and shoulder dystocia.

The most common type of brachial plexus palsy affects the upper trunk (C5 and C6) and is known as *Erb palsy*. This palsy has the characteristic waiter's tip appearance due to shoulder internal rotation, elbow extension, forearm pronation, and wrist flexion (Fig. 11.181). With complete plexus involvement, the neonate's limb is often totally flaccid and may be associated with Horner syndrome (ptosis, miosis, and enophthalmos) of the ipsilateral eye when the sympathetic chain is affected.

The management of brachial plexus palsies remains controversial. Typically as few as 1 out of 10 infants with plexus palsies at birth will require surgical intervention, so the goal of initial management is to maintain passive range of motion while motor function is recovering. Historically, brachial plexus exploration with or without nerve grafting has been recommended if there is no recovery in biceps function between 3 and 6 months. A recent study, however, has suggested that there are patients with no biceps recovery by 3 months who can eventually achieve adequate biceps and shoulder function without surgery. Children with persistent late deformity are best treated by various techniques to improve shoulder rotation since the fixed internal rotation position markedly inhibits hand function. Release of the pectoralis major and subscapularis muscles can often improve external rotation. The L'Episcopo procedure, which is a transfer of the teres major and latissimus dorsi to a lateral position, produces a similar effect. Some authors prefer external rotation osteotomy of the humerus because of more reliable outcomes. Before executing any of these procedures, care must be taken to ensure that the humeral head is well located in the glenoid because a number of children will develop posterior shoulder dislocations from prolonged internal rotation contracture. Although most of the late sequelae are the result of contracture, a small number of children are afflicted by a pure flaccid paralysis. In this situation, the only options are shoulder arthrodesis and elbow flexorplasty.

Congenital Dislocation of Radial Head

Perhaps the major significance of this rare condition is in the differentiation between it and an acquired dislocation of the radial head, which can occur after an unrecognized Monteggia fracture dislocation. The congenitally dislocated radial head is more often convex or flattened as opposed to the normal radial head, which is concave with a central depression (Fig. 11.182). The child with a congenital dislocation of the radial head often presents after minor trauma when the parents notice a prominent "bump" on the lateral side of the elbow. Some restriction in pronation or supination may be seen, but this condition rarely causes any functional limitations.

Treatment of congenital dislocation of the radial head usually consists of benign neglect. Attempts at surgical reduction are fraught with complications. The vast majority redislocate, frequently leaving the elbow stiffer than it otherwise would have been. After physeal closure, one can consider excision of the radial head in cases of severe cosmetic deformity.

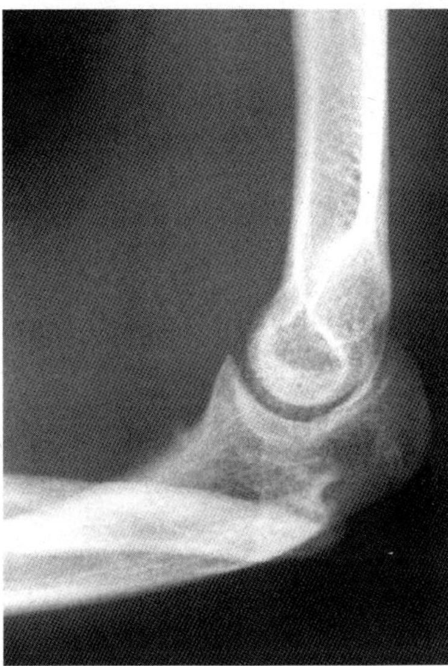

Figure 11.182 Lateral radiograph of a congenital posterolateral dislocation of the radial head. Note that the radial head appears small and dome-shaped. (*Reproduced with permission from* Morrissy RT, Weinstein SL. *Lovell and Winter's Pediatric Orthopaedics*. Philadelphia, PA: Lippincott Williams & Wilkins, 2006.)

Congenital Radioulnar Synostosis

This abnormal fusion between the radius and ulna may occur proximally, distally, or in both locations (Fig. 11.183). It is often bilateral and is inherited as an autosomal dominant condition. Typically, it is identified in the older child when some mild functional impairment, especially in throwing sports, is recognized. Most children adapt well to the limited motion in the forearm by compensating at the shoulder and the wrist. As a result, surgery is usually not necessary. Procedures designed to resect the synostosis have notoriously poor results. Usually no increase in pronation or supination can be achieved; in fact, should myositis ossificans develop, further loss of function will occur. Occasionally, an osteotomy can be useful to place the hand in a more functional position. For example, a forearm fixed in supination can be made more functional by being rotated into slight pronation, which improves writing and keyboard use.

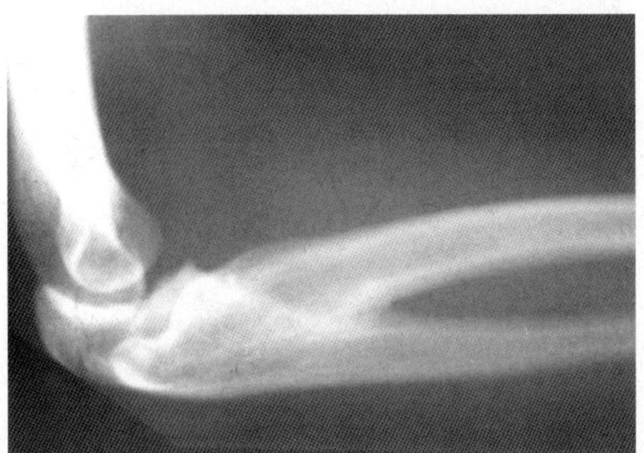

Figure 11.183 Lateral radiograph of the elbow showing a proximal congenital radioulnar synostosis. (*Reproduced with permission from* Morrissy RT, Weinstein SL. *Lovell and Winter's Pediatric Orthopaedics*. Philadelphia, PA: Lippincott Williams & Wilkins, 2006.)

HAND AND WRIST

Madelung Deformity

True Madelung deformity is a congenital anomaly that results from arrest of the ulnar and volar portions of the distal radial growth plate (Fig. 11.184). As a result, a unique carpal deformity results, referred to as a triangulation defect of the distal radius. The distal radius and ulna appear V-shaped, with the carpus having migrated somewhat centrally. The condition is transmitted as an autosomal dominant trait, is more common in females, and frequently is bilateral.

When the anomaly is primarily cosmetic, little or no treatment is required. In more severe cases, surgical options include epiphysiodesis of the remaining distal radial physis to minimize progression, osteotomy of the distal radius to correct deformity, resection of the distal ulna, and ultimately wrist fusion. An acquired type of Madelung deformity can be seen following damage to the distal radial physis from osteomyelitis or trauma.

Syndactyly

Webbing or fusion of two or more fingers is the most common congenital anomaly of the hand. It results from a failure of differentiation between adjacent fingers. The most common connection occurs between the long and ring finger. Males are affected twice as often as females, with a familial incidence of 25%. It is important to determine the extent of soft tissue and bony involvement. Syndactyly that involves only skin and soft tissue is referred to as *simple syndactyly*, whereas those with bony fusions are referred to as *complex syndactyly* (Fig. 11.185). As with radial deficiency syndromes, it is important to be sure that these are isolated phenomena. Numerous syndromes and anomalies have been associated with syndactyly, including Apert syndrome and Poland syndrome.

Surgical separation typically improves finger and hand function. If left uncorrected, syndactyly will cause the longer of the two fingers to deviate; therefore, surgical intervention is generally recommended within the first year of life.

Polydactyly

Extra digits are usually obvious at birth (Fig. 11.186). The supernumerary digit may be postaxial (on the ulnar side of the hand) or preaxial (on the radial side of the hand).

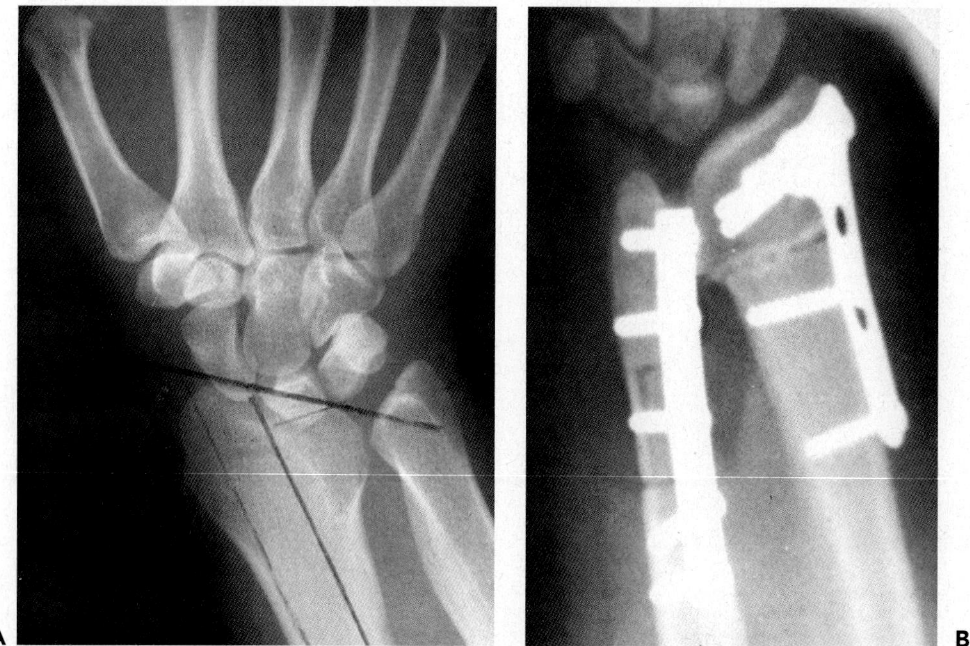

Figure 11.184 **(A)** Anteroposterior view of the wrist demonstrating the characteristic Madelung deformity from incompetence of the ulnar and volar portions of the distal radial growth plate. **(B)** Postoperative radiograph after corrective osteotomy of the distal radius and ulna. (*Reproduced with permission from* Morrissy RT, Weinstein SL. *Lovell and Winter's Pediatric Orthopaedics*. Philadelphia, PA: Lippincott Williams & Wilkins, 2006.)

Again, it is important to confirm whether or not the extra digit is soft tissue or bony, and if bony, whether it contains only phalanges or its own metacarpal.

Polydactyly is 10 times more common in the African American population than in Caucasians and most commonly postaxial. Small finger duplications are rarely associated with other anomalies and are inherited as an autosomal dominant trait. Duplicated thumbs, however, can be associated with other abnormalities. Soft tissue polydactylies and "nubbins" can be easily ligated in the newborn nursery. Removal of bony duplications and extra thumbs are somewhat more complex procedures and should be performed in the operating room.

Congenital Trigger Thumb

Congenital trigger thumb is one of the more common hand problems in children. Typically, the child presents with

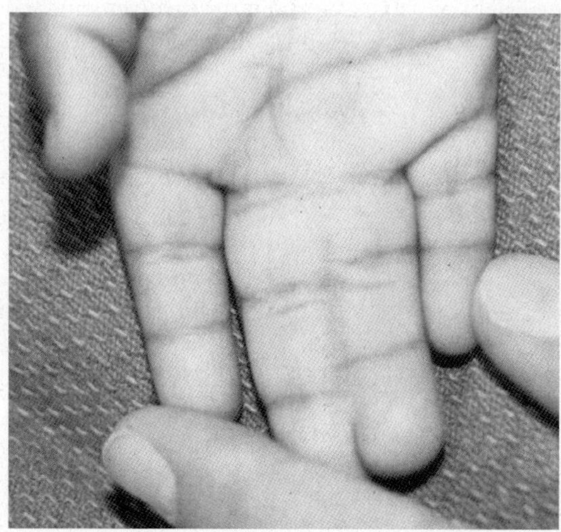

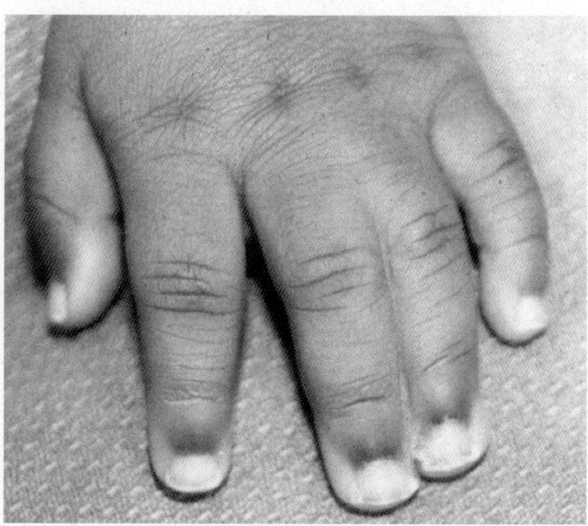

Figure 11.185 **(A** and **B)** A 1 year-old child with complete simple third web-space syndactyly. (*Reproduced with permission from* Morrissy RT, Weinstein SL. *Lovell and Winter's Pediatric Orthopaedics*. Philadelphia, PA: Lippincott Williams & Wilkins, 2006.)

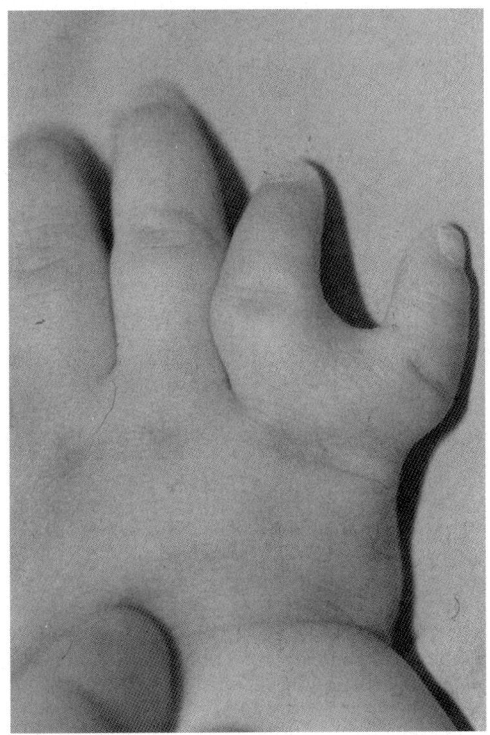

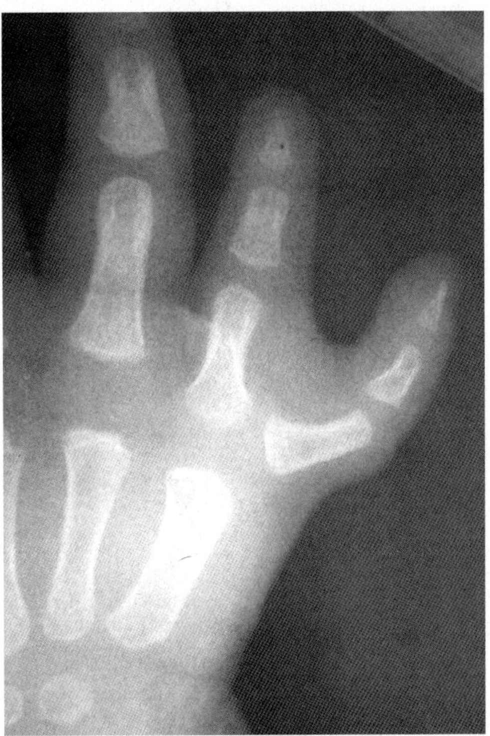

Figure 11.186 **(A)** Complete postaxial polydactyly with phalangeal duplication and a conjoined metacarpal. **B**: Radiographs of the same patient. (*Reproduced with permission from* Morrissy RT, Weinstein SL. *Lovell and Winter's Pediatric Orthopaedics*. Philadelphia, PA: Lippincott Williams & Wilkins, 2006.)

"locking" of the interphalangeal joint of the thumb. Usually the deformity is fixed and the "clicking," typical in adults, is rarely seen in children. Depending on the age of presentation, many will resolve spontaneously. As a result, it is best to simply observe children throughout the first year of life. Those who continue to have issues into childhood are best treated by tenolysis through the A1 pulley.

MISCELLANEOUS CONDITIONS

Limb Length Discrepancy

Frequently, orthopaedic surgeons are asked to evaluate the child with a limb length discrepancy. There are numerous congenital and acquired causes for this, and the treatment will need to be individualized on the basis of the cause and the extent of the inequality. Modest limb length discrepancies are relatively common: one study of healthy military recruits demonstrated a 32% incidence of leg length discrepancies between 0.5 and 1.5 cm. Although there are some contradictory reports in the literature, the general consensus is that small discrepancies (<2 cm) do not increase the risk of future back or hip problems. These minimal discrepancies can be well tolerated by the individual and require essentially no treatment. On the other hand, extensive differences may require significant procedures to overcome the otherwise-anticipated disability.

Etiology

Many different conditions can cause a leg length inequality. Congenital causes such as PFFD and fibular hemimelia have been previously discussed. DDH with a high dislocation can similarly cause a difference in limb lengths. Acquired conditions such as juvenile rheumatoid disease, damage to the physis following trauma or infections, and obscure etiologies such as radiation and burns are all capable of producing unequal limb lengths. Even neuromuscular conditions such as CP can produce a limb length discrepancy.

Evaluation

The history of a child with limb length discrepancy should be screened for both congenital and acquired causes. Family history may be helpful for identifying inherited disorders. Birth history and the time that the discrepancy was first noted are also important: discrepancies present at birth are almost certainly due to congenital hypoplasia or DDH.

On physical examination, absolute leg length inequality can be determined by comparing the length of the two legs from the anterior superior iliac spine to the medial malleolus. This technique does not account for angular changes or for deformities of the foot and ankle. Apparent discrepancy is measured from the umbilicus to the medial malleolus; this is also a less useful measure since it can be influenced by hip adduction contractures, pelvic obliquity, and

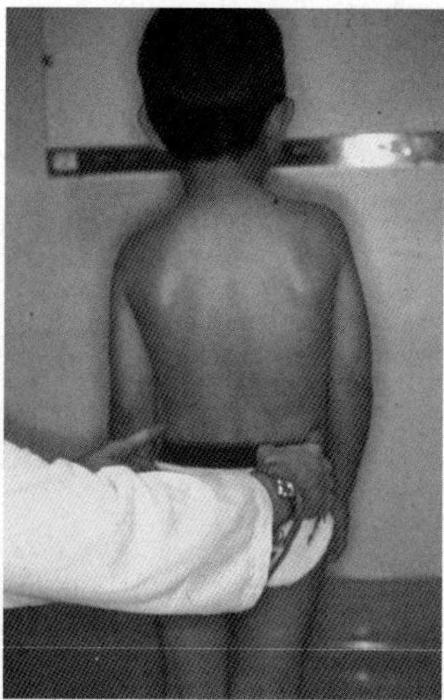

Figure 11.187 Limb lengths can be accurately assessed by placing your fingers on the iliac crests and using blocks to level the pelvis. (*Reproduced with permission from* Skaggs DL, Flynn JM. *Staying Out of Trouble in Pediatric Orthopaedics.* Philadelphia, PA: Lippincott Williams & Wilkins, 2006.)

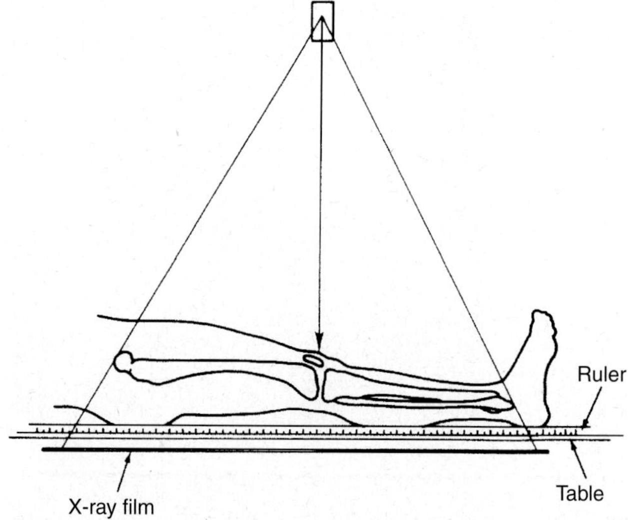

Figure 11.188 The teleoroentgenogram takes a single exposure of the hips to ankles and is subject to the errors of magnification. However, it is probably the best technique for children who cannot reliably comply with instructions to remain still for multiple exposures. (*Reproduced with permission from* Morrissy RT, Weinstein SL. *Lovell and Winter's Pediatric Orthopaedics.* Philadelphia, PA: Lippincott Williams & Wilkins, 2006.)

positioning. The most accurate and efficient way to clinically evaluate a leg length discrepancy is to have the child stand on measured blocks until the pelvis is level (as judged by a finger placed on each iliac crest) (Fig. 11.187). This technique is the most functional measure as it accounts for both angular malalignment and foot deformity. It is also important to observe the child walking, to look for compensatory movements and to determine the functional effect of the discrepancy. In most cases, children vault over the long leg, walk with the knee of the long leg flexed, and/or toe-walk on the short side.

Accurate radiographs, including scanograms and teleoroentgenograms, are essential in the evaluation of limb length discrepancies. A teleoroentgenogram is a single AP radiograph of both lower extremities (including hips, knees, and ankles) taken on top of a ruler. An advantage of this film is visualization of the entire lower extremity and the single exposure (since children often have difficulty staying still) (Fig. 11.188). A major disadvantage, especially in larger children, is magnification error because the same x-ray beam strikes the hips, knees, and ankles at different angles. Scanograms minimize this error by moving a smaller cassette beneath the patient and obtaining multiple orthogonal exposures of the hip, knees, and ankles (Fig. 11.189). Although more accurate, this technique requires that the patient lay still between exposures (Fig. 11.190). In addition, scanograms do not allow visualization of the femoral and tibial diaphyses nor do they account for foot deformity in the overall measurement of leg length discrepancy. Both teleoroentgenograms and scanograms can give false readings in children with hip or knee contractures or rotational malalignments. In these cases, CT scanograms are a more accurate option.

Skeletal growth typically ends around 14 years of age in girls and 16 years of age in boys. Although chronologic age provides some information about a child's skeletal maturity, there can be significant variability from child to child, depending on the onset of puberty. A more accurate way to estimate skeletal maturity is to determine the child's bone age. This is done by obtaining a posteroanterior radiograph of the hand and wrist and comparing the findings to a

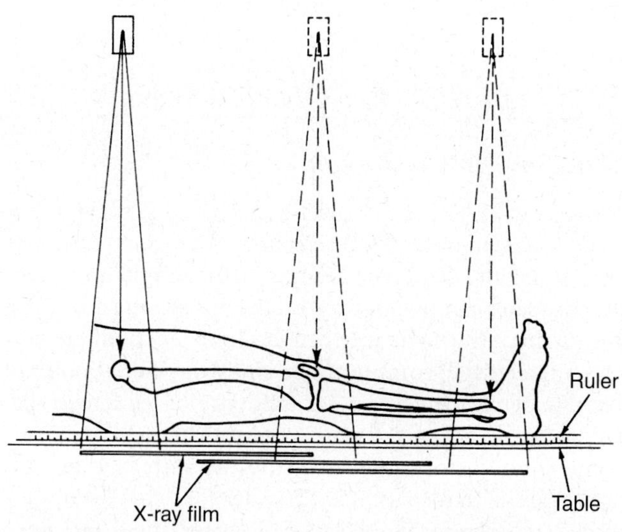

Figure 11.189 The scanogram technique avoids magnification error by exposing each joint individually. The child must remain still for each exposure. (*Reproduced with permission from* Morrissy RT, Weinstein SL. *Lovell and Winter's Pediatric Orthopaedics.* Philadelphia, PA: Lippincott Williams & Wilkins, 2006.)

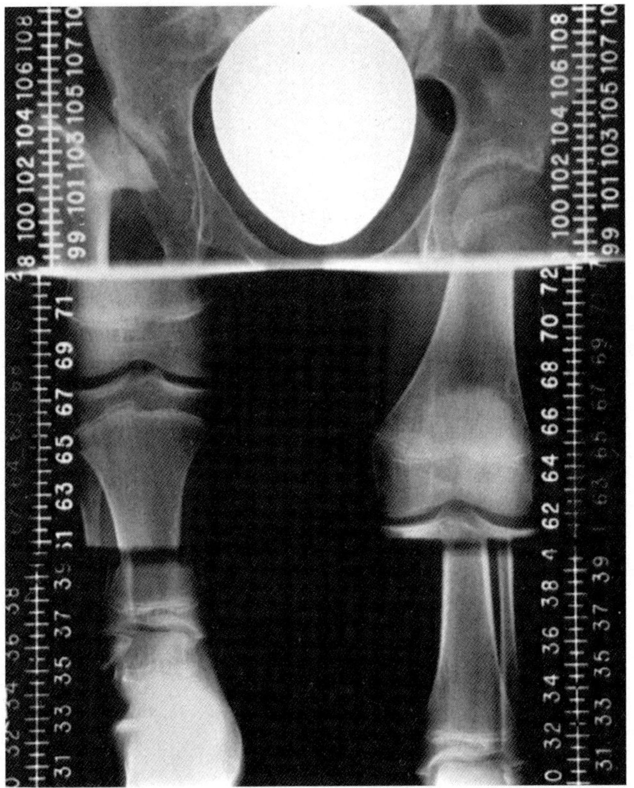

Figure 11.190 Scanogram allows the images of the three joints to be captured on a radiograph of convenient size by moving the radiograph beneath the patient between exposures. (*Reproduced with permission from* Morrissy RT, Weinstein SL. *Lovell and Winter's Pediatric Orthopaedics.* Philadelphia, PA: Lippincott Williams & Wilkins, 2006.)

reference atlas. These bone age measurements are usually accurate to within 6 months but are notoriously inaccurate in children younger than 6 years.

Management

It is important to remember that the focus of treatment is not the presenting leg length discrepancy but rather the predicted leg length discrepancy at skeletal maturity. As a result, proper management of a growing child with a limb length discrepancy depends on accurate prediction of the discrepancy at skeletal maturity. There are four commonly used techniques for predicting limb length discrepancy, each with a different level of accuracy and complexity. These include the arithmetic method, growth-remaining method, multiplier method, and the straight-line method. Regardless of the technique, the potential accuracy of these predictive methods is improved by longitudinal data. Therefore, repeated leg length measurements at 6- to 12-month intervals provide more information from which to base these future predictions.

The arithmetic method of Menelaus, also known as the rule-of-thumb method, is the most straightforward method for predicting leg length inequality. The technique is based on the following assumptions regarding growth: (1) girls stop growing at age 14, (2) boys stop growing at age 16, (3) the distal femoral physis grows 10 mm a year, and (4) the proximal tibial physis adds 6 mm of growth a year. By comparing the patient's current chronologic age to these assumptions, one can estimate the amount of growth remaining. This technique is useful only for the few years preceding skeletal maturity and, although simple, is considered the most inaccurate.

The growth-remaining method is based on growth tables published by Green and Anderson (Fig. 11.191). Growth percentiles can be calculated by comparing a child's leg lengths and age to the tables. Other graphs allow the prediction of growth remaining and the effects of epiphysiodesis. Although it is the longest-standing technique for predicting leg length discrepancy, many find the method cumbersome as it requires referral to two separate sets of graphs. The multiplier method is based on the same Green and Anderson data but allows prediction of leg length discrepancy without the need for bone age or graphing. Based on the child's gender and chronologic age, the final leg length discrepancy can be determined by multiplying the existing discrepancy by a factor determined from a reference table. Although accurate for congenital discrepancies, some authors believe that the multiplier method underestimates the importance of skeletal age in predicting final discrepancies. The Moseley straight-line method is considered the most accurate technique for predicting leg length differences but requires multiple measurements and graphic interpretation (Fig. 11.192). The straight-line method is also based on the Green and Anderson growth data: bone age and leg lengths are used to determine growth percentile, and the growth of both limbs are expressed graphically by two straight lines. By comparing the difference in the slopes of both lines, one can predict the leg length discrepancy at maturity.

Treatment options depend on the magnitude of the predicted leg length discrepancy (Table 11.5). Since leg length discrepancies less than 2 cm are well tolerated, treatment is usually not necessary. For noticeable differences, a shoe lift or orthotic can be helpful. For predicted discrepancies between 2 to 6 cm, treatment options include larger shoe lifts, acute shortening, or epiphysiodesis. Generally, lifts larger

TABLE 11.5
GUIDELINES FOR THE TREATMENT OF LEG LENGTH DISCREPANCY

Discrepancy	Treatment
<2 cm	No treatment or shoe lift
2–6 cm	Shoe lift, acute shortening, or epiphysiodesis
6–20 cm	Lengthening
>20 cm	Amputation and prosthetic fitting

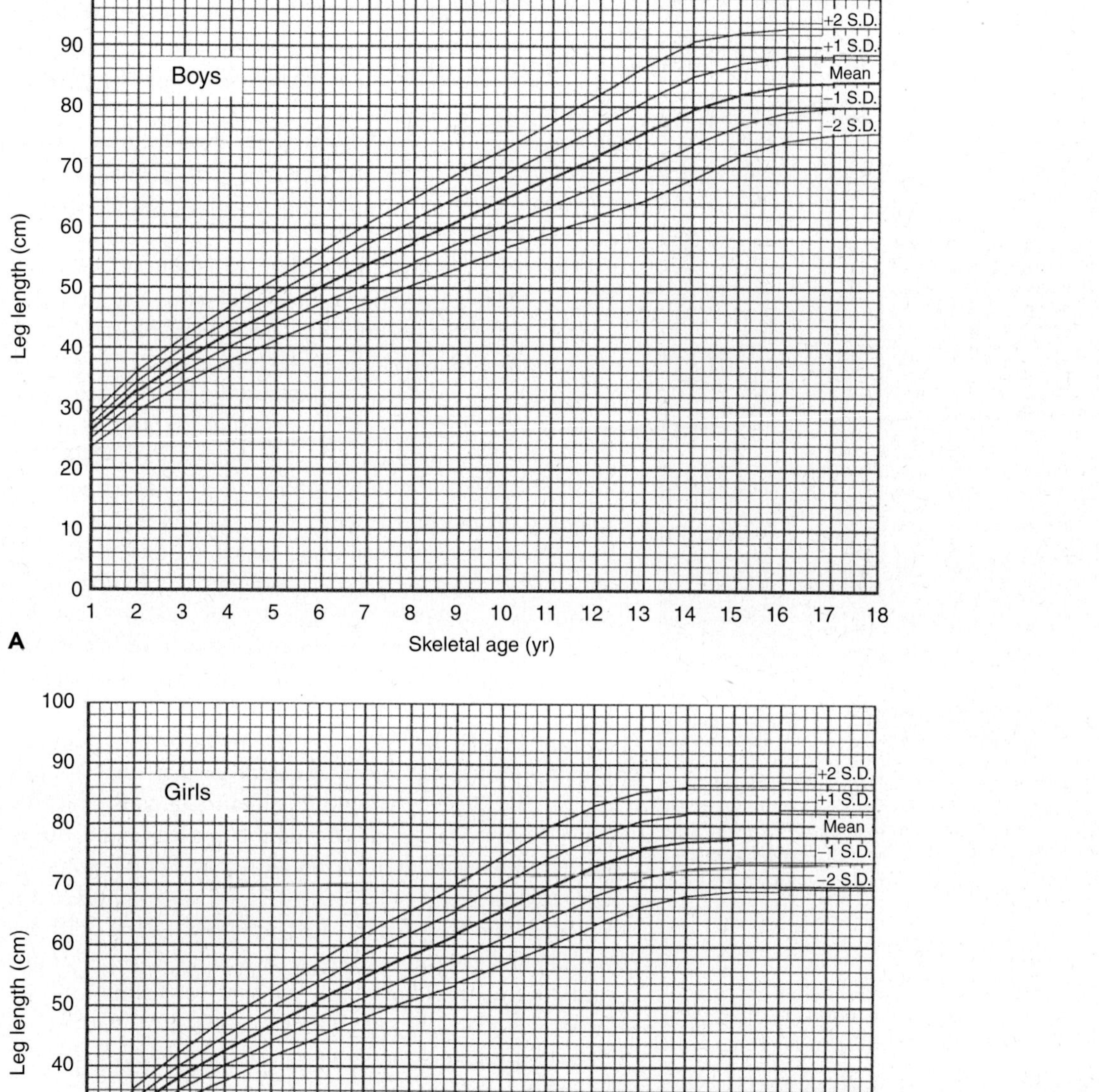

Figure 11.191 **(A)** Graph showing total leg length versus skeletal age for boys allows a specific boy to be related to the population by plotting his leg length as a function of his skeletal age. **(B)** Equivalent plot for girls. (*Reproduced with permission from* Morrissy RT, Weinstein SL. *Lovell and Winter's Pediatric Orthopaedics.* Philadelphia, PA: Lippincott Williams & Wilkins, 2006.)

than 5 cm are poorly tolerated because of ankle instability and frequent sprains, as well as the heaviness of lifts of such size. Acute femoral shortening is indicated for discrepancies less than 5 to 6 cm in which there is insufficient growth remaining for an epiphysiodesis to work. Surgery can be performed using an intramedullary nail or plate for fixation. A major disadvantage of this technique is quadriceps weakness due to the disrupted length–tension relationship of the muscle. The best treatment option for a moderate leg length discrepancy in a child with sufficient growth remaining is a well-timed epiphysiodesis (Fig. 11.193). On the basis of the method of prediction, one can estimate when to close the growth in the distal femoral physis and/or the proximal tibial physis of the longer leg so that the leg lengths roughly equalize by the time the child finishes growing. In general, it is better to aim for slight undercorrection since small discrepancies are well tolerated and families are often unhappy if the long leg is shortened too much. Surgery is

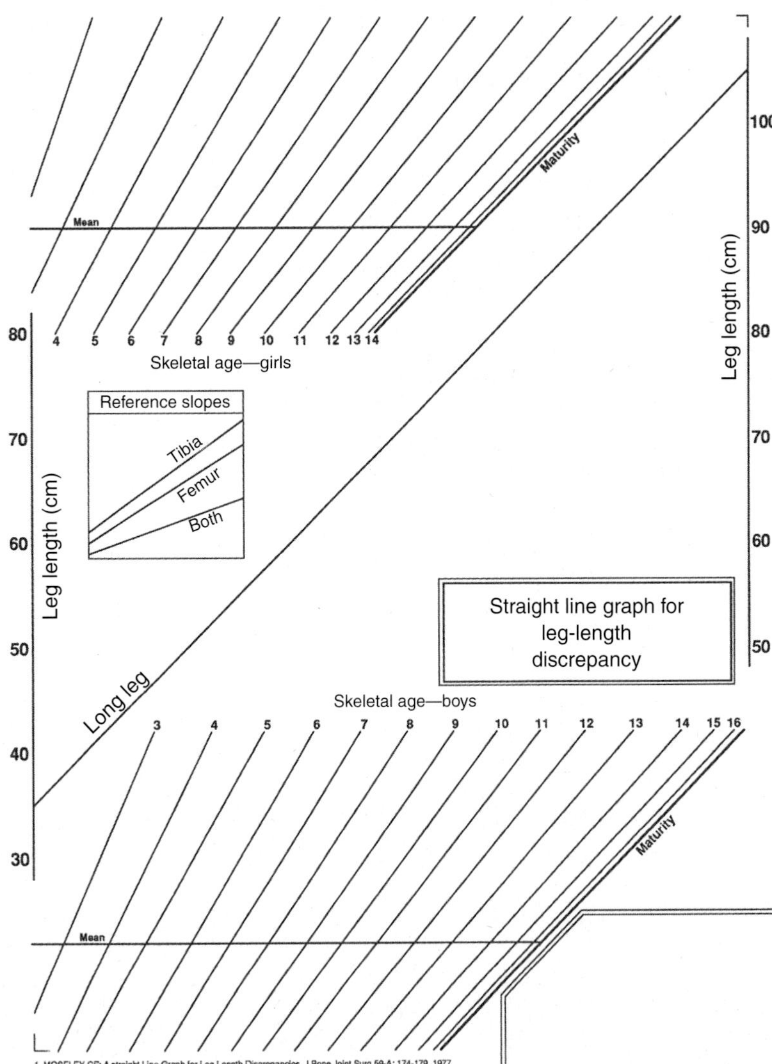

Figure 11.192 The straight-line graph comprises three parts: the leg length area with the predefined line for the growth of the long leg, the areas of sloping lines for plotting skeletal ages, and reference slopes to predict growth following epiphysiodesis. (*Reproduced with permission from* Morrissy RT, Weinstein SL. *Lovell and Winter's Pediatric Orthopaedics*. Philadelphia, PA: Lippincott Williams & Wilkins, 2006.)

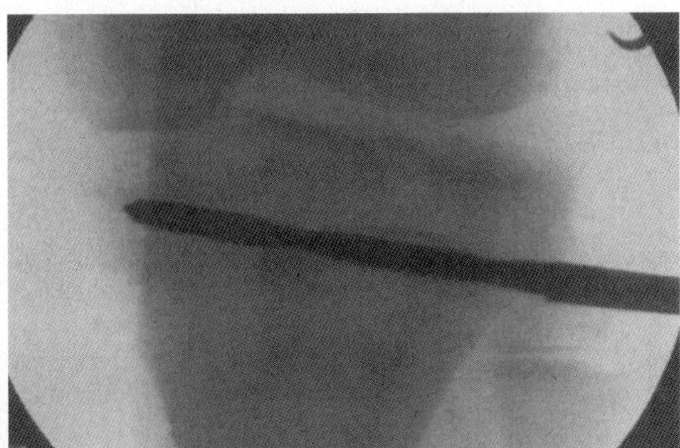

Figure 11.193 Example of a percutaneous epiphysiodesis performed on the proximal tibial physis. The physis is ablated with a drill followed by a curette. (*Reproduced with permission from* Morrissey RT, Weinstein SL. *Atlas of Pediatric Orthopaedic Surgery*. Philadelphia, PA: Lippincott Williams & Wilkins, 2006.)

typically performed in a percutaneous fashion using a drill and curette to scrape out the physis. Although the surgery is technically straightforward, it is important to double-check growth calculations as the operation is permanent.

Larger predicted leg length discrepancies (6–20 cm) may be amenable to limb lengthening. Several techniques exist, but most involve a minimally invasive osteotomy followed by gradual incremental distraction using an external fixator (Fig. 11.194). Typically, the bone is lengthened 1 mm a day. After the goal length is achieved, the fixator is maintained in place until the regenerated bone consolidates. Controversy exists over what is the maximum achievable lengthening, but most authors agree that it is the condition of the soft tissues, not the bone, that determines the endpoint of treatment. Although limb lengthening can produce some impressive results, it is vital that families and physicians understand that the process is long and arduous, often taking a physical and psychological toll on both the patient and the caregiver. Complications should be expected and include joint contracture, joint subluxation or dislocation,

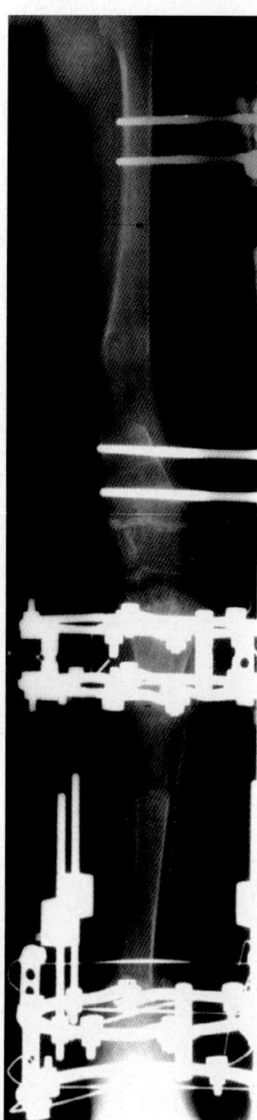

Figure 11.194 Example of a circular external fixator (tibia) and a monorail fixator (femur) used to achieve gradual lengthening of both bones. Note the regenerate bone at the site of both lengthenings. (*Reproduced with permission from* Morrissy RT, Weinstein SL. *Lovell and Winter's Pediatric Orthopaedics*. Philadelphia, PA: Lippincott Williams & Wilkins, 2006.)

muscle weakness, neurovascular injury, refracture through regenerate bone, and pin-site infection. For even larger predicted discrepancies (>15–20 cm), amputation and prosthetic fitting is usually the best option. Although difficult to accept, amputation offers an easier treatment course and superior long-term function compared with a heroic lengthening.

The Limping Child

A limp is a common reason for a child to present to an orthopaedic surgeon. Although this is a relatively common problem, evaluation can be difficult. Multiple etiologies, the child's difficulty in localizing pain, and a vague history make it essential that the physician have a systematic approach to this problem.

History and Physical Examination

Although the differential diagnosis for a limp may be long, a careful history will narrow the possible diagnoses and help focus diagnostic testing. The age of the child provides the first clue to the diagnosis as certain conditions are far more prevalent in certain age groups (Table 11.6). A history of trauma or recent illness is important to elicit as it suggests fracture or infection as a possible etiology. Likewise, a history of failing to meet developmental milestones or, worse, a deterioration in motor ability suggests a metabolic or neuromuscular cause. Parents, and children if possible, should be asked about the character of the limp, the presence or absence of pain, and the timing and duration of symptoms. A painful limp is more likely due to trauma, infection, or malignancy, whereas a painless limp is more often caused by a metabolic, congenital, or neuromuscular abnormality. In addition, the character of the pain itself can provide useful information. Pain with acute onset is probably caused by fracture or infection; pain that gradually worsens over time is more likely caused by mechanical, inflammatory, or neoplastic conditions. Morning pain is suggestive of an inflammatory condition such as JRA. Pain after activities is associated with mechanical and overuse injuries. Night pain is characteristic of malignant conditions.

The most important step in the physical examination of a child with a limp is observing the child walk. Children should be dressed in a gown or gym shorts so that the lower extremities can be adequately visualized. Because of the small size of most examining rooms, it is usually better to have the patient walk in a nearby hallway. Several "laps" may be needed so that each aspect of the gait (i.e., hips, knees, ankles) can be evaluated sequentially. Normal gait occurs in two phases—stance and swing. The stance phase begins with initial contact for a given limb and terminates with toe-off of that extremity. Stance accounts for approximately 60% of the gait cycle, normally leaving 40% of the cycle for swing. The swing phase begins when the foot leaves the ground and ends at initial contact of the contralateral limb. Most children learn to walk between 12 and 18 months of age. Early gait is characterized by short stride lengths, fast cadence, and a widened stance. Adult-like gait develops by the age of 7.

There are several specific types of limps that deserve mention. An antalgic gait is caused by pain in the affected extremity. This leads to a shortened stance phase on the painful side and a shortened stride length on the contralateral side (as children transfer their weight back to the good leg as quickly as possible). Antalgic gaits are seen in children with fracture, infection, or foreign bodies in the foot. A Trendelenburg gait results from weakness of the hip abductors. During stance on the affected side, the contralateral pelvis drops because of the muscle's inability to stabilize the pelvis. To maintain balance, children will often lean their torsos over the affected side. Common causes of this type of gait include developmental hip dysplasia, Legg-Calvé-Perthes disease and slipped capital femoral epiphysis. A

TABLE 11.6
DIFFERENTIAL DIAGNOSIS OF A LIMPING CHILD

<4 Years of Age	4–10 Years of Age	>10 Years of Age
Fracture	Fracture	Fracture
Osteomyelitis, septic arthritis, diskitis	Osteomyelitis, septic arthritis, diskitis	Osteomyelitis, septic arthritis, diskitis
Juvenile rheumatoid arthritis	Juvenile rheumatoid arthritis	Apophysitis (e.g., Osgood–Schlatter disease)
Lyme disease	Lyme disease	Tumor
Discoid meniscus	Discoid meniscus	Cerebral palsy
Foreign body in the foot	Transient synovitis	Osteochondritis dissecans
Tumor	Tumor	Legg–Calvé–Perthes disease
DDH	DDH	Muscular dystrophy
Cerebral palsy	Cerebral palsy	Slipped capital femoral epiphysis
Leg length discrepancy	Leg length discrepancy	Tarsal coalition
	Osteochondritis dissecans	Accessory tarsal navicular
	Legg–Calvé–Perthes disease	
	Muscular dystrophy	
	Slipped capital femoral epiphysis	
	Accessory tarsal navicular	
	Sever apophysitis	

DDH, developmental dysplasia of the hip.
(*Adapted from* Flynn JM, Widmann RF. The limping child: evaluation and diagnosis. *J Am Acad Orthop.* 2001;9(2): 89–98.)

child with a short leg limp may manifest one of many compensatory mechanisms to account for the leg length inequality. Some children will circumduct the long leg to improve foot clearance; others will vault with the short leg or toe-walk to achieve functional equalization of their leg lengths.

In addition to observing the child's limp, the examiner should carefully range every major joint and palpate the lower extremities to determine a point of maximum tenderness. By localizing the source of the symptoms, one can narrow the differential diagnosis and drastically reduce the need for excess imaging. A Gowers test should be performed on almost every child to minimize the chance of missing a muscular dystrophy.

Diagnostic Studies

The choice of diagnostic studies should be guided by information garnered from the history and physical examination. Normally, high-quality plain radiographs are the first imaging modality that should be obtained. For children who can localize their symptoms, orthogonal views should be taken of the region including the joint above and the joint below the point of maximal tenderness. Oblique views, especially in the foot and ankle, are helpful to identify subtle fracture lines or minor physeal widening. Bone scans are an excellent test for evaluating a limping child in whom the history and physical examination are unable to localize the anatomic region that is affected. Sensitive, but not specific, bone scans can identify fracture, infection, or malignancy. Ultrasonography is the diagnostic study of choice for the evaluation of hip joint effusions. Ultrasonography is noninvasive, does not require sedation, and can be used to guide aspiration. MRI, while not appropriate as a first-line test, is extremely useful in the workup of suspected stress fractures and malignancies.

Laboratory testing is indicated for children with constitutional symptoms including fever, malaise, or weight loss. Appropriate tests include a complete blood cell count with differential count, an ESR, and a CRP. White blood cell counts may be elevated only in 20% to 30% of children with osteomyelitis, but a left shift in the differential is more sensitive for infection. Extremely elevated counts can be seen in both JRA and leukemia. ESR and CRP are nonspecific inflammatory markers that are excellent screening tests for infection and autoimmune disease. The ESR is somewhat less useful than CRP because it is slow to rise in the early phase of an acute process and remains elevated for up to 3 weeks in spite of appropriate treatment. When suspected on the basis of the history and physical examination, laboratory tests for autoimmune disease (rheumatoid factor and antinuclear antibodies) and Lyme disease (ELISA) should be performed.

Diagnosis

Making the diagnosis in a limping child depends on integrating information obtained from the history, physical examination, and diagnostic studies. In particular, the child's age, the presence or absence of pain, and the type of limp are important initial clues to the diagnosis and can help guide the diagnostic workup. For example, a painful, antalgic limp following trauma in an adolescent is most likely due to fracture; plain radiographs of the affected extremity are usually sufficient to make the diagnosis. In contrast, an antalgic gait in a toddler with hip pain, fever, and malaise raises the suspicion of infection. An elevated ESR and CRP level should prompt an ultrasound of the hip, which may reveal a septic effusion. Like these examples, most limps can be accurately diagnosed with a careful history and physical examination, followed by appropriate diagnostic studies.

RECOMMENDED READINGS

Alman BA. Duchenne muscular dystrophy and steroids: pharmacologic treatment in the absence of effective gene therapy. *J Pediatr Orthop*. 2005;25(4):554–556.

Chung SM. The arterial supply of the developing proximal end of the human femur. *J Bone Joint Surg Am*. 1976;58:961–970.

Flynn JM, Miller F. Management of hip disorders in patients with cerebral palsy. *J Am Acad Orthop*. 2002;10:198–209.

Flynn JM, Widmann RF. The limping child: evaluation and diagnosis. *J Am Acad Orthop*. 2001;9(2):89–98.

Gillingham BL, Sanchez AA, Wenger DR. Pelvic osteotomies for the treatment of hip dysplasia in children and young adults. *J Am Acad Orthop*. 1999;7(5):325.

Heath CH, Staheli LT. Normal limits of knee angle in white children—genu varum and genu valgum. *J Pediatr Orthop*. 1993;13(2):259–262.

Herring JA, Kim HT, Browne R. Legg-Calve-Perthes disease, II: prospective multicenter study of the effect of treatment on outcome. *J Bone Joint Surg Am*. 2004;86-A(10):2121–2134.

Johnston CE. Congenital pseudarthrosis of the tibia: results of technical variations in the Charnley-Williams procedure. *J Bone Joint Surg Am*. 2002;84:1799–1810.

Kay RM. Lower extremity surgery in children with cerebral palsy. In: Skaggs DL, Tolo VT, eds. *Master Techniques in Orthopaedic Surgery*. Philadelphia, PA: Lippincott Williams & Wilkins; 2008.

Lincoln TL, Suen PW. Common rotational variations in children. *J Am Acad Orthop*. 2003;11:312–320.

Misra M, Pacaud D, Petryk A, et al. Vitamin D deficiency in children and its management: review of current knowledge and recommendations. *Pediatrics*. 2008;122:398–417.

Moseley CF. Assessment and prediction in leg-length discrepancy. *Instr Course Lect*. 1989;38:325–330.

Ponseti IV. Growth and development of the acetabulum in the normal child: anatomical, histological, and roentgenographic studies. *J Bone Joint Surg Am*. 1978;60:575.

Rauch F, Glorieux FH. Osteogenesis imperfecta. *Lancet*. 2004;363: 1377–1385.

Skaggs DL, Flynn JM. *Staying Out of Trouble in Pediatric Orthopaedics*. Philadelphia, PA: Lippincott Williams & Wilkins; 2006.

Stout JL, Gage JR, Schwarz, et al. Distal femoral extension osteotomy and patellar tendon advancement to treat persistent crouch gait in cerebral palsy. *J Bone Joint Surg Am*. 2008;90:2470–2484.

Section 2 Pediatric Spine

Wudbhav N. Sankar David L. Skaggs

The pediatric spine presents several issues that differ from those in adults. Deformity, rather than degeneration, is the common complaint. Scoliosis or kyphosis can be due to idiopathic, neuromuscular, or congenital causes. Certain cervical spine anomalies are congenital and usually present during childhood; these include Klippel–Feil syndrome and torticollis. One common complaint between adults and children is back pain, and a careful workup should be performed before the diagnosis of mechanical back pain can be made. In particular, one must rule out spondylolysis and spondylolisthesis as these conditions often affect adolescents. Children have physical differences that make them more prone to spine trauma; proper evaluation and treatment of these injuries is essential to ensure a positive outcome.

IDIOPATHIC SCOLIOSIS

Scoliosis can be due to a number of different etiologies, including neuromuscular disease, congenital vertebral anomalies, collagen disorders, neurofibromatosis, and spinal cord injury. Idiopathic scoliosis is the most common form of scoliosis and is a diagnosis of exclusion, implying that no other underlying condition is present.

Pathophysiology

Scoliosis refers to coronal or frontal plane curvature of the spine greater than 10 degrees. It is a complex three-dimensional (3-D) deformity not only including the obvious abnormality in the frontal plane but also involving alteration in sagittal plane balance and rotation in the transverse plane (Fig. 11.195). This combination of abnormalities in three planes leads to the cosmetically apparent aspects of the deformity including shoulder and pelvis asymmetry, hypokyphosis, and rotational prominence of the rib or flank. Although the etiology of idiopathic scoliosis remains unknown, potential causes include abnormalities in platelet dysfunction, muscle imbalance, collagen structure, growth plate mechanics, and the central nervous system (CNS). Idiopathic scoliosis is thought to be polygenetic; a history of scoliosis in a first-degree relative significantly increases an individual's risk.

Classification

Idiopathic scoliosis can be divided into infantile (younger than 3 years), juvenile (3–10 years), and adolescent (older than 10 years) forms. Infantile scoliosis is extremely rare, more common in boys than in girls, and more often characterized by left thoracic curve patterns. Juvenile scoliosis

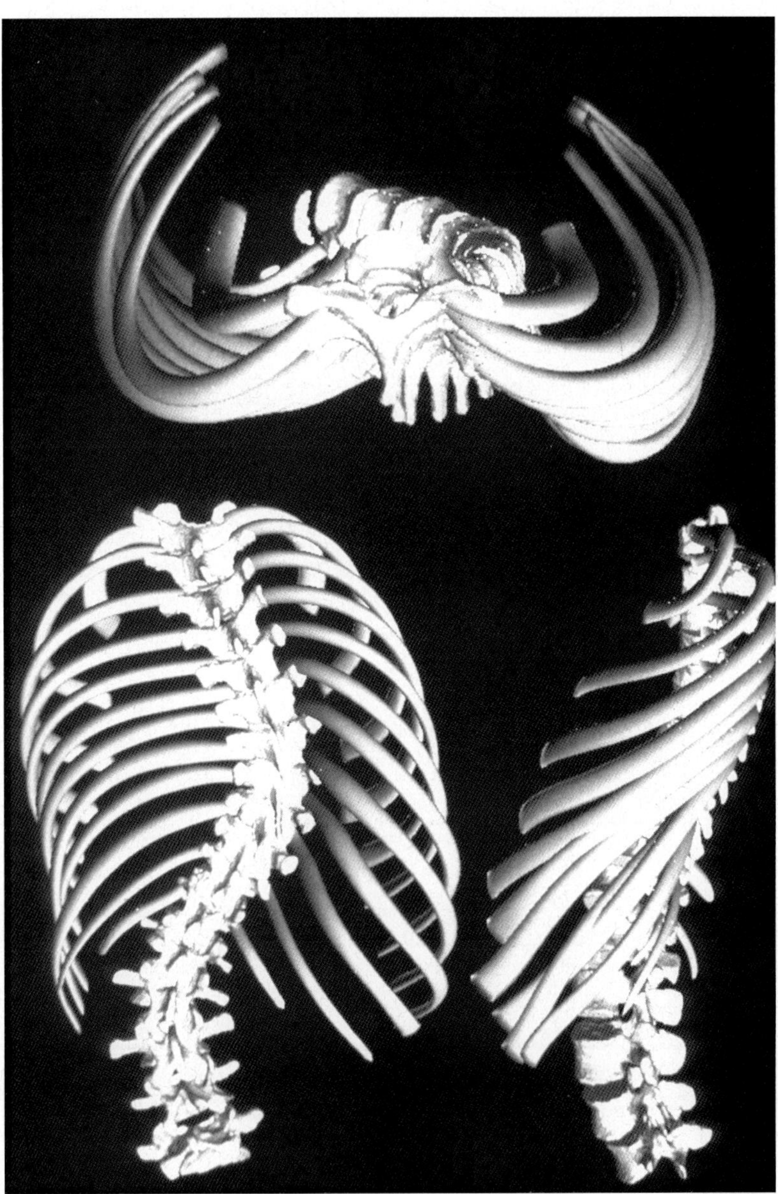

Figure 11.195 A three-dimensional reconstruction of a scoliotic spine demonstrating the three planes of deformity. The torsional deformity is maximal at the apex of the curvature. (*Reproduced with permission from* Morrissy RT, Weinstein SL. *Lovell and Winter's Pediatric Orthopaedics*. Philadelphia, PA: Lippincott Williams & Wilkins, 2006.)

comprises between 12% and 16% of all scoliosis patients and has similar demographics and presentation to adolescent scoliosis. Adolescent idiopathic scoliosis (AIS) is the most common form of idiopathic scoliosis, with a prevalence of 2% to 3% in the teenage population. Historically, AIS has been classified by the King–Moe classification. This radiographic classification is based on the location of the frontal plane deformity and the relative size and flexibility of the thoracic and lumbar components. In 2001, the Lenke classification for AIS was described (Fig. 11.196). This system is more complete and accounts for the location of the major curve, the relative magnitudes of the lesser curves, deviation of the apical lumbar vertebrae from the midline, and the sagittal profile. Six patterns have been described: primary thoracic, double thoracic, double major (thoracic/lumbar), triple major, thoracolumbar/lumbar, and thoracolumbar/lumbar with a structural thoracic curve. These patterns are then modified on the basis of the deviation of the apical lumbar vertebra from the midline (central sacral vertical line [CSVL]) and the sagittal balance.

Presentation

AIS occurs more frequently in girls than in boys, by a 10:1 ratio. Patients are usually asymptomatic, although adolescents may occasionally complain of mild back pain. Pain severe enough to require frequent medication or causing missed time from school should be thoroughly investigated for another etiology. Patients more often present with complaints about their body image due to their trunk shift or rib hump. Alternatively, trunk asymmetry

Curve Type

Type	Proximal Thoracic	Main Thoracic	Thoracolumbar / Lumbar	Curve Type
1	Nonstructural	Structural (Major*)	Nonstructural	Main Thoracic (MT)
2	Structural	Structural (Major*)	Nonstructural	Double Thoracic (DT)
3	Nonstructural	Structural (Major*)	Structural	Double Major (DM)
4	Structural	Structural (Major*)	Structural	Triple Major (TM)
5	Nonstructural	Nonstructural	Structural (Major*)	Thoracolumbar/Lumbar (TL/L)
6	Nonstructural	Structural	Structural (Major*)	Thoracolumbar/Lumbar - Main Thoracic (TL/L–MT)

*Major = Largest Cobb Measurement, always structural
Minor = all other curves with structural criteria applied

STRUCTURAL CRITERIA
(Minor Curves)

Proximal Thoracic:–Side Bending Cobb ≥ 25°
–T2 - T5 Kyphosis ≥ +20°

Main Thoracic:–Side Bending Cobb ≥ 25°
–T10 - L2 Kyphosis ≥ +20°

Thoracolumbar/Lumbar:–Side Bending Cobb ≥ 25°
–T10 - L2 Kyphosis ≥ +20°

LOCATION OF APEX
(SRS definition)

CURVE	APEX
THORACIC	T2 - T11-12 DISC
THORACOLUMBAR	T12 - L1
LUMBAR	L1-2 DISC - L4

Modifiers

Lumbar Spine Modifier	CSVL to Lumbar Apex
A	CSVL Between Pedicles
B	CSVL Touches Apical Body(ies)
C	CSVL Completely Medial

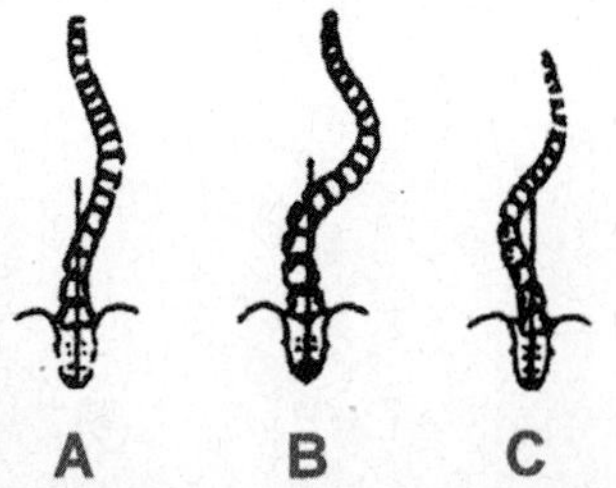

A B C

Thoracic Sagittal Profile T5–T12		
–	(Hypo)	<10°
N	(Normal)	10°–40°
+	(Hyper)	>40°

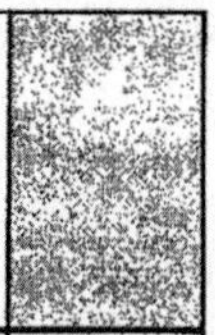

Curve Type (1–6) + Lumbar Spine Modifier (A, B, or C) + Thoracic Sagittal Modifier (-, N, or +)
Classification (e.g. 1B+):__________

Figure 11.196 Synopsis of the Lenke classification for adolescent idiopathic scoliosis. SRS, Scoliosis Research Society; CSVL, central sacral vertical line. (*Reproduced with permission from* Lenke LG, Betz RR, Harms J, et al. Adolescent idiopathic scoliosis: a new classification to determine the extent of spinal arthrodesis. *J Bone Joint Surg Am.* 2001;83:1169–1181.)

or uneven shoulder heights may be incidentally noted by parents or pediatricians (Fig. 11.197). Often, adolescents with no complaints are identified in school screening and referred for evaluation. Patients with idiopathic scoliosis usually do not present with neurologic symptoms.

History and Physical Examination

History should focus on confirming the diagnosis of idiopathic scoliosis and assessing the degree of physical maturity. Patients should be questioned about paresthesias, weakness, stumbling or clumsiness, and bowel or bladder dysfunction. Other important aspects of the history include any family history of spinal deformity, the patient's overall medical condition, and the patient's physiologic maturity, including the presence of pubic hair (Tanner stage) and the onset of menarche.

Patients should be examined in a gown (open in the back), with shoes and socks removed. The skin should be examined for midline defects, clefts, dimples, hairy patches, or café au lait spots. In the standing position, symmetry of the shoulders, scapula, and pelvis should be assessed, as should the overall coronal and sagittal balance. The Adams forward bending test, in which patients bend over to touch their toes, reveals the degree of rotational deformity (rib hump) and is helpful in detecting subtle cases of scoliosis (Fig. 11.198). The lower extremities should be evaluated for hamstring tightness, asymmetric muscular girth, and foot deformity; abnormal findings may be evidence of an underlying intraspinal abnormality. A popliteal angle of greater than 50 degrees implies very tight hamstrings and suggests an underlying neurologic or muscular pathology. This finding is very sensitive but not very specific. A thorough neurologic testing should be performed, including an evaluation of light touch sensation,

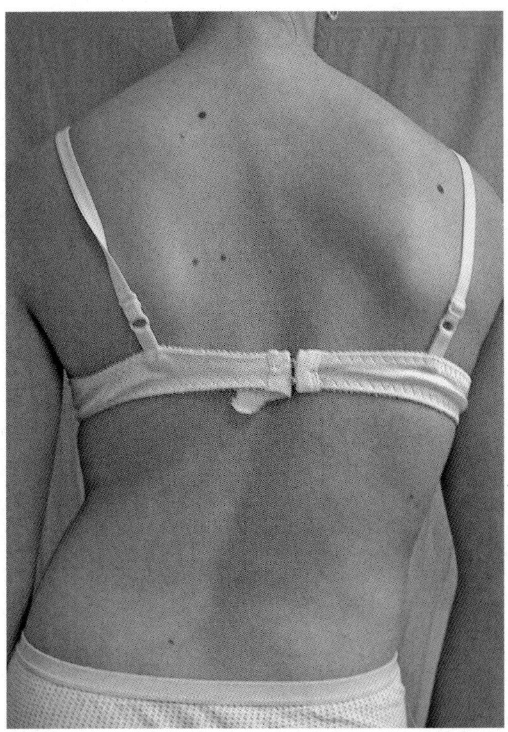

Figure 11.197 Careful examination of the back is required to identify the physical features of scoliosis. These include asymmetry of the scapulae, shift of the trunk, and asymmetry of the waistline, as well as asymmetry in the level of the shoulders. (*Reproduced with permission from* Morrissy RT, Weinstein SL. *Lovell and Winter's Pediatric Orthopaedics.* Philadelphia, PA: Lippincott Williams & Wilkins, 2006.)

motor strength, lower extremity tone, and deep tendon reflexes. Babinski sign should be sought and the abdominal reflex routinely tested. This latter reflex is assessed by lightly stroking the abdomen on either side of the umbilicus with a blunt instrument; a normal response consists of a symmetric unilateral contraction of the abdominal muscles toward the side being stimulated. Any evidence of upper motor neuron pathology or asymmetry in findings from one leg to the other calls into question the diagnosis of idiopathic scoliosis and should be investigated further.

Radiographs

Initial radiographic evaluation of a patient with spinal deformity consists of standing posteroanterior (PA) and lateral views on a single, long cassette. Generally, the PA view is preferred over the anteroposterior (AP) view to limit the amount of radiation exposure to the breast tissue. The frontal view is repeated at regular intervals (usually 3–6 months) depending on the age and growth velocity of the child to determine curve progression; an increase of at least 5 degrees is generally accepted as evidence of curve progression. Lateral views are important initially to assess the sagittal balance and to look for coexisting spondylolysis but are not necessary at each follow-up visit. Bending x-rays are helpful for assessing curve flexibility and planning fusion levels but are indicated only as preoperative studies (Fig. 11.199).

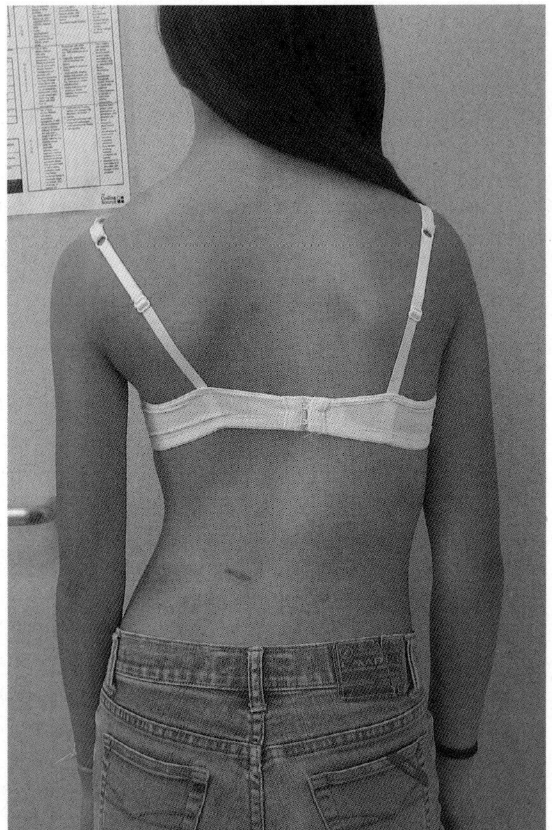

A

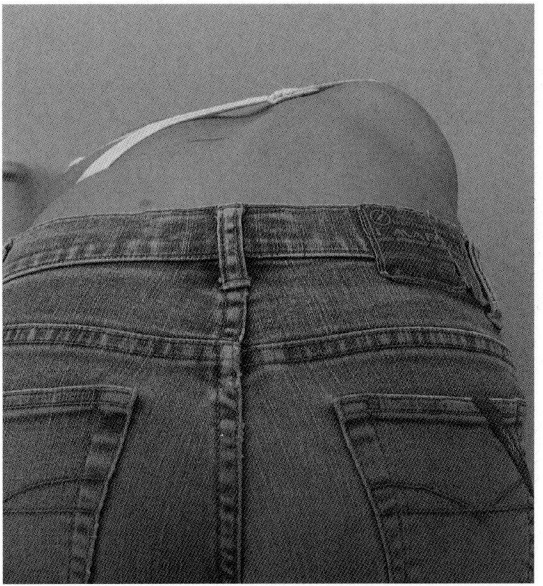

B

Figure 11.198 **(A)** Viewed from the back, the deformity associated with this girl's scoliosis appears mild. **(B)** The Adams forward bending test reveals the rotational deformity. (*Reproduced with permission from* Children's Orthopaedic Center, Los Angeles, CA.)

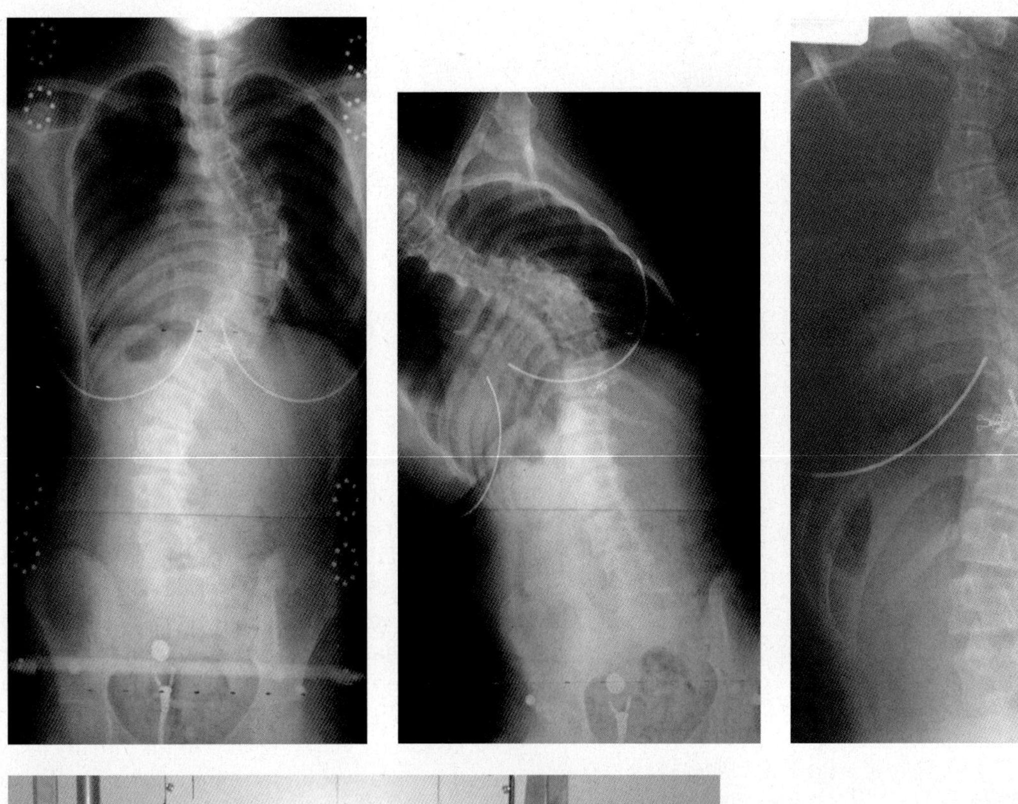

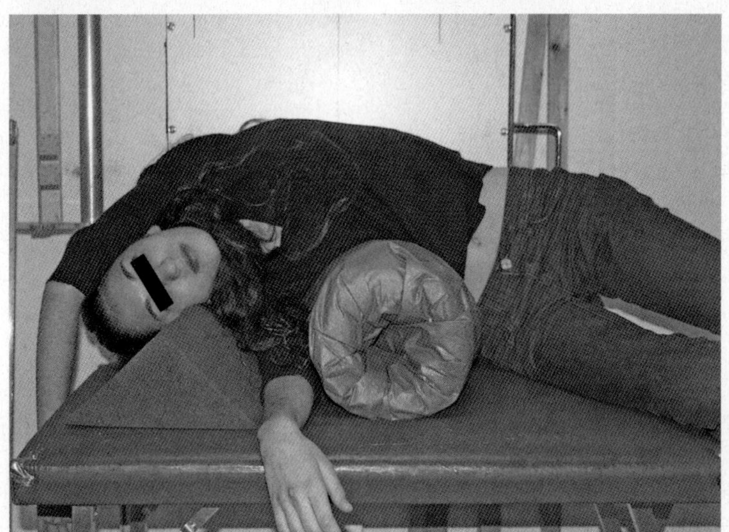

Figure 11.199 The standing posteroanterior radiograph demonstrates right thoracic scoliosis with moderate left lumbar scoliosis. **(B)** The flexibility of the left upper thoracic and left lumbar curves was assessed via the left-side-bending radiograph. **(C)** The flexibility of the right thoracic curve was evaluated using the bolster side-bending technique. **(D)** The bolster side-bending film is taken with the trunk laterally flexed on a bolster positioned under the ribs that correspond to the apex of the deformity. (*Reproduced with permission from* Morrissy RT, Weinstein SL. *Lovell and Winter's Pediatric Orthopaedics*. Philadelphia, PA: Lippincott Williams & Wilkins, 2006.)

Curve magnitude is quantified by measuring the Cobb angle of a given curve (Fig. 11.200). Typical idiopathic curves are right thoracic and left lumbar. Coronal balance can be determined by evaluating the position of the CSVL relative to the spine. In a balanced spine, the CSVL should meet the C7 plumb line. In the sagittal plane, Cobb measurements can also be used to determine the degree of thoracic kyphosis and lumbar lordosis. Normal values for thoracic kyphosis are 20 degrees to 45 degrees and lumbar lordosis is normally between 30 and 60 degrees. Generally, idiopathic scoliosis results in hypokyphosis of the thoracic spine. Transverse plane deformities are more difficult to assess on 2-D images, but the Nash–Moe technique tries to quantify the degree of rotation by evaluating the amount of overlap between the pedicles and the vertebral bodies. The Risser sign is a measure of skeletal maturity and is based on the degree of ossification of the iliac crest apophysis, which proceeds from lateral to medial (Fig. 11.201).

In infantile idiopathic scoliosis, it is important to measure the rib vertebral angle difference (RVAD) of Mehta (Fig. 11.202) as this can help predict the risk of curve progression. An RVAD of less than 20 degrees has been shown to be strongly predictive of curve resolution, whereas an RVAD greater than 20 degrees is more likely to progress. Mehta has also reported that overlapping of the rib head with the vertebral body is a poor prognostic sign.

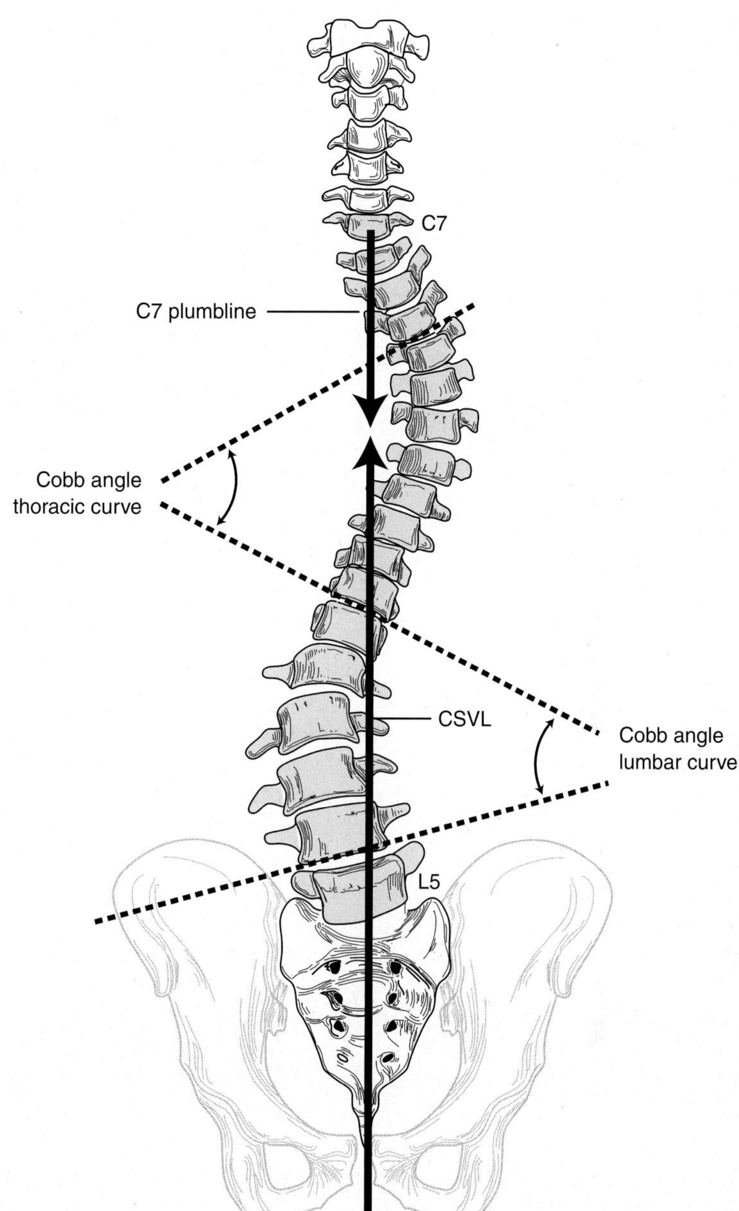

Figure 11.200 Schematic of Cobb angle measurements and central sacral vertical line (CSVL). Coronal compensation exists when the C7 plumb line and the central sacral vertical line meet. The stable vertebrae are bisected by the CSVL. (*Adapted from* Mason DE, Carango P. Spinal decompensation in Cotrel-Dubousset instrumentation. *Spine* 1991;16(suppl 8):S394–S403.)

Special Tests

Computed tomography (CT) scans are generally unnecessary in idiopathic scoliosis but are useful for other diagnoses such as congenital scoliosis and osteoid osteoma. Magnetic resonance imaging (MRI) is the diagnostic modality of choice for all intraspinal anomalies and spinal cord tumors. Most surgeons obtain an MRI of the full spine in young patients (younger than 10 years), patients with a history of significant pain, and those children with objective findings of neurologic dysfunction to rule out an underlying neural axis abnormality. In addition, atypical curve patterns (e.g., left thoracic curves, hyperkyphosis) and rapidly progressive curves should be evaluated with an MRI.

Differential Diagnosis

Idiopathic scoliosis is a diagnosis of exclusion and implies that no other underlying condition is present. Other potential causes of scoliosis include neuromuscular disease, congenital vertebral malformations, collagen disorders, neurofibromatosis, and spinal cord injury. A careful history and physical examination should be sufficient to identify other causes for scoliosis, although an MRI may be necessary to rule out underlying conditions.

Natural History

The risk of deformity progression depends on the amount of growth remaining and the size of the curve. During

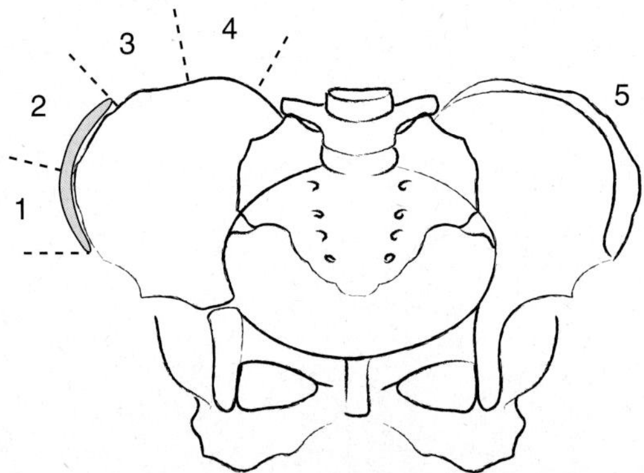

Figure 11.201 Risser sign. The iliac apophysis ossifies in a predictable manner beginning laterally and progressing medially. The capping of the iliac crest is correlated with slowing and completion of growth, generally occurring over a period of 18 to 24 months. (*Reproduced with permission from* Morrissy RT, Weinstein SL. *Lovell and Winter's Pediatric Orthopaedics*. Philadelphia, PA: Lippincott Williams & Wilkins, 2006.)

periods of rapid growth velocity, such as the adolescent growth spurt, curves can progress an average of 1 degree per month. As a result, age at menarche, Tanner stage, Risser sign, and other assessments of physical maturity are important for predicting the behavior of a curve and for planning appropriate treatment. Increasing curve magnitude also raises the risk for progression; double curves are more likely to progress than single curves. In general, curves less than 50 degrees tend to remain stable after skeletal maturity, whereas curves greater than 50 degrees continue to progress 1 degree per year through adulthood. Natural history studies have demonstrated that untreated AIS results in a slightly higher incidence of back pain and altered body image later in adulthood compared with controls. Altered pulmonary function (based on pulmonary function tests) can be seen in curves greater than 60 degrees to 70 degrees and life expectancy may be decreased in curves greater than 100 degrees.

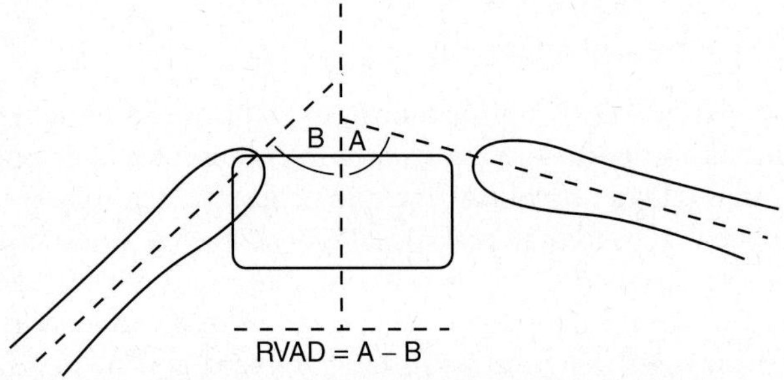

Figure 11.202 The rib vertebral angle difference (RVAD) is measured by determining the angle of the right and left ribs at the apical vertebra. The slope of the ribs relative to the transverse plane is measured for each rib. The difference in the angle between the right and left sides is the RVAD. (*Reproduced with permission from* Morrissy RT, Weinstein SL. *Lovell and Winter's Pediatric Orthopaedics*. Philadelphia, PA: Lippincott Williams & Wilkins, 2006.)

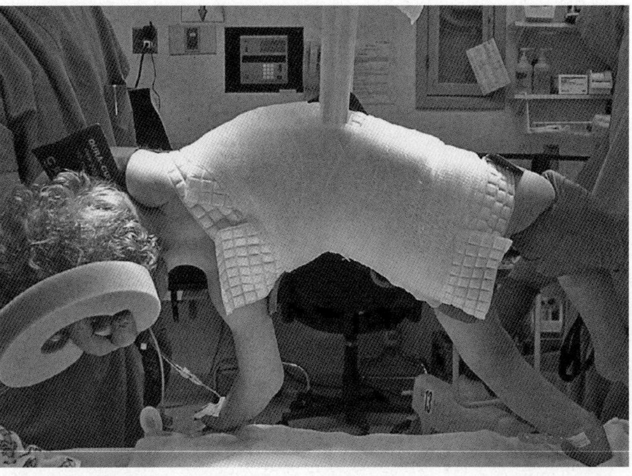

Figure 11.203 Serial casting is often used for the treatment of progressive infantile idiopathic scoliosis. This demonstrates a method of applying a bending force by suspending the trunk with muslin before rolling a Gore-tex lined fiberglass cast. (*Reproduced with permission from* Morrissy RT, Weinstein SL. *Lovell and Winter's Pediatric Orthopaedics*. Philadelphia, PA: Lippincott Williams & Wilkins, 2006.)

Treatment

Infantile idiopathic scoliosis with an RVAD less than 20 degrees is typically observed, although treatment is often instituted if a progression beyond 30 degrees is noted. Children with progressive infantile scoliosis or an RVAD greater than 20 degrees may be treated with serial corrective casting under general anesthesia (Fig. 11.203). These growing children usually require cast changes every 3 months. When the curve has been corrected and maintained at less than 10 degrees, full-time bracing is instituted. In juvenile scoliosis, several studies have shown continued curve progression in spite of brace use. In certain cases, however, bracing may limit the rate of curve progression and may be effective in delaying the need for surgical intervention. As a result, bracing of juveniles is often continued even in larger curves to allow further trunk growth, recognizing that surgical treatment will be needed in the future. In children with progressive infantile and juvenile scoliosis that have failed nonsurgical treatment, early long segment spinal fusion is generally avoided because it can drastically affect trunk height and pulmonary function. Instead, most surgeons favor the use of "growing" instrumentation without fusion, which allows serial lengthenings in the operating room to achieve increased spinal length (Fig. 11.204).

The primary goal of treatment in AIS is to control curve progression and allow children to enter adulthood with a stable spine. Observation is indicated for patients with smaller curves (<25 degrees) and older adolescents (Risser III, IV, or V) with limited growth remaining. Observation is also appropriate for adolescents with significant curves who may have gone beyond the suitable range for bracing but are not yet candidates for surgical treatment.

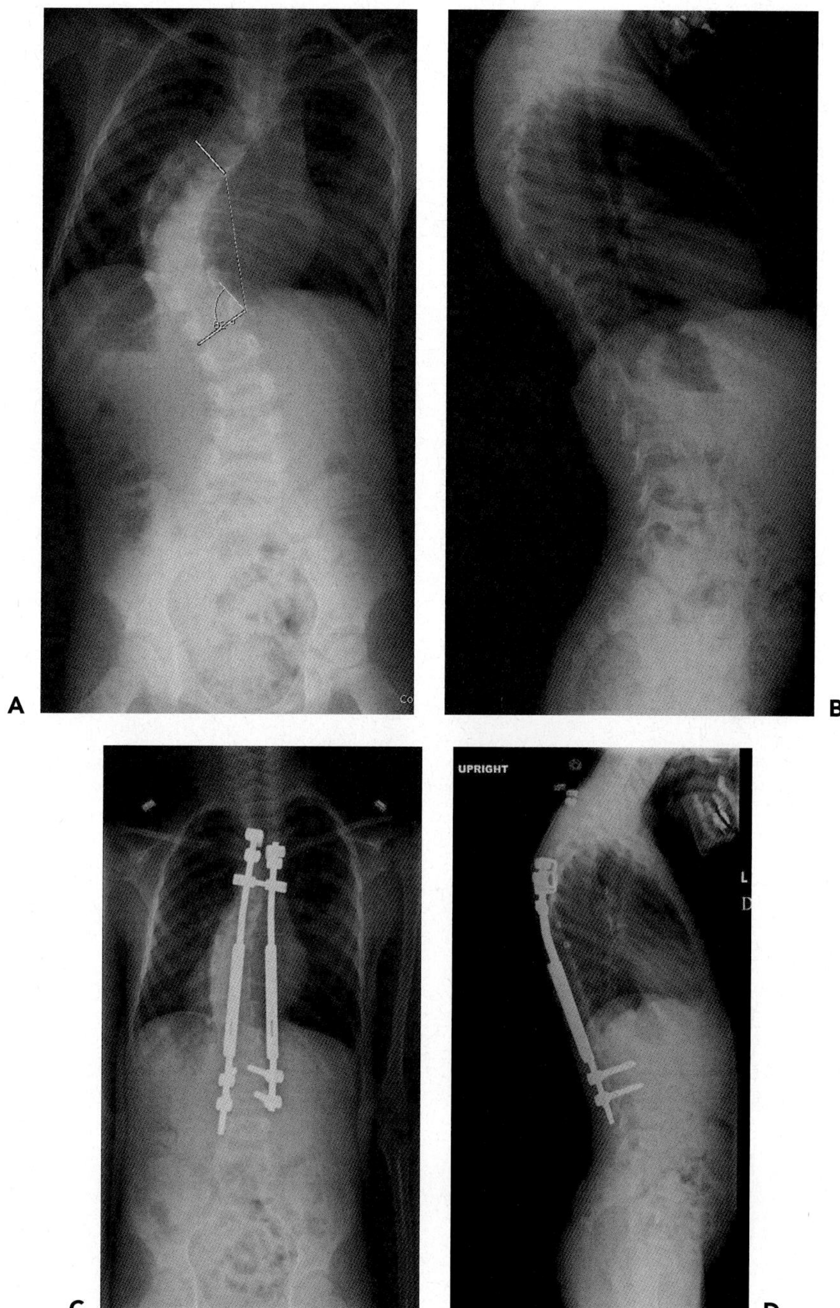

Figure 11.204 **(A, B)** Posteroanterior (PA) and lateral radiograph of a 5-year-old boy with juvenile idiopathic scoliosis and an 82-degree spinal deformity. **(C, D)** PA and lateral radiographs after treatment with growing rod spinal instrumentation. (*Reproduced with permission from* Children's Orthopaedic Center, Los Angeles, CA.)

This would include curves of approximately 40 degrees or 45 degrees in skeletally mature adolescents (Risser III, IV, or V), curves that have not been documented to progress, or well-balanced double major curves between 40 degrees and 50 degrees that are cosmetically unobjectionable in a patient who is near the end of growth. Patients being observed should be followed closely for curve progression, especially during times of rapid growth.

Bracing as a treatment for AIS remains controversial. Previous studies have been limited by unpredictable compliance, variable spinal orthoses, and uncontrolled study designs. Nevertheless, bracing is still the most common nonsurgical treatment modality for AIS. Spinal orthoses provide a three-point mold to achieve curve correction and require continued growth to gradually control spinal deformity. The goal of treatment is to prevent the deformity from worsening; improvement of the curve, while it can occur, should not be expected. Braces are generally prescribed for curves between 25 degrees and 40 degrees in adolescents who are still growing (Risser 0, I, II). A wide variety of braces and bracing protocols exist. Most surgeons favor an underarm thoracolumbosacral orthosis (TLSO) and recommend that it be worn up to 23 hours a day, allowing some time out of the brace for bathing and participation in sports.

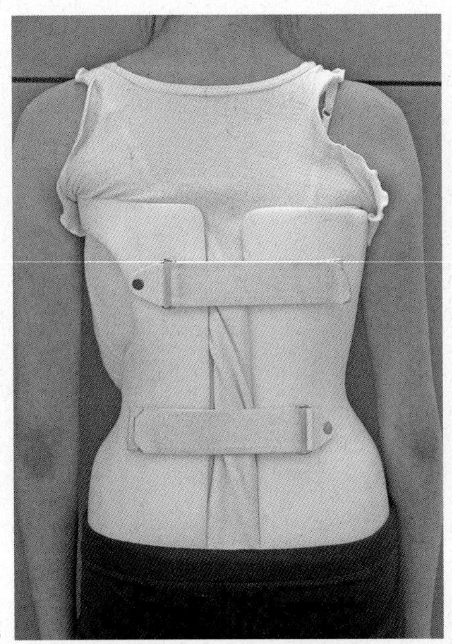

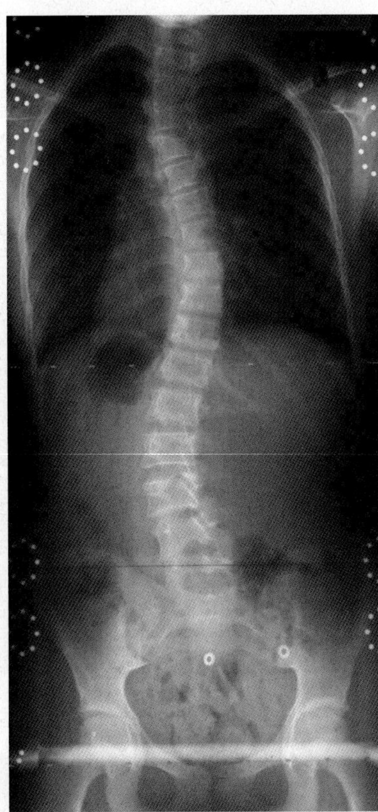

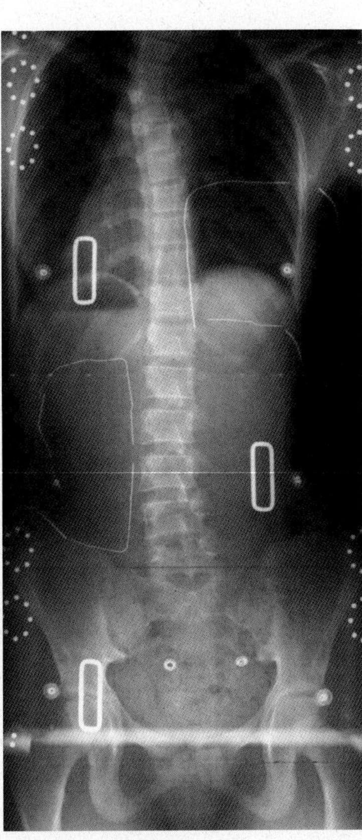

A,B C

Figure 11.205 **(A)** Thoracolumbosacral orthosis underarm brace. **(B)** Posteroanterior radiograph demonstrates a right thoracic and left lumbar curve pattern in an adolescent with remaining growth. **(C)** The in-brace radiograph demonstrates a reduction of both the thoracic and lumbar curves. (*Reproduced with permission from* Morrissy RT, Weinstein SL. *Lovell and Winter's Pediatric Orthopaedics.* Philadelphia, PA: Lippincott Williams & Wilkins, 2006.)

After the brace has been worn for 1 month, a radiograph should be taken in the brace to determine the amount of curve correction since the prognosis for ultimate success is dependent on the initial response to bracing (Fig. 11.205). Bracing is discontinued when curves reach surgical dimensions (45 degrees–50 degrees) or when skeletal maturity has been reached.

Surgery is generally indicated for skeletally immature patients who, despite bracing, have documented progression beyond 45 degrees and for skeletally mature adolescents with curves greater than 50 degrees. These guidelines are based on clear evidence that untreated curves greater than 50 degrees will continue to progress through adulthood while those less than 50 degrees will likely remain stable.

For adolescents at or near skeletal maturity, the standard of care is segmental posterior spinal instrumentation and fusion (Fig. 11.206). The selection of fusion levels depends on the curve pattern, the magnitude of the curve, and the flexibility of the minor curves. Instrumentation generally spans the entire fusion, usually on both sides of the spine. Hooks, wires, or pedicle screws can be used to achieve segmental fixation. The placement of instrumentation posterior to the axis of the spine can create a lordosing effect; as a result, care should be taken to release sufficient tissue and appropriately bend the rods to preserve thoracic kyphosis. Correction of 50% or more with a pseudarthrosis rate of 2% to 3% and a 0.5% risk of neurologic complications can be expected. Release of the anterior longitudinal ligament and discs (either open or thoracoscopically) can be used as an adjunct to posterior spinal fusion in larger, stiffer curves, although the use of modern pedicle screw instrumentation has reduced the need for this.

Anterior fusion with anterior instrumentation has been proposed for certain thoracolumbar and lumbar curves as a means of "saving" distal fusion levels (Fig. 11.207). This approach requires a flexible major curve and a flexible minor curve with documented ability of the distal fusion level to approach horizontal on bending radiographs. Thoracic curves can also be treated by anterior instrumentation and fusion through either an open thoracotomy or a thoracoscopic approach. Concerns about the pulmonary impact of both exposures have quelled some of the enthusiasm for this technique. *Crankshaft phenomenon* is defined as continued progression of the scoliotic deformity due to persistent anterior growth after a posterior-only spinal fusion.

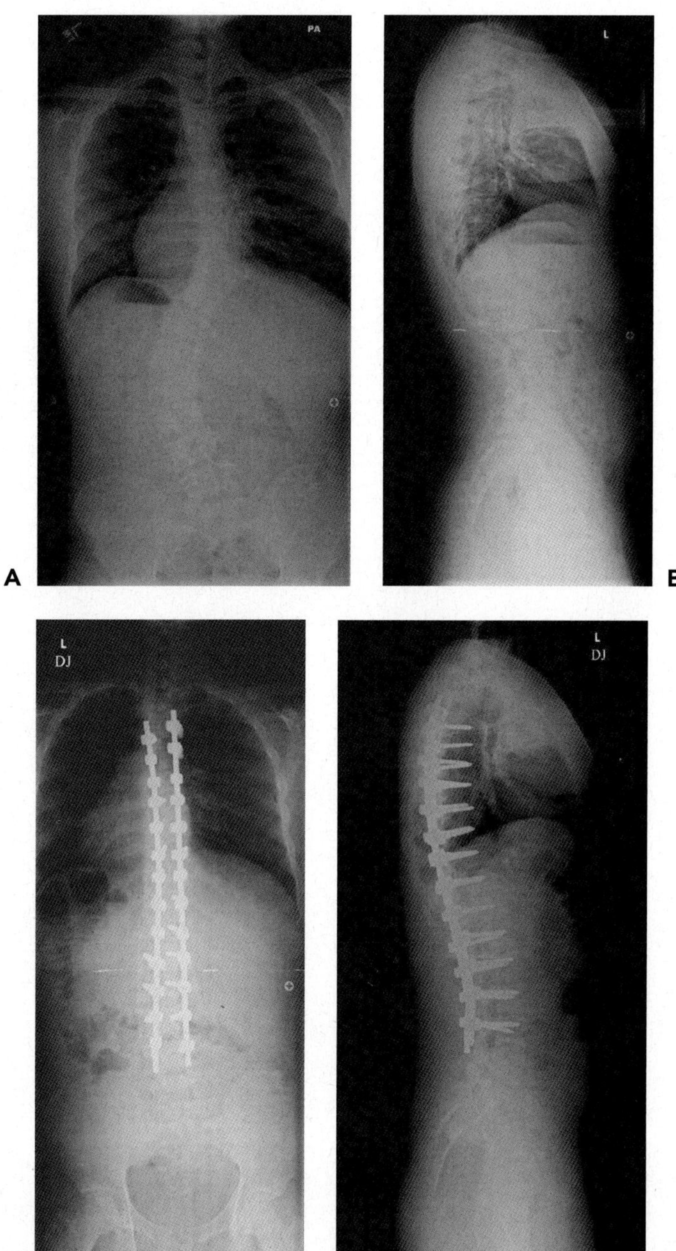

Figure 11.206 **(A, B)** Posteroanterior (PA) and lateral radiographs of a 16-year-old boy with Lenke 3 adolescent idiopathic scoliosis. The thoracic curve measures 53 degrees and the lumbar curve measures 60 degrees. **(C, D)** Postoperative PA and lateral radiographs after posterior spinal instrumentation and fusion. (*Reproduced with permission from* Children's Orthopaedic Center, Los Angeles, CA.)

Combined anterior fusion and posterior fusion and instrumentation have classically been indicated for severe curves and in children younger than 10 years to minimize the risk of crankshaft. The use of modern pedicle screw instrumentation allows for greater curve correction and may decrease the risk of crankshaft with a posterior-only approach.

NEUROMUSCULAR SCOLIOSIS

A number of neuromuscular conditions are seen in which scoliosis is common and contributes significantly to the functional deterioration of the patient. Recognition of the risk of spinal deformity, knowledge of the natural history, and integration of these with patients' overall function and prognosis lead to appropriate decision making.

Pathophysiology and Classification

The exact etiology of neuromuscular scoliosis is poorly understood and likely depends on the underlying condition. In most cases, abnormal muscle forces about the spine from increased spasticity (e.g., cerebral palsy) or muscle weakness (e.g., spinal muscular atrophy, muscular dystrophy)

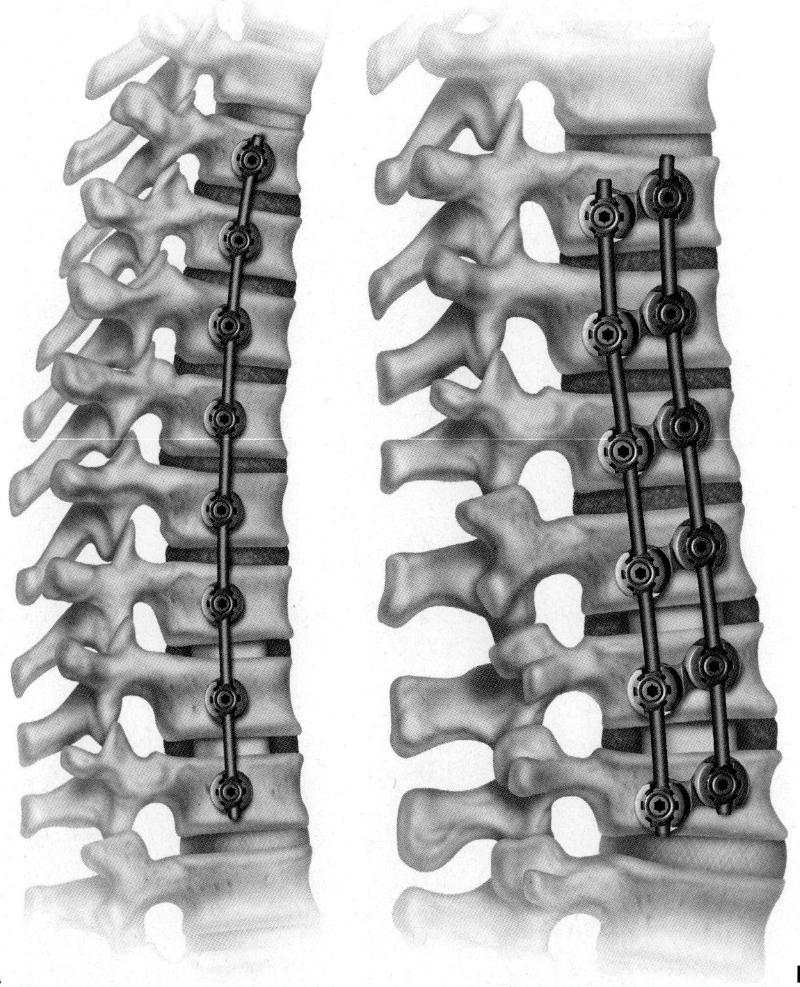

Figure 11.207 **(A)** Schematic of a single-rod anterior construct used for thoracic scoliosis correction. Note the structural grafting of the lower two levels. **(B)** Dual-rod constructs are generally preferred for thoracolumbar scoliosis. (*Reproduced with permission from* Morrissy RT, Weinstein SL. *Lovell and Winter's Pediatric Orthopaedics*. Philadelphia, PA: Lippincott Williams & Wilkins, 2006.)

lead to progressive deformity. Neuromuscular scoliosis has been classified by the Scoliosis Research Society as either neuropathic or myopathic. Neuropathic conditions include upper motor neuron or lower motor neuron abnormalities. The most common upper motor neuron conditions include Friedrich ataxia, Charcot–Marie–Tooth disease, and abnormalities of the spinal cord such as syringomyelia and spinal cord tumors or trauma. Lower motor neuron conditions include poliomyelitis and spinal muscular atrophy. Myopathic conditions include arthrogryposis, congenital hypotonia, and, most importantly, muscular dystrophy.

Presentation

Neuromuscular scoliosis may be diagnosed early in children who are followed for other orthopaedic issues related to their underlying condition. Alternatively, patients may present later with more advanced deformity. These patients generally complain of difficulty sitting due to truncal imbalance and/or pelvic obliquity. In severe cases, ischial ulcers can occur from asymmetric loading. In children with normal cognition, the ability to freely use the upper extremities and function independently in a wheelchair may be compromised by worsening scoliosis. Families with highly involved children often complain that transfers, positioning, and bathing are difficult. Pain may or may not be associated with neuromuscular scoliosis and is often difficult to assess, particularly in patients with cerebral palsy.

History and Physical Examination

Evaluation of a patient with neuromuscular spinal deformity includes assessment of the patient's intellectual skills, communication skills, and sitting capabilities. The presence of contractures, particularly about the hip, or pelvic obliquity should be noted. The skin is carefully assessed for turgor and for any areas of skin breakdown, especially in the ischium. It is essential to evaluate the impact of the curve on the child's ability to sit (Fig. 11.208). In addition to

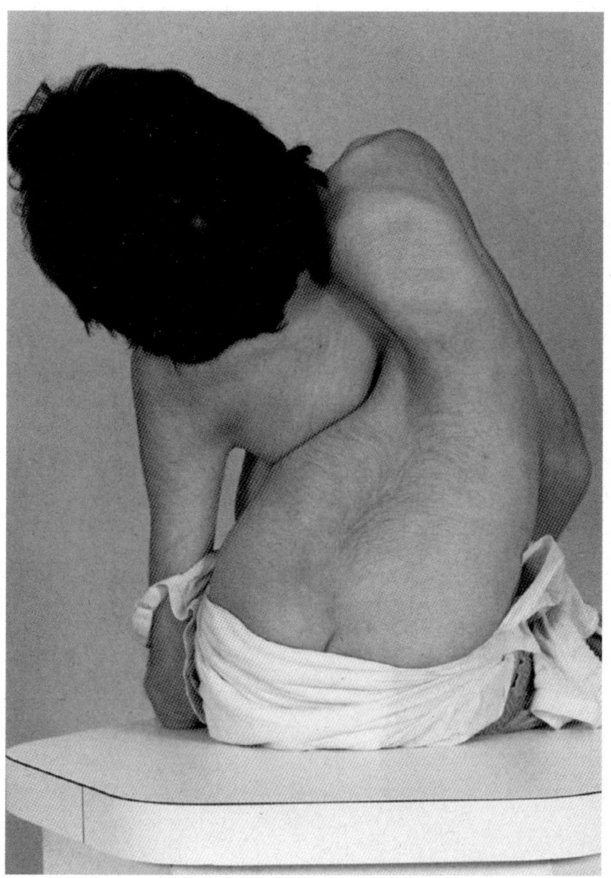
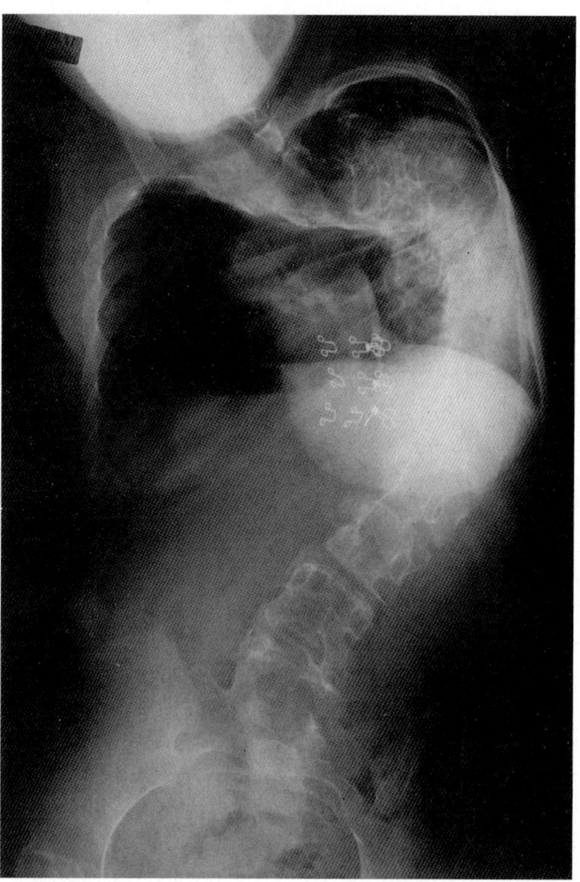

Figure 11.208 Clinical **(A)** and radiographic **(B)** images of a girl with neuromuscular scoliosis due to cerebral palsy. Note the sitting imbalance and pelvic obliquity. (*Reproduced with permission from* Morrissy RT, Weinstein SL. *Lovell and Winter's Pediatric Orthopaedics*. Philadelphia, PA: Lippincott Williams & Wilkins, 2006.)

examining the coronal sitting balance and pelvic obliquity, careful attention must be paid to sagittal plane problems when seated; many patients with poor muscle tone lack head and trunk control and have a tendency to fall forward. The magnitude of the deformity in both the frontal and sagittal plane should be assessed clinically, as should the flexibility of the curve.

It is important when evaluating a child with neuromuscular scoliosis to assess the cardiopulmonary function and the nutritional status. Patients with neuromuscular curves are at risk for, or already have, cardiopulmonary dysfunction. This is frequently exacerbated by alterations in the chest cage seen with scoliosis. These children should be referred for cardiac and pulmonary evaluations to accurately assess the risk of complications and prolonged intubation after surgery. Formal consultation with a nutritionist, if there is any question about the patient's protein balance and caloric intake, is frequently very helpful. Potential surgery should be deferred until a positive nitrogen balance has been achieved to help avoid catastrophic wound complications. At times, this may require the placement of a gastrostomy tube to aid in nutrition prior to spine surgery.

Radiographs

As in cases of idiopathic scoliosis, long-cassette AP and lateral radiographs are necessary to evaluate neuromuscular spinal deformity. Often these patients are nonambulatory, so radiographs must be performed in the seated position (Fig. 11.209). This is preferred over supine radiographs, which can drastically underestimate the degree of spinal deformity. In addition to using the Cobb angle to quantify the severity of the curve, one should assess pelvic obliquity by measuring the angle between the horizontal and a line tangential to the iliac crests (Fig. 11.210). Flexibility is best assessed with traction radiographs since bending radiographs are often difficult to obtain in this patient population.

Special Tests

CT scans are usually not necessary unless there is a suspicion of a congenital vertebral anomaly. Occasionally, CT scans can be helpful in cases of myelodysplasia to determine the presence or absence of posterior elements.

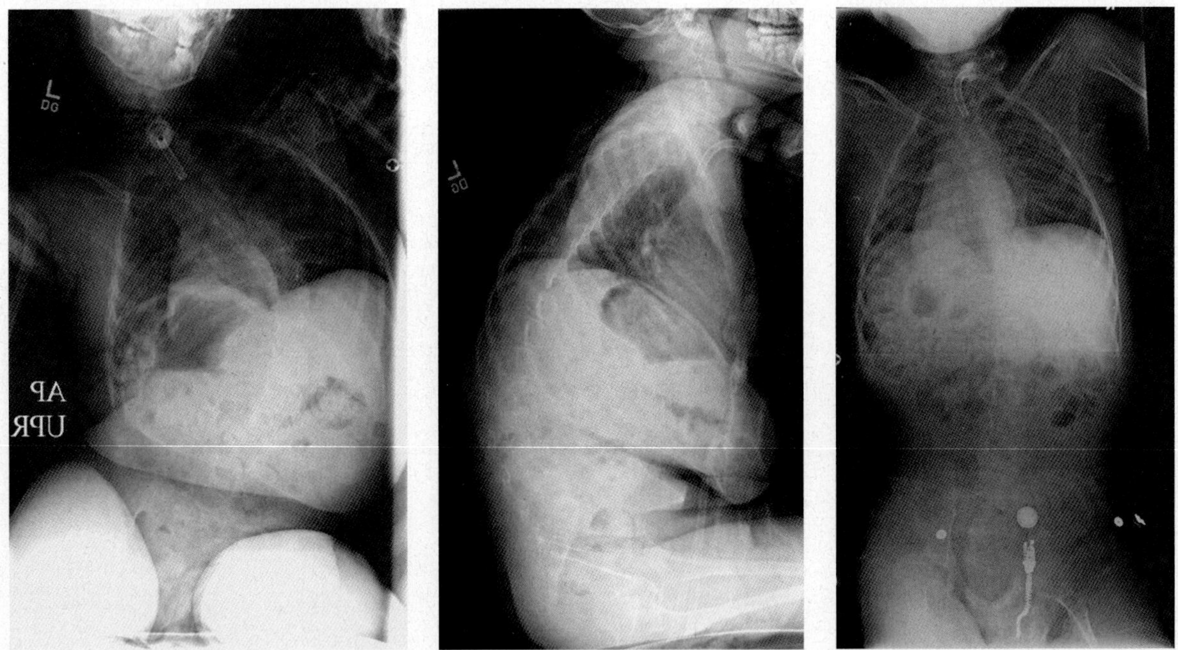

Figure 11.209 **(A, B)** Seated posteroanterior and lateral radiographs of a 10-year-old boy with a mitochondrial disorder and neuromuscular scoliosis. Note the severe thoracolumbar scoliosis and pelvic obliquity. **(C)** In these patients, traction x-rays are superior to bending x-rays to assess curve flexibility. (*Reproduced with permission from* Children's Orthopaedic Center, Los Angeles, CA.)

MRI is indicated for neural axis abnormalities (e.g., syringomyelia) and for cases with more rapid curve progression than would otherwise be suspected for the particular condition.

Differential Diagnosis

The differential diagnosis for neuromuscular scoliosis includes idiopathic scoliosis, congenital scoliosis, and spinal deformity due to connective tissue disorders (e.g., Marfan syndrome, Ehlers–Danlos syndrome). Any spinal deformity in the presence of an underlying neuromuscular disorder can be diagnosed as neuromuscular scoliosis.

Treatment

Nonoperative treatment may include observation, seating support systems, or bracing. Observation is appropriate for mild curves without functional impairment. These children, however, should be closely followed, as most are at relatively high risk for progression. The risk of progression is greatest in patients with spastic quadriplegia, particularly those who are nonambulators. Seating support systems are extremely useful for managing mild to moderate deformities. A well-made support system can accommodate pelvic obliquity, minimize the risk of skin complications, provide assistance in sitting balance, and even assist with head control (Fig. 11.211). Bracing is controversial for neuromuscular spinal deformity. It is generally accepted that bracing is ineffective for correcting spinal deformity. Occasionally, however, curve progression can be halted or at least slowed by a spinal orthosis. More commonly, bracing is employed for young children and for those who need some assistance to sit upright.

Surgical treatment is indicated for progressive curves greater than 60 degrees that are adversely affecting a child's quality of life. In children with Duchenne muscular dystrophy, the cardiopulmonary system can deteriorate rapidly with worsening spinal deformity. As a result, surgery is indicated for curves greater than approximately 30 degrees before the patients are too compromised to tolerate spinal surgery.

Surgical treatment of neuromuscular scoliosis consists of a posterior spinal fusion with segmental instrumentation. The issues to be addressed by the surgeon include whether or not to extend the fusion to the pelvis, the type of segmental instrumentation utilized, and whether or not circumferential fusion is necessary. Fusion to the pelvis is indicated in neuropathic curves such as cerebral palsy in the presence of fixed pelvic obliquity. Fusion to the pelvis should be avoided in ambulators if possible, as this may decrease the patient's ambulatory status. Several options exist for achieving pelvic fixation, including the Galveston technique (custom bent rod with pelvic limbs), unit rod (prebent continuous rod with pelvic limbs), and iliac bolts (Fig. 11.212). Circumferential anterior and posterior fusion has traditionally been advocated for curves at risk for the development of crankshaft phenomenon, for nonunion, and for curves that are very large (greater than 90 degrees–100 degrees), very rigid, or involve significant kyphosis such

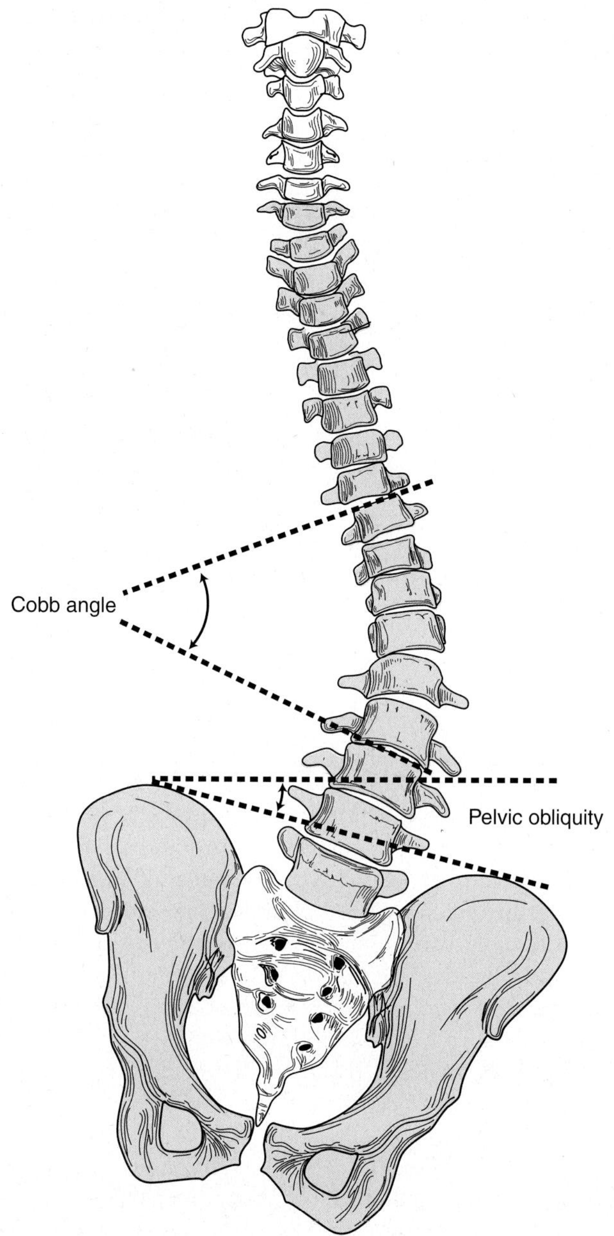

Figure 11.210 Measurement of pelvic obliquity.

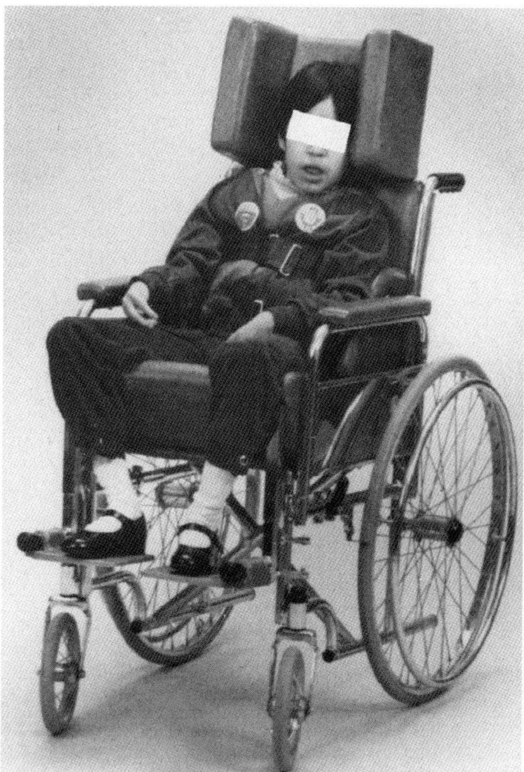

Figure 11.211 An appropriately fitted wheelchair provides proper body positioning, including head control. (*Reproduced with permission from* Morrissy RT, Weinstein SL. *Lovell and Winter's Pediatric Orthopaedics.* Philadelphia, PA: Lippincott Williams & Wilkins, 2006.)

that posterior instrumentation alone is unlikely to result in adequate alignment.

The results of surgery for neuromuscular spinal deformities have varied among authors and are dependent on the underlying disorder. Curve correction between 50% and 75% has been reported for patients with cerebral palsy; with the use of banked allograft bone, a pseudarthrosis rate of 5% to 10% may be expected. Fusion to the pelvis generally results in long-lasting improvement in fixed pelvic obliquity and sitting balance in most patients. Complications are not uncommon in these patients, however, and include wound breakdown, deep infection, and nonunion leading at times to instrumentation failure.

CONGENITAL SPINAL ANOMALIES

Congenital anomalous vertebrae may lead to the development of spinal deformities. These deformities range from mild to severe and are among the types of spinal deformity that are most likely to lead to neurologic impairment and even paraplegia. Because of the propensity for certain types of congenital spinal deformity to progress rapidly, because of the risk of neurologic impairment and intraspinal anomalies, and because of the association of congenital spinal deformity with congenital anomalies of other organ systems, all orthopaedic surgeons should be aware of the implications of congenital deformity of the spine when recognized.

Pathophysiology and Classification

The specific etiology of congenital spine deformities remains largely unknown. Vertebral malformations are thought to arise from a gene disruption during somatogenesis, the process by which the axial skeleton is formed during embryogenesis, or from environmental insults sustained during gestation. Congenital deformities of the spine are categorized by the plane of deformity (scoliosis, kyphosis, or kyphoscoliosis) and the specific type of

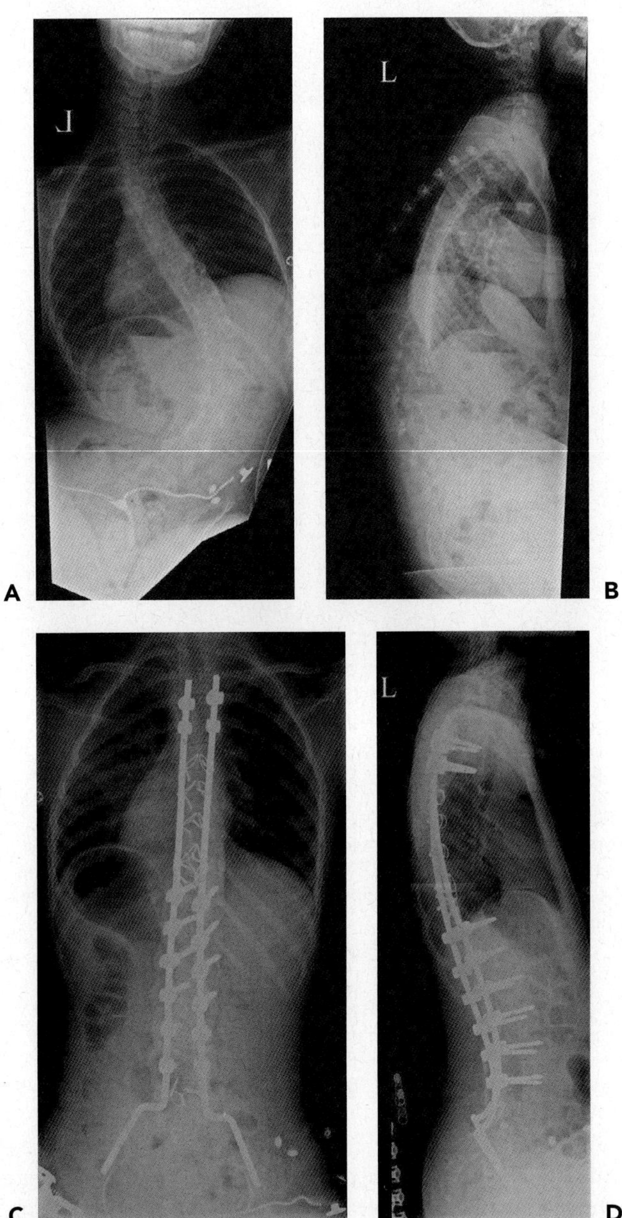

Figure 11.212 **(A, B)** Seated posteroanterior (PA) and lateral radiographs of a 13-year-old boy with neuromuscular scoliosis and pelvic obliquity due to Duchenne muscular dystrophy. **(C, D)** PA and lateral radiographs after posterior spinal instrumentation and fusion using the Galveston technique for pelvic fixation. (*Reproduced with permission from* Children's Orthopaedic Center, Los Angeles, CA.)

vertebral anomaly or anomalies. Vertebral malformations are classified as either failure of formation (type I), failure of segmentation (type II), or mixed anomalies (type III) (Fig. 11.213). Failure of formation usually leads to a hemivertebra. Hemivertebrae can be completely segmented, meaning there is disk tissue separating the anomalous vertebra from both the vertebra above and below it; semisegmented, meaning disk tissue is present either above or below the hemivertebra; or nonsegmented, meaning it is attached to both the vertebra above and below. Hemivertebrae can also be described as incarcerated if the lateral border of the hemivertebra is in line with or medial to a line drawn along the lateral border of the vertebral body above and below. Type II anomalies (failure of segmentation) lead to a fibrous or bony bar between adjacent vertebrae. Bilateral failure of segmentation results in a block vertebra; unilateral segmentation defects result in a unilateral bar on the concave side of the curve. Mixed anomalies (type III) are the most common type of congenital spinal deformity.

Presentation

The incidence of congenital scoliosis in the general population is estimated between 1% and 4%; congenital kyphosis is even rarer. Most children with congenital spine deformities present at an early age, and most are asymptomatic. Young children may present with a mild deformity or with anomalies that were found incidentally on radiographs taken for other reasons. In advanced cases (especially severe congenital kyphosis), patients may present with neurologic deficits.

History and Physical Examination

Physical examination should include evaluation of spine and shoulder symmetry, overall balance, and cervical, thoracic, and lumbar flexibility. Neck range of motion and scapular height should be assessed because of the strong association of congenital spinal deformity with Klippel–Feil syndrome and Sprengel deformity. A careful neurologic examination including sensation, motor strength, and reflexes is warranted in all children with congenital spine deformity. Neurologic deficits can be due to the vertebral anomalies themselves or from an associated spinal dysraphism that exists in 20% to 40% of children with congenital spinal deformity. The most common neural axis abnormality is a tethered cord, but Chiari type I malformations, diastematomyelia, syringomyelia, or a low conus can also be seen. Physical findings associated with an intraspinal anomaly include a cavus foot, hairy patches, dimples, nevi, or asymmetrical or absent abdominal reflexes.

In addition to the association with neural axis abnormalities, congenital spinal deformity is frequently associated with defects in other organ systems. The incidence of coexisting congenital heart disease (particularly ventricular or atrial septal defects and patent ductus arteriosus) is approximately 10%. As a result, all patients with congenital spinal deformity should be referred for a cardiac evaluation and an echocardiogram if indicated. Approximately 25% to 40% of patients with congenital spine deformity have anomalies of the genitourinary (GU) tract, the most common of which is unilateral renal agenesis. An MRI of the kidneys or renal ultrasound should, therefore, be performed on most patients.

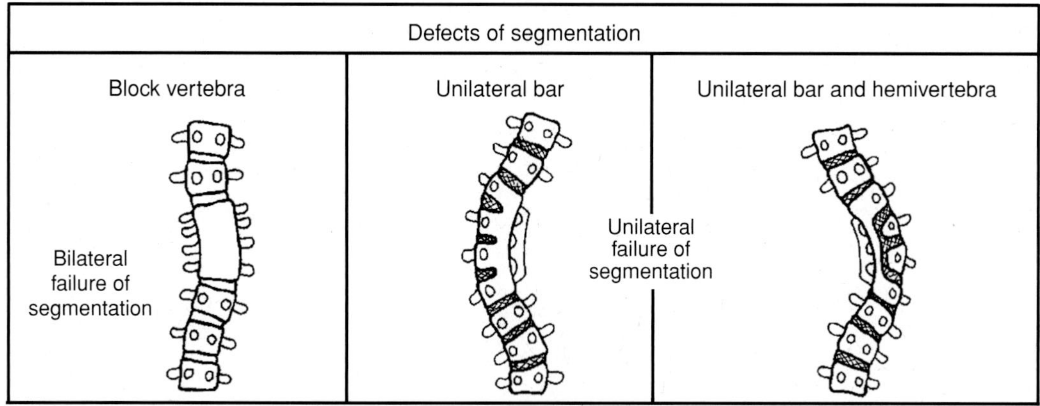

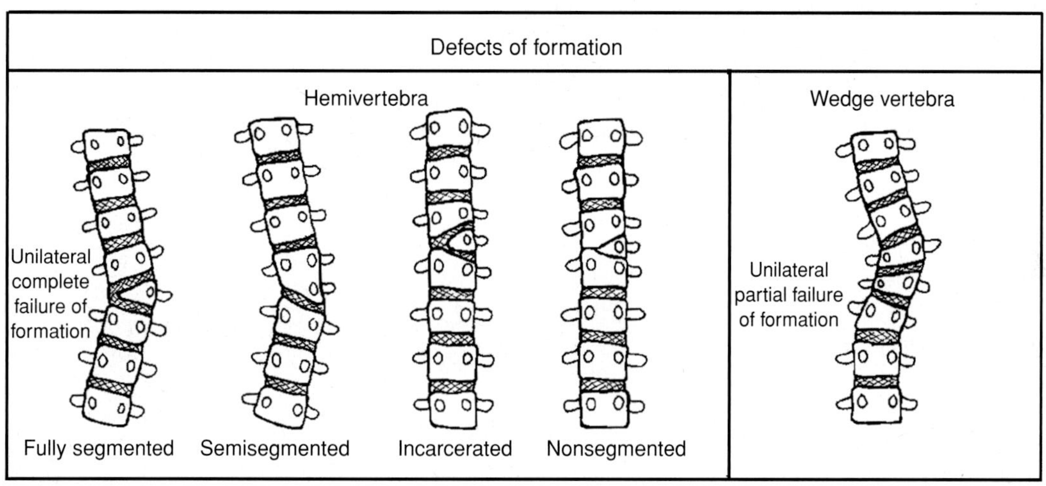

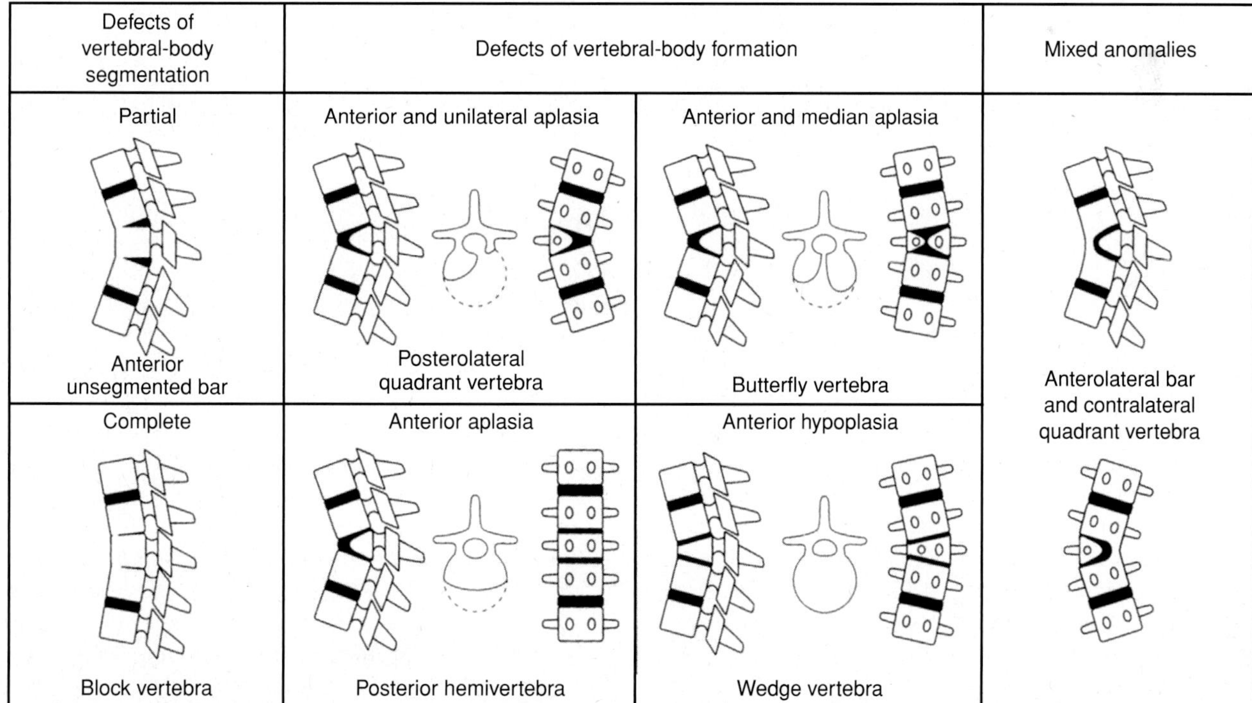

Figure 11.213 Classification of congenital scoliosis. (*Reproduced with permission from* Morrissy RT, Weinstein SL. *Lovell and Winter's Pediatric Orthopaedics.* Philadelphia, PA: Lippincott Williams & Wilkins, 2006.)

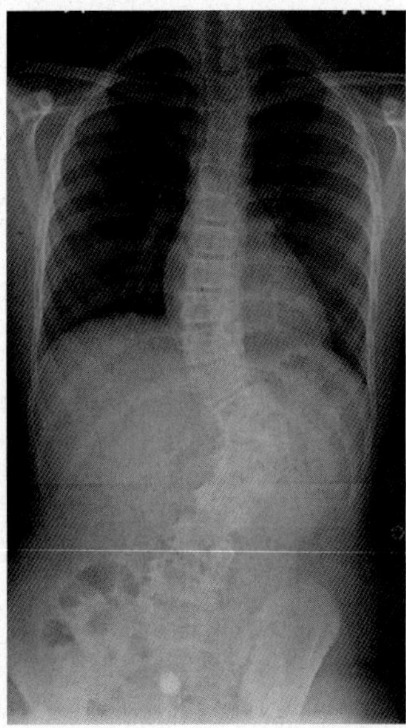

A

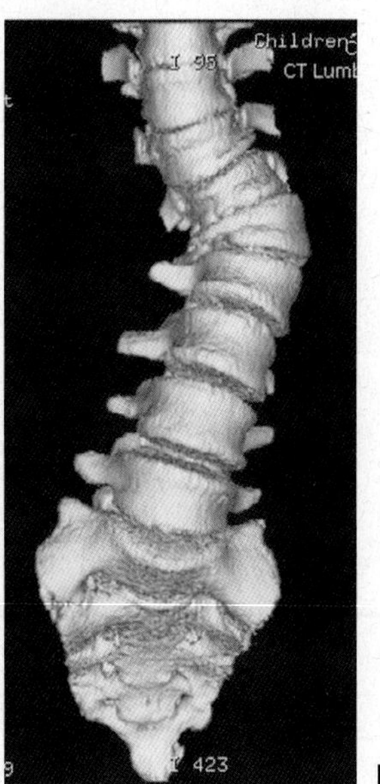

B

Figure 11.214 **(A)** Anteroposterior spinal radiograph demonstrating a L1 hemivertebra. **(B)** Three-dimensional computed tomography reconstruction more clearly defines the nature of the hemivertebra. (*Reproduced with permission from* Children's Orthopaedic Center, Los Angeles, CA.)

Radiographs

The initial diagnostic tests of choice are high-quality radiographs of the entire spine. Careful evaluation of the vertebrae and disk spaces is important to define the area of spine involvement and to determine the specific pattern of deformity (Fig. 11.214). Identifying one vertebral anomaly should prompt a search for other contiguous and noncontiguous malformations. The overall radiographic balance of the spine should be assessed. For example, contralateral hemivertebrae can result in a relatively balanced curve and a stable spine deformity. In addition to evaluating the coronal plane deformity, it is essential to obtain lateral radiographs to adequately examine the sagittal plane. Kyphosis, not scoliosis, is the most concerning type of congenital spinal deformity due to its high risk for neurologic complications.

Special Tests

CT scan is the diagnostic modality of choice for evaluating bony anatomy and is extremely useful for elucidating vertebral malformations that can often be difficult to define on the basis of plain radiographs. In particular, CT scans with 3-D reconstructions can be very helpful for understanding abnormal anatomy and planning corrective surgery. MRI is indicated in all children with congenital spinal deformity to rule out an intraspinal anomaly (Fig. 11.215). As mentioned, renal ultrasound and echocardiogram may be necessary to look for coexisting GU or cardiac abnormalities.

Differential Diagnosis

The differential diagnosis of isolated congenital scoliosis includes scoliosis due to syndromes and idiopathic scoliosis. VATER syndrome (Vertebral anomalies, Anorectal anomalies, TracheoEsophageal fistula, and Renal and vascular abnormalities) and Goldenhar syndrome (ocular, auricular, and vertebral defects) can both be associated with vertebral body malformations and scoliosis. Usually, the presence of the associated organ system anomalies helps distinguish isolated congenital scoliosis from these other diagnoses. Idiopathic scoliosis, especially infantile and juvenile forms, can occur in a similar age group as congenital scoliosis. In idiopathic scoliosis, however, radiographs do not demonstrate any defects in vertebral segmentation or formation. The differential diagnosis of kyphosis in young children includes postinfectious kyphosis, achondroplasia, Scheuermann kyphosis, and trauma.

Treatment

Treatment of congenital spinal deformity is determined by the natural history of the specific anomalies present, an assessment of the potential for curve progression, and the risk of neurologic deterioration. McMaster and Ohtsuka, in a large review, demonstrated significant progression in 75% of their patients. Both the region of the spine and the type of anomaly impacted on the risk of progression (Table 11.7). The worst prognosis was seen in patients with a unilateral unsegmented bar opposite a hemivertebra, although an isolated unilateral unsegmented bar was also at significant risk for progression. The best prognosis was seen with isolated hemivertebra, particularly incarcerated, semisegmented, and nonsegmented hemivertebrae. Defects at the thoracolumbar junction had a higher risk of progression than elsewhere; however, because of the impact on shoulder balance, defects in the upper thoracic and cervicothoracic spine resulted in the most readily apparent clinical deformities seen.

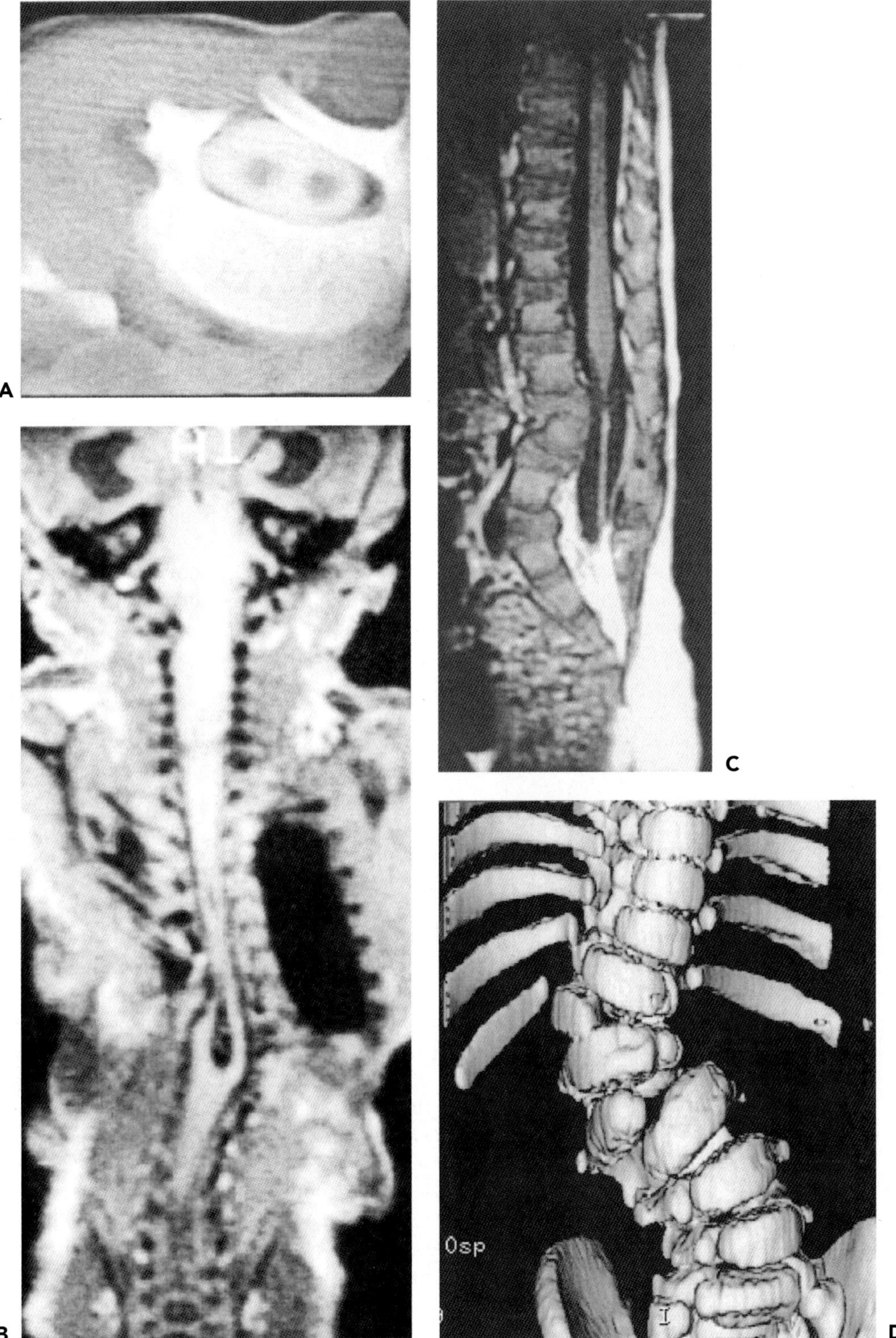

Figure 11.215 **(A)** Intraspinal anomalies accompanying vertebral anomalies are common. Indications for magnetic resonance imaging include planned surgical intervention, abnormalities found on neurologic examination, and progressive curvature in the unaffected section of the spine. Diplomyelia is visible in this computed tomography (CT) myelogram. **(B)** Diastematomyelia, diplomyelia, tethered spinal cord, and other anomalies are present in this infant with multiple vertebral anomalies. **(C)** Tethered spinal cord with thickened filum terminale. **(D)** A CT scan with three-dimensional reconstruction is helpful to understand the details of congenital vertebral anomalies. Two lumbar hemivertebrae are readily visible here. (*Reproduced with permission from* Morrissy RT, Weinstein SL. *Lovell and Winter's Pediatric Orthopaedics.* Philadelphia, PA: Lippincott Williams & Wilkins, 2006.)

TABLE 11.7

LIKELIHOOD OF PROGRESSION OF CONGENITAL SCOLIOSIS ASSOCIATED WITH DIFFERENT VERTEBRAL ANOMALIES, BASED ON ANNUAL RATE OF PROGRESSION

	Type of Congenital Anomaly					
			Hemivertebra			
Site of Curvature	**Block Vertebra**	**Wedge Vertebra**	**Single**	**Double**	**Unilateral Unsegmented Bar**	**Unilateral Unsegmented Bar and Contralateral Hemivertebrae**
Upper thoracic	<1°–1°	*–2°	1°–2°	2°–2.5°	2°–4°	5°–6°
Lower thoracic	<1°–1°	2°–3°	2°–2.5°	2°–3°	5°–6.5°	6°–7°
Thoracolumbar	<1°–1°	1.5°–2°	2°–3.5°	5°–*	6°–9°	>10°–*
Lumbar	<1°–*	<1°–*	<1°–1°	*	>5°–*	*
Lumbosacral	*	*	<1°–1.5°	*	*	*

☐ No treatment required ▣ May require spinal surgery ☐ Require spinal fusion * Too few or no curves.
Ranges represent the degree of derotation before and after 10 years of age.

The natural history of congenital kyphosis also depends on the type of vertebral anomalies and the age of the patient. Type III (mixed anomalies) malformations usually result in the most rapid curve progression, followed by type I malformations. Of all congenital spinal deformities, congenital kyphosis has the highest risk of neurologic compromise (Fig. 11.216).

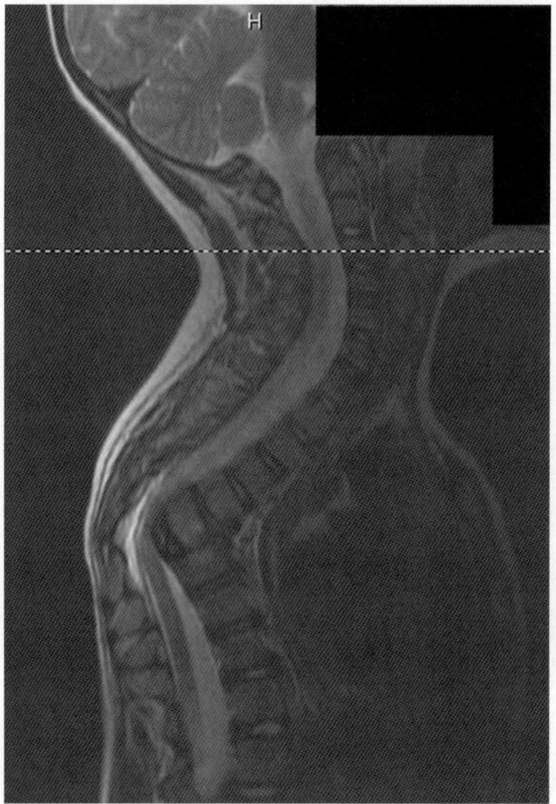

Figure 11.216 Congenital kyphosis has the highest risk of neurologic impairment. Sagittal magnetic resonance imaging view of a 4-year-old boy who presented with myelopathy. The spinal cord is draped across the apex of the deformity. (*Reproduced with permission from* Children's Orthopaedic Center, Los Angeles, CA.)

Children with mild spinal deformity and a favorable natural history can be followed with serial radiographs until skeletal maturity. The frequency of radiographic evaluation depends on the risk of curve progression and the patient's age. Congenital curves are usually less flexible than idiopathic curves; and therefore, bracing is rarely effective in controlling the primary curve. Occasionally, bracing can be helpful for managing compensatory curves.

In congenital scoliosis, surgery is indicated to halt progressive deformity and spinal imbalance. All surgical procedures involve some amount of spinal fusion and can potentially decrease the overall spine length in these growing children. The risks of limiting growth potential, however, must be compared with the risks of continued asymmetric growth and worsening spinal deformity. Early, limited in situ fusion can stop curve progression with relatively low risk of complications. For younger children, a combined anterior and posterior arthrodesis should be considered to minimize the risk of crankshaft phenomenon. In smaller children, postoperative immobilization can consist of a cast or brace. Instrumentation can be used to stabilize the arthrodesis and achieve more curve correction; however, the neurologic risks of instrumentation are higher in children with congenital scoliosis than in children with idiopathic scoliosis. For children younger than 5 years with progressive deformity due to a fully segmented hemivertebra, convex anterior and posterior hemiepiphysiodesis may allow for continued growth on the concave side of the curve, thereby causing some gradual improvement of the deformity. In more severe deformities, hemivertebra excision can be performed (Fig. 11.217). This procedure allows for greater correction but does carry an increased risk of neurologic complications.

Because of their tendency to progress and the high risk for neurologic deterioration, most cases of congenital kyphosis warrant surgery. Posterior fusion alone can be performed in children younger than 5 years with curves less than 55 degrees, as this can allow for some improvement in

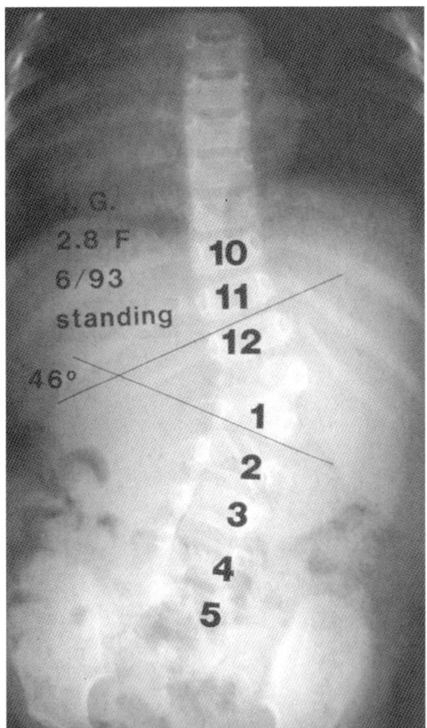

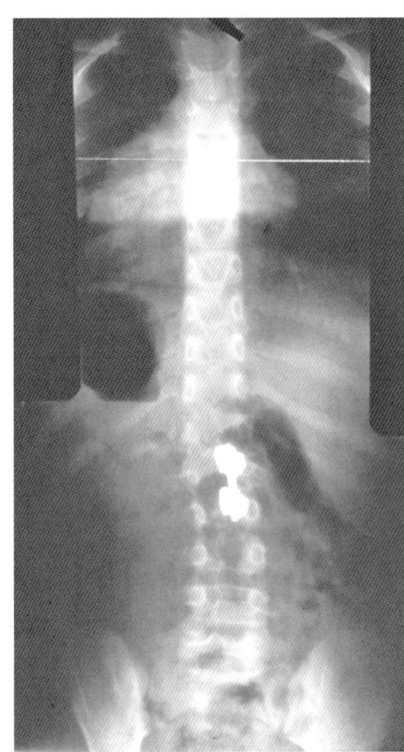

Figure 11.217 **(A)** Posteroanterior (PA) radiograph showing a hemivertebra between T12 and L1 that has caused scoliosis. **(B)** Final PA radiographs after excision of the hemivertebra and correction of the deformity. (*Reproduced with permission from* Skaggs DL, Tolo VT. *Master Techniques in Orthopaedic Surgery: Pediatrics.* Philadelphia, PA: Lippincott Williams & Wilkins, 2008.)

the deformity with anterior spinal growth. Instrumentation is often used primarily for stabilization rather than for correction because of the neurologic risk associated with large correction. Anterior and posterior fusion is often necessary in older patients and in kyphosis greater than 55 degrees.

SCHEUERMANN KYPHOSIS

While scoliosis refers to deformities in the coronal plane, kyphosis is measured in the sagittal plane. The normal thoracic spine has slight kyphosis ranging from 20 degrees to 45 degrees (Fig. 11.218). The thoracolumbar spine should be relatively straight between T10 and L2, and the lumbar spine below L2 should have more lordosis than the thoracic spine has kyphosis. Abnormal thoracic kyphosis can be due to multiple etiologies, but Scheuermann kyphosis is one of the most classic causes in an adolescent.

Pathophysiology

The etiology of Scheuermann kyphosis continues to be debated. Mechanical and metabolic factors have been suggested, and disruption of the cartilage ring apophysis, abnormalities of the endplates leading to Schmorl node formation (herniation of disk material through the endplate), and genetic factors have all been implicated. These endplate disturbances cause anterior wedging of the vertebral bodies and the resultant kyphosis.

Presentation

Scheuermann kyphosis occurs in 0.4% to 8.3% of the population and is more common in boys than in girls. Unlike juvenile forms of scoliosis, Scheuermann kyphosis is rarely diagnosed prior to age 10, typically presenting during later teenage years. Patients are usually brought to a surgeon because of concerns on the part of the parents about hunched posture. Mild to moderate thoracic back pain is more common in more severe deformities or in deformity of the thoracolumbar junction or upper lumbar spine. Natural history studies have shown that although affected patients seem to have more back pain than health controls, their ability to perform activities of daily living or maintain gainful employment is not altered.

Physical Examination

Typical patients with Scheuermann kyphosis have rigid hyperkyphosis of the midthoracic or lower thoracic spine. There is often compensatory hyperlordosis of the lumbar spine. This rigidity distinguishes Scheuermann kyphosis from more benign causes such as postural kyphosis and can be assessed by positioning the prone patients on the examining table and asking them to hyperextend the back and lift the head. The sagittal profile during a forward bending test often appears more sharply angulated compared with the gentle roundness of postural kyphosis (Fig. 11.219). Associated hamstring tightness is common and should be evaluated by measuring the popliteal angles (Fig. 11.220).

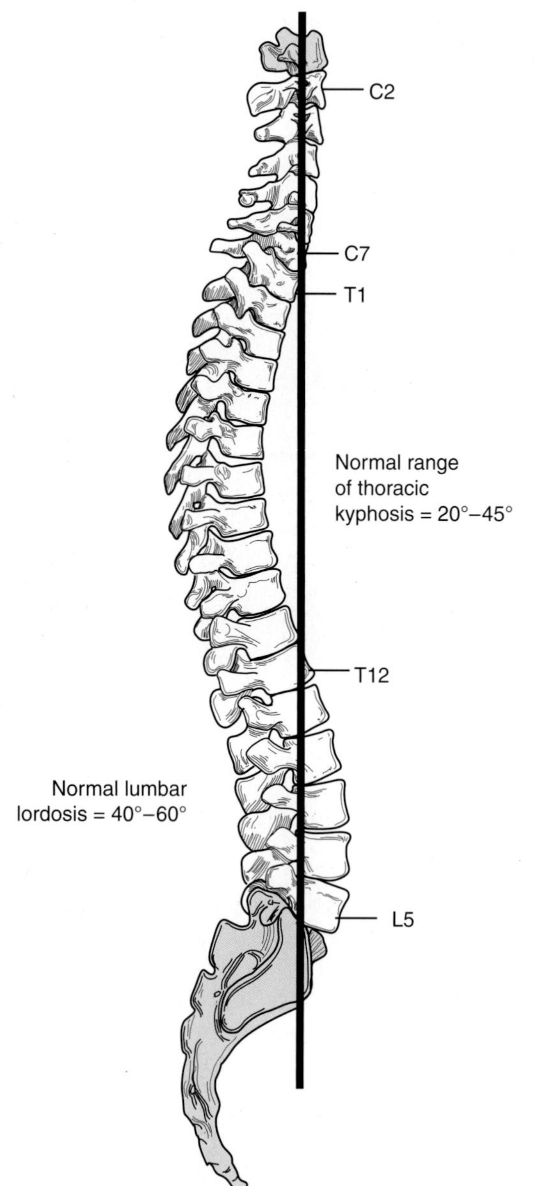

Figure 11.218 Normal sagittal alignment of the spine. (*Adapted from* Abel MF. *Orthopaedic Knowledge Update: Pediatrics.* Rosemont, IL: American Academy of Orthopaedic Surgeons, 2006.)

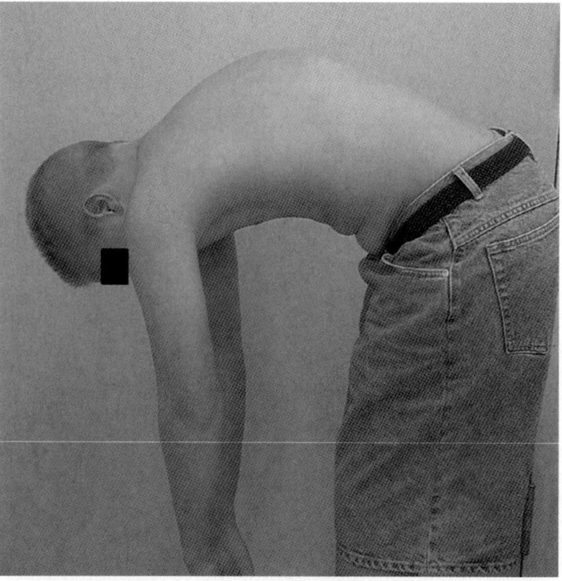

Figure 11.219 In Scheuermann kyphosis, the sagittal profile appears more sharply angulated than the gentle "roundness" of postural kyphosis. (*Reproduced with permission from* Children's Orthopaedic Center, Los Angeles, CA.)

As with any condition of the spine, a thorough neurologic examination including strength, sensation, and reflexes is warranted.

Radiographs

The classic radiographic criteria for diagnosing Scheuermann kyphosis are (1) wedging of three adjacent vertebrae of 5 degrees or more, (2) endplate irregularity, and (3) Schmorl node formation (Fig. 11.221). Many consider changes in a single vertebral body especially in the thoracolumbar or lumbar spine to be forms of Scheuermann kyphosis, even though these patients do not meet the strict definition of the disease. Long-cassette radiographs should also be obtained in the AP plane to evaluate for a concomitant scoliotic deformity. A coexisting spondylolysis should be ruled out on lateral radiographs as these occur in increased frequency in patients with Scheuermann kyphosis.

Special Tests

MRI is indicated as a preoperative study to rule out any spinal cord abnormalities. In addition, MRI is useful to evaluate the health of lumbar disks, because the presence of disk degeneration may be the underlying cause of the patient's symptoms and can alter the extent of fusion.

Differential Diagnosis

The differential diagnosis for abnormal kyphosis includes postural kyphosis, congenital kyphosis, and posttraumatic kyphosis among others. The most common kyphotic disorder seen by the orthopaedist is the adolescent with postural round back. Long-standing complaints of "poor posture" are common and may have been present in other members of the family. An appreciation of the tendency of some adolescents going through puberty to habitually stand with rounded shoulders may explain the perceived increase in kyphosis. Postural roundback may be differentiated from Scheuermann kyphosis by the lack of characteristic endplate changes on radiographs, increased flexibility of the spine, and more generalized rounding in the sagittal plane compared with the more localized, angular appearance of

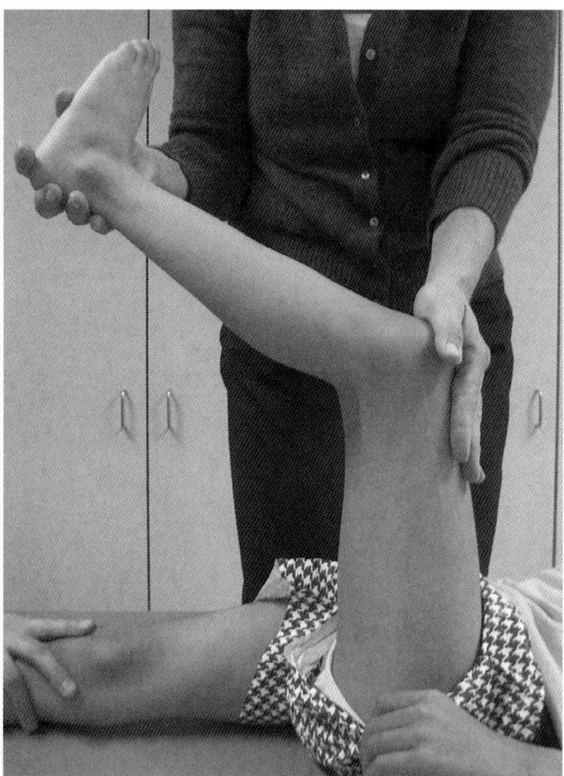

Figure 11.220 The popliteal angle is measured by flexing the hip to 90 degrees and extending the knee. The popliteal angle is the angle formed between the leg and the vertical.

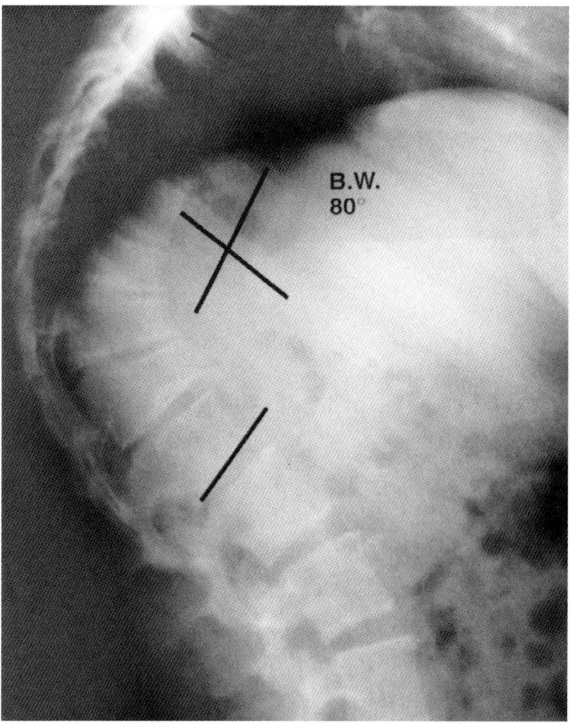

Figure 11.221 Lateral radiograph of a patient with Scheuermann kyphosis demonstrates the kyphotic deformity seen with this disorder. Note the irregularity of the vertebral endplates, Schmorl node formation, and the anterior vertebral wedging. (*Reproduced with permission from* Morrissy RT, Weinstein SL. *Lovell and Winter's Pediatric Orthopaedics.* Philadelphia, PA: Lippincott Williams & Wilkins, 2006.)

Scheuermann kyphosis. Patients with postural kyphosis can be treated with observation or an exercise program focusing on core strengthening. Congenital kyphosis can often be difficult to distinguish from Scheuermann kyphosis, especially in those children with failure of segmentation whose boney bars do not appear until later in adolescence. Congenital kyphosis, however, tends to present at younger ages compared with Scheuermann kyphosis. Additional studies such as MRI, and possibly CT scans, are usually sufficient to distinguish the diagnoses.

Treatment

Nonoperative treatment is classically indicated for growing children with kyphosis greater than 45 degrees to 50 degrees. Physical therapy can be useful to improve symptoms and reduce hamstring tightness but is not capable of improving the deformity. Bracing is helpful only in patients with somewhat flexible deformities and at least a year of growth remaining. Long-term results are best in curves less than 75 degrees and when the more extensive Milwaukee brace is used. Underarm orthoses, such as the TLSO, are at a mechanical disadvantage in most cases of Scheuermann kyphosis but may be utilized for curves with an apex below T9, particularly for disease occurring at the thoracolumbar junction.

The indications for surgical treatment of Scheuermann kyphosis are not well defined. Generally, surgery can be considered for patients with kyphosis greater than 75 degrees, persistent pain recalcitrant to nonoperative treatment, and certainly for any cases with neurologic impairment. Unlike scoliosis, the effect of severe kyphosis on pulmonary function is mild: in most cases, pulmonary function tests are either normal or even increased. As a result, the decision for surgery should be made on an individual basis for those adolescents who have failed bracing and who have a sufficiently objectionable cosmetic appearance as perceived by the patient, the parent, and the surgeon. Surgical treatment consists of posterior spinal fusion with instrumentation (Fig. 11.222). Anterior release of the thickened and shortened anterior longitudinal ligament (either open or thoracoscopic) is classically indicated for curves that do not correct to less than 50 degrees on forced hyperextension lateral radiographs. However, the advent of modern segmental instrumentation with pedicle screws combined with multiple posterior osteotomies has reduced the need for anterior surgery. It is important when undertaking surgery to select the appropriate fusion levels including an appreciation of the uppermost kyphotic segment and extending the fusion distally, not only to the

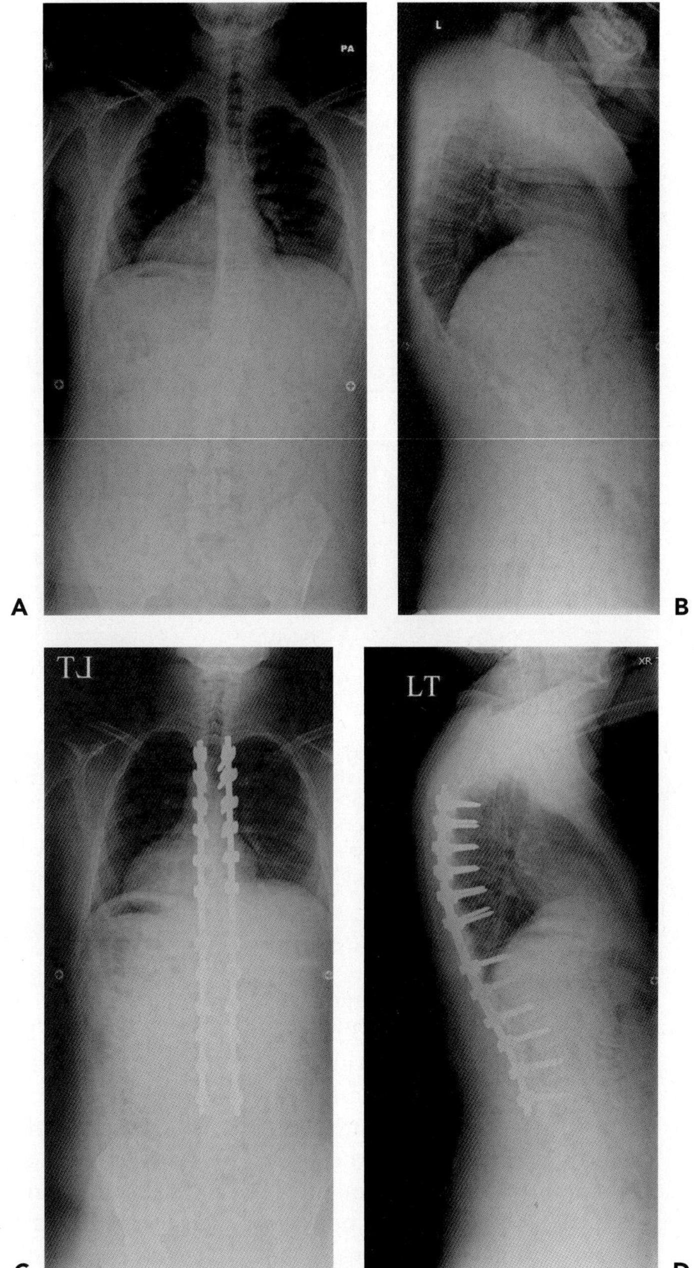

Figure 11.222 **(A, B)** Posteroanterior (PA) and lateral radiographs of a 17-year-old boy with symptomatic Scheuermann kyphosis and 80 degrees of sagittal plane deformity. **(C, D)** PA and lateral radiographs 1 year after posterior spinal instrumentation and fusion. (*Reproduced with permission from* Children's Orthopaedic Center, Los Angeles, CA.)

lowest involved level but also to and across the first lordotic disk space. This may require extending the fusion down as low as L2 or L3 but is necessary to reduce the risk of junctional kyphosis.

CERVICAL SPINE DISORDERS

Klippel–Feil Syndrome

In 1912, Klippel and Feil described massive congenital fusion of the cervical spine in a 46-year-old tailor with multiple associated anomalies. Since then, the classic triad of Klippel–Feil syndrome has consisted of a short neck, low posterior hairline, and marked limitation of motion of the neck. Most surgeons now consider any case of congenital fusion of cervical vertebrae to constitute an example of Klippel–Feil syndrome and to suggest that the patient is at risk for associated anomalies (Fig. 11.223).

The etiology of Klippel–Feil syndrome continues to be disputed. Theories include primary vascular disruption, fetal insult, primary neural tube abnormality, and a primary genetic etiology. The incidence of this condition has never been determined, but reasonable estimates vary from 0.2 to 7 per 1000.

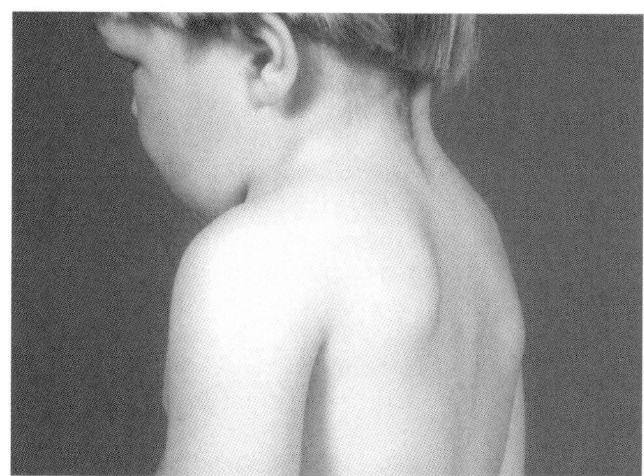
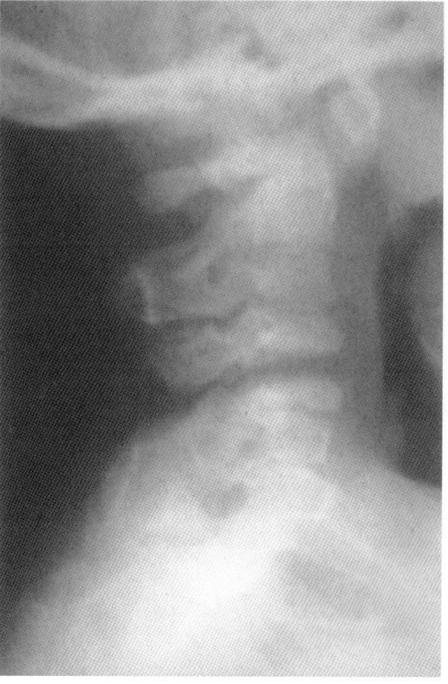

Figure 11.223 A 3-year-old boy with Klippel–Feil syndrome. **(A)** Note the short neck and low posterior hair line. **(B)** The lateral cervical spine radiograph demonstrates complete fusion of the posterior elements of C2–C3, with reduced disc height anteriorly. Note the reduced space between C3 and C4, which most likely represents a cartilage fusion between C3 and C4 that will probably progress to an osseous fusion later in life. (*Reproduced with permission from* Morrissy RT, Weinstein SL. *Lovell and Winter's Pediatric Orthopaedics.* Philadelphia, PA: Lippincott Williams & Wilkins, 2006.)

Probably the most important aspect of the Klippel–Feil syndrome is its association with other syndromes and anomalies. Congenital cervical fusion has been reported in fetal alcohol syndrome, as well as in Goldenhar syndrome. The most common associated musculoskeletal anomaly is scoliosis, which is most often congenital. Sprengel deformity, cervical ribs, thoracic outlet syndrome, and torticollis are also seen. The most common associated craniofacial anomaly is hearing loss, reported in 15% to 36% of patients. CNS anomalies include synkinesis (involuntary paired movement of the hands and arms), syringomyelia, and diastematomyelia. An increased incidence of congenital cervical spinal stenosis is a well-known phenomenon; this may be complicated by the development of instability adjacent to the congenital fusion, which is also common in Klippel–Feil syndrome. GU anomalies are present in 25% to 35% of patients. Distribution is similar to that of congenital scoliosis, and the most common anomaly is unilateral renal agenesis. As with congenital spine deformity, routine screening of the GU tract with ultrasound has been recommended for patients with Klippel–Feil syndrome.

Congenital cervical spine fusion is, in many individuals, asymptomatic. On the other hand, progressive instability may develop secondary to abnormal stresses on motion segments above or below the areas of congenital fusion. This instability, particularly in individual with preexisting stenosis, may lead to clinically significant spinal cord or nerve root compression. Three fusion patterns have been defined that may identify patients with Klippel–Feil syndrome who are at particular risk for neurologic injury. These include two sets of adjacent block vertebrae with one or two intervening open disk spaces, occipitalization of the atlas with a congenital fusion below C2, creating a risk for C1–C2 instability, and congenital fusion with associated cervical stenosis.

The literature generally advocates a conservative approach for asymptomatic patients with minimal instability. Patients with any evidence of myelopathy or significant instability warrant surgical stabilization to minimize the risk of a catastrophic neurologic injury.

Os Odontoideum

Os odontoideum is an anomaly of the cervical spine in which the normal odontoid process is replaced by an ossicle with smooth circumferential cortical margins that has no osseous continuity with the body of the axis. The etiology has been debated; many believe that os odontoideum results from unrecognized trauma that leads to nonunion of the fractured dens. Others believe that os odontoideum has a congenital origin.

On radiographic evaluation, the os is typically seen as a hypoplastic, sclerotic ossicle that may be anterior to, at, or

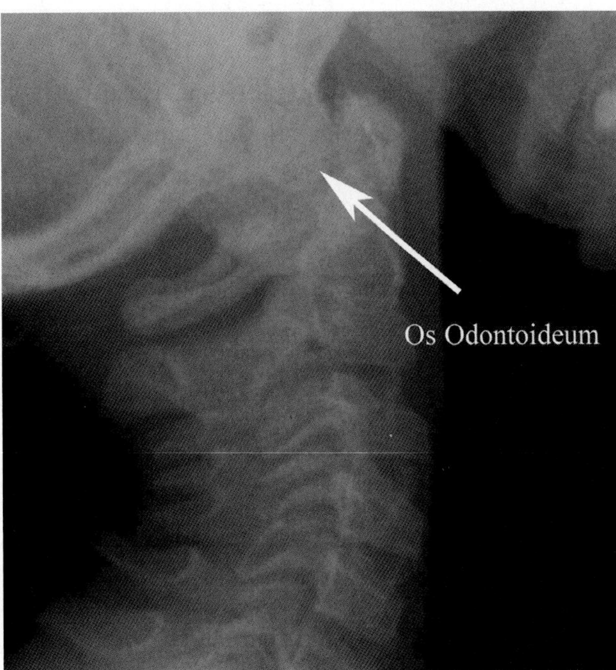

Figure 11.224 Lateral cervical spine radiograph demonstrating an ossicle with well-circumscribed cortical margins and open posterior ring of C1. (*Reproduced with permission from* Sankar WN, Wills BP, Dormans JP, et al. Os odontoideum revisited: the case for a multifactorial etiology. *Spine*. 2006;31:979–984.)

posterior to the typical location of the dens (Fig. 11.224). CT scans may be necessary to adequately visualize the ossicle. Flexion/extension views of the cervical spine are important to check for atlantoaxial instability. In children with neurologic changes or if there is any suspicion for associated spinal cord anomalies, an MRI is warranted.

Os odontoideum has been reported to cause neurologic compromise and even sudden death. Any patient with a history of neurologic impairment or neurologic symptoms should undergo surgical stabilization. A more controversial issue is the appropriate treatment for the asymptomatic child with os odontoideum. Generally, surgical treatment is indicated in cases of documented instability (>4 mm of motion at C1–2 on flexion/extension views). In the absence of instability, the child may be followed with serial dynamic radiographs; any evidence of increasing motion, pain, or neurologic sequelae warrants surgery.

Atlantoaxial Rotatory Displacement

Atlantoaxial rotatory displacement may be seen following minor trauma, an upper respiratory infection, or head and neck surgery. An acute torticollis is seen with a classic "cocked robin" appearance, in which the head is rotated in one direction but tilted toward the other direction. Neck discomfort is usually present, but in nontraumatic cases, neurologic involvement is rare.

The diagnosis of fixed rotatory displacement of C1 on C2 is made radiographically. Plain lateral radiographs can be used to assess for anterior subluxation of the atlas on the axis, which may be absent, mild, or marked. Subtle malalignment of the head or the posterior arch of C1 may also be seen. The most definitive test is dynamic CT scanning. Axial cuts through the C1–C2 complex with the head rotated 45 degrees to the right and 45 degrees to the left will identify failure of the atlas to rotate normally around the axis, even when the head appears to be turned (Fig. 11.225). This finding is diagnostic of atlantoaxial rotatory displacement, or fixed rotatory subluxation as it is sometimes called.

Treatment of rotatory subluxation depends on the duration of symptoms and the presence of C1–C2 subluxation. Individuals with less than 1 week of symptoms are usually treated with a soft cervical collar, oral muscle relaxants, and rest. In patients who fail to respond or in whom symptoms have persisted for more than 1 week, hospitalization with the use of cervical halter traction is indicated. When symptoms have been present for more than 1 month, halo traction can be used, although there is a relatively high risk of redisplacement even after reduction.

Surgery is warranted for atlantoaxial rotatory displacement that has persisted for more than 3 months, that has recurred following adequate reduction, or in patients with neurologic changes. C1–C2 arthrodesis is performed with halo immobilization. Residual deformity usually resolves spontaneously over time in the presence of a solid fusion.

Congenital Muscular Torticollis

Although strictly speaking it is not a disorder of the cervical spine, congenital muscular torticollis (CMT) is a common cause of neck deformity, especially in young children. CMT is a painless deformity that results from contracture of the sternocleidomastoid muscle and is the most common cause of torticollis in newborns. The etiology remains controversial but is most likely from intrauterine or perinatal compartment syndrome that causes fibrosis of the sternocleidomastoid muscle. Risk factors include breech position and difficult delivery; associated conditions include DDH and metatarsus adductus.

The clinical appearance is characteristic with the child's head tilted toward the involved muscle and the chin rotated toward the contralateral shoulder (Fig. 11.226). A mass (often likened to an olive) can sometimes be felt in the body of the sternocleidomastoid during the first 3 months of life. This mass often disappears during early infancy but is replaced with a tight fibrous band over the length of the sternocleidomastoid as the muscle fibroses.

Initial treatment consists of a stretching program which is successful in the majority of cases if started in the first 6 months of life. Infants that do not have a palpably tight sternocleidomastoid muscle or those that do not respond

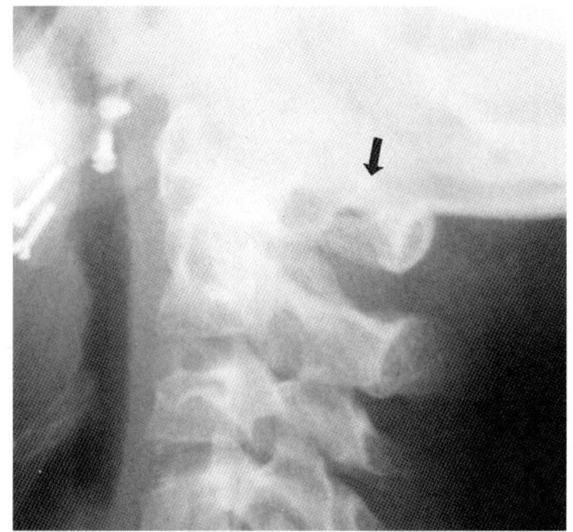

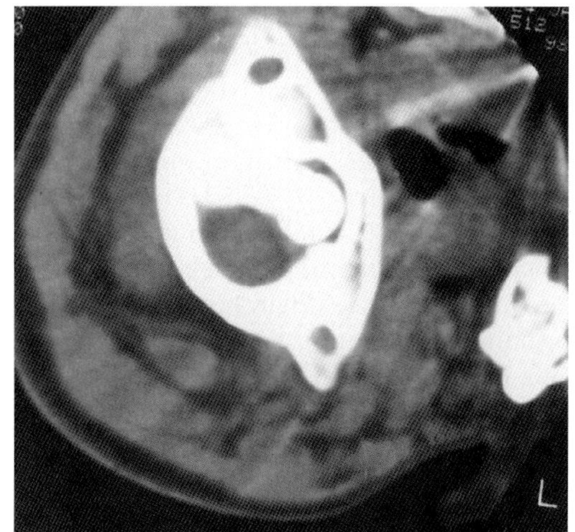

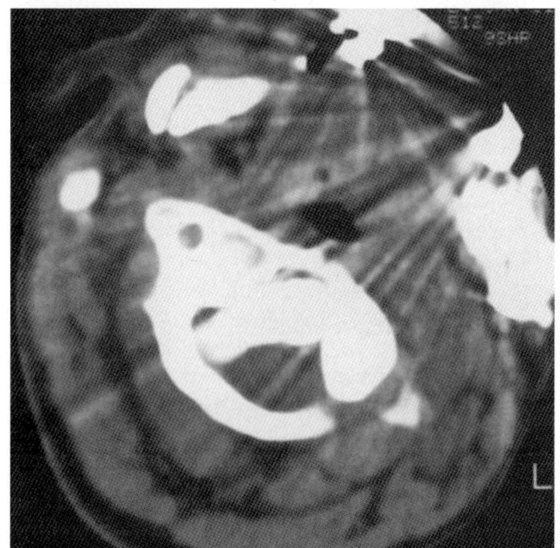

Figure 11.225 Radiographic findings in atlantoaxial rotatory subluxation. **(A)** The lateral cervical spinal radiograph demonstrating that the posterior arches fail to superimpose because of the head tilt (*arrow*). **(B)** Dynamic computed tomography scans in a 9-year-old girl with a fixed atlantoaxial rotatory displacement, with the head maximally rotated to the left. **(C)** Her head maximally rotated to the right, in this case, does not reach the midline. The ring of C1 is still in the exact relation to the odontoid as in **B,** indicating a fixed displacement. (*Reproduced with permission from* Morrissy RT, Weinstein SL. *Lovell and Winter's Pediatric Orthopaedics.* Philadelphia, PA: Lippincott Williams & Wilkins, 2006.)

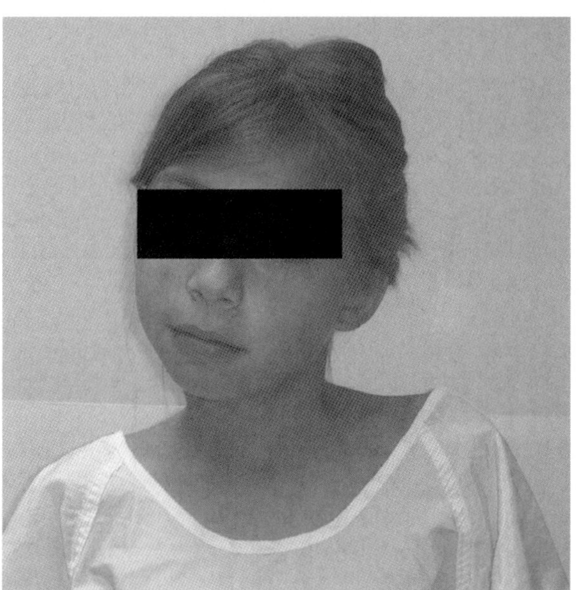

Figure 11.226 Clinical photograph of a young girl with left-sided congenital muscular torticollis. Note the tight left sternocleidomastoid muscle. (*Reproduced with permission from* Children's Orthopaedic Center, Los Angeles, CA.)

to months of diligent physical therapy should be imaged with plain radiographs or if needed CT to rule out a congenital cervical spine anomaly. Children who present at an older age and those patients with torticollis refractory to therapy may occasionally require surgery. Options include unipolar or bipolar release of the sternocleidomastoid, resection of the muscle, and Z-plasty lengthening.

Down Syndrome

Upper cervical involvement in Down syndrome (trisomy 21) has been reported in an alarmingly high proportion of affected children and adults. Both occipitocervical and atlantoaxial instability have been reported, with estimates as high as 60% and 20%, respectively. An increased incidence of cervical spine anomalies, such as os odontoideum, has been reported in individuals with Down syndrome and C1–C2 instability.

The natural history of atlantoaxial instability in Down syndrome has not been clearly defined. There is a tendency toward gradual progression in some individuals, and it has been reported that progressive instability and neurologic impairment is more likely in male patients and after the age of 10 years. Most individuals are asymptomatic, however, and screening radiographs taken for the Special Olympics lead in most cases to diagnosis, evaluation, and questions about appropriate treatment.

Because most children with Down syndrome and C1–C2 instability are asymptomatic, the appropriate role for surgical treatment is unclear. An exceedingly high complication rate, including nonunion, infection, neurologic worsening, and even death, has been reported with C1–C2 fusion in these patients, and there is only anecdotal evidence that atlantoaxial instability is associated with neurologic catastrophe. Because of the high complication rate, most surgeons favor a fairly conservative approach. For children with C1–C2 instability and more than 4 to 5 mm of motion, restriction from high-risk sports such as gymnastics, diving, and soccer is recommended. Surgery can be considered for asymptomatic individuals with atlantoaxial instability of 10 mm or more. The only definite indication for surgery is a child with a clear-cut history of neurologic impairment or evidence of myelopathy on physical examination along with documented atlantoaxial instability. The significance and treatment of occipitocervical instability is even less clearly defined.

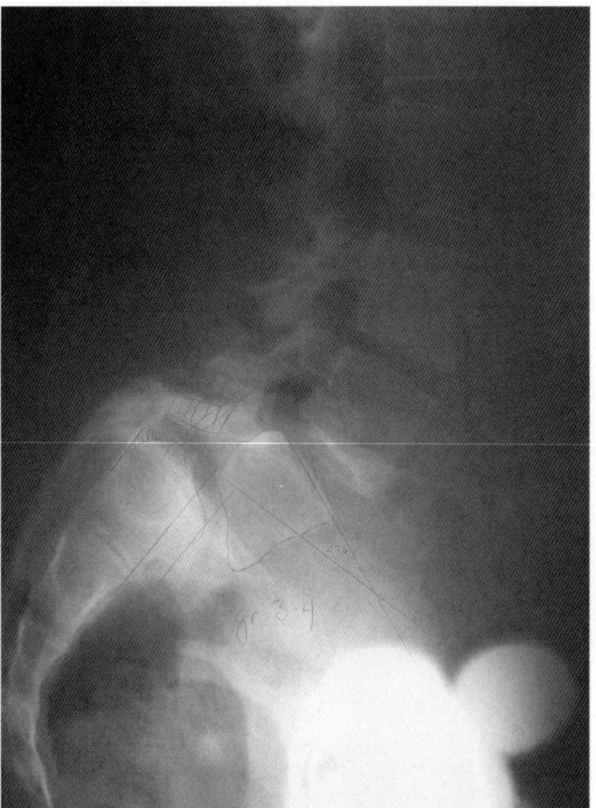

Figure 11.227 An 18-year-old girl with high-grade spondylolisthesis. Note the anterior translation of L5 relative to the body of S1.

SPONDYLOLYSIS AND SPONDYLOLISTHESIS

Spondylolysis is a stress fracture of the pars interarticularis of the lumbar spine. Spondylolisthesis refers to the forward slippage of one vertebra on another. The overall incidence in adolescents is 5% to 6% by the end of skeletal growth. Male patients are more commonly affected than female patients, by a 6:1 ratio.

Pathophysiology and Classification

Spondylolysis is a stress fracture that is thought to result from repetitive hyperextension stresses in genetically predisposed individuals. Spondylolysis is more common in athletes who incur repetitive hyperextension forces in the lower lumbar spine such as gymnasts or interior linemen in football. In some cases, spondylolysis can progress to a spondylolisthesis. Spondylolisthesis refers to the forward slippage of one vertebra on another (Fig. 11.227). Wiltse and others have classified spondylolisthesis into six types based on etiology. In children, class I (congenital) and II (isthmic) are most common. Congenital or dysplastic spondylolisthesis is the result of a congenital defect at the L5–S1 articulation. Typically, the defect consists of hypoplastic facets or abnormal facet orientation that allows the superior vertebral body to slip over the inferior vertebral body. The pars interarticularis may be dysmorphic but is intact. Progression is common in this type of spondylolisthesis. Class II, or isthmic, spondylolisthesis is the most common type seen in children. In this case, the spondylolisthesis occurs because of a defect in the pars interarticularis (spondylolysis). Approximately 80% to 90% of cases involve the L5–S1 level, with 5% to 15% affecting L4–L5. The remaining types of spondylolisthesis (which rarely affect children) include degenerative, traumatic, pathologic, and postoperative. Progression of spondylolisthesis has been associated with the adolescent growth spurt, lumbosacral kyphosis, and greater degree of initial slip on presentation.

Presentation

Spondylolysis and spondylolisthesis are some of the most common causes of back pain in the pediatric population, and patients present typically with pain in the low back, occasionally radiating into the buttocks or posterior thigh. This back pain is largely mechanical and is worsened by activity and improved by rest. In advanced cases of spondylolisthesis, anterior translation of the superior vertebral body can result in foraminal stenosis of the exiting nerve root and can present as radiculopathy.

Physical Examination

In spondylolysis, the pain is usually aggravated by hyperextension and rotation. Tight hamstrings (as evidenced by an increased popliteal angle) are common. High-grade slips can also result in the typical appearance of lumbar hyperlordosis (balancing the lumbosacral kyphosis), crouched posture, and waddling gait.

Radiographs

A number of radiographic findings have been described in spondylolysis and spondylolisthesis. Most defects of the pars interarticularis can be seen on spot lateral radiographs of the lumbosacral spine. In some cases, further definition of the defect can be seen on oblique radiographs, where the characteristic "collar" on the neck of the "Scotty dog" is seen (Fig. 11.228). Lateral radiographs also allow grading of spondylolisthesis. The two most important radiographic measures are the percent slip (Meyerding classification) and the slip angle. The Meyerding classification is based on the percentage of translation of the superior vertebral body across the inferior vertebral body. The superior endplate of the inferior vertebrae is divided into quadrants, and the amount of translation is graded between I and IV. Grade V or translation over 100% is termed *spondyloptosis* (Fig. 11.229). The slip angle quantifies the amount of kyphosis that results from the L5 vertebral body sliding forward over the sacrum. The slip angle is measured by drawing a line perpendicular to a line drawn along the posterior aspect of the vertebral body and measuring the angle between that and a line parallel to the inferior endplate of L5 (Fig. 11.230). Slip angles greater than 35 degrees to 40 degrees are at risk for progression.

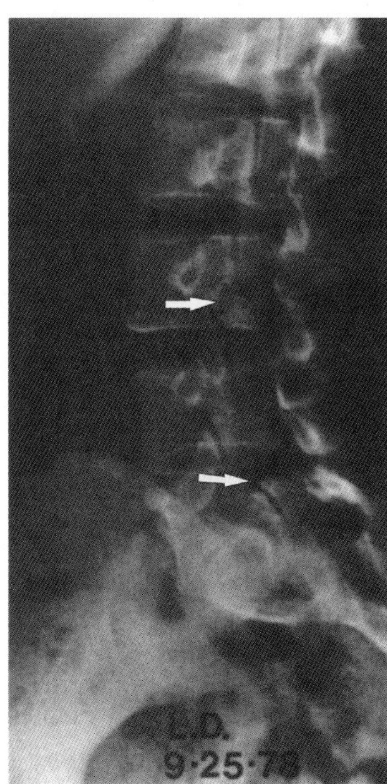

Figure 11.228 Oblique radiograph demonstrating spondylolysis (*white arrows*) at L3 and L5. The location of the stress fracture is the neck of the "Scotty dog." (*Reproduced with permission from* Weinstein SL. *The Pediatric Spine.* Philadelphia, PA: Lippincott Williams & Wilkins, 2001.)

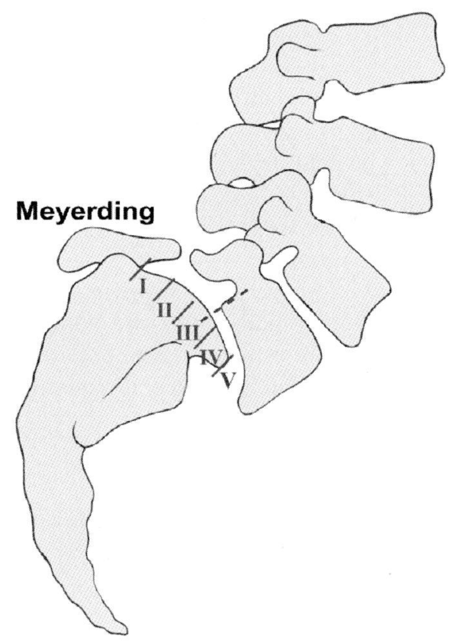

Figure 11.229 Meyerding system for grading spondylolisthesis. (*Reproduced with permission from* Morrissy RT, Weinstein SL. *Lovell and Winter's Pediatric Orthopaedics.* Philadelphia, PA: Lippincott Williams & Wilkins, 2006.)

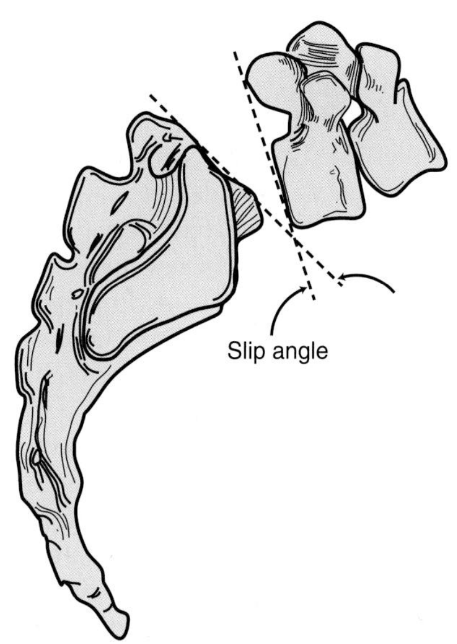

Figure 11.230 Slip angle helps quantify the amount of local kyphosis. (*From* Wiesel SW, Delahay JN. *Essentials of Orthopaedic Surgery.* 2nd ed. Philadelphia, PA: WB Saunders, 1997.)

Special Tests

In certain cases of spondylolysis, plain radiographs (including obliques) are nondiagnostic. Bone scans can show increased uptake in patients with new spondylolytic lesions but may be cold in those who have had long-term symptoms. CT scans are more sensitive than either plain radiographs or bone scans and allow for multiplanar reconstructions. Single-photon emission CT (SPECT) scans have greater sensitivity and specificity for diagnosing spondylolysis compared with radiographs and bone scans. MRI is useful for ruling out other causes of back pain and for evaluating stenosis as part of preoperative planning.

Differential Diagnosis

The differential diagnosis for spondylolysis and spondylolisthesis is similar to that of back pain (see later). Neoplasms, muscular strains, infections, and psychosomatic back pain can all present similar to spondylolysis/spondylolisthesis. Usually, radiographs or advanced imaging techniques are diagnostic.

Treatment

Many cases of spondylolysis are found incidentally, are asymptomatic, and require no treatment. In patients who present with symptomatic spondylolysis, the mainstay of treatment is nonsurgical. Usually this involves activity restriction, nonsteroidal anti-inflammatory drugs (NSAIDs), and physical therapy focusing on core strengthening and hamstring stretching. In patients suffering from acute spondylolysis, bracing can be useful. It is important to note that the resolution of symptoms does not necessarily correlate with healing of the pars defect. The goal of treatment is pain resolution and return to full activity; as a result, patients should be managed on the basis of their clinical response, not the radiographic findings. Patients with spondylolysis who are still symptomatic after conservative treatment may be candidates for direct repair of the pars defect. Various techniques have been described including wiring, screw fixation, and screw hook constructs usually with autogenous bone grafting. In patients with disk degeneration or any degree of segmental instability, posterolateral fusion with or without instrumentation is the treatment of choice.

Treatment of spondylolisthesis depends on the grade of the slip and the presence or absence of symptoms. Asymptomatic patients with grade I spondylolisthesis are typically treated with observation alone without activity restriction; routine radiographic follow-up is recommended on an annual basis to monitor for slip progression. Asymptomatic patients with higher grades of spondylolisthesis are usually restricted from high-risk activities such as gymnastics or contact sports. Symptomatic patients with grade I or II spondylolisthesis are treated conservatively in a similar manner as for patients with spondylolysis. The role of prophylactic fusion in higher-grade but asymptomatic spondylolisthesis is somewhat controversial. Because of the risk of further progression and the development of significant back pain in adulthood, most surgeons recommend fusion in an asymptomatic child or adolescent if the percent slip is greater than 50% (grade III or more). Harris and Weinstein, however, have reported a series of adults with high-grade spondylolisthesis treated nonoperatively and compared them with individuals who had undergone fusion. Although pain was not uncommon, there was a relatively high level of function in individuals with grades III and IV spondylolisthesis who had not undergone surgery, suggesting that observation may be reasonable in these patients, particularly if they are followed closely for progression.

In general, surgery is indicated for patients who have persistent back pain despite 6 to 12 months of aggressive nonoperative treatment (regardless of grade) and for most patients with spondylolisthesis greater than 50%. Arthrodesis is usually performed with the most common approach in the pediatric population being posterior fusion (Fig. 11.231). In higher-grade slips, the fusion is usually extended to L4 and an anterior fusion may be used with or without dowel grafting or interbody structural support. Noninstrumented procedures are effective in reducing symptoms but have a lower fusion rate than do instrumented techniques. Historically, patients were immobilized in a spica cast after noninstrumented fusion; however, some surgeons use a TLSO with a thigh extension during the postoperative period. Most surgeons now prefer posterior segmental instrumentation and fusion for patients with spondylolisthesis. As mentioned, instrumentation increases fusion rates and also allows correction of the slip angle, which can improve body posture and mechanics. Another advantage of instrumentation is that it allows for full neural decompression, which is vital in cases of foraminal stenosis.

Reduction of high-grade spondylolisthesis is controversial. Patients with high-grade disease have significant cosmetic deformity and abnormal body mechanics. In addition, high-grade spondylolisthesis creates an environment in which the fusion mass (even if extended up to L4) is under tension and is therefore at significant risk for nonunion, bending, and continued progression. For these theoretical reasons, reduction has its advantages. Techniques include traction and casting, combined anterior and posterior approaches, posterior instrumentation and reduction, and circumferential L5 body resection with reduction. Although success has been reported for all these techniques, reduction of high-grade spondylolisthesis has a significant risk of complications including loss of fixation, loss of correction, and, most importantly, a worrisome rate of neurologic deficits (up to 20%–30% in some series). As a result, many surgeons prefer in situ fusion.

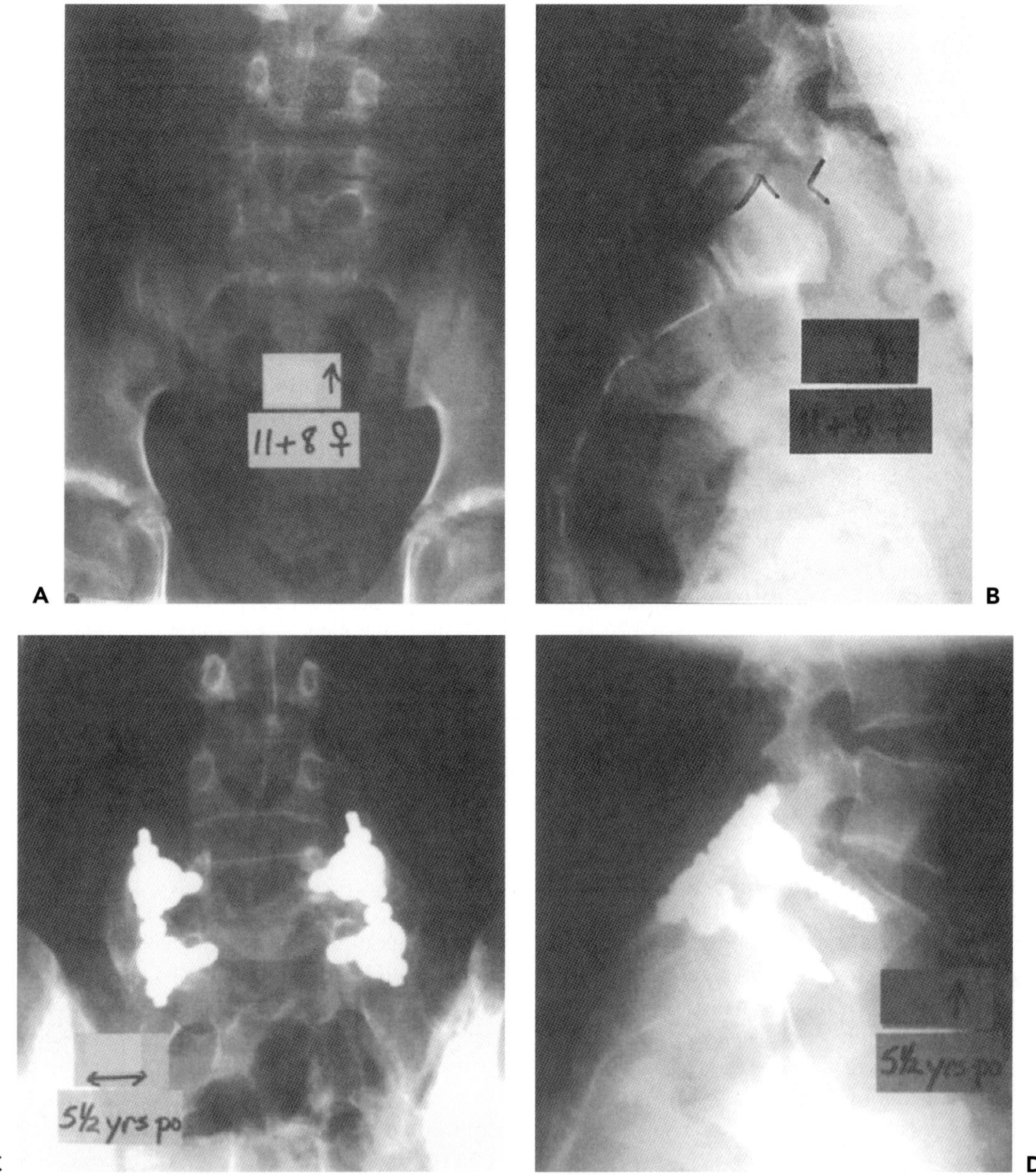

Figure 11.231 **(A, B)** This 11-year-old girl underwent posterior decompression and instrumented posterolateral fusion from L5 to sacrum, using autogenous iliac crest graft laterally. **(C)** At 5 years 6 months postoperatively, she had an excellent arthrodesis on the posteroanterior view. **(D)** The lateral view shows stability at L5–S1. (*Reproduced with permission from* Morrissy RT, Weinstein SL. *Lovell and Winter's Pediatric Orthopaedics.* Philadelphia, PA: Lippincott Williams & Wilkins, 2006.)

BACK PAIN

Back pain in adults is so common that it is almost a normal variant. Although bothersome and at times incapacitating, most patients and family members accept the fact that a backache is a routine occurrence, frequently difficult to diagnose, and often resistant to treatment. When significant back pain occurs in children, however, a certain anxiety level is seen on the part of family members and referring physicians. Most of this concern stems from the fact that back pain has traditionally been considered a rare finding in the pediatric population. In reality, back pain is relatively common in adolescents and children. Recent studies indicate that more than 50% of children will experience back pain by age 15 and roughly 24% of adolescent girls complain of back pain more than once a week. It is unclear what has caused this apparent increase in incidence, although sedentary lifestyles, increased sports participation, and backpack use have all been thought to play a role. Pediatric back pain can be caused by a variety of conditions some of which require prompt treatment. As a result, an organized approach with a thorough history, physical examination, and appropriate diagnostic studies is necessary when evaluating back pain. A diagnosis of mechanical back pain should be considered only after other more serious pathologies have been ruled out.

Presentation

A careful detailed history should be obtained from both the child and the parent. The age of the patient at presentation is important in the evaluation of low back pain. The prevalence of back pain in children younger than 10 years is less common than in adolescents and is more likely to have an organic etiology such as an infection or a tumor. The onset of symptoms should be explored, including any inciting trauma, as well as the location of the pain and sites of radiation. Pain at rest is concerning and is classically associated with neoplasms. The severity of pain is often best assessed by asking about the child's ability to participate in sports and other recreational activities. It is not at all uncommon for adolescents to complain of relatively mild back pain with no specific cause; this is particularly true if the diagnosis of scoliosis has recently been made. On the other hand, pain that is of sufficient magnitude to interfere with activities such as attending school or participating in organized sports is more worrisome. Patients should be questioned about neurologic symptoms such as radiculopathy or paresthesias in the legs and recent changes in bowel or bladder habits. An inquiry should be made about the child's general medical status, including a thorough review of systems and specific questioning about constitutional symptoms (e.g., fever, chills). Finally, it is important to remember that psychological factors can play a role in back pain, especially in teenagers. It is therefore important to assess the social history for family dysfunction and other sources of psychological stress.

Physical Examination

Physical examination is performed with the patient in an examining gown, disrobed down to underwear with shoes and socks removed. Skin should be assessed for café au lait spots, dimples, or hairy patches. Balance and posture should be evaluated in the standing position to determine thoracic kyphosis, lumbar lordosis, and overall alignment. Gait should be evaluated for evidence of weakness or pain. Flexibility can be assessed by examining forward bending, rotation, and extension—pain with the latter can be suggestive of spondylolysis. The spinous processes and paraspinal muscles should be palpated to determine the location of the pain. Back pain that is well localized (positive "finger test" in which the patient points to one particular spot as the source of pain) over bone is particularly indicative for underlying pathology, whereas pain over a broad distribution is likely to be standard mechanical back pain. Intraabdominal and retroperitoneal pathology can be ruled out with a careful abdominal examination. The straight leg raising test can help diagnose radiculopathy, and the popliteal angle should be measured to determine the degree of hamstring tightness. The presence of a cavus foot or claw toes, particularly unilateral, is suggestive of intraspinal pathology. Finally, a thorough neurologic examination is mandatory including an assessment of motor strength, sensation, and deep tendon reflexes.

Radiographs

Adolescents with mechanical back pain (without any red flags in the history and physical examination) often do not require radiographic evaluation. Symptomatic treatment including rest, physical therapy, and judicious use of NSAIDs is usually sufficient, but follow-up examinations are important to ensure improvement with these measures. Children younger than 10 years and any patients with persistent symptoms, night pain, or constitutional complaints should be imaged at the initial visit. Plain AP and lateral radiographs of the spine should be obtained, and dynamic films are helpful if instability is suspected. Oblique films of the lumbosacral spine can be obtained if spondylolysis is being considered but are not routinely ordered. Standing views of the full spine are utilized for cases of spinal deformity.

Special Tests

Bone scans are a sensitive but relatively nonspecific modality that will identify most spinal column and pelvic conditions such as tumors, infections, and spondylolysis. The sensitivity and specificity can be enhanced with SPECT scanning, particularly when the diagnosis of spondylolysis is an issue. CT scans are the best imaging modality for evaluating boney anatomy, and are extremely useful in cases where a bone tumor (such as osteoid osteoma) is suspected (Fig. 11.232). The presence of neurologic findings usually warrants an MRI of the spine. MRI is more sensitive and specific in the diagnosis of tumor or infection and is the imaging modality of choice for disk abnormalities including herniation and diskitis. Laboratory testing is occasionally indicated in the child or adolescent with back pain and is more commonly utilized in this setting than in the adult. Urinalysis and complete blood cell count may be obtained, and the sedimentation rate and C-reactive protein level are good screening tests for neoplasm or infection. Several blood tests are available to complement the search for underlying rheumatologic disorders, but this testing is usually deferred to the rheumatologist.

Differential Diagnosis and Treatment

Multiple diagnoses can result in back pain. Some clue as to the underlying nature of the condition may be apparent

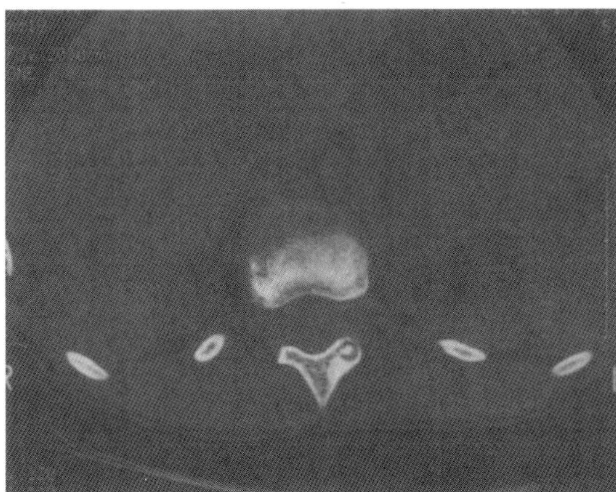

Figure 11.232 A computed tomographic scan of a 13-year-old boy with back pain demonstrates a nidus consistent with an osteoid osteoma in the posterior elements of the spine. (*Reproduced with permission from* Weinstein SL. *The Pediatric Spine.* Philadelphia, PA: Lippincott Williams & Wilkins, 2001.)

based on the history and physical examination, but it is usually the radiographic workup that will ultimately lead to the diagnosis. Since neoplasia and infection are the most ominous conditions associated with back pain, it is important to consider these diagnoses and rule them out in a timely fashion before considering more mechanical or psychosomatic etiologies.

Neoplasms are rare but are a concerning cause of back pain in children and adolescents. Most bone tumors are benign and have a predilection for the posterior elements of the spine. The most common tumors of the posterior elements include osteoid osteoma, osteoblastoma, and aneurysmal bone cyst. Langerhans cell histiocytosis (or eosinophilic granuloma) usually affects the anterior column and can lead to vertebral body collapse and the characteristic vertebra plana (Fig. 11.233). Malignant bone tumors such as Ewing sarcoma or osteosarcoma are rare. In younger children, leukemia can first present as back pain. Neuroblastoma can also be seen in this age group. Intraspinal tumors may manifest as back pain, and compression of neural elements can lead to leg symptoms, atrophy, or bowel and bladder dysfunction. Tumors are classically associated with night pain and can be associated with a variety of constitutional complaints such as fever and weight loss. Plain radiographs may reveal lytic or blastic lesions, but further workup with a CT or an MRI is usually necessary. Biopsy may be necessary, and treatment is dependent on the nature of the specific lesion.

Spine infections in children are usually due to diskitis or vertebral osteomyelitis, and the mean age of presentation is 6 years of age. In addition to back pain, patients can complain of abdominal pain and lower extremity discomfort. Children often refuse to walk, stand, or even sit. Fever is common on presentation and the sedimentation rate and C-reactive protein level are usually elevated. Radiographs early in the disease course may be nondiagnostic; eventually disk space narrowing and endplate irregularities will develop. Prior to the appearance of these radiographic changes, a bone scan or MRI may be necessary to make the diagnosis (Fig. 11.234). Patients with diskitis or osteomyelitis are usually treated empirically without biopsy because the predominant offending organism is *Staphylococcus aureus.* A short course of intravenous antibiotics followed by transition to an oral regimen is a typical treatment algorithm.

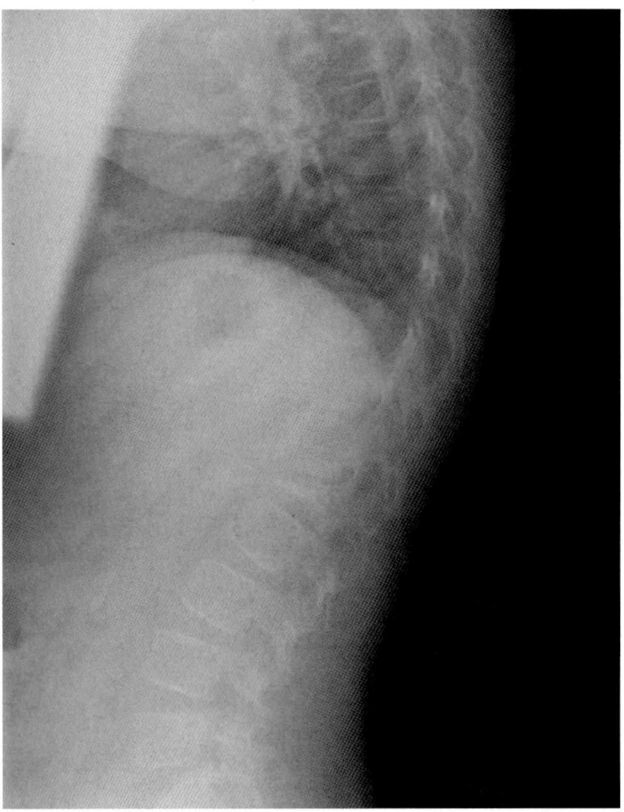

Figure 11.233 Lateral view of the spine demonstrating complete collapse of the L1 vertebral body (vertebra plana) from Langerhans cell histiocytosis. (*Reproduced with permission from* Children's Orthopaedic Center, Los Angeles, CA.)

Spinal deformity can be associated with some degree of back pain. Thoracolumbar Scheuermann kyphosis is a common source of pain in adolescents and probably results from mechanical overuse. Diagnosis is apparent on lateral radiographs and treatment usually consists of core strengthening, and occasional use of NSAIDs (see previous section). Idiopathic scoliosis is not thought to be a painful condition but can be associated with mild complaints from time to time. Generally, advanced imaging is not necessary unless the pain is so severe as to interfere with school attendance or recreational activities, a neurologic abnormality is seen, or in the setting of scoliosis there is rapid curve progression or an atypical curve pattern.

Spondylolysis and spondylolisthesis are a common cause of back pain in children and adolescents and have been discussed in a previous section. Diagnosis is usually

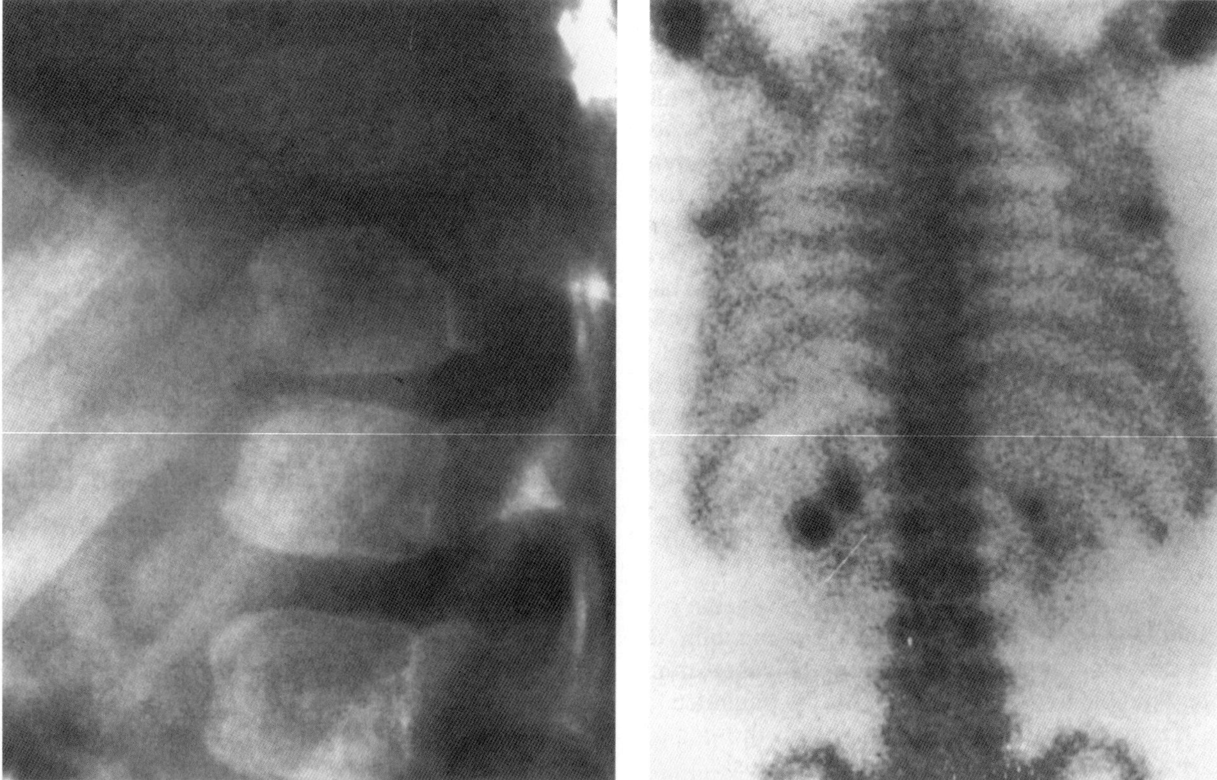

Figure 11.234 **(A)** Lateral radiograph of a 4-year-old child with diskitis demonstrating disc space narrowing. **(B)** A positive bone scan with increased uptake at T11 and T12 confirms inflammatory involvement on both sides of the disc. (*Reproduced with permission from* Weinstein SL. *The Pediatric Spine*. Philadelphia, PA: Lippincott Williams & Wilkins, 2001.)

made on spot lateral radiographs of the lumbosacral spine. Low-grade disease is managed conservatively with core strengthening and occasional use of NSAIDs; high-grade conditions may require surgery.

Disk herniation is a much less common entity in children than in adults. The straight leg raising test correlates well with presence of a herniation, but MRI is the gold standard for making the diagnosis. One should keep in mind that MRI can be "overread" and that most findings of bulging discs in children are not clinically relevant. This condition should be distinguished from vertebral apophyseal ring fractures, which do not occur in adults. Patients with apophyseal injuries typically present with a sudden onset of pain (with or without associated radiculopathy) after trauma or lifting a heavy object. Male weight lifters are most commonly affected. The mechanism of injury is flexion and axial loading of the spinal column. Under an axial load, the disk bulges and places traction on the posteroinferior apophysis. This apophysis can avulse and displace into the spinal canal, causing neural compression. CT or MRI can be diagnostic, although both are often needed to confirm this relatively rare diagnosis, and surgical excision of the fragment may be necessary for pain relief.

Mechanical or activity-related back pain is common among adolescents, especially those who are active in sports. Most pain is due to soft tissue strains or overuse fatigue. Characteristically, the pain is diffuse, is exacerbated by activity, and is relieved by rest. Radiographs are usually not required but should be ordered if other conditions need to be ruled out. It is important to remember that while the diagnosis of mechanical back pain in adolescents is common, the surgeon must not miss a more concerning underlying diagnosis. Any red flags in the history or physical examination should prompt a more thorough diagnostic workup. This is particularly true in children younger than 10 years, in whom one can almost always find a specific diagnosis when persistent back pain is present. Most acute soft tissue strains will resolve over 4 to 6 weeks with appropriate activity modifications. Overuse back pain is generally treated by avoiding the offending activity, physical therapy focusing on stretching, core strengthening and aerobic conditioning, and appropriate use of NSAIDs. Patients who have persistent symptoms in spite of conservative management should undergo further diagnostic imaging.

In a significant number of patients, no discrete etiology may be found for back pain in spite of a thorough diagnostic workup. Several studies have shown that adolescents suffering from psychological stress, either from unstable home environments or from peer pressure, can manifest somatic complaints such as headache, fatigue, and back pain. The diagnosis of psychosomatic back pain is one of exclusion, and it is essential that all other organic causes of back pain be ruled out. A multidisciplinary approach consisting of physicians, psychologists, and therapists is recommended when treating this subgroup of patients. In general, treatment should focus on mental counseling and physical conditioning and should avoid the use of muscle relaxants and opioids.

SPINE TRAUMA

Spine fractures constitute approximately 1% of all pediatric fractures. The cervical spine is the most typical location of injury, accounting for 60% of all pediatric spinal injuries.

Mechanisms of Injury

Motor vehicle accidents are the most common mechanism of spinal injury in children. Other mechanisms vary by the age of the patient. In newborns, birth trauma or child abuse should be considered as an etiology. In school-aged children, spine injuries often result from falls; in adolescents, athletic trauma is more common.

Unique Factors in Pediatric Spine Injuries

Several factors make pediatric spine injuries unique compared with those in adults. The head of a child is proportionately larger than that of an adult. In addition, children have weaker paraspinal muscles to provide head control. The result is an increased relative risk of cervical spine injury in children. Because of their larger head-to-body ratio, immobilization on a standard adult spine board will flex the neck and could exacerbate any cervical spine injury (Fig. 11.235). Children should therefore be immobilized and transported on pediatric spine boards that have recesses for the head or that elevate the body in relation to the head. Children also have increased ligamentous laxity in their necks and more horizontally shaped facet joints, both of which put them at increased risk for cervical spine instability. Finally, the pediatric spinal column has increased elasticity compared with that in adults; as a result, spinal cord injury without radiographic abnormality (SCIWORA) can occur.

Physical Examination

Because children are often difficult to examine, all children with potential trauma to the spine should be treated as a spinal injury until proven otherwise. In patients sustaining high-energy trauma, initial evaluation consists of ensuring the standard ABCs of airway, breathing, and circulation. After completion of the primary survey and stabilization of the patient, the secondary survey is conducted similar to standard adult trauma protocols. As mentioned, patients should be immobilized and transported using modified spine boards.

After initial stabilization, all children with suspected spine injuries should undergo a careful neurologic examination. Strength, sensation, and deep tendon reflexes in both the upper and lower extremities should be evaluated. A rectal examination may be indicated.

Radiographs

Initial evaluation should consist of standard AP and lateral radiographs of the involved area. If an injury is identified, radiographs should be performed of the entire spine to rule out a noncontiguous injury. It is important to be aware that several radiographic findings in the immature spine can be misinterpreted as pathologic when in fact they are normal. As in other parts of the body, pediatric spine bones can be incompletely ossified and growth centers can be mistaken for fractures. For example, in the young child,

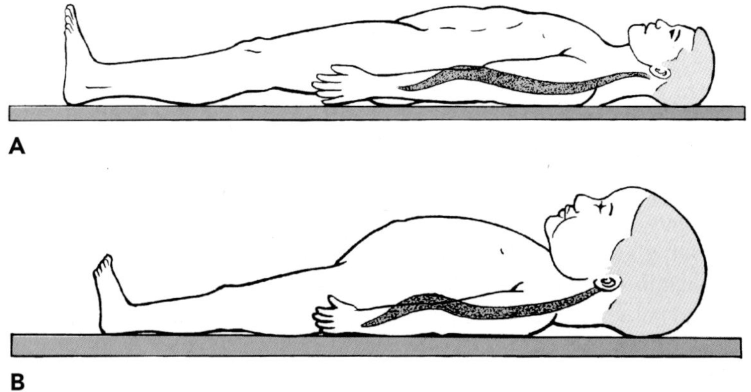

Figure 11.235 **(A)** Adult immobilized on a standard backboard. **(B)** Young child on a standard backboard. The relatively large head flexes the neck and forces the cervical spine into a kyphotic position. (*Reproduced with permission from* Beaty JH, Kasser JR. *Rockwood and Wilkins' Fractures in Children.* 6th ed. Philadelphia, PA: Lippincott Williams & Wilkins, 2006.)

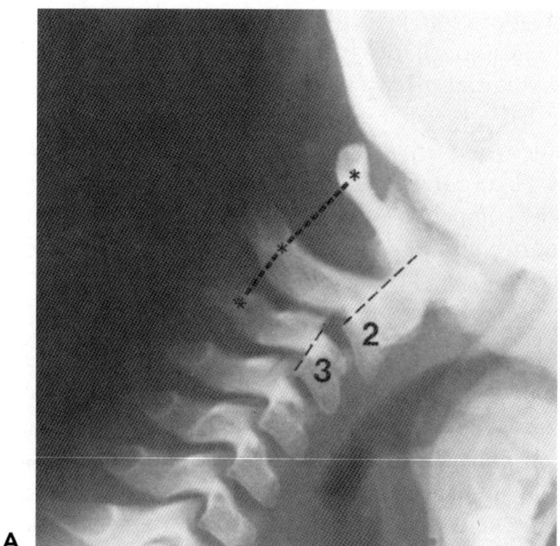

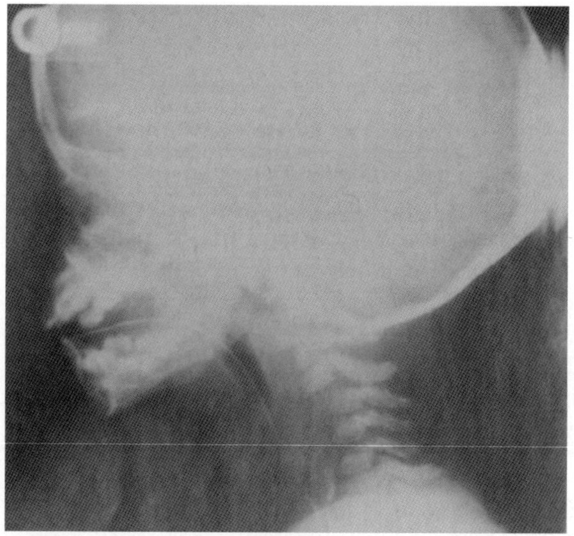

Figure 11.236 **(A)** Pseduosubluxation of C2 on C3. In flexion, the posterior element of C2 should normally align itself with the posterior elements of C1 and C3. The relationship of the body of C2 with the body of C3 gives the appearance of subluxation; however, the alignment of the posterior elements of C1–C3 confirms pseudosubluxation. **(B)** True subluxation. (*Reproduced with permission from* Beaty JH, Kasser JR. *Rockwood and Wilkins' Fractures in Children.* 6th ed. Philadelphia, PA: Lippincott Williams & Wilkins, 2006.)

cervical vertebral bodies often appear wedged with deficient anterosuperior margins. The atlantodens interval is often increased compared with adults because of the presence of cartilage around the immature odontoid process; generally, an interval less than 5 mm is considered normal in a child. Perhaps the most common mistake is diagnosing pseudosubluxation as true cervical spine instability. Pseudosubluxation is the apparent anterior displacement of C2 on C3 (or less commonly C3 on C4), which occurs in 9% of children (Fig. 11.236). It is believed to be facilitated by the more horizontal orientation of the upper cervical facet joints, which become more vertical as the child ages; as a result, pseudosubluxation is rarely seen after the age of 8 years. Pseudosubluxation can be distinguished from true cervical injury by the absence of a history of sufficient trauma to explain the injury, by spontaneous reduction of C2 on C3 when the head is extended, and by alignment of the spinolaminar line (Swischuk's line) (Fig. 11.237).

Special Tests

CT scans are extremely useful in pediatric spine trauma. In patients who have inadequate radiographs or in whom the diagnosis is uncertain, CT is an excellent screening tool with a high sensitivity for boney injury. In addition, CT is the diagnostic modality of choice to visualize the upper cervical spine including the occipitocervical junction. MRI is indicated for cases of suspected soft tissue injury such as ligamentous tears or herniated disks. MRI is also the best test for evaluating spinal cord injury.

Treatment

The majority of pediatric spine fractures are stable and can be treated with simple immobilization (cervical collar or TLSO). Displaced cervical spine fractures that require reduction and upper cervical spine instability may necessitate

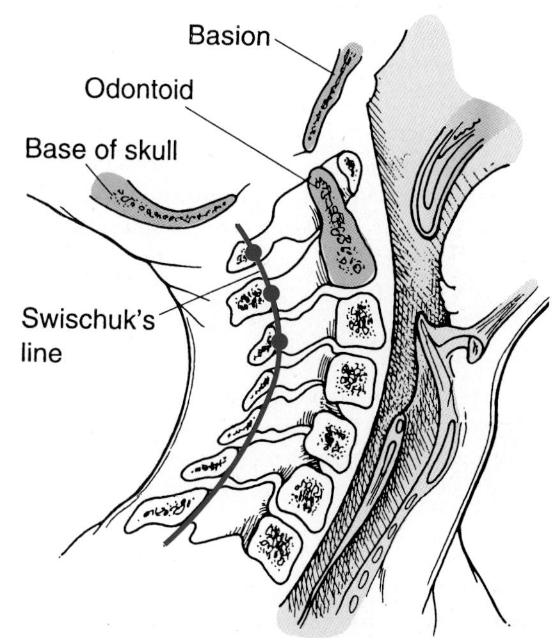

Figure 11.237 The spinolaminar line (Swischuk's line) should remain aligned in the presence of pseudosubluxation of C2 on C3. (*Reproduced with permission from* Beaty JH, Kasser JR. *Rockwood and Wilkins' Fractures in Children.* 6th ed. Philadelphia, PA: Lippincott Williams & Wilkins, 2006.)

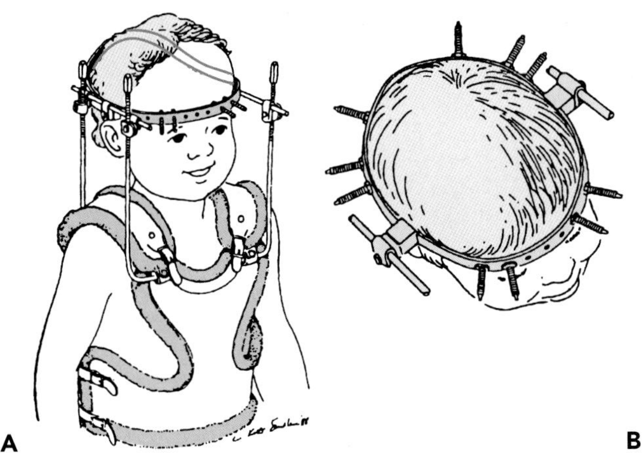

Figure 11.238 **(A)** Custom halo vest and superstructure. **(B)** In the multiple pin, low-torque technique, 10 pins can be used for an infant halo attachment. Usually four pins are placed anteriorly, avoiding the temporal region, and the remaining six pins are placed in the occipital area. (*Reproduced with permission from* Beaty JH, Kasser JR. *Rockwood and Wilkins' Fractures in Children.* 6th ed. Philadelphia, PA: Lippincott Williams & Wilkins, 2006.)

halo immobilization with or without cervical fusion. Use of halo is well accepted for pediatric patients older than 1 year. Because children have thinner skulls, application techniques are slightly different than for adults. In children younger than 8 years, multiple pins (often as many as 8–12) should be placed at lower torque. Usually, four pins are placed anteriorly with the remaining pins in the occiput (Fig. 11.238). Unlike adult pins that are routinely tightened to 8 inch-pounds, pins in young children should be "finger-tight" (approximately 2–4 inch-pounds). Retightening of pins after the initial application is not recommended to minimize the chance of skull penetration. Similar to adults, the halo ring should be positioned below the equator of the head, approximately 1 cm above the ears and eyebrows. Anterior pins should be placed above the lateral half of the orbit to avoid injury to the supraorbital and supratrochlear nerves. In children younger than 1 year, Minerva casts can be used to immobilize the spine.

SPECIFIC PEDIATRIC SPINE INJURIES

Occipitocervical Injuries

Occipitocervical dissociations are purely ligamentous injuries and are associated with an extremely high mortality rate (Fig. 11.239). Injuries can be classified as anterior, vertical, or posterior on the basis of the displacement of the occiput in relation to the cervical spine. Early diagnosis and treatment are critical because patients are at a high risk for neurologic injury or sudden death. If radiographs are nondiagnostic, an urgent MRI is warranted. Reduction should be performed under fluoroscopic guidance; traction should be avoided as it can exacerbate axial displacement. Patients can be temporarily immobilized in a halo vest, but definitive treatment consists of occipitocervical fusion with instrumentation.

Fractures of C1

Fractures of the atlas ring constitute roughly 10% of all cervical spine injuries (Fig. 11.240). The mechanism of injury is an axial load; neurologic injury is rare because, when fractured, the ring of C1 expands, creating more space for the spinal cord. Posterior arch fractures are stable and can

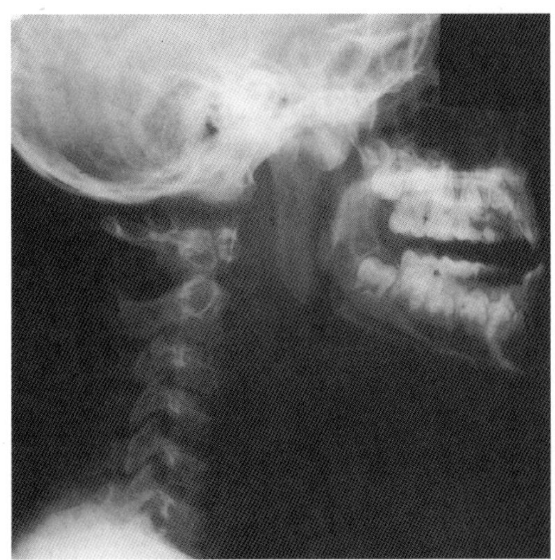

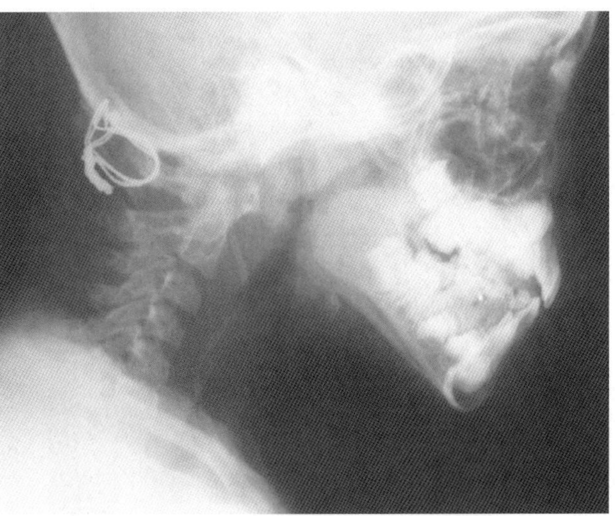

Figure 11.239 **(A)** Lateral radiograph of a patient with atlanto-occipital dislocation. Note the increase in the facet condylar distance. **(B)** Lateral radiograph after occipital-C1 arthrodesis. (*Reproduced with permission from* Beaty JH, Kasser JR. *Rockwood and Wilkins' Fractures in Children.* 6th ed. Philadelphia, PA: Lippincott Williams & Wilkins, 2006.)

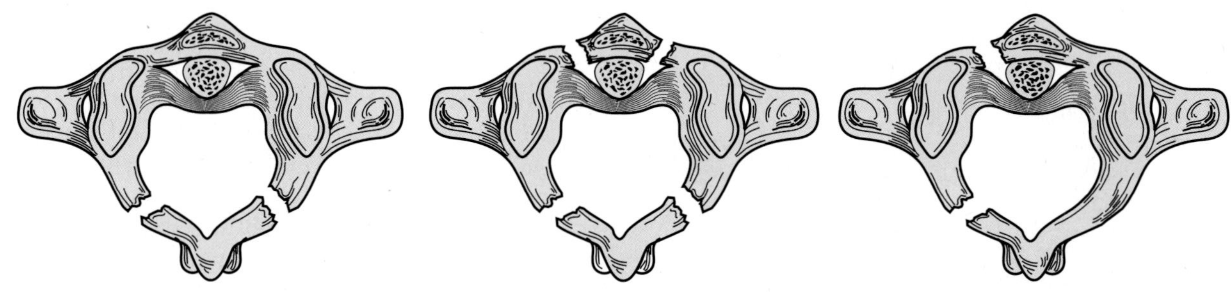

Figure 11.240 There are three common types of atlas fractures: posterior arch fractures, in which the lateral masses do not spread; burst or Jefferson fractures, in which the lateral masses will spread and displace laterally; and lateral mass fractures, in which displacement of the lateral mass occurs on the fractures side. (*Reproduced with permission from* Jackson RS, Banit DM, Rhyne AL, et al. Upper cervical spine injuries. *J Am Acad Orthop Surg*. 2002;10:271–280.)

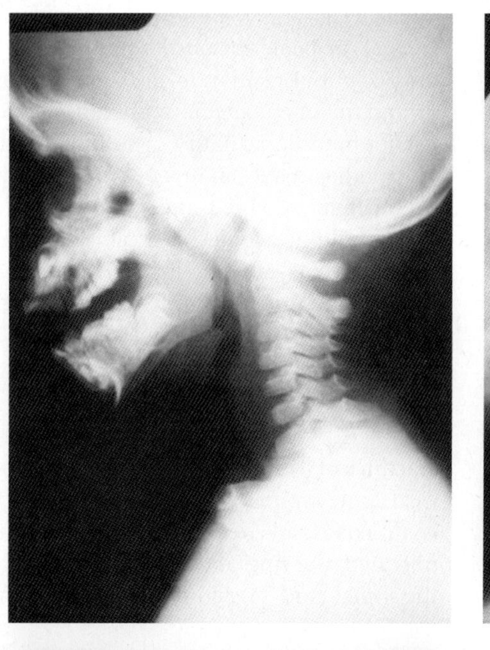

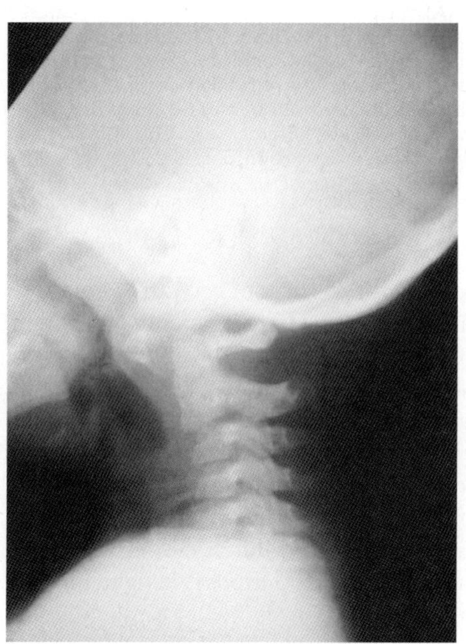

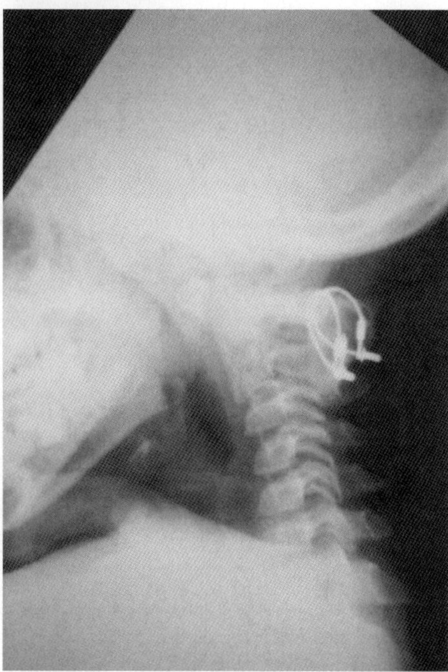

Figure 11.241 **(A)** Lateral radiograph of traumatic C1–C2 instability. **(B)** Note the increase in the atlantodens interval on the dynamic lateral radiograph. **(C)** Lateral radiograph after C1–C2 arthrodesis. (*Reproduced with permission from* Beaty JH, Kasser JR. *Rockwood and Wilkins' Fractures in Children*. 6th ed. Philadelphia, PA: Lippincott Williams & Wilkins, 2006.)

be treated with collar immobilization for 10 to 12 weeks. Burst fractures or lateral mass fractures with more than 6.9 mm of overhang on the open mouth odontoid view imply injury to the transverse ligament. Because of the resultant atlantoaxial instability, these injuries usually require C1–C2 arthrodesis. Fractures with less than 5 mm of displacement can be treated with a halo vest for 3 months.

Atlantoaxial Injuries

Atlantoaxial injuries are almost always ligamentous. Normally, the transverse ligament is the primary stabilizer of the C1–C2 articulation, with additional stability provided by the apical and alar ligaments. Rupture of this ligamentous complex can occur from excessive flexion forces. Lateral flexion/extension views of the cervical spine are usually diagnostic (Fig. 11.241). In children, an atlantodens interval more than 5 mm is considered abnormal. MRI can also be helpful to delineate the ligamentous injury. Confirmed cases of instability should be treated with posterior arthrodesis of C1–C2.

Odontoid Fractures

In children, a synchondrosis, exists at the base of the odontoid process, which closes around the age of 5 years. The majority of pediatric dens fractures occur through this physeal area due to a flexion moment to the cervical spine (Fig. 11.242). Lateral cervical radiographs are usually diagnostic but can be inconclusive in nondisplaced injuries. In these cases, MRI can be helpful to make the definitive diagnosis. Most fractures can be treated by reduction and halo immobilization for 8 to 12 weeks.

Traumatic spondylolisthesis of C2 (Hangman Fracture)

Fractures through the pedicle of C2 are referred to as *Hangman fractures* and result from hyperextension injuries. The diagnosis is usually apparent on lateral cervical spine radiographs, as there is often displacement at the fracture site with some forward subluxation of C2 on C3 (Fig. 11.243). Neurologic injury is rare because (similar to C1 ring fractures) more space is created for the spinal cord from displacement of the fracture. Treatment should be symptomatic with immobilization in a halo or Minerva cast for approximately 8 to 12 weeks. For nonunions and fractures with significant angulation, posterior or anterior arthrodesis of C2–C3 may be indicated.

Subaxial Cervical Spine Injuries

The subaxial cervical spine refers to C3–C7; injuries in this region are rare in young children and usually occur in adolescents. Several patterns of injury have been described in the subaxial cervical spine including ligamentous disruptions, facet dislocations, compression fractures, and burst fractures. Posterior ligamentous disruptions result from flexion or distraction mechanisms (Fig. 11.244). Patients usually complain of posterior tenderness at the site of injury; often, the only radiographic evidence of injury is subtle widening of the spinous processes. MRI can be helpful to confirm the presence of ligamentous damage. Patients can be initially managed with a cervical orthosis; however, any sign of instability is an indication for posterior arthrodesis.

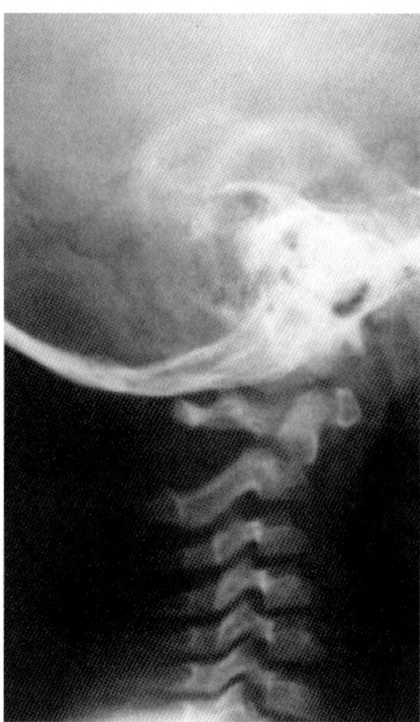

Figure 11.242 Lateral radiograph in an almost 3-year-old boy demonstrates an odontoid fracture through the dentocentral synchondrosis with anterior angulation and translation. (*Reproduced with permission from* Morrissy RT, Weinstein SL. *Lovell and Winter's Pediatric Orthopaedics*. Philadelphia, PA: Lippincott Williams & Wilkins, 2006.)

Similar to other subaxial cervical spine injuries, unilateral and bilateral facet dislocations are more common in adolescents. Diagnosis is usually apparent on lateral radiographs. Reduction should be performed by traction if possible or open reduction if closed methods are unsuccessful. Either way, definitive treatment consists of posterior arthrodesis.

Compression fractures are the most common subaxial spine fracture in children. The mechanism of injury is flexion and axial loading. Lateral cervical spine films will demonstrate loss of vertebral body height. These injuries are almost always stable and can be treated with a cervical collar for 3 to 6 weeks. Flexion/extension radiographs should be obtained 2 to 4 weeks after injury to confirm stability of the cervical spine.

Burst fractures are caused by an axial load. Although radiographs are usually sufficient to make the diagnosis, CT scans are helpful in determining the amount of spinal canal

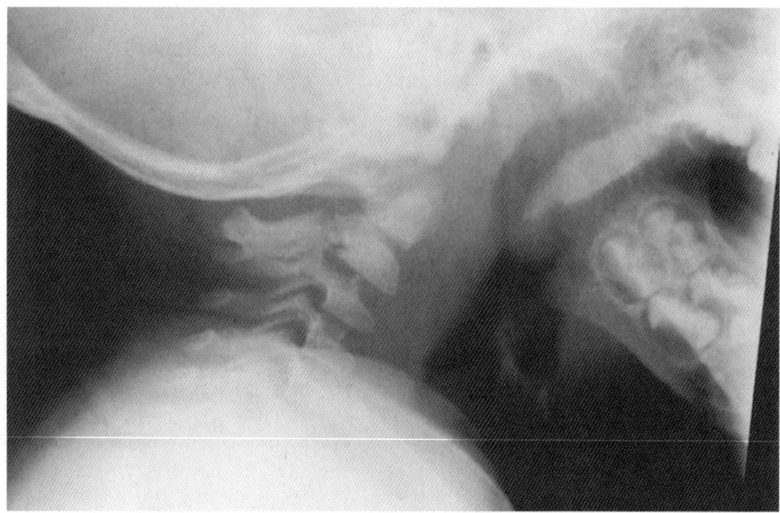

Figure 11.243 Lateral radiograph of a child with traumatic C2 spondylolisthesis (Hangman fracture). (*Reproduced with permission from* Beaty JH, Kasser JR. *Rockwood and Wilkins' Fractures in Children.* 6th ed. Philadelphia, PA: Lippincott Williams & Wilkins, 2006.)

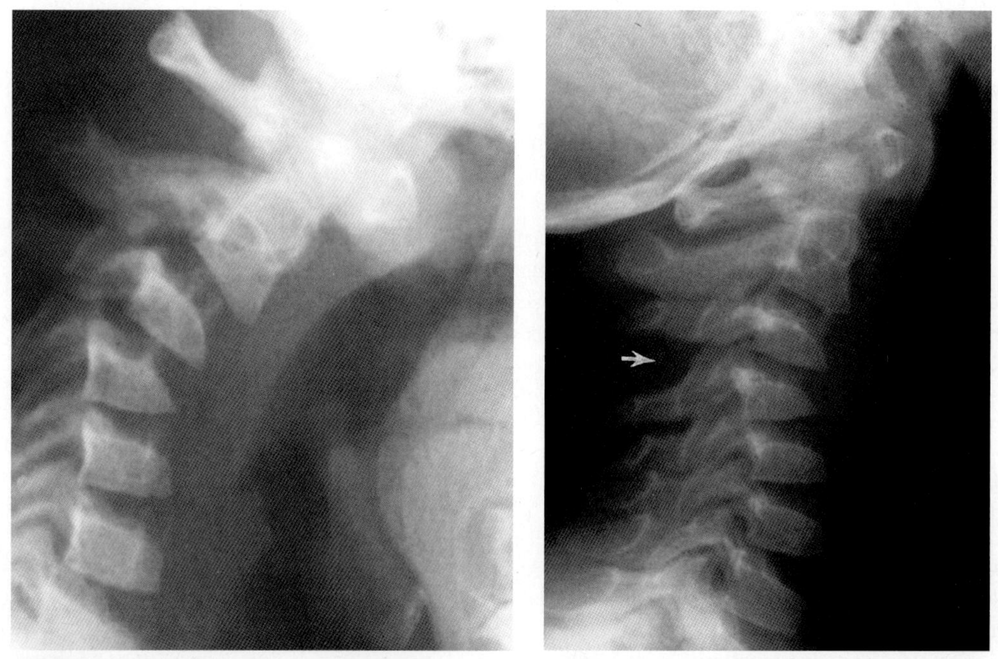

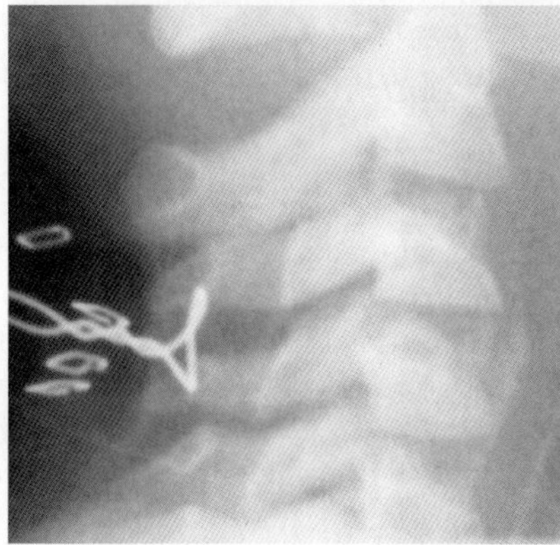

Figure 11.244 **(A)** Lateral flexion radiograph showing significant instability at the C3–C4 interspace. **(B)** The instability does not completely reduce in extension. Note the widening of the spinous processes (*arrow*). **(C)** The patient was treated with posterior fusion with iliac crest bone grafting and interspinous wiring. (*Reproduced with permission from* Morrissy RT, Weinstein SL. *Lovell and Winter's Pediatric Orthopaedics.* Philadelphia, PA: Lippincott Williams & Wilkins, 2006.)

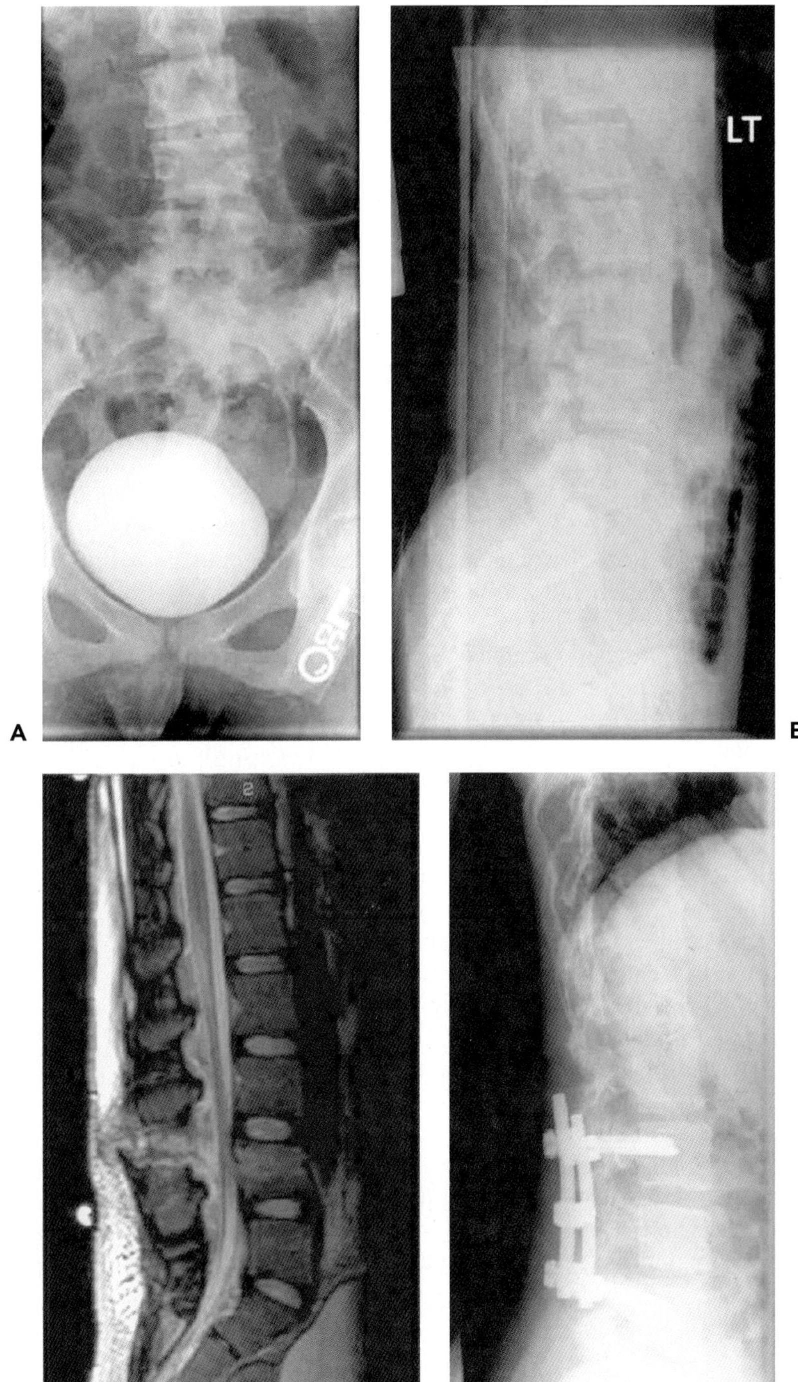

Figure 11.245 Chance fracture with bony and ligamentous injury. **(A, B)** Anteroposterior and lateral radiographs of a 14-year-old girl who sustained a high-speed motor vehicle accident. She was a front-seat, restrained passenger. Radiographs demonstrate a probable injury at L4. **(C)** Sagittal magnetic resonance imaging shows fracture through the L4 vertebral body and complete disruption of the posterior ligamentous complex. **(D)** Lateral radiograph taken after the patient was treated with posterior spinal instrumentation and fusion. (*Reproduced with permission from* Morrissy RT, Weinstein SL. *Lovell and Winter's Pediatric Orthopaedics*. Philadelphia, PA: Lippincott Williams & Wilkins, 2006.)

compromise from retropulsed fragments. The majority of fractures do not cause neurologic impairment and have minimal canal compromise; these injuries can be treated with a halo for 6 to 8 weeks, followed by flexion/extension radiographs to document stability. Those fractures associated with neurologic deficits or significant canal compromise may require surgical decompression and stabilization.

Thoracolumbar Fractures

Compression fractures occur due to an axial load with some degree of flexion. In these injuries, the anterior vertebral body collapses more than the posterior wall, resulting in anterior wedging of the vertebrae. Falls are the most common mechanism of injury. Fractures can occur at single or multiple levels depending on the severity of injury. Usually, diagnosis is straightforward given the radiographic findings and complaints of localized pain. For those cases in which the acuity of injury is uncertain, MRI can be useful. Most compression fractures are stable and can be treated symptomatically with a TLSO for 6 to 8 weeks. Rarely, local kyphosis can be severe enough (>40 degrees) to warrant posterior instrumentation and fusion.

Burst fractures occur from similar mechanisms as compression fractures but result from higher-energy injuries. In addition to affecting the anterior column, the fracture extends through the posterior wall of the vertebral body. Neurologic injury can result from spinal canal encroachment by retropulsed bony fragments. Determining the stability of these fractures can be difficult but usually relies on an intact posterior ligamentous complex. Stable fractures without neurologic impairment can be treated with brace immobilization for 2 to 4 months. Unstable fractures and any injuries associated with neurologic deficits require surgical decompression and stabilization through an anterior or posterior approach.

Chance fractures are ligamentous or bony injuries that occur from a flexion-distraction mechanism. Classically, Chance fractures occur from lap belt injuries sustained during motor vehicle accidents. During a frontal impact, the torso is driven forward and flexes over the restraining belt. The axis of rotation is anterior to the spine resulting in posterior distraction injuries and variable degrees of anterior compression; as a result, all three columns of the spine are affected. A high percentage of Chance fractures are associated with intraabdominal injuries. The plane of injury can be entirely through bone, soft tissue, or a combination of the two (Fig. 11.245). Bony injuries are readily diagnosed on lateral radiographs. If the injury is purely ligamentous, however, the only radiographic finding may be subtle widening of the spinous processes. MRI is usually indicated to assess the spinal cord and the integrity of the posterior ligamentous complex. Pure bony injuries can be treated with extension bracing or casting (often with thigh extension). Chance fractures with ligamentous components, significant abdominal injury, or neurologic impairment should be treated with posterior instrumentation and fusion.

Spinal Cord Injury without Radiographic Abnormality

The acronym SCIWORA refers to Spinal Cord Injury Without Radiographic Abnormality and is almost exclusively a pediatric injury. As its name implies, SCIWORA is characterized by a spinal cord injury in a patient with normal radiographs. The injury is thought to result from greater elasticity of the spinal column relative to the spinal cord that can allow for spinal cord stretch. Vascular insults to the cord have also been suggested as a possible etiology. Neurologic injury can be partial or complete, and the onset of symptoms can be delayed. MRI is the diagnostic modality of choice and can reveal edema, hemorrhage, or contusion of the spinal cord. Treatment consists of immobilization to prevent further neurologic deficit.

RECOMMENDED READINGS

Cavalier R, Herman MJ, Cheung EV, et al. Spondylolysis and spondylolisthesis in children and adolescents, I: diagnosis, natural history, and nonsurgical management. *J Am Acad Orthop.* 2006;14:415–424.

Cheung EV, Herman MJ, Cavalier R, et al. Spondylolysis and spondylolisthesis in children and adolescents, II: surgical management. *J Am Acad Orthop.* 2006;14:488–498.

Guille JT, Sherk HH. Congenital osseous anomalies of the upper and lower cervical spine in children. *J Bone Joint Surg Am.* 2002;84:277–288.

Hedequist D, Emans J. Congenital scoliosis. *J Am Acad Orthop.* 2004; 12:266–275.

Lenke LG, Betz RR, Harms J, et al. Adolescent idiopathic scoliosis: a new classification to determine the extent of spinal arthrodesis. *J Bone Joint Surg Am.* 2001;83:1169–1181.

McMaster MJ, Ohtsuka K. The natural history of congenital scoliosis: a study of 251 patients. *J Bone Joint Surg Am.* 1982;64:1128–1147.

Newton PO, ed. *Adolescent Idiopathic Scoliosis Monograph.* Rosemont, IL: American Academy of Orthopaedic Surgeons; 2004.

Skaggs DL, Flynn JM. *Staying Out of Trouble in Pediatric Orthopaedics.* Philadelphia, PA: Lippincott Williams & Wilkins; 2006.

Weinstein SL, Dolan LA, Spratt KF, et al. Health and function of patients with untreated idiopathic scoliosis: a 50-year natural history study. *JAMA.* 2003;289:559–567.

Section 3 Pediatric Musculoskeletal Trauma

Wudbhav N. Sankar John M. Flynn

Orthopaedic injuries in children differ from those in adults for both biologic and mechanical reasons (Table 11.8). Fractures in children are more common and more likely to occur after seemingly insignificant trauma. Although most fractures in children are easier to manage because of the rapidity and certainty of bony union and the ability of the child's bones to remodel, several specific fractures can be problematic and require proper understanding and treatment to achieve an optimal result.

TABLE 11.8
BIOLOGIC AND MECHANICAL DIFFERENCES BETWEEN CHILDREN AND ADULTS

Children	Adults
Active skeletal growth	Skeletal maturity
Thick, osteogenic periosteum	Thin, less osteogenic periosteum
Improved vascular supply	Inferior blood supply
Bones less brittle	Bones more brittle
Physis at risk for fracture	Ligaments more likely to fail
High remodeling potential	Low remodeling potential

CHARACTERISTICS OF THE IMMATURE SKELETON INFLUENCING PEDIATRIC INJURIES

One major biologic difference between adults and children is the phenomenon of active skeletal growth. In children, the machinery for skeletal growth is already "turned on," and this results in rapid remodeling of fractures from both physeal and appositional growth. The periosteum is the second major biologic difference between child and adult. In the adult, the periosteum is a relatively thin fibrous membrane that is not actively osteogenic. In the child, however, this periosteum is extremely thick, highly vascular, and osteogenic. In fact, the periosteum of the child is dual layered, with an outer fibrous layer and an inner osteogenic (cambial layer). This dual layer reflects its two purposes: the inner "biologic" layer facilitates fracture healing and the outer "mechanical" layer acts as a thick skin, which minimizes fracture displacement.

Another biologic difference is that the blood supply to the bone in children is reportedly richer, leading to more rapid and certain union. However, in certain areas, the circulation is as tenuous as in the adult. The femoral head and the lateral condyle of the distal humerus are two examples of anatomic regions that are highly vulnerable to avascularity and necrosis due to a fragile blood supply.

Mechanical differences also exist between the young and aging skeleton. Immature bone is less brittle than mature bone. As a result, a child's bone can deform plastically under a given load without necessarily fracturing completely through (Fig. 11.246). Unlike adults, incomplete fractures are not uncommon in this age group. Greenstick and torus fractures are examples of this unique ability of the child's bone to plastically deform.

The ultimate mechanical difference in the child is the presence of a "flaw" in the long bone. This flaw, the physis, is the weakest segment in a child's bone, and as a result, it is often the first point of failure during the application of excessive load. As a general principle, children less commonly sustain ligamentous injuries because the growth plate usually fails first (Fig. 11.247). An injury that would produce a sprain or dislocation in an adult is more likely to result in a physeal fracture in a child. These fractures may be subtle, and stress radiographs or more sophisticated imaging may be required to document the fracture if the initial radiographs are inconclusive. A typical example is the distal fibular physeal fracture, which can often be mistakenly diagnosed as an ankle sprain.

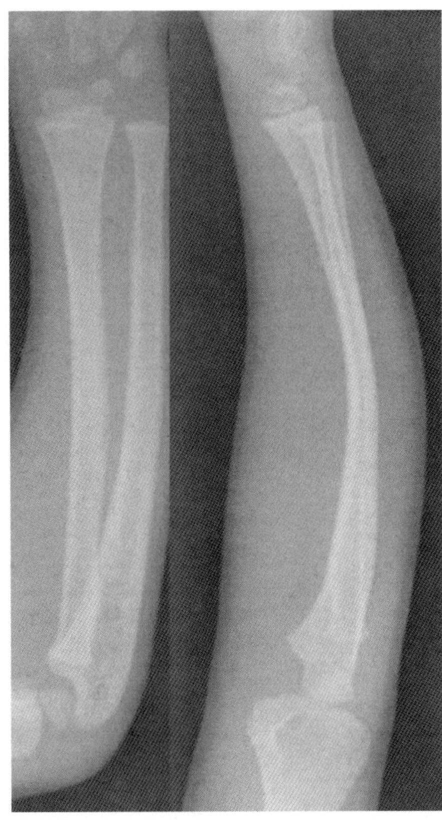

Figure 11.246 Plastic deformation of the forearm, resulting in approximately 15 degrees of apex dorsal angulation. (*Reproduced with permission from* Beaty JH, Kasser JR. *Rockwood and Wilkins' Fractures in Children.* 6th ed. Philadelphia, PA: Lippincott Williams & Wilkins, 2006.)

Fifteen to thirty percent of all skeletal injuries in children involve the physis. Although physeal fractures are classically thought to occur through the zone of provisional calcification (within the hypertrophic zone), they can actually occur through all four zones. Depending on the entrance and exit of the fracture line, physeal fractures can be classified according to the Salter–Harris classification (Fig. 11.248). It is worth mentioning that in Salter–Harris type II fractures, the metaphyseal fragment is also known as the *Thurston–Holland fragment.* In certain cases, this fragment is large enough to accept fixation and is often used to guide fracture reduction.

Although an open physis certainly contributes to the rapid healing of children's fractures, it also provides a source of unique complications compared with adults. Injury to the physis can result in a partial or complete growth arrest. Should the arrest be complete, the resulting

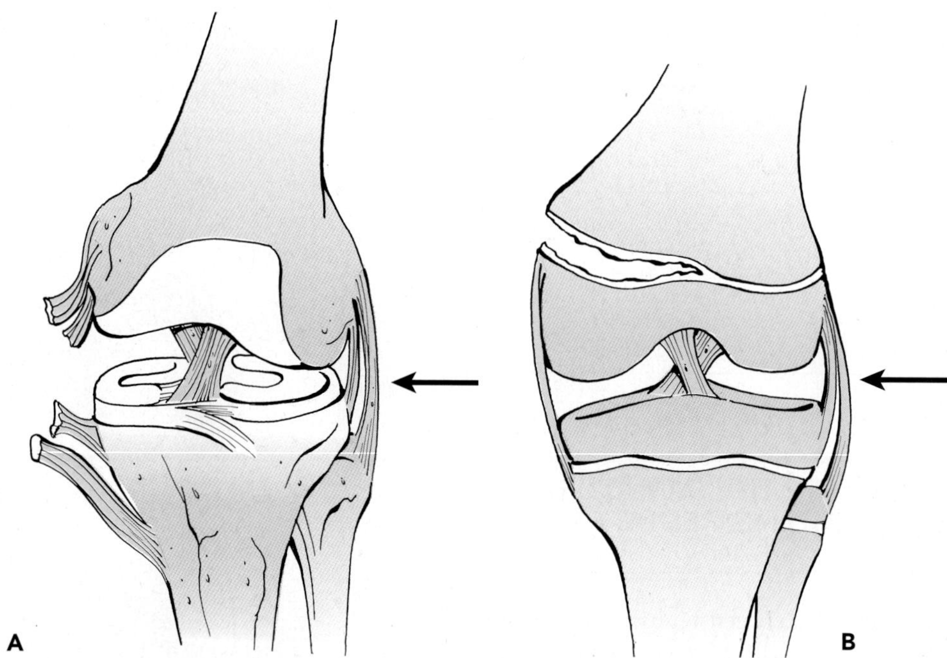

Figure 11.247 **(A)** In skeletally mature patients with closed physes, tensile failure usually occurs across the ligament. **(B)** In skeletally immature patients with open physes, failure usually occurs across the physis. (*Reproduced with permission from* Beaty JH, Kasser JR. *Rockwood and Wilkins' Fractures in Children.* 6th ed. Philadelphia, PA: Lippincott Williams & Wilkins, 2006.)

growth slowdown could result in a limb length discrepancy. If the arrest is partial, one side of the growth plate could shut down and an angular deformity may develop as the child grows asymmetrically. After a physeal fracture, follow-up radiographs should be carefully assessed for premature physeal closure and divergent Park–Harris growth lines (Fig. 11.249). These lines appear in the metaphysis after temporary periods of slowed growth (e.g., trauma, illness). Resumption of normal growth is marked by a parallel progression of the Park–Harris line away from the physis. Lack of progression may indicate a complete arrest, and an oblique Park–Harris line implies a partial arrest.

Finally, because of the "turned on machinery," the active periosteum, and (usually) improved blood supply, children's fractures have a superior remodeling potential compared with adults. As a result, the orthopaedic surgeon is frequently able to accept reductions in a child that would be considered completely inadequate in the adult. Depending on the anatomical region, a certain amount of displacement, overriding, and angulation (especially in the plane

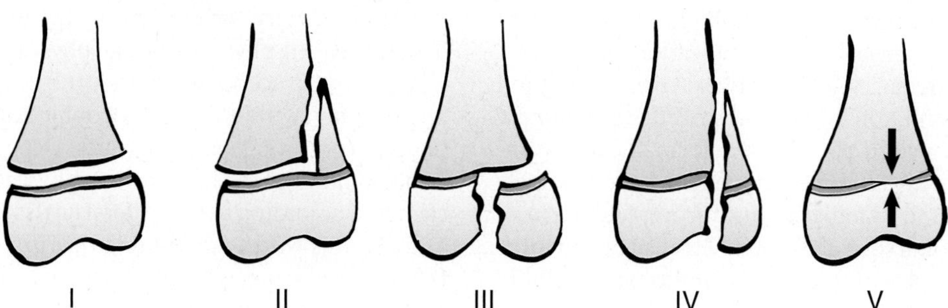

Figure 11.248 Salter–Harris classification of physeal fractures. In Salter–Harris type I fractures, the fracture line is entirely within the physis. In Salter–Harris type II fractures, the fracture line extends from the physis into the metaphysic; in Salter–Harris type III fractures, the fracture enters the epiphysis from the physis and almost always exits the articular surface. In Salter–Harris type IV injuries the fracture extends across the physis from the articular surface and epiphysis, to exit in the margin of the metaphysic. Salter–Harris type V fractures were described by Salter and Harris as a crush injury to the physis with initially normal radiographs with late identification of premature physeal closure. (*Reproduced with permission from* Beaty JH, Kasser JR. *Rockwood and Wilkins' Fractures in Children.* 6th ed. Philadelphia, PA: Lippincott Williams & Wilkins, 2006.)

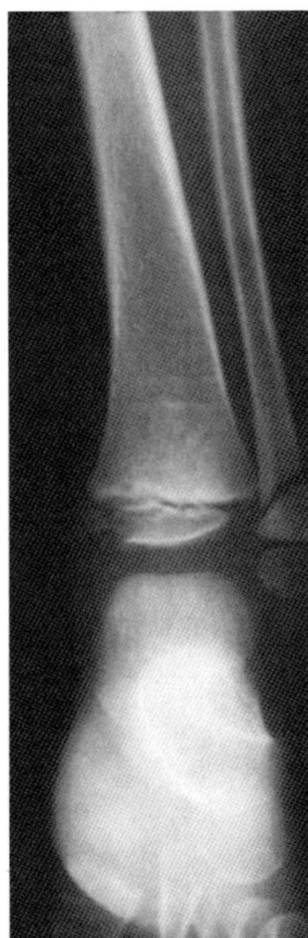
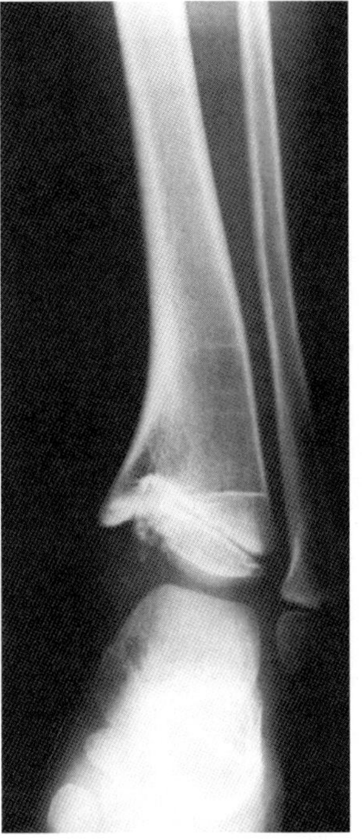

Figure 11.249 Distal tibial growth arrest. **(A)** Distal tibial physeal Salter–Harris type IV injury treated with cast immobilization without reduction. **(B)** Two years later, there is varus angulation to the distal tibia from a medial physeal bar. The Park–Harris growth arrest line is not parallel to the distal physis and indicates a partial arrest. (*Reproduced with permission from* Morrissy RT, Weinstein SL. *Lovell and Winter's Pediatric Orthopaedics.* Philadelphia, PA: Lippincott Williams & Wilkins, 2006.)

of joint motion) will be corrected by this remodeling phenomenon (Fig. 11.250). There is a limit to the amount of remodeling that can be achieved; for example, rotational deformities are rarely amenable to this type of correction. It is important to remember that remodeling depends on the presence and proximity of an active physis; therefore, adolescents with closing physes have decreased remodeling potential and should be treated more like adults.

GENERAL TREATMENT PRINCIPLES

On the basis of the improved biology of fracture healing, more pediatric fractures can be treated with cast immobilization (with or without reduction) than adult fractures. Children have higher activity levels than do adults and are often less compliant with activity restrictions. These issues should be considered before discontinuing immobilization. In spite of the predominance of nonoperative treatment for children's fractures, certain injuries necessitate operative intervention. Open fractures should be treated with formal irrigation and debridement in the operating room, followed by appropriate fracture specific treatment. Intraarticular fractures with any significant degree of displacement (>2 mm) should be treated with adult principles of anatomic reduction and internal fixation. Physeal fractures with any concerning degree of displacement should be reduced gently to minimize trauma to the growth plate. Depending on the anatomic region, the physis may need to be stabilized with internal fixation. If it is necessary to cross the physis with hardware to achieve adequate fixation, smooth pins are usually used to minimize the possibility of growth arrest.

PEDIATRIC POLYTRAUMA

Approximately 10% of all pediatric trauma patients admitted to the hospital are victims of multiple injuries. Trauma is the leading cause of death in children, accounting for more fatalities and disabilities than all other causes combined in children older than 1 year. Motor vehicle accidents involving the child as a passenger, pedestrian, or bicyclist are the most common mechanisms of pediatric polytrauma.

An aggressive team approach for these severely injured children is required, including input from general surgeons, neurosurgeons, pediatricians, and emergency department physicians. Initial management consists of ensuring the standard ABCs (airway, breathing, and circulation). After completion of the primary survey and stabilization of the patient, the secondary survey is conducted in a manner similar to standard adult trauma protocols.

Certain differences in the anatomy and physiology of pediatric patients can provide unique challenges. Compared with adults, children have relatively large tongues, smaller mouths, and smaller larynxes, which can make intubation more difficult. The head of a child is proportionately larger; as a result, immobilization on a standard adult spineboard will flex the neck and could exacerbate any cervical spine injury. The protuberant abdomen in children offers less protection to vital organs from either the rib cage or the pelvis, consequently pediatric patients have a higher incidence of intraabdominal injuries. Children and adults also have physiologic differences that impact their care as polytrauma patients. In the pediatric population, tachycardia is able to compensate for large intravascular volume losses; therefore, decreased blood pressure is usually a late sign of hypovolemic shock. Hypothermia is also more prevalent in children due to the large surface area to body weight ratios.

Outcomes in children can be predicted by using the modified injury severity scale (MISS), as described by Mayer (Table 11.9). This has proved to be useful in predicting morbidity and mortality rates in the pediatric age group. The MISS employs the Glasgow coma scale for grading the neurologic injury; in addition, it reviews damage to individual body areas, such as the face and neck, the chest, the abdomen, and the extremities. Rapid evaluation of the pediatric polytrauma patient can be assessed also by using the Pediatric Trauma Score (Table 11.10). Several components such as size, airway integrity, central nervous system

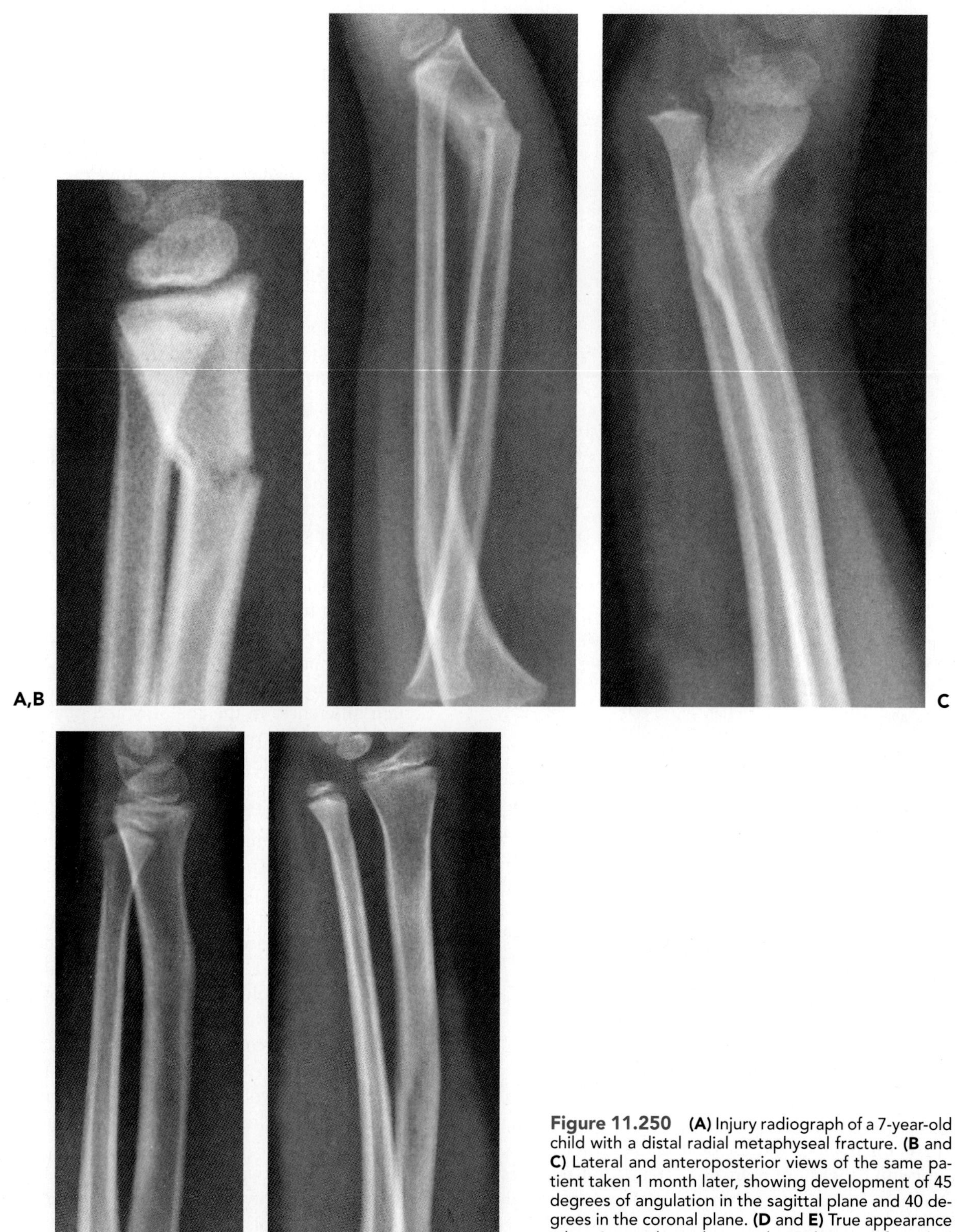

Figure 11.250 **(A)** Injury radiograph of a 7-year-old child with a distal radial metaphyseal fracture. **(B** and **C)** Lateral and anteroposterior views of the same patient taken 1 month later, showing development of 45 degrees of angulation in the sagittal plane and 40 degrees in the coronal plane. **(D** and **E)** True appearance taken 4 years later shows only 10 degrees of residual angulation in the sagittal plane and full correction of coronal plane angulation. The patient had full range of motion, equal to that of the opposite extremity, and was asymptomatic. (*Reproduced with permission from* Beaty JH, Kasser JR. *Rockwood and Wilkins' Fractures in Children.* 6th ed. Philadelphia, PA: Lippincott Williams & Wilkins, 2006.)

TABLE 11.9

THE MODIFIED INJURY SEVERITY SCALE (MISS) FOR MULTIPLE INJURY CHILDREN

Body Area	1—Minor	2—Moderate	3—Severe, Not Life-Threatening	4—Severe, Life-Threatening	5—Critical, Survival Uncertain
Neural	GSC 13-14	GSC 9-12	GSC 9-12	GSC 5-8	GSC 4
Face and neck	Abrasion or contusions of ocular apparatus or lid Vitreous or conjuctival hemorrhage Fractured teeth	Undisplaced facial-bone fracture Laceration of eye, disfiguring laceration Retinal detachment	Loss of eye, avulsion of optic nerve Displaced facial fracture "Blow-out" fracture of orbit	Bone or soft-tissue injury with minor destruction	Injuries with major airway obstruction
Chest	Muscle ache or chest-wall stiffness	Simple rib or sternal fracture	Multiple rib fractures Hemothorax or pneumothorax Diaphragmatic rupture Pulmonary contusion	Open chest wounds Pneumomediastinum Myocardial contusion	Lacerations, tracheal hemomediastinum Aortic laceration Myocardial laceration or rupture
Abdomen	Muscle ache, seat-belt abrasion	Major abdominal-wall contusion	Contusion of abdominal organs Retroperitoneal hematoma Extraperitoneal bladder rupture Thoracic or lumbar spine fractures	Minor laceration of abdominal organs Intraperitoneal bladder rupture Spine fractures with paraplegia	Rupture or severe laceration of abdominal vessels or organs
Extremities and pelvic girdle	Minor sprains Simple fractures and dislocations	Open fractures of digits Non-displaced long-bone or pelvic fractures	Displaced long-bone or multiple hand or foot fractures Single open long-bone fracture Pelvic fractures with displacement Laceration of major nerves or vessels	Multiple closed long-bone fractures Amputation of limbs	Multiple open long-bone fractures

GSC = Glasgow Comma Scale.
(*Adapted from* Mayer T, Matlak ME, Johnson DG, Walker ML: The Modified Injury Severity Scale in pediatric multiple trauma patients. *J Pediatr Surg.* 1980;15:719; and *from* Green NE, Swiontkowski MF: Skeletal Trauma in Children, Vol 3. Philadelphia, WB Saunders, 1998.)

TABLE 11.10
PEDIATRIC TRAUMA SCORE

Variable	+2	+1	−1
Weight (kg)	>20	10–20	<10
Airway patency	Normal	Maintained	Unmaintained
Systolic blood pressure (mm Hg)	>90	50–90	<50
Neurologic	Awake	Obtunded	Comatose
Open wound	None	Minor	Major
Skeletal trauma	None	Closed	Open or multiple

(*Reprinted with permission from* Morrissy RT, Weinstein SL. *Lovell and Winter's Pediatric Orthopaedics*. Philadelphia, PA: Lippincott Williams & Wilkins, 2006.)

integrity, systolic blood pressure, the presence or absence of open wound, and the amount of skeletal damage can be used to rapidly assess these patients. Total point counts greater than 8 predict an excellent prognosis for survival; scores less than 0 indicate a very high risk of death.

When evaluating orthopaedic injuries in the polytrauma patient, it is important to remember that children tend to be better able to survive extremely severe injuries and frequently respond better to a given injury than do adults. As a result, care must be taken not to overlook musculoskeletal injuries or to delay treatment any longer than absolutely necessary in the multiply injured child, as this can result in future problems. A common example is the head-injured child with a supracondylar elbow fracture who receives late treatment for his elbow injury because of prolonged concerns for the safety of the brain. One year later, the child has made a full neurologic recovery and his only complaint is about the malunion of his elbow and the resulting loss of elbow motion. Good communication between orthopaedic surgeons, trauma surgeons, and neurosurgeons is essential to ensure safe and timely treatment of all injuries.

UPPER EXTREMITY

Shoulder and Arm Injuries

Clavicle Fractures and Dislocations

Fractures of the clavicle occur in all age groups, from the neonate to the adult. Birth fractures of the clavicle are the most common fracture in the newborn. Frequently, the diagnosis can be made in the nursery when the child develops pseudoparalysis of the involved limb and an asymmetric Moro reflex. It is important to evaluate the child for associated brachial plexus palsy as both conditions can result from a difficult delivery. Treatment for these clavicle injuries should be simple immobilization of the extremity with a soft wrap of cast padding or stockinette. Healing is rapid, and long-term sequelae are virtually nonexistent.

In older patients, diaphyseal fractures are the most common injury to the clavicle. Typically, these fractures result from a fall onto the point of the shoulder, and the diagnosis is straightforward: patients have tenderness along the clavicular shaft, associated with pain on motion of the upper extremity. Standard treatment is brief immobilization in a sling or figure-of-8 dressing. Rapid healing in 3 to 6 weeks is expected, with restoration of full motion, function, and strength in most patients. Parents should be warned about the "bump" or mass of callus that can form around these fractures. This mass resolves with normal growth and remodeling. Recent concerns in adults regarding malunion, nonunion, and refracture have caused a trend toward open reduction and internal fixation of markedly displaced midshaft clavicle fractures. The indications for operative fixation in adolescents are somewhat unclear but may have a role in severely displaced fractures in older adolescents.

Fractures of the medial end of the clavicle are quite rare, accounting for fewer than 10% of clavicular fractures. Equally rare are true sternoclavicular dislocations. The clavicle is the first bone to ossify; however, the medial physis does not close until approximately 25 years of age. As a result, most medial injuries to the clavicle are actually physeal fractures that can mimic a sternoclavicular dislocation. In patients with these injuries, plain radiographs are often difficult to interpret, and computed tomography (CT) scans are usually needed to make the diagnosis. Posterior injuries are of particular concern because they can compress the trachea, esophagus, or great vessels (Fig. 11.251). Closed reduction in the operating room with vascular or thoracic surgery support has traditionally been advocated for these fractures. Because of concerns about recurrent instability after closed reduction, many surgeons are starting to prefer open reduction of these injuries. Usually the medial clavicle is approached anteriorly. The fracture is reduced under direct visualization, and suture is used to repair the sternoclavicular joint capsule and ligaments to preserve a stable reduction.

Fractures of the distal end of the clavicle also are frequently physeal separations. The distal physis remains open until approximately 19 years of age. The persistence of this open physis along with the presence of a thick periosteal sleeve around the distal clavicle makes physeal fractures more common than true lateral clavicular fractures. Once the physis closes, an acromioclavicular separation is the usual injury. Again, the injury typically results from a fall onto the point of the shoulder and simple radiographs are usually adequate to make the diagnosis. Short-term sling immobilization is sufficient for most of these injures.

Fractures of the Proximal Humerus and Humeral Shaft

Proximal humerus fractures can be either physeal or metaphyseal but usually are Salter–Harris type I or type II injuries. Physeal separations have been described in

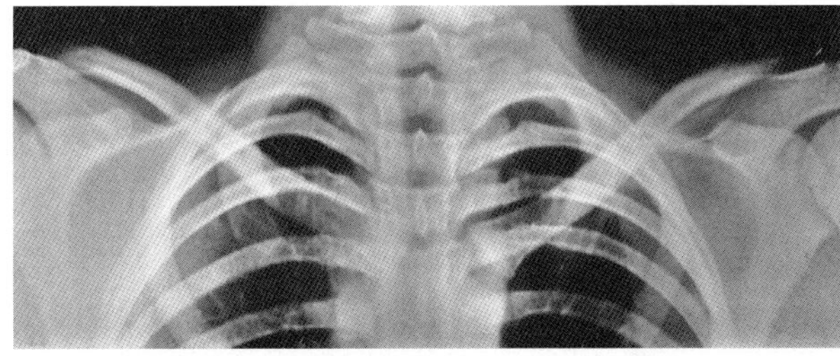
A

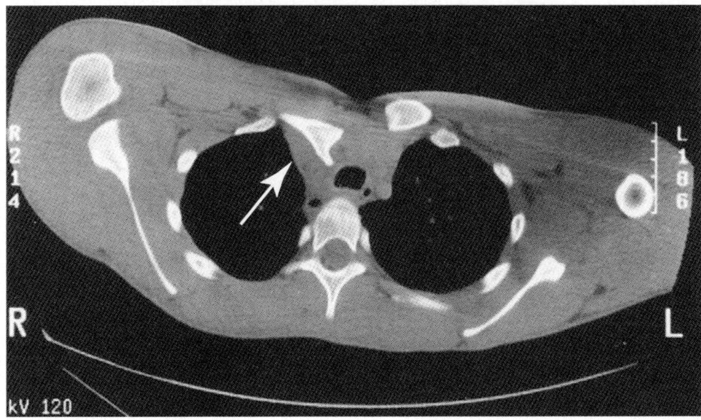

B

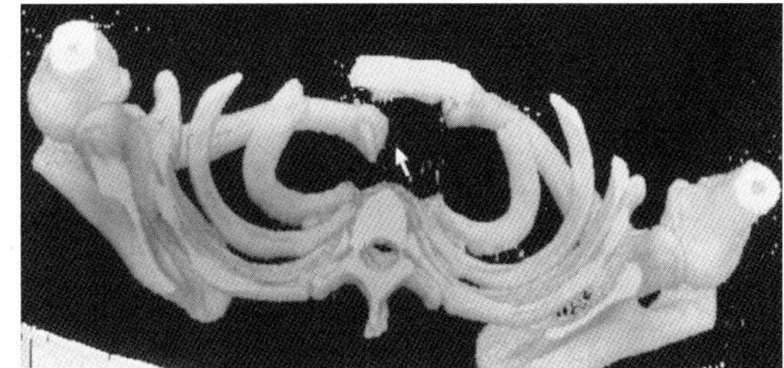
C

Figure 11.251 Sternoclavicular separation. This 14-year-old boy sustained an injury to the right clavicle during a wrestling match when his shoulder was compressed against his chest wall. He complained of shortness of breath, especially when he extended his neck. **(A)** The anteroposterior radiograph demonstrates asymmetry of the sternal position of the clavicle. **(B)** The computed tomographic scan demonstrates posterior displacement of the medial end of the right clavicle, which is near the trachea (*arrow*). **(C)** A three-dimensional reconstruction, with a cephalic projection, demonstrates the posterior and midline displacement of the clavicle. (*Reproduced with permission from* Morrissy RT, Weinstein SL. *Lovell and Winter's Pediatric Orthopaedics.* Philadelphia, PA: Lippincott Williams & Wilkins, 2006.)

neonates, but most injuries occur in adolescents. The geometry of the proximal humeral physis is not planar but rather "tent shaped," with the apex located posteromedially. Before closing between the ages of 14 and 18, the proximal humeral physis contributes 80% of the growth of the total humerus. Because of this large growth potential, a tremendous amount of deformity can be accepted and expected to remodel (Fig. 11.252). Furthermore, the vast range of motion of the glenohumeral joint permits adequate compensation for any residual deformity. As a result, closed treatment with sling immobilization is recommended for almost all pediatric patients with either a metaphyseal or physeal fracture of the proximal humerus. Closed reduction and percutaneous pin fixation is generally not necessary unless a child has greater than 40 degrees of malalignment and is nearing skeletal maturity. One definite indication for open reduction and internal fixation is a biceps tendon entrapped in the fracture site.

Fractures of the humeral shaft are uncommon in children; when seen, the child is usually older than 12 years or younger than 3 years. It is critically important to recognize the association between spiral fractures of the humeral shaft and child abuse. In children younger than 3 years, an acute torsional injury to the upper extremity typically produces this unique spiral lesion. If there is an inconsistent history of injury, delay in presentation for care, or associated injuries in these children, additional investigation into possible abuse is warranted. Humeral shaft fractures have also been reported in neonates following difficult delivery and, much like clavicle fractures, are heralded by pseudoparalysis of the upper extremity (Fig. 11.253). Because of compensatory shoulder and elbow range of motion, up to 30 to 40 degrees of malalignment is acceptable. As a result, the vast majority of humeral shaft fractures can be treated by closed methods, such as collar and cuff, functional brace, or sling immobilization. Most fractures are "sticky" by 4 weeks, and mobilization can occur at this time. Select polytrauma victims (usually adolescents) may be candidates for operative treatment. In these rare cases, both titanium elastic nails and plate fixation have been used with good success.

Radial nerve injuries associated with humeral shaft fractures are usually due to a contusion sustained during initial fracture displacement. These palsies are classically associated with fractures at the junction of the middle and distal third (Holstein–Lewis fractures). True entrapment of the radial nerve in the fracture site is rare; therefore, almost all children with radial nerve injuries should be observed with the expectation of full recovery. If the radial nerve fails to recover by 3 to 4 months, electrodiagnostic studies and surgical exploration are warranted.

Elbow Injuries

No injury generates as much anxiety for orthopaedic surgeons unaccustomed to treating children as do elbow fractures. There is good reason for this: a small swollen elbow is difficult to examine, neurovascular structures are often at risk, and radiographs can be difficult to interpret because of multiple evolving ossification centers. The anatomy of the child's elbow differs dramatically from that of the adult. At birth, no epiphyseal structures are present. The first secondary ossification center to appear is that of the capitellum, usually observed at 6 months of age. Following that, in order of appearance, the ossification centers of the radial head, medial epicondyle, trochlea, olecranon, and the lateral epicondyle are seen (Fig. 11.254). Initially, these are all parts of one large chondroepiphysis. With rapid differential

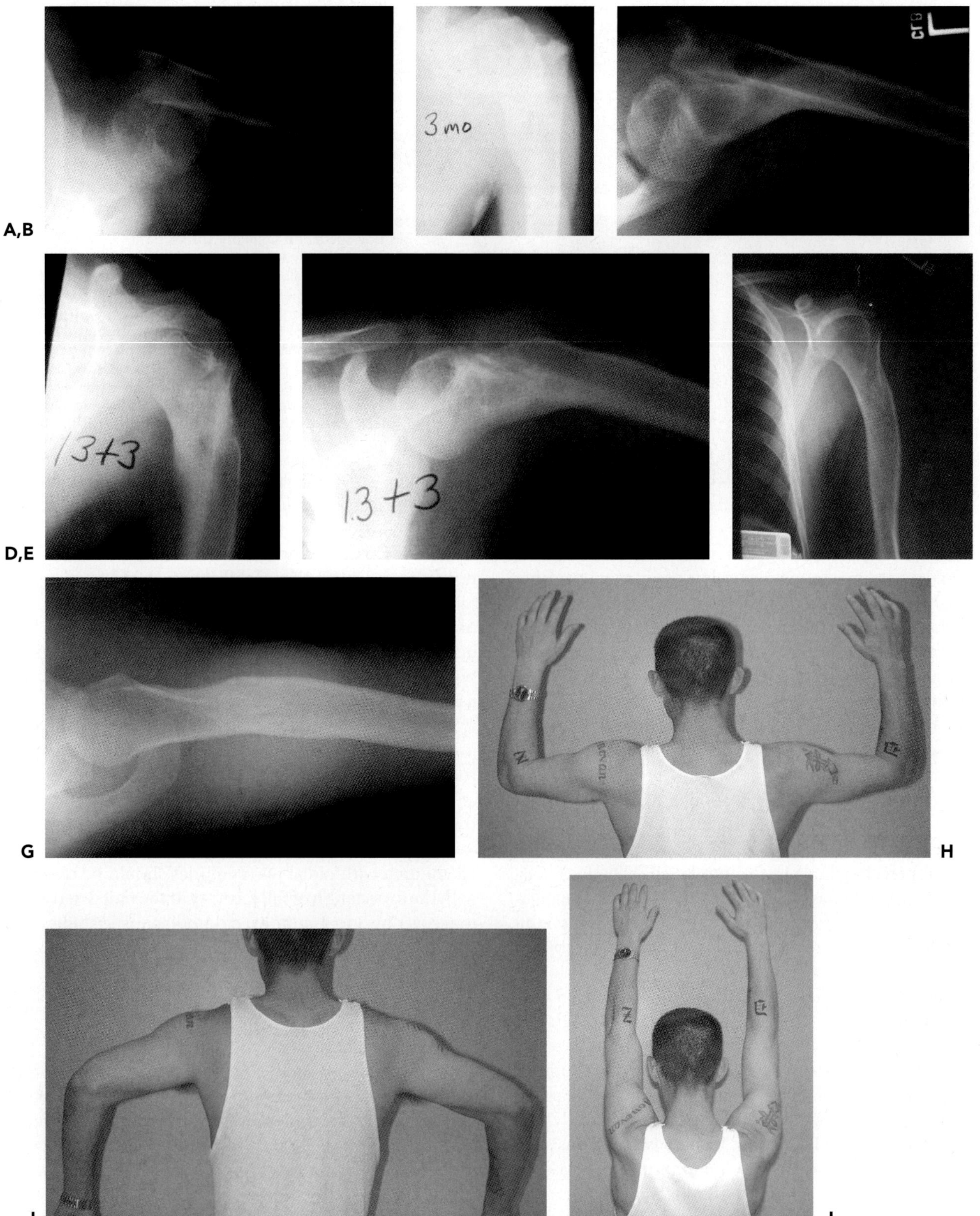

Figure 11.252 Proximal humeral fracture in a 12-year-old boy. **(A)** the initial fracture was treated with a sling and swathe. **(B** and **C)** Three months after injury, healing and early remodeling are evident. **(D** and **E)** One year after injury, remodeling continues. **(F** and **G)** Four years after injury, remodeling is complete. **(H–J)** The patient has recovered full range of motion but has a 1 cm arm length discrepancy. (*Reproduced with permission from* Morrissy RT, Weinstein SL. *Lovell and Winter's Pediatric Orthopaedics*. Philadelphia, PA: Lippincott Williams & Wilkins, 2006.)

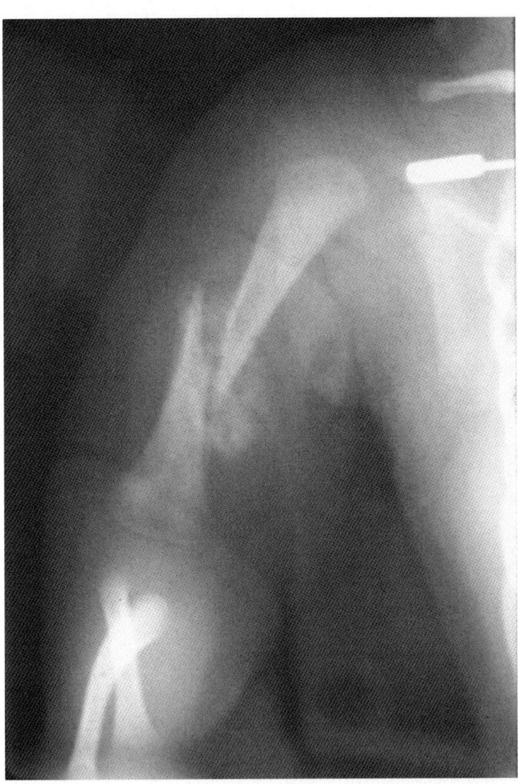

Figure 11.253 Fracture of the humeral shaft sustained at birth demonstrates significant callus by the age of 14 days and was probably comfortable enough in 7 days to obviate the need for any immobilization. (*Reproduced with permission from* Skaggs DL, Flynn JM. *Staying Out of Trouble in Pediatric Orthopaedics.* Philadelphia, PA: Lippincott Williams & Wilkins, 2006.)

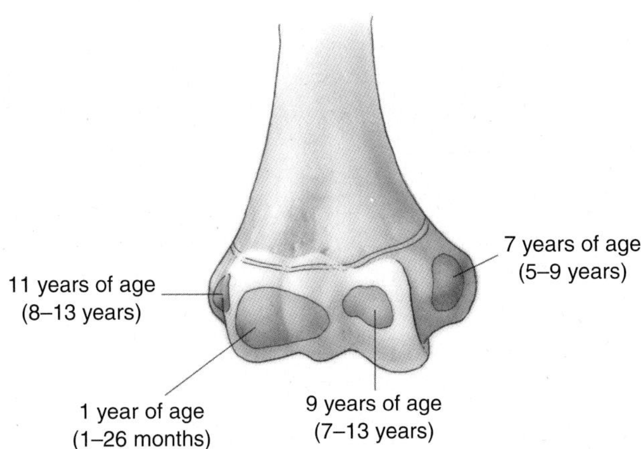

Figure 11.254 Ossification of the secondary centers of the distal humerus. The average ages are specified, and the age ranges are indicated. The ossification ranges are earlier for girls than for boys. The lateral epicondyle, capitellum, and trochlea coalesce between 10 and 12 years of age, subsequently fusing to the distal humerus between 13 and 16 years of age. This is about the time that the medial epicondyle fuses to the proximal humerus. (*Reproduced with permission from* Morrissy RT, Weinstein SL. *Lovell and Winter's Pediatric Orthopaedics.* Philadelphia, PA: Lippincott Williams & Wilkins, 2006.)

growth, the medial epicondyle forms its own ossification center, and the capitellum, trochlea, and lateral epicondyle become one center. Proper understanding of the sequence, timing, and appearance of these secondary ossification centers is essential for interpreting pediatric elbow injuries. Even with this knowledge, it is still often difficult to distinguish a subtle fracture from a normal ossification center, and radiographs of the contralateral elbow can provide much needed clarity. If the diagnosis remains uncertain, ultrasound, arthrography, or magnetic resonance imaging (MRI) may be necessary to avoid missing an important injury.

Supracondylar Humerus Fractures

If elbow injuries as a group generate the most anxiety for orthopaedic surgeons, then supracondylar humerus fractures are certainly the biggest culprit. The complications of this injury, as well as the treatment, are legendary in the pediatric orthopaedic literature. Satisfactory long-term outcomes are not guaranteed even with anatomic reduction. However, techniques and practices that have advanced over the last two decades have significantly reduced the number of serious complications.

Supracondylar fractures are the most common elbow fractures in children, accounting for roughly 60% of all pediatric elbow injuries. The incidence of supracondylar fractures is correlated with age as it is almost exclusively an injury of the immature elbow; the peak incidence of these fractures is between the ages of 5 and 7 years. Boys are more affected than girls, by a 3:2 ratio. There are two general groups of supracondylar fractures: extension type (95%) and flexion type (5%) (Fig. 11.255). Each results from different mechanisms of injury.

In the supracondylar region of the humerus, there are two strong columns of bone: one medial and one lateral. Between them is a central "wafer" of bone, which is often no thicker than 1 mm. Because of this dramatic decrease in anteroposterior (AP) diameter and the acute change in cross-sectional geometry (from cylindrical to flattened), the supracondylar region is mechanically vulnerable (Fig. 11.256). With hyperextension loading, the olecranon levers against the olecranon fossa and creates a bending moment. This can cause tensile failure of the anterior surface of the distal humerus, resulting in the classic extension-type injury. The fact that hyperextension loading is so common accounts for the preponderance of these injuries. The few flexion-type injuries seen typically result from a direct fall on the olecranon, thereby bending the supracondylar region in the opposite direction.

The classification most widely accepted is that proposed by Gartland in 1959. A type I fracture is nondisplaced and is often diagnosed by a positive posterior fat pad sign (Fig. 11.257). Type II injuries are displaced but have an intact posterior hinge of periosteum and bone, usually making them stable in external rotation. Type III fractures are completely displaced and can be further subdivided into those

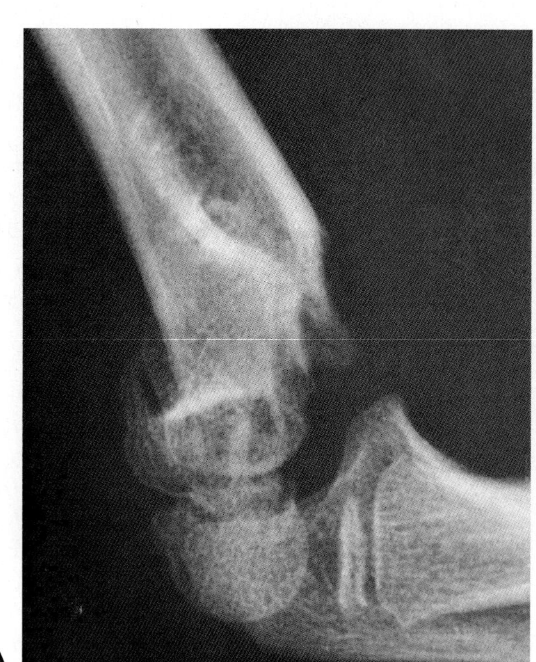

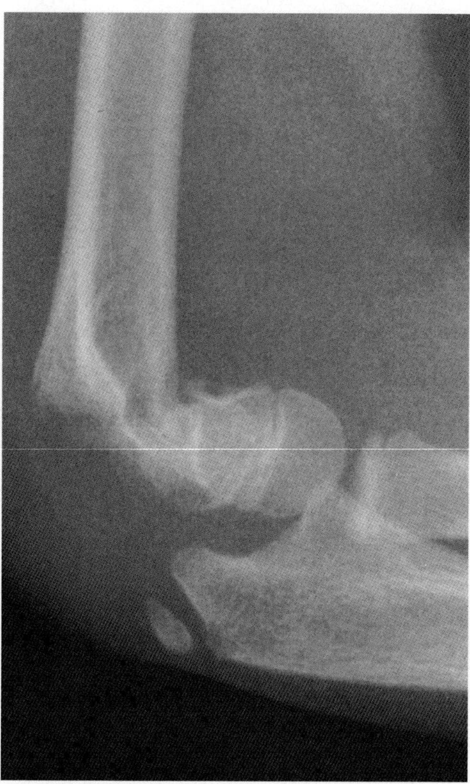

Figure 11.255 **(A)** Lateral radiograph showing an extension-type supracondylar humerus fracture. **(B)** Lateral radiograph demonstrating a flexion-type fracture. (*Reproduced with permission from* Beaty JH, Kasser JR. *Rockwood and Wilkins' Fractures in Children*. 6th ed. Philadelphia, PA: Lippincott Williams & Wilkins, 2006.)

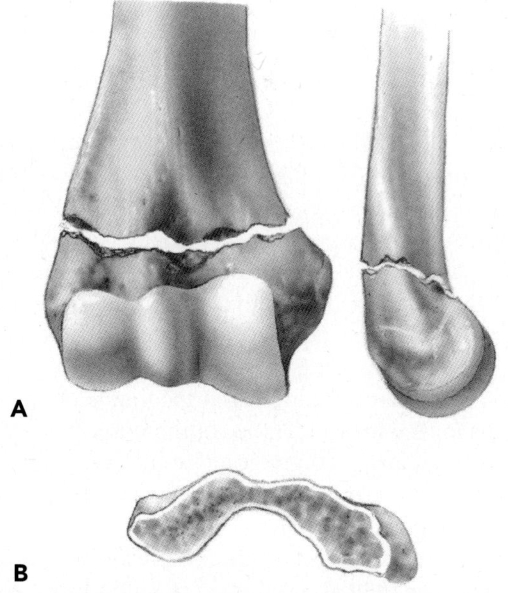

Figure 11.256 **(A)** The typical orientation of the fracture line in a supracondylar fracture. **(B)** A cross-sectional view through the fracture demonstrates the thin cross-sectional area of bone that is mechanically vulnerable. (*Reproduced with permission from* Morrissy RT, Weinstein SL. *Lovell and Winter's Pediatric Orthopaedics*. Philadelphia, PA: Lippincott Williams & Wilkins, 2006.)

displaced posterolaterally and those displaced posteromedially; the latter account for approximately 75% of the total. It is important to note the direction of displacement, because it frequently has an impact on management. A more recent type IV fracture has been described by Skaggs et al., in which the periosteum has been stripped circumferentially and the fracture is, therefore, unstable in both flexion and extension.

In addition to the Gartland classification, there are several radiographic measurements that are essential when evaluating a supracondylar humerus fracture. The single most important measurement is drawn on the lateral view by extending a line down the anterior surface of the humerus through the elbow joint (Fig. 11.258). If the line intersects any part of the capitellar ossification center, then the reduction (at least in the sagittal plane) is deemed acceptable. If, however, the anterior humeral line falls anterior to the ossification center, it indicates extension at the fracture site and the need for reduction. On the AP view, the most important measurement is Baumann angle, which is formed between a line perpendicular to the axis of the humerus and a line paralleling the metaphysis on the lateral side of the distal humerus (Fig. 11.259). The normal angle varies between 9 and 26 degrees. A measurement less than this indicates that the fracture is in varus,

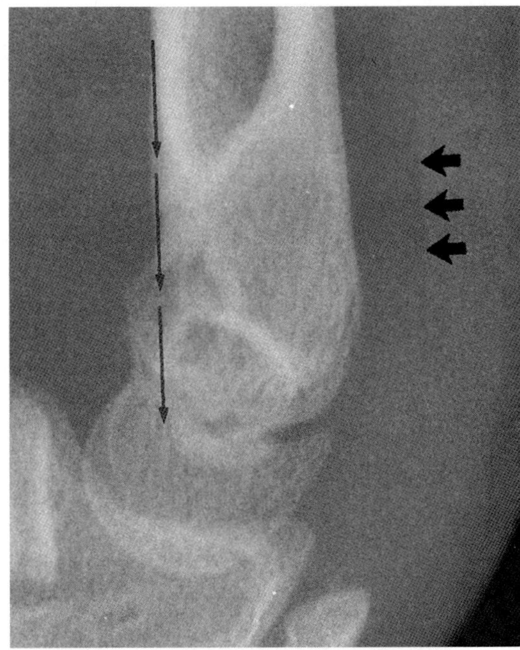

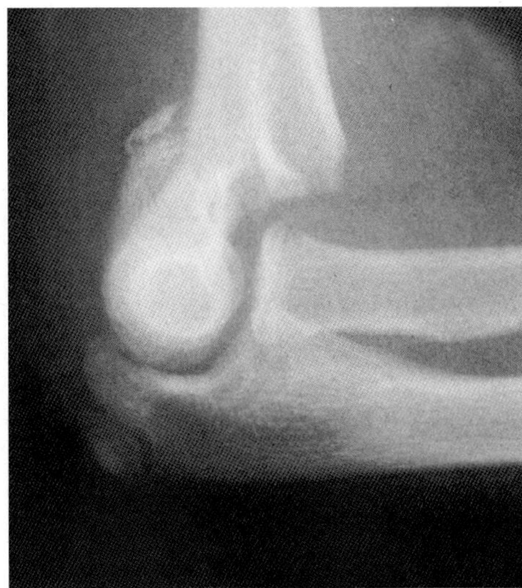

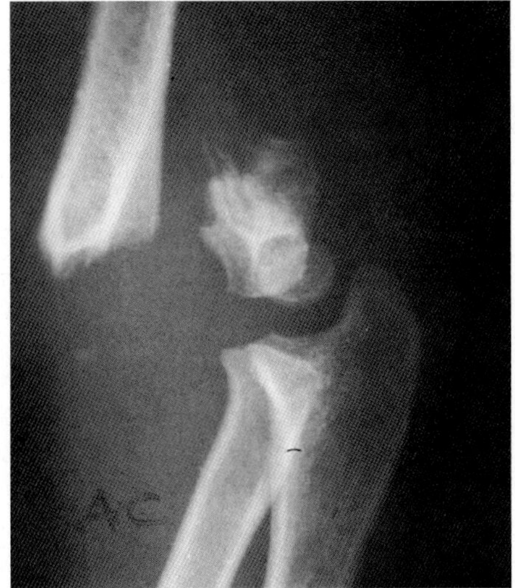

Figure 11.257 Types of supracondylar fractures. **(A)** Type I fracture is nondisplaced. Often the only evidence is posterior displacement of the olecranon fat pad due to intraarticular blood (*large arrows*). **(B)** Type II fracture. Lateral view demonstrates a displaced supracondylar fracture with the posterior cortex intact. **(C)** Type III fracture is totally displaced. (*Reproduced with permission from* Beaty JH, Kasser JR. *Rockwood and Wilkins' Fractures in Children.* 6th ed. Philadelphia, PA: Lippincott Williams & Wilkins, 2006.)

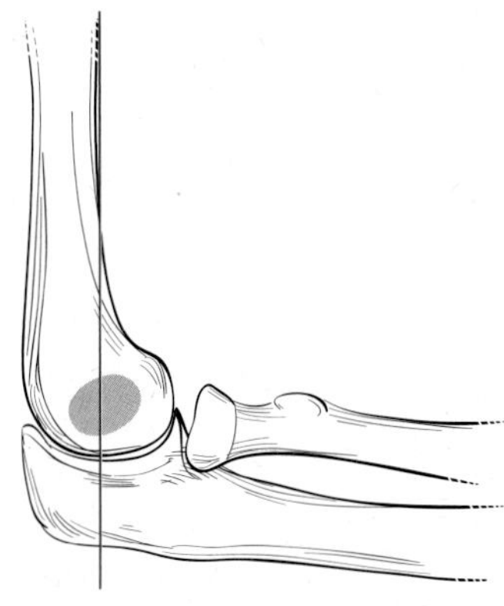

Figure 11.258 In the normal elbow, the anterior humeral line should intersect the capitellum. (*Reproduced with permission from* Skaggs DL, Flynn JM. *Staying Out of Trouble in Pediatric Orthopaedics.* Philadelphia, PA: Lippincott Williams & Wilkins, 2006.)

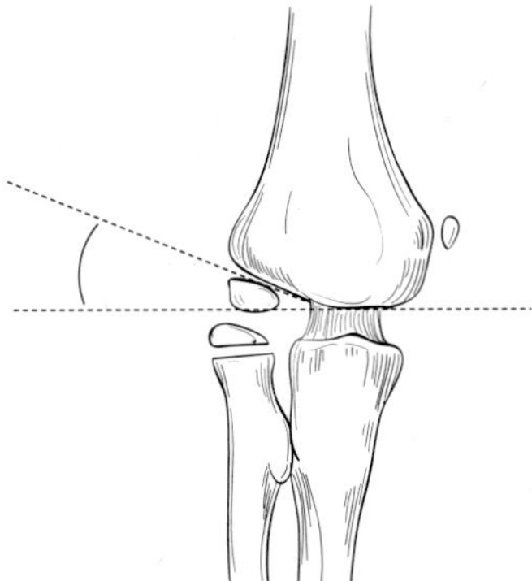

Figure 11.259 Baumann angle is formed between a line perpendicular to the axis of the humerus and a line paralleling the metaphysis on the lateral side of the distal humerus. The normal angle varies between 9 and 26 degrees. (*Reproduced with permission from* Skaggs DL, Flynn JM. *Staying Out of Trouble in Pediatric Orthopaedics.* Philadelphia, PA: Lippincott Williams & Wilkins, 2006.)

whereas a measurement greater than normal implies a valgus malalignment.

Because of the high rate of complications associated with these fractures, it is imperative that the initial evaluation of these children include a thorough physical and neurologic examination (and documentation of results). Although these patients experience pain and anxiety as a result of the injury, it is usually possible, even in small children, to conduct an accurate motor function examination. Evaluation should include testing of the median, ulnar, and radial nerves (including the anterior interosseus nerve and the posterior interosseus nerve). The radial pulse should be palpated, and the overall perfusion of the hand (i.e., warm and pink vs. cool and white) should be assessed. The skin should carefully be evaluated for signs of open fracture, tenting from buttonholed fracture fragments, and excessive bruising. The extremity should be examined for compartment syndrome by palpation and compartment pressure measurement if indicated.

Treatment of these fractures is generally based on the type. The major pitfall surrounding type I injuries is failure to recognize that a given fracture is actually type II. Type I injuries are truly nondisplaced. Care should be taken to ensure that the fracture does not have subtle varus impaction; Baumann angle is often helpful in the evaluation of this deformity. If the injury is truly a type I, then the application of a long arm cast, usually for 3 weeks, is sufficient treatment. Type II injuries again can suffer from too casual an approach by the treating surgeon. Although the posterior cortex is intact by definition, angulation (and progressive extension) can and does occur. If the anterior humeral line does not intersect the capitellum, then reduction is necessary. Although this reduction can be achieved by hyperflexion of the elbow, maintenance of the reduction requires immobilization in this position. It is well understood that hyperflexion of the elbow reduces perfusion to the hand; and therefore, the vast majority of surgeons prefer closed reduction and percutaneous pinning (CRPP) in the operating room (followed by immobilization at less than 90 degrees of flexion) for type II injuries. All type III injuries require CRPP. The initial displacement, whether it be posteromedial or posterolateral, will indicate the location of the intact periosteal hinge. The hinge is typically intact on the side of displacement. For example, in the more common posteromedially displaced injury, the periosteal hinge is medial. Therefore, pronation, which closes the lateral side and tightens the medial hinge, is generally employed (along with elbow flexion) to reduce these injuries. Likewise, supination and flexion are usually necessary for posterolaterally displaced fractures. If the fracture is difficult to reduce, the proximal fragment may be entrapped in the brachialis muscle. Manipulating the brachialis by "milking" it distally is usually successful in extracting the muscle away from the metaphyseal spike. Intraoperatively, fluoroscopy should be used to assess the quality of reduction by using both the anterior humeral line and Baumann angle. Rotational and translational residual deformities are less critical than residual varus or valgus tilt. Late deformities, which complicate the treatment of these injuries, result primarily from residual tilt in the coronal and sagittal plane that have minimal remodeling potential. Open reduction is reserved for those few cases of open injuries, compartment syndrome, or irreducible fractures.

Controversy still exists over the optimal number and configuration of pin placement. Although crossed medial and lateral pins have been shown to be more stable biomechanically, more surgeons are beginning to prefer lateral entry pin fixation because of the decreased risk of ulnar nerve injury (Fig. 11.260). In general, two lateral entry pins are sufficient for type II fractures, whereas three pins are usually necessary for type III fractures. As long as the pins engage both fracture fragments and have bicortical fixation and adequate spread at the fracture site, lateral-entry pins have been shown to be as clinically effective as crossed pins. If a medial pin is used, it should be placed after lateral pin placement, with the elbow extended to reduce the risk of anterior subluxation of the ulnar nerve. After percutaneous pinning, children should be immobilized in a cast or splint (depending on the amount of soft tissue swelling) at no more than 90 degrees of flexion for 3 to 4 weeks. At that point, pins are usually removed on an outpatient basis, and children are allowed to gradually return to their normal activities.

Complications of supracondylar fractures are acute nerve and vascular injuries and the late development of deformity. Nerve palsies have been reported in approximately 7% of patients. Although it was traditionally thought that the posterior interosseous nerve (PIN) was the most common to be damaged, recent data suggest that the anterior interosseous nerve (AIN) is actually the most commonly injured nerve. The ulnar nerve is the most common nerve injured during flexion-type fractures and as an iatrogenic result of percutaneous pinning (1%–5% incidence). The vast majority of nerve injuries sustained at the time of the fracture will resolve between 3 and 6 months and should therefore be observed. Ulnar nerve injuries as a result of medial pinning or other nerve palsies clearly sustained during CRPP should be explored and undergo revision pinning if necessary.

Vascular injuries are also associated with supracondylar humerus fractures. Often the brachial artery is tented over the metaphyseal fragment and tethered by its supratrochlear branch (Fig. 11.261). True injury to the artery occurs in 0.5% of cases. Cases of a cold, pulseless hand represent a surgical emergency and should undergo immediate reduction and stabilization. In most fractures, the vascularity of the hand will be restored after reduction. If arterial flow is still poor, immediate surgical exploration of the brachial artery (often with the help of a vascular consultant) is necessary. Not uncommonly, a child's hand is warm but pulseless on initial evaluation. This is usually the result of excellent peripheral and collateral blood flow

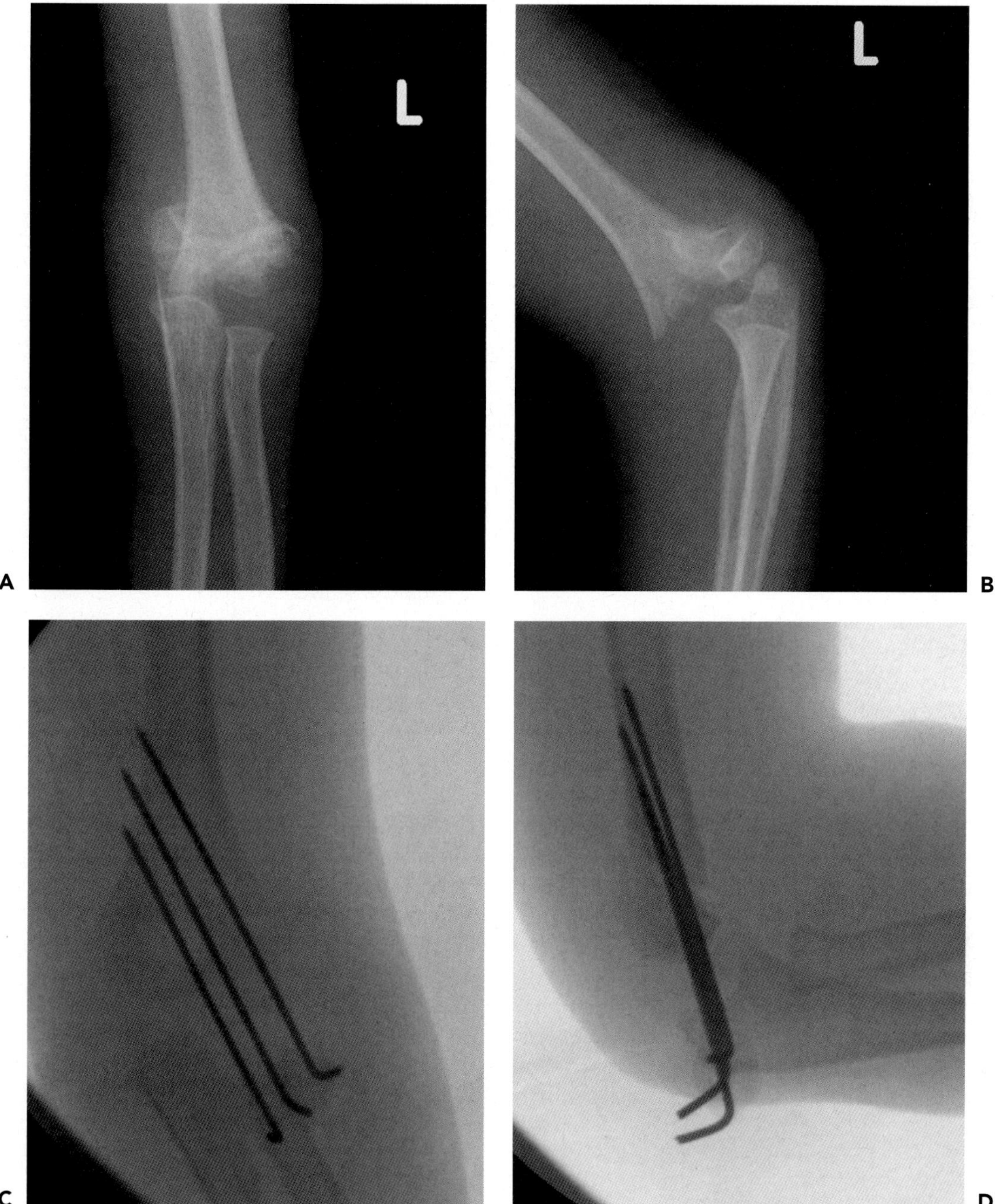

Figure 11.260 **(A** and **B)** Anteroposterior and lateral radiographs of a 4-year-old boy with at type III supracondylar humerus fracture. **(C** and **D)** Intraoperative AP and lateral view after closed reduction and percutaneous pinning. (*Reproduced with permission from* Children's Orthopaedic Center, Los Angeles, California.)

around the elbow. These children should undergo CRPP in a timely fashion but do not truly constitute a vascular emergency as most authors have demonstrated good results in these patients after treatment with careful observation and expedited CRPP without vascular exploration. Compartment syndrome can exist in the presence of a pulse, and conversely, the absence of a pulse does not necessarily mandate exploration of the vessel. Recognition of the clinical signs of compartment syndrome is essential including inordinate levels of pain, pain with passive motion, and alterations in temperature and hand function. The most common sign, however, of impending compartment syndrome in pediatric patients is increased narcotic requirements. If indicated, compartment pressures should be measured and fasciotomies performed. Failure to appropriately treat a compartment syndrome results in irreversible myonecrosis and subsequent contracture. This contracture of the volar musculature of the forearm and the resulting

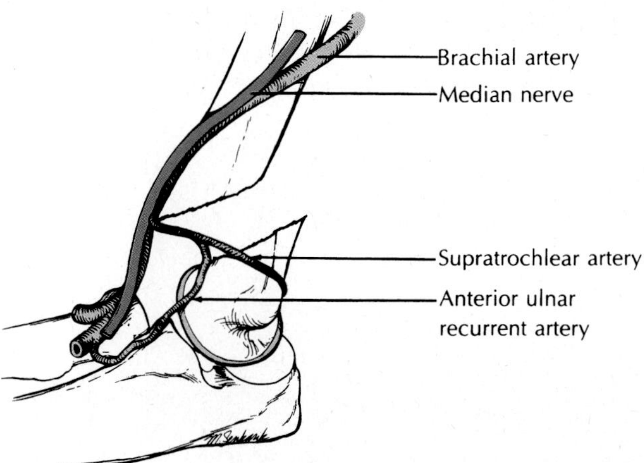

Figure 11.261 The brachial artery can be tented over the sharp end of the proximal fragment and tethered by the supratrochlear branch. (*Reproduced with permission from* Beaty JH, Kasser JR. *Rockwood and Wilkins' Fractures in Children*. 6th ed. Philadelphia, PA: Lippincott Williams & Wilkins, 2006.)

deformity of the hand have been identified for many years as Volkmann ischemic contracture (Fig. 11.262).

Late deformity resulting from these fractures is usually due to malunion in the coronal or sagittal plane. In the coronal plane, this residual tilt results in changes to the carrying angle of the arm. Cubitus varus (resulting from residual varus) is the most common angular deformity and is classically referred to as the *gunstock* deformity (Fig. 11.263). Although the deformity is primarily cosmetic, there is often a great deal of parental pressure to correct the unsightly appearance. For significant deformities, performing a supracondylar osteotomy is appropriate, although it is best delayed until adolescence to minimize the risk of recurrence. Valgus deformity, on the other hand, tends to cause a functional problem. In certain cases, a tardy ulnar nerve palsy can develop. As a result, early surgical correction is warranted to minimize the risk of irreversible ulnar nerve injury.

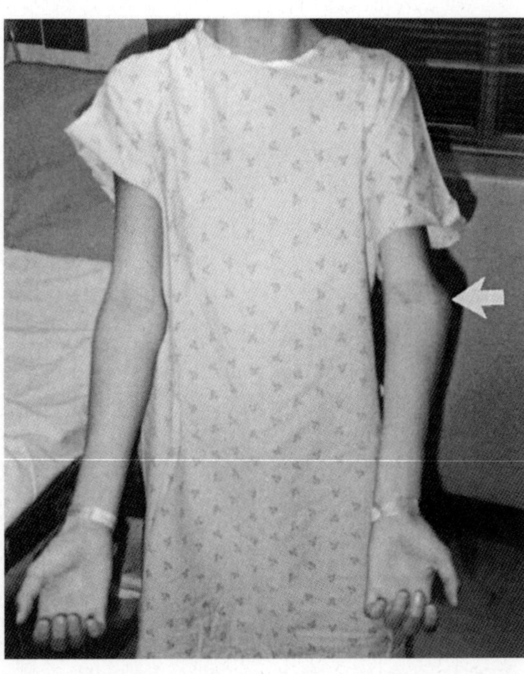

Figure 11.263 Cubitus varus from a supracondylar malunion causing a "gunstock" deformity, which is mostly cosmetic. (*Reproduced with permission from* Beaty JH, Kasser JR. *Rockwood and Wilkins' Fractures in Children*. 6th ed. Philadelphia, PA: Lippincott Williams & Wilkins, 2006.)

Lateral Condyle Fractures of the Humerus

Lateral condyle fractures account for approximately 20% of elbow fractures in children. There is some debate as to whether the mechanism is avulsion or compression, but most authors agree that the fracture results from a varus stress to the extended elbow and supinated forearm. These fractures are classified according to the Milch classification, which depends on the location of the fracture line through the distal part of the humerus (Fig. 11.264). In a Milch type I (Salter–Harris type IV) injury, the fracture line is lateral to the trochlear groove and the elbow tends to remain stable.

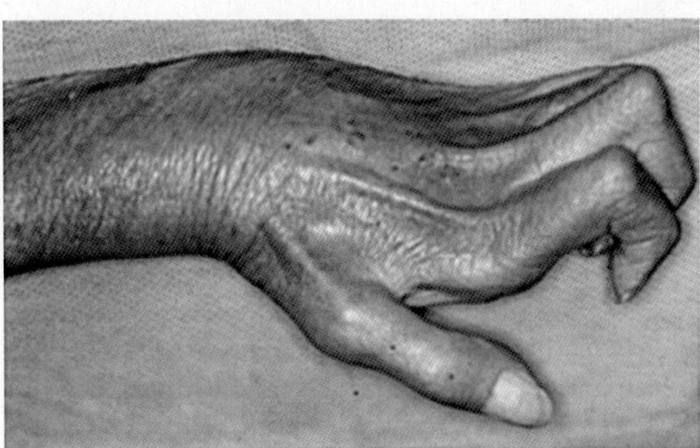

Figure 11.262 Volkmann ischemic contracture caused by a supracondylar fracture of the humerus. (*Reproduced with permission from* Berger RA, Weiss AP. *Hand Surgery*. Philadelphia, PA: Lippincott Williams & Wilkins, 2004.)

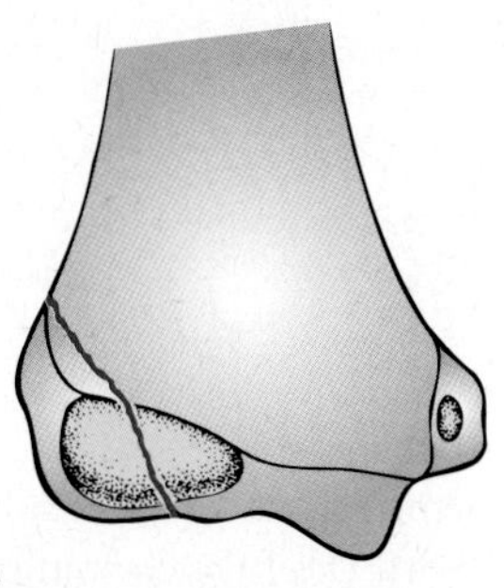

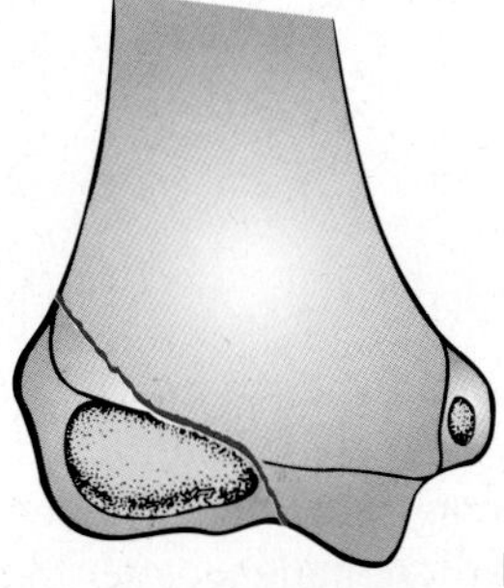

Figure 11.264 Physeal fractures of the lateral condyle. **(A)** Milch type I injury with the fracture line lateral to the trochlear groove. **(B)** Milch type II fracture extending medial to the ossific nucleus of the lateral condyle. (*Reproduced with permission from* Beaty JH, Kasser JR. *Rockwood and Wilkins' Fractures in Children*. 6th ed. Philadelphia, PA: Lippincott Williams & Wilkins, 2006.)

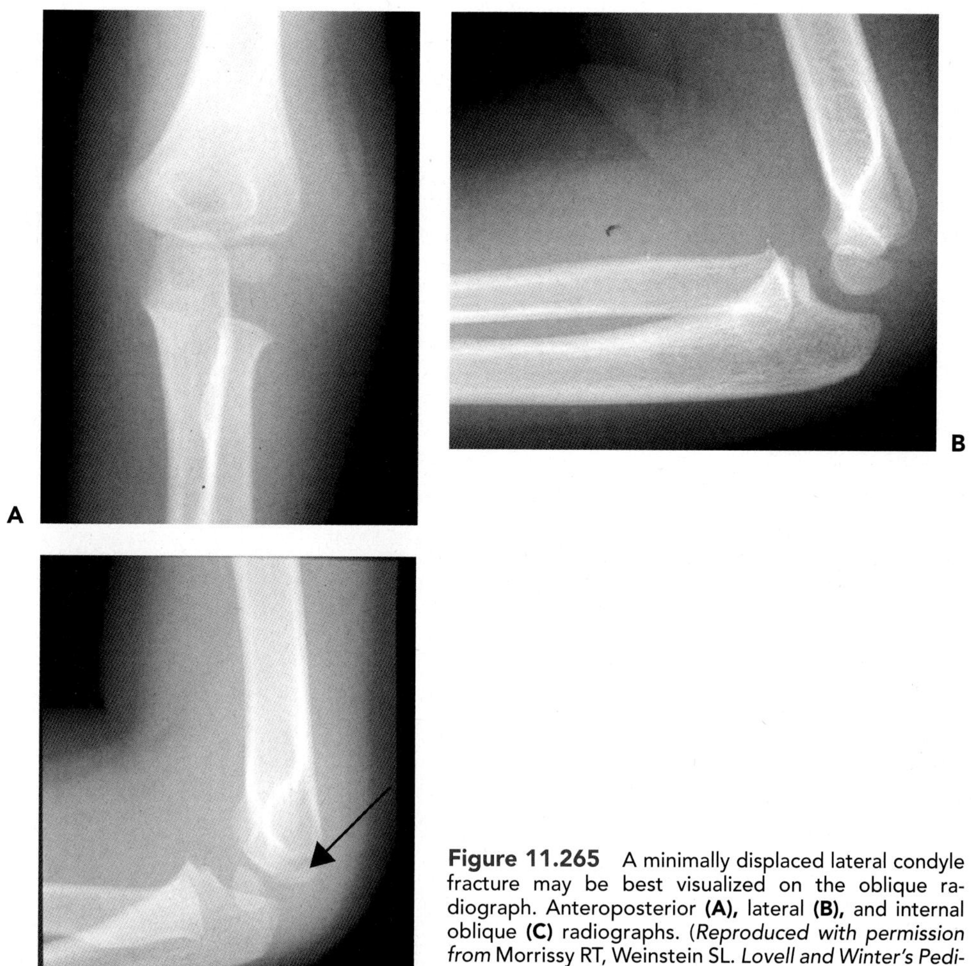

Figure 11.265 A minimally displaced lateral condyle fracture may be best visualized on the oblique radiograph. Anteroposterior **(A)**, lateral **(B)**, and internal oblique **(C)** radiographs. (*Reproduced with permission from* Morrissy RT, Weinstein SL. *Lovell and Winter's Pediatric Orthopaedics*. Philadelphia, PA: Lippincott Williams & Wilkins, 2006.)

In a Milch type II (Salter–Harris type II) injury, the fracture line extends medial to the trochlear groove, and because of the loss of the trochlear buttress, the ulna and radius often displace laterally.

Great care must be taken in assessment of fracture displacement, as the full extent of the fracture line can be difficult to perceive on standard plain radiographs. There is a tendency to think that many of these fractures are nondisplaced, when actually there is a small amount of rotation or translation. Oblique radiographs or arthrograms are useful in determining the degree of displacement (Fig. 11.265). On the basis of displacement, fractures can be categorized as type I (<2 mm displacement), type II (2–4 mm displacement), and type III (>4 mm displacement). In all cases, the goal of treatment is anatomic alignment and healing since these fractures not only involve the physis but are also intraarticular.

Treatment of type I fractures is somewhat controversial. Truly nondisplaced fractures are at low risk for displacement in a cast and can, therefore, be treated with cast immobilization for 3 to 6 weeks. However, even minimally displaced type I fractures (<2 mm) can displace late, with an increased risk of nonunion, in up to 10% of cases. As a result, any lateral condyle fracture treated conservatively in a cast should be monitored closely to avoid loss of articular and physeal alignment (Fig. 11.266). Type II and III fractures with more significant displacement (>2 mm) are usually treated with reduction and stabilization. For some type II fractures without malrotation, CRPP can be performed. In most cases, arthrography is used to confirm articular congruity at the time of the pinning. For more displaced type II fractures and all type III fractures, open reduction and internal fixation is the standard of care. The fracture site is exposed through the interval between the brachioradialis and the triceps, with care taken not to strip the posterior soft tissue attachments to the condyle, as this would disrupt the blood supply to the capitellum. Anterior exposure of the joint allows for anatomic reduction, and then two or three K-wires are used to maintain the reduction for 3 to 6 weeks. It is not uncommon for patients to develop a lateral spur on the lateral condyle as a result of periosteal disruption; warning parents about this "bump" ahead of time can prevent unnecessary worry.

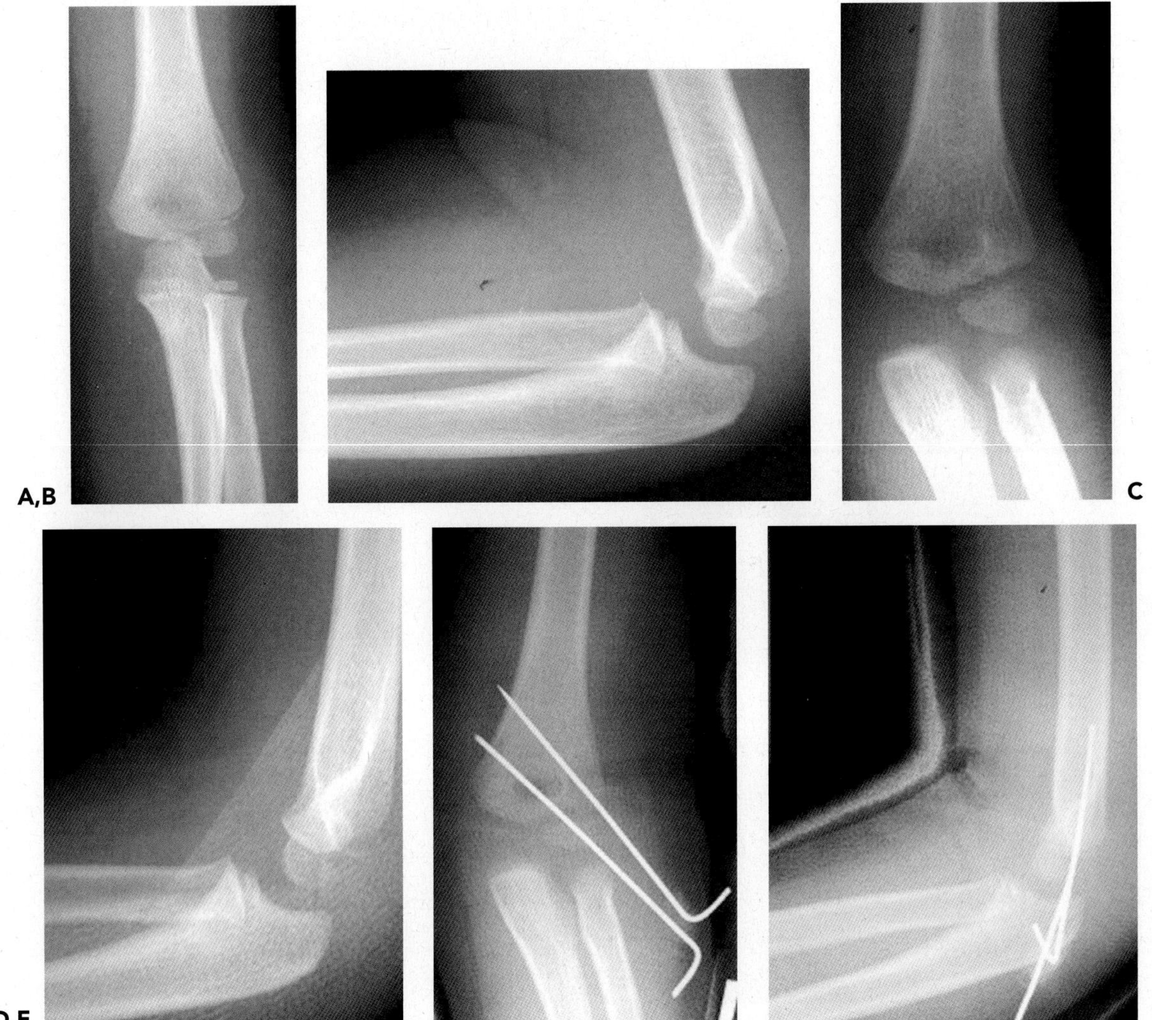

Figure 11.266 The drifting lateral condyle fracture. **(A** and **B)** Anteroposterior (AP) and lateral radiographs at presentation. This lateral condyle fracture had only approximately 2 mm of displacement on the AP view. No displacement is noted on the lateral view. The child was placed in a long arm cast and a follow-up 1 week later was recommended. **(C** and **D)** AP and lateral radiographs taken 1 week after injury show further displacement of the lateral condyle fracture, with 5 mm of separation of the lateral condyle from the distal humerus. Open reduction and pinning was performed. **(E** and **F)** Radiographs taken in the cast 4 weeks after open reduction and pinning show anatomic alignment and early healing. (*Reproduced with permission from* Morrissy RT, Weinstein SL. *Lovell and Winter's Pediatric Orthopaedics.* Philadelphia, PA: Lippincott Williams & Wilkins, 2006.)

Similar to supracondylar humerus fractures, lateral condyle fractures have their own share of complications. Growth arrest is uncommon but can occur across the distal humeral physis, causing a "fishtail" deformity of the distal humerus. Cubitus varus can result from malunion, lateral column overgrowth, or trochlear osteonecrosis and undergrowth. Nonunion can occur perhaps because of the tenuous blood supply or because the fragment is bathed in synovial fluid. Treatment is difficult and is often dictated by the degree of displacement. Fractures displaced less than 1 cm can be treated with in situ screw fixation and bone grafting. Because of the high risk of osteonecrosis with excessive dissection, nonunions displaced more than 1 cm may be better off observed. Cubitus valgus can occur as a result of nonunion and collapse of the lateral column. A tardy ulnar nerve palsy can develop from this deformity and may require corrective osteotomy and ulnar nerve transposition.

Medial Epicondyle Fractures

Accounting for 10% of elbow fractures and occurring in an older age group, medial epicondyle fractures are associated with elbow dislocations in up to 50% of cases. The application of valgus stress can avulse the medial epicondyle and subsequently cause the elbow to dislocate. The flexor–pronator muscle mass originates partly from the epicondyle and acts to displace the fracture further as it shortens. In general, the extent of displacement is the criteria for treatment. Nondisplaced fractures and fractures displaced

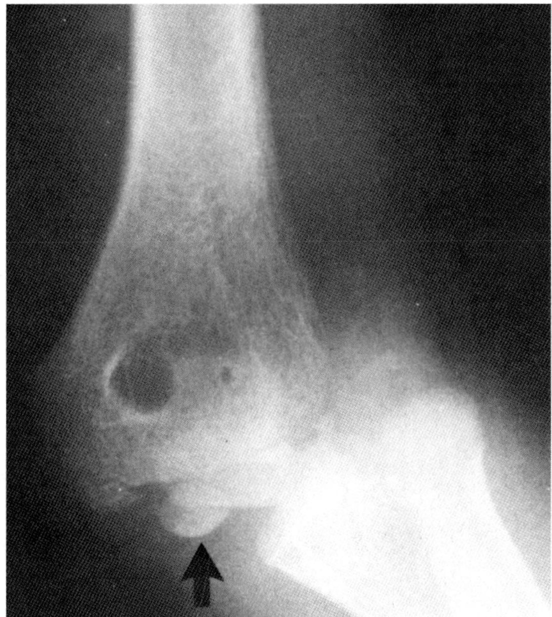

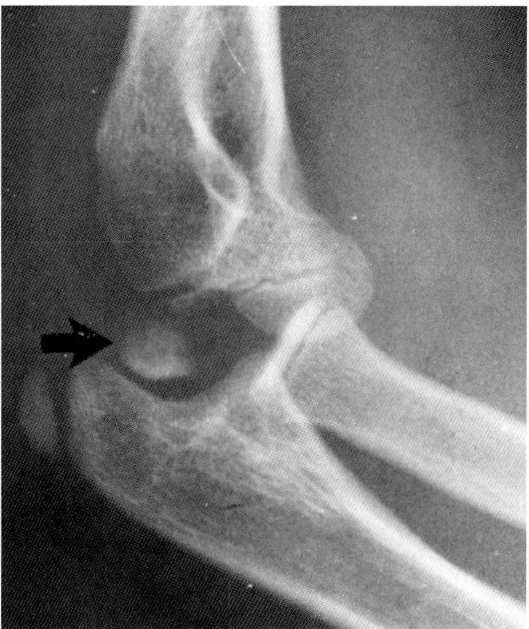

Figure 11.267 **(A)** Anteroposterior view showing an elbow dislocation with an incarcerated medial epicondyle fracture within the joint (*arrow*). **(B)** Lateral view of the same elbow demonstrates the fragment (*arrow*) between the humerus and olecranon. (*Reproduced with permission from* Beaty JH, Kasser JR. *Rockwood and Wilkins' Fractures in Children.* 6th ed. Philadelphia, PA: Lippincott Williams & Wilkins, 2006.)

less than 5 mm are generally treated by short-term immobilization followed by early range-of-motion exercises to minimize the risk of elbow stiffness. Surgical treatment for fractures displaced more than 5 mm is extremely controversial since studies have shown that fibrous unions and nonunions cause little functional deficits. Some surgeons favor open reduction and internal fixation for these fractures in those patients who participate in repetitive valgus stress activities (pitching and gymnastics). The only definite indication for operative treatment is a displaced medial epicondyle fragment, which is incarcerated in the joint (Fig. 11.267). Surgical dissection proceeds through a medial approach. The ulnar nerve is identified and protected, and the fragment is reduced by flexing the elbow. Rigid internal fixation using a compression screw is preferred to allow early mobilization and prevent elbow flexion contracture.

Because of its proximity to the fracture fragment, ulnar nerve injury is relatively common, occurring in 10% to 16% of cases. Some loss of terminal extension is common after treatment but can be minimized by early mobilization. Nonunions may occur in over 50% of patients treated conservatively, but as previously mentioned, this appears to have little functional consequence.

Fractures of the Distal Humeral Physis

Fractures through the distal humeral physis are rare and most often occur before the age of 6 or 7 years. The mechanism of injury is unknown but most likely involves rotatory forces on the elbow, often from child abuse or birth trauma. DeLee classified these fractures as group A, occurring in children up to 12 months of age, before the appearance of capitellum ossification center. These injuries are usually Salter–Harris type I fractures and are difficult to diagnose because of the lack of ossification centers in the distal fragment. Group B fractures occur in children between 12 months and 3 years of age when there is definite ossification of the lateral condylar epiphysis. These, too, are usually Salter–Harris type I fractures. Group C fractures occur in older children (3–7 years of age) and are associated with a large metaphyseal fragment. Group C fractures can be distinguished from a low supracondylar fracture by the smooth outline of the distal humerus.

A distal humeral physeal separation should be considered in any child younger than 18 months with a swollen elbow. Radiographic diagnosis can be difficult, especially in group A, because of the lack of ossification centers. One key concept to remember is that in a distal humeral physeal fracture, the relationship of the ulna to the radius is maintained but both are displaced posteromedially in relation to the distal humerus (Fig. 11.268). Although these injuries are often confused with elbow dislocations, it is important to remember that dislocations are exceedingly rare in children of this age. In an elbow dislocation, the displacement of the proximal radius and ulna is almost always posterolateral, and the relationship between the proximal radius and lateral condylar epiphysis (when it appears) is disrupted. If diagnosis is still uncertain, ultrasound or arthrography can be used to outline the epiphysis of the humerus.

Neonates and extremely small infants can be treated with closed reduction and cast immobilization at

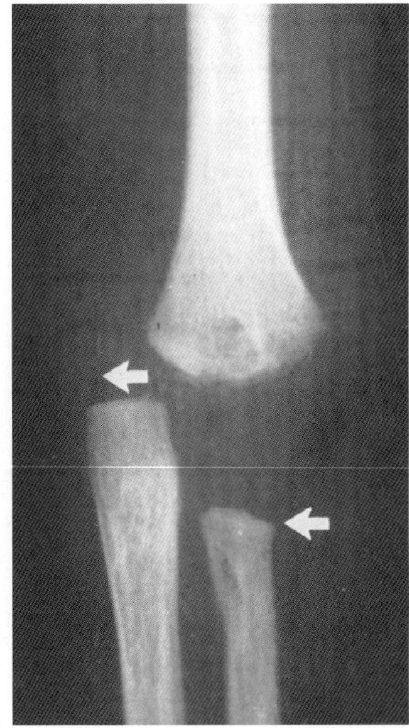
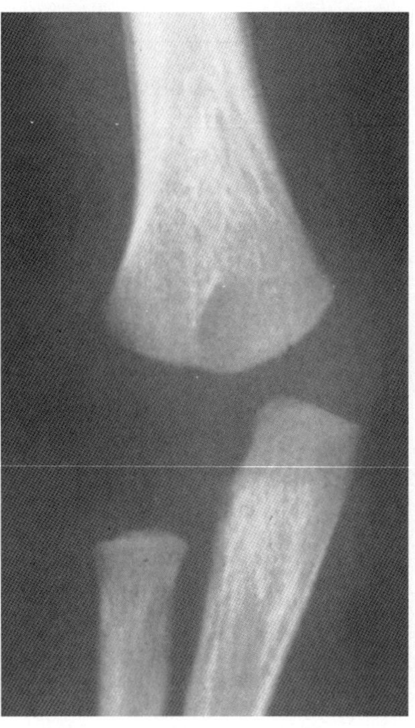

Figure 11.268 **(A)** Anteroposterior view of a distal humeral physeal fracture. Note that the proximal radius and ulna are displaced medially as a unit. **(B)** Normal elbow for comparison. (*Reproduced with permission from* Beaty JH, Kasser JR. *Rockwood and Wilkins' Fractures in Children.* 6th ed. Philadelphia, PA: Lippincott Williams & Wilkins, 2006.)

90 degrees of elbow flexion with the forearm pronated. Closed reduction and pinning (with concomitant arthrogram) are preferred for older children and for those fractures with significant displacement.

T-condylar Fractures of the Distal Humerus

T-condylar fractures are rare in children and predominantly affect older adolescents. They usually occur by the same hyperextension mechanism that causes supracondylar fractures but with higher energy. It has also been postulated that a fall directly on the elbow causes the olecranon to act as wedge, splitting the trochlea. If the fracture is nondisplaced, the fracture can be treated similar to a supracondylar fracture. If there is intraarticular displacement of greater than 2 to 3 mm, then open reduction is required. In younger children, K-wires can be used to hold the condylar fragments to each other and to the humeral shaft. In adolescents, rigid internal fixation using bicolumn plating or 90–90 plating is essential to allow early motion (Fig. 11.269). Surgical exposure can be achieved from a posteromedial (Bryan–Morrey) approach, olecranon osteotomy, or triceps splitting technique. Since intraarticular comminution is rare in adolescents, an olecranon osteotomy is rarely needed to anatomically reduce the articular surface. Both ulnar and radial nerve injures have been associated with T-condylar fractures. During surgical exposure, the ulnar should be identified and transposed.

Olecranon Fractures

Fractures of the olecranon are relatively uncommon and can occur at any age. The mechanism of injury is either a fall directly on the olecranon or avulsion injury from triceps pull. Metaphyseal fractures are usually minimally displaced and can be treated with immobilization in a long arm cast for 3 to 6 weeks. Radiographs should be obtained after 5 to 7 days to be sure that there has not been any displacement of the proximal fragment. If there is more than 3 mm of intraarticular displacement or gapping of the fracture with elbow flexion, then open reduction and internal fixation is indicated (Fig. 11.270). Similar to the treatment in adults, fixation in children is achieved with a tension band construct. Contrary to adults, in whom stainless steel wire is recommended, either absorbable or nonabsorbable suture can be used for the tension band in children. This reduces irritation from hardware and avoids the need for later wire removal. Apophyseal fracture separation is less common than metaphyseal fracture, although it occurs through a similar mechanism. Diagnosis can sometimes be difficult because the secondary ossification center of the olecranon is often irregular and sometimes bipartite; radiographs of the contralateral elbow are often extremely useful to distinguish between a fracture and normal ossification. Most apophyseal fractures can be treated nonoperatively, although operative treatment may be indicated for persistent pain or wide displacement. Of note, apophyseal fractures of the olecranon have been classically associated with the diagnosis of osteogenesis imperfecta.

Fractures of the Proximal Radius

Fractures of the upper end of the radius account for approximately 10% of fractures about the elbow. Most of these fractures involve the metaphyseal neck or the physis and usually occur in children between 8 and 12 years of age. Intraarticular injury is rare; however, these fractures

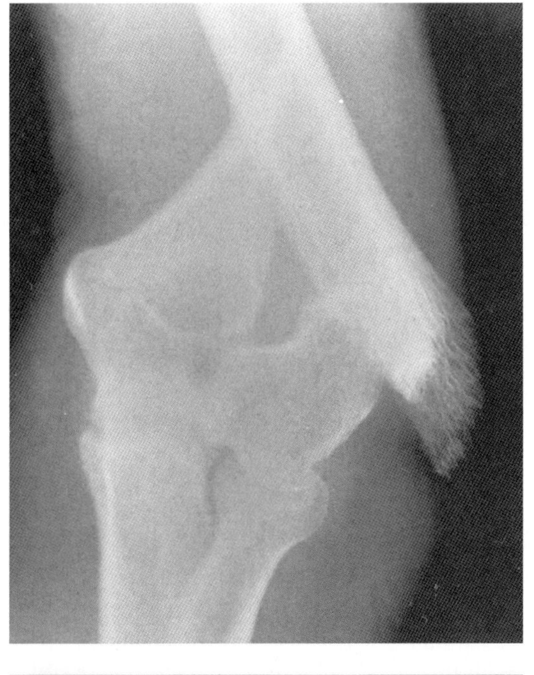

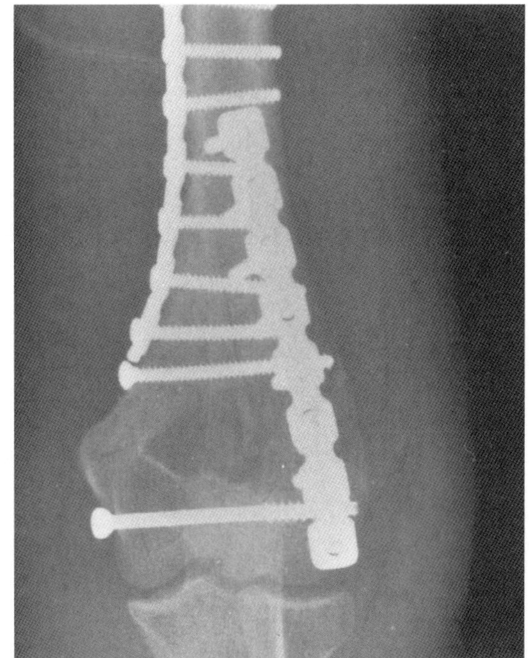

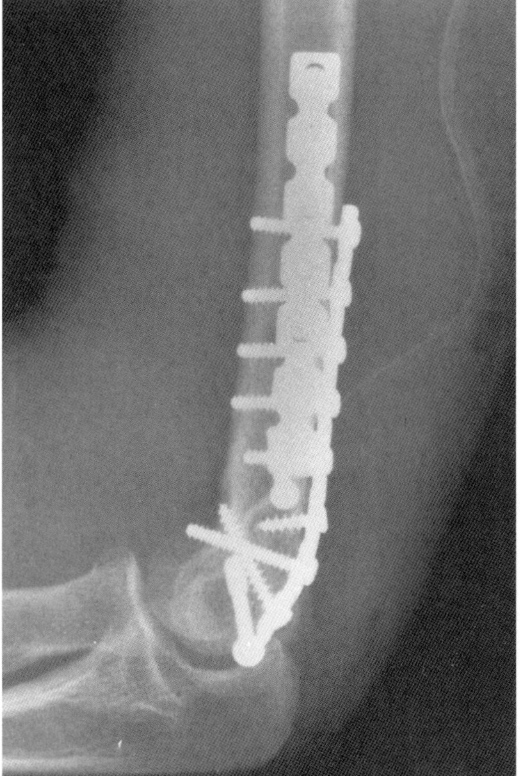

Figure 11.269 **(A)** T-condylar fracture in a 16-year-old boy. Note the intraarticular split and the dissociation of the shaft from the metaphysic. **(B** and **C)** Anteroposterior and lateral radiographs after open reduction of the articular surface and internal fixation with 90–90 plates. (*Reproduced with permission from* Beaty JH, Kasser JR. *Rockwood and Wilkins' Fractures in Children*. 6th ed. Philadelphia, PA: Lippincott Williams & Wilkins, 2006.)

are often associated with other injuries about the elbow, including olecranon fractures, medial epicondyle fractures and elbow dislocations. Mechanism of injury involves a fall on an outstretched hand with a valgus stress to the elbow. Diagnosis can be difficult in the younger patient with a more cartilaginous epiphysis. In these cases, ultrasound, MRI, or arthrography may be required to define the injury. Treatment is dictated by the amount of displacement and angulation. In general, reduction is acceptable when there is less than 4 mm of translation and less than 30 degrees of angulation. Fractures with greater displacement or angulation should be treated in a stepwise fashion, starting with the least invasive techniques before moving to more aggressive modalities. The reason for this treatment progression is that more aggressive treatment (i.e., open reduction) is associated with higher rates of postoperative stiffness,

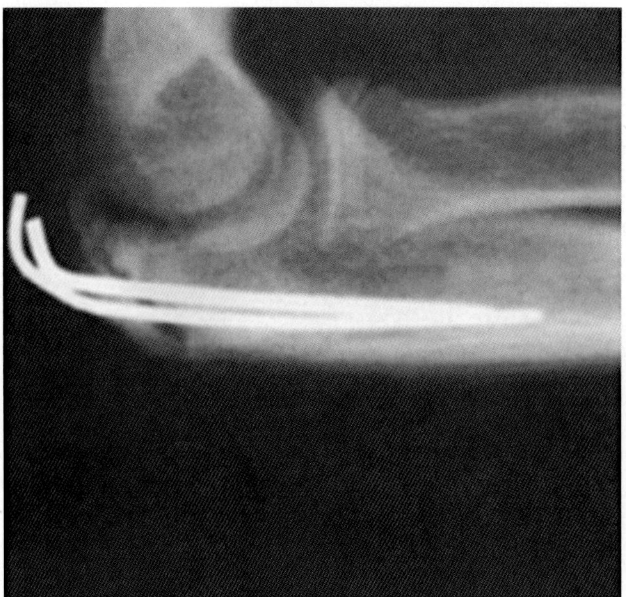

Figure 11.270 **(A)** Lateral radiograph demonstrating an internal tension band technique using axial wires plus absorbable suture for a displaced olecranon fracture. (*Reproduced with permission from* Beaty JH, Kasser JR. *Rockwood and Wilkins' Fractures in Children.* 6th ed. Philadelphia, PA: Lippincott Williams & Wilkins, 2006.)

osteonecrosis, and nonunion compared with closed or percutaneous methods. Closed reduction using the Israeli technique of flexion, pronation, and direct pressure on the radial head or the Patterson technique of extension, varus, and direct pressure should be attempted first. If closed reduction is unsuccessful, percutaneous reduction with a K-wire or a Freer elevator should be attempted (Fig. 11.271). Care should be taken to note the location of the PIN nerve to minimize the risk of inadvertent injury. Recently, Metaizeau has described the use of a titanium elastic nail inserted through the distal radius to "catch" the radial head and rotate it into a better position. Only after all attempts at closed and percutaneous reduction have failed should open reduction be attempted. After performing a standard lateral approach to the elbow, the fracture should be reduced with care taken to preserve the annular ligament and other soft tissue attachments. If needed, an oblique K-wire can be placed anterograde through the head and into the metaphysis. Transcapitellar pin placement is associated with an unacceptable rate of pin breakage. Unlike adults, excision of the radial head is never indicated in children.

The most important complications associated with the treatment of radial neck fractures are osteonecrosis and loss of motion, particularly in pronation and supination. Complications are most common after open reduction, but it is difficult to say whether this is due to the more aggressive treatment method or the severity of the initial injury.

Forearm and Wrist Injuries

Monteggia Fracture–Dislocations

Monteggia fracture–dislocations refer to a fracture of the proximal ulna with an associated dislocation of the radiocapitellar joint. The direction of the radial head dislocation generally follows the apex of the ulnar fracture and forms the basis of the Bado classification (Fig. 11.272). Diagnosis can often be subtle, and for this reason, many Monteggia fractures are mistakenly diagnosed as simple ulna fractures. In the normal forearm, a line drawn along the axis of the radius should bisect the capitellum on every radiographic view (Fig. 11.273). It is, therefore, imperative that elbow radiographs be obtained in all cases of forearm fractures so that this relationship can be adequately assessed. If this relationship is violated in the setting of an ulna fracture, then a Monteggia injury is present.

As a general principle, it is the alignment and stability of the ulnar fracture reduction that dictates the stability of the radial head reduction. Therefore, treatment of Monteggia injuries is guided by the ulnar fracture pattern. Plastic deformation of the ulna and incomplete (greenstick) fractures are treated with closed reduction and long arm cast

A,B

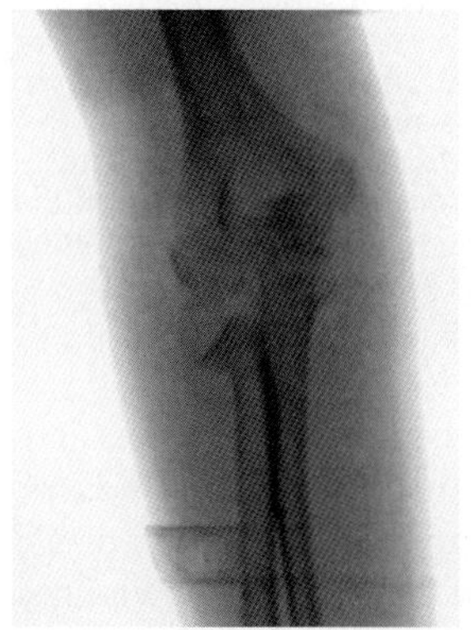

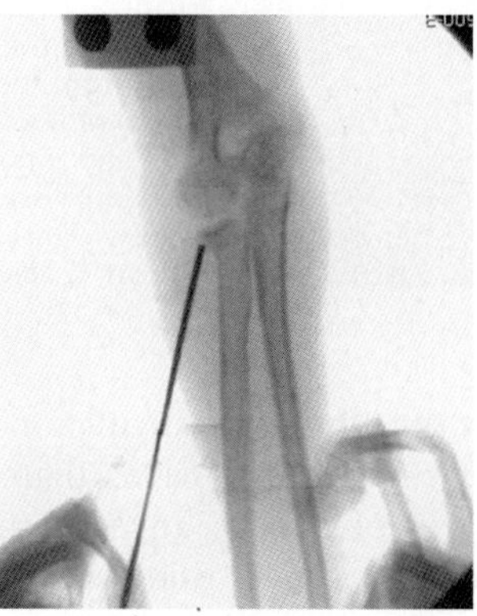

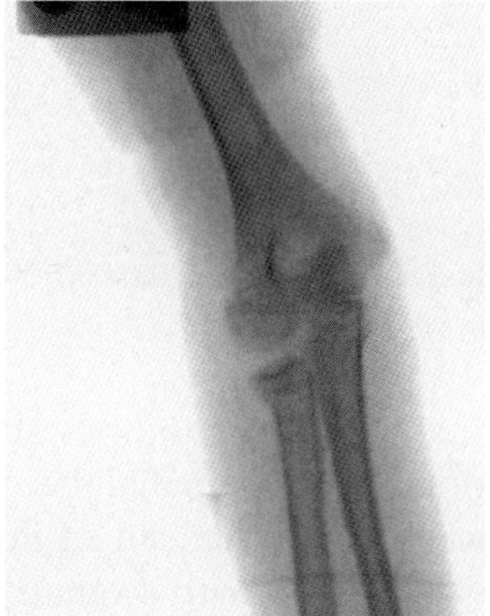

C

Figure 11.271 **(A)** Displaced radial neck fracture in an 11-year-old girl. **(B)** Percutaneous reduction with a K-wire. **(C)** Final image showing near-anatomic reduction. (*Reproduced with permission from* Skaggs DL, Flynn JM. *Staying Out of Trouble in Pediatric Orthopaedics.* Philadelphia, PA: Lippincott Williams & Wilkins, 2006.)

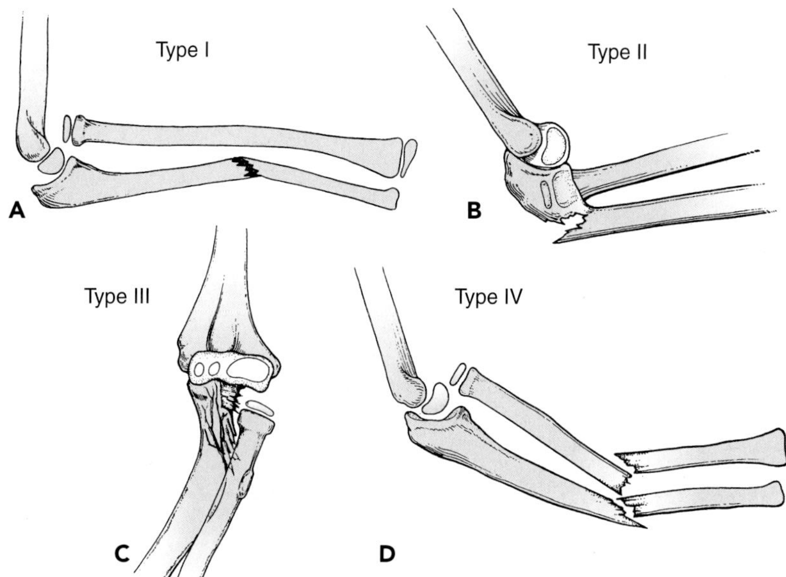

Figure 11.272 Bado classification. **(A)** Type I: apex anterior ulna fracture with anterior dislocation of the radial head. **(B)** Type II: apex posterior ulna fracture with posterior dislocation of the radial head. **(C)** Type III: apex lateral ulna fracture and lateral dislocation of the radial head. **(D)** Type IV: fracture of both the ulna and radius with anterior dislocation of the radial head. (*Reproduced with permission from* Beaty JH, Kasser JR. *Rockwood and Wilkins' Fractures in Children*. 6th ed. Philadelphia, PA: Lippincott Williams & Wilkins, 2006.)

immobilization. The forearm is usually supinated and the elbow flexed 90 degrees (although elbow extension may be necessary for Bado type II fracture patterns). Complete transverse or short oblique fractures of the ulna are usually treated by closed reduction and intramedullary nail fixation. Long oblique fractures or comminuted injuries are best treated with open reduction and plate fixation. Regardless of treatment method, it is important that these fractures be followed closely to prevent loss of radial head reduction.

Chronic Monteggia fracture–dislocations result from missed diagnosis or loss of reduction after treatment. In late cases, the ulna may have remodeled significantly so that the only apparent injury is an "isolated" radial head dislocation. Normally, the posterior border of the ulna should be completely straight. Usually, careful review of the forearm radiographs will demonstrate subtle bowing of the posterior ulnar border indicating the site of the original fracture (Fig. 11.274). An additional challenge is

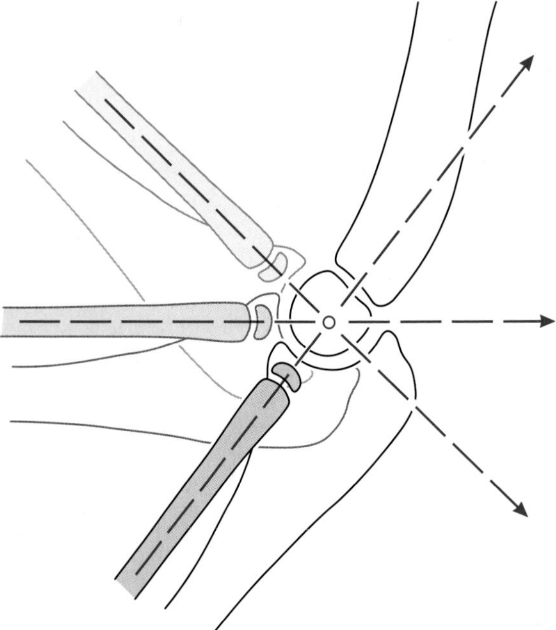

Figure 11.273 A line drawn down the long axis of the radius should bisect the capitellum in any view. (*Reproduced with permission from* Beaty JH, Kasser JR. *Rockwood and Wilkins' Fractures in Children*. 6th ed. Philadelphia, PA: Lippincott Williams & Wilkins, 2006.)

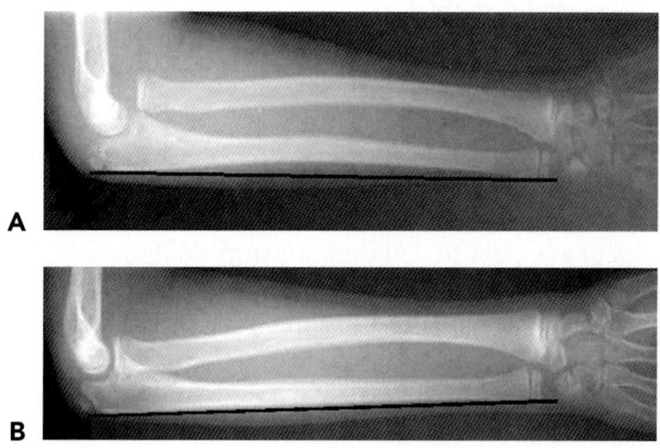

Figure 11.274 Monteggia injury. **(A)** A 10-year-old boy with a radial head dislocation and a plastically deformed ulna (note the anterior bow of the ulna demonstrated by a line drawn along its subcutaneous border). **(B)** Contralateral, uninjured arm. Note the straight subcutaneous border. (*Reproduced with permission from* Morrissy RT, Weinstein SL. *Lovell and Winter's Pediatric Orthopaedics*. Philadelphia, PA: Lippincott Williams & Wilkins, 2006.)

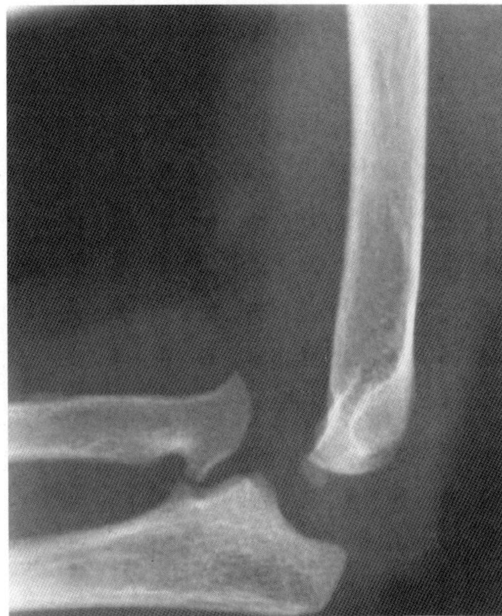

Figure 11.275 Lateral radiograph of a congenital radial head dislocation. Note the dysplastic shape of the radial head. (*Reproduced with permission from* Beaty JH, Kasser JR. *Rockwood and Wilkins' Fractures in Children.* 6th ed. Philadelphia, PA: Lippincott Williams & Wilkins, 2006.)

distinguishing a chronic Monteggia injury (with remodeled ulna) from a congenital radial head dislocation. Unlike the radial head in Monteggia injuries, the congenitally dislocated radial head is small, convex, and usually associated with a hypoplastic capitellum (Fig. 11.275). Treatment of chronic Monteggia injuries is challenging and often necessitates shortening ulnar osteotomy, open reduction of the radiocapitellar joint, and annular ligament reconstruction. Loss of pronation after this late reconstruction should be expected.

Diaphyseal Fractures

Diaphyseal forearm fractures are divided into three categories based on fracture pattern: plastic deformation, greenstick, and complete fractures. Plastic deformation results when the forces applied to the young child's forearm exceed the elastic limit of bone but fall short of its ultimate strength. Excessive plastic deformation (usually >20 degrees of angulation) can limit forearm rotation, so closed reduction is indicated for any of these injuries. Reduction is obtained by applying a sustained three-point load over the apex of the deformity until the deformity gradually improves (usually under general anesthesia), and the arm is immobilized in a well-molded long arm cast. Greenstick fractures are incomplete fractures and usually have both angular and rotational displacement. Most of these fractures can also be treated with closed reduction and placement of a well-molded long arm cast. Reduction must correct both components of the deformity and is performed according to the "rule of thumbs." In this maneuver, the thumb is rotated toward the apex of the deformity as the angulation is corrected. For example, to reduce an apex dorsal fracture, the wrist is supinated and a volarly directed force is applied at the fracture site.

Complete fractures occur in older children and by definition are more inherently unstable. Cast immobilization (with a proper mold) is indicated for those patients who can achieve and maintain an adequate reduction. In general, 20 degrees of angulation and bayonet apposition can be accepted in children younger than 8 years. No more than 10 degrees of angulation should be accepted in children older than 10 years. Although it has been suggested that 30 degrees of rotational malalignment can be tolerated, it is important to remember that malrotation does not remodel and should be corrected whenever possible. Operative treatment is indicated for unstable fractures, unacceptable alignment, refractures, and neurovascular or soft tissue compromise. In younger patients, intramedullary nail fixation (with a K-wire or titanium elastic nail) is the preferred treatment method (Fig. 11.276). Since these devices do not control rotation, postoperative cast immobilization is necessary. Patients with comminuted fractures or less than 1 year of skeletal growth remaining can be treated similar to adults with open reduction and plate fixation.

Distal Radius Fractures

Approximately 75% of all forearm fractures involve the distal radius, and the location of the injury can be either metaphyseal or physeal. Metaphyseal fractures of the distal radius include buckle (torus) fractures and bicortical fractures. Buckle fractures are inherently stable because the cortex fails in compression, and simple immobilization in a splint or short arm cast for 3 weeks is sufficient treatment. Bicortical fractures are generally treated with cast immobilization after closed reduction of the fracture (if necessary) (Fig. 11.277). Because of the proximity of these fractures to the distal radial physis, a tremendous amount of remodeling potential exists, and therefore, substantial residual angulation and displacement can be accepted. Generally, 20 to 25 degrees of angulation in the sagittal plane is acceptable in children younger than 12 years. Approximately 10 to 15 degrees of sagittal angulation can be accepted in older patients. Although two randomized controlled trials support the use of short arm casts alone, most orthopaedic surgeons still use long arm casts for 3 weeks followed by short arm casts until healing. Surgical indications include irreducible or unstable fractures, open fractures, neurovascular injuries, and excessive soft tissue swelling. The most common technique is percutaneous pinning with one or two smooth pins; plate fixation has limited indications primarily in older patients.

Distal radial physeal fractures are usually Salter–Harris type I or II injuries and are treated in a similar fashion as metaphyseal fractures. Reduction maneuvers should be performed gently under adequate sedation to minimize undue trauma to the physis. Multiple attempts at reduction

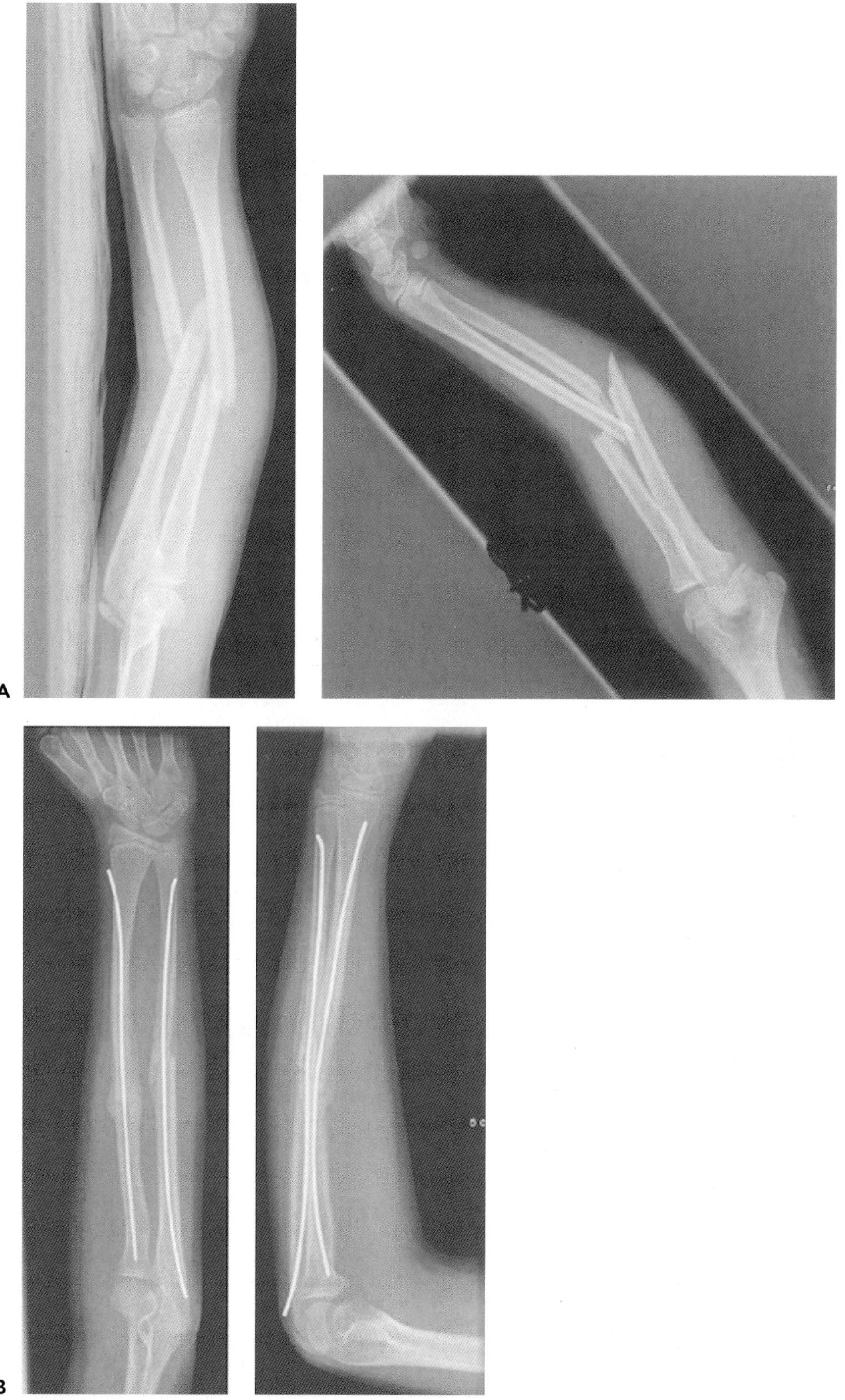

Figure 11.276 A 12 year-old girl with complete midshaft forearm fracture. **(A)** AP and lateral injury radiographs demonstrating marked displacement of both the radius and ulna. **(B)** Post operative AP and Lateral films demonstrating reduction of both bones and fixation with titanium elastic nails. (*Reproduced with permission from* Beaty JH, Kasser JR. *Rockwood and Wilkins' Fractures in Children.* 6th ed. Philadelphia, PA: Lippincott Williams & Wilkins, 2006.)

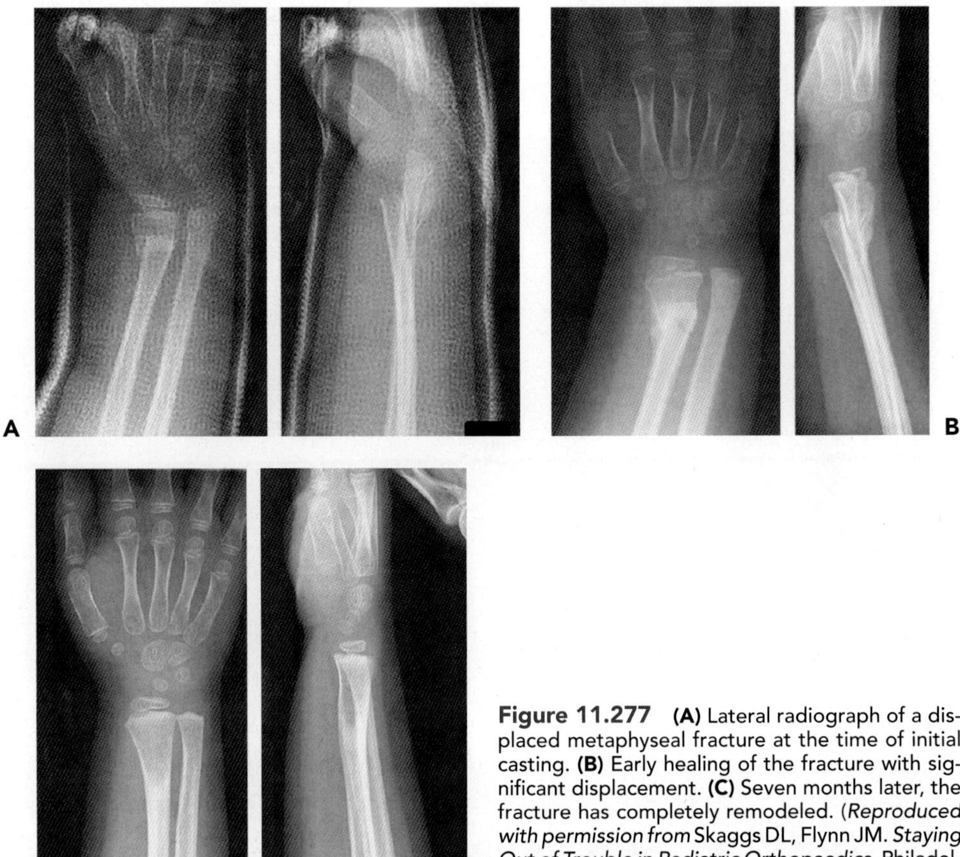

Figure 11.277 **(A)** Lateral radiograph of a displaced metaphyseal fracture at the time of initial casting. **(B)** Early healing of the fracture with significant displacement. **(C)** Seven months later, the fracture has completely remodeled. (*Reproduced with permission from* Skaggs DL, Flynn JM. *Staying Out of Trouble in Pediatric Orthopaedics*. Philadelphia, PA: Lippincott Williams & Wilkins, 2006.)

should be avoided, as this can increase the risk of a growth arrest. For the same reasons, manipulation should not be attempted after 7 to 10 days. Overall, the incidence of growth arrest after distal radial physeal fracture has been reported to be roughly 4%. Similar to metaphyseal fractures, operative intervention usually consists of percutaneous pinning and is indicated for unstable injuries, neurovascular compromise, and severe soft tissue swelling.

Hand Injuries

Most metacarpal and phalangeal fractures in children are nondisplaced and require minimal treatment. The majority of displaced fractures can be adequately reduced closed and immobilized, using simple splints or casts. It is important to immobilize fingers in the position of function to prevent unnecessary stiffness. As is so often the case, when the vast majority of injuries are benign, it is easy to overlook the problem hand and finger fractures. Therefore, several specific injuries are worthy of note. Condylar fractures, especially if intraarticular (in either the middle or proximal phalanx), require anatomic reduction and fixation. As in adults, degenerative changes and deformity will result if they are not treated appropriately. Physeal fractures occur typically at the base of the proximal phalanx; these are usually Salter–Harris type II injuries. Because angulation typically is out of the plane of the motion of the joint (usually medial or lateral), remodeling is minimal at best. Therefore, reduction of these injuries is essential; once reduced, they are usually stable with simple buddy taping to the adjacent digit with a small splint. Adolescents who sustain metacarpal fractures and fractures of the thumb as a result of aggressive behavior should be managed in a manner similar to their adult counterparts.

PELVIC FRACTURES

The pelvis in a child is far more flexible than that of the adult. Because of the presence of significantly more cartilage, the pediatric pelvis is able to absorb more energy prior to failure. Unfortunately, the abdominal contents are not necessarily as pliable; thus, with the relative lack of protection provided by the immature pelvis, they are more likely to be damaged. Although associated genitourinary injuries and head trauma are common, the mortality of pelvic fractures is only one-third the rate reported for adults. Pelvic trauma in children is indicative of a high energy injury and primarily results from pedestrian versus motor vehicle accidents. Lower energy avulsion injuries can be secondary to athletic trauma.

Initial evaluation of children with pelvic trauma follows standard trauma protocols (see the section on "Pediatric Polytrauma"), with the first priority being securing the airway and ensuring hemodynamic stability. Given the association with other injuries, it is imperative that all major organ systems are thoroughly checked for the presence of injury. Workup for the pelvic fracture includes a rectal examination and inspection of the perineum to rule out an open injury, as well as proper imaging (either inlet/outlet views or CT scan) to define the fracture pattern.

Pediatric pelvic fractures are classified in a manner similar to adult pelvic fractures. One major difference, however, is that children can experience a single break to the pelvic ring. Avulsion injuries are treated nonsurgically with rest, activity modification, rehabilitation, and protected weight bearing. More significant pelvic fractures are still treated nonoperatively unless they are significantly unstable. In these rare cases, external fixation or open reduction and internal fixation with reconstruction plates may be indicated.

Unique to this age group is damage to the open triradiate cartilage. Should this occur, the normal height and depth of the acetabulum may not be achieved. Premature closure of this physis could result in acetabular dysplasia and progressive hip subluxation. Late osteotomies of the pelvis are usually required to treat this unfortunate complication.

LOWER EXTREMITY

Fractures of the Hip and Thigh

Hip Fractures

Unlike osteoporotic hip fractures in the elderly, which result from relatively low loads, hip fractures in children are nearly always the result of high-energy trauma. Mechanism of injury is usually a motor vehicle accident or fall from height, and associated injuries include head trauma, long bone fractures, and visceral injuries. The high-energy nature of these injuries can jeopardize the vascular anatomy of the hip in the growing child, leading to avascular necrosis (AVN) of the femoral head. Urgent anatomic reduction and stabilization is necessary to restore blood flow to the femoral head and decompress the fracture hematoma.

Pediatric hip fractures are classified according the system of Delbet (Fig. 11.278). Type I fractures are transphyseal and are, therefore, similar to an acute slipped capital

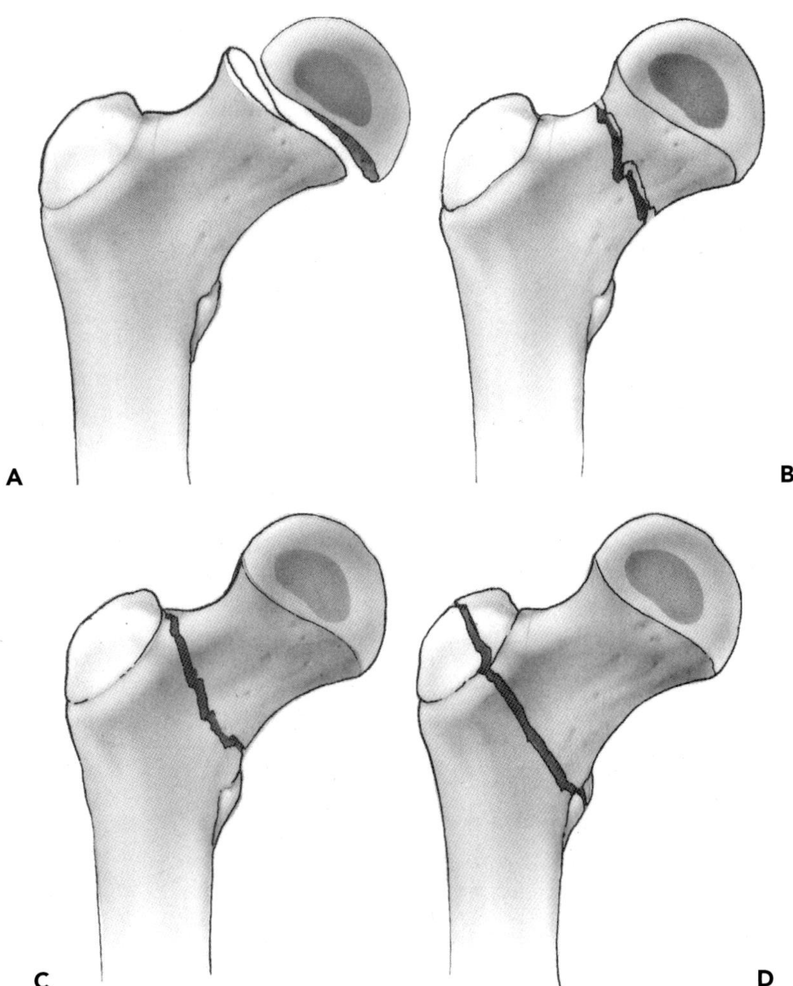

Figure 11.278 Delbet classification for proximal femur fractures. **(A)** Type I is transepiphyseal. **(B)** Type II is a transcervical fracture. **(C)** Type III is a basicervical fracture. **(D)** Type IV is an intertrochanteric fracture. (*Reproduced with permission from* Morrissy RT, Weinstein SL. *Lovell and Winter's Pediatric Orthopaedics*. Philadelphia, PA: Lippincott Williams & Wilkins, 2006.)

femoral epiphysis. These fractures are rare, accounting for less than 10% of all hip fractures. Unfortunately, they also have the highest rate of AVN, at nearly 90%. As a result, it is imperative that type I fractures be reduced and stabilized in an emergent fashion. Only one or two attempts should be made to gently close reduce this fracture, as repeated attempts can increase the risk of osteonecrosis and premature physeal closure. If the fracture cannot be reduced closed, or if there is any question about the adequacy of the reduction, the fracture site should be exposed through an anterior approach to directly visualize the reduction. To obtain stable fixation, multiple smooth pins should be used to cross the physis. It is the general consensus that the stability of reduction supercedes the preservation of the physis, since AVN is a much more difficult complication to treat than a leg length discrepancy. Children younger than 10 years should be protected in a spica cast postoperatively.

Delbet type II fractures are transcervical with the fracture line running across the middle of the femoral neck. The risk of AVN from these injuries is roughly 50%. Type III fractures are basicervical and have a lower rate of AVN, reported between 20% and 30%. For nondisplaced fractures and those fractures in which an anatomic reduction can be achieved closed, percutaneous fixation can be used. If sufficient bone exists between the fracture and the physis, cannulated screws or threaded pins can be used to achieve fixation (Fig. 11.279). If the physis must be crossed, smooth pins should be used to minimize the risk of growth arrest. Similar to type I fractures, one should have a low threshold to open the fracture site if there is any question as to the adequacy of the reduction. In younger patients, a spica cast is generally used to protect the reduction after surgery.

A

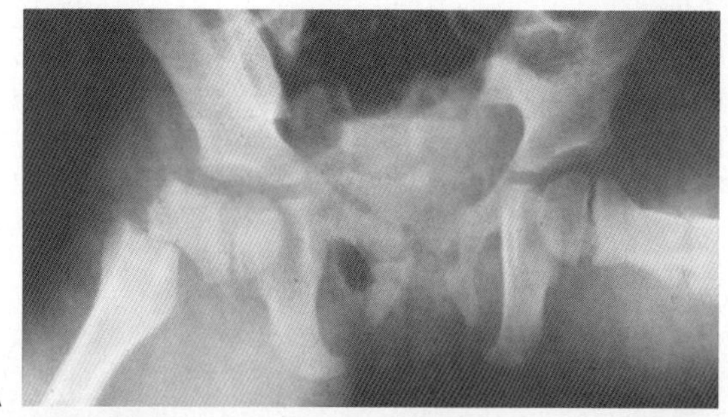

B

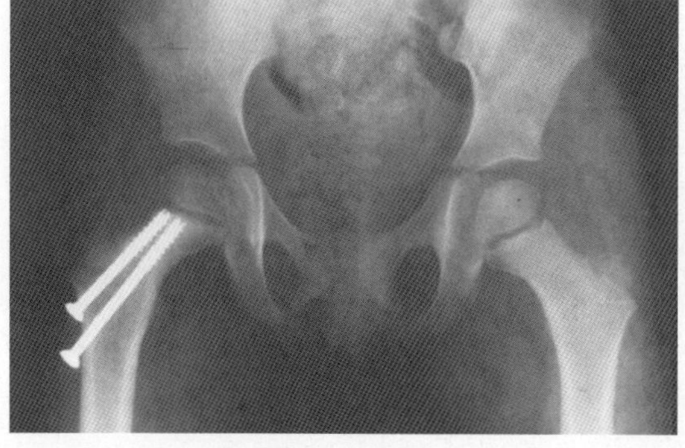

Figure 11.279 **(A)** Approximately 5-year-old boy with a type III femoral neck fracture. **(B)** Three months after anatomic open reduction and internal fixation with two screws sparing the physis. (*Reproduced with permission from* Beaty JH, Kasser JR. *Rockwood and Wilkins' Fractures in Children*. 6th ed. Philadelphia, PA: Lippincott Williams & Wilkins, 2006.)

Delbet type IV injuries are intertrochanteric fractures. Since they are extracapsular, the blood supply to the femoral head is rarely disrupted, and these fractures have the lowest rate of AVN (10%). Children younger than 6 years can usually be treated with closed reduction and spica casting. In older children and in those younger children with unstable fractures, percutaneous fixation with screws or pins should also be used. Again, hardware should be left short of the physis to minimize the risk of a growth arrest. Open reduction should be performed whenever the fracture cannot be reduced anatomically through closed means. In older children or adolescents, a screw and side plate or blade plate can be used for fixation. These techniques obviate the need for a postoperative spica cast.

As previously mentioned, the most devastating complication of pediatric hip fractures is osteonecrosis. AVN usually develops within 6 months, although it can be seen as late as 2 years after the initial injury (Fig. 11.280). Early treatment consists of protected weight bearing. After collapse, proximal femoral osteotomies can be used to rotate intact portions of the femoral head into the weight-bearing zone. Another complication of hip fractures is varus deformity (coxa vara) either from malunion or growth disturbance; the incidence of this has been reported between 20% and 30%. Coxa vara is best prevented by obtaining an anatomic reduction at the time of surgery with rigid fixation. Severe deformities may require a subtrochanteric valgus producing osteotomy. Nonunions occur most often with displaced type II fractures and can be seen in 5% to 10% of hip fractures overall. Treatment usually consists of valgus intertrochanteric osteotomy with bone grafting. Premature physeal arrest usually occurs in type I fractures or other fractures in which hardware was placed across the growth plate. The incidence of growth arrest has been reported anywhere between 5% and 65% in the literature; if the arrest results in a significant leg length discrepancy, a contralateral epiphysiodesis may be indicated.

Diaphyseal Femur Fractures

Fractures of the femoral shaft constitute approximately 2% of childhood fractures. In children younger than 1 year, who are not yet walking, femur fractures should be thoroughly worked up for the possibility of child abuse. However, after the walking age, femur fractures are not uncommon and can result from motor vehicle accidents, falls from height, and sports injuries.

The remodeling potential for femur fractures is greatest in children younger than 10 years, fractures close to the physis, and malalignments in the plane of joint motion. As a general guideline, in children younger than 10 years, up to 15 degrees of coronal plane angulation, 20 degrees of

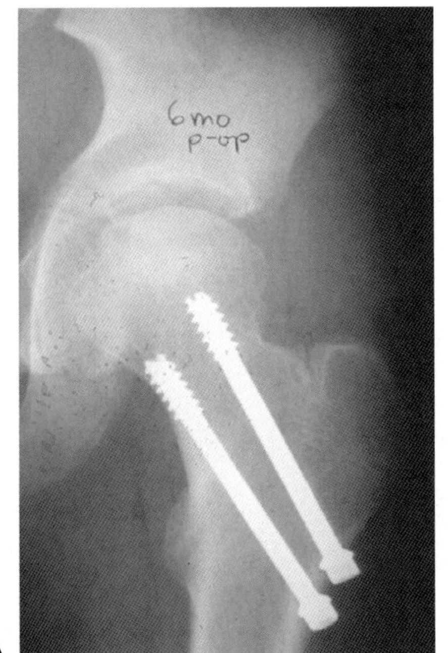

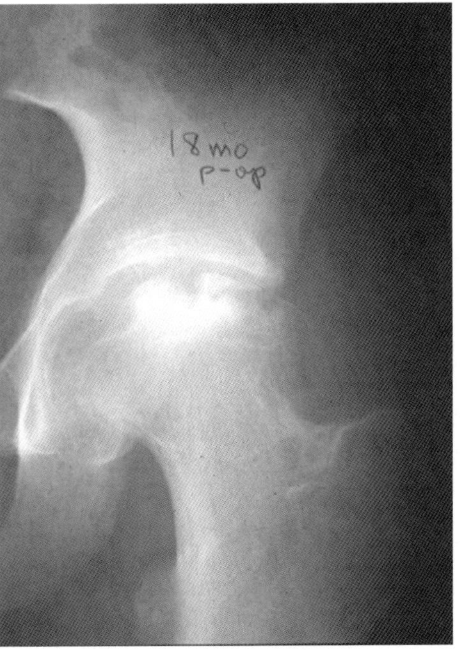

Figure 11.280 **(A)** Anteroposterior radiograph taken 6 months after screw implantation. **(B)** Another radiograph taken after screw removal at 18 months shows avascular necrosis of the femoral head. (*Reproduced with permission from* Skaggs DL, Flynn JM. *Staying Out of Trouble in Pediatric Orthopaedics.* Philadelphia, PA: Lippincott Williams & Wilkins, 2006.)

sagittal plane angulation, and 30 degrees of malrotation can be accepted. Overgrowth of the involved femur is common and should be discussed with the family. In children between the ages of 2 and 10 years, the overgrowth averages 0.9 cm. As a result, shortening in children of this age group of 1.5 to 2.0 cm at union can be accepted. In older children, with less potential for overgrowth, no more than 1 cm of shortening is recommended.

Based on improved surgical techniques and a better understanding of the social impact of prolonged immobilization in children, there has been a recent trend toward more operative treatment for pediatric femur fractures. The specific choice of treatment, however, depends on the age and size of the patient as well as the fracture pattern. In children younger than 1 year, a Pavlik harness or soft roll spica cast can be used to immobilize the child. Healing is rapid and immobilization can usually be discontinued by 4 weeks. For children between the ages of 1 and 6 years, early spica casting is preferred for all but the most unstable fractures. There are recent reports of compartment syndromes as a result of excessive traction during spica cast application. It is currently recommended that a long leg cast be rolled first with care taken not to apply excessive force to the posterior calf or popliteal area. After ensuring a proper valgus mold, the rest of the cast can be extended up to the nipple line. For those high-energy injuries with unstable fracture patterns, a period of skeletal traction may be necessary prior to the spica cast to prevent unacceptable shortening.

Multiple treatment options exist for the school-aged child with open physes. As previously mentioned, there has been an evolving trend toward operative treatment in this age group, as it allows earlier mobilization and minimizes the social impact of prolonged immobilization. Flexible intramedullary nailing is the treatment of choice for most diaphyseal fractures in the school-aged child (Fig. 11.281). Flexible nails provide load-sharing fixation that allows for sufficient motion at the fracture site to generate abundant callus. The incidence of malunion and refracture are rare; the most common complication is soft tissue irritation at the nail entry site. For very proximal or distal fractures, comminuted fractures, or other patterns that are "length-unstable," external fixators have many advantages over flexible nails. Benefits of external fixation include rapid application, ability to achieve length and alignment, minimal blood loss, and low risk of physeal damage or osteonecrosis. Complications include pin-site irritation, knee stiffness, delayed union, and an increased risk of refracture after fixator removal. An alternative treatment option for the proximal, distal, and length-unstable fractures is plate fixation. Submuscular techniques allow plates to be placed through percutaneous incisions with less soft tissue stripping and no need for postoperative immobilization.

Older adolescents with closed physes can be treated in a manner similar to that in adults. Usually this consists of a rigid, reamed intramedullary nail. Advantages include rapid mobilization, a predictably high union rate, and a low risk of malalignment. Rigid intramedullary nails are not advised in the skeletally immature because of the risk of femoral head AVN. Insertion through the piriformis fossa can disrupt the lateral ascending branches of the medial

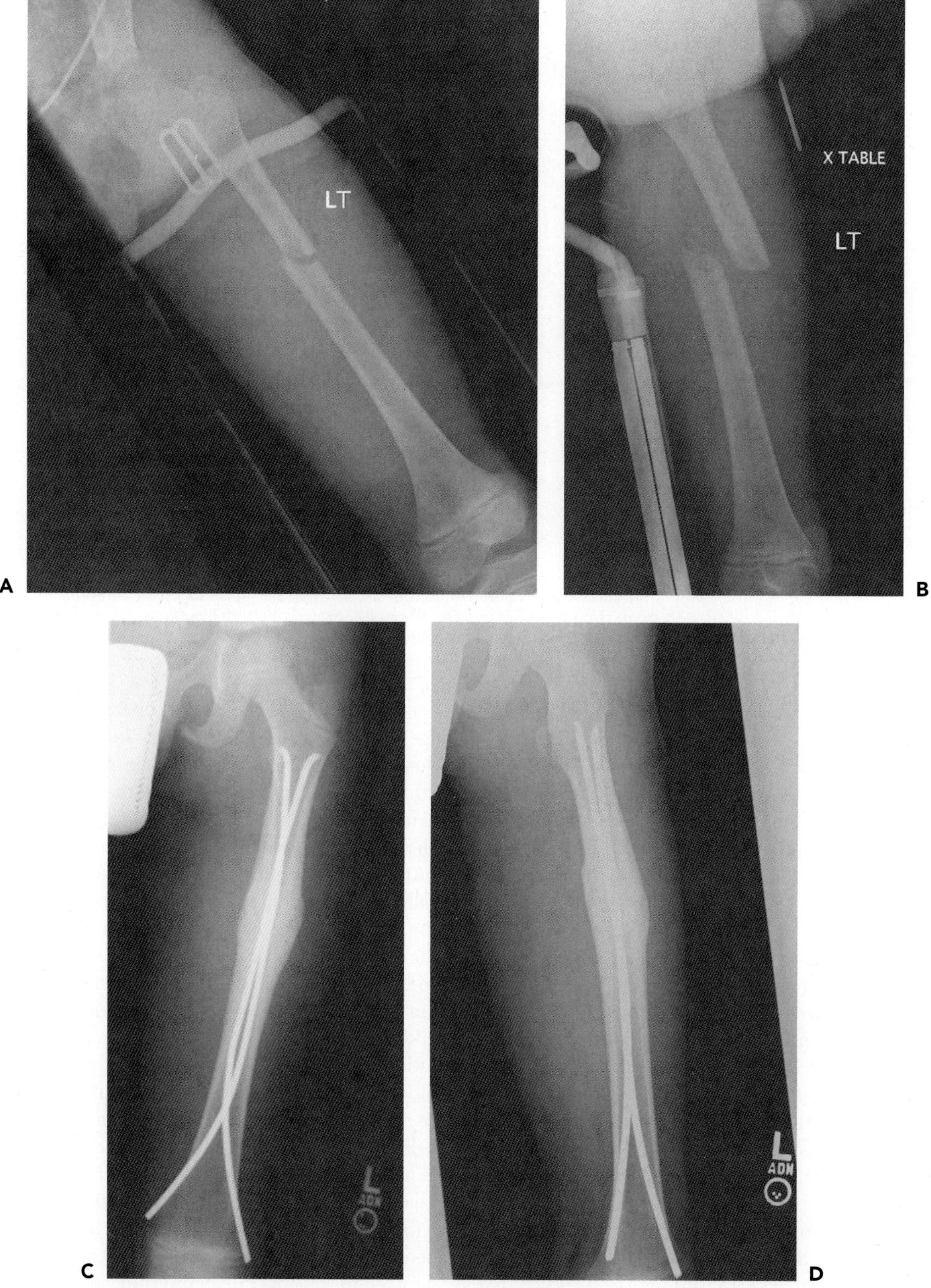

Figure 11.281 **(A** and **B)** Injury radiographs demonstrating a short oblique femoral shaft fracture in an 8-year-old boy. **(C** and **D)** Anteroposterior and lateral radiographs 4 months after treatment with flexible intramedullary nails. Note the abundant callus at the fracture site. (*Reproduced with permission from* Skaggs DL, Tolo VT. *Master Techniques in Orthopaedic Surgery: Pediatrics*. Philadelphia, PA: Lippincott Williams & Wilkins, 2008.)

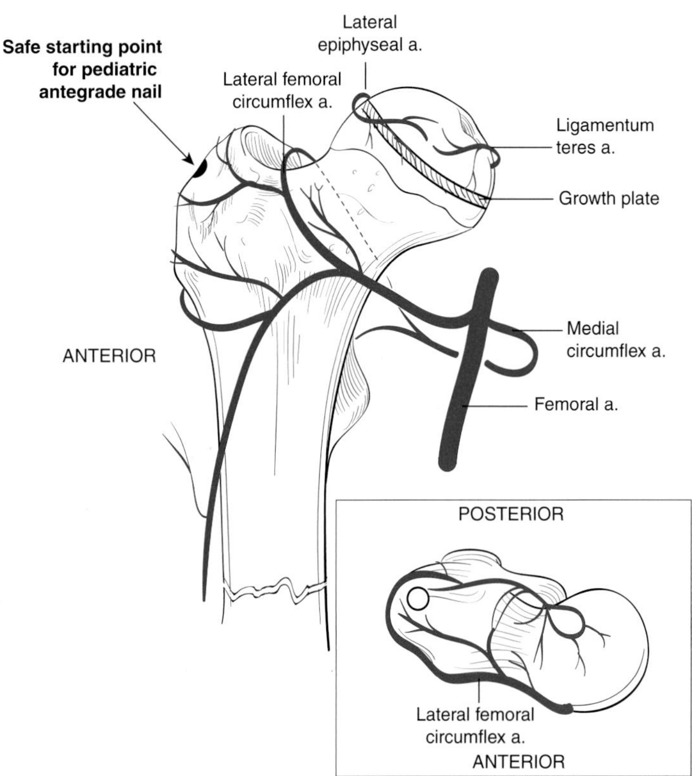

Figure 11.282 Blood supply of the proximal femur. Note the safe entry site for an antegrade nail. (*Reproduced with permission from* Skaggs DL, Flynn JM. *Staying Out of Trouble in Pediatric Orthopaedics.* Philadelphia, PA: Lippincott Williams & Wilkins, 2006.)

circumflex artery compromising the circulation of the femoral epiphysis (Fig. 11.282). While trochanteric entry nails may have a lower risk of osteonecrosis, growth disturbances of the proximal femur have been reported.

Fractures About the Knee

Distal Femoral Physeal Fractures

Fractures through the distal femoral physis do not have a unique classification and are usually described by the Salter–Harris classification. The distal femoral physis is not planar but has a complex undulating shape that actually matches four mammillary processes in the distal femoral metaphysis; this arrangement provides some resistance to shear. Unfortunately, when a fracture does occur, this configuration reduces the odds of a clean cleavage plane and increases the risk of partial or complete physeal arrest. The diagnosis is usually evident based on swelling about the knee and plain radiographs. In more subtle cases, it is important to remember that in patients with open growth plates, physeal injuries are more likely than ligamentous injuries. In these cases, stress radiographs are often helpful to diagnose nondisplaced fractures.

The goal of treatment should be anatomic reduction. Nondisplaced fractures and those fractures that are stable after closed reduction can be treated with immobilization in a long leg cast. For fractures that do not reduce easily and unstable fractures, closed or open reduction with percutaneous fixation (followed by casting) is the preferred form of treatment. Crossed smooth pins can be inserted either retrograde or anterograde. While retrograde insertion is technically easier, anterograde pin placement allows one to keep the hardware out of the joint, thereby reducing the risk of intraarticular sepsis. Salter–Harris type II fractures with large Thurston–Holland fragments can be stabilized with cannulated screws placed across the metaphyseal spike (Fig. 11.283). Salter–Harris type III and IV fractures can be treated with screws placed across the epiphysis.

In spite of proper treatment, 50% of distal femoral physeal fractures will develop a partial or complete growth arrest. These arrests can rapidly result in significant deformities since the distal femoral physis is the most active physis in body, generating roughly 0.9 cm/yr of growth. If there is any suspicion of physeal damage, MRI is indicated to evaluate the health of the growth plate. Depending on the nature and location of the arrest, options include bar resection, completion of the epiphysiodesis, contralateral epiphysiodesis, or corrective osteotomy (plus lengthening if needed).

Tibial Eminence Fractures

Tibial eminence fractures are the pediatric equivalent of an anterior cruciate ligament (ACL) injury as it is the site of the ACL insertion. The injury typically occurs in children aged 8 to 12 years and is usually the result of a hyperextension load. Not surprisingly, most of these result from athletic

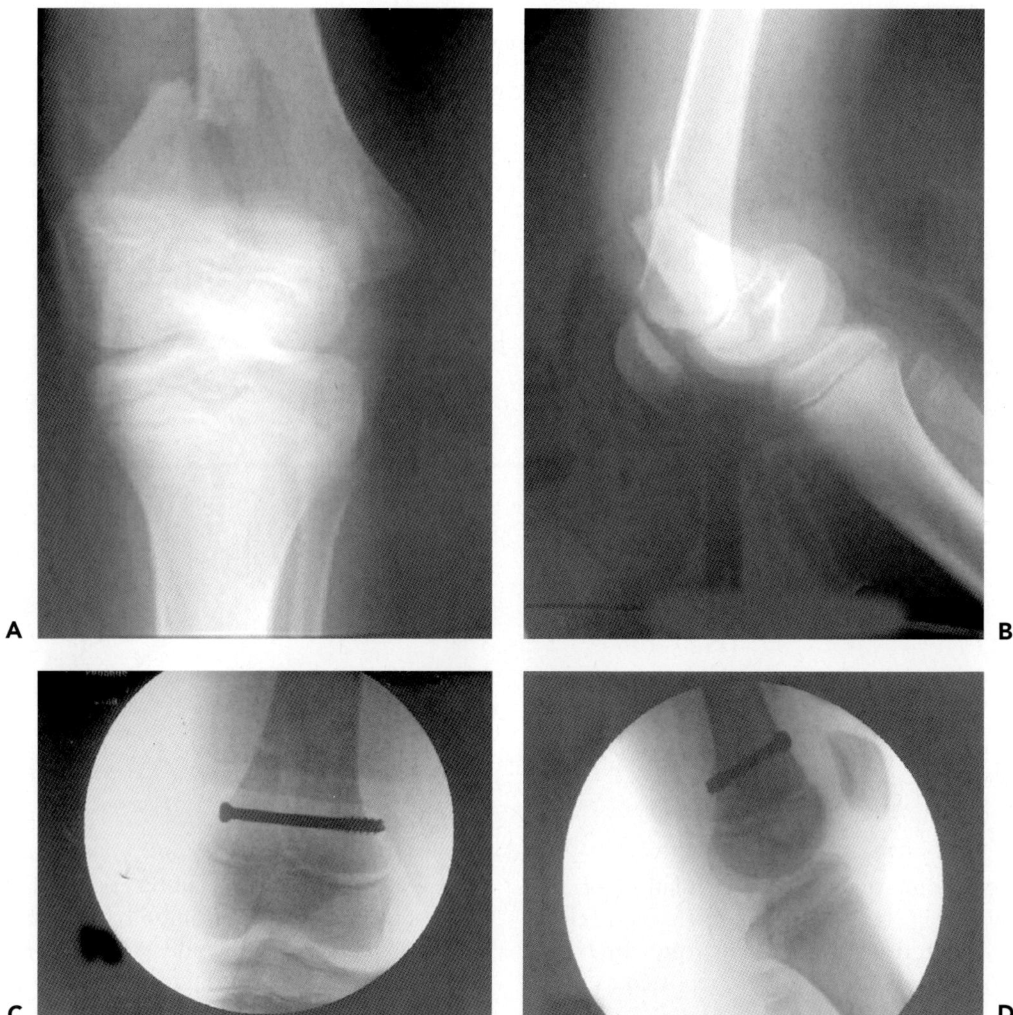

Figure 11.283 (**A** and **B**) AP and lateral radiographs of a 13-year-old boy with a Salter–Harris type II distal femoral physeal fracture. Note the size of the Thurston–Holland fragment. (**C** and **D**) Intraoperative radiographs after reduction and fixation with a 7.3-mm cannulated screw. (*Reproduced with permission from* Morrissy RT, Weinstein SL. *Lovell and Winter's Pediatric Orthopaedics*. Philadelphia, PA: Lippincott Williams & Wilkins, 2006.)

trauma. Meyers and McKeever classified these fractures into type I (nondisplaced), type II (anterior elevation with an intact posterior hinge), and type III (completely displaced) (Fig. 11.284). Type I injuries can be treated closed with 6 weeks of cast immobilization. An attempt can be made to reduce type II injuries by extending the knee, followed by immobilization for 6 weeks. Irreducible type II injuries and all type III fractures require open or arthroscopic reduction and fixation. Fixation can be achieved by an epiphyseal screw or by passing sutures through the base of the ACL and tying over the front of the tibia. Stable fixation and early mobilization can reduce the risk of arthrofibrosis.

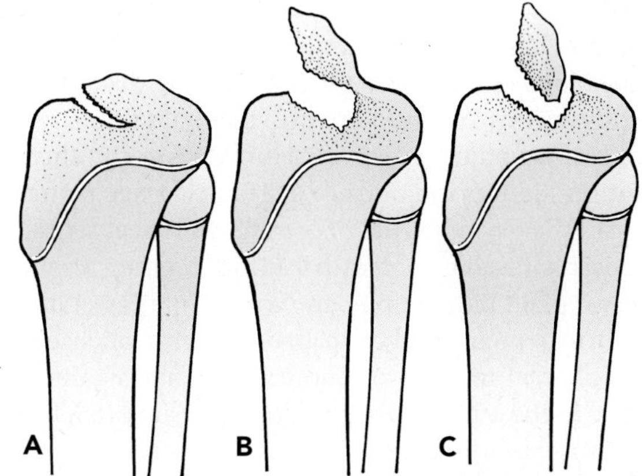

Figure 11.284 Classification of tibial spine fractures. **(A)** Type I—minimal displacement. **(B)** Type II—hinged posteriorly. **(C)** Type III—completely displaced. (*Reproduced with permission from* Beaty JH, Kasser JR. *Rockwood and Wilkins' Fractures in Children*. 6th ed. Philadelphia, PA: Lippincott Williams & Wilkins, 2006.)

Tibial Tubercle Avulsions

Tibial tubercle avulsions occur through the physis of the tubercle and most often occur in children who are nearing skeletal maturity. Most injuries are due to the eccentric

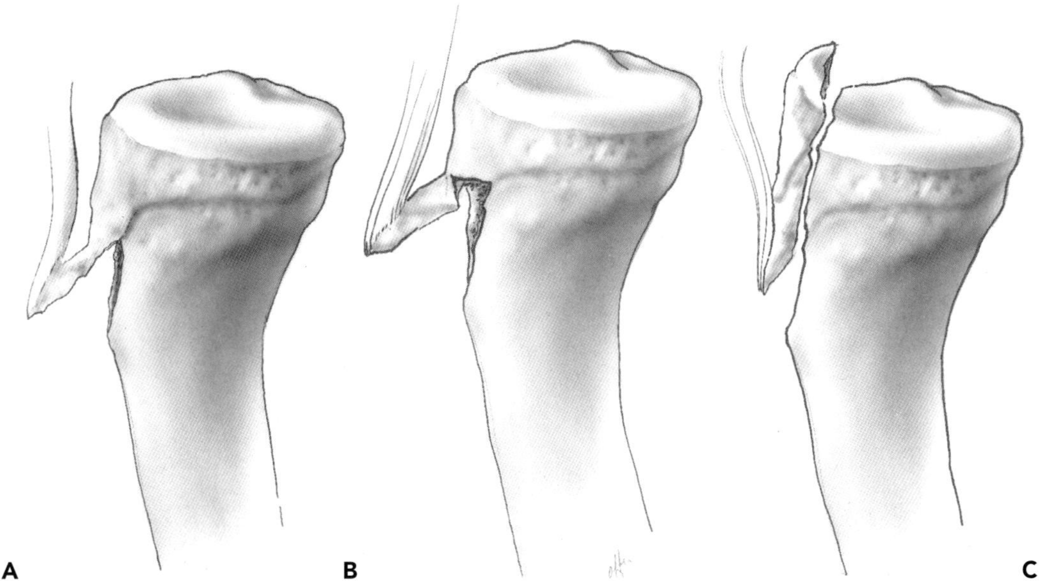

Figure 11.285 Classification of tibial tuberosity fractures. **(A)** Type I fracture through the secondary ossification center. **(B)** Type II fracture located at the junction of the primary and secondary ossification centers. **(C)** Type III fracture is an intraarticular fracture (Salter–Harris type III). (*Reproduced with permission from* Morrissy RT, Weinstein SL. *Lovell and Winter's Pediatric Orthopaedics.* Philadelphia, PA: Lippincott Williams & Wilkins, 2006.)

loading of the quadriceps during jumping or landing. Ogden has classified these fractures into three types: type I is a small avulsion of the distal part of the tubercle, type II is a larger avulsion up to the transverse level of the tibial epiphysis, and type III is a complete avulsion that extends through the epiphysis and into the joint (Fig. 11.285). Small, nondisplaced fractures can be treated by casting the leg in extension. Displaced type I fractures can be fixed with suture weaved through the patellar tendon and tied over a post. Type II and III fractures usually require open reduction and screw fixation into the metaphysis. Since most fractures occur in children with closing physes, growth disturbance is rare following tibial tubercle avulsions. In those rare injuries in patients younger than 11 years, genu recurvatum can occur.

Proximal Tibial Fractures

Proximal tibial physeal fractures are similar to growth plate injuries of the distal femur. The mechanism is most often the result of force applied to the planted leg. This fracture has been described as the pediatric equivalent of a knee dislocation, and neurovascular injury has been reported in up to 10% of these fractures, especially those with an apex posterior angulation. As a result, careful assessment for vascular insufficiency and compartment syndrome is mandatory in these injuries (Fig. 11.286). Nondisplaced fractures can be treated in a long leg cast. Unstable fractures are best treated with CRPP. As with distal femoral physeal injuries, approximately 40% of these fractures are complicated by partial or complete growth arrest.

Proximal tibial metaphyseal fractures usually present in children between 2 and 10 years of age. These fractures often appear relatively benign, with only a minimal gap on the medial side of the proximal tibial metaphysis. Treatment consists of closed reduction with varus stress, followed by immobilization in a long leg cast for at least 6 weeks. Occasionally, soft tissue can be interposed in this gap and can prevent anatomic reduction; in these cases, open exploration and reduction is indicated. In spite of an adequate reduction, parents should be warned that these fractures can develop a late valgus deformity (usually within 12–18 months). Most authors believe that this results from asymmetrical growth after fracture healing. The vast majority of these malalignments will spontaneously correct within 3 years of the injury. As a result, corrective osteotomy is usually not necessary. Premature osteotomies are often complicated by recurrent deformity.

Leg and Ankle Injuries

Tibial Diaphyseal Fractures

Tibial shaft fractures are the most common lower extremity fractures in children, accounting for 5% of all pediatric fractures. The most likely mechanism of injury depends on the age of the patient. In children between 1 and 6 years of age, fractures usually result from torsional stresses on the tibia that occur during running, jumping, and other seemingly innocuous activities. These injuries have been termed *toddler* fractures and are frequently so subtle that radiographs may be interpreted as normal (Fig. 11.287). Oblique radiographs and bone scans can help to identify occult fractures.

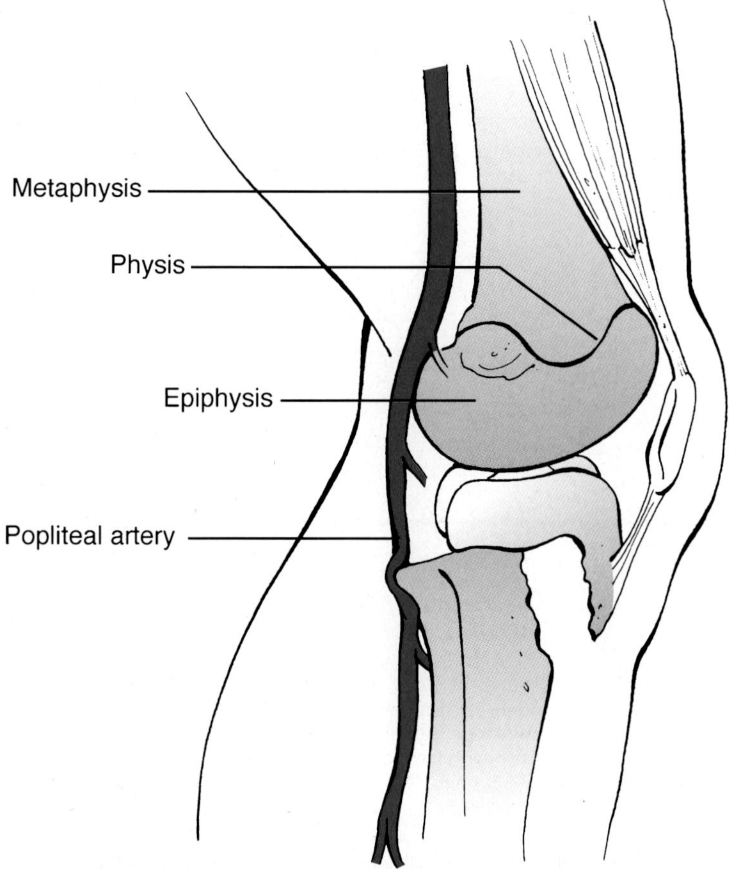

Figure 11.286 Posterior displacement from a proximal tibial physeal fracture can cause arterial injury. (*Reproduced with permission from* Skaggs DL, Flynn JM. *Staying Out of Trouble in Pediatric Orthopaedics*. Philadelphia, PA: Lippincott Williams & Wilkins, 2006.)

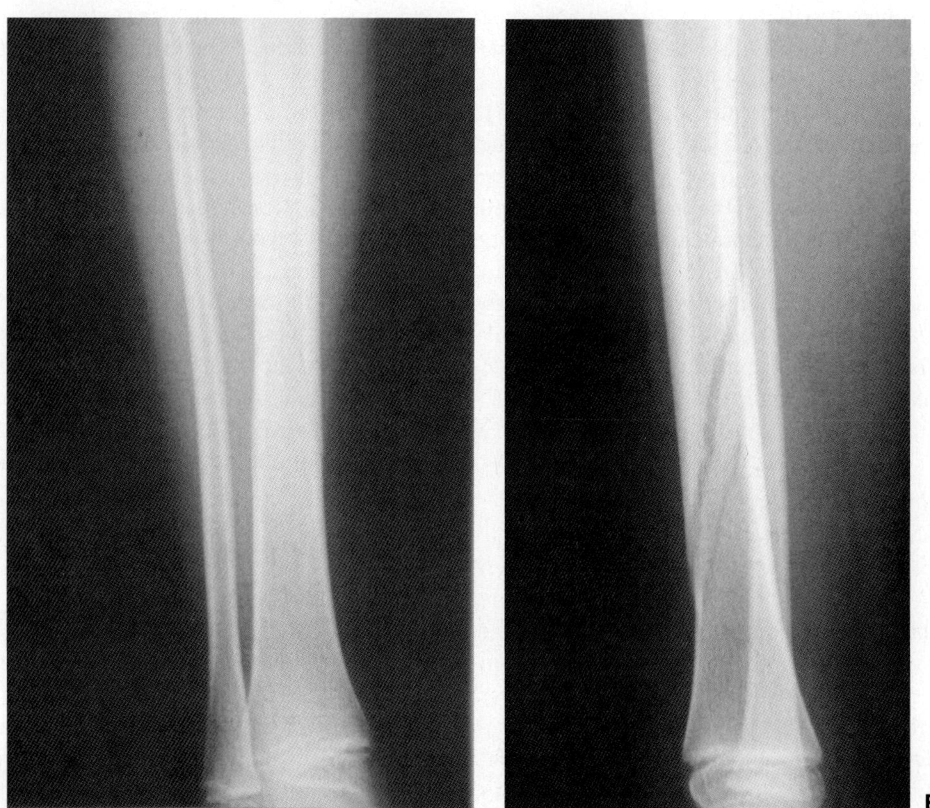

Figure 11.287 **(A** and **B)** Toddler fractures are often difficult to appreciate on a single radiographic view. The lateral view demonstrates the spiral fracture. (*Reproduced with permission from* Skaggs DL, Flynn JM. *Staying Out of Trouble in Pediatric Orthopaedics*. Philadelphia, PA: Lippincott Williams & Wilkins, 2006.)

However, diagnosis can usually be made on the basis of a careful physical examination, which demonstrates localized tenderness over the shaft of the tibia. In older adolescents, the mechanism of injury is more often motor vehicle accidents, falls from height, or athletic trauma. Standard radiographs in these patients are usually diagnostic.

The majority of toddler fractures can be treated conservatively. These fractures are usually spiral in nature and nondisplaced because of the presence of dense, thick periosteum, which holds its position. Immobilization in a long leg cast for 3 to 4 weeks is more than adequate treatment. For older children, the guidelines for acceptable reduction are less than 10 degrees of coronal or sagittal angulation and less than 10 degrees of malrotation. Unlike femoral fractures, overgrowth in the tibia is quite variable, so most authors recommend that no more than 1 cm of shortening be accepted. As long as these criteria are met, conservative treatment is appropriate. Surgery is indicated in cases of open fracture, compartment syndrome, polytrauma, irreducible fracture, and loss of reduction during conservative treatment. Flexible intramedullary nails are an excellent treatment choice for length-stable fractures (transverse or short oblique) in the middle third of the tibia. As in the femur, flexible nails result in predicable union rates with a low risk of complications. External fixators are an effective tool for restoring length and alignment when comminution is present or in cases of very distal or proximal fractures. External fixation is also the treatment of choice for severe open fractures or significant soft tissue injury.

Ankle Fractures

Pediatric ankle fractures are relatively common injuries, and usually affect children between 8 and 15 years of age. The mechanism of injury is usually indirect trauma from a twisting injury although direct trauma from motor vehicle accidents, falls, or contact sports can be responsible. Proper evaluation includes AP, lateral, and mortise radiographs of the involved extremity. The mortise view, in particular, is important as some pediatric physeal fractures cannot be readily visualized on standard AP and lateral radiographs. Accessory ossification centers including the os subtibiale, os subfibulare, and os trigonum are common and can often be confused with acute fractures. Careful physical examination, radiographs of the contralateral extremity, and a bone scan (if necessary) can distinguish these anatomic variants from acute injuries. A CT scan is useful in cases of suspected intraarticular injury. In these instances, plain radiographs often underestimate the degree of displacement, and CT scans can be invaluable for determining the need for and extent of surgery.

Most injuries are physeal and can be classified according to the Salter–Harris system. Salter–Harris type I fractures of the distal tibia or fibula are often misdiagnosed as ankle sprains since there can be minimal or no displacement at the fracture site. It is important to remember that in children, the physis is weaker than the surrounding ligaments and, therefore, more susceptible to injury. In the distal tibia, acceptable reduction in children with more than 2 years of growth remaining consists of no more than 15 degrees of plantar tilt in the sagittal plane, no more than 10 degrees of valgus malalignment, and no varus. For older adolescents with less growth remaining, acceptable alignment is reduced to less than 5 degrees in all planes. For nondisplaced fractures of the distal tibia and those fractures that can be adequately reduced, treatment consists of long leg cast immobilization for 4 weeks, followed by transition to a short leg walking cast for an additional 2 weeks. Open reduction may be necessary if there is interposed periosteum or soft tissue that blocks adequate reduction. Isolated Salter–Harris type I fractures of the distal fibula are usually nondisplaced and can be treated with a short leg walking cast for 3 to 4 weeks. Salter–Harris type II fractures are the most common distal tibial physeal injuries in children. The criteria for reduction is the same as for Salter–Harris type I fractures as is the treatment for nondisplaced and reducible injuries. When necessary, operative treatment consists of clearing interposed soft tissue from the fracture site, stabilizing the fracture with smooth pins, and applying a long leg cast.

Because of their intraarticular nature and their propensity for causing a growth arrest, most Salter–Harris type III and IV fractures of the distal tibia and medial malleolus require surgery. Achieving anatomic reduction with adequate stabilization is the best means of minimizing the risk of growth disturbance. Closed treatment can be successful for fractures with minimal articular displacement (2–3 mm); however, open reduction, including an arthrotomy to visualize the joint surface, is usually necessary. Fixation most commonly consists of interfragmentary screws place parallel to the physis (Fig. 11.288). If necessary, smooth pins can be placed across the physis. After healing, routine radiographs should be taken at 6-month intervals for 2 years after injury to ensure normal growth. Premature physeal closure and angular deformity will usually be apparent by that time.

Two unique ankle fractures are seen in the preadolescent and adolescent age groups. These fractures have been referred to as *transitional* fractures, because they result from the specific anatomy of the closing physis. Closure of the distal tibial physis begins at approximately 12 in girls and 13 years in boys and generally takes 18 months to complete. Physeal closure does not occur uniformly but rather occurs centrally, then medially, and finally laterally. The anterolateral portion of the physis is, therefore, the last region to close. During this closure period, transition zones between fused and unfused areas of the physis represent areas of relative weakness that are susceptible to fracture. Tillaux fractures are Salter–Harris type III avulsions of the anterolateral epiphysis that result from pull of the anterior inferior tibiofibular ligament (Fig. 11.289). As mentioned earlier, this is the last region of the physis to close. Radiographs

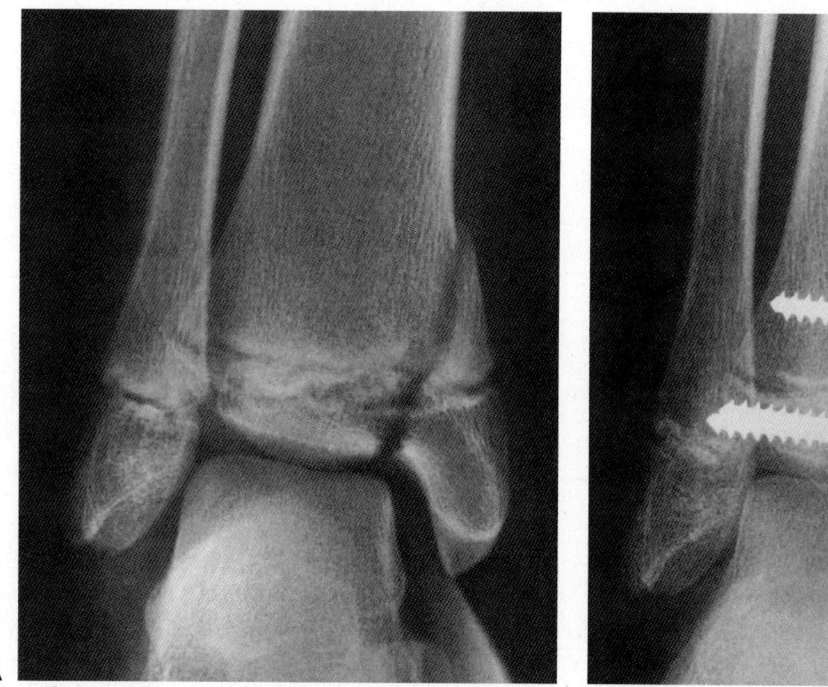

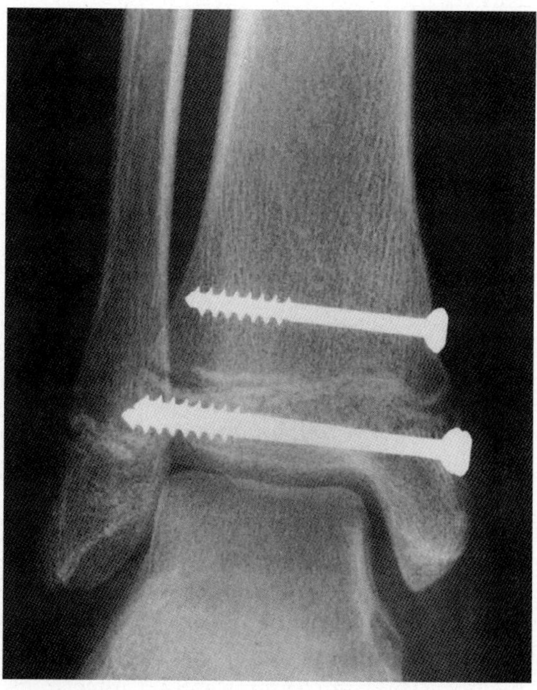

Figure 11.288 **(A)** Salter–Harris type IV distal tibia fracture in a 12-year-old girl. **(B)** Anteroposterior radiograph after open reduction and fixation with screws placed parallel to the physis. (*Reproduced with permission from* Beaty JH, Kasser JR. *Rockwood and Wilkins' Fractures in Children.* 6th ed. Philadelphia, PA: Lippincott Williams & Wilkins, 2006.)

usually make the diagnosis, but CT scans may be necessary to elucidate the full extent of articular involvement. Similar to other Salter–Harris type III injuries, treatment consists of anatomic reduction of the articular surface usually with internal fixation. Since these injuries occur in patients with closing physes, growth disturbance is not a concern. Triplane fractures are complex Salter–Harris type IV fractures that, as their name implies, have multiple planes of involvement. On AP and mortise views, triplane fractures appear to be Salter–Harris type III injuries (Fig. 11.290). In the lateral view, however, the fracture often looks more like a Salter–Harris type II injury with a posterior metaphyseal fragment. Because the fracture is difficult to visualize in three dimensions, CT scans with sagittal and coronal reconstructions are usually indicated. Similar to other intraarticular fractures, the goal of treatment is anatomic reduction of the joint surface. An articular step-off of more than 2 mm or fracture gap of more than 2 to 3 mm is an indication for open reduction with an arthrotomy to visualize the articular surface. Fixation usually consists of interfragmentary screws placed across the epiphysis from a lateral to medial direction and across the metaphysis from anterior to posterior. Similar to Tillaux injuries, triplane fractures occur in patients nearing skeletal maturity; as a result, the risk of growth disturbance is minimal and fixation may cross the physis if necessary. Patients should be placed into a non–weight-bearing cast for approximately 6 weeks.

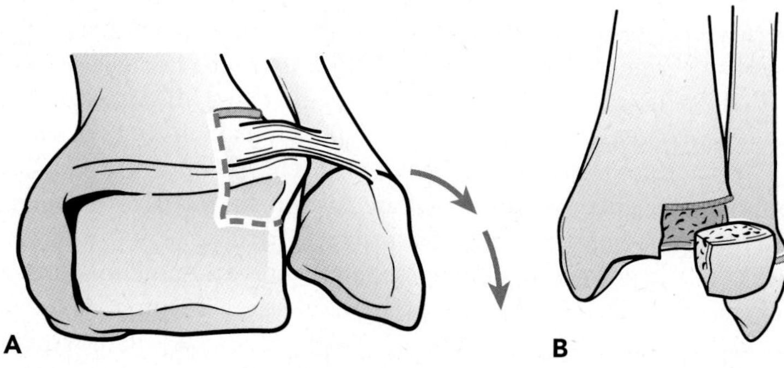

Figure 11.289 Juvenile Tillaux fracture. **(A** and **B)** Mechanism of injury is due to avulsion of a fragment of the lateral epiphysis by the anteroinferior tibiofibular ligament. (*Reproduced with permission from* Beaty JH, Kasser JR. *Rockwood and Wilkins' Fractures in Children.* 6th ed. Philadelphia, PA: Lippincott Williams & Wilkins, 2006.)

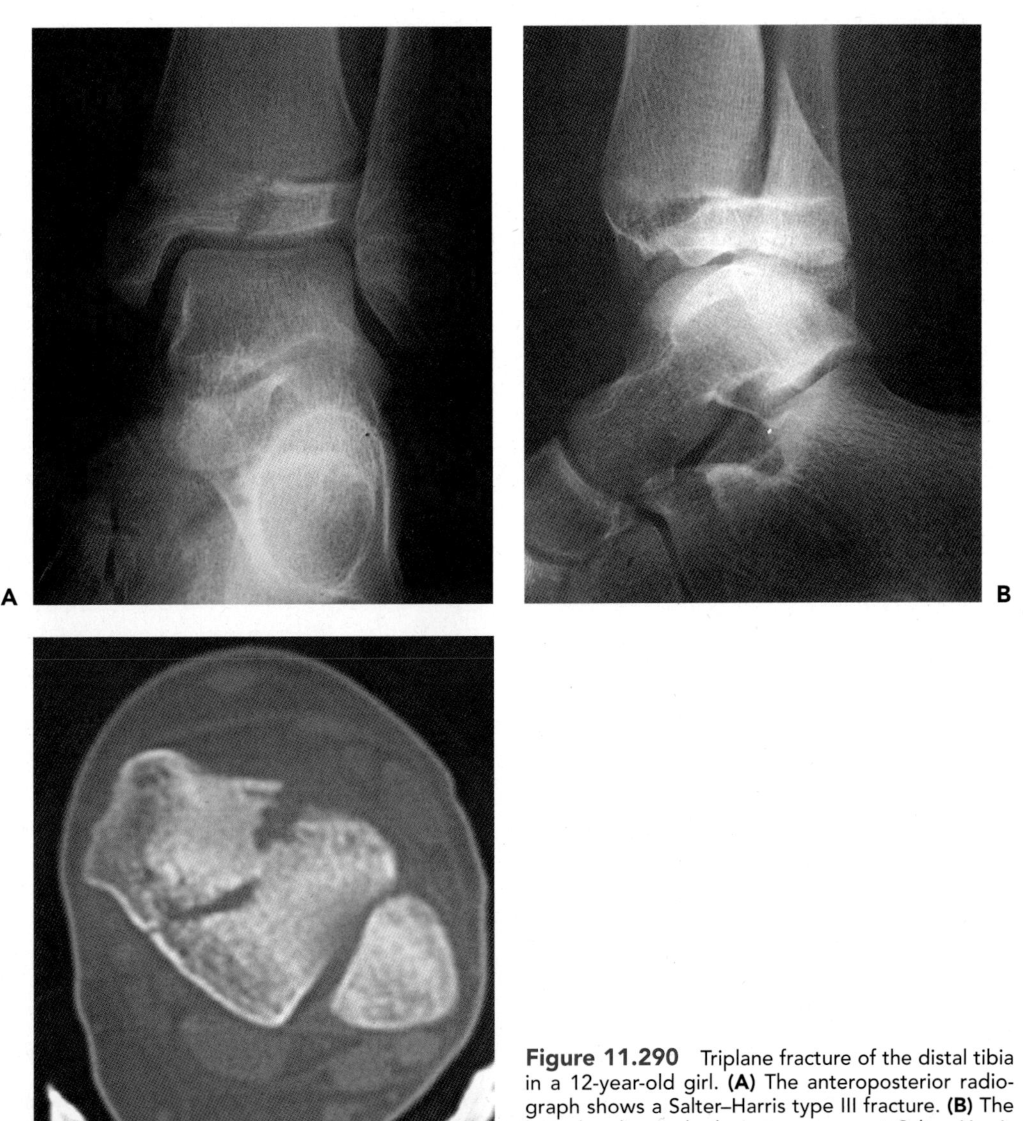

Figure 11.290 Triplane fracture of the distal tibia in a 12-year-old girl. **(A)** The anteroposterior radiograph shows a Salter–Harris type III fracture. **(B)** The lateral radiograph shows an apparent Salter–Harris type II fracture. **(C)** Computed tomography through the epiphysis helps assess the true displacement of the fracture. (*Reproduced with permission from* Morrissy RT, Weinstein SL. *Lovell and Winter's Pediatric Orthopaedics*. Philadelphia, PA: Lippincott Williams & Wilkins, 2006.)

Foot Fractures

Fractures of the foot in children are very similar, both in mechanism and management, to those in adults. Fractures of the metatarsals and phalanges are almost ubiquitously managed nonoperatively. Excellent results are usually anticipated. One injury unique in this age group is the stress fracture of the calcaneus. Frequently, the child who presents with heel pain is diagnosed with Sever disease. This osteochondrosis of the calcaneal apophysis is common in young children. However, should the tenderness be more distal in the body of the calcaneus and the symptoms be more intense, a stress fracture of the calcaneus should be considered. A bone scan is usually adequate to make the diagnosis, because radiographs are often normal. A short leg cast for 3 to 4 weeks is usually an adequate treatment.

Child Abuse

Approximately 2 million children experience child abuse every year. Approximately 25% of these children are physically abused, resulting in more than 1,000 deaths per year. Half of the children are younger than 2 years, and 40% are between 2 and 5 years of age. It is widely recognized that early diagnosis is important. Green has stated that should an abused child be returned to his or her home without appropriate intervention, approximately 50% to 70% are at risk for further injury, and 10% are at risk for death. Parents (including the mother) are commonly at fault, as are stepfathers and other male partners of the mother who are not the biologic father.

Orthopaedic surgeons are frequently called upon to evaluate musculoskeletal injuries and to weigh in on the likelihood that a given fracture resulted from nonaccidental trauma. Many large pediatric hospitals have dedicated, multidisciplinary "abuse" teams that are responsible for the evaluation of suspected cases of child abuse. In many situations, however, decisions must be made by the treating physician, whether it be the pediatrician, emergency department physician, or the orthopaedic surgeon. The diagnosis rests on the finding of a constellation of symptoms, that, when viewed collectively, point to child abuse. Usually a vague or inconsistent history is offered by the caregiver that does not explain the child's injuries. Most children are withdrawn and anxious while being evaluated by a doctor. Assessment of the skin for bruises and burns is essential as 60% of physically abused children have only soft tissue injuries. Multiple bruises of different colors suggest that multiple injuries have occurred at different points in time. Bruising on the buttocks, trunk, and back of legs are all highly suspicious for intentional injuries. In addition, bruise patterns from common objects can occur from belt buckles and coat hangers and other household devices. Multiple, small burns of different ages suggest the use of cigarettes or matches to punish the child.

Non skeletal trauma is common and should be evaluated by the appropriate specialists. Retinal hemorrhages can occur from violent shaking of small infants. Visceral injury can result from an impact with a thick object, such as a wall. The most common intraabdominal injury is a liver laceration; however, kidney injuries, ruptured intestines, and rectal perforations can occur. Head injury is the most frequent cause of death and implies a significant mechanism of injury. Skull fractures involving multiple sites with complex configurations are usually nonaccidental. In particular, nonparietal skull fractures are suspicious for abuse.

Common skeletal injuries from child abuse include diaphyseal long bone fractures, injuries to the metaphysis/epiphysis, and rib fractures. Certain diaphyseal fractures are highly suggestive of nonaccidental trauma including spiral fractures of the humerus in children younger than 2 years. In addition, femur fractures in children before the walking age are extremely concerning for abuse. Metaphyseal "corner" fractures seen in the distal femur, proximal tibia, and distal humerus and bucket-handle fractures in which the entire peripheral metaphyseal rim is avulsed are considered characteristic abuse injuries (Fig. 11.291). Rib fractures are very common and can occur from vigorous squeezing of a child or following a kicking injury. Multiple rib fractures, in various stages of healing, again suggest battery.

If child abuse is suspected, hospital admission is mandatory. Proper medical care should be provided, and child protection services should be notified. Virtually all state and local jurisdictions now have mandatory laws requiring the reporting of suspected cases of battered child syndrome; in fact, the physician may be held liable for failure to do so.

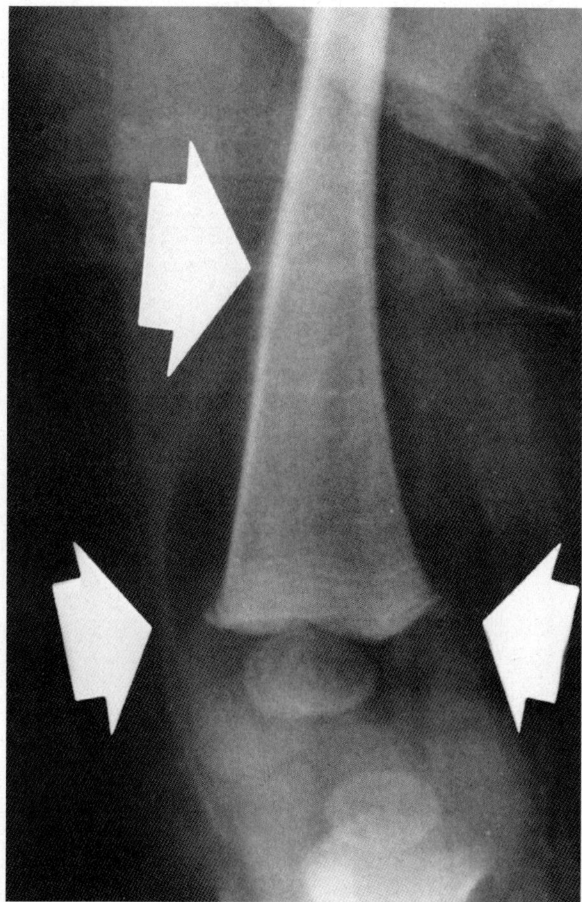

Figure 11.291 An 11-month-old girl with thigh swelling. Radiograph of the distal femur shows corner or "chip" fractures in the metaphysis (*bottom arrow*). Faint periosteal calcification is also visible along the lateral cortex (*top arrow*). Such fractures raise suspicion for child abuse. (*Reproduced with permission from* Beaty JH, Kasser JR. *Rockwood and Wilkins' Fractures in Children.* 6th ed. Philadelphia, PA: Lippincott Williams & Wilkins, 2006.)

RECOMMENDED READINGS

Flynn JM, Sarwark JF, Waters PM, et al. The operative management of pediatric fractures of the upper extremity. *J Bone Joint Surg Am.* 2002;84:2078–2089.

Flynn JM, Skaggs DL, Sponseller PD, et al. The operative treatment of pediatric fractures of the lower extremity. *J Bone Joint Surg Am.* 2002;84:2288–2300.

Kay RM, Matthys GA. Pediatric ankle fractures: evaluation and management. *J Am Acad Orthop.* 2001;9:268–279.

Kocher M, Kasser JR. The orthopaedic aspects of child abuse. *J Am Acad Orthop.* 2000;8:10–20.

Omid R, Choi PD, Skaggs DL. Current concepts review: supracondylar humerus fractures in children. *J Bone Joint Surg Am.* 2008;90:1121–1132.

The Spine

12

William Postma Steven Scherping William Lauerman
Sam W. Wiesel

INTRODUCTION

All orthopedic surgeons need to be able to effectively evaluate and treat the patients with back or neck pain regardless of their subspecialty as symptoms surrounding the spine represent one of the most common reasons for visiting physicians, and disease entities encompassing the spine often masquerade as problems involving other areas of the body. This chapter will provide an introduction to the most common problems involving the adult spine. The chapter will begin focusing on trauma before moving onto degenerative disorders and other associated entities including adult scoliosis. Finally, a brief discussion on spine pathology, including tumor and infection, will ensue. The purpose of this chapter is to provide the reader with a broad, solid basis for understanding and treating spinal conditions.

SPINE TRAUMA

Spinal Cord Injury

Spinal cord injury (SCI) is without a doubt the most devastating condition encountered by the orthopedic surgeon. No other injury or condition is as disruptive physically, emotionally, or economically or has such a high rate of premature death and associated complications. Described originally in the time of Pharaohs, there is a long and pessimistic history of the response of SCI to treatment. Labeled by ancient Egyptian physicians as "an ailment not to be treated," it is only in the latter half of the twentieth century, with the evolution of special SCI units, that an improvement in the functional prognosis of SCI patients has been reported.

The tragedy of SCI is highlighted by its predilection for young, healthy individuals. The incidence of SCI is between 30 and 50 cases per million people per year with little change over the last quarter of a century despite advances in car safety, technology, and laws regulating automotives. This estimates about 11,000 cases of SCI admitted to emergency departments per year. These numbers do not include the approximate 20 cases per million people per year involving SCI with death at the scene of the accident. The majority (around 60%) of these patients are between the ages of 16 and 30, with men affected four times more commonly than women. The most common time of year for injury is during the summer months, with motor vehicle accidents (MVAs) estimated to be the cause approximately 50% of the time. Following MVAs, falls, gunshot wounds, and sports-related injuries are all responsible for around 15% of SCI. In the United States alone, over 200,000 patients live with quadriplegia or tetraplegia secondary to the effects of SCI.

SCIs span a pattern of injury ranging from complete SCI to isolated nerve root injury. Complete SCI implies complete physiologic, although rarely anatomic, disruption of the spinal cord below the level of injury. With the exception of root sparing, which may be seen one or two levels distal to the cord injury, any function further distally is evidence of incomplete SCI by definition. The distinction is important prognostically as complete SCI has a bleak prognosis with functional recovery distal to the lesion being highly unlikely if not impossible. On the other hand, incomplete SCI carries with it a potential for functional recovery to be made.

When making the distinction between complete and incomplete lesions, it is important to ensure that the patient is not suffering from spinal shock because patients with spinal shock can appear to have a complete lesion, when in actuality, once the shock resolves (generally over 48–72 hours), the patient can be noted to have an incomplete injury. The bulbocavernosus reflex is used to determine whether a patient is in spinal shock and its recovery marks the resolution of spinal shock and the point at which prognostication can be made. The bulbocavernosus reflex is performed by placing the examiner's finger in the patient's rectum and squeezing the glans penis or tugging on the Foley catheter, resulting in a reflexive contraction of the sphincter. This is a normal finding. If this test is performed on an SCI patient and is absent, diagnosis of the type of injury (i.e., complete vs. incomplete) should be postponed until return of the reflex, denoting the end of spinal shock.

Incomplete injuries are further divided into several categories depending on the portion of the cord affected. Incomplete syndromes include anterior cord syndrome, central cord syndrome, Brown–Sequard syndrome, posterior cord syndrome, and cauda equina syndrome. Anterior cord syndrome involves injury to the anterior horn cells, resulting in disruption of the corticospinal or motor tract, most commonly in the cervical region. Because of the level at which these generally occur (i.e., cervical) and because the motor tract is involved, these patients have the worst prognosis of all incomplete SCI syndromes. These patients mimic complete injury secondary to disruption of the motor tract, although they generally have patchy distal sparing, thus differentiating the two. Poor outcome is the norm with anterior cord syndrome.

Central cord syndrome offers a better prognosis than anterior cord syndrome and has a much more variable presentation. The classic description is a hyperextension injury in an older individual with a preexisting, long-standing spondylosis. The cord injury results from either central hemorrhage within the cord or from contusion leading to central edema during the hyperextension injury. The patients present with significantly greater impairment of upper extremity function than lower extremity function with a variable amount of sensory disturbance. Bladder and bowel function are variably affected, though usually return to function if affected, and perianal sensation is retained. Lower extremity return of function generally precedes upper extremity return of function. Clumsiness of hands and a wide-based gait remain frequent long-term sequelae.

Brown–Sequard syndrome describes functional hemisection of the cord, generally from penetrating trauma, leading to ipsilateral paralysis or paresis, with contralateral loss of pain and temperature sense (spinothalamic tract), classically two levels below the lesion. The posterior tract generally evades disruption, although with full hemisection, ipsilateral loss of vibration and proprioception should be observed. The syndrome is rare and almost never occurs in its pure sense. Generally, a picture of incomplete hemisection of the cord is seen.

Posterior cord syndrome describes sole involvement of the posterior column, thereby clinically producing loss of sense of vibration and proprioception. This is extremely rare following trauma.

Cauda equina syndrome describes injury to the nerve roots distal to the termination of the spinal cord, and the cord itself is not affected. The spinal cord typically terminates at L1-L2, whereas the nerve roots to the lower extremity typically exit the cord itself two or three rows proximal to this level and traverse the remaining distance until they exit the canal essentially as peripheral nerves. Therefore, injury to this area results in a lower motor neuron-type lesion with peripheral nerve impingement or damage. As such, prognosis for recovery is typically better than would be expected for an equivalent cord injury, and more aggressive surgical management should be employed.

Evaluation

Evaluation of these patients begins with evaluation and stabilization of the entire medical condition following the advanced trauma life support (ATLS) guidelines. The details of ATLS are beyond the scope of this article. Any patient that has suffered a significant trauma should be assumed to have a spinal injury until proven otherwise. Therefore, all polytrauma patients at the minimum should receive lateral radiographs of the cervical spine with visualization of the superior end plate of T1.

When possible, a detailed history should be obtained either from the patient or any observers present focusing on the mechanism of injury as well as any transient loss of neurologic function at the time of the injury. A convincing history of transient loss of motor or sensory function may suggest the occurrence of an incomplete SCI that has resolved rapidly and may affect treatment decision making if a fracture is identified.

Regarding the spine physical examination, the entire spine must be inspected and palpated with the patient logrolled while maintaining in-line traction of the neck. Ecchymosis, tenderness, or a palpable gap between spinous processes suggests injury to the posterior elements, and supplemental radiographic information must therefore be obtained. Neurologic examination must be detailed, systematic, and documented. It should be repeated at regular intervals. Most SCI centers utilize the American Spinal Injury Association (ASIA) guidelines for classification and documentation, which is then entered in the patient's chart, facilitating accurate identification of neurologic status, prognostication, and in many cases treatment. The Frankel grading system or a modification of it is also utilized to classify the extent of function following neurologic injury:

- Frankel A: complete SCI
- Frankel B: sensory incomplete
- Frankel C: motor incomplete, motor useless
- Frankel D: motor incomplete, motor useful
  - D1: nonambulatory
  - D2: ambulatory
- Frankel E: normal

In addition to documenting intact or absent levels of sensation, motor function must be clearly defined and graded on a 0 to 5 scale. By convention, the spinal level applied to the injury level (i.e., C6 quadriplegia) refers to the lowest level with intact, at least antigravity, strength. It is also important, when performing the neurologic examination, to diligently search for evidence of sacral sparing, such as retained toe flexion, perianal sensation, and so on. Rectal examination and evaluation of the bulbocavernosus reflex are routinely carried out as described earlier.

Radiographic assessment begins with a routine lateral cervical view and proceeds as indicated per physical examination findings. If the lateral cervical view is negative, and the patient is awake and alert without any neck pain subjectively or on physical examination, no other views are necessary. If the patient has neck pain, but the lateral view is negative, additional films include an AP, oblique views, and an open-mouth odontoid view. Of note, 80% of injuries can be identified on the lateral view. Flexion and extension views can be obtained in the neurologically normal patient under physician supervision, but these have largely been supplanted by computed tomography (CT) scanning that can be obtained quickly in most emergency departments. CT can be used if T1 is not visualized on plain film, to look for an injury not present on plain film, or to further evaluate a fracture/dislocation that is apparent on plain film. It offers better definition of bony injury and can more accurately assess canal compromise. Magnetic resonance imaging (MRI) is utilized to assess for intrinsic cord damage, to evaluate possible cases of posterior ligamentous injury, or to assess the presence of a herniated disk in a patient with a subluxation or dislocation. The major disadvantage of MRI is logistic, including difficulty introducing an intubated patient or a patient with tongs into the scanner, as well as the time it takes to scan with an MRI as opposed to the CT scan.

The identification of *any* fracture or dislocation of the spine mandates AP and lateral radiographs of the entire spine (or CT scan) due to the high incidence of associated noncontiguous injuries, which is as high as 20%. As alluded to earlier, the identification of a fracture in the cervical, thoracic, or lumbar spine is typically followed by CT scanning of the area to better define bony disruption and determine the presence and extent of spinal canal compromise. MRI scanning is less commonly utilized but is most helpful for identifying injury to the posterior ligamentous complex to better ascertain stability.

Management

As soon as the possibility exists for an SCI injury, the patient should be immobilized with a backboard. It must be emphasized that the backboard or spine board should be used for transportation purposes only, and the patient should be safely transferred to a bed while protecting the spine and maintaining immobilization as soon as the patient arrives at the hospital. Aside from protecting the spine from further injury, management of the patient with SCI begins with medical stabilization. This is usually accomplished with the help of a general surgery trauma team, an intensive care unit team, and an orthopedic trauma team following the ATLS algorithm and protocols as mentioned earlier. Of note, during this treatment, it is important to keep the patient's blood pressure elevated to a normal level to adequately perfuse the spine and prevent ongoing injury from further ischemia.

With regards specifically to the spine, the most effective and important early step in treating SCI is realignment of the spine. In most cases, the application of skeletal traction represents the first step in realignment, generally with the use of Gardner–Wells tongs, which are readily available, inexpensive, and easy to apply. Initial application of 20 lb of traction with increasing weight also serves to immobilize the spine as realignment is accomplished. It must be emphasized that there are certain injuries in which traction is contraindicated, which will be addressed under those specific injuries in future sections, but as a general rule, the application of skeletal traction should be carried out once a spinal injury is recognized.

After the spine has been realigned, the presence of ongoing compression on the cord or cauda equina, as demonstrated by a persistent neurologic deficit, suggests that decompression should be considered. Most SCI patients suffer from neurologic injury as a result of either malalignment of the canal or anterior compression from retropulsed bone. If a deficit persists after realignment, a source of ongoing compression should be sought and is usually identified on CT scanning or MRI. The role of decompression in incomplete injuries is now well accepted with patients who have plateaued neurologically responding well to anterior decompression and stabilization. This is true even in cases of late decompression. With complete injury, the role of decompression is less clear and controversial, although we favor an aggressive approach as some patients do respond with partial recovery.

The next step is determining stability of the injury, which will be discussed later in further detail. If an injury pattern is unstable, surgery should be considered to provide stabilization, whereas a stable injury pattern can be treated nonoperatively. Because the modern approach to SCI management includes early participation in rehabilitation, an increasingly aggressive approach to surgical stabilization is undertaken in most SCI centers for patients who are neurologically impaired. Even in the presence of complete SCI, surgical stabilization minimizes or eliminates the need for external immobilization, facilitates early transfer to a rehabilitation center, and may minimize the risk of medical complications such as pneumonia, skin breakdown, and sepsis.

Halo brace immobilization is commonly utilized in the treatment of injuries to the cervical spine, either with or without neurologic deficit. It has been demonstrated repeatedly to provide markedly increased rigidity when compared with other external orthoses. The halo is routinely used for immobilization of upper cervical spine injuries with some use in subaxial injuries as well. Complications include pin tract infections as well as paradoxical motion or "snaking" of the lower cervical spine.

One of the most controversial topics regarding spinal cord trauma is the use of high-dose methylprednisolone in the acute setting, although it is routinely used in most trauma centers. Methylprednisolone first showed promising results in 1990 when Bracken et al. reported on the results of its use in a multicenter, randomized, double-blind study of patients with complete and incomplete SCI. Patients with incomplete cord injuries showed significant improvement. The dose used was an initial bolus of 30 mg/kg followed by an infusion rate of 5.4 mg/kg/hr. Following Bracken's 1990 study (termed National Acute Spinal Cord Injury Study [NASCIS] 2), it became standard practice to use this dose of steroids. In 1997, Bracken was involved with another study, NASCIS 3, which again was a multicenter, double-blind, randomized, controlled trial evaluating high-dose methylprednisolone. It again showed promising results that have since become scrutinized. Furthermore, the groups who were treated with high-dose steroids had an increased incidence of wound infection, sepsis, and gastrointestinal (GI) bleeding. Though there is no consensus nationwide, the current recommendations are that patients presenting less than 3 hours status post a blunt SCI may be considered for an initial bolus followed by 23 hours of treatment at 5.4 mg/kg/hr. Patients presenting between 3 and 8 hours may be considered for an initial bolus followed by 48 hours of treatment. Those presenting after 8 hours should not be treated with steroids.

Finally, one of the most important aspects of the increased success with the treatment of SCI is the development of specialty SCI rehabilitation centers for the long-term management of these injuries. This movement was started and developed at the time of and after World War II by, among others, Sir Ludwig Guttmann. He proposed a list of guidelines, which are still followed today when dealing with these injuries. Guttmann's guidelines are as follows:

- Transfer to a specialized unit as early as possible
- Management supervised by a physician knowledgeable in SCI care
- A team of allied health professionals trained in SCI management and complications
- Commitment to vocational rehabilitation
- Commitment to addressing psychosocial and recreational needs
- Provision for lifetime follow-up care of the SCI patient

An ongoing federally sponsored system of SCI rehabilitation centers based on Guttmann's guidelines was begun in the United States in 1970 and has without a doubt greatly improved patients' functional and emotional outcomes.

SPINAL STABILITY

When deciding upon treatment for particular injuries to the vertebral column, one needs to understand the stability of the spine and essentially what makes an injury stable or unstable. White and Panjabi defined spinal stability as the ability of the spinal motion segment to resist forces, either acutely or chronically, so as to prevent the development of neurologic injury, pain, or spinal deformity. The different regions of the spine have differences in anatomy and various forces applied, thus contributing to differences in the stability. This must be considered when determining which injury patterns are stable and which are unstable. For example, the cervical spine is more inherently unstable than the thoracic spine since the thoracic spine has the added stability of the ribs and less motion is allowed through the thoracic spine. Therefore, although a good definition of stability has been provided, the question remains how to determine whether an injury is stable as this will ultimately guide management.

Although one would think that such an important concept would have firm guidelines, there have been many propositions of criteria for the establishment of stability, but all have flaws and none are universally accepted. White and Panjabi attempted to provide firm guidelines defining the concept of "clinical stability" of the spine, which highlights the important concepts one needs to consider. They devised a checklist assigning points to various aspects of the injury including radiographic criteria, neurologic status, and anticipated physiologic loads. Critics of this system note difficulty in applying it to clinical situations and lack of validation. Although not perfect, it is a very useful tool when determining spinal stability.

Conceptually important and easier to apply is the proposition of Denis with his "three-column theory" for the stability of the thoracolumbar spine (Fig. 12.1). He divides the thoracolumbar spine into three columns and suggests that instability occurs when two of the three columns are disrupted. Although this theory considers only radiographic criteria, it is easy to understand and also establishes an important concept for evaluating spinal images. The anterior column consists of the anterior longitudinal ligament and the anterior half of the vertebral body. The middle column consists of the posterior half of the vertebral body and posterior longitudinal ligament (PLL). The posterior column comprises the remaining bony and ligamentous structures, specifically the posterior bony arch (pedicles, lamina, spinous processes), the facet joints, the ligamentum flavum, the interspinous ligament, and the supraspinous ligaments. A similar system was proposed in JBJS 2007 by Anderson et al. for the cervical spine. They broke the cervical spine into four columns and assigned numeric values to the degree of disruption of each column. Their proposed system is termed the cervical spine injury severity score (CSISS).

Although there have been numerous systems proposed for defining stability without any being completely accepted, it is important to understand what factors contribute to the stability. These include the injury pattern, neurologic status, patient's overall health status, associated

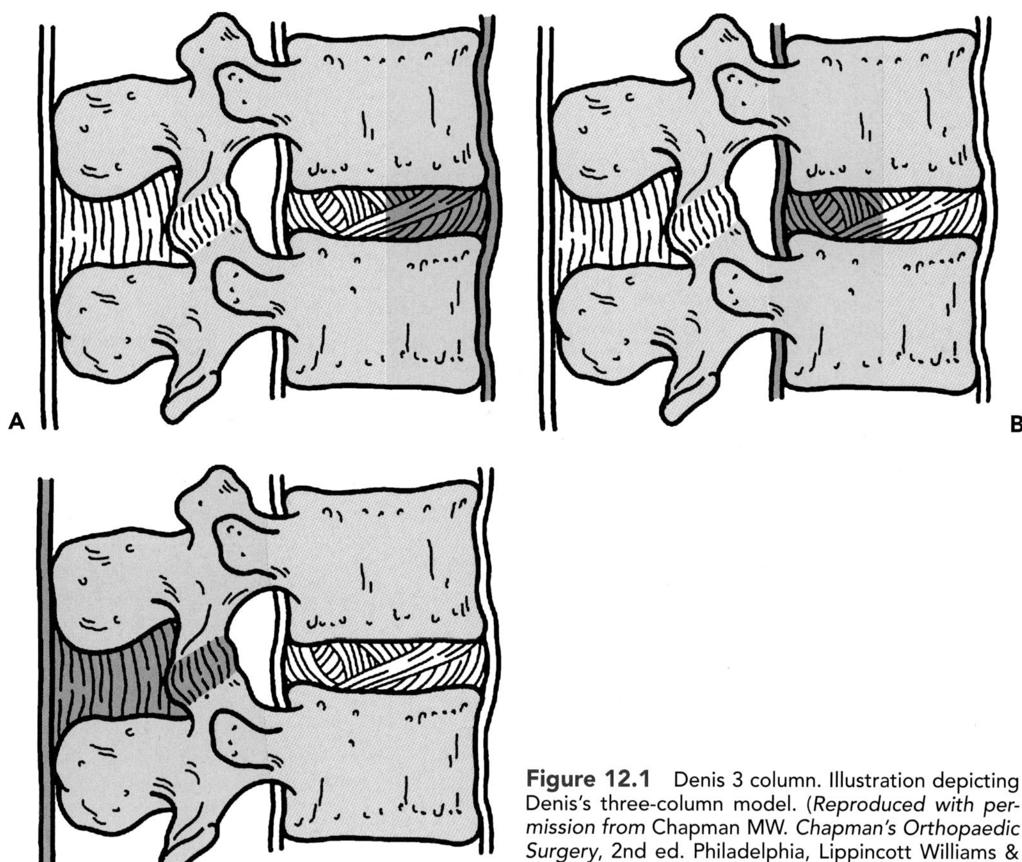

Figure 12.1 Denis 3 column. Illustration depicting Denis's three-column model. (*Reproduced with permission from* Chapman MW. *Chapman's Orthopaedic Surgery*, 2nd ed. Philadelphia, Lippincott Williams & Wilkins, 1993.)

injuries, and potential for healing of the injury. Specific injuries will be discussed in future sections and the stability of each lesion will be discussed as well to better grasp this difficult concept.

CERVICAL SPINE ANATOMY

The cervical spine consists of the region between the cervicocranium junction and the C7–T1 articulation. The cervical spine can essentially be divided into two separate areas: the upper cervical spine and the subaxial spine. The upper cervical spine consists of the region between the base of skull and C2, the axis. This area is unique from the remainder of the cervical spine in that each articulation has its individualized anatomy, whereas the subaxial spine has little variation between articular segments.

As previously mentioned, the upper cervical spine consists of three important structures and their articulations: the base of the skull, the atlas (C1), and the axis (C2). The base of the skull articulates with the atlas through two large condyles projecting from the base of the skull and conforming with the two lateral masses of the atlas, essentially holding up the skull. The anterior and posterior arches of the atlas connect the lateral masses forming a large central hole, allowing the passage of the spinal cord in this region. The articulating surfaces are further stabilized by ligamentous and capsular attachments.

C1 subsequently articulates with C2, the axis, through three separate articulations. The first is through the superior projection of C2, the dens, articulating with the posterior aspect of the anterior arch, and the other two are through the paired facets of the atlas and axis. The axis additionally has a bifid spinous process that can be helpful when trying to identify it. The unique C1–C2 anatomy allows a significant amount of controlled rotation to occur through the atlantoaxial articulation, whereas the occipital-C1 articulation provides a substantial degree of flexion and extension.

The upper cervical spine is further stabilized by ligamentous attachments both extrinsic to the canal and within the spinal canal itself. The attachments external to the canal include the ligamentum flavum, anterior longitudinal ligament, intervertebral disks, and the joint capsules. The stronger ligamentous attachments within the canal include the tectorial membrane, the cruciate ligaments (including the transverse atlantal ligament), and the odontoid ligaments, specifically the alar and apical ligaments (Fig. 12.2). These ligaments provide the majority of stability to the upper cervical spine.

The subaxial cervical spine consists of the vertebral segments of C3–C7, which all have very similar anatomy. The

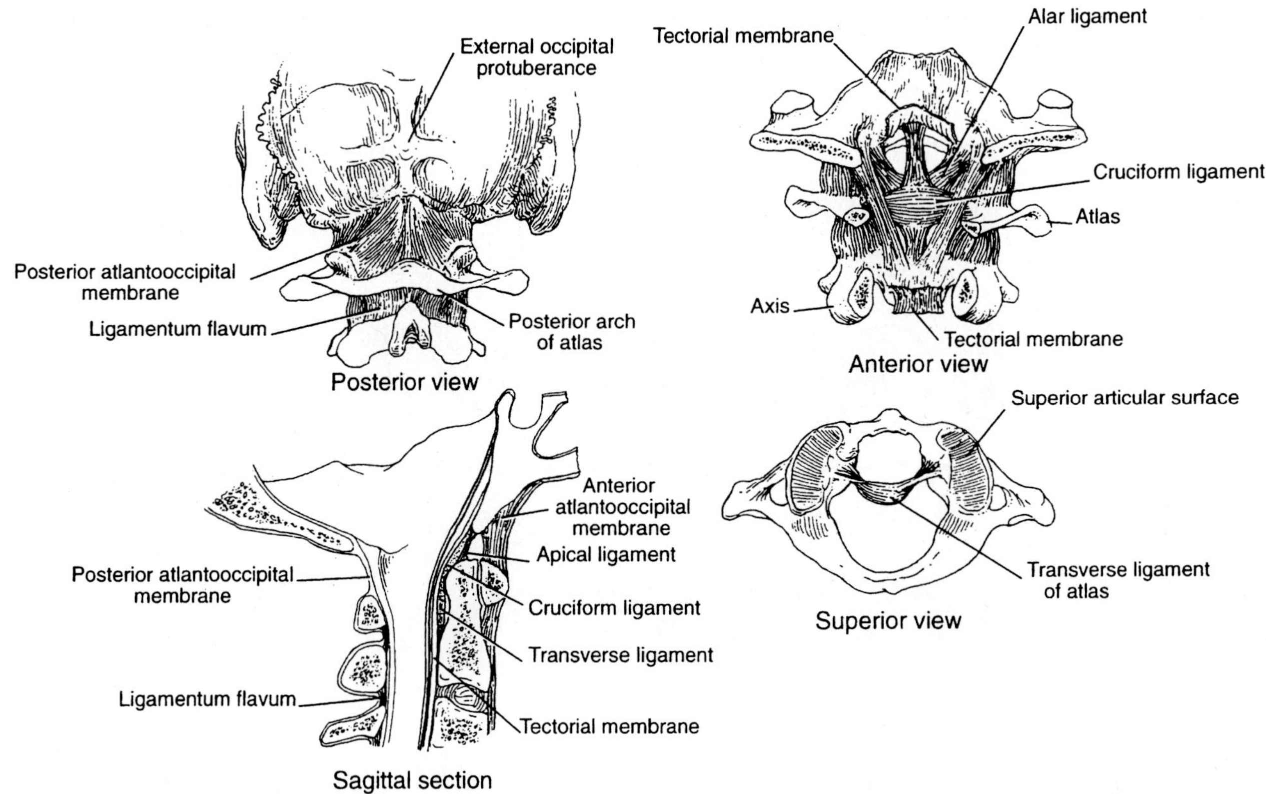

Figure 12.2 Upper cervical spine ligamentous anatomy. Illustration depicting the ligamentous anatomy in the occipitocervical region from posterior, anterior, sagittal, and superior views. (*Reproduced with permission from* Frymoyer JW, Wiesel SW, An HS, et al. *The Adult and Pediatric Spine*, 3rd ed. Philadelphia: Lippincott Williams & Wilkins, 2003.)

vertebral bodies have a slightly oval shape with the coronal distance larger than the sagittal distance. The pedicles project from the body in a posterolateral direction with the facets subsequently arising from the posterior portions of the pedicles. The superior facets of the inferior segment articulate with the inferior facets of the superior vertebral segment, comprising the diarthrodial facet joints. The superior facets face posteriorly and lie anterior to the inferior facets, whereas the inferior facets face anteriorly and lie posterior to the superior facets. In the cervical spine, there is a 45-degree inclination of the facet joint, while there is no facet angulation in the coronal plane (the facets face directly anterior/posterior).

The area of bone between the superior and inferior facets in a single segment is referred to as the lateral mass, and the lamina subsequently arise from these structures. The laminae are oriented posteromedially and combine to close the posterior ring of the spinal canal and continue posteriorly forming the spinous processes. Typically, the spinous processes of C2–C6 are bifid, differentiating themselves from C7 and the remaining spinous processes that have a single projection.

The transverse processes of the subaxial cervical spine are unique in that they have a foramen that allows passage of the vertebral artery. The vertebral artery typically enters into the transverse processes above C7 and thus the foramens of C6–C1 transmit passage through the neck. Classically, the C7 foramen does not house the vertebral artery but one of the vertebral veins.

There are several soft-tissue structures in the subaxial cervical spine, which help maintain stability and dissipate forces. The important elements anteriorly are the anterior longitudinal ligament, the PLL, and the intervertebral disk that lies between the anterior and PLLs. The longitudinal ligaments lie anterior and posterior to the vertebral bodies the entire length of the spinal column. Posterior stability is maintained by the ligamentum flavum, facet joint capsule, interspinous ligaments, and supraspinous ligaments, also known as the ligamentum nuchae in the cervical region. These structures provide stability mainly with flexion.

Finally, it is important to understand the cervical nerve roots and how they are numbered in relation to the vertebral level as this is the basis for understanding and locating cervical root pathology. The roots are numbered for the vertebral level below them in the cervical spine as they exit. Therefore, the C5 nerve root exits between C4 and C5. Unlike the lumbar spine, in the cervical spine, a herniated disk or disk pathology impinges on the exiting nerve root the vast majority of the time. Therefore, a herniated disk between C4 and C5 impinges on the C5 nerve root, the exiting root, resulting in a C5 radiculopathy. Following the same pattern, a C5–C6 disk affects the C6 root; the C6–C7 disk affects the C7 root; and the C7–T1 disk affects the C8 root. It should be recognized that as there is no C8 vertebral body, the numbering of the nerves changes to the vertebral level above the exiting root in the thoracic spine. Of note, the most common areas of disk herniation in the cervical spine are C5–C6 affecting the C6 nerve root and C6–C7 affecting C7.

Radiographs of the Cervical Spine

The timing and indications for ordering different radiographs is very important to understand and is covered in different sections in this article. Equally important is the ability to read radiographs, CT, and MRI scans. An in-depth discussion on this subject is beyond the scope of this article, but this section will discuss the basics of reading plain radiographs and CT scans with emphasis on the trauma setting. Radiographic assessment of the cervical spine starts with an image of the lateral cervical spine and proceeds as indicated. Typically, a lateral, AP, and open-mouth odontoid views will be obtained of the cervical spine, followed by a CT scan if an abnormality is found or suspected. For the lateral view to be adequate, it must allow visualization of the superior end plate of T1. If adequate visualization is lacking, a swimmer's view can be obtained, but most will obtain a CT scan to ensure visualization. Many institutions will get a CT scan with the initial workup or in lieu of plain radiographs secondary to the speed and ease with which CT scans can now be done. CT scans provide very good detail of the bony anatomy and relationships and excellent visualization of the occipital cervical region and cervicothoracic junction that can be difficult to evaluate with plain films. Additionally, sagittal and coronal reconstructions, which are routinely done with CT scanning, allow a clearer picture of the injury. It must be noted, however, that axial CT images alone can miss injuries that are in the plane of the cut.

When reading radiographs of the cervical spine, it is very important to have a systematic approach, especially when first beginning, to decrease the likelihood of missing an injury. The lateral radiograph or sagittal CT scan is not only the easiest to evaluate but also provides the most information. Approximately 80% of injuries can be picked up on the lateral radiograph. Alignment should first be evaluated by following the smooth progression of four longitudinal lines along the anterior vertebral body, posterior vertebral body, lamina (spinal laminar line), and spinous processes. A smooth curvilinear relationship should exist. If there is a disruption in any of these lines, an injury likely exists and the radiograph should be scrutinized carefully for fracture or dislocation. Prevertebral swelling should also be noted on the lateral radiographs as increased swelling often indicates an underlying occult fracture. Prevertebral swelling is evaluated by observing the prevertebral soft tissue shadow.

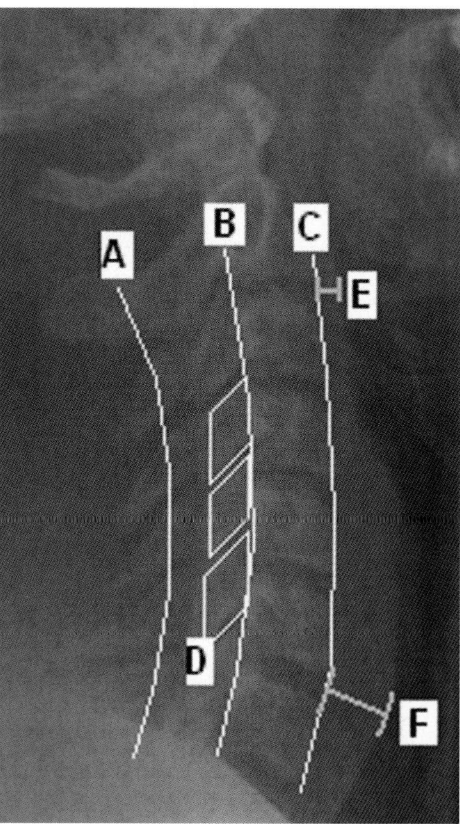

Figure 12.3 Lateral cervical spine radiographic lines. X-ray lines, landmarks, and measurements using a lateral cervical spine film. The spinolaminar line **(A)**, posterior vertebral line **(B)**, and anterior vertebral line **(C)** are normally unbroken. On a perfect lateral view the facet joints should appear as stacked parallelograms **(D)**. The prevertebral soft tissue shadow is measured at the C2–C3 **(E)** and C6–C7 **(F)** disk spaces. More than 6 to 7 mm at C2–C3 or 21 mm at C6–C7 is strongly suggestive of underlying spinal injury. (*Reproduced with permission from* Bucholz RW, Heckman JD, Court-Brown C, et al. *Rockwood and Green's Fractures in Adults*, 6th ed. Philadelphia, Lippincott Williams & Wilkins, 2005.)

If this shadow is greater than 7 mm at the C2–C3 junction or more than 21 mm at the C6–C7 junction, a high likelihood for an underlying injury exists and further workup should be done (Fig. 12.3).

Aside from the relationships discussed previously, there are several specific relationships and measurements in the upper cervical spine that should be evaluated as well. Several measurements and relationships have been described, and there are different proponents for all. The following will be discussed briefly: Wackenheim's line, atlantodens interval (ADI), space available for the cord (SAC), anterior spinal laminar line, and Powers ratio. Wackenheim's line describes an imaginary line representing the extension of the clivus distally. In the normal spine, the tip of the odontoid should fall within 2 mm of this imaginary line. One should be suspicious for possible occipitocervical injury should this relationship be skewed. The ADI is the distance from the posterior portion of the anterior arch of C1 to the anterior portion of the dens as it articulates with C1. This

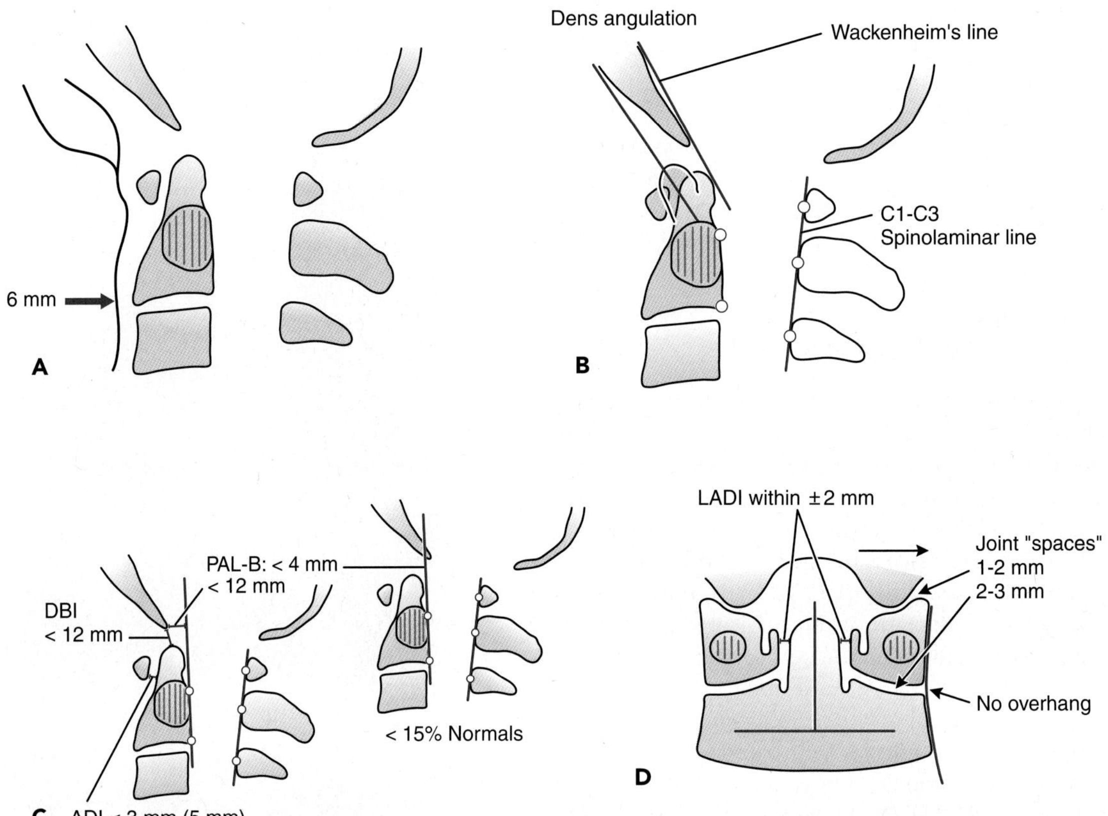

Figure 12.4 Upper cervical spine lines. **(A)** Prevertebral shadow at C2–C3 should not exceed 6 mm in a healthy patient without an endotracheal tube in place. **(B)** Bony screening lines and dens angulation. The anterior cortex of the odontoid should parallel the posterior cortex of the anterior ring of the atlas. Any deviation should be viewed with suspicion for an odontoid fracture or injury the TAL. Wackenheim's line is drawn as a continuation of the clivus caudally. The tip of the odontoid should fall within 1 to 2 mm of this line. The C1–C3 spinolaminar lines should fall within 2 mm of one another. **(C)** Ligamentous injury reference lines. The ADI should be less than 3 mm in adults. The SAC is measured as the distance from the posterior cortex of the odontoid tip to the anterior cortex of the posterior arch of the atlas and should measure greater than 13 mm typically. The dens-basion interval (DBI) is the distance between the odontoid tip and the basion. It should be less than 12 mm in the adult. The posterior axis line (PAL-B) should not be more than 4 mm anterior and less than 12 mm posterior to the basion. **(D)** Bony screening lines. The left and right lateral atlantodens interval (LADIs) should be symmetric to one another (within 2 mm of deviation). The bony components of the atlanto-occipital joints should be symmetric and should not be spaced more than 2 mm apart on AP images. The combined lateral overhang of the lateral masses should also not exceed 7 mm. (*Reproduced with permission from* Bucholz RW, Heckman JD, Court-Brown C, et al. *Rockwood and Green's Fractures in Adults*, 6th ed. Philadelphia, Lippincott Williams & Wilkins, 2005.)

distance should be less than 3 mm. Fractures of the odontoid and C1–C2 dislocation/subluxation can cause this distance to be greater. The SAC represents the region from the posterior aspect of the dens or the posterior aspect of the vertebral bodies to the anterior aspect of the posterior arch. In the cervical spine, this distance will typically be greater than 13 mm in the average adult. The anterior spinal laminar line is an imaginary line from the opisthion along the anterior aspect of the posterior arch of C1 and the laminae of C2, C3, and the remaining subaxial cervical spine as mentioned earlier. This line should remain smooth and curvilinear. Any deviation from the norm of the relationships described earlier should alert the physician to probable fracture or dislocation and further evaluation should be done. Finally, the Powers ratio is the ratio of the distance between the basion (or clivus) and the posterior arch of C1 to the distance between the opisthion and the anterior arch of C1. Normally, this ratio should be less than 1. A ratio greater than 1 suggests the likelihood of an occipitocervical dislocation. These relationships are not inclusive of the described radiographic measurements of the cervical spine but rather provide the most common measurements utilized or discussed (Figs. 12.4 and 12.5).

The AP radiograph and the open-mouth odontoid views provide less information than the lateral radiograph, but there are several important relationships that need to be evaluated. On the AP view, the pedicles should be evaluated and the interpedicular distance should be symmetric throughout the cervical spine. Widening of the interpedicular distance suggests a fracture, typically a burst fracture.

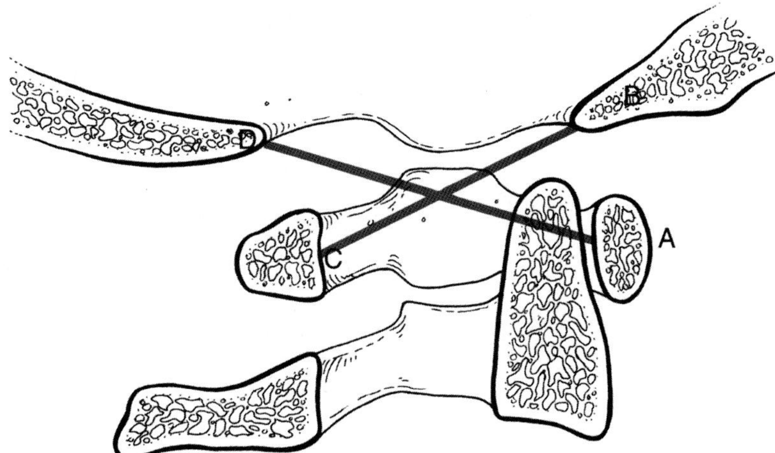

Figure 12.5 Powers Ratio If BC:DA >1, then an antero-occipitoatlantal dislocation exists. Ratios less than 1 are normal except in posterior dislocations, associated fractures of the odontoid process or ring of the atlas, and congenital anomalies of the foramen magnum. (*Reproduced with permission from* John W Frymoyer, Sam W. Wiesel, et al. *The Adult and Pediatric Spine.* Philadelphia: Lippincott Williams & Wilkins, 2004.)

On the open-mouth odontoid, the odontoid should be well visualized as well as the lateral masses of C1. The odontoid should be symmetric between the lateral masses of C1. The lateral masses of C1 should also articulate symmetrically inferiorly with C2. Any asymmetry should alert the physician to probable ligamentous injury or fracture of the ring of C1. If there is asymmetry or widening of the lateral masses, one should evaluate the combined lateral spread or overhang of the lateral masses of C1 (Fig. 12.4). The combined extension laterally of the lateral masses of C1 over C2 should be less than 7 mm. Greater than 7 mm of combined spread is associated with transverse atlantal ligament (TAL) disruption.

Whenever an injury is suspected or identified, a CT scan is usually obtained. As mentioned earlier, the CT scan shows detailed bony anatomy, and sagittal and coronal reconstructions allow evaluation in three planes. The same relationships discussed earlier with plain films can be used to evaluate CT scans with their respective counterparts (i.e., AP to coronal recons and lateral to sagittal recons). Additionally, fractures throughout the cervical spine are much easier to appreciate on CT scan, especially to the untrained eye. The discussion of MRI is beyond the scope of this article, but it should be appreciated that MRI evaluates the soft tissues better than CT but does not provide as clear a picture of the bony anatomy. Therefore, herniated disks, cord/nerve root impingement, and ligamentous injuries, amongst other pathology, are best evaluated with this modality, while CT scan better visualizes bony structure.

UPPER CERVICAL SPINE TRAUMA

Craniocervical Dissociation

Craniocervical dissociation is a rare, commonly fatal condition in which the ligamentous structures connecting the occiput to the atlas become disrupted with subluxation or dislocation of the occiput. The most common mechanism of injury results from motor vehicle accidents. For patients who do survive, they may have subtle or no neurologic deficits because a dissociation resulting in neurologic compromise essentially results in death. These patients have a highly unstable injury despite their preserved neurologic function, and thus a high degree of suspicion and prompt recognition of the injury is essential as neurologic function can decline rapidly if these patients are not immobilized. It must be noted that children, particularly those under the age of 8, are predisposed to these injuries secondary to their relative ligamentous laxity and larger head size. As these injuries are purely ligamentous in nature, there will be no fracture seen on plain films, so one needs to look for more subtle radiographic findings, including prevertebral soft-tissue swelling (should not exceed 6 mm in adults), increased Powers ratio, and abnormality of Wackenheim's line. Following recognition of this injury or if the injury is suspected, immediate immobilization in a halo vest should be considered prior to further imaging studies.

Once the diagnosis is established prompt, aggressive treatment is indicated. Typically a craniocervical fusion will be performed after initial halo-vest immobilization. Nonoperative treatment will almost always result in persistent instability as the injury is usually a purely soft-tissue injury.

C1 Ring Injury-Fractures of the Atlas

Fractures of C1 are relatively common injuries, accounting for approximately 10% of all cervical spine injuries. The fractures themselves generally occur without neurologic sequelae because C1 is in the shape of a ring, and a fracture generally results in expansion of the ring with more room available for the cord. These fractures also have a high rate of associated injuries, so close examination of the remaining vertebral column is essential, especially radiographically. Common associated injuries, as might be expected secondary to their intimate relationship to C1, include odontoid fractures, Hangman's fractures (C2), and TAL disruption.

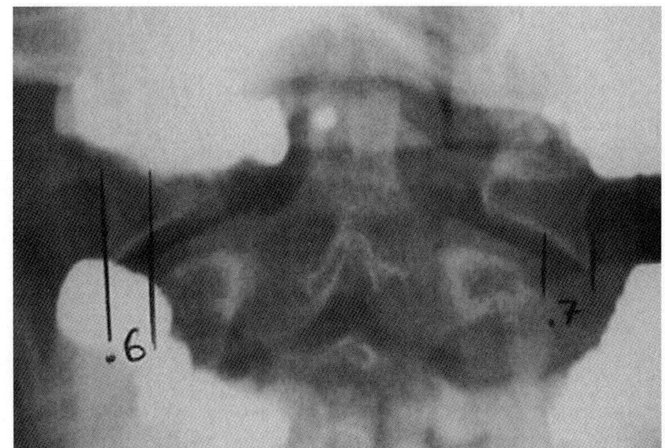

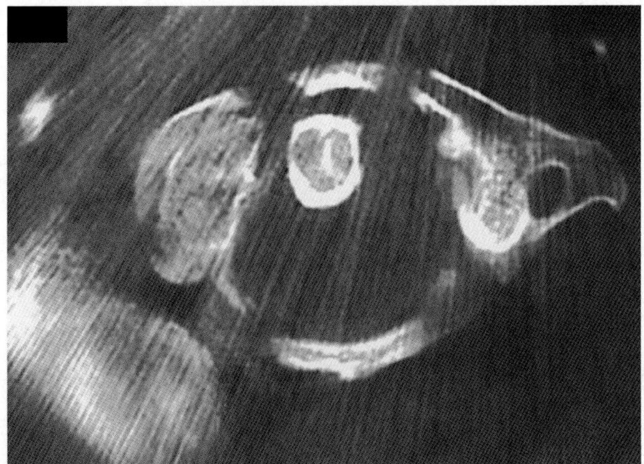

Figure 12.6 Jefferson Fracture **(A)** The open-mouth odontoid view shows bilateral overhang of the C1 lateral masses relative to the C2 facets, with combined lateral displacement measuring 13 mm. **(B)** Axial CT image shows a true Jefferson fracture in the form of a four-part burst fracture of the atlas. This fracture is unstable secondary to the associated TAL disruption. (*Reproduced with permission from* Bucholz RW, Heckman JD, Court-Brown C, et al. *Rockwood and Green's Fractures in Adults*, 6th ed. Philadelphia, Lippincott Williams & Wilkins, 2005.)

Fractures of the ring of C1 may occur anteriorly, posteriorly, and/or laterally and may consist of one to four fracture lines. The classic mechanism of injury is a direct hit to the top of the head producing a pure axial load compressing C1, resulting in the well-known eponym, the "Jefferson fracture," which classically describes a burst fracture resulting in disruption of both the anterior and posterior arches producing four different fractures. There are several other fracture patterns depending on the degree and direction of flexion/extension of the neck and resultant vector of the force producing the fracture. For example, a hyperextended neck with a concomitant posterior load can cause a posterior arch fracture alone or vice versa for a hyperflexed neck resulting in an isolated anterior arch fracture. The degree of force applied dictates whether the TAL will be disrupted, which is the key to the stability of the fracture.

When evaluating these fractures radiographically, routine radiographs of the cervical spine often reveal no evidence of fractures even in the case of multiple fractures. It is therefore essential to obtain an open-mouth odontoid view to look for spread of the lateral masses of C1, which is evidence for C1 ring disruption. Spence et al. found that combined extrusion of both lateral masses of 7 mm or more to be consistent with TAL disruption. Further evaluation of these injuries should be done using a CT scan with fine cuts to visualize the full extent of the injury and help with decision making regarding the treatment (Fig. 12.6).

Nonoperative treatment is indicated for the vast majority of these fractures and patients generally do well, as demonstrated by the series of patients of Levine and Edwards. Minimally displaced fractures can be treated in either a cervical orthosis or a halo vest, depending on the injury, for a period of around 3 months. Displaced fractures require reduction with traction or prolonged traction followed by halo vest. Cases treated nonoperatively need to be followed up regularly with radiographs to ensure that reduction has been maintained. Surgical treatment is occasionally needed for severely displaced fractures, which consists of C1–C2 fusion or occasionally C2-occiput fusion. Associated injuries complicate matters, and management must be individualized in these situations.

Odontoid Fractures

Odontoid fractures account for 15% to 20% of all cervical spine fractures and are the most common fracture of the axis. These fractures are particularly common in the very young and the elderly, ages in which failure to recognize the injury, always a common problem, is even more likely. The most common mechanism of injury depends on the population involved with falls accounting for the majority of the cases in the elderly and pediatric population, and MVAs accounting for the vast majority in young adults and middle-aged population.

The bony, ligamentous, and vascular anatomy surrounding the odontoid (dens) is unique and pertinent for understanding the mechanism of injury, management, and complications of these fractures. The odontoid consists of a broad base with a toothlike projection extending from the body of the axis that articulates with the posterior portion of the anterior arch of the atlas providing inherent bony stability through this configuration. The intricate ligamentous complex encompassing the odontoid greatly enhances stability. The TAL of the cruciate complex (Fig. 12.2) forms a sling around the posterior portion of the dens and serves as the primary restraint to anterior translation of C1 on C2 and the primary stabilizer of atlantoaxial motion. Secondary stabilizers include the apical and alar ligaments originating from the base of the skull and inserting on the tip of the dens. Because of these insertions on the dens,

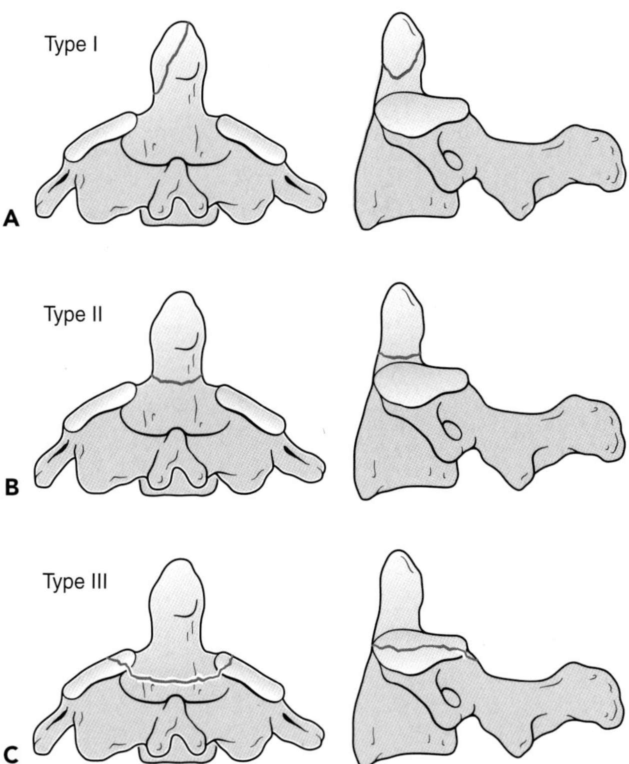

Figure 12.7 Anderson and D'Alonzo odontoid fracture classification. **(A)** Type I fracture-alar ligament avulsions. **(B)** Type II fracture-odontoid waist fractures. **(C)** Type III fracture extends into the body of C2. (*Reproduced with permission from* Bucholz RW, Heckman JD, Court-Brown C, et al. *Rockwood and Green's Fractures in Adults*, 6th ed. Philadelphia, Lippincott Williams & Wilkins, 2005.)

soft-tissue tension may create a traction force to distract the fracture through the waist and contributes to nonunion.

As one moves down to the base of the dense, there is relative thinning of the bone before reaching the cortical margins of the vertebral body of C2, rendering this region susceptible to fracture, accounting for the majority of odontoid fractures (Type II fractures). Once thought to be due to its lack of blood supply in this region, the high rate of nonunion in this region is most likely due more to distraction than ischemia. Studies have now demonstrated a rich anastomosis from contributions by the vertebral and carotid arteries. Although this blood supply may be temporarily disrupted, it is not thought to contribute to nonunion assuming adequate reduction. The most widely used classification for odontoid fractures was devised in 1974 by Anderson and D'Alonzo, which divides the fractures into three types (Fig. 12.7). The classification stood the test of time as it is easy to use, guides treatment, and informs of prognosis, which are the marks of a good classification system. Type I fractures occur through the tip of the odontoid, superior to the insertion of the TAL, and commonly represent an avulsion of the alar ligament. These are the least common odontoid fracture and are quite stable in isolation; however, one needs to rule out craniocervical dissociation as this can be associated with this type of fracture. Type II fractures, as previously pointed out, occur through the base of the odontoid and are the most common fracture pattern. The reported rate of nonunion has ranged from 15% to 85% with nonoperative treatment and around 10% with operative treatment. In actuality, for all cases, the rate is around 30% to 40%. Risk factors for nonunion include initial displacement of 5 mm or greater (most important), patient age, posterior displacement, angulation at the fracture site, and delay in diagnosis. If one has persistent distraction at the fracture site, the fracture will almost assuredly result in nonunion. Finally, Type III fractures extend into the body of C2, thereby providing a greater surface area and greater involvement of cancellous bone, both of which promote fracture healing, making nonunion much less likely than with Type II injuries.

Although low-energy mechanisms account for fractures in the elderly, most odontoid fractures occur as a result of high-energy injury, and as such, associated injuries are common. Therefore, as with other spinal trauma, a thorough evaluation is mandatory. Patients generally complain of neck pain and pain around the base of the skull. Neurologic deficit is uncommon occurring in less than 10% of the cases because there is generally a large amount of SAC in this region. However, as one might expect, those patients with posterior subluxation are at increased risk. On physical examination, one can typically elicit pain with palpation at the base of the skull, and muscle spasm is common.

Radiographic examination begins with the standard cervical spine trauma radiographs. Close examination of these radiographs is warranted as these fractures can be easily missed, especially in the elderly with preexistent degenerative changes obscuring the fracture. Failure to recognize the fracture is not uncommon and most assuredly will result in nonunion if not more catastrophic instability. The two most important images for identification of an odontoid fracture are the lateral and the open-mouth odontoid views. If there is any question at all, or if a fracture is identified, a CT scan of the cervical spine should be obtained with thin cuts. It must be noted, however, that it is possible to miss a fracture on the CT scan if the CT image is obtained in the plane of the fracture, even with coronal and sagittal reconstructions. MRI can be used if an occult odontoid fracture is suspected or to evaluate associated ligamentous injuries.

The treatment depends on the type of fracture as alluded to earlier. Isolated Type I fractures are best treated symptomatically with bracing for comfort with rare complications. However, if there is associated craniocervical dissociation, it should be treated accordingly. Treatment of Type II fractures is more controversial secondary to the high incidence of nonunion. Those patients with nondisplaced or minimally displaced fractures reduced adequately via closed means can be successfully treated nonoperatively with halo-vest immobilization for a period of 12 weeks. This treatment would include fractures with less than 4 mm

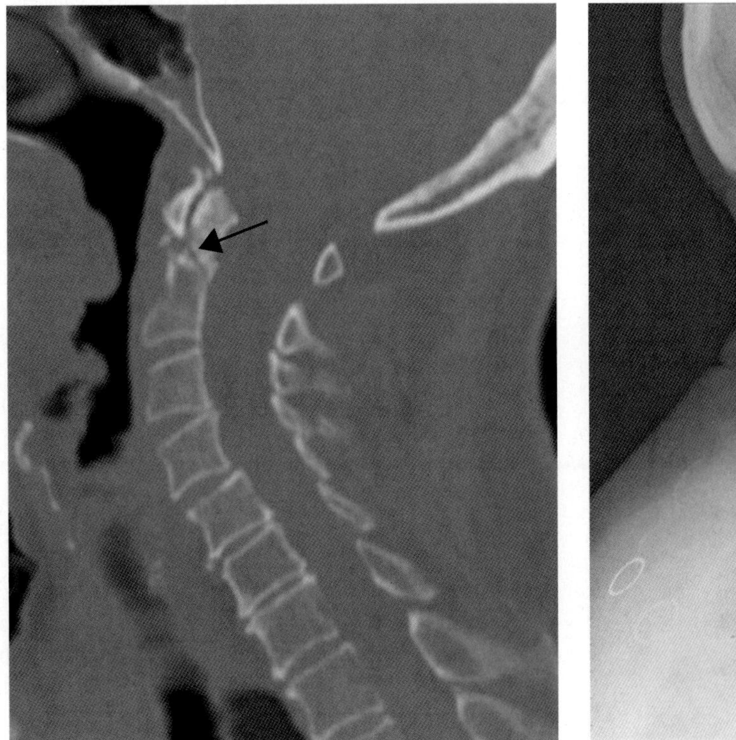

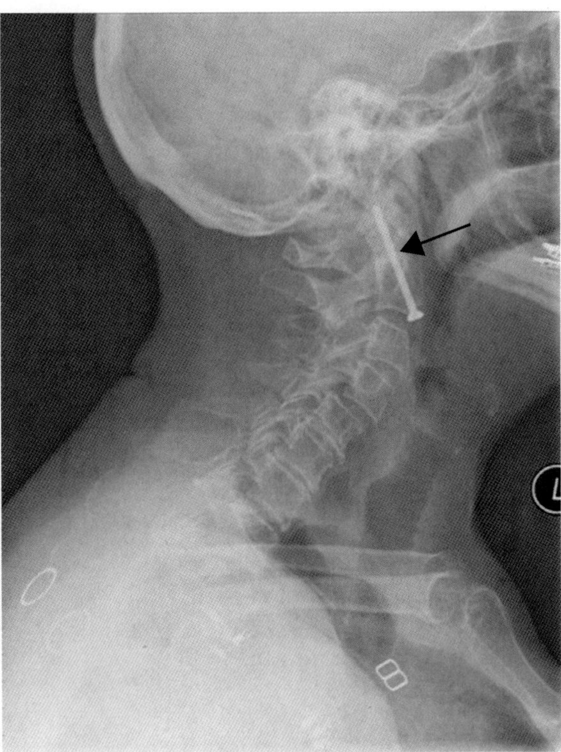

Figure 12.8 Odontiod fracture treated with anterior screw fixations. **(A)** Saggital CT scan image demonstrating a Type II odontiod fracture sustained in a fall. **(B)** Post-operative films demonstrating fixation with a single anterior screw.

of displacement, angulation less than 10 degrees, younger patients with good bone quality, anatomic reduction, and early recognition of the fracture (within 7–10 days). Collar immobilization is inadequate as it does not control atlantoaxial motion and will result in nonunion. After 12 weeks, the halo is removed and the patient is reimaged. If the fracture has healed adequately, no additional treatment is necessary. If there is evidence of nonunion, dynamic (flexion/extension) views should be obtained to look for displacement at the nonunion site. If negative, the patient can be followed with radiographs at 1 month, 3 months, and 1 year to verify a stable nonunion. If motion does occur, surgical intervention may be required.

Surgical intervention is necessary for many Type II odontoid fractures. Relative indications include displaced fractures (>4 mm), angulation greater than 10 degrees, delayed presentation (typically >10–14 days), associated injuries, elderly patients who cannot tolerate a halo, and other risk factors for nonunion. Traditional surgical treatment involves a posterior C1–C2 fusion. Another popular method is primary fixation with placement of an anterior odontoid screw(s) (Fig. 12.8). Proper patient selection is necessary for successful treatment including noncomminuted fracture, transverse fracture or fracture line angled from anterior-superior to posterior-inferior to allow screw placement perpendicular to the fracture, good bone quality, reducible fracture, and a non-obese patient (large body habitus prevents proper drill orientation when attempting to obtain the proper angle for screw insertion). Typically one or two 3.5-mm screws are placed. It must be noted that this is a technically demanding procedure and should not be performed by surgeons without the proper experience.

Finally, Type III fractures, secondary to their abundant blood supply and relative fracture stability, rarely go onto nonunion and therefore rarely require surgical stabilization. However, these fractures should be treated with halo immobilization as nonunion can occur with cervical orthosis only. Operative stabilization, though uncommonly needed for these fractures, does play a small role. The mainstay of operative treatment is posterior C1–C2 fusion as primary screw fixation has resulted in high failure rates. Relative indications are similar to those for Type II fractures; however, displacement is less commonly seen in comparison with Type II fractures.

Traumatic Spondylolisthesis of the Axis (Hangman's Fracture)

Traumatic spondylolisthesis of the axis accounts for approximately 15% of all cervical spine fractures and is the second most common fracture of C2 accounting for approximately 35%. There is a significant fascination with this injury among physicians from all specialties secondary to its unique historical significance. When judicious hanging was refined sufficiently so that instant death was achieved without avulsing the subject's skull, the submental knot used resulted in a bipedicular fracture of C2, which is now immortalized as the Hangman's fracture. The pars interarticularis of the axis represents a zone of transition from the anteriorly placed facet joints of the occiput to C2 to the posteriorly placed facet joints of the subaxial cervical and thoracolumbar spine. The relatively thin pars at this site is therefore susceptible to injury, particularly from a hyperextension force. Subsequent flexion is believed to disrupt the PLL and the disk, resulting in anterior displacement in more unstable injuries. The typical mechanism seen today occurs as result of MVAs with hyperextension and an axial load (rather than the historical hyperextension/distraction), resulting in a fracture of the pars. The subsequent rebound flexion described earlier with PLL and C2–C3 disk disruption occurs by the same mechanism. It must be noted that Hangman's fractures have a high mortality rate at the scene of the accident, anywhere from 25% to 70%, although once the treatment is initiated, the mortality rate falls to about 2%. On those surviving the initial accident, neurologic injury occurs in only 5% to 10% of patients.

The classification of Hangman's fractures was first proposed by Effenti and has subsequently been modified by Levine and Edwards and then by Starr and Eismont who added Type IA (Fig. 12.9). The classification is based upon

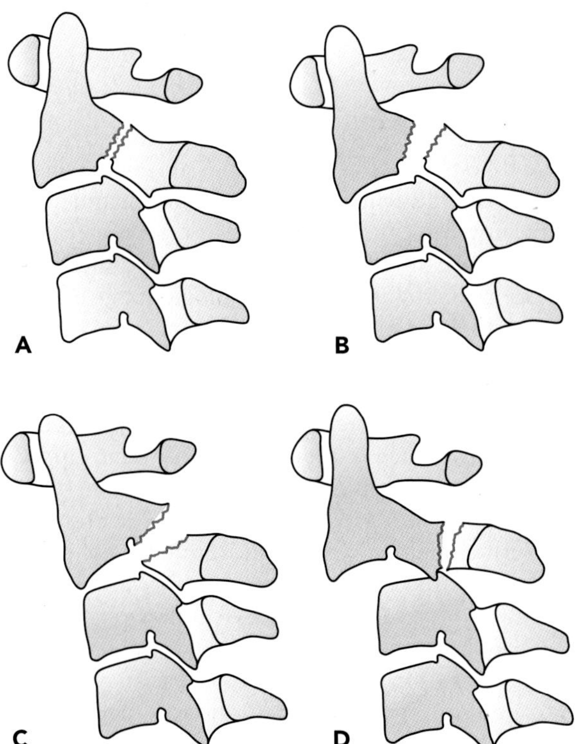

Figure 12.9 Levine and Edwards classification of traumatic spondylolisthesis of the axis (Hangman's fracture). **(A)** Type I-nondisplaced fracture of the pars interarticularis. **(B)** Type II-displaced fracture of the pars interarticularis. **(C)** Type IIa-displaced fracture of the pars with disruption of the C2–C3 discoligamentous complex. **(D)** Type III-dislocation of the C2–C3 facets with fracture of the C2 pars interarticularis. (*Reproduced with permission from* Bucholz RW, Heckman JD, Court-Brown C, et al. *Rockwood and Green's Fractures in Adults*, 6th ed. Philadelphia, Lippincott Williams & Wilkins, 2005.)

the angulation and translation resulting from the fracture, which indirectly demonstrates the degree of ligamentous injury associated with the fracture. Type I fractures occur from a hyperextension injury with axial load, as previously discussed, with no secondary flexion injury. This results in a fracture through the pars (majority bilateral) with minimal translation (<2–3 mm) and no angulation. These fractures are stable as the PLL and the C2–C3 disk remain intact. The Type IA subclassification results from a similar injury and describes a fracture line that enters into the body of C2 oftentimes accompanied by a unilateral pars fracture with minimal displacement and angulation. Type IA injuries have a higher association with neurologic deficit and vertebral artery injury because the foramen is commonly involved. These injuries, however, are typically stable.

Type II injuries occur from a similar mechanism of injury; however, a subsequent rebound flexion injury results in disruption of the PLL, the C2–C3 disk, and often strips the anterior longitudinal ligament off of C3. The result is translation and angulation of varying degrees, which can be quite large. It must be noted, however, that most of the Type II injuries do not result in neurologic injury secondary to the large size of the canal at this level and by the fact that anterior displacement of C2 actually enlarges the canal (although the posterior ring of C1 is brought anteriorly and the posterior superior corner of C3 is left in place, posing an eventual risk for cord injury). The much less common subcategory, Type IIA, differs from Type II in that the fracture line is oblique or more horizontal than the typical vertical fracture line of Type II and is thought to result from a flexion–distraction injury. There typically is minimal translation but marked angulation secondary to the obliquity of the fracture (Fig. 12.10). From a clinical standpoint, the importance of differentiating the two fractures lies in the fact that traction tends to distract Type IIA injuries and should be avoided, whereas it is the proper treatment of Type II fractures. If one has a difficult time differentiating between the two, initial traction of 10 lb can be applied. If distraction occurs, the fracture represents a Type IIA and further traction should be avoided.

Type III fractures are the final category in the classification system and refer to a fracture of the pars in combination with bilateral (rarely unilateral) C2–C3 facet dislocation. These are unusual and extremely unstable fracture dislocations that are generally not suitable for closed reduction, and operative intervention is required. Associated SCI with Type III fractures is around 60%.

The treatment of Hangman's fractures depends on the severity or type of fracture. Type I and IA fractures are stable by definition and can be treated successfully in a cervical orthosis. Flexion/extension views should be obtained under physician guidance to verify that no further displacement or angulation occurs. Type II fractures are treated differently than Type IIA fractures as the latter are made worse with traction, although both require reduction followed by immobilization. Type II fractures are reduced with gentle traction in extension in 5- to 10-lb increments (initially starting

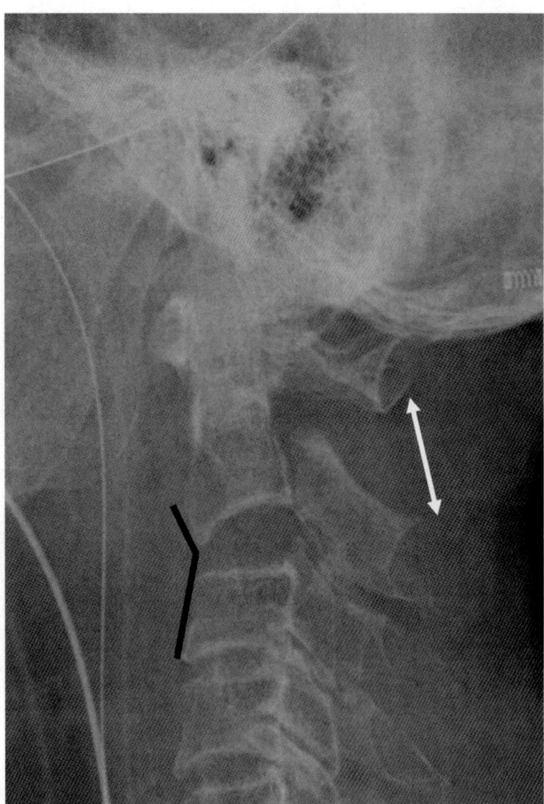

Figure 12.10 Type IIa traumatic spondylolisthesis (Hangman's fracture). Lateral cervical spine film demonstrates angulation predominating over translation (*black lines*), which is pathognomonic for Type IIa C2 arch fractures. The causative flexion–distraction mechanism is thought to result in progressive tensile failure of the posterior atlantoaxial membrane (*white arrow*), the posterior longitudinal ligament (PLL), posterior annulus, and intervertebral disk. The anterior annulus and anterior longitudinal ligament (ALL) are thought to remain intact. (*Reproduced with permission from* Bucholz RW, Heckman JD, Court-Brown C, et al. *Rockwood and Green's Fractures in Adults*, 6th ed. Philadelphia, Lippincott Williams & Wilkins, 2005.)

with 10 lb), followed by either immediate immobilization in a halo vest once fracture reduction is confirmed radiographically or by 4 to 6 weeks of skeletal traction followed by immobilization in a halo vest. Total treatment time is generally 10 to 12 weeks. These fractures typically heal by virtue of spontaneous ankylosis of the C2–C3 disk space underneath the anterior longitudinal ligament, which has been stripped off of the body of C3. Alternative treatment for widely displaced fractures (>5 mm) is primary osteosynthesis utilizing compression screw fixation across the pars or C2–C3 arthrodesis. Type IIA fractures cannot be treated by traction as discussed earlier and are subsequently reduced in a halo ring under extension and compression with halo-vest immobilization for approximately 12 weeks. Finally, Type III injuries cannot generally be reduced by closed means, and open reduction is necessary followed by fusion of C2–C3 with primary osteosynthesis across the pars or by extension of the fusion to include C1.

Subaxial Cervical Spine Trauma

Subaxial cervical spine trauma describes injuries from the region of C3 to the upper border of T1. Subaxial cervical injuries account for around 70% of cervical spine trauma. As discussed earlier, when viewing radiographs of the cervical spine, it is absolutely necessary to be able to visualize the upper section of the vertebral body of T1 as fractures and fracture dislocations in the C7 region account for 15% to 20% of subaxial cervical injuries. Subaxial cervical spine injuries can be classified in reference to mechanism or according to anatomic location. In 1982, Allen and Ferguson devised a classification for subaxial cervical spine injuries on the basis of the mechanism of injury and the severity of injury. This classification helps better understand the mechanism of injury, fracture severity, prognosis, and treatment. There are six different groups: compressive flexion, vertical compression, distractive flexion, compression extension, distractive extension, and lateral flexion. The descriptive classification simply divides fractures into vertebral body fractures and facet fractures/dislocations among others. This section will focus on the descriptive classification but will describe mechanisms of injury with each fracture. Of note, injuries that will not be discussed but can occur include isolated lamina fractures, pedicle fractures, facet fractures (without dislocation), and anterior tension band injuries.

Vertebral Body Fractures

Vertebral body fractures in the subaxial cervical spine are common injuries whose evaluation and treatment differ significantly from those of injuries to the upper cervical spine. Variables affecting the treatment include fracture pattern, associated injuries, and neurologic status of the patient. Fracture patterns include compression fracture, burst fracture, and "teardrop fracture," describing a more unstable variant. Not only does the fracture pattern guide decision making, the presence of multiple fractures at contiguous levels, which is not uncommonly seen, guides decision making as well. As with all cervical spine injuries, close attention needs to be paid to the presence/absence of associated injuries, specifically injuries to the posterior ligamentous structures as this renders a given fracture significantly more unstable. Finally, neurologic status weighs heavily on treatment decisions, with particular attention to a declining neurologic status as this marks an absolute reason to perform operative stabilization to prevent further deterioration.

The mechanism of vertebral body fractures involves axial compression with varying degrees of flexion producing the various fracture patterns described. Stability of these injuries is highly variable as some of these fractures are very unstable with the potential for quick neurologic deterioration. Burst fractures by definition result from a purely axial compression load, while compression fractures have a flexion component with an asymmetrical compression load beginning in the anterior half of the vertebral body with subsequent tensioning of the posterior structures. Depending on the force of the applied load, the anterior elements can be compressed very little with overall maintenance of vertebral height, or compression can be quite significant with substantial loss of height. In the same manner, tensile forces can leave the posterior elements virtually without injury or they can be completely disrupted making the injury grossly unstable. An important concept to remember is that the posterior elements fail under tension secondarily as the anterior vertebral body fails under the initial compressive forces.

Compression fractures (classified as compression flexion injuries by Allen and Ferguson), therefore, need to be classified as stable or unstable as there is such a vast continuum of injury characteristics. While one can gather the degree of disruption to some extent by physical examination, more concrete evidence is gained by radiographic studies, initially plain films. A stable compression fracture is generally defined as a fracture with less than 40% loss of anterior height, without disruption of the posterior cortex of the body or disruption of the posterior ligamentous complex, in a neurologically intact patient (Fig. 12.11).

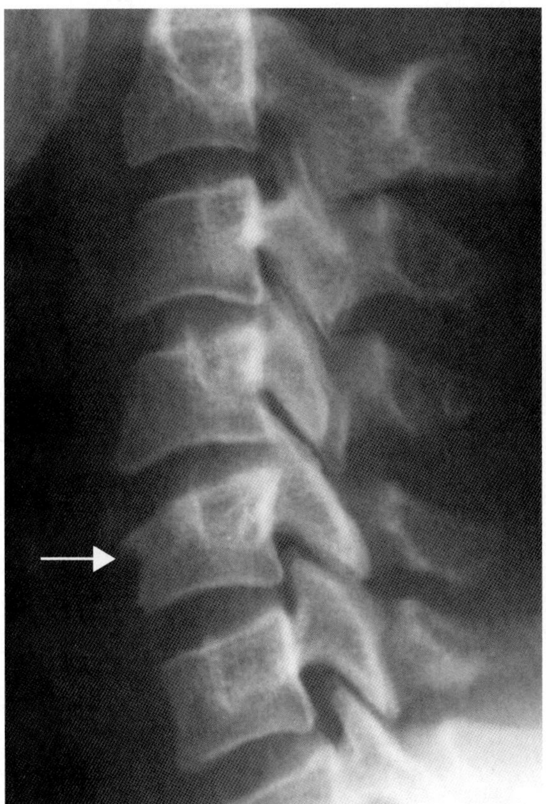

Figure 12.11 Lateral cervical x-ray of a stable compression fracture. There is minimal appreciable kyphosis, no translation, no facet joint gapping, and minimal evidence of interspinous widening. (*Reproduced with permission from* Bucholz RW, Heckman JD, Court-Brown C, et al. *Rockwood and Green's Fractures in Adults*, 6th ed. Philadelphia, Lippincott Williams & Wilkins, 2005.)

Stable fractures can generally be treated nonoperatively with use of a cervical orthosis only. Determination of posterior stability can be inferred from plain films by the degree of kyphosis between segments. Kyphosis between segments greater than 11 degrees suggests probable disruption of the posterior elements and therefore instability. Other markers of posterior disruption include posterior tenderness/ecchymosis on physical examination and the additional radiographic findings of interspinous widening or facet subluxation. CT can help with the bony evaluation as well and is almost always obtained after an injury is identified. If there is still question as to whether the posterior elements are disrupted or intact, an MRI can be obtained to help guide decision making. Of note, more severe compression fractures involving greater than 40% of the anterior height, with intact posterior ligaments, in a neurologically intact patient can be treated with a halo vest. A halo vest is typically not used for definitive treatment if there is a ligamentous disruption, however, as a high rate of failure will ensue.

Burst fractures as previously discussed result from a pure axial compression injury and are classified as vertical compression fractures under the Allen and Ferguson classification scheme. These injuries generally are the result of a high-energy injury producing posterior vertebral body comminution, often with a fragment of retropulsed bone into the spinal canal. As such, SCIs are common secondary to canal compromise. Since these fractures are caused by pure axial compression, theoretically the posterior ligamentous elements should remain intact. However, there often is some degree of flexion, so the posterior structures can be damaged as the result of secondary distraction. As with compression fractures, assessment of stability as well as the patient's neurologic status must be considered when discussing optimal treatment. The indications for surgical treatment of burst fractures are less clear than other fractures, especially in a patient who is neurologically intact. Absolute indications for surgery are incomplete neurologic injury, and most would argue complete neurologic injury, regardless whether the posterior structures are intact if there is persistent cord compression from retropulsed bone. The typical surgery involves anterior decompression/corpectomy with anterior strut grafting and fusion with or without posterior fusion, depending on the stability of the posterior elements.

The treatment of burst fractures in the patient with no neurologic deficit is less clear. The elements one examines are the degree of loss of height, kyphotic deformity, canal compromise, and evidence of posterior ligamentous disruption, which are determined by the same findings as discussed under compression fractures: interspinous widening, facet subluxation, and physical examination. CT evaluation is the norm with these injuries with attention being paid to the retropulsed fragment of bone and the amount of canal compromise secondary to the fragment (Fig. 12.12). Compromise of 20% or more should generally

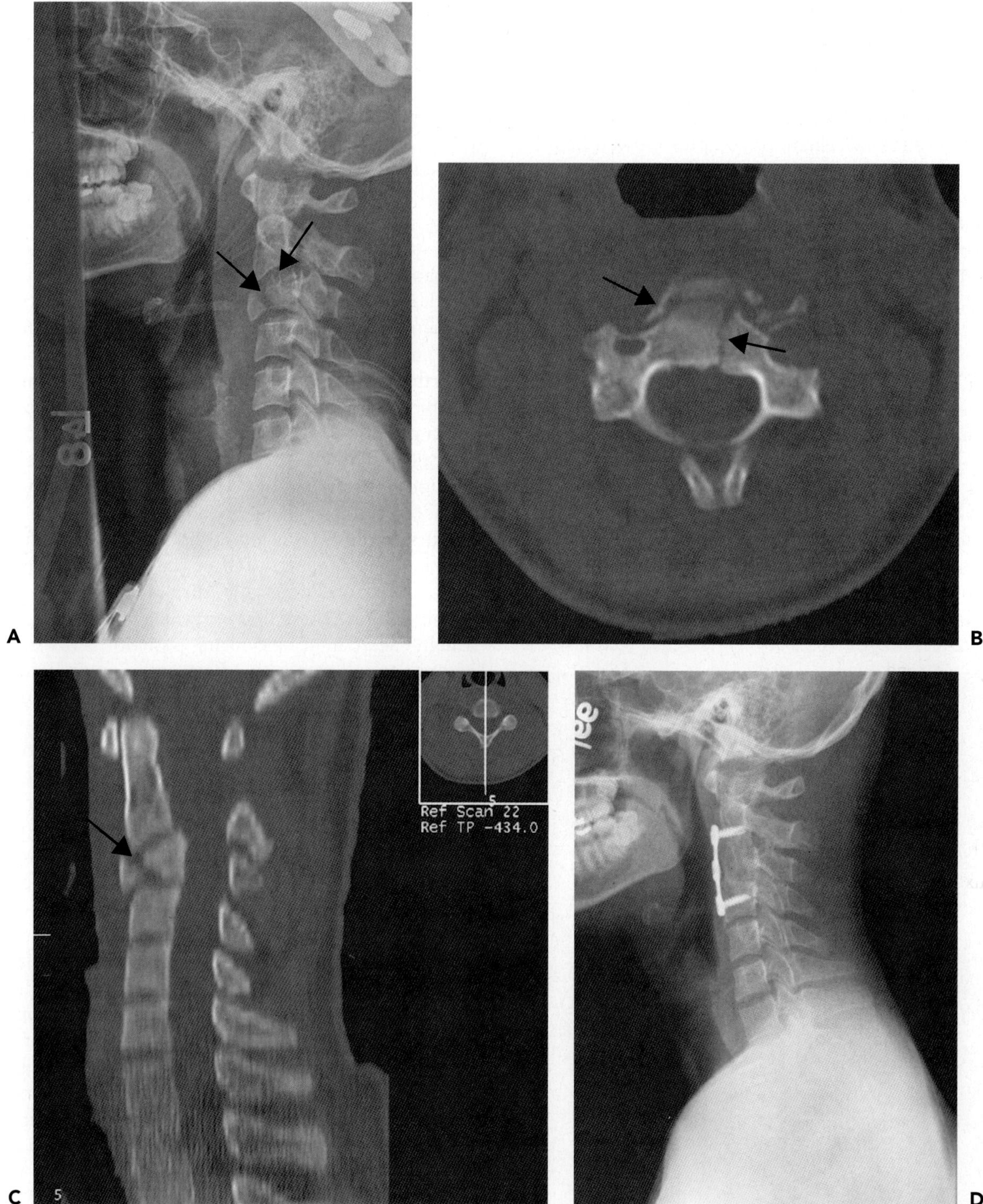

Figure 12.12 C3 burst fracture. **(A)** Preoperative lateral view. **(B)** Preoperative axial CT scan. **(C)** CT reconstruction. **(D)** Healing after anterior corpectomy and plating. (*Reproduced with permission from* Frymoyer JW, Wiesel SW, An HS, et al. *The Adult and Pediatric Spine,* 3rd ed. Philadelphia: Lippincott Williams & Wilkins, 2003.)

be treated operatively, with lesser degrees perhaps undergoing nonoperative management (provided that the patient is neurologically intact). MRI can provide further information if necessary, examining the cord itself as well as the posterior elements. MRI should not be ordered unless it will provide additional information to guide decision making. If one decides upon nonoperative management, typical treatment involves a halo vest, or occasionally a rigid cervical orthosis. Regardless of the type of immobilization, close follow-up is necessary to ensure that the fracture is adequately stabilized.

The infamous "teardrop" variant of compression (Allen and Ferguson compressive flexion Type III) fractures needs to be discussed briefly as there is such a high incidence of neurologic injury with this fracture, and surgery is almost always indicated. The mechanism of injury is the same as discussed earlier with compression fracture, but there is such a high degree of flexion with compression that an anterior fragment of bone separates from the remainder of the body (anterior extrusion of a fragment from the anterior lip of the body) often with retrolisthesis of the remainder of the posterior body or posterior displacement of the posteroinferior corner of the involved vertebral body. The commonality of neurologic injury results from the posterior displacement of either the body or the posteroinferior corner, and as such surgery is generally indicated. In the case of neurologically intact patients, surgical decision making follows the same algorithm as with other types of compression fractures with close attention to any evidence of posterior instability.

Facet Subluxation and Dislocation

Subluxation, dislocation, and fracture dislocation of the facet joints of the subaxial spine represent a spectrum of injuries resulting from a mechanism of flexion–distraction with or without an element of rotation. Appropriate treatment of these relatively common injuries requires appreciation of the exact pathologic anatomy as well as the patient's current neurologic status and the expected natural history of the injury. The variation in injury patterns includes unilateral or bilateral subluxation, dislocation, dislocation with varying degrees of displacement, and facet fractures associated with any of the above (most commonly associated with dislocation). If fracture does occur, the most common fracture pattern is that of the superior facet of the caudad level, although fracture of the inferior facet of the cephalad level is seen as well. An important consideration when assessing this injury is the associated disruption of the ligamentous anatomy of the spine as this determines stability. As with any dislocation, disruption of the joint capsule is seen, but with these injuries, disruption of the ligamentum flavum, interspinous ligament, and the PLL may also be present, contributing further to instability. Finally, and most importantly, consideration needs to be paid to the neurologic status of the patient. As one should expect, neurologic injury is common following these injuries and correlates roughly with the degree of sagittal translation present since this determines the SAC. Kang et al. demonstrated that the risk of injury is also highly dependent on the preexisting sagittal canal diameter of the cervical spine, which is intuitive considering there is very little room for the cord to displace without causing cord impingement. Neurologic injury can range from isolated root deficit to complete cord injury.

As mentioned earlier, virtually all facet injuries occur following a flexion injury, most commonly with distraction and various degrees of rotation. C5–C6 is the most common injury level seen, but the possible presence of C6–C7 and even C7–T1 injury mandates thorough radiographic evaluation down to the superior end plate of T1. In most cases, displacement is readily apparent on lateral radiographs (Fig. 12.13) with disruption in the alignment of the facet joints. On the AP view, offset of the spinous processes can sometimes be visualized depending on the rotational component involved, and subluxation or dislocation can also be visualized on the oblique or pillar views. CT scanning after identification of the fracture is the norm, and CT provides more specific information including the degree of displacement and associated fractures that may not have been appreciated on plain films.

MRI is also useful, especially when evaluating for the potential of an associated herniated disk as this can cause worsening neurologic compromise with subsequent reduction (Fig. 12.13B). Although this risk is recognized, the timing of MRI is difficult as the study takes time to perform and not all facilities have instant access to MRI. Therefore, when an MRI should be performed is an area of much debate. Most would agree that an MRI should be obtained prior to closed reduction in the patient who has a normal examination as the risks of causing potential harm outweigh the benefits of immediate reduction when the patient is neurologically intact. Conversely, most would agree that patients with a complete SCI should undergo immediate skeletal traction and closed reduction and, if unsuccessful, should then undergo MR imaging prior to determination of definitive intervention. These patients already have a complete injury and benefit from decompression as soon as possible. The difficult patient population is those with an incomplete injury who would benefit most from urgent reduction but at the same time are at risk for further neurologic deterioration. Most would agree that these patients should undergo skeletal traction and closed reduction rather than await MRI provided they are awake, alert, and can cooperate with serial examinations. The patient can then provide feedback during the reduction so that any signs of neurologic worsening can be noted, at which time closed reduction should be ceased. Any evidence of neurologic worsening during reduction should result in neuroimaging and treatment as indicated. If closed reduction is unsuccessful in a patient with an incomplete SCI, MRI is obtained prior to any attempt at open reduction. If at any point along this algorithm a disk

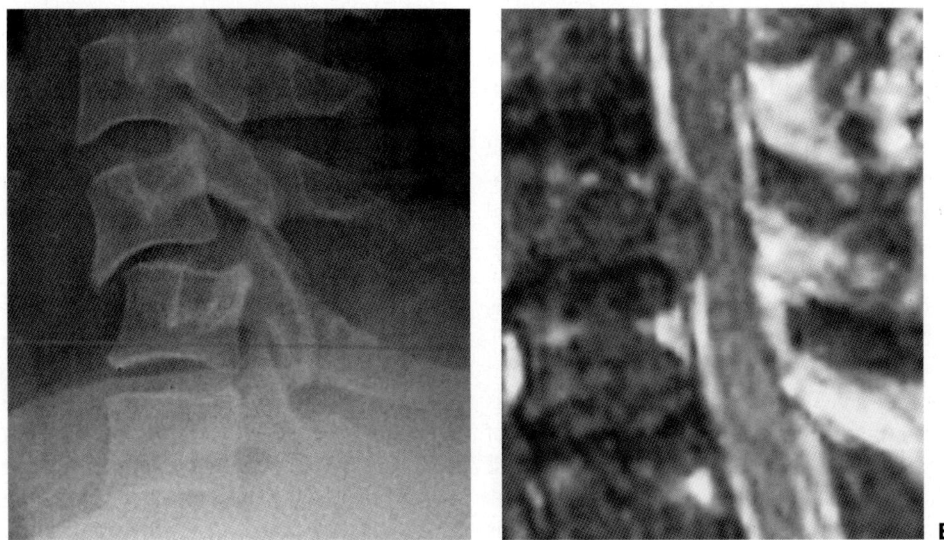

Figure 12.13 Bilateral facet subluxation. **(A)** Lateral plain film. **(B)** Postreduction MRI shows a herniated disk present. (*Reproduced with permission from* Bucholz RW, Heckman JD, Court-Brown C, et al. *Rockwood and Green's Fractures in Adults*, 6th ed. Philadelphia, Lippincott Williams & Wilkins, 2005.)

herniation is appreciated on MRI, its significance must be assessed. Of note, plain films can pick up a massive, clinically significant disk herniation by a complete loss of disk height on the lateral radiograph. On MRI, the presence of an extruded disk fragment posterior to the posteroinferior corner of the cephalad vertebral body, a relatively rare occurrence, represents a risk following closed reduction and should therefore be addressed. Anterior discectomy is carried out in this setting prior to any reduction, followed by reduction, fusion, and stabilization, generally anteriorly, but sometime via a combined approach.

Given the foregoing considerations, the diagnosis of a facet subluxation or dislocation requires reduction and stabilization. In the presence of a neurologic deficit, other than an isolated nerve root injury, reduction is an emergency and is obtained with the application of skeletal traction with skull tongs. Once reduction is obtained, stabilization can be carried out more electively, usually in the first 48 to 72 hours after the injury. Failure to achieve a closed reduction in a patient with a neurologic injury merits urgent open reduction and stabilization.

Neurologic considerations aside, the optimal means of stabilizing these injuries depends on the spectrum of soft-tissue and bony injury present. Nonoperative treatment plays a very limited role and is reserved for those with a mild subluxation, a unilateral dislocation with unremarkable neurologic examination (these we generally recommend for operative treatment), and those who are too sick to undergo operative treatment. Nonoperative treatment involves a cervical orthoses for a period of 10 to 12 weeks as halo-vest immobilization has been shown to be much less reliable than in the upper cervical spine. Halo-vest immobilization has a high risk of redisplacement because of paradoxical motion of the subaxial vertebral bodies. Because of the risk of redisplacement, even unilateral dislocations are generally treated by operative means as there is not a good method of adequately immobilizing the injury nonoperatively.

Bilateral facet dislocations commonly occur in conjunction with significant disruption of the interspinous ligament, ligamentum flavum, and often the PLL and are therefore highly unstable. Ligamentous disruption with unilateral facet dislocation is generally less severe, with the PLL spared much more commonly. This constitutes the reason why some surgeons attempt to treat unilateral dislocations nonoperatively. Our preference for either injury is surgical stabilization due to the inconsistent results following nonoperative management and the unstable nature of the injuries. With operative management, the neurologically normal patient is returned much more quickly to normal activity with minimal risk of long-term sequelae, while the neurologically impaired patient is ready to aggressively undergo rehabilitation following surgery without the need for prolonged external immobilization. Operative treatment involves stabilization and fusion, which can be done anteriorly, posteriorly or with a combined approach and depends on associated injuries (i.e., herniated disk treated with discectomy and anterior fusion, generally). With no neurologic injury or no need for removal of elements from the canal, a posterior approach is generally used.

Thoracolumbar Trauma

Thoracolumbar injuries encompass injuries from T1 to L5 and range in severity from mild to life threatening. The initial management has been covered in the previous sections but includes initially following ATLS protocol with specific attention paid to the protection of the spinal column. A thorough physical examination should be performed with particular attention to neurologic deficits followed by appropriate radiographic examination. All patients with suspected thoracolumbar trauma should initially receive at least an AP and lateral of the entire region with close inspection at each level. If there is any question about the injury following plain films, or if a closer examination is needed, CT is obtained for further evaluation. Additionally, MRI is utilized if there is any neurologic deficit, a need to evaluate ligamentous disruption, and/or before surgical intervention. This section will focus on specific injuries and injury patterns.

There are many classification schemes for thoracolumbar injuries, and as one might expect, none are universally agreed upon. Therefore, the classic and easiest way to discuss these injuries is by a descriptive classification based on the three-column theory of the thoracolumbar spine popularized by Denis in 1983 (Fig. 12.1). The anterior column consists of the ALL and the anterior two-thirds of the vertebral body; the middle column consists of the posterior one-third of the vertebral body; the posterior column consists of the remaining posterior structures including the facet joints, interspinous ligament, supraspinous ligament, and the ligamentum flavum. As discussed previously, Denis defined instability as disruption of at least two columns. In the following sections, these columns will be referred to when discussing injury patterns and mechanisms of injury. The injuries will be divided into compression fractures, burst fractures, flexion–distraction injuries (Chance injuries), and fracture dislocations.

Compression Fractures

Compression fractures make up the majority of traumatic injuries to the thoracic and lumbar spine, even after pathologic fractures through osteoporotic bone have been excluded. The mechanism of injury involves axial compression combined with mild degrees of forward flexion producing compressive failure of the anterior aspect of the vertebral body (Denis's anterior column). By definition, a compression fracture involves only the anterior column with preservation of the middle and posterior columns. The isolated involvement of the anterior column differentiates them from burst fractures, which result in compression of the middle column as well. Compression fractures generally result from low-energy trauma in the elderly but can be secondary to much higher-energy mechanisms in the younger population. True compression fractures represent stable injuries; however, many times it is difficult to differentiate a compression fracture from its more serious counterpart, the burst fractures, or even a flexion–distraction injury, involving tension failure, or distraction, of the posterior elements.

Differentiation of these injuries is important as more serious injuries often require surgical intervention, while compression fractures can generally be treated nonoperatively. The differentiation lies in the radiographic examination. On the lateral view, loss of height of the anterior column and the degree of kyphosis should be assessed with true compression fractures having less than 40% loss of height, and less than 30 degrees of kyphosis, making them stable (Fig. 12.14). Many still consider fractures with loss of height greater than 50% to be compression fractures if only the anterior column is involved; however, with this amount of loss of height, it can be argued that the posterior column is disrupted and by definition should be considered a flexion–distraction injury. Additionally, kyphosis greater than 30 degrees represents an unstable fracture with likely disruption of the posterior elements to some extent. Of note, an additional finding on the lateral film that is suggestive of a burst fracture rather than a compression fracture is an increase to greater than 100-degree angle between the superior end plate and the posterior cortical line at the posterosuperior corner of the vertebral body. Increase in this angle indicates probable loss of height in the middle column. On the AP view, an increase in interpedicular distance suggests disruption of the posterior cortex, splaying of the pedicles, and the presence of a burst fracture. If there is any question regarding the differentiation, a CT scan should be obtained as there can be disastrous consequences for misdiagnosis and subsequent mistreatment. Ballock and colleagues reported a misdiagnosis rate of 25% in attempting on plain radiography to differentiate compression fractures from burst fractures and recommended the routine use of CT scanning in the case of compression fractures to avoid this error. If after physical examination, plain films, and CT scanning, one is still uncertain of posterior ligamentous stability, an MRI can be obtained to evaluate the soft tissue stability of the posterior column. Of note, physical examination findings suggestive of tension failure of the posterior columns, and by definition, not a simple compression fracture (rather a flexion distraction injury), include marked midline tenderness at fracture site, ecchymosis, or a palpable gap between spinous processes as in the cervical spine.

Most compression fractures do not result in neurologic injury. However, compression fractures, particularly in the upper thoracic spine between T2 and T10, can result in neurologic compromise. Although the rib cage and sternum provide an added degree of stability to fractures in this region, their presence should be understood to imply an even greater degree of energy required to produce the injury. This factor, in addition to the relatively low spinal canal–spinal cord ratio in the midthoracic spine, as well as the sensitivity of the spinal cord to minor trauma, all contribute to a significant risk of injury at this level.

As mentioned previously, compression fractures can generally be treated nonoperatively, as they are by Denis's definition stable because only one column is disrupted. Nonoperative treatment generally consists of an external orthosis prescribed for 2 to 3 months for most patients

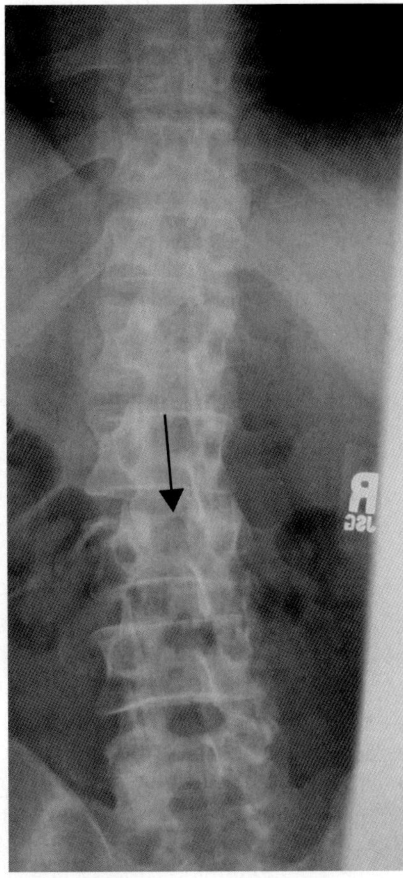

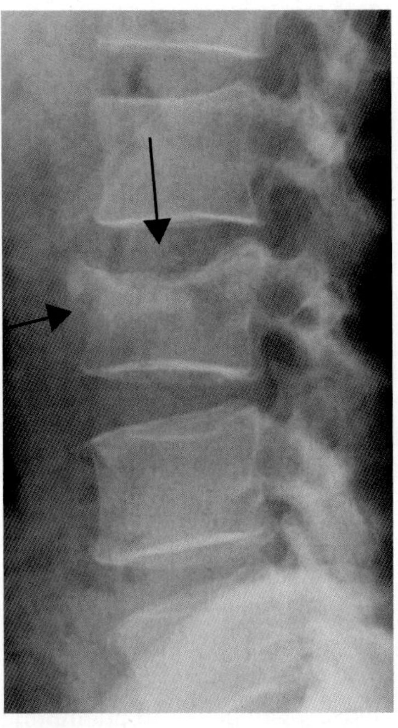

Figure 12.14 Stable L3 compression fracture. AP **(A)** and lateral **(B)** radiographs showing a stable compression fracture. (*Reproduced with permission from* Bucholz RW, Heckman JD, Court-Brown C, et al. *Rockwood and Green's Fractures in Adults*, 6th ed. Philadelphia, Lippincott Williams & Wilkins, 2005.)

with close radiographic follow-up. Those patients with less than 10% loss of vertebral height can be treated without external support. These injuries need to be followed closely with radiographs to ensure that further loss of height does not occur. Finally, those fractures with greater than 50% loss of height and/or greater than 30 degrees of kyphosis should be treated operatively with posterior stabilization.

Burst Fractures

Sir Frank Holdsworth was the first to use the term "burst fracture" to describe what is today recognized as one of the most common injuries to the thoracolumbar spine and one whose treatment continues to be hotly debated. Part of the reason for the confusion surrounding the treatment of burst fractures stems from differences in definitions among various authors. Most reports are consistent with Holdsworth's original description of a fracture that results from the cephalad disk exploding through the upper end plate into the vertebral body, causing a fracture of both the anterior and posterior cortices. Therefore, with burst fractures one observes compression of both the anterior and middle column, as opposed to compression fractures in which only the anterior column is disrupted. Secondary to the mechanism and usual high-energy injury, there is typically a retropulsed burst fragment extruded into the canal at the level of the pedicles, often causing neural element compression and neurologic injury. Most surgeons agree with Denis who noted that the posterior column is either intact in a burst fracture or sustains a greenstick-type fracture of the lamina or spinous process but that tension failure of the ligamentous components of the posterior column is not present.

Radiographic evaluation of these injuries is similar to that described in the previous section for compression fractures, with most of the information gathered from plain film and CT. On plain films, one looks for the extent of loss of vertebral height, whether the loss is both anteriorly and posteriorly in the vertebral body, and the acute kyphotic angulation. Additionally, with CT scan, one can also determine the presence of a retropulsed fragment, the extent of canal compromise as a percentage of the cross sectional area (which many will base a surgical decision upon), the presence of a laminar fracture, and the integrity of the facet joints (Fig. 12.15). Finally, the extent of posterior soft-tissue injury can be evaluated with MRI, which helps many surgeons to decide upon operative versus nonoperative treatment.

After taking all of these radiographic measurements into account as well as the patient's neurologic status, one tries to decide upon fracture stability and hence operative versus nonoperative management. It is the topic of stability wherein the confusion and disagreement lies with this

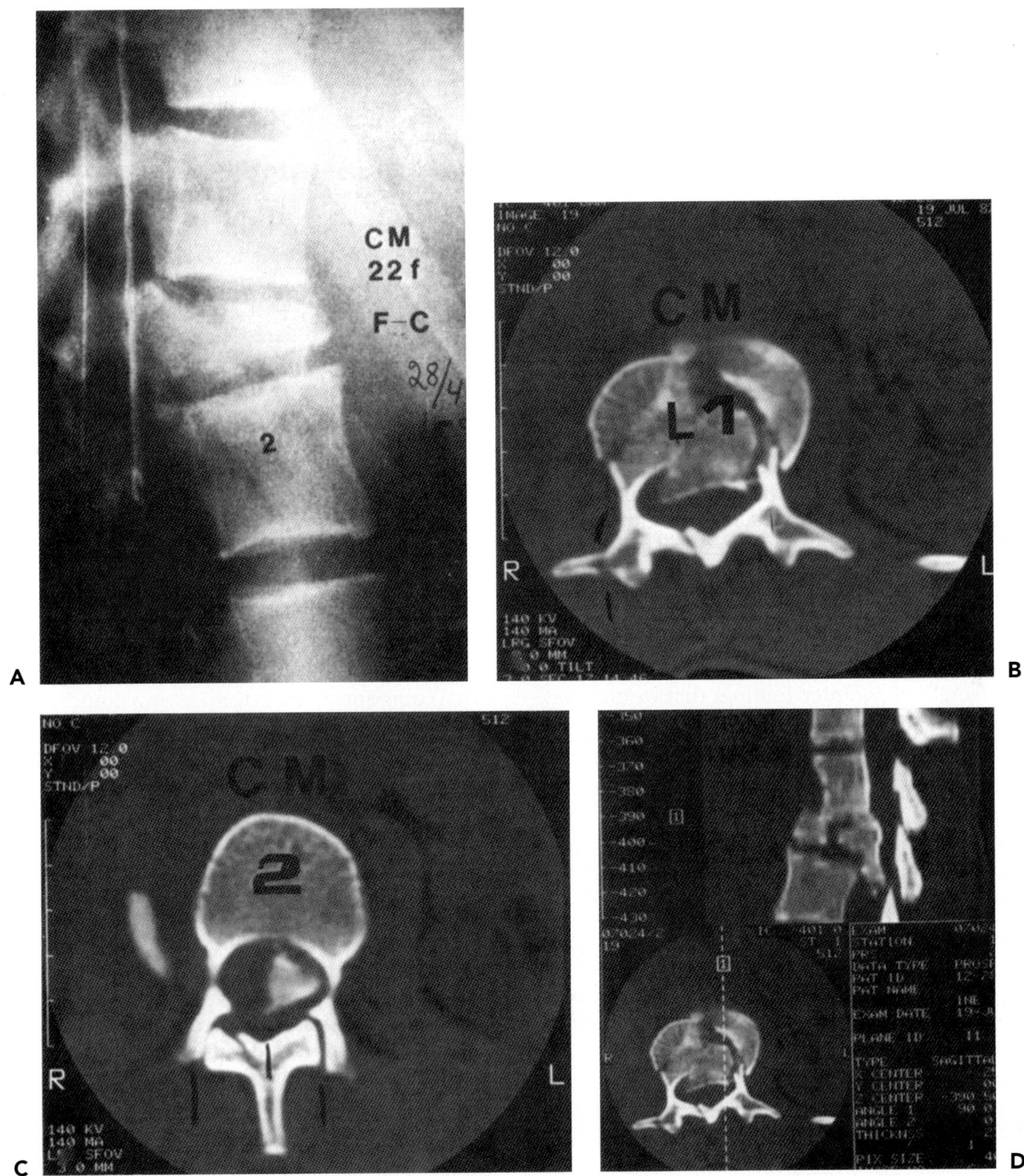

Figure 12.15 Burst Fx L1. This patient was a 19-year-old female who sustained a burst fracture of L1 following an MVA. **(A,B)** The fracture on CT scan was judged to compromise about 60% of the canal diameter. **(C,D)** Notice the large fragment seen on the CT scan at L2. By proper examination and sagittal reconstruction via CT scanning, this fragment was noted to still be in continuity with L1 and as such did not have to be removed during surgery as it reduced to L1 with height restoration. (*Reproduced with permission from* Chapman MW. *Chapman's Orthopaedic Surgery*, 2nd ed. Philadelphia, Lippincott Williams & Wilkins, 1993.)

particular injury. Holdsworth originally defined the burst fracture as a stable injury because of the slight risk of progressive deformity and neurologic deficit. Denis, on the other hand, utilizing his three-column theory, would define all burst fractures as unstable since two of the three columns are disrupted. McAfee and colleagues in 1982 proposed criteria for an unstable burst fracture, including a progressive neurologic deficit, disruption of the posterior ligamentous complex (which many authors feel would exclude such an injury from classification as a burst fracture), acute kyphosis greater than 20 degrees with a neurologic deficit, 50% loss of vertebral height in the presence of facet joint subluxation, and/or the presence of retropulsed bone causing neural element compromise in association with an incomplete neurologic injury. Bradford and McBride have stressed, on the other hand, the importance of a neurologic deficit as a clinical indicator of instability at least as it pertains to the appropriateness of surgical stabilization.

Though there remains a great deal of controversy surrounding the appropriate management, most authors favor surgical decompression and fusion for the patient who is neurologically impaired, and all would agree on surgical intervention for the patient with an incomplete neurologic injury as decompression has been shown to have favorable results with neurologic improvement. Patients with complete neurologic injury are commonly treated surgically to facilitate early return to rehabilitation. In general, patients requiring decompression are treated with an anterior approach to adequately decompress the cord followed generally by strut grafting, stabilization (generally anteriorly), and fusion. Laminectomy alone does not contribute to decompression of the cord or cauda equine in the presence of a burst fracture.

Surgery is not reserved only for those with a neurologic deficit, however. In the patient who is neurologically intact, one makes the decision of surgical intervention on radiographic findings that suggest structural instability. As alluded to earlier, there are no concrete rules stating when to operate and when not to operate. However, we will provide some general radiographic findings that would sway most surgeons toward operative intervention in the patient who is neurologically intact. These include acute kyphotic angulation of 25 to 30 degrees or greater than the norm at a particular level, greater than 50% loss of vertebral height, greater than 50% compromise of the spinal canal by retropulsed bony fragment(s), and tension failure of the posterior ligamentous complex. The neurologically normal patient who undergoes surgery for potential instability is usually treated posteriorly with posterior instrumentation and fusion. In general, the posterior approach is less morbid than the anterior approach with fewer serious complications. However, posterior instrumentation provides less support than anterior instrumentation as it is unable to reconstitute the anterior support. Therefore, posterior instrumentation is more likely to fail with increasing kyphosis/compression, especially in fractures with severe kyphosis and/or loss of height. Success rates have been similar when comparing anterior and posterior instrumentations and fusion for burst fractures.

Following the trend with the treatment of burst fractures, the number of levels fused varies from surgeon to surgeon. Prior to pedicle screw fixation, Harrington rod instrumentation was mostly used with instrumentation and fusion three levels above and two or three levels below the fractured vertebrae. As this requires a fairly extensive fusion, the advent of pedicle screw fixation has allowed better three-point fixation, and hence less levels needed for fusion. Currently, most surgeons advocate pedicle screw fixation and fusion either one or two levels (our personal preference) above and one or two levels below the compression fracture depending on the severity of the fracture and associated ligamentous disruption. Another option is adding anterior instrumentation and fusion, and therefore, less need for fusion more than one level above and one level below as the construct is more stable.

Chance Injuries

In 1948, G.Q. Chance provided the first description of an injury to the lumbar spine involving flexion and distraction of the posterior elements, what we know today as Chance fractures or injuries. The most common cause of flexion–distraction injuries today are lap belt injuries from MVAs, even though Chance's original description predated the use of lap belts. The lap belt scenario, although not always the cause, helps one to visualize and understand the mechanism of injury and the forces involved. Following an MVA, the individual sitting in the back seat is wearing a lap belt and the sudden deceleration injury forces the patient forward over the lap belt. The lap belt causes blunt trauma to the abdominal viscera in its course to the spine as the victim continues to move forward. The belt essentially acts as a fulcrum over which the spine rotates around an axis of rotation centered on the anterior cortex or anterior longitudinal ligament of the spine. The classic description is a pure flexion–distraction injury, but there often is a rotational component to it as well. As one would imagine, there is a very high rate of associated abdominal injuries, quoted around 50%, which one needs to keep in mind when evaluating lap belt injuries from either the orthopedic or the trauma surgery standpoint. Patients will typically present with the "seatbelt sign" with a band of ecchymosis across the abdomen where the patient hinged over the belt during deceleration.

The standard Chance injury may be a pure bony injury, extending through the spinous process, lamina, pedicle, and vertebral body; a pure soft-tissue injury, extending through the interspinous ligament, ligamentum flavum, facet joint capsule, and disk; or mixed, with variable involvement of bone and soft tissue (Fig. 12.16). The common finding among all three is the marked distraction of the posterior elements, moderate distraction of the middle column, and classically a neutral appearance of the far anterior column, reflecting an instantaneous axis of rotation in or about the ALL (Fig. 12.17). It is not uncommon to see mild-to-moderate wedging of the vertebral body reflecting an element of axial loading in addition to pure flexion. Burst-type fractures of the vertebral body may also be seen, reflecting a mechanism of injury that changes from axial loading to sudden flexion such as in a fall from a height.

Neurologic injury is uncommon but not rare in injuries of this type. As with other areas of the spine, the presence of a neurologic injury is initially treated with realignment either through an operative or nonoperative approach, followed by stabilization. Reduction involves various hyperextension maneuvers. If the patient recovers neurologic status following reduction, the treatment can then be operative or nonoperative, but in that situation, most surgeons would likely elect operative intervention for reliable stability. If

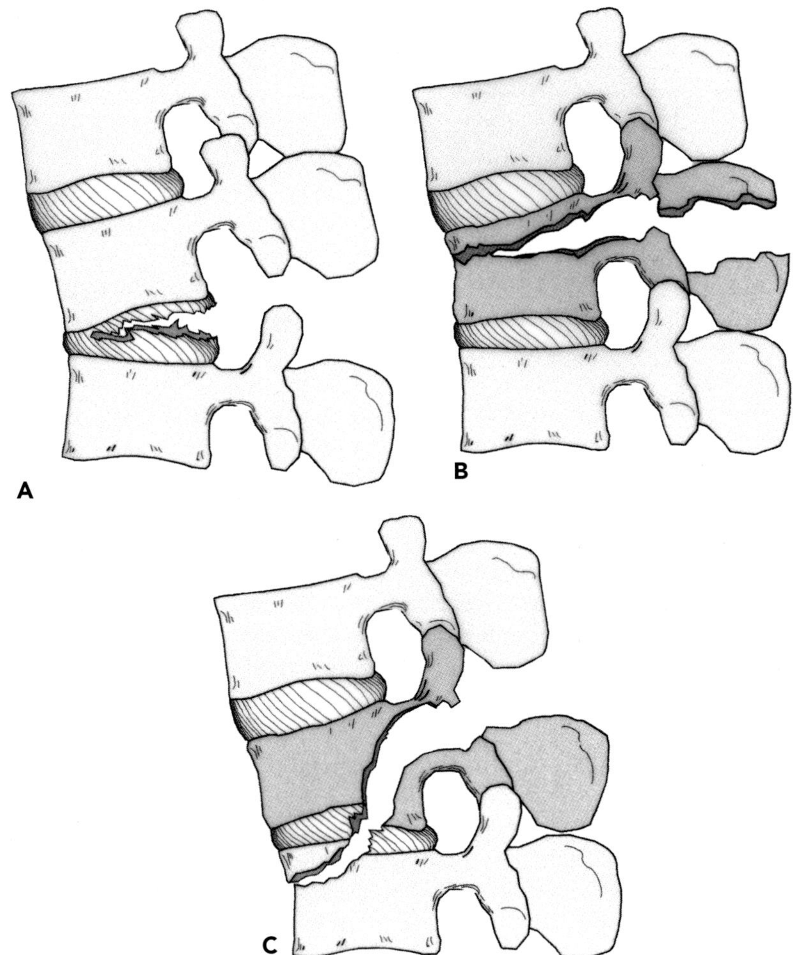

Figure 12.16 Chance fracture. **(A)** Pure soft-tissue injury. **(B)** Pure bony chance fracture. **(C)** Mixed injury. (*Reproduced with permission from* Frymoyer JW, Wiesel SW, An HS, et al. *The Adult and Pediatric Spine*, 3rd ed. Philadelphia: Lippincott Williams & Wilkins, 2003.)

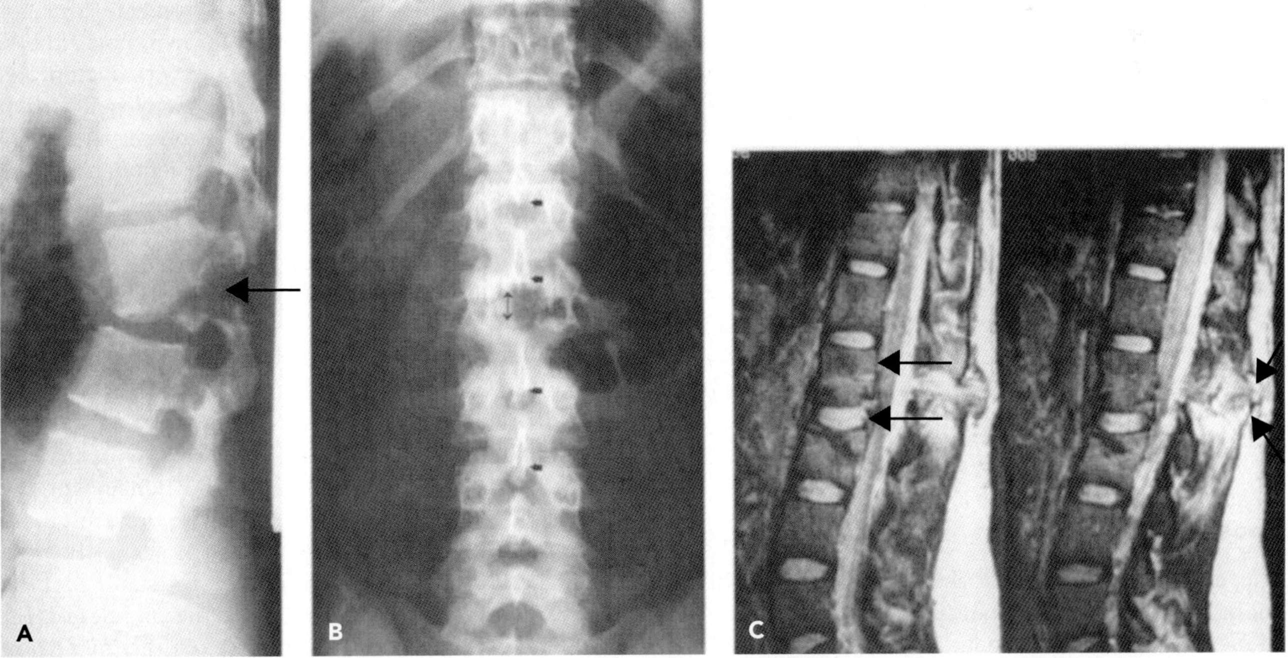

Figure 12.17 Radiographic characteristics of Chance injury. **(A)** Lateral radiograph of a severe flexion–distraction injury status post MVA. **(B)** AP radiograph shows wide spacing between spinous processes at the level of the injury. **(C)** MRI confirms extensive soft-tissue disruption. (*Reproduced with permission from* Frymoyer JW, Wiesel SW, An HS, et al. *The Adult and Pediatric Spine*, 3rd ed. Philadelphia: Lippincott Williams & Wilkins, 2003.)

after reduction, the patient maintains a neurologic deficit, suggesting continued compression on either the cord or the cauda equina, formal operative decompression should be performed, usually from a posterior approach. Chance injuries are highly unstable and are therefore not amenable to anterior stabilization as the disruption occurs posteriorly. If anterior decompression is required, a circumferential approach is recommended. Preoperative CT and MRI are recommended to further evaluate the fracture, to recognize all associated injuries, and to evaluate the possibility of a herniated disk protruding into the canal as this may require anterior decompression.

The treatment for the patient who is neurologically intact depends on the type of injury, that is, bony, ligamentous, or mixed. Pure bony Chance fractures are amenable to nonoperative treatment provided one can maintain reduction through bracing or casting. These tend to heal well as bony union can be obtained incurring stability to the spinal column. These injuries are by definition unstable as tension failure has occurred posteriorly. Reduction is accomplished through hyperextension and then maintained through hyperextension casting or bracing. Casting is more reliable as compliance is not an issue. If there is any worry about maintenance of reduction, one should proceed to operative intervention.

The majority of the injuries are not pure bony chance fractures, and as such, nonoperative intervention is likely to fail, since ligamentous healing in the spine is suboptimal. Pure ligamentous injuries, or primarily ligamentous injuries, should be stabilized operatively. Again, preoperative CT scanning and MRI are warranted to fully evaluate the injury and look for the possibility of a herniated disk. Provided there is no herniated disk to suggest a need for anterior decompression, a posterior approach is recommended as the primary mode of injury is distraction through the posterior elements. With a pure flexion distraction injury with no involvement of compression at the anterior column, spinal instrumentation in the form of pedicle screw fixation and a single-level fusion is employed. If there is an element of anterior compression, more complicated measures may have to be employed in the form of a three-point bending type of system to restore lordosis with a touch of distraction to restore height. Of note, distraction in most flexion–distraction injuries is inappropriate as this will increase the distraction between the posterior elements.

Fracture Dislocation of the Thoracolumbar Spine

The most ominous and most unstable of all injuries of the thoracolumbar spine is the fracture dislocation. There are numerous mechanisms depending on the resultant dislocation, but the hallmark of all injuries is translation in the coronal and/or sagittal planes. If translation, even when mild, is observed either on the AP or lateral radiograph, its importance should not be overlooked. As with any dislocation or subluxation, the displacement of the spine may be reduced by the time of radiographic assessment, and may therefore be missed, which underscores the importance of taking a careful look at even the mildest of translations, since fracture dislocations are serious injuries with life-threatening consequences when missed.

Fracture dislocations of the spine are high-energy injuries resulting in extremely unstable fracture patterns with a high rate of associated severe neurologic deficits. As alluded to earlier, a combination of mechanisms of injury occur including flexion, extension, rotation, compression, and shear (Fig. 12.18). A few of the classic mechanisms will be discussed later, but keep in mind that this is not an all-inclusive set of mechanisms. Holdsworth first described the "slice fracture," referring to a flexion-rotation injury at the thoracolumbar junction with translation in both the AP and lateral planes, and frequently paraplegia. Translation is the most striking feature radiographically and may be associated with fracture of the vertebral body and/or facet fracture. In this injury, the ALL is usually intact, although it is typically stripped off of the anterior aspect of the inferior vertebral body. Another common mechanism is the severe variant of the flexion–distraction injury discussed in the previous section, differentiated by translation, typically seen only on the lateral radiograph, which can be severe at times. The mechanism is typically the same and can involve an element of rotation (as can Chance injuries) as well. The ALL again is usually intact but may be stripped off of the anterior aspect of the inferior vertebral body as well. The importance of distinguishing between the standard flexion–distraction injury and the more severe fracture dislocation variant lies in the greater extent of energy involvement, the greater risk for neurologic injury, and the greater degree of instability seen with fracture dislocations. Therefore, again, one needs to pay close attention to any degree of translation. The final mechanism of injury that will be discussed involves a pure translational force applied to the spine in the form of hyperextension and shear forces, typically at the thoracolumbar junction. The classic example is the lumberjack that is struck directly on the back by a falling log. These shear-type injuries are the most unstable variant of the fracture dislocations as they typically involve failure of the ALL rendering the spine grossly unstable. As expected, these injuries have a very high rate of associated neurologic deficits.

To fully appreciate the injury, one needs to understand the pathoanatomy of the region, which will help with the proper reduction maneuvers needed. The thoracolumbar junction is the most frequently involved region because it represents a transition zone between the stable thoracic region enclosed by the rib cage and the mobile lumbar region. There is also a transition between the orientation of the thoracic facet joints to the lumbar facet joints, further rendering this region prone to injury.

Upon presentation, one should follow the guidelines laid out for all spinal trauma, and attention needs to be

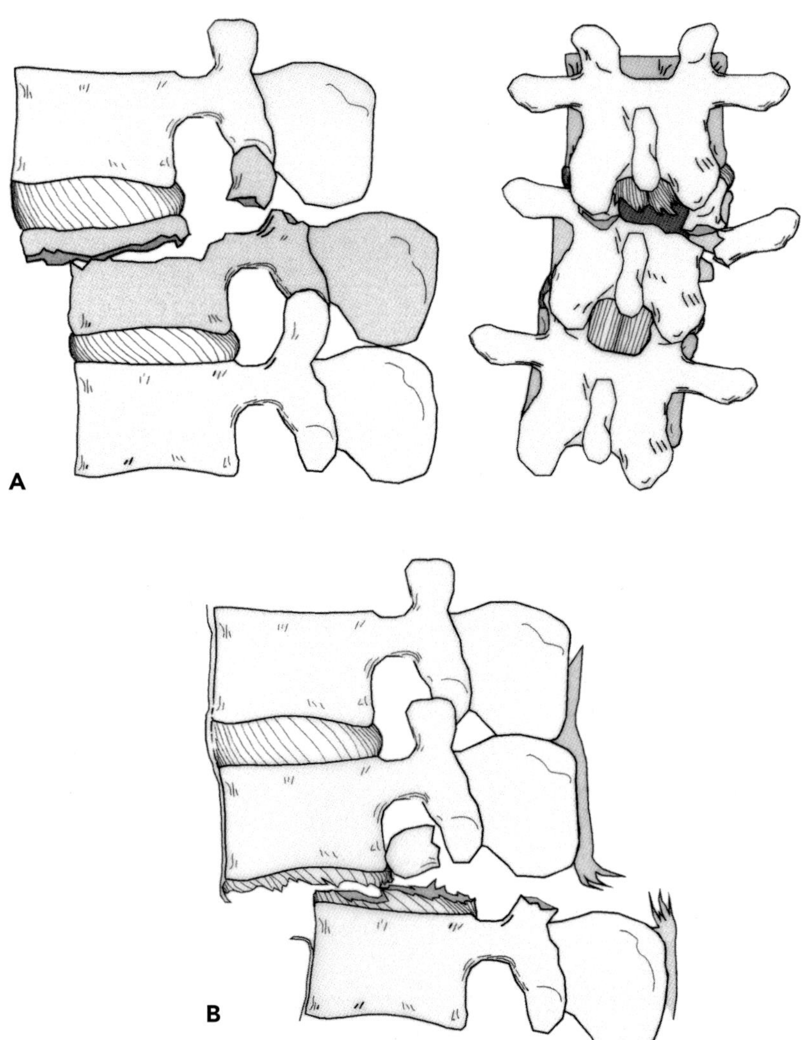

Figure 12.18 Fracture dislocations. **(A)** Flexion rotation. **(B)** Shear. **(C)** Flexion–distraction. (*Reproduced with permission from* Frymoyer JW, Wiesel SW, An HS, et al. *The Adult and Pediatric Spine*, 3rd ed. Philadelphia: Lippincott Williams & Wilkins, 2003.) (*Continued*)

paid to the serious associated injuries with fracture dislocations including trauma to the thorax, mediastinum, and abdomen, as well as blunt trauma to the aorta. Neurologic injury is the norm that unfortunately is frequently complete or near-complete resulting in paraplegia. Dural tears occur around half of the time as well. Careful evaluation of sacral sparing should be carried out. Radiographic evaluation begins with standard AP and lateral radiographs followed by CT scanning with sagittal and coronal reconstructions and MRI evaluation once the injury is identified.

As stressed earlier, recognition of this very serious injury stems from recognizing the radiographic hallmark, translation. Once the diagnosis is made, all of these fractures require operative stabilization as all three columns are disrupted and thus the only stability that is maintained is by the ALL if it is intact. These represent the most unstable of all spine injuries, and patient mobilization for improved pulmonary function and general medical care in these patients should be deferred until definitive treatment of the spine is performed. Therefore, these injuries should be definitively stabilized as soon as possible, preferably in the first 48 hours after injury. Because of the inherent instability of these injuries, it is important to accept that rigid segmental instrumentation should be employed and strategies designed to minimize the number of levels fused that are used with other injuries are generally inappropriate for these cases. Most advocate long fusions extending three levels above and at least two, if not three levels below the fracture with pedicle screw instrumentation. There are reports of less aggressive fusion with good results; however, long fusion is still recommended. Other methods aside from pedicle screw fixation and instrumentation include sublaminar wiring, interspinous wiring, and segmental and non-segmental hook fixation. These methods are often combined with anterior instrumentation to obtain even more stability.

Reduction should be obtained in all cases, even in complete neurologic injury, as anatomic reduction restores significant inherent stability and thus lessens the stress on surgical implants and may contribute to a lesser degree of postoperative pain. Additionally, there still exists the remote possibility of some degree of neurologic recovery.

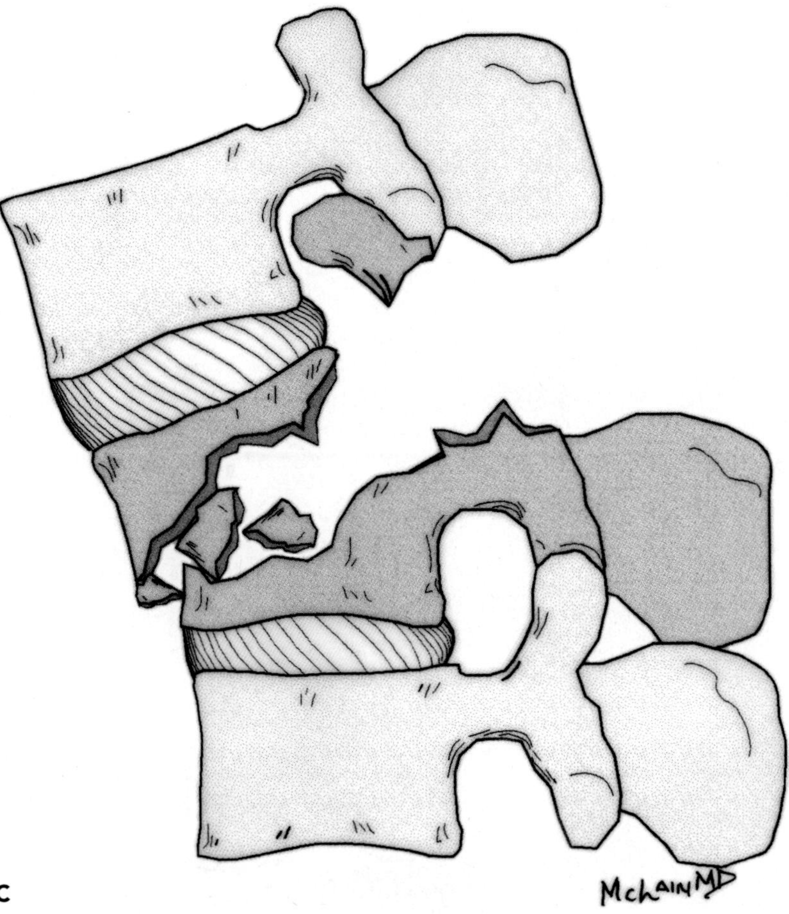

Figure 12.18 *(continued)*

In cases of incomplete neurologic injury, reduction is the primary means of decompression and should be accomplished expeditiously. Stabilization is carried out, and the patient is then reassessed for any persistent canal compromise anteriorly. The presence of persistent bone or disk in the canal can then be treated through a separate anterior approach with structural anterior grafting to maintain height. In general, these highly unstable injuries are not amenable to anterior stabilization alone, and it is therefore our preference to proceed with reduction and rigid fixation through a posterior approach prior to any consideration for anterior surgery.

DEGENERATIVE DISORDERS OF THE SPINE

A major proportion of the adult population is affected by degenerative conditions of the spine. These disorders have a major impact on the cost of health care delivery. Every physician should have a working knowledge of these pathologic conditions and should be able to recognize a serious problem when it arises. In both the cervical spine (myelopathy) and the lumbar spine (cauda equina compression), disastrous sequelae such as paralysis can occur if these are overlooked.

Spondylosis (osteoarthritis) is the technical term that describes the sequence of degenerative changes that occurs throughout the spine with increasing age. Everyone develops spondylosis, but only a subgroup will complain of symptoms. The physician needs to accurately diagnose the specific etiology for each patient and prescribe the appropriate treatment.

This section will focus on degenerative conditions in the cervical, thoracic, and lumbar spine. In each area, the appropriate history, physical findings, and diagnostic studies will be reviewed. Additionally, an algorithm will be described for the treatment of cervical and lumbar conditions.

CERVICAL SPINE

Before discussing individual entities of the cervical spine, we will first discuss the history and physical examination of the cervical spine followed by sections on the definition, symptoms, and physical examination findings of radiculopathy and myelopathy that often occur in conjunction with many cervical spine degenerative conditions. Additionally, we will discuss common conditions that can present with radiculopathy and myelopathy. In the sections following the radiculopathy and myelopathy overviews, individual disease entities will be discussed in further detail.

History and Physical Examination

Prior to the physical examination of the cervical spine, a thorough history should be obtained with specific focus on symptoms (pain, numbness, etc.), length of time of the symptoms, radiation of the symptoms, quality, associated symptoms, history of trauma, and whether the condition has been progressive. Only after a careful history has been obtained, one should move to the actual physical examination. The majority of the time the diagnosis can be made with history alone and the physical examination is used to confirm the diagnosis.

As with the physical examination on any portion of the body, the physical examination of the cervical spine should be conducted in a structured, systematic way, thus allowing efficiency and comprehensiveness. Inspection is the first step, looking for asymmetry, muscular atrophy, and injuries (ecchymosis, lacerations, etc.), especially when discussing trauma, in not only the cervical spine but also in the shoulders, arm, and forearms. Atrophy in a specific muscular group may be a sign of nerve root impingement, whereas abrasions/ecchymosis would lead the examiner down another path.

Palpation follows inspection, with careful attention to any areas of bony tenderness and step-off between spinous processes (especially in trauma). Paraspinal tenderness is quite common and much less specific and less worrisome for a severe injury than bony tenderness. Bony tenderness or step-off warrants a radiographic workup, whereas paraspinal tenderness often does not.

Following palpation, a careful neurologic examination should be performed with a thorough motor, sensory, and reflex testing. The motor examination generally provides the most specific information, so it is important to isolate each myotome and test each area individually. Comparison of both sides is vital as well. Muscle strength is graded on a scale from 0 to 5 with 5 representing normal strength, 4 representing strength against resistance but not normal, 3 represents movement against gravity only, 2 represents movement with gravity taken out of the equation, 1 represents evidence of contraction but no active movement, and 0 represents no evidence of contractility.

Following the motor examination, sensation should be tested in all dermatomes with specific attention to whether there is a level below which testing becomes abnormal. The sensory examination is much less specific than the motor examination, although it does provide additional helpful information. Following the sensory examination, deep tendon reflex testing should be done; this essentially consists of the biceps (C5/6), brachioradialis (C6), and triceps (C7). The Hoffman's test (an upper motor neuron test) should also be done, which, if positive, shows evidence of a myelopathic picture.

After careful focus in the upper extremities, the lower extremities need to be examined as well because cervical spine myelopathy usually has positive findings in the upper and lower extremities. Specifically, the patient's gait should be observed, which is classically described as a wide, broad-based gait with myelopathy. Additionally, strength and reflex testing should be examined. The most common abnormal lower extremity myelopathic signs are weakness, spasticity, and hyperreflexia. One may find a positive Babinski's sign as well with myelopathy. Finally, atrophy can be observed in the lower extremities but is less common and denotes a much longer standing problem. As will be discussed in the next sections, myelopathy tends to affect the upper and lower extremities, while radiculopathy only affects the upper extremities; thus, the lower extremity examination should be normal in the face of a pure radiculopathy.

Cervical Radiculopathy

Cervical radiculopathy is defined as pain or symptomatology in the distribution of one of the cervical roots. This is typically radiating pain from the neck into the arm, although the classic dermatomal distribution is not always seen. It is caused by compression of a cervical nerve root, generally as it exits from the spinal cord, which can be secondary to a variety of reasons ranging from herniated disks to degenerative changes. It is the compression of the nerve itself that differentiates radiculopathy from myelopathy, which is compression of the cord as a whole rather than of an individual nerve root.

History

Patients will generally present secondary to pain in the neck region that radiates into the arm. This radiating pain from the neck into the arm is the hallmark of radicular pain. The patient typically describes the pain as shooting, burning, or a deep ache. Many times, they will describe paresthesias down the arm as well. It must be noted, however, that there are radiculopathies that radiate no further than the shoulder, and the predominating complaint of patients will be shoulder pain rather than the classic presentation.

Physical Examination

When dealing with the physical examination for a suspected radiculopathy, the typical examination of the cervical spine should be done as previously discussed, with specific attention on certain parts of the physical examination. As mentioned earlier, the underlying abnormality is irritation on the affected root from a site of compression. Keeping this in mind, there are maneuvers described that further irritate the nerve to elicit the patient's symptoms. The classic test is Spurling's sign. In this test, the patient's head is flexed laterally, slightly rotated toward the symptomatic side, and then compressed to elicit reproduction or aggravation of the radicular symptoms. Another test described that has the opposite effect is the abduction relief

TABLE 12.1
CERVICAL RADICULOPATHY

C2–C3 Disk: C3 Nerve Root Pain: Back of neck, mastoid process, pinna of ear Sensation: Back of neck, mastoid process, pinna of ear Motor: None Reflex: None	**C5–C6 Disk: C6 Nerve Root** Pain: Neck, shoulder, medial scapula, lateral arm, dorsal forearm Sensation: Thumb and index finger Motor: Biceps, wrist extension Reflex: Brachioradialis
C3–C4 Disk: C4 Nerve Root Pain: Back of neck, levator scapula, anterior chest Sensation: Back of neck, levator scapula, anterior chest Motor: None Reflex: None	**C6–C7 Disk: C7 Nerve Root** Pain: Neck, shoulder, medial scapula, lateral arm, dorsal forearm Sensation: Index and middle fingers Motor: Triceps, Wrist flexion Reflex: Triceps
C4–C5 Disk: C5 Nerve Root Pain: Neck, tip of shoulder, anterior arm Sensation: Deltoid area Motor: Deltoid, biceps Reflex: Biceps	**C7–T1 Dicks: C8 Nerve Root** Pain: Neck, medial scapula, medial arm/forearm Sensation: Ring and little finger Motor: Intrinsic muscles of hand Reflex: None

sign. The arm is abducted overhead decreasing the tension on the affected nerve and thereby the severity of the radicular symptoms.

The major focus of the examination is directed at finding a neurologic deficit (Table 12.1). The most likely objective finding is a motor deficit or diminished deep tendon reflex in the distribution of the affected nerve. It is in this way that the specific root affected can be identified. It is important to isolate each group of muscles rather than test gross strength with actions that involve a combination of muscle groups. Sensory changes are inconsistently present and should not bare the brunt of the physical examination but rather provide additional information when present. One must keep in mind that the physical examination is not always precise as crossover between myotomes and dermatomes exists. It must also be noted that radiculopathy and myelopathy can coexist, and physical examination findings can mirror this.

Diagnostic Studies

It must be emphasized that the core of the information obtained should be from the history and physical examination, and diagnostic studies should be used to confirm the clinical impression. Many of these studies are overly sensitive and relatively nonspecific and therefore should not be used for screening purposes. When interpreting the information gained from these studies, the clinical picture needs to be correlated with the findings in the study, and the studies should never be interpreted in isolation.

Plain Radiographs

As discussed previously, the typical plain films of the cervical spine should include AP, lateral, oblique, and odontoid views. Plain films provide important information regarding degenerative changes and can suggest the specific level of the cervical spine involved. The generally accepted radiographic signs of cervical disk disease include loss of height of the disk space, osteophyte formation, secondary encroachment of the intervertebral foramina, and osteoarthritic changes in the apophyseal joints. Alignment and listhesis (slipping) of one vertebral body on another should be examined as well.

It must be stressed that the identification of "some pathology" on plain cervical films does not necessarily indicate the cause of the patient's symptoms as several studies have shown that a large percentage of asymptomatic individuals have radiographic evidence of degenerative changes on x-ray.

MRI

MRI is currently the study of choice when evaluating root compression (or cord compression in the case of myelopathy). MRI is excellent at clearly visualizing the cord and roots and stenosis or compression of both. It is best at identifying soft tissues, so herniated intervertebral disks (soft disks) (Fig. 12.19) causing root compression are better visualized than osteophytes (hard disks) causing compression, but both can be appreciated. Foraminal stenosis is also well visualized. Additionally, MRI is safe (does not use ionizing radiation and rarely uses contrast agents) and is currently becoming cheaper, although it is still a much more expensive test than CT. The only caution is the prevalence of findings in asymptomatic patients is very high (19%), and results should therefore be strictly correlated with the history and physical examination.

CT

The use of CT scanning in the spine, as with any other place in the body, visualizes the bony anatomy much better than the soft tissues and is thus limited in detecting soft-tissue pathology causing impingement. However, CT does visualize bony causes of impingement better than MRI. In general, it is used for those patients who cannot undergo MRI or in those in which the MRI is equivocal. The addition of myelography (injection of dye into the spinal canal prior to imaging) may be necessary if surgical treatment is considered. In general, CT with or without myelography is used as a backup test to MRI in the evaluation of a radiculopathy.

Electromyography

Electromyography (EMG) is an electrical test that confirms the interaction of nerve to muscle. It is performed by placing needles into specific muscles to determine if there is an intact nerve supply to that muscle. EMG is particularly useful in localizing a specific abnormal nerve root. However, it

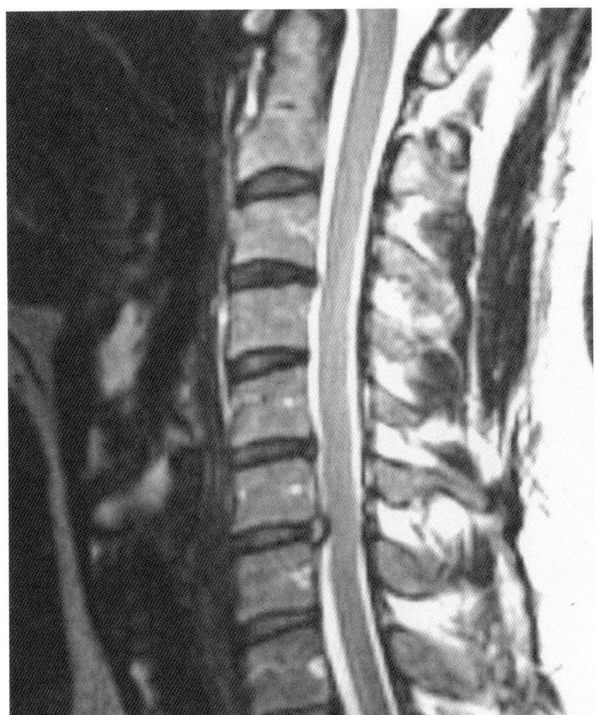

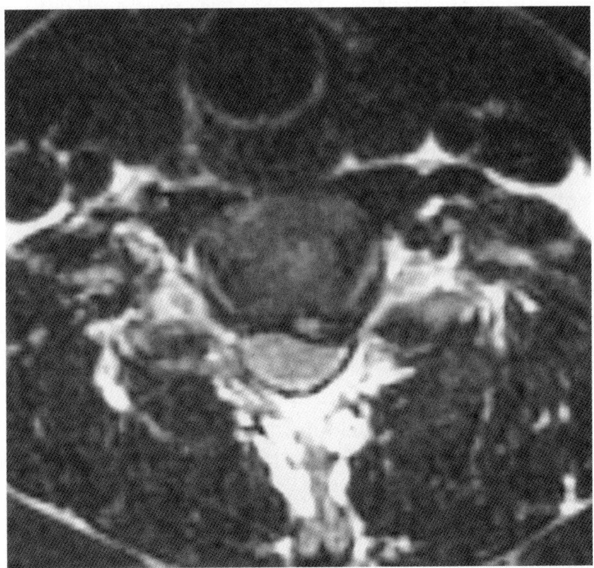

Figure 12.19 Disk herniation. Midsagittal **(A)** and axial **(B)** T2-weighted MRI depicting left paracentral herniation extending into the neuroforamen. (*Reproduced with permission from* Frymoyer JW, Wiesel SW, An HS, et al. *The Adult and Pediatric Spine*, 3rd ed. Philadelphia: Lippincott Williams & Wilkins, 2003.)

takes at least 21 days from the time of nerve impingement for an EMG to show up as abnormal. Before that period of time, the EMG may be unremarkable as the nerve has not experienced enough pressure to show signs of denervation.

The accuracy of EMG is around 80% to 90% in establishing the diagnosis of cervical radiculopathy. Reasons for false negatives include sensory root involvement only and timing of the study. If only the sensory portion of the nerve is affected, the EMG will be negative as EMG tests motor innervation. As previously mentioned, the study will also read as negative if performed too early. Therefore, a negative study should be repeated 3 weeks later if symptoms still persist and a diagnosis has not been made. It must be noted that EMG is not part of the routine evaluation of the cervical spine and should be used to confirm one's clinical suspicion or to rule out other pathologies such as peripheral or compressive neuropathies.

Natural History

Generally speaking, the natural history of cervical radiculopathy is favorable with the majority resolving with nonoperative treatment. Lees and Turner studied the natural history in 51 patients and showed that 45% had only 1 episode with resolution, while 25% reported persistent symptoms. The remainder had mild symptoms, and no patient progressed to myelopathic symptoms. Therefore, nonoperative management is the initial treatment of choice. The question remains as to whether methods of nonoperative treatment actually improve the course of the disease or whether nonoperative treatment provides symptomatic relief only. There is limited information comparing nonoperative treatments, and it remains surgeon preference as to which method to use. The different methods of treatment are discussed in the individual sections on the pathologies causing radiculopathy (i.e., herniated disk, cervical spondylosis) as well as in the treatment algorithm for cervical pathology.

Cervical Myelopathy

Cervical Myelopathy is defined as compression of the spinal cord, which is usually due to degenerative changes. The compression occurs on the cord itself, which differentiates it from radiculopathy, where compression is on the individual root.

History

Myelopathy typically presents in those over the age of 50 with males predominating over females. The onset is generally insidious with symptoms worsening over time. Common presenting symptoms include numbness and paresthesias in the hands, clumsiness of the fingers, weakness (greatest in the lower extremities), and gait/balance disturbances. Abnormalities of micturition can occur and indicate more severe or progressed cord involvement. Sensory abnormalities are also common and may show a patchy distribution. Spinothalamic tract (pain and temperature) deficits can be seen throughout and are classically described as being in a stocking or glove distribution. Posterior column deficits (vibration and proprioception) also commonly occur in the hands and feet. The patient typically complains of globally diminished appreciation of touch or sensation. It must be noted that a significant amount of patients will present with radiculopathic symptoms in addition to myelopathic symptoms thus clouding the presentation.

Physical Examination

The myelopathic physical examination will generally have nonspecific findings in addition to findings specific to cord compression. One nonspecific but important finding is limited neck extension on examination secondary to pain from the narrowed canal. Especially important with myelopathy is a full neurologic examination with particular attention paid to weakness, muscle atrophy, and clumsiness in both the upper and lower extremities. There are various specific maneuvers described for hand/finger clumsiness including rapidly opening and closing the hands, which is often slowed. In the lower extremities, the usual findings are spasticity and weakness, in addition to atrophy (pyramidal tract signs).

On the reflex examination, hyperreflexia, clonus, and a positive Babinski's sign are often positive in the lower extremities, while hyperreflexia and a positive Hoffman's sign may be observed in the upper extremities. Sensory examination should be documented but is much less sensitive. Usually there is no gross sensory dysfunction but rather a patchy decrease in light touch and pin prick. The sensory examination does not make the diagnosis but can support the diagnosis.

Finally, it is important to assess the patient's gait. The classic myelopathic gait is described as a wide-based gait and further testing may show difficulty with toe walking, heel walking, and/or heel–toe gait. Additionally, the Romberg's test can be positive, demonstrating a disturbance in balance secondary to dysfunction in the posterior column.

Diagnostic Studies

Again, it must be emphasized that the core of the information obtained should be from the history and physical examination, and diagnostic studies should be used to confirm the clinical impression. Many of these studies are overly sensitive and relatively nonspecific and therefore should not be used for screening purposes as they can identify pathology in asymptomatic individuals for which no treatment is necessary. Therefore, when interpreting the information gained from these studies, the clinical picture needs to be correlated with the findings in the study, and the studies should never be interpreted in isolation.

Plain Films

Radiographs of the cervical spine in myelopathic patients typically show changes consistent with advanced degenerative disease. Findings include disk-space narrowing, end plate sclerosis, facet joint arthrosis, osteophytosis with spinal canal narrowing/foraminal narrowing, and instability. Congenital cervical stenosis, defined as a canal less than 13 mm in diameter, is frequently seen and predisposes the patient to myelopathy.

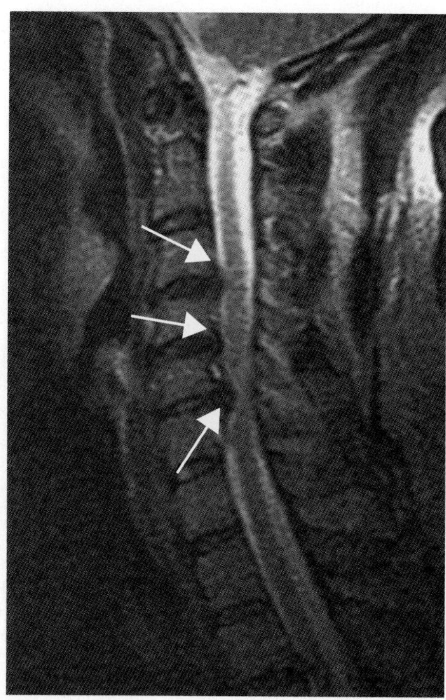

Figure 12.20 Multilevel disk herniation causing cord compression with myelopathy. Note multiple disk herniations (*arrows*). (*Reprinted with permission from* Ross JS. *MRI of the Spine*, 2nd ed. Philadelphia: Lippincott Williams & Wilkins, 2000.)

MRI

In a patient with a physical examination consistent with myelopathy, an MRI is the next step after plain films. The MRI findings can be very impressive as it images the cord/soft tissue extremely well, thereby allowing one to visualize cord impingement closely (Fig. 12.20). The typical findings are cord compression at multiple levels, disk herniation, facet hypertrophy, buckling/hypertrophy of the ligamentum flavum, and soft-tissue changes. It must be stressed again to correlate findings with the physical examination as MRI is often positive in asymptomatic individuals.

Natural History

The natural history for cervical myelopathy is not as favorable as for radiculopathy, but it is not an absolute indication for surgery. Patients typically experience plateau periods followed by exacerbations of the disease. It differs from radiculopathy in the sense that generally speaking it is progressive. The rapidity of progression varies from patient to patient with most eventually requiring surgery.

Management

There remains a limited role for nonoperative treatment initially, but once further deterioration is observed, surgery is clearly indicated. Conservative management involves immobilization and rest with a cervical orthosis. To our knowledge, there are no good clinical trials indicating that conservative treatment alters disease progression, although it offers an option for those who are not good operative candidates and those who have minor symptoms. The absolute indications for surgery are not clearly defined and vary from surgeon to surgeon. However, most would agree that neurologic deterioration marks a need for surgical intervention. The goals of surgery are decompression of the cord with prevention of further cord compression and vascular compromise.

Cervical Spine Clinical Conditions

Many conditions may present as neck pain, radiculopathy, myelopathy, or any combination in any particular individual. Those that are most common will be presented in detail below.

Neck Sprain (or Strain) and Neck Ache

Neck sprain, while a misnomer, describes a clinical condition involving a nonradiating discomfort or pain about the neck area associated with a concomitant loss of neck motion (stiffness). Although the clinical syndrome may present as a headache, most often the pain is located in the middle to lower part of the back of the neck with various patterns of referred pain that may be present in addition to or instead of the typical pattern. A history of injury is rarely obtained, but the pain may start after a night's rest or simply on turning the head. The infamous traumatic form of neck sprain, the whiplash injury, is a cervical acceleration–deceleration injury from an MVA in which a car is rear ended, resulting in cervical hyperflexion followed by hyperextension causing a neck sprain. This condition is somewhat different from the more common atraumatic (or minimally traumatic) forms, and will not be discussed further, but the same structures are involved resulting in similar pain patterns. The natural history of traumatic neck strain, however, may be different for a variety of reasons, including litigation, which is beyond the scope of this chapter.

There is debate about the actual source(s) of the pain with a cervical sprain, but it is commonly believed to be the ligaments about the cervical spine and the facet joints, as well as the surrounding musculature. The ligaments contain nerve endings resulting in pain sensation, while the musculature surrounding the damaged area tends to contract to essentially protect or splint the involved area resulting in a myofascial pain syndrome. Additionally, axial pain may be produced by small annular tears within the disk without actual disk herniation.

The pain most often associated with a neck sprain is a dull aching pain, which is exacerbated by neck motion and abated by rest or immobilization. The pain may be referred to other mesenchymal structures derived from a similar sclerotome during embryogenesis. Common referred pain patterns include the scapular area, the posterior shoulder, the occipital area, or the anterior chest wall (cervical angina pectoris). Those referred pain patterns do not connote a true radicular pattern and are not usually mechanical in origin.

Physical examination of patients with neck ache usually reveals nothing more than a locally tender area(s) just lateral to the spine in the area of the paraspinal musculature with or without loss of motion secondary to pain. The intensity of the pain is variable, and the loss of cervical motion correlates directly with the pain intensity. The presence of true spasm, defined as a continuous muscle contraction, is rare except in severe cases when the head may be tilted to one side (torticollis). There are no examination findings suggestive of radiculopathy or myelopathy.

Radiographs with a neck ache or sprain are usually normal and, therefore, are not warranted on the initial visit when the working diagnosis is neck ache. If the pain continues for more than 2 weeks or the patient develops other physical findings, radiographs should be taken to rule out more serious causes for the clinical picture, such as instability or neoplasm.

The prognosis for patients with neck ache is excellent—the natural history is one of complete resolution of the symptoms over several weeks. The mainstay of therapy includes rest and immobilization, possibly in a soft cervical orthosis for comfort. NSAIDs and muscle relaxants will aid in comfort as well; however, none of these treatments seem to alter the duration of the natural history of this disorder.

Acute Herniated Disk

A herniated disk is defined as the protrusion of the nucleus pulposus through the fibers of the annulus fibrosis. This generally occurs around the fourth decade when the nucleus is still gelatinous. Older patients will rarely have an acute disk herniation secondary to the loss of water content in the nucleus pulposus, which leads to an inability of the nucleus pulposus to protrude through the annulus. Most herniations occur posterolaterally, although central and intraforaminal protrusion can occur as well. The higher incidence of posterolateral protrusion is thought to be secondary to the relative weakness of the PLL just lateral to the midline with subsequent protrusion through perforations in the region. The most common areas of cervical disk herniation are C5–C6 and C6–C7, whereas C7–T1 and C3–C4 occur infrequently, and C2–C3 herniation is extremely rare.

The disk herniation in the cervical spine generally results in a radiculopathy secondary to root impingement, but unlike the lumbar spine, findings of myelopathy may be present as well. The herniation will cause pressure on the local nerve root in addition to pressure on the cord in the region, with the amount of cord pressure depending on the laterality of the herniation. More central herniations are more likely to result in significant cord compression. Cervical disk herniation usually affects the root numbered lowest for the given disk level as that is the nerve that eventually exits through the foramen at that level. For example, a C3–C4 disk affects the C4 root, C4–C5 affects the C5 root,

C5–C6 affects the C6 root, C6–C7 affects the C7 root, and C7–T1 affects the C8 root.

Herniated disks result in a wide array of symptomatology from asymptomatic to debilitating pain with neurologic symptoms. The presence of symptoms depends on the spinal reserve capacity or size of the canal (amount of space available for the nerve/cord to be displaced prior to impingement), presence of inflammation, size of the herniation, and concomitant disease such as associated osteophyte formation. Generally, the patient's major complaint is arm pain, with minor complaints of neck pain. The pain is often perceived as starting in the neck area and radiating from this point down the shoulder to the arm, forearm, and often the hand in a dermatomal distribution. The onset is usually gradual, although sudden onset can occur often with a snapping sensation. As mentioned earlier, the severity of the arm pain varies from incapacitating to a dull ache. The pain is generally enough to awaken the patient at night.

The physical examination varies depending on the root involved as well as the amount, if any, of cord impingement. Nonspecific physical examination findings include limited range of motion, pain with range of motion, positive Spurling's sign, pain with valsalva maneuver, and pain with spine extension secondary to narrowing of the intervertebral foramen. The most important or helpful finding on examination is a positive neurologic finding as this will allow one to pinpoint the area of impingement. To be significant, the neurologic examination must show objective signs of reflex diminution (in comparison with the opposite side), motor weakness, and/or atrophy in a myotomal region. Subjective sensory findings are difficult to interpret, and sensory changes alone are not enough to make a firm diagnosis. Additionally, findings of clonus, hyperreflexia, Babinski's sign, Hoffman's sign, and/or other myelopathic signs are significant as they are manifestations of cord impingement. However, they are less helpful in pinpointing the exact area of involvement.

After the provisional diagnosis of a herniated disk is made by the history and physical examination, radiologic studies are done to confirm the diagnosis and to evaluate the extent and level(s) of involvement. Plain films are obtained first, although they are often of little diagnostic utility. Their value largely lies in excluding other causes of neck and arm pain. The most useful information will be obtained from MRI, but MRI should only be used as a confirmatory study as around 10% of asymptomatic individuals under 40 years of age will have evidence of a herniated disk on MRI. MRI is excellent at visualizing the disks and the cord and thus is excellent at confirming herniated disks and the amount of impingement present. As discussed previously, positive findings on MRI should be correlated with the physical examination and the patient should be treated according to the physical findings rather than the findings on MRI. The most helpful MR images are on the sagittal and axial views showing protrusion of the disk into the canal with impingement on the cord and/or nerve roots (Fig. 12.19). Other studies such as EMG/NCS can be done to show evidence of nerve root involvement, but they are less sensitive and specific than MRI and as such are used less often.

The treatment for most patients with a herniated disk is nonoperative, and the majority of patients respond over a period of months. The efficacy of the nonoperative approach depends heavily on the doctor–patient relationship with open communication for the patient to understand the natural history of the disease. If a patient is well informed, insightful, and willing to follow instructions, the chances for a successful nonoperative outcome are greatly improved.

The cornerstone to management of a cervical herniated disk is rest and immobilization, possibly in a cervical orthosis for pain relief. The use of a cervical orthosis greatly increases the likelihood that the patient will rest. Patients should markedly decrease their physical activity for at least 2 weeks while the symptoms are most acute. After the acute pain begins to abate, patients should gradually increase their activity. Most patients will be able to return to work, or at least to light activities, in a month.

Pharmaceutical therapy is an important adjunct to rest and immobilization. Anti-inflammatory medication, analgesic medications, and muscle relaxants have been used historically in the acute setting. Because it is believed that the radicular pain is in part inflammatory, the use of NSAIDs seems appropriate. Much more controversial is the role of narcotics and muscle relaxants. Many believe that narcotics should only be used if the pain is severe and the patient has failed a trial of anti-inflammatory medications. Others are much more liberal with narcotic prescriptions. We believe that there is a limited role for narcotics and only in the acute setting only. They should be used sparingly, and it should be made clear that they are not for extended treatment. Long-term use should be prohibited secondary to the addictive properties of the medications, as there are many patients who suffer from this if continued use is allowed. Rarely a patient may need to be admitted to the hospital for a short period of time for pain relief.

Surgical treatment is reserved for patients with unremitting radicular symptoms after an adequate period of conservative therapy. What constitutes an adequate period of conservative therapy is controversial. The presence of an isolated neurologic finding, such as an absent bicep reflex, is not an indication for surgery. The goal of surgery is to relieve pain. Return of an isolated neurologic deficit is unpredictable. The results of surgery for pain relief are quite good (over 90%) when the history, physical examination, and diagnostic studies are confirmatory. Surgery generally involves anterior cervical discectomy and fusion (ACDF), although laminoforaminotomy with or without discectomy may be a reasonable alternative. Disk replacement is a newer technique that has shown some promise, although the long-term results are not known. Proponents for disk replacement over fusion site that range of motion is maintained, possibly diminishing the amount of segmental disease at the levels above and below the fusion site.

Cervical Spondylosis

Once commonly referred to as "cervical degenerative disk disease," cervical spondylosis is a chronic process defined as the development of osteophytes and other stigmata of degenerative arthritis as a consequence of age-related disk disease. This process may produce a wide array of symptoms from neck pain to symptoms of a radiculopathy and/or myelopathy.

The process begins with disk degeneration from age-related changes resulting in a change in the proteoglycan and collagen content of the disk as well as loss of water content. Ultimately, these changes lead to desiccation of the nucleus pulposus, loss of annular elasticity, and narrowing of the disk space with or without disk protrusion or rupture. The changes within the disk and the loss of disk height disrupt the biomechanics in the vertebral column, resulting in progressive degeneration and motion between segments. Increased motion between segments results in overriding facets, facet hypertrophy, inflammation of the synovium, osteophyte formation, hypertrophy of the ligamentum flavum and/or PLL, and even microfractures. Depending on the location of these changes within the spine, a variety of clinical syndromes can occur including spondylosis, ankylosis, central or foraminal spinal stenosis, radiculopathy, myelopathy, or spinal segmental instability.

The typical patient with spondylosis alone (i.e., without radiculopathy and/or myelopathy) is over the age of 40 with a primary complaint of neck pain. Not infrequently, however, these patients will have little neck pain and will present with referred pain patterns: occipital headaches or as pain in the shoulder, suboccipital, interscapular areas, and/or the anterior chest wall. In patients with predominantly referred pain, a previous history of neck pain is usually obtained. These patients have nonspecific physical examination findings.

The patient with spondylosis and radiculopathy and/or myelopathy will often have little neck pain but rather present mainly with radicular and/or myelopathic symptoms. Radiculopathy results from irritation of the nerve root from a bony protuberance (osteophytes, facet joint hypertrophy) or less commonly soft disk herniation as the nerve root is exiting the canal. This is commonly referred to as foraminal stenosis. Myelopathy can result from a similar process; however, the cord is impinged from central rather than foraminal stenosis. Central stenosis occurs from disk bulging (less common), uncovertebral hypertrophy, vertebral end plate osteophytes, and/or ligamentum flavum hypertrophy. Posterior osteophytes causing cord impingement are commonly referred to as "hard disks" that delineates them from intervertebral disk herniation, "soft disks." Commonly, radiculopathy and myelopathy will coexist in these patients, referred to as myeloradiculopathy.

Myelopathy occurs in less than 5% of patients with spondylosis, but it is the most serious sequelae and the most difficult to treat effectively. The symptoms are generally gradual, and patients typically notice loss of dexterity in their hands and more difficulty with gait. They may exhibit the typical stooped, wide-based, and somewhat jerky gait of chronic myelopathy. Physical examination may demonstrate hyperreflexia, Hoffman's sign, Babinski's sign, clonus, and/or other findings previously discussed in the myelopathy section.

Radiographs of patients with cervical spondylosis will show varying degrees of changes depending on the severity of the disease including disk space narrowing, osteophytosis, foraminal narrowing, facet hypertrophy, and instability (Fig. 12.21). In patients without radicular and/or myelopathic findings, further diagnostic testing is unnecessary. In patients with these findings, however, one should pursue further imaging preferably with an MRI.

Treatment of cervical spondylosis varies, again, depending on the severity of the disease. Spondylosis alone is treated with nonoperative measures. The mainstay of treatment for the acute pain superimposed on the chronic problem is rest and immobilization in addition to anti-inflammatory medications, which often will need to be taken long term. Additionally, trigger point injections can be performed and many times will provide substantial relief. Trigger point injections contain a local anesthetic combined with a corticosteroid administered in the points or areas of maximal tenderness. Patients may also begin a program of physical therapy emphasizing isometric exercises aimed at toning debilitated musculature in the cervical region with the benefit of adding more stabilization to the cervical region. Finally, patients should be counseled regarding sleeping position, automobile driving, and work. It should be noted that axial neck pain alone does not respond well to surgical stabilization, and thus surgery is rarely employed.

Patients with radiculopathy should follow the same conservative management pathway with the addition of selective nerve root blocks and epidural steroid injections. If conservative management fails, surgical intervention can then be employed with success rates of over 90%. The type of surgery performed depends on the location of the pathology with surgical options including posterior laminoforaminotomy for isolated purely foraminal stenosis but more commonly ACDF as isolated disease is the exception rather than the norm.

Spondylosis with myelopathy is a surgical disease but is not an absolute indication for surgical decompression. Conservative therapy as discussed earlier offers the myelopathic patient, who is not a good operative risk, a viable option. Depending on the aggressiveness of the surgeon, the indications for operative treatment vary slightly as there is a lack of absolute definitive clinical data. If the disease progresses despite a trial of conservative therapy, surgery is clearly indicated to prevent further progression. The

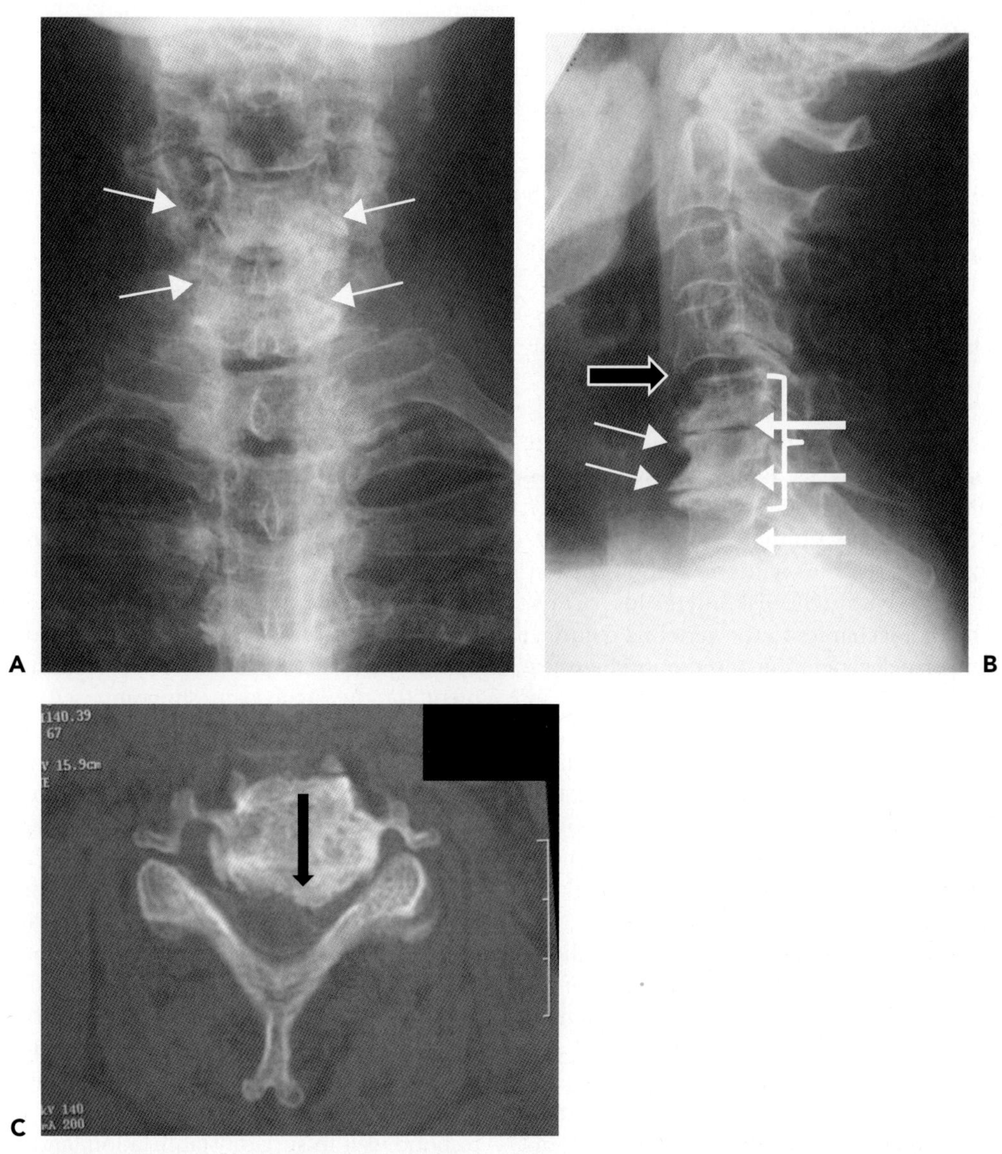

Figure 12.21 Spondylosis with myelopathy. A 78-year-old woman presenting with myelopathy including myelopathic hand, broad-based gait, and positive Hoffman's sign on left. **(A)** AP radiograph demonstrates severe uncovertebral joint narrowing (*arrows*) and sclerosis characteristic of advanced osteolysis. **(B)** Lateral radiograph demonstrates anterolisthesis of C4 on C5 (*open arrow*) with severe disk space narrowing of C5–C6, C6–C7, and C7–T1 (*closed arrows*). Note also the anterior osteophytes (*small arrows*) and concomitant loss of the normal cervical lordosis. **(C)** Transaxial CT scan at the C5–C6 disk level demonstrates a large posterior hard disk (*arrow*) protruding into the spinal canal with associated uncovertebral joint osteophytes. (*Reproduced with permission from* Frymoyer JW, Wiesel SW, An HS, et al. *The Adult and Pediatric Spine*, 3rd ed. Philadelphia: Lippincott Williams & Wilkins, 2003.)

goals of surgery in the myelopathic patient are decompression of the spinal cord and prevention of further neurologic deterioration. ACDF is used in the majority of cases, although with multilevel disease, laminoplasty may be indicated.

Rheumatoid Arthritis

Rheumatoid arthritis (RA) is an autoimmune inflammatory arthropathy affecting around 2% of the population with cervical spine involvement becoming symptomatic in around 60% of rheumatoid patients and radiographic involvement occurring as high as 85% of patients. As with other areas in the body, chronic synovial inflammation eventually leads to destruction of the ligaments, joints, and bone causing instability and pain in the cervical region. If left untreated, severe pain, neurologic deterioration, and death can occur. With the significant improvement of the medical management of RA through disease modifying anti-rheumatoid drugs, the number and severity of cases should continue to decline.

Cervical spine involvement secondary to the erosive inflammatory changes of RA is divided into three main

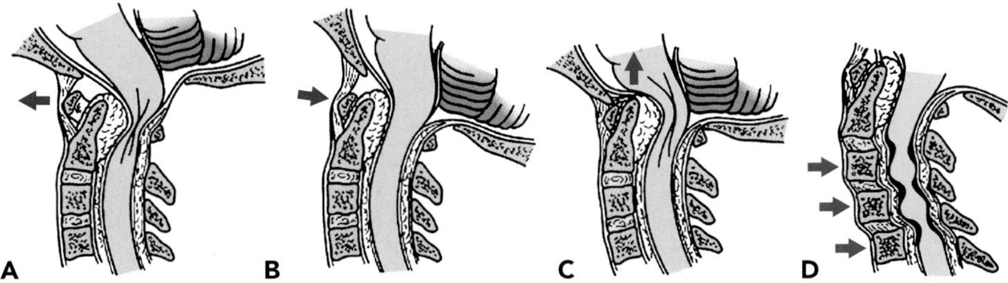

Figure 12.22 Patterns of cervical spine instability secondary to rheumatoid arthritis. **(A,B)** Atlantoaxial instability. **(C)** Cranial settling (basilar invagination). **(D)** Subaxial instability. (*Reproduced with permission from* Chapman MW. *Chapman's Orthopaedic Surgery*, 3rd ed. Philadelphia, Lippincott Williams & Wilkins, 2000.)

categories: (1) atlantoaxial instability, (2) basilar invagination, and (3) subaxial instability (Fig. 12.22). Atlantoaxial instability is the most common form of instability accounting for approximately 70% of the cases. Inflammation and pannus formation lead to weakening of the ligamentous structures about C1 and C2, eventually resulting in anterior subluxation of C1 on C2. Subluxation results in cord impingement as the SAC decreases. Basilar invagination refers to the cephalad migration of the odontoid secondary to involvement of the atlantoaxial and atlanto-occipital joints, resulting in impaction of the odontoid on the brainstem with severity depending on the amount of migration. This is the least common yet most feared complication of RA of the cervical spine as severe neurologic deficits can occur, and death from compression on the respiratory center at the brainstem is possible. Subaxial instability occurs in approximately 25% of the cases, resulting in decreased SAC via the same mechanism as in atlantoaxial instability.

Symptomatic patients with cervical spine involvement typically complain of neck pain in the middle, posterior neck, and occipital area with varying complaints of weakness about the neck itself and/or in the extremities. Physical examination should start with a careful neurologic examination, which often can be difficult with the associated changes in the appendicular skeleton. Range of motion of the neck is often decreased and crepitus or a feeling of instability may be elicited.

Plain radiographs are the first step after the physical examination with AP, lateral, odontoid, and lateral flexion/extension views obtained. Certain radiographic parameters are critical in evaluating the rheumatoid cervical spine. On the lateral view, these include the anterior atlantodents interval (aADI), the posterior atlantodental interval (pADI), odontoid migration in relation to McGregor's line, and the spinolaminar line (Fig. 12.4). An aADI 3 mm or greater is significant for atlantoaxial instability, while a pADI less than 14 mm signifies a decreased SAC with an indication for surgical fixation. Basilar invagination is defined as migration of the odontoid tip more than 4.5-mm cephalad to McGregor's line (line from hard palate to caudal surface of the basiocciput). Subaxial instability appears as a stepladder appearance of the spinolaminar line known as "stepladder" vertebrae. Flexion/extension views are obtained to analyze the extent of atlantoaxial instability as the patient can exhibit an increased aADI and a decreased pADI on the flexion view in comparison to the extension view, as well as subaxial instability highlighting the stepladder appearance on the flexion view, which may not be present on neutral or extension films. Additional radiographic findings include osteopenia, facet erosion, and disk space narrowing. CT is very helpful following plain films to more accurately determine the measurements mentioned earlier as well as for surgical planning. The addition of MRI evaluates the amount of cord compression and visualizes the amount of pannus formation at the odontoid as well as other soft-tissue inflammation, resulting in canal space narrowing that cannot be appreciated on plain films or CT scan (Fig. 12.23).

The majority of these patients, despite dramatic disease patterns, can be successfully managed nonoperatively. Although the natural history of RA predicts a high incidence of cervical involvement with progression (the spine does not stabilize itself over time), few patients die from medullary compression, and only approximately 10% of patients with atlantoaxial disease exhibit neurologic compression. The mainstay of nonoperative management is a cervical orthosis along with patient education and

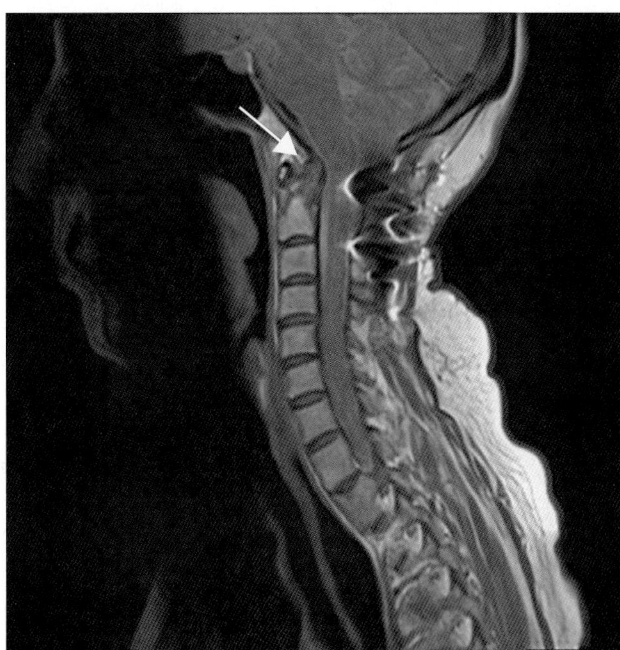

Figure 12.23 Rheumatoid arthritis pannus formation at odontoid. This is a 55-year-old female with rheumatoid arthritis with atlantoaxial instability with an MRI showing large pannus formation (*arrow*) at the odontoid.

communication with the rheumatologist to maximize medical therapy. Finally, patients should be followed with serial radiographs to evaluate for radiographic progression, which may place the patient at severe risk for neurologic compromise.

The surgical indications for the treatment of RA in the cervical spine are progressive neurologic deficit, axial neck pain unresponsive to nonoperative management, and radiographic parameters that place the patient at risk for severe neurologic deterioration. The following are radiographic parameters that have been shown through studies to place patients at risk for significant deterioration: pADI $\leq$14 mm in patients with atlantoaxial instability, cephalad migration of the odontoid $\geq$5 mm above McGregor's line representing significant basilar invagination, and sagittal canal diameter $\leq$14 mm in patients with subaxial instability. Of note, as previously addressed, uncontrollable axial neck pain with no neurologic symptoms may be an indication for surgery in the rheumatoid patient as these patients do well following surgical stabilization for pain control. This is in contradistinction to nonrheumatoid patients presenting solely with axial pain. Surgical stabilization generally involves a posterior spinal fusion of all unstable segments.

Cervical Spine Algorithm

The task of the physician, when confronted with the cervical spine patient, is to integrate the patient's complaints into an accurate diagnosis and to prescribe appropriate therapy. Achieving this goal depends on the accuracy of the physician's decision-making ability. Although specific information is not available for every aspect of neck pain, there is a large body of data to guide us in handling these patients. Using this knowledge, which has already been presented, an algorithm for neck pain has been designed.

Webster defines an algorithm as "a set of rules for solving a particular problem in a finite number of steps." It is, in effect, an organized pattern of decision-making and thought processes. In this instance, we present an algorithm for approaching the universe of cervical spine patients. The algorithm can be followed in sequence (Fig. 12.24).

The primary objective for the physician is to return patients to normal function as quickly as possible. In the course of achieving this goal, the physician must be concerned with other circumstances, which include making efficient and precise use of diagnostic studies, minimizing the use of ineffectual surgery, and making therapy available at a reasonable cost to society. The algorithm follows well-delineated rules, established from the consensus of a broad segment of qualified spine surgeons. It allows the patient to receive the most helpful diagnostic and therapeutic measures at optimal times.

The algorithm begins with the universe of patients who are initially evaluated for neck pain, with or without arm pain. Patients with major trauma, including fractures, are excluded from this algorithm. After an initial history and physical examination—and assuming that the patient's symptoms are originating from the cervical spine—the first major decision is to rule out the presence of a cervical myelopathy.

The character and severity of myelopathy depend on the size, location, and duration of the lesion. Ventrolateral lesions encroach on the nerve roots and lateral aspects of the spinal cord, producing all of the manifestations accompanying nerve root compression. These lesions will therefore give a mixed presentation with weakness and loss of tone in the upper extremities as well as pyramidal tract signs and spasticity in the lower extremities (these may also be seen in the upper extremities as well, such as a positive Hoffman's sign).

Midline lesions intrude on the central aspect of the anterior portion of the spinal cord. They produce no signs of nerve root compression. Both lower extremities are primarily involved, and the most common problem relates initially to gait disturbance, though clumsiness of the hands often follows. As the disease progresses, bowel and bladder control may be affected.

Once a diagnosis of cervical myelopathy is made, surgical intervention should be considered, although many will advise a short course of conservative treatment. An MRI should be performed for confirmation of the diagnosis, determination of the number of levels involved, and for preoperative planning. The timing of surgery is a matter of judgment. If nonoperative management is tried, progression of the disease signifies failure of management and warrants surgical intervention.

After cervical myelopathy has been ruled out, the remaining patients, who constitute an overwhelming majority, should be started on a course of conservative management. At this stage of the patient's care, the specific diagnosis, whether it be a herniated disk, degenerative disk disease, or neck strain, is not important because the entire group is treated in the same fashion.

Conservative Treatment

The primary mode of therapy in both acute and chronic cervical spine disease is immobilization. In acute neck injuries, immobilization allows for healing of torn and attenuated soft tissues, whereas in chronic conditions immobilization is aimed at reduction of inflammation in the supporting soft tissues and around the nerve roots of the cervical spine.

Immobilization is best achieved by the use of a soft collar. It needs to be properly fitted and comfortable on the patient. Initially, the collar is worn 24 hours a day. The patient must understand that during sleep the neck is totally unprotected from awkward positions and movements, and therefore collar wear is most important.

Drug therapy is the other mainstay of initial treatment. It is directed at reducing inflammation, especially in the soft tissues. A variety of anti-inflammatory medications are

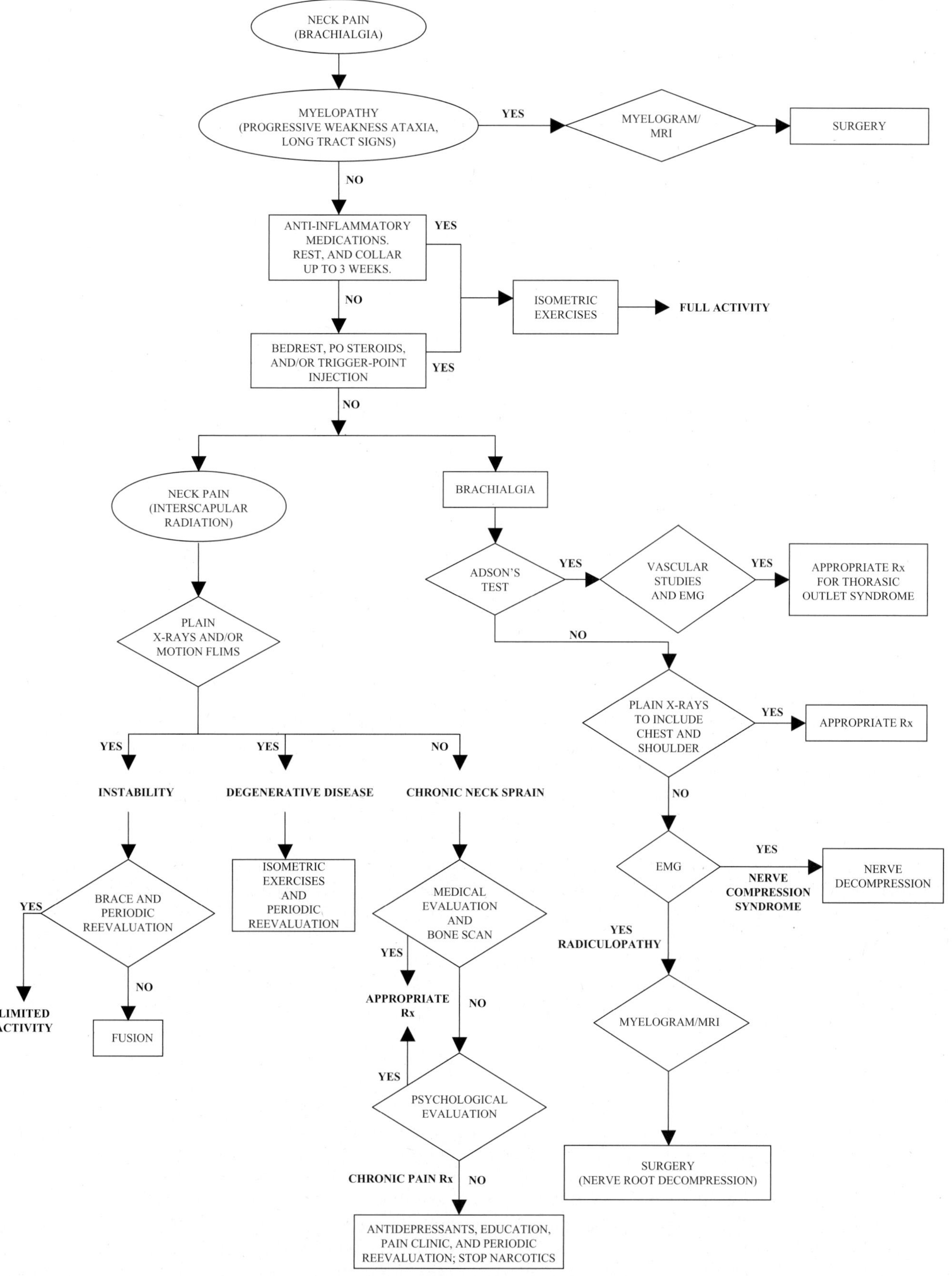

Figure 12.24 Cervical algorithm.

available, with preference often depending on the surgeon's preference, although patients with a history of gastric ulcers or severe reflux should probably be on a COX-II inhibitor or else should take another medication to counteract or alleviate the GI side effects of traditional NSAIDs. That being said, we prefer naproxen initially as we have had good success with this medication. The efficacy of this treatment regimen is predicated on the patient's ability to understand the disease process and the role of each therapeutic modality. The vast majority of patients will respond to this approach in the first 10 days, but a certain percentage will not heal rapidly.

If the patient is not improving at this juncture, a trigger point injection should be considered. A trigger point injection is an injection combining an anesthetic (lidocaine) with 1 mL of a steroid into the areas of maximal tenderness around the paravertebral musculature and trapezii. These areas of maximal tenderness are referred to as "trigger points." The objective is to decrease the inflammation in a specific anatomic area, thereby relieving pain. The more localized the trigger point, the more effective therapy will be. Often patients exhibit marked relief of symptoms.

The patient should be treated conservatively for up to 6 weeks at which time the majority of patients will be better and should be encouraged to gradually increase their activities. The goal is for the patient to return to his/her normal lifestyle. An exercise program should be directed at strengthening the paravertebral musculature, not at increasing the range of motion.

The pathway along this top portion of the algorithm is reversible. Should regression occur with exacerbation of symptoms, the physician can resort to more stringent conservative measures. These measures may include additional bed rest and stronger anti-inflammatory medication. The majority of patients with neck pain will respond to therapy and return to a normal life pattern within 2 months of the beginning of their problem. If the initial conservative treatment regimen fails, symptomatic patients are divided into two groups. The first group comprises patients who have neck pain as a predominant complaint, with or without interscapular radiation. The second group is made up of those who complain primarily of arm pain (brachialgia).

Neck Pain Predominance

After 6 weeks of conservative therapy with no symptomatic relief, plain roentgenograms are taken and carefully examined for abnormalities. Patients then fall into a subgroup on the basis of the plain film findings. One group of patients will have objective evidence of instability. In the subaxial cervical spine, instability is identified by horizontal translation of one vertebra on another of more than 3.5 mm or a kyphotic angulation of more than 11 degrees. The majority of patients with instability will respond to further nonoperative measures, including thorough education about the problem and symptomatic bracing and medications. If these measures fail, surgical fusion may be required in some cases.

Another group of patients with predominantly neck pain will show evidence of degenerative changes on plain films including loss of disk height, osteophyte formation, foraminal stenosis, and facet hypertrophy. The difficulty is not in identifying the abnormalities on the radiographs but rather in determining their significance. Degeneration in the cervical spine can be a normal part of the aging process. In a study of matched pairs of asymptomatic and symptomatic patients, it was concluded that large numbers of asymptomatic patients show roentgenographic evidence of advanced degenerative disease. The most significant roentgenographic finding relevant to symptoms was found to be narrowing of the intervertebral disk space, particularly between C5–C6 and C6–C7. There was no difference between the two groups as far as changes at the apophyseal joints, intervertebral foramina, or posterior articular processes.

These patients should be treated symptomatically with anti-inflammatory medications, support and trigger point injections as required. In the quiescent stages, they should be placed on isometric exercises. Finally, they should be reexamined periodically because some will develop myelopathy and should then be treated appropriately.

The majority of patients with neck pain predominance will have normal roentgenograms. The diagnosis for this group of patients is neck strain. At this point, with no objective findings, other pathologic conditions must be considered. These patients should be considered for a more thorough medical evaluation with consideration for early tumors and infection. A thorough medical search may also reveal problems missed in the early stages of neck pain evaluation. If a medical cause for the symptoms is identified, the patient should be treated appropriately.

If the workup is negative, the patient should have a thorough psychosocial evaluation. This is predicated on the belief that the patient's disability is related not only to his/her pathologic anatomy but also to his/her perception of pain, and his/her stability in relation to his/her sociologic environment. Drug habituation, alcoholism, depression, and other psychiatric problems are frequently seen in association with neck pain. If the evaluation reveals this type of pathology, proper measures should be instituted to overcome the disability.

Should the outcome of the psychosocial evaluation prove to be normal, the patient can be considered to have chronic neck pain. One must be aware that other outside factors such as compensation or litigation can influence a patient's perception of his subjective pain. Patients with chronic neck pain need encouragement, patience, and education from their physicians. They need to be detoxified from narcotics and placed on an exercise regimen. Many will respond to antidepressant medications such as amitriptyline (Elavil). All of these patients need periodic reevaluation to avoid missing any new or underlying pathology.

Arm Pain Predominance (Brachialgia)

Patients who have pain radiating into their arm may be experiencing their symptoms secondary to mechanical pressure and inflammation of the involved nerve roots. This mechanical pressure may arise from a ruptured disk (soft disk) or from a bony protuberance (hard disk) secondary to degenerative changes. Other pathologic causes of arm pain should be carefully considered. Extrinsic pressure on the vascular structures or the peripheral nerves are the most likely imitators of brachialgia. Pathologic involvement in the chest and shoulder should also be ruled out.

A careful physical examination should be conducted. If there is any question about these findings, appropriate roentgenograms and an EMG should be obtained. If any of these are positive for peripheral pressure on the nerves or other pathology, the appropriate therapy should be administered. If the patient has a positive neurologic deficit on examination or a positive EMG, an MRI should be obtained to evaluate for nerve root impingement.

If the MRI is positive, that patient is considered a candidate for surgical treatment, although conservative therapy should first be attempted for a period of 6 weeks. If the patient has not improved with nonoperative treatment after 6 weeks, and the symptoms are consistent with the examination and diagnostic studies, surgical decompression should be considered.

It has been repeatedly documented that for surgery to be effective, unequivocal evidence of nerve root compression must be found at surgery. One must have a strong confirmation of mechanical root compression from the history, neurologic examination, and a confirming study (i.e., MRI) before proceeding with surgery. If the patient does not have these, there is inadequate clinical evidence of root compression to proceed with surgery, regardless of the radiographic findings. For individuals who have met these criteria for surgical decompression, the results will usually be satisfactory: 95% of them can expect good or excellent outcomes.

LUMBAR SPINE

Low-back pain occurs much more commonly than neck pain. The lifetime incidence of low-back pain is estimated to be 65%. Every physician will be either personally affected or professionally challenged by this problem.

History

A general medical review, especially in the older patient, is imperative. Metabolic, infectious, and malignant disorders may initially present to the physician as low-back pain.

The location of the pain is one of the most important historical points. The majority of patients just have back pain with or without referral into the buttocks or posterior thigh. Referred pain is defined as pain in structures that have the same mesodermal origin. These patients have a localized injury, and the referral of pain does not signify any compression of the neural elements. This type of pain is described as dull, deep, and/or boring.

Another group of patients complains of pain that originates in the back and travels below the knee into the foot. It is described as sharp and shooting or lancinating. It may be accompanied by numbness and tingling. This pain is termed "radicular pain" or a "radiculopathy." A radiculopathy, as discussed in previous sections, is defined as a mechanical compression of a nerve root where the pain travels along the anatomic course of the nerve. The compression can be secondary to soft-tissue or bony impingement. The most common nerve roots affected are L5 and S1—levels that account for pain traveling below the knee.

Finally, one should inquire about changes in bowel or bladder habits. Occasionally, a large midline disk herniation may compress several roots of the cauda equina, resulting in cauda equina syndrome. Urinary retention or incontinence of bowel and bladder (always bladder) are, along with severe pain, the major symptoms. Cauda equina is considered a surgical emergency as spontaneous recovery has not been observed.

Physical Examination

The physical examination is directed at finding the location of the pain and any associated neurologic findings. All patients with low-back pain can have nonspecific findings that vary in degree, depending on the severity of the condition. These findings include a list to one side, tenderness to palpation and percussion, and a decreased range of motion of the lumbar spine and can be present in both radiculopathic and referred pain patients. Their presence denotes that there is a problem but does not identify the etiology or level of the problem.

The neurologic examination may yield objective evidence of nerve root compression. If such evidence is present, a thorough neurologic evaluation of the lower extremities should be conducted, particularly to check the reflexes and motor findings. Sensory changes may or may not be present, but because of the overlap in the dermatomes of spinal nerves, it is difficult to identify specific root involvement.

In patients with radiculopathies, there are several maneuvers that tighten the sciatic nerve and in so doing, further compress an inflamed lumbar root against a herniated disk or bony spur. These maneuvers are generally termed "tension signs" or a "straight leg raising test" (SLRT). The conventional SLRT is performed with the patient supine. The examiner slowly elevates the leg by the heel with the knee kept straight. This test is positive when the leg pain below the knee is reproduced or intensified; the production of back pain or buttock pain does not constitute a positive finding. The reliability of the SLRT is age dependent. In a young patient, a negative test most probably excludes the possibility of a herniated disk. After the age of 30, however, a negative SLRT no longer reliably excludes the diagnosis.

Finally, the physical examination should evaluate some specific problems that can present as low-back pain. This includes a peripheral vascular examination, hip joint evaluation, and abdominal examination.

There are certain indications for radiographic studies, which will be discussed in the section regarding the lumbar spine algorithm, but for the most part, radiographs are unnecessary on the initial visit. If the patient returns and there has been no change in the pain or worsening, plain films should be obtained to rule out more serious causes for low-back pain, including tumor. If the patient is having neurologic symptoms, one can consider an MRI to evaluate for disk herniation. Again, the specific timing for obtaining these studies will be discussed in further detail later.

Lumbar Spine-Clinical Entities

Back Strain

Pain localized to the back or buttocks region with no radiation further down the leg is typically classified as lower back pain, lower back strain, and/or lumbar strain, and they are all describing the same phenomenon. Approximately 80% of the population, perhaps up to 95%, will experience this clinical entity at some point during their lifetime. The exact source of the pain is not completely understood in many cases and is probably a combination of sources that vary between patients, but the potential pain generators include the paraspinal musculature, ligaments, facet joints, sinuvertebral nerve inflammation, and intervertebral disks. The history of pain varies from an acute mechanism where the patient suddenly experiences a severe pain from lifting or while bending over, to awakening from sleep with pain, to a slowly progressive, insidious onset of back pain. The severity of the pain differs as well, with some patients experiencing debilitating pain to others having mild pain.

Low-back pain can conveniently be divided into three categories: mild, moderate, and severe. Those placed in the mild group have subjective pain without objective findings and should be able to return to customary activity in less than a week. The moderate group is characterized by a limited range of motion and paravertebral muscle spasm as well as pain, and these patients should be able to return to activities in less than 2 weeks. The severe group includes those patients who are tilted forward or to the side. They have trouble ambulating and can take up to 3 weeks to become functional again.

Physical examination of these patients usually finds mild paravertebral nonspecific tenderness, limited range of motion, and no neurologic findings. Because no findings on plain films is the norm for these patients, radiographs are not initially obtained if the physician is comfortable with the diagnosis; however, if the response to the treatment does not proceed as expected, films should be taken to rule out other more serious problems, such as spondylolisthesis or tumor. The authors' usual recommendation is that if a patient fails to respond to conservative treatment for an acute attack of low-back pain after a period of 2 weeks, a routine lumbosacral spine x-ray series is clinically indicated.

The authors' preferred treatment for low-back strain is the functional restorative approach. For an acute strain, NSAIDs and a brief period of activity modification or rest is indicated to calm down the inflammatory, painful phase. Additionally, patients should be educated regarding proper postural mechanics to promote a healthy lower back. Once the acute pain subsides following a short period of activity modification, patients should begin a controlled physical therapy program either formally or, for reliable and motivated patients, on their own. The focus of the physical activity is trunk flexibility and strengthening exercises. Often, particularly in the obese patient with weak abdominal muscles, a lightweight lumbosacral corset is useful in helping mobilize those encumbered by low-back strain.

Herniated Disk

A herniated disk can be defined as the protrusion of the nucleus pulposus through the torn fibers of the annulus fibrosus. Most disk herniations occur during the third and fourth decades of life while the nucleus pulposus is still gelatinous. The perforations usually arise through a defect just lateral to the posterior midline where the PLL is weakest. The two most common levels for disk herniation are L4–L5 and L5–S1, accounting together for 95% of all lumbar disk herniations.

Because disk herniations are generally posterolateral as discussed earlier, the herniation generally affects the nerve traversing the region rather than the exiting nerve root. The spinal cord ends around L1/L2, so the nerve roots of the lumbar spine exit the cord well above that level where they exit the canal. They, therefore, have a long way to travel before exiting through the foramen, unlike in the cervical spine. The nerves begin moving laterally and inferiorly from a proximal direction rather than exiting almost in a straight lateral direction like the cervical spine. For this reason, by the time the nerve root reaches its exiting level, it is already so far lateral from its descent that a herniated disk at the level where the nerve root exits will not disrupt it unless the herniation is the much less common far lateral type. Therefore, a herniated disk will impinge upon the traversing nerve that exits at the next level down, rather than the exiting nerve, which differs from a cervical disk herniation that impinges upon the exiting nerve root. However, because the nerves in the lumbar spine exit below their respective vertebra, the same rule applies for the likely nerve impinged, which is the nerve named for the lowest vertebral segment (i.e., L4–L5 disk herniation impinges upon L5). This concept is difficult to understand initially but is a very important one to grasp conceptually.

Therefore, disk herniations at L5–S1 usually compromise the first sacral nerve root; L4–L5 herniations affect L5; L3–L4 herniations affect L4; and so forth. As alluded to earlier, variations do in fact exist in that far lateral herniations can affect the nerve exiting at the same level as the disk herniation (i.e., L4–L5 affecting L4), and other likely more central herniations can affect the nerves exiting two levels below the herniation (i.e., L4–L5 affecting the S1 root).

There are a variety of clinical presentations and histories regarding disk herniations, and not everyone with a disk herniation experiences pain. A large disk herniation in a patient with a capacious canal may not experience any symptoms at all as the nerves have room to be displaced and avoid compression. On the other end of the spectrum, a patient with a small canal may experience debilitating pain from a relatively small disk herniation as there is not enough room to accommodate the disk and the nerve root.

Clinically, the patient's major complaint is pain. Although there may be a prior history of intermittent episodes of localized low-back pain, this is not always the case. The pain not only is present in the back but radiates down the leg in the distribution of the affected nerve root. It will usually be described as sharp, or lancinating, progressing from the top downward in the involved leg. Its onset may be insidious or sudden and associated with a tearing or snapping sensation in the spine. Occasionally, when sciatica develops, the back pain may resolve because once the annulus has ruptured, it may no longer be under tension. Finally, the sciatic pain may vary in intensity as well; it may be so severe that patients will be unable to ambulate and will feel their back is "locked." Conversely, the pain may be limited to a dull ache that increases in intensity with ambulation.

On physical examination, there is usually a decreased range of motion in flexion, and patients will tend to drift away from the involved side with a bend that expands the area of the involved side and hence put less pressure on the nerve. On ambulation, the patients walk with an antalgic gait, holding the involved leg flexed so as to put as little weight as possible on the extremity.

Although neurologic examination may yield objective evidence of nerve root compression, these findings are not dependable because the involved nerve is often still functional. In addition, such a deficit may have little temporal relevance if it is related to a prior attack at a different level. To be significant, reflex changes, weakness, atrophy, or sensory changes must conform to the rest of the clinical picture.

The different physical findings that can be present are summarized in Table 12.2. Involvement of the first sacral nerve can show calf atrophy, weak plantar flexion or inability to repeatedly rise on toes, and/or diminished Achilles reflex in comparison to the opposite side. Fifth lumbar root involvement can lead to weak great toe extension and less often weak eversion and/or dorsiflexion. Compression of the fourth lumbar root can result in weak knee extension secondary to quadriceps involvement with or without quadriceps atrophy along with a diminished patellar reflex. Of note, it is important to compare both sides, especially when evaluating reflexes as many people, especially older individuals, have natural hyporeflexia. Therefore, a diminished reflex is generally only significant if it is unilateral.

Nerve root sensitivity can be elicited by any maneuver that creates tension, which most often consists of the SLRT. For the test to be positive, it must reproduce the leg pain (below the knee), not the back pain, as previously highlighted.

The diagnosis of a lumbar disk herniation is made by history and physical examination. Therefore, plain x-rays or MRI do not need to be obtained on an initial visit. If the patient fails conservative treatment, plain films should be obtained to rule out other causes of pain such as tumor or infection. MRI can be used to confirm the diagnosis (Fig. 12.25) as well as for surgical planning, but it should never be used as a screening tool as many asymptomatic pathologies that do not warrant treatment can be demonstrated on MRI and skew the examiner and the patient as to what is actually causing the symptoms. Further guidance, timing, and indications for radiologic studies will follow in the lumbar algorithm section.

The treatment for most patients with a herniated disk is nonoperative; eighty percent of them will respond to conservative treatment when followed over a period of five years. The efficacy of nonoperative treatment, however, depends upon a healthy relationship between a capable

TABLE 12.2
LUMBAR DISK HERNIATION-CLINICAL FEATURES

L3–L4 Disk: L4 Nerve Root	
■ Pain	Lower back, hip, posterolateral thigh, across patella, anteromedial leg
■ Numbness	Anteromedial thigh and knee
■ Weakness	Knee extension
■ Atrophy	Quadriceps
■ Reflexes	Patella reflex diminished
L4–5 Disk: L5 Nerve Root	
■ Pain	SI region, hip, posterolateral thigh, anterolateral leg
■ Numbness	Lateral leg, first webspace
■ Weakness	Dorsiflexion of great toe and foot
■ Atrophy	Minimal anterior calf
■ Reflexes	None
L5–S1 Disk: S1 Nerve Root	
■ Pain	SI region, hip, posterolateral thigh/leg
■ Numbness	Back of calf; lateral heel, foot, and toe
■ Weakness	Plantar flexion of foot and great toe
■ Atrophy	Gastrocnemius and soleus
■ Reflexes	Ankle jerk diminished

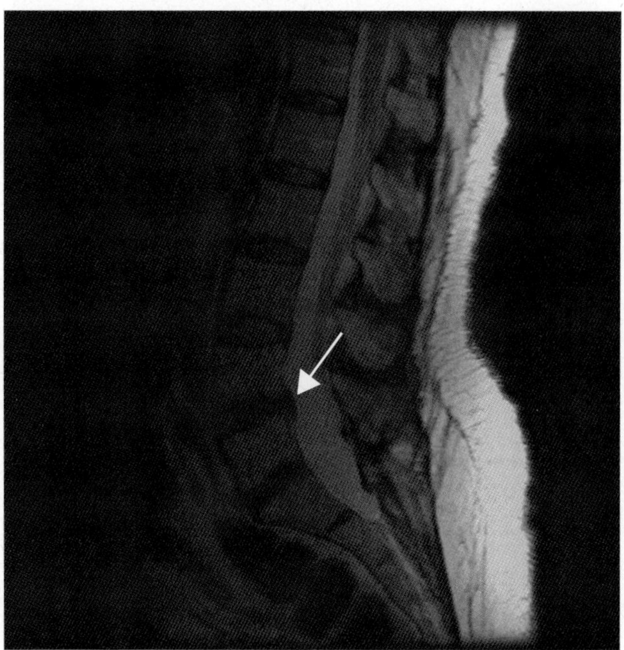

Figure 12.25 Lumbar herniated disk. Sagittal MRI of a 35-year-old female complaining of back pain with radiation to right ankle. MRI shows a disk herniation (*arrow*) at L5–S1.

physician and a well-informed patient. If a patient has insight into the rationale for the prescribed treatment and follows instructions, the chances for success are greatly increased.

One of the most important elements in nonoperative treatment is controlled physical activity. Patients should markedly decrease their activity in the acute stages. This will occasionally require bed rest and in most cases can be accomplished at home. An acute herniation usually takes about 2 weeks of rest before the pain substantially eases.

Drug therapy is another important part of the treatment, and three categories of pharmacologic agents are commonly used: anti-inflammatory drugs, analgesics, and muscle relaxants. Inasmuch as the symptoms of low-back pain and sciatica result from an inflammatory reaction as well as a mechanical compression, the authors feel that anti-inflammatory medication in the form of aspirin or NSAIDs taken regularly should be included with rest. We prefer naproxen 500 mg twice daily, although we have had success with aspirin or other NSAIDs as well. For those with GI intolerance, celecoxib or a buffering agent can be used.

Analgesic medication is rarely needed if the patient truly follows the nonoperative protocol of resting. Occasionally, narcotics will be needed to overcome the initial hump, although it should be made clear that narcotics will not be used long term and are not the answer to the problem. Rarely, a patient may need to be admitted to the hospital for pain control with IV narcotics.

There is some question as to whether there actually is a muscle relaxant; all drugs that are designated as such probably act to some degree as tranquilizers. If one is required, cyclobenzaprine is probably the most frequently used and is well tolerated with side effects of sedation and drowsiness occurring less often than with some of the other medications, though they do occur. Other choices include methocarbamol, carisoprodol, and valium, although valium is not recommended secondary to its depressant qualities, which can often add to the patient's psychological problems.

Eighty percent of those who follow the above regimen will markedly improve, but this regimen requires patience because frequently at least 6 weeks will have passed before any additional therapy is indicated. Though results are satisfying in the end, patients need to be well aware of the time constraints from the beginning to understand the rationale and to prevent frustration and depression, which often accompanies this disorder. If these conservative measures fail, patients should be considered for an injection such as a selective nerve root block, which have good efficacy in preventing surgical intervention. If the patient has no relief with injections, surgery should be considered.

The indications for surgery are less clear as there have been studies that show equal efficacy of operative and nonoperative treatment with long-term follow-up. Currently, surgery should be considered for patients with unremitting pain despite an adequate course of conservative therapy, which is at least 6 weeks. These patients need to have symptoms of leg pain, not merely back pain, for predictably good surgical results. Prior to surgery, an MRI (or CT myelogram for those who cannot have an MRI) should be obtained if not already done to confirm the diagnosis of a herniated disk. In the properly selected patient, with the appropriate history, physical examination, and confirming MRI or the equivalent, surgery is over 90% successful. Surgery involves discectomy or microdiscectomy at the affected level.

The long-term prognosis for disk herniation is quite good. It has been shown that between 85% and 90% of surgically and nonsurgically treated patients are asymptomatic at 4 year. Less than 2% of both groups remained symptomatic after 10 years.

Spinal Stenosis

Spinal stenosis can be defined as a narrowing of the spinal canal secondary to degenerative, developmental, or congenital conditions. The degree of mechanical pressure on the neural elements within the canal depends directly upon the degree of narrowing. It must be realized that every person will have some degree of narrowing with age secondary to osteoarthritis; however, not everyone will have symptoms.

The most common form of spinal stenosis is degenerative stenosis secondary to the effects of osteoarthritis on the aging spine. The stenosis is due to a combination of changes in osseous anatomy as well as soft-tissue hypertrophy. The typical sequence of events results from disk degeneration due to loss of water content that leads to segmental instability as loss of disk height results in motion within the spinal column secondary to a disruption of the biomechanics. Segmental instability, or motion between vertebral levels, leads to overriding facets, facet joint hypertrophy, osteophyte formation, hypertrophy of the ligamentum flavum and other ligamentous structures, and/or microfractures. The ultimate result is narrowing of the cord secondary to osteophytes and/or soft-tissue hypertrophy. This usually results in nerve root impingement or symptomatic stenosis at the lateral recess, though less commonly impingement can occur in the neural foramen and centrally.

Spinal stenosis affects around 2% to 10% of the population. The typical patient with lumbar stenosis is over the age of 50 when they first experience symptoms beginning with vague pains in the lower back, which slowly progress to dysesthesias and paresthesias down the legs during ambulation. The symptoms gradually increase in nature with worsening pain and/or pain after minimal walking to pain while standing. These neurogenic claudication symptoms will abate when the patient sits or lies down, though the pain usually takes more time to abate than claudication secondary to peripheral vascular disease. Ambulation and standing typically exacerbate the symptoms because those actions result in hyperextension of the lumbar spine, which further narrows an already diseased region. Sitting or lying supine results in a more kyphotic lumbar spine and thus relieves the pressure by enlarging the stenotic regions. For this reason, many of these patients will walk with their shoulder hunched forward over or anterior to the pelvis, thereby increasing kyphosis.

With maturation of the syndrome, symptoms may even occur at rest. Muscle weakness, atrophy, and asymmetric reflex changes may then appear; however, as long as the symptoms are only aggravated dynamically, neurologic changes will occur only after the patient is stressed. For this reason, most of these patients will have an absent SLRT as opposed to patients with an acute herniated disk. The physical examination of these patients will therefore be unremarkable other than nonspecific findings in the majority of cases. The following stress test can be used in an outpatient clinic; after a neurologic examination has been performed on the patient, he/she is asked to walk up and down the corridor until symptoms occur or the patient has walked 300 feet. A repeat examination is then done, and in many cases, the second examination will be positive for a focal neurologic deficit when the first was negative. While helpful if positive, this test does not rule out stenosis if negative.

Plain x-rays should be obtained when one suspects spinal stenosis and generally are helpful in visualizing stenosis, especially if it is degenerative. The typical findings are intervertebral disk degeneration or loss of height, decreased interpedicular distance, a decreased sagittal canal diameter, and facet degeneration. These are also visualized well on CT scan (Fig. 12.26). If a patient fails conservative treatment and becomes a surgical candidate, the location and degree of neurologic compression can be assessed with MRI and/or CT scan, depending on whether the compression is osseous or of soft tissue origin. Typically, preoperative planning will consist of both if the patient is able to obtain all vital pieces of information before proceeding.

The majority of patients with spinal stenosis can be treated nonoperatively with NSAIDs or the application of a lumbosacral corset. These patients also need to be educated about the natural history of their disease and activity modification. Nonoperative treatment is preferable as long as the pain is tolerable for the patient. Indications for surgery include intractable pain, worsening neurologic deficit, and inability to cope with functional limitations. Surgical intervention includes laminectomy, laminoplasty, limited laminotomy, and posterior fusion of varying levels.

Spondylolisthesis

Spondylolisthesis refers to the forward displacement of one vertebra on another. It can occur from a variety of causes and thus can be classified as congenital, isthmic, degenerative, traumatic, pathologic, and postoperative. The most frequent causes are degenerative and isthmic, though degenerative most commonly occurs in adulthood. Isthmic spondylolisthesis, on the other hand, begins in childhood and adolescence, although many times it will not present until adulthood.

Isthmic spondylolisthesis occurs secondary to spondylolysis, which means a defect in the area of the vertebra known as the pars interarticularis. Approximately 5% to 6% of the population has a defect in the pars. The reason for this is not completely understood, although it is believed to result from a fatigue-type fracture that develops in childhood. Some of these patients will remain asymptomatic, though some will progress to develop spondylolisthesis secondary to a degree of instability from the pars defect with subsequent subluxation or anterior displacement (listhesis) of one vertebra onto another. The most common areas affected are L5–S1, followed by L4–L5, and L3–L4. As alluded to earlier, spondylolysis occurs in childhood, while the eventual development and manifestations of spondylolisthesis can occur in childhood, adolescence, or adulthood.

The correlation between spondylolysis or spondylolisthesis and back pain is not clear, and there are conflicting findings in the literature. Sarasate et al. found radiographic evidence of disk degeneration and a slip of greater than 10 mm correlated positively with symptoms as did a low lumbar index, increased lumbar lordosis, and spondylolysis at L4. It is important to be aware when evaluating the patient with back pain and radiographic evidence of spondylolisthesis, however, that this condition may be non-painful and that there are many other potential sources of pain. Leaping to the conclusion that spondylolisthesis, as seen on plain films, is the source of the patient's pain may lead to unsuccessful treatment. Pain in the adult patient with spondylolisthesis has several potential sources, and each should be considered before determining that the pain is secondary to the slip.

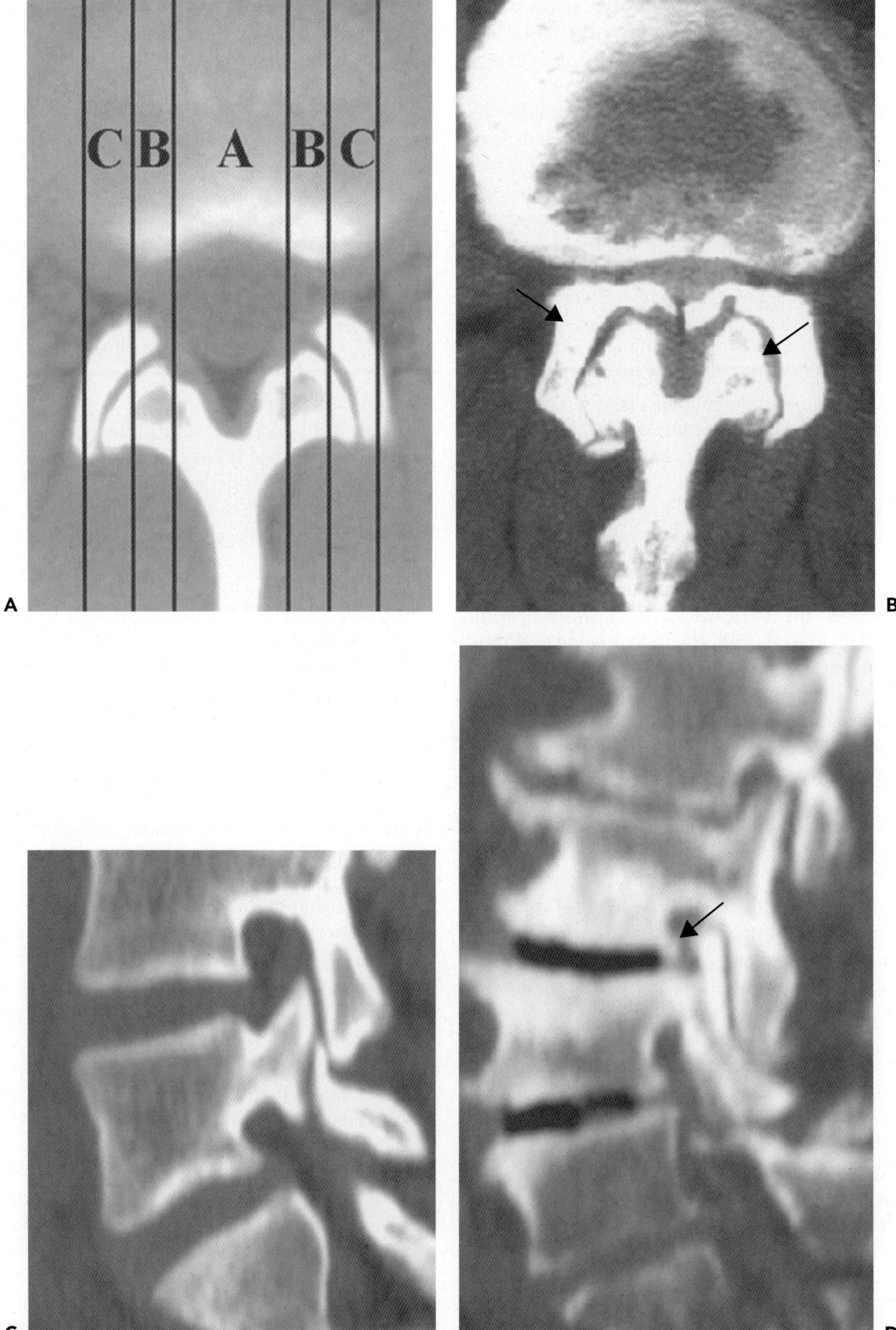

Figure 12.26 Spinal stenosis. **(A)** Axial CT scan showing the central region **(A)**, lateral recess **(B)**, and foraminal regions **(C)**. **(B)** Axial CT scan showing facet degeneration with hypertrophy and resultant lateral recess stenosis. **(C)** Normal sagittal CT scan showing foraminal dimensions. **(D)** Sagittal CT scan showing foraminal encroachment due to degenerative changes. (*Reproduced with permission from* Frymoyer JW, Wiesel SW, An HS, et al. *The Adult and Pediatric Spine*, 3rd ed. Philadelphia: Lippincott Williams & Wilkins, 2003.)

The reason for pain secondary to spondylolisthesis is unclear, but suggested sources include segmental instability and disk degeneration. Disk degeneration is more common in individuals with isthmic spondylolisthesis, at the level of the slip, and is associated with the presence of low-back pain in these patients. Leg pain is frequently present in the adult population with isthmic spondylolisthesis. Narrowing of the intervertebral foramen due to disk bulging, hypertrophy of the fibrous reparative tissue at the lysis, and a bony beak extending into the foramen from the proximal stump of the pars all contribute to foraminal stenosis and compression of the exiting nerve root, resulting in radicular symptoms.

Degenerative spondylolisthesis is most common at the L4–L5 level and is seen in the same patient population as spinal stenosis as both entities have the same underlying etiology, though with somewhat different end results. Interestingly, as opposed to spinal stenosis, spondylolisthesis occurs more commonly in women, which is thought to be secondary to increased ligamentous laxity. The degenerative changes in spondylolisthesis eventually render the vertebral column unstable to varying degrees, resulting in the displacement of one vertebra over another. It must be noted that anterolisthesis or forward displacement occurs most commonly, though retrolisthesis can occur as well. Following the common theme with spinal conditions, patients with spondylolisthesis present in a variety of ways, from completely asymptomatic to suffering from debilitating pain. The most common presenting symptoms with degenerative spondylolisthesis are lower back pain, neurogenic claudication, and radiculopathy. As many patients are asymptomatic with degenerative spondylolisthesis, again, it is absolutely essential to consider the possibility of another source of pain. Also, as with isthmic spondylolisthesis, the reason this condition is painful is not entirely clear, but likely secondary to segmental instability and disk degeneration. Radiculopathy and neurogenic claudication, on the other hand, result from narrowing of the intervertebral foramen due to disk protrusion, soft-tissue hypertrophy, or a change in osseous anatomy, as discussed in previous sections.

The history and physical examination of these patients regardless of the type of listhesis should focus on the exact location, source, and radiation patterns of the patient's pain. Patients often report a catching pain in the lower back when rising from a chair. On physical examination, this represents one of the most common findings reproduced as limited extension with a painful catch on forced extension in patients with isthmic spondylolisthesis, while there is full forward flexion. Other findings on physical examination that can be useful include a stooped posture, hip flexion contracture, and spinal muscle atrophy. Additionally, some patients will have a palpable step-off from the displacement on one segment to another. Physical examination may reveal mild L5 findings in the patient with L5–S1 spondylolisthesis, although the neurologic examination is frequently normal and SLRT is rarely positive. It must be kept in mind that many times the physical examination will be nonspecific, but ideally the history, examination, and radiographic findings should all correlate.

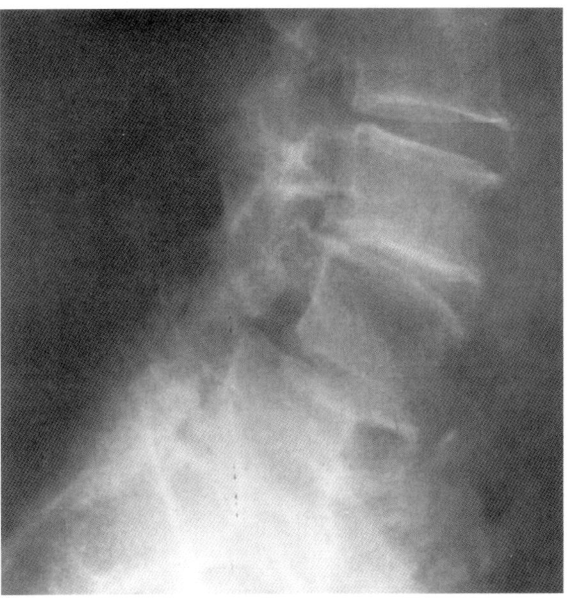

Figure 12.27 Degenerative spondylolisthesis lateral upright lumbar radiographs demonstrating instability at L4–L5 with approximately 30% slip of L4 anteriorly on L5. (*Reproduced with permission from* Chapman MW. *Chapman's Orthopaedic Surgery*, 2nd ed. Philadelphia, Lippincott Williams & Wilkins, 1993.)

Radiographic evaluation initially includes standing AP and lateral radiographs that demonstrate variable subluxation of one segment (Fig. 12.27) on another and/or a pars defect in the case of isthmic spondylolisthesis. Eighty percent of pars defects can be visualized on plain lateral radiographs, and the presence and extent of forward slippage is best defined on this view. Often, flexion and extension views are then obtained to assess the stability of the slip by evaluating for movement with each view. Myerding proposed the following classification to assess slip severity: Grade I—25% slip; Grade II—50% slip; Grade III—75% slip; and Grade IV—100% slip or greater. Complete slips (Grade IV) are referred to as spondyloptosis. Additionally, CT scan, myelography, and MRI can be used for further evaluation with MRI being the modality of choice as it provides the most information about the soft tissues. MRI accurately defines the intervertebral foramen, nerve roots, hydration status of the disks adjacent to proposed fusion sites, disk herniations, and any occult defects in the pars. MRI and often CT, to better define bony changes, are used prior to surgical consideration and for preoperative planning.

The natural history of the disease varies with the initial clinical presentation. Most patients who present with back pain do not progress and can be treated nonoperatively, while those presenting with claudication and radiculopathy often progress and will eventually need surgery. An initial regimen of nonoperative therapy is indicated for almost all patients, except those with significant neurologic deficits. Nonoperative treatment consists of NSAIDs, activity modification, and physical therapy with a focus on back strengthening, aerobic conditioning, and, especially, flexion exercises. A significant number of patients will respond to this regimen, although some will ultimately fail to find relief and require surgical intervention.

The indications for surgical intervention include persistent and intolerable back or leg pain despite a trial of nonoperative therapy; worsening neurologic symptoms; and bowel/bladder symptoms, suggestive of cauda equina syndrome. There are multiple surgeries depending on the type and severity of dysfunction with all having the common theme of arthrodesis. Standard practice is to fuse *in situ* without reduction, unless the patient is experiencing neurologic compromise or the patients has a complete slip (spondyloptosis). However, there are those who now have trended toward reducing lesser slips.

The results of fusion are affected by smoking status, degree of slippage, type of fusion selected, and the use of either internal or external immobilization. Kim and associates reported a significantly higher success rate when anterior and posterior fusion were performed and when cast immobilization was used following surgery. Improved functional outcome was reported by Hanley and Levy in adults with isthmic spondylolisthesis in noncompensation cases, women, patients with back pain only, nonsmokers, and absence of a pseudarthrosis.

Cauda Equina Syndrome

Cauda equina syndrome is a highly discussed, though uncommon, condition resulting from a large acute compression of the nerve roots in the lumbar spine that make up the cauda equina resulting in a clinical syndrome with variable amounts of back pain, sciatica, lower extremity weakness, saddle anesthesia, numbness, and bowel/bladder dysfunction. For the diagnosis to be made, the patient must have urinary symptoms that usually begin as retention, followed by incontinence. The compression generally results from a mechanical compression often by a large herniated disk most commonly at L4–L5 but can also result from compression from epidural hematoma, epidural abscess, trauma, and tumor to name a few. Additional damage to the roots can occur by venous congestion and ischemia as well.

The signs and symptoms of cauda equina syndrome are a complex mixture of low-back pain, bilateral motor weakness of the lower extremities, bilateral sciatica, saddle anesthesia, and occasionally frank paraplegia with bowel and bladder incontinence or urinary retention. As mentioned previously, urinary retention or incontinence must be present for a diagnosis of cauda equina syndrome. These patients should undergo an immediate definitive diagnostic test, usually an MRI, and, if it is positive, surgical decompression within 24 to 48 hours, usually as emergently as possible. There, however, have been no studies showing improved results from decompression within the first 24 hours compared within the first 48 hours, but there have been multiple studies showing improved results within the first 48 hours compared with more than 48 hours from the onset of symptoms.

The principal reason for prompt surgical intervention is to arrest the progression of the neurologic loss with hopeful return of function, although this is variable and often incomplete. Although the incidence of cauda equina syndrome in the entire back pain population is very low, it is the only event that requires immediate operative intervention; if its diagnosis is missed, the consequences can be devastating resulting in loss of bowel and bladder function, paraplegia, and even death.

LUMBAR SPINE ALGORITHM

As with patients with neck pain, the task of the physician when confronted with low-back pain patients is to integrate their complaints into an accurate diagnosis and to prescribe appropriate therapy. This problem (the universe of low-back pain patients) has been formulated into an algorithm, the aim of which is to select the correct diagnostic category and proper treatment avenues for each patient with low-back pain. A specific patient may fall outside of the limits of the algorithm and require a different approach, and the physician must constantly be on the alert for exceptions. The algorithm can be followed in sequence (Fig. 12.28).

The information necessary to use the algorithm initially is obtained through the history and physical examination. The key points in the history are differentiation of back pain that is mechanical in nature from nonmechanical pain that is present at rest, detecting changes in bowel or bladder function, and defining the precise location and quality of the pain. The physical examination must be oriented toward ruling out other medical causes of low-back pain, assessing neurologic function, and evaluating for the presence of tension signs.

Following the low-back pain algorithm, the first major decision is to make a ruling on the presence or absence of cauda equina syndrome. Mechanical compression of the cauda equina, with truly progressive motor weakness, is the only surgical emergency in lumbar spine disease. This compression, often from a massive rupture of the L4–L5 disk in the midline, is usually due to pressure on the caudal sac, through which pass the nerves to the lower extremities, bowel, and bladder. Patients thought to have cauda equina syndrome need emergent imaging (MRI) followed by surgical intervention within the first 24 to 48 hours.

The remaining patients make up the overwhelming majority. They should be started on a course of conservative therapy, regardless of the diagnosis. At this stage, the specific diagnosis, whether a herniated disk or simple back strain, is not important to the therapy because the entire population is treated in a similar way. A few of these patients will eventually need an invasive procedure, but at

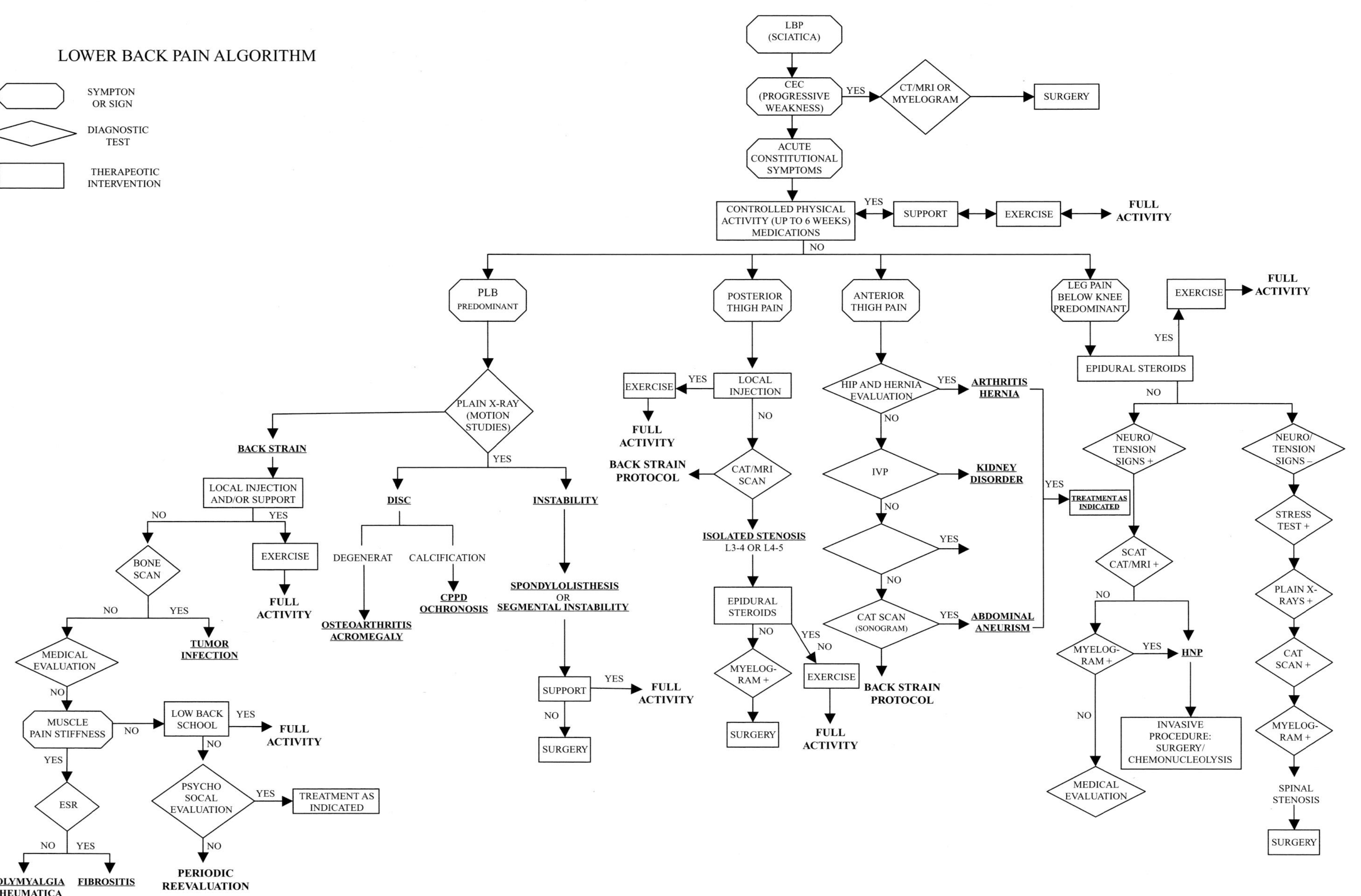

Figure 12.28 Lumbar algorithm.

this point, there is no way to predict which individuals will respond to conservative therapy and which will not.

Conservative Treatment

The vast majority in this initial group have nonradiating low-back pain, termed lumbago or back strain. The etiology of back strain is not clear. There are several possibilities, including ligamentous or muscular strain, continuous mechanical stress from poor posture, facet joint irritation, or a small tear in the annulus fibrosis. Patients usually complain of pain in the low back, often localized to a single area. On physical examination, they demonstrate a decreased range of lumbar spine motion, tenderness to palpation over the involved area, and paraspinal muscle spasm. Their roentgenographic examinations are usually normal, but if therapy is not successful, films should be obtained to rule out other possible etiologic factors. Two exceptions to this rule are patients younger than 20 years and patients over 60 years; x-rays are important early in the diagnostic process for these patients because they are more likely to have a diagnosis other than back strain (tumor or infection). Other situations warranting x-rays sooner rather than later include a history of serious trauma, known cancer, unexplained weight loss, or fever.

The early stage of treatment of low-back pain (with or without leg pain) is a waiting game. The passage of time, the use of anti-inflammatory medication, and controlled physical activity are the modalities that have proved safest and most effective. The vast majority of these patients will respond to this approach within the first 10 days, although a small percentage will not. In today's society with its emphasis on quick solutions and "high technology," many patients are pushed too rapidly toward more complex (i.e., invasive) management. This "quick fix" approach has no place in the treatment of low-back pain. The physician treats the patient conservatively and waits up to 6 weeks for a response. As already stated, most of these patients will improve within 10 days, although a few will take longer.

Once the patients have achieved approximately 80% relief, they should be mobilized with the help of a lightweight, flexible corset. After they become more comfortable and have increased their activity level, they should begin a program of isometric lumbar exercises and return to their normal lifestyles. The pathway along this section of the algorithm is a two-way street; should regression occur with exacerbation of symptoms, the physician can resort to more stringent conservative measures. The patient may require further bed rest. Most acute low-back pain patients will proceed along this pathway, returning to a normal life pattern within 2 months of the onset of symptoms.

If the initial conservative regimen fails and 6 weeks have passed, symptomatic patients are sorted into four groups. The first group comprises those with low-back pain predominating. The second group complains mainly of leg pain, defined as pain radiating below the knee and commonly referred to as sciatica. The third group has anterior thigh pain and the fourth group has posterior thigh pain. Each group follows a separate diagnostic pathway.

Refractory Patients with Low-Back Pain

Patients who continue to complain predominantly of low-back pain for 6 weeks should have plain x-rays carefully examined for abnormalities. Spondylolysis with or without spondylolisthesis is the most common structural abnormality to cause significant low-back pain. Approximately 5% of the population has this defect, thought to be caused by a combination of genetics and environmental stress. In spite of this defect, most people are able to perform their activities of daily living with little or no discomfort. When symptoms are present, these patients will usually respond to nonoperative measures, including a thorough explanation of the problem, a back support, and exercises. In a small percentage of such cases, conservative treatment fails and a fusion of the involved segments becomes necessary. This is one of the few times primary fusion of the lumbar spine is indicated, and it must be stressed that it is a relatively infrequent occurrence.

The vast majority of patients with pain predominantly in the low back will have normal plain films. The diagnosis at this point is back strain. Before there is any additional workup, a local injection of steroids and lidocaine may be tried at the point of maximum tenderness, known as a trigger point injection. This medication can be quite successful, and if there is a good response, the patient is begun on exercises, with gradual resumption of normal activity. In some instances, if there are no objective findings, a "trigger point" injection can be considered as early as the third week after onset of symptoms.

Should the patient not respond to local injection, other pathology must be seriously sought. A bone scan or an MRI, along with a general medical evaluation, should then be obtained. The bone scan is an excellent tool, often identifying early bone tumors or infections not visible on routine radiographic examination. It is particularly important to obtain one or both of these studies in the patient with nonmechanical back pain. If the pain is constant, unremitting, and unrelieved by postural adjustments, more often than not the correct diagnosis will be one of an occult neoplasm or metabolic disorder not readily apparent from other testing.

Approximately 3% of cases of apparent low-back pain that present at orthopedic clinics are attributed to extraspinal causes. A thorough medical search frequently reveals problems missed earlier such as a posterior penetrating ulcer, pancreatitis, renal disease, or an abdominal aneurysm. If these diagnostic studies are positive, the patient should be transferred into a nonorthopedic treatment mode and would no longer be in the therapeutic algorithm.

Patients who have no abnormality on their bone scan or MRI and do not show other medical disease as a cause for their back pain are then referred to another type of therapy—the low-back school. It is believed that many of these patients are suffering from discogenic pain or facet joint pain syndrome. The low-back school concept has as its basis the belief that patients with low-back pain, given proper education and understanding of their disease, can often return to a productive and functional life. Ergonomics, the proper and efficient use of the spine in work and recreation, is stressed. Back school need not be an expensive proposition. It can be a one-time classroom session with a review of back problems and a demonstration of exercises with patient participation. This type of educational process has proved to be very effective. It is most important, however, that before they are referred to this type of program, patients are thoroughly screened. One does not want to be in the position of treating a metastatic tumor in a classroom.

If low-back school is not successful, the patient should undergo a thorough psychosocial evaluation in an attempt to explain the failure of the previous treatments. This is predicated on the knowledge that a patient's disability is related not only to his or her pathologic anatomy but also to his/her perception of pain and stability in relation to the social environment. It is quite common to see a stable patient with a frank herniated disk continue working, regarding the disability as only a minor problem, while a hysterical patient takes to bed at the slightest twinge of back discomfort.

Drug habituation, depression, alcoholism, and other psychiatric problems are seen frequently in association with back pain. If the evaluation suggests any of these problems, proper measures should be instituted to overcome the disability. There are a surprising number of ambulatory patients addicted to commonly prescribed medications using complaints of back pain as an excuse to obtain these drugs. Oxycodone, hydrocodone, and diazepam are the most popular offenders. Oxycodone and hydrocodone are truly addictive; diazepam is both habituating and depressing. Because the complaint of low-back pain may be a common manifestation of depression, it is counterproductive to treat such patients with diazepam.

Approximately 2% of patients who initially present with low-back pain will fail treatment and elude any diagnosis. There will be no evidence of any structural problem in the back or criteria for an underlying medical disease or psychiatric disorder. This is a very difficult group to manage. The authors' strategy has been to discontinue narcotics, reassure the patients, and periodically reevaluate them. Over time, one-third of these patients will be found to have an underlying medical disease; thus, one cannot abandon this group and discontinue treatment. For the remainder, as much physical activity as possible should be encouraged.

Refractory Patients with Sciatica

The next group of patients is those with sciatica that is pain radiating below the knee. These patients usually experience their symptoms secondary to mechanical pressure and inflammation of the nerve roots that originate in the back and extend down the leg. The etiology of the mechanical pressure can be soft tissue, such as a herniated disk, or bone, or a combination of the two.

At this point in the algorithm, the patient has had up to 6 weeks of controlled physical activity and medication but still has persistent leg pain. The next therapeutic step is an epidural steroid injection, which is performed on an outpatient basis. An epidural injection is worth trying; the chance of success is around 40% and the morbidity rate is low, particularly compared with the next step—surgery. The maximum benefit from a single injection is achieved at 2 weeks. The injection may have to be repeated once or twice, and 4 to 6 weeks should pass before its success or failure can be judged.

If epidural steroids are effective in alleviating the patient's leg pain or sciatica, the patient is begun on a program of back exercises and encouraged to return promptly to as normal a lifestyle as possible. Should the epidural steroids prove ineffective, and 3 months have passed since the initial onset of symptoms without relief of pain, some type of invasive treatment should be considered. The patient group is then divided into those with probable herniated disks and those with symptoms secondary to spinal stenosis or degenerative disease.

The physician must now carefully reevaluate the patient for a neurologic deficit and for a positive tension sign or SLRT. For those who have either a neurologic deficit or positive tension signs along with continued leg pain, an MRI scan should be obtained. If the MRI is clearly positive and correlates with physical findings, testing is done and surgical intervention can then be considered. If there is any question about the findings, one should proceed with either a CT scan or a myelogram to further evaluate.

As in the cervical spine, there is repeated documentation that for surgery to be effective in the treatment of a herniated disk, the surgeon must find unequivocal operative evidence of a nerve root compression. Accordingly, nerve root compression must be firmly substantiated preoperatively, not only by neurologic examination but also by radiographic data. There is no place for "exploratory" back surgery. Many asymptomatic patients have been found to have abnormal myelograms, EMGs, CT scans, and MRI scans. If the patient has neither a neurologic deficit nor a positive SLRT, regardless of radiographic findings, there is not enough evidence of root compression to proceed with surgery. These patients without objective findings are the ones who have poor results.

If there are no objective findings, the physician should avoid surgery and proceed to psychosocial evaluation. Exceptions should be few and far between. When sympathy for the patient's complaints outweighs the objective evaluation, surgery is fraught with difficulties. For those who meet these specific criteria for surgery, results will be satisfactory; 95% of these patients can expect to have a good to excellent result.

The second group of patients whose symptoms are on the basis of mechanical pressure on the neural elements are those with spinal stenosis. The diagnosis of spinal stenosis usually can be inferred from the plain x-rays, which will demonstrate facet degeneration, disk degeneration, decreased interpedicular distance, and decrease sagittal canal diameter as previously reviewed. A CT scan or MRI scan can confirm the diagnosis. If symptoms are severe, and there is radiographic evidence of spinal stenosis, surgery is appropriate. Age alone is not a deterrent to surgery; many elderly people who are in good health except for a narrow spinal canal will benefit greatly from adequate decompression of the lumbar spine.

Refractory Patients with Anterior Thigh Pain

A small percentage of patients will have pain that radiates from the back into the anterior thigh. This usually is relieved by rest and anti-inflammatory medication. If the discomfort persists after 6 weeks of treatment, a workup should be initiated to search for an underlying disorder. Although an upper lumbar radiculopathy can cause anterior thigh pain, several other entities must be considered.

A hip problem or hernia can be ruled out with a thorough physical examination. If the hip examination is positive, radiographs should be obtained. An IV pyelogram is useful to evaluate the urinary tract because kidney stones often may present as anterior thigh pain. Peripheral neuropathy, most commonly secondary to diabetes, also can present initially with anterior thigh pain; a glucose tolerance test and EMG will reveal the diagnosis. Finally, a retroperitoneal tumor can cause symptoms by mechanically pressing on the nerves that innervate the anterior thigh. A CT scan or MRI scan or the retroperitoneal area will eliminate or confirm this possibility.

If any of the entities reviewed here is diagnosed, the patient is treated accordingly. If no physical cause can be found for anterior thigh pain, the patient is treated for recalcitrant back strain by the method already outlined.

Refractory Patients with Posterior Thigh Pain

This final group of patients will complain of back pain with radiation into the buttock and posterior thigh. Most of them will be relieved of their symptoms with 6 weeks of conservative therapy. However, if their pain persists after the initial treatment period, they can be considered to have back strain and given a trigger point injection in the area of maximum tenderness. If the injection is unsuccessful, it is necessary to distinguish between referred and radicular pain.

As noted earlier, referred pain is the pain in mesodermal tissues of the same embryologic origin. The muscles, tendons, and ligaments of the buttocks and posterior thigh have the same embryologic origin as the lower back. When the lower back is injured, pain may be referred to the posterior thigh, where it is perceived by the patient. Referred pain from irritated soft tissues cannot be cured with a surgical procedure.

Radicular pain is caused by compression of an inflamed nerve root along the anatomic course of the nerve. A herniated disk or spinal stenosis in the high lumbar area can cause radiation of pain into the posterior thigh. An MRI or CT scan and an EMG may be used in this situation to differentiate radicular etiology from referred pain or a peripheral nerve lesion. If the studies are within normal limits, the patient is considered to have low-back strain and treated according to the algorithm. If a radicular abnormality is found, the patient is diagnosed as having mechanical compression on the neural elements either from a herniated disk or spinal stenosis. Epidural steroids should be tried first; if these drugs do not provide adequate relief, surgery should be contemplated.

This group of patients with unexplained posterior thigh pain is very difficult to treat. The biggest mistake is the performance of surgery on people thought to have radicular pain but who actually have referred pain. Again, referred pain in this setting is not responsive to surgery.

In most instances, the treatment of low-back pain is no longer a mystery. The algorithm described here presents a series of easy-to-follow and clearly defined decision-making processes. Use of this algorithm provides patients with the most helpful diagnostic and therapeutic measures at the optimal time. It neither denies them helpful surgery nor subjects them to procedures that are useless technical exercises.

ADULT SCOLIOSIS

Scoliosis is described as a coronal plane curvature occurring most commonly in the thoracic, thoracolumbar, and lumbar spine. Although the frontal curve is the most commonly recognized aspect of the deformity, scoliosis is a three-dimensional abnormality with alterations not only in the frontal plane but also in the sagittal and axial planes, all contributing significantly to the cosmetic deformity and morbidity seen with this condition. Adult scoliosis refers to scoliosis in the skeletally mature individual, in most series, beyond the age of 20.

The prevalence of scoliosis, as well as the severity of the curves identified, increases with increasing age. Kostuik and Bentivoglio reported on 5,000 patients undergoing IV pyelography, noting 3.9% of these individuals to have thoracolumbar or lumbar curves greater than 10 degrees. They also noted that the overall prevalence was probably somewhat higher, but chest radiographs were not included. Many authors have noted the potential for *de novo* development of scoliosis in middle-aged and older patients secondary to degenerative changes, as well as the tendency for mild-to-moderate curves in adolescence to progress slowly during adulthood, leading to increasing prevalence and severity as older patients are surveyed.

When treating an adult patient with scoliosis, the etiology of the curve is frequently related to the age of the patients. Young and middle-aged adults frequently present with idiopathic scoliosis that may have been diagnosed in adolescence or may be newly identified. Older patients will be more likely to have newly diagnosed scoliosis secondary to degenerative disease. In fact, the most common form of scoliosis is degenerative in nature.

Patient presentation again varies with adult scoliosis, and often depends on the type of scoliosis, that is, idiopathic versus degenerative. Some patients have no complaints, and scoliosis is discovered as an incidental finding, for example, on a chest x-ray. The most common presenting complaint for the adult patient with idiopathic scoliosis is back pain, and it is incumbent on the physician to clearly identify the location of the pain, in particular whether it is related to the curve or is the more typical low-back pain. It is important to recognize that there is no clear-cut correlation between the presence of idiopathic scoliosis and back pain. The vast majority of the pediatric population with idiopathic scoliosis present with painless deformity. A certain percentage of adults with idiopathic scoliosis will develop persistent, at times worsening pain that is clearly related to their curve and are good candidates for either nonsurgical or surgical treatment. On the other hand, many patients with scoliosis present with nonspecific low-back pain. In these individuals, treatment directed at the curve, especially surgical treatment, is unlikely to be effective. Curve progression may occur even in adulthood and is more likely in curves that are greater than 50 degrees at the time of skeletal maturity, particularly right thoracic curves. Slow progression is seen, so it is important to compare curve measurements over a period of 5 or even 10 years to accurately identify possible curve progression. Although pulmonary symptoms, and even respiratory failure, have been reported in scoliosis, the incidence of objective respiratory insufficiency is really quite low. Finally, cosmesis is a significant concern of many patients with idiopathic scoliosis. This is particularly true in the adult, although many patients are reluctant to identify this to the physician as a reason for seeking treatment.

The second and more extensive group of patients presents with degenerative scoliosis. These patients are typically older and have only recently been diagnosed with scoliosis. The etiology of degenerative scoliosis is uncertain, but it probably related to preexisting small curves that progress as a response to asymmetric degeneration and collapse in the posterior facets and anterior disk thereby essentially destabilizing the column. Significant spondylotic changes are seen with associated rotation, coronal plane curvature, and frequently loss of lumbar lordosis. Central, lateral recess, and foraminal stenosis are common, thereby leading to possible nerve root compression in the concavity of either the primary lumbar or the lumbosacral fractional curve (opposite the primary curve). These patients therefore usually have a history of long standing, gradually worsening low-back pain and seek treatment secondary to a newer onset of symptoms typical of spinal stenosis secondary to nerve root compression.

Evaluation

Evaluation of the patient with scoliosis includes history, physical examination, and radiographic studies. The history should focus on determining the chief complaint of the patient, whether it is back pain, neurogenic claudication, loss of balance, or deformity. If pain is the presenting complaint, one must obtain a clear, detailed description of the exact location of the pain as well as radiation. Evidence of curve progression, such as loss of height or a notable change, over the last few years, in the fit of clothing, is important. It is also important to ask about the patient's subjective sense of balance.

Physical examination should follow the typical spine physical examination with focus on gait, balance, and range of motion. The presence of a rotational rib, flank deformity, or a leg length discrepancy should be noted. Neurologic testing seeking both upper and lower motor neuron findings is carried out; it should be noted that idiopathic scoliosis, as opposed to degenerative scoliosis, never results in spinal cord compression or paraplegia, and the presence of upper motor neuron findings such as clonus or a positive Babinski's sign should trigger a search for intraspinal pathology.

Radiographic evaluation includes standing PA (Fig. 12.29) and lateral radiographs of the full spine, bending films when surgery is contemplated, and may include supine views of the lumbar region to better define degenerative changes. The Cobb angle is used to measure curve severity and document progression. MRI should be obtained in cases of rapid progression, any upper motor neuron finding, or a history suggestive of lumbar stenosis. It should be noted that the abnormal three-dimensional anatomy seen in scoliosis secondary to rotation and curvature superimposed on the spondylotic changes present with degenerative scoliosis may make accurate diagnosis of the site and severity of stenosis difficult on MRI. Therefore, CT is often obtained as well to better delineate the bony anatomy.

Treatment

Many patients with scoliosis present for evaluation and treatment of their backs, but only rarely is surgical treatment necessary. Accurate identification of the patient's major source of concern will in many cases lead to observation as the appropriate form of management. When treatment is indicated, many patients either have low-back pain, leading to nonoperative management in most cases, or have mild-to-moderate curve-related pain, which will frequently respond to nonoperative treatment as well.

Nonoperative treatment for low-back pain related to scoliosis essentially follows the treatment protocol outlined earlier. Usually a program of weight reduction, aerobic

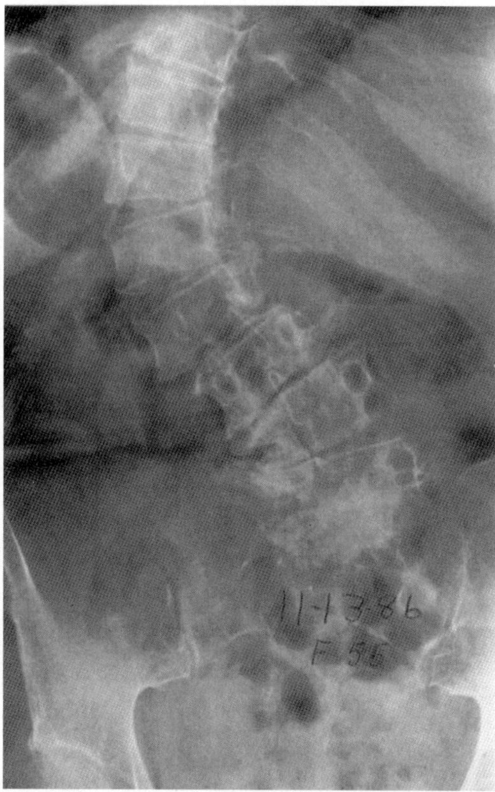

Figure 12.29 Adult degenerative scoliosis. Note the coronal plane curvature. The curve is secondary to degenerative changes from spondylosis. (*Reproduced with permission from* Chapman MW. *Chapman's Orthopaedic Surgery*, 2nd ed. Philadelphia, Lippincott Williams & Wilkins, 1993.)

exercise, and back stretching and strengthening exercises will relieve symptoms when combined with NSAIDs. Other nonoperative options used less frequently are injections (i.e., trigger point, facet joint, or epidural steroid injections), transcutaneous electrical nerve stimulation (TENS), and medical management of any metabolic abnormalities associated with scoliosis such as osteoporosis. Some advocate the use of tricyclic antidepressants for help with night pain and gabapentin or pregabalin for neurogenic pain, though success with these medications is less consistent. The use of narcotics, as highlighted in previous sections, is limited and should be prescribed only for short-term use, if at all. Occasionally a custom-molded thoracolumbosacral orthosis (TLSO) is utilized in an individual who is a poor surgical candidate. It should be noted that orthoses do not stop progression of the curve and are used primarily to control symptoms.

There are no standardized indications on when to operate on these patients, but for the most part, surgery is reserved for patients with documented curve progression, intractable pain clearly related to the curve itself, or a persistent, unacceptable pain pattern secondary to stenosis in a patient with degenerative scoliosis. Cosmesis is rarely identified as the primary indication for surgical treatment, although many patients will attest to its importance when questioned following surgery.

The goals of surgery depend on the reason for the operation but usually involve decompression and fusion, curve correction and fusion, or a combination of the two, with emphasis on the need for fusion in these patients to control pain and prevent subsequent curve progression following surgery. Virtually, all modern scoliosis surgery includes fusion and instrumentation utilizing pedicle screws, multiple hooks, sublaminar wires, or combinations with the addition of bone graft. Approaches include posterior, anterior, or a combination.

Posterior fusion with instrumentation is indicated for moderately severe curves, particularly flexible curves, and is most often employed in isolated thoracic curves. When a curve exceeds 60 to 70 degrees, is particularly rigid, or extends into the thoracolumbar and lumbar spine, isolated posterior fusion is inadequate leading to a high rate of pseudarthrosis. In these cases, a combined anterior approach is best utilized. Anterior instrumentation and anterior fusion is commonly used in isolation in younger patients with flexible thoracolumbar or lumbar curves in an attempt to save a distant fusion level. It is most commonly utilized in combination with a posterior approach, especially with more rigid curves.

Results of surgery for scoliosis in the adult depend on a number of factors, including curve etiology, severity, patient age, and the patient's presenting complaint. Pain is the most common indication for surgery in adult scoliosis, but pain relief frequently is inadequate. Careful correlation of the patient's complaints with their spinal deformity, as well as establishing realistic goals for the surgery, offers the best hope for minimizing this problem. Curve correction is certainly less in adults than in adolescents, although this can be improved utilizing a combined anterior and posterior approach, in which case curve correction of 40% to 50% is routinely reported. Patients have an overall high satisfaction with cosmetic results, and this is particularly important to many patients, although may not be their primary reason for obtaining surgery. Complications from surgery occur approximately 20% of the time and include a wide array of problems from major to minor. Neurologic complications can occur, although they are rare. Complications include pseudarthroses, wound infection, respiratory complications, urinary tract infections, hardware failure, junctional kyphosis, and neurologic injury, amongst others. Overall, surgery can be successful in the properly selected patient, but proper patient education and understanding of the goals, limitations, and risks of surgery must be established prior to embarking on surgical treatment.

TUMORS OF THE SPINE

The overwhelming majority of neoplastic afflictions of the spine are metastatic. The skeleton is the third most common site of metastatic deposit (after the lung and liver), and the spine is the most common skeletal location for metastatic disease. It has been estimated that up to 70% of patients with disseminated cancer will have evidence of skeletal metastasis on autopsy, and symptomatic disease of the spine is the most frequent clinically significant manifestation. Primary tumors of the spine, on the other hand, are exceedingly rare. Their occurrence, however, extends over the entire age spectrum, and pain, deformity, and paralysis can occur as a result of either benign or malignant primary neoplasms. For this reason, despite their relatively infrequent appearance, these lesions merit review.

Pain is the most common presenting complaint of patients with tumor of the spine. Back pain almost always precedes neurologic involvement, and a common progression of back pain, followed by radicular pain, followed by cord compression, and dysfunction is seen. Other than the age of the patient, very little in history or physical examination serves to differentiate the presence of a primary from a metastatic tumor. Historical points that should serve to alert the physician to the possibility of metastatic disease as the cause for a patient's pain include age over 50; constitutional symptoms such as unexplained weight loss, fever, and so on; night pain; and a history of prior malignancy. Specific questioning about a previous diagnosis of cancer is necessary, even though many would assume such information to be an obvious point in routine questioning about past medical history. Additionally, one must be aware of the distinct possibility of late presentation of skeletal metastases, particularly in cancer of the breast.

When evaluating the patient with a known primary lesion of the spine, some generalizations can be made regarding the differentiation between benign and malignant disease. Younger patients are more likely to have a benign spinal neoplasm, whereas, after the age of 21, over 70% of primary tumors are malignant. As the age group extends into older patients, it becomes apparent that the risk of malignancy, either primary or secondary, is markedly increased. Additionally, the location of the lesion also gives a clue as to its histology. Most lesions of the vertebral body are malignant including primary and metastatic tumors, whereas disease involving the posterior elements is more likely to be benign.

Evaluation of the patient with a possible spinal tumor begins with the history, concentrating on the points just described. Careful questioning about the location and extent of the pain as well as activities and positions that exacerbate and ameliorate the symptoms is essential. In addition, constitutional symptoms are reviewed, and questioning about bowel and bladder function is carried out; bowel and bladder dysfunction may be seen in cases of cord compression and may, on occasion, precede back pain. On physical examination, tenderness, spasm, deformity, and the presence of a mass are sought. Most important, a careful neurologic examination is performed. This assessment must include sensory and motor testing along the trunk to determine a subtle sensory pinprick level. The presence or absence of upper motor neuron findings should be ascertained.

Radiographic evaluation includes plain films, scintigraphy, CT scanning, and MRI. Plain radiographs are routinely obtained, although they are relatively insensitive to the presence of either primary or secondary neoplasm. Plain film findings that may be present include pathologic compression fracture, lysis of a vertebral body, or deformity. On AP views, involvement of a pedicle, with destruction of its cortical bone, may lead to the "winking owl sign." Although most metastatic lesions arise from the vertebral body, it has been well documented that plain radiographic evidence of bony destruction in the vertebral body is not apparent until somewhere between 30% and 50% of the trabecular bone has been destroyed. In many cases, the tumor spreads before this point into the pedicle, where destruction of the mostly cortical bone leads to early radiographic identification of the absent pedicle.

For the reasons discussed earlier, plain films are not very sensitive at screening for tumors. On the other hand, technetium-99 bone scanning is a highly sensitive test for screening the skeleton for metastatic or any neoplastic disease. These lesions appear as increased uptake on bone scanning with the exception of multiple myeloma and other aggressively lytic lesions that may appear cold. Although relatively nonspecific in differentiating tumor from infection or fracture, routine bone scanning is used as a surveillance method to detect early metastases. Metastatic lesions will appear on a bone scan from 3 to 18 months prior to plain films. Bone scans also provide the added benefit of scanning the whole body to see if there are other lesions. Because of its lack of specificity, bone scanning has largely been replaced by MRI, but there still remains a large benefit from bone scanning especially when screening for distant metastatic lesions.

CT scanning with or without myelography can be used to more clearly delineate the cross-sectional bony anatomy and extent of bony destruction involved, while to a lesser extent evaluate the extent of cord compression or neural impingement. MRI has largely supplanted CT in the evaluation of most metastatic disease of the spine, but CT can be very helpful in evaluating primary tumors, particularly those involving the posterior elements, and most clearly defines the pathologic bony anatomy. Additionally, CT can be very helpful for preoperative planning.

MRI has evolved as the gold standard for imaging of the spine. Advantages include the lack of ionizing radiation, noninvasiveness, and the ability to identify marrow replacement patterns, soft-tissue masses, and neurologic compression. MRI is the most sensitive radiologic means of evaluating neoplastic disease, and it is certainly the most specific modality for differentiating tumor from infection. This common question is resolved, primarily, by involvement of the disk. Relatively resistant to metastatic spread by its lack of vascularity, the disk is typically spared on plain radiography as well as on MRI in cases of metastatic disease.

On the other hand, infection, which usually arises in the vertebral body, rapidly spreads into the disk, and extensive destruction of the disk is commonly seen on plain radiographs and MRI. Additionally, although not necessary in all cases, MRI can be enhanced with addition of gadolinium contrast to evaluate the soft tissue, the spinal canal, and the epidural space.

Primary Benign Tumors

Primary tumors of the spine can be differentiated on the basis of tissue origin, location, and age of the patient. Soft-tissue or bony tumors may be seen, and these lesions may arise primarily in the vertebral body or in the posterior elements. It is important to know that benign tumors of the spine arise primarily in the posterior elements, while malignant lesions arise primarily in the vertebral body. In addition, the age of the patient has been demonstrated in several series to provide predictive value as to whether a benign or malignant tumor is present, with adults much more likely to suffer from primary malignancy than children.

Osteoid Osteoma/Osteoblastoma

Osteoid osteoma and osteoblastoma are tumors of bony origin that commonly arise in the spine, almost exclusively in the posterior elements. These tumors can be differentiated from each other on the basis of size, with osteoid osteoma consisting of a nidus less than 2 cm and osteoblastoma being greater than 2 cm. Approximately 40% of osteoid osteoma and 30% of osteoblastomas occur in the spine, with both occurring most commonly in the second and third decades. Both present as back pain, usually unrelated to activity. Osteoid osteomas occur most commonly in the lumbar spine, while osteoblastomas occur most commonly in the cervical spine, though both can be found throughout the spine. Radiographic demonstration, particularly with the smaller osteoid osteoma, is difficult and x-rays often appear normal. When this lesion is suspected and films are normal, technetium bone scanning enables localization of the lesion that is then better defined by CT (Fig. 12.30). Both of these lesions can result in painful scoliosis, which is usually rapidly progressive and rigid, and these should be considered when pain is the presenting complaint in a patient with a spinal deformity. Osteoid osteoma more commonly results in scoliosis than osteoblastoma. As mentioned earlier, back pain is the most common complaint with 30% of these patients experiencing the pain at night. Classically, the pain in osteoid osteoma is relieved with aspirin or NSAIDs, though this occurs only about 30% of the time in the spine.

Excision is the preferred treatment for both of these lesions, though asymptomatic patients with osteoid osteoma can be monitored. Intralesional curettage and bone grafting as needed result in excellent pain relief with small recurrence rates in osteoid osteoma, while recurrence rates

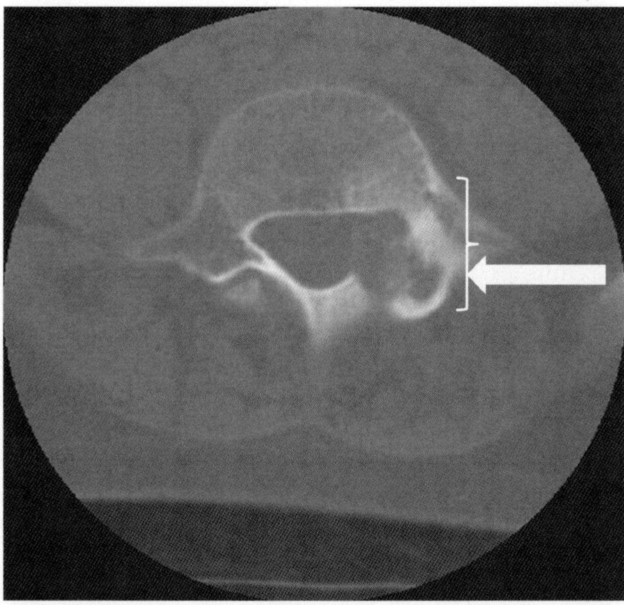

Figure 12.30 Osteoblastoma. Radiographic appearance of an osteoblastoma (cross-sectional CT scan through the L5 lesion). The lesion is larger than the osteoid osteoma, and there is a significant soft-tissue mass extending into the spinal canal. (*Reproduced with permission from* Frymoyer JW, Wiesel SW, An HS, et al. *The Adult and Pediatric Spine*, 3rd ed. Philadelphia: Lippincott Williams & Wilkins, 2003.)

tend to be higher with this treatment for osteoblastoma. Therefore, most osteoblastomas are treated by wide excision if possible. The best indication for successful excision of these lesions is the relief of pain following treatment. On occasion, an osteoblastoma will destroy enough of the posterior arch and associated facet joint so as to require stabilization, particularly when seen at the thoracolumbar junction, but this is relatively uncommon. Finally, when recognized early, painful scoliosis resulting from these entities will usually resolve. If scoliosis persists, surgical indications and techniques mirror those for idiopathic scoliosis.

Aneurysm Bone Cyst

Aneurysmal bone cyst is a less common lesion affecting the spine. Most lesions arise in the posterior elements, but up to 40% extend into the vertebral body. Pain is the typical presentation occurring in approximately 95% of patients. Radiographically, a lytic, fairly extensive lesion is seen, and it may involve more than one level. MRI with gadolinium contrast typically shows septa with fluid–fluid levels. The treatment involves excision that, in many cases, consists of intralesional curettage following embolization, with recurrence rates of approximately 10% to 15%. Recurrence is treated with repeat curettage.

Hemangioma

At autopsy, approximately 10% of individuals will have evidence of hemangioma somewhere in the spinal column, making hemangioma the most common benign neoplasm of the spine. Most of these lesions are silent clinically, and the correlation between the presence of a hemangioma and back pain is therefore uncertain. Though most benign lesions occur in the posterior elements, hemangioma most commonly occurs in the vertebral body, though approximately 10% appear in the posterior elements. The diagnosis of vertebral body hemangioma is typically made on plain radiographs, in which increased trabecular striations and a "jailhouse vertebrae" appearance may be seen. Differentiation from Paget's disease, wherein the vertebral body will actually be enlarged, should be possible on plain radiography. CT and MRI scan will show, on axial images, a punctuate appearance to the thickened trabeculae with the addition of a high signal seen on T2-weighted MR images. Occasionally, a hemangioma will present with a soft-tissue mass, although neurologic impairment is rare.

Hemangiomas are treated symptomatically. Therefore, most do not require any therapy. In those with symptomatic hemangiomas, we have had success with alcohol sclerotherapy in which ethanol is injected into the lesion via CT guidance. Additionally, radiation therapy succeeds in relieving pain in approximately 50% to 80% of cases. Others have reported success with vertebroplasty in which bone cement is injected into the vertebral body, essentially filling the lesion. Because of the risk of hemorrhage, surgery should be reserved for cases of pathologic fracture and/or neurologic injury. Prior to surgery, embolization of the lesion should be done to minimize the risk of bleeding.

Giant Cell Tumor

Giant cell tumor is occasionally seen in the spine and typically involves young adults. It is the second most common benign neoplasm of the spine occurring in the sacrum the vast majority of the time. Usually arising in the vertebral body, extensive destruction and expansion of the bone may be seen. As with most other vertebral tumors, pain is the most common presenting complaint, followed by neurologic impairment. MRI is vital in demonstrating the extent of disease and in helping guide surgical treatment. Because of the aggressive nature of these lesions, surgical treatment involves wide excision with reconstruction. Despite aggressive treatment, recurrence is common with a rate between 10% and 50%.

Primary Malignant Neoplasms of the Spine

Multiple Myeloma, Plasmacytoma, and Lymphoma

Hematogenous malignancies of the spine include multiple myeloma, plasmacytoma, and lymphoma. Multiple myeloma and plasmacytoma represent two ends of a spectrum of B-cell lymphoproliferative diseases. Solitary plasmacytoma involves an isolated lesion that commonly occurs in the spine, whereas in multiple myeloma, as the name implies, the disease is disseminated and the prognosis bleak. Anemia is common with multiple myeloma, and the presence of an osteopenic compression fracture in a patient who is anemic should alert the physician to the possibility of myeloma. Although plasmacytoma is considered a precursor to disseminated myeloma, the natural history is significantly better; McLain and Weinstein reported a 5-year survival rate of 60% with solitary plasmacytoma of the spine, whereas the 5-year survival rate in patients with multiple myeloma was only 18%. Both diseases occur equally in men and women presenting most commonly between the sixth and eighth decades. Diagnosis can generally be suspected by radiographs showing lytic lesions in the case of multiple myeloma or a solitary lesion in the case of plasmacytoma. Confirmation occurs with a monoclonal gammopathy on serum and urine electrophoresis. Local treatment of these lesions consists of radiation in most cases. The exquisite radiosensitivity of this condition usually renders operative treatment unnecessary, and surgery is reserved for pathologic fractures with spinal instability or neurologic deficit that worsens despite radiation. Mild or moderate degrees of cord compromise due to soft-tissue spread of myeloma can usually be treated with radiation.

Lymphoma, either primary or metastatic, can occur as an isolated spinal lesion. Approximately 10% of cases of lymphoma of bone, either primary or secondary, involve the spine with predilection for the thoracic spine. Local treatment consists of radiotherapy with adjuvant chemotherapy if multifocal disease is present. Surgery is reserved for cases of pathologic fracture with instability or neurologic compromise not responding to radiation therapy.

Osteosarcoma

The spine is a rare site for primary osteogenic sarcoma (only 3% of all primary osteosarcomas), and the treatment of osteosarcoma in this location represents a particularly challenging undertaking with a poor prognosis. Most patients present with pain, although neurologic deficits are present over 50% of the time as well. Most cases arise in the vertebral body, usually with extensive soft-tissue masses or extra-compartmental disease at the time of diagnosis. A variety of radiographic appearances may be seen from blastic to lytic or a combination, both generally involving cortical destruction. CT is useful to show the pathologic bony anatomy, while MRI is useful in delineating the soft-tissue pathology. Although prognosis is poor, an aggressive attempt at chemotherapy prior to en bloc excision and reconstruction followed by adjuvant radiotherapy is generally recommended.

Ewing's Sarcoma

As with osteosarcoma, Ewing's sarcoma rarely presents in the spine, accounting for approximately 5% of all cases. It also has a predilection for the vertebral body and is most common in the sacrum (50% of the time). Again, patients present most commonly with pain, although neurologic deficits are common with Ewing's sarcoma. Secondary soft-tissue extension is typical, and it is commonly present at the time of diagnosis. These tumors are generally lytic in nature with evidence of soft-tissue extension on MRI. Diagnosis is generally not made until after biopsy showing small round blue cells. The radiosensitivity of Ewing's sarcoma makes high-dose radiotherapy with adjuvant chemotherapy the treatment of choice for most lesions. Surgery is undertaken for pathologic fracture with instability or neurologic compromise. Although better than for osteosarcoma, the prognosis for patients with Ewing's sarcoma of the spine is worse than for extremity disease, and 5-year survival rates are around 30% with proper treatment.

Chordoma

Chordoma is a slow growing malignancy arising from the residual notochord in the midline of the spine and skull base. These tumors are most common in the sacrum and the clivus (skull base) but can occasionally be seen in the lumbar, thoracic, and cervical spine as well. It is twice as common in men compared with women and commonly presents between the fifth and seventh decades of life. Secondary to its indolent nature, symptoms develop slowly, and patients frequently have a large paraspinal or presacral mass present at the time of diagnosis. Many times, the mass may be palpated on examination through the rectum. Radiographs typically show a lytic lesion with variable amounts of calcification. MRI is the imaging of choice to evaluate these lesions as there is usually a significant soft-tissue component at the time of diagnosis (Fig. 12.31). Though the tumor is slow growing, high recurrence rates are seen without wide surgical excision. True cure of the patient with chordoma is rare, but long-term survival can be achieved with local disease control. Aggressive surgical excision should be undertaken, even if sacrifice of sacral nerve roots is the price; functional disability related to sacral nerve

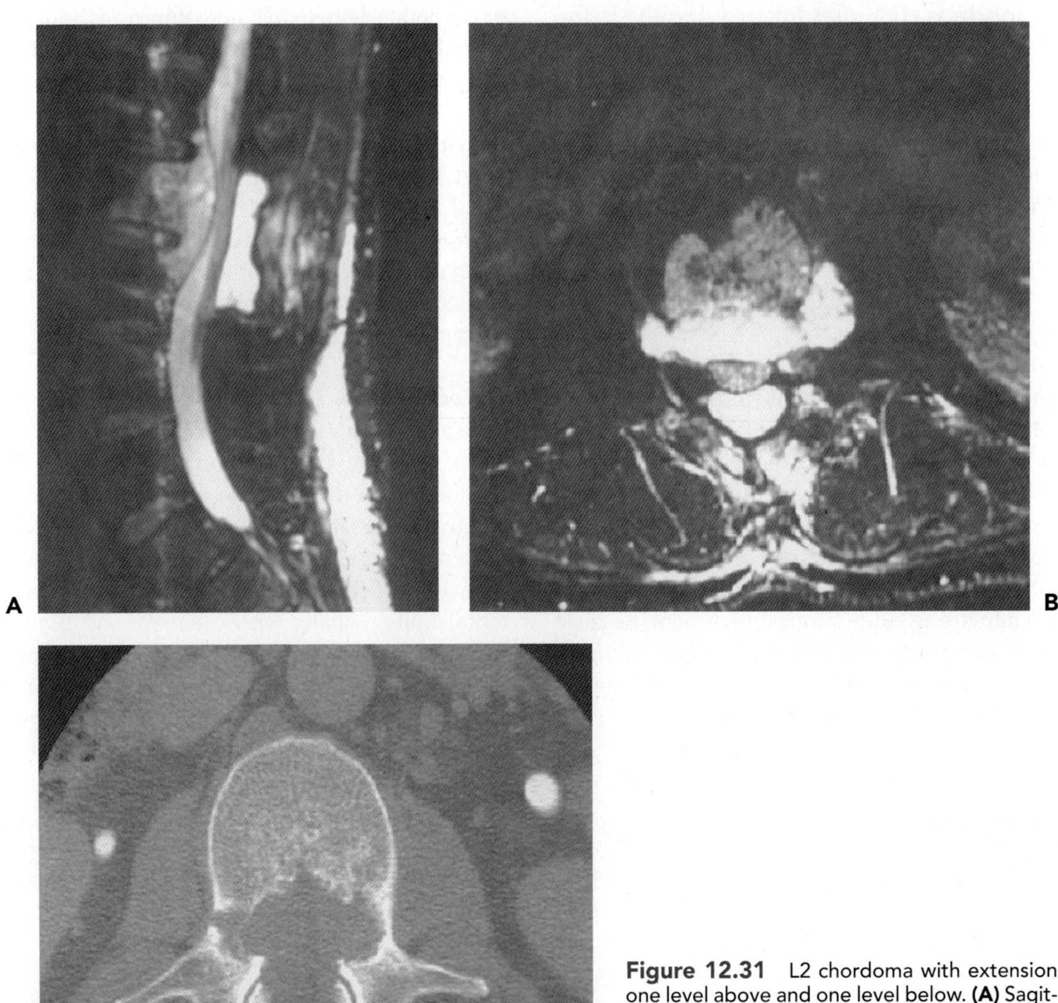

Figure 12.31 L2 chordoma with extension one level above and one level below. **(A)** Sagittal MRI shows epidural extension into adjacent bodies. **(B)** Axial MRI shows canal compromise. **(C)** CT scan showing bone destruction. (*Reproduced with permission from* Frymoyer JW, Wiesel SW, An HS, et al. *The Adult and Pediatric Spine*, 3rd ed. Philadelphia: Lippincott Williams & Wilkins, 2003.)

root resection has been acceptable in most series when compared with the prospect of disease control.

Metastatic Disease of the Spine

The overwhelming majority of spinal tumors represent metastatic lesions, particularly in patients over the age of 40. A history of persistent back pain, unrelieved by rest, particularly in a patient with a known history of cancer should alert the physician about the possibility of a metastatic deposit in the spine. Primary malignancies that most commonly metastasize to the spine include breast, lung, prostate, kidney, and thyroid cancers. Advances in supportive care for patients with these and other types of malignancies as well as advances in awareness, imaging, and surgical technique have greatly increased the number of patients presenting for surgical treatment of metastatic disease of the spine.

The spine is the third most common site for metastasis in the body, and symptomatic spinal metastasis are the presenting complaint in approximately 15% of new cancer diagnosis. Approximately 90% of metastatic deposits in the spine originate in the vertebral body where the trabecular bone acts as a filter to blood-borne metastases (Fig. 12.32). It is hypothesized that the red marrow of the trabecular bone of the vertebra provides a favorable environment for deposition and proliferation of tumor. Once deposited, tumor cells are capable of forming a protective fibrin sheath and of secreting osteoclast activating factors and possibly lytic prostaglandins, which furthers their spread. Patients present primarily with pain, which according to Harrington, may be due to cortical expansion with microfracturing and invasion of paravertebral soft tissues, compression of adjacent nerve roots, pathologic fracture with instability, or compression of the cord. The history of back pain in a patient with a prior diagnosis of cancer should be viewed as worrisome, even with a remote history of a malignancy presumed to be cured; this is particularly true for carcinoma of the breast.

The diagnosis of metastatic disease of the spine is made radiographically and confirmed by the pathologist. Plain films are relatively insensitive because of the extent of vertebral body destruction that is necessary before a radiographic abnormality is seen (50%). The test of choice is MRI, although bone scan is sensitive, but nonspecific, for metastatic lesions. MRI demonstrates early lesions, accurately defines soft-tissue spread, images neural compression, and is very specific in differentiating metastatic disease from infection. One common quandary for which MRI is the most helpful noninvasive modality is differentiating a pathologic fracture caused by osteopenia from metastatic disease. In our experience, most pathologic fractures caused by metastatic deposits display a pattern of diffuse marrow replacement, have involvement at more than

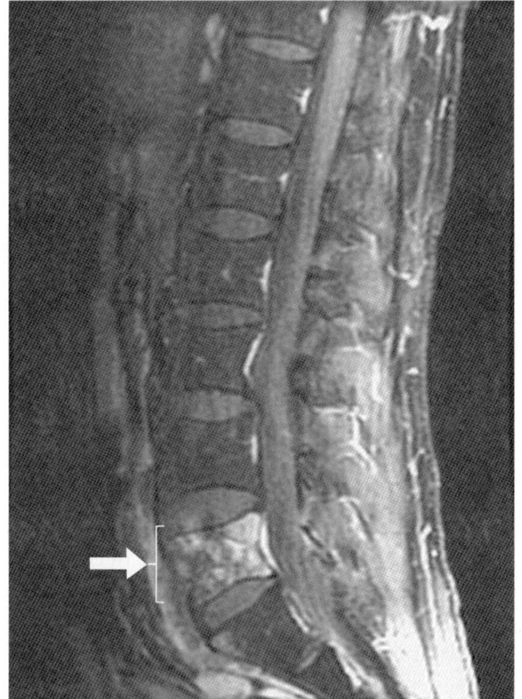

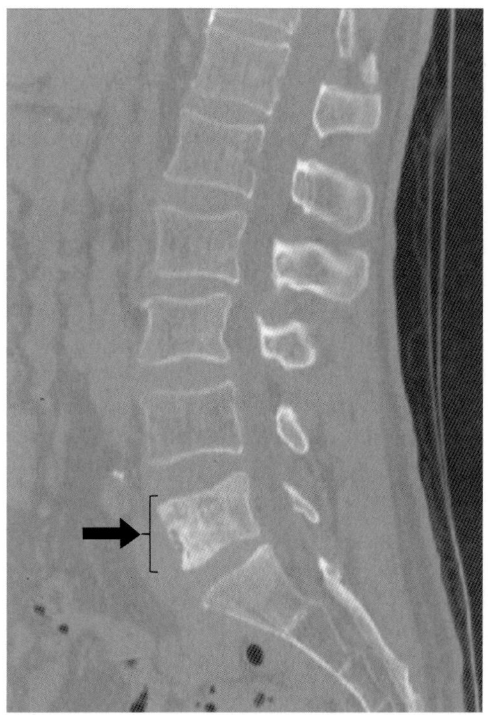

Figure 12.32 Metastatic disease. **(A)** Sagittal MRI scan of a 58-year-old man with isolated colon adenocarcinoma metastasis to L5 with low-back pain. **(B)** Sagittal CT reconstruction showing mixed blastic and lytic regions within L5. (*Reproduced with permission from* Frymoyer JW, Wiesel SW, An HS, et al. *The Adult and Pediatric Spine*, 3rd ed. Philadelphia: Lippincott Williams & Wilkins, 2003.)

one level, or have an associated paraspinal soft tissue mass. Finally, CT scan can be very helpful as well, especially when evaluating the amount of bony destruction by the lesion. Once all imaging that is necessary has been completed, CT-guided biopsy is the test of choice in almost all cases for accurately establishing the diagnosis before proceeding to treatment.

Treatment of metastatic disease of the spine may be systemic, local, or both. Systemic treatment consists usually of chemotherapy, as appropriate for the involved tumor. Because of the complexity of treatment for most of these cancers, the treatment should involve a multidisciplinary team including a medical oncologist, a radiation oncologist, orthopedic oncologist, and/or orthopedic spine surgeon familiar with treating spinal tumors. Patients whose disease is amenable to chemotherapy alone rarely come under the treatment of an orthopedic surgeon, but chemotherapy as the primary mode of treatment should be considered for cancers such as prostate or breast in which metastatic deposit is seen without collapse or neurologic compromise, as well as for certain hematopoietic malignancies.

Local treatment may consist of radiotherapy, bracing, or surgery. Radiotherapy is the treatment of choice for the large majority of metastatic lesions of the spine. The efficacy of radiotherapy is highly dependent upon the radiosensitivity of the tumor present. The most radiosensitive tumors, such as myeloma, lymphoma, Ewing's sarcoma, and to a lesser extent carcinoma of the breast, respond highly favorably to radiotherapy, which should be considered in virtually all such cases unless clear-cut spinal instability is present. On the other hand, radioresistant lesions such as carcinoma of the lung or prostate, GI cancers, or renal cell carcinoma have a much less favorable response and surgery should be undertaken in these diseases if there is vertebral collapse with pain, borderline instability, or impending neurologic compromise. Obviously, this relatively aggressive surgical approach would be tempered by the overall extent of patient disease, associated medical problems, and the presence of multiple levels of spinal involvement.

Bracing may be used as an adjunct to radiotherapy. Custom-molded thoracolumbosacral or lumbosacral orthoses frequently provide excellent short-term pain relief and may be particularly advantageous in patients with limited life expectancy. Halo-vest immobilization should be considered in patients with radiosensitive metastatic lesions in the cervical spine where short-term prophylaxis against neurologic catastrophe is needed, pending disease ablation with either radiotherapy or chemotherapy.

Another means of treating pain from compression fractures secondary to metastatic lesions is through vertebroplasty or kyphoplasty in which cement is injected into the vertebral body providing stability and preventing further collapse. Kyphoplasty involves insufflations of the vertebral segment prior to PMMA injection and theoretically results in greater correction of collapse in comparison to vertebroplasty. It must be noted that these are symptomatic treatments only but offer a minimally invasive alternative for many patients that are not suitable for larger surgical procedures. Currently, this is an off-label use for vertebroplasty/kyphoplasty, but these procedures do provide patients with significant pain relief.

The final method of local treatment is surgery. The indications for surgical intervention in metastatic disease of the spine include (1) the need for tissue for diagnosis; (2) a radioresistant tumor with local collapse or impending neurologic impairment; (3) persistent or recurrent pain or neurologic deficit despite radiotherapy; (4) neurologic deterioration during radiotherapy; (5) neurologic deficit due to bone or disk retropulsion; and (6) spinal instability, either present or impending. All but item 6 are relatively straightforward. The definition of spinal instability in metastatic disease is the source of significant debate. We feel that lesions that result in greater than 50% collapse of the vertebral body, particularly at the thoracolumbar junction, any translational deformity on either AP or lateral radiographs, segmental kyphosis of greater than 20 degrees above that expected at the involved level, and lesions that involve both the anterior and posterior columns should be considered potentially unstable. A highly radiosensitive tumor fulfilling one of those criteria is occasionally treated first with radiotherapy, but surgery performed before radiotherapy is more likely to preserve neurologic function, relieve pain, and preserve overall function while minimizing the risk of operating through previously radiated tissue.

The surgical approach for metastatic lesions can be anterior, posterior, or combined. Because most metastatic lesions arise anteriorly and result in destruction of the anterior column of the spine, with anterior cord or cauda equina compression, our preferred approach is usually anterior. This approach allows safe and thorough decompression of the spinal canal as well as mechanically sound reconstruction of the anterior column of the spine. There are multiple forms of instrumentation and stabilizing devices that can be used such that the anterior approach alone can be used in the majority of situations.

Alternatively, the posterior approach or posterolateral approach can be used. Laminectomy alone is relatively inefficient at decompressing the spinal canal and should be avoided in most cases. However, posterolateral decompression has been used with success with results comparable with the anterior approach. Finally, depending on the stability needed or the amount of decompression needed, these procedures can be combined with the downside of a much larger surgery with greater morbidity.

Overall, aggressive surgical treatment has gained widespread acceptance for the treatment of metastatic spinal disease in patients that fit the criteria outlined. This reflects our experience that, in the properly selected patient, surgical treatment of metastatic disease of the spine is highly predictable for pain relief, restoration and protection of neurologic function, and an acceptably low complication rate.

SPINE INFECTIONS

Infections of the spine occupy a perversely important place in the history of orthopedic surgery in general and spine surgery in particular. Percival Pott's description of tuberculosis (TB) and associated paralysis gave rise to the enduring eponym "Pott's paraplegia." Many of this century's seminal advances in spine surgery including the development of posterior fusion of the spine by Hibbs and Albee related to the treatment of tuberculous spondylitis. Hodgson pioneered anterior surgery of the spine, currently in widespread use for numerous conditions, as the treatment for spinal TB. We now see infections of the spine in numerous settings and caused by a variety of organisms, but despite significant technologic and medical advances in our treatment, the underlying principles of the treatment of infection of the spine are still largely based on lessons learned from TB.

Pyogenic Infection

The incidence of pyogenic vertebral osteomyelitis appears to be increasing with an increase in medical and social conditions that lead to immunosuppression. The spine is the site for up to 7% of all cases of osteomyelitis and certainly is the area with the greatest potential for morbidity. Prior to the current antibiotic era, the mortality secondary to vertebral osteomyelitis reached 20% to 25%. With the advent of current antibiotic treatment and advances in spinal surgical techniques, the mortality rate is less than 10%, with a significant drop in morbidity as well, but the consequences can still be devastating.

The pathophysiology of vertebral osteomyelitis arises from three potential sources: direct inoculation, contiguous spread from another source, and the most common, hematogenous spread. Direct inoculation can occur via penetrating trauma or from iatrogenic inoculation through procedures ranging from surgical intervention to percutaneous procedures. Contiguous spread as the name implies occurs from another infection in the region of the affected area, generally a retroperitoneal abscess or possibly from the spinal canal itself. The vast majority of cases are the result of hematogenous spread from a distant source, with the most common locations being the genitourinary tract, the skin and soft tissues, and the upper respiratory tract. Approximately 50% of patients with an infection of the spine will give a history of a preceding infection elsewhere. The infection seeds the metaphyseal region of the vertebral body through the rich anastomotic network in the area. Once the infection reaches the vertebral body, it locally spreads and commonly violates the vertebral end plate to involve the avascular intervertebral disk, which commonly distinguishes infection from metastases on plain film and MRI. Because of the avascularity of the disk, bacteria thrive in this region and quickly degrade the disk, allowing entrance into the adjacent vertebral body. Instability often ensues secondary to degradation of the disk and the vertebral body. The infection can then further spread to adjacent vertebrae or into the soft tissues including the prevertebral fascia in the neck and retroperitoneal structures such as the psoas muscle in the lumbar region. If left untreated, eventually, patients can develop neurologic compromise secondary to instability and collapse with subsequent impingement of neural structures, pathologic fractures, or direct impingement from the infection itself in the form of an epidural abscess. Death can subsequently ensue from neurologic compromise, although most commonly results from septicemia.

Although infection of the spine may occur in any age group, there appears to be two peaks: children/adolescents and patients greater than 50 years of age. This article will focus on infections in the adult population, but as an aside, the pediatric population generally is affected by bloodborne diskitis secondary to their unique blood supply to the vertebral region. In adults, most, but not all, cases of vertebral osteomyelitis occur in immunosuppressed patients and the elderly, with males being more commonly affected than females. Immunosuppressive disorders such as RA and diabetes, the use of immunosuppressive medication following surgery, immunosuppressive states such as AIDS, and a history of IV drug abuse are all frequently associated with spine infection.

The causative organisms seen in most infections of the spine have evolved over time. In the pre-antibiotic era, *Staphylococcus aureus* predominated. More recently, the incidence of *S. aureus* has dropped significantly, although the incidence of methicillin-resistant *S. aureus* is on the rise. They both still account for approximately 50% of infections. Gram-negative infections are increasing in number, likely from the increasing rate of pseudomonas infection in IV drug users, although these are the usual organisms from genitourinary tract infections as well. Not uncommon are indolent infections caused by low virulence organisms such as *Staphylococcus epidermidis* and *Streptococcus* species. Finally, anaerobic organisms can also be found particularly in diabetic patients.

The primary manifestations of pyogenic infection of the spine include pain, neurologic impairment, and signs and symptoms of sepsis, with the most common complaint being pain. Carragee et al. reviewed a large series of patients with pyogenic infections and found that over 90% presented with pain. A history of pain at night should alert the physician to a condition more serious than run of the mill back pain. A number of authors have demonstrated the tendency toward delay in diagnosis; as many as 50%

of patients have pain for 3 months or longer prior to the correct diagnosis of spinal sepsis. Greater awareness and improved imaging techniques appear to be lessening this problem. Fever is less common than pain and is seen only in about 50% of patients. Fifteen to 20% of patients will present with evidence of neurologic involvement, with predisposing factors including diabetes, RA, increasing age, and a more cephalad level of involvement. Finally, approximately 15% of patients will present with atypical symptoms such as hip pain, abdominal or chest pain, or testicular discomfort. These atypical complaints are more common in infections in the lumbar spine and contribute significantly to prolonged delay in diagnosis.

The importance of recognizing the patient at risk for spinal infection as well as recognizing the common presenting complaint is highlighted by the paucity of specific physical findings suggesting infection. Abscesses are now quite rare but are seen more commonly in infections of the cervical or thoracic spine. Significant paraspinal spasm may be seen, and pain on percussion in the midline, at the affected level, is the most specific finding. An infection with a subsequent psoas abscess will have pain with hip extension. Other physical findings can relate to neurologic findings, but no physical examination maneuvers are particularly specific for infection.

Laboratory studies are a very important aspect for the workup of possible infection, especially when considering the lack of specificity of the physical examination, although laboratory values may even further confuse the clinical picture. A white blood cell (WBC) count, erythrocyte sedimentation rate (ESR), and C-reactive protein (CRP) should be obtained in all patients suspected of having an infection. The most sensitive test of all of these is the ESR that is elevated over 90% of the time, with the CRP being the next most sensitive. Both of these tests are nonspecific but should not be elevated in a patient with nonspecific back pain, and therefore, further studies are warranted should one or both of these be elevated. The WBC count, on the other hand, is only elevated approximately 50% of the time and is therefore less useful. Once an infection has been diagnosed, treatment response can be followed by monitoring the CRP, which drops much more quickly than the ESR. Finally, blood cultures should be obtained.

Radiographic evaluation is vital in cases of infection and should begin with plain films. Unfortunately, plain films are relatively insensitive in early infections of the spine, and normal routine x-rays of the back are of limited value in ruling out infection. The most common early finding, frequently seen only retrospectively, is soft-tissue swelling including loss of the psoas shadow or widening of the retropharyngeal clear space in the neck. Three to 4 weeks following the establishment of infection, disk space narrowing may be seen. Although disk space narrowing can be due to a number of causes, irregularity and destruction of the bony end plate are not present in degenerative disorders of the spine and should heighten suspicion of infection. Finally, at about 6 weeks, destructive changes in the vertebral body, including collapse and lysis anteriorly, are seen.

Much more sensitive than plain films, scintigraphy offers an excellent method of detecting early spinal infection. The most sensitive and frequently used method is technetium-99 m bone scan with sensitivities greater than 90%, though specificity is low. However, it remains very useful especially as a screening test when infection is suspected and plain films are negative. Other methods include gallium scanning and indium-111-labeled leukocyte scanning, both of which are less sensitive, with leukocyte scanning the least sensitive. Prior to the emergence of MRI, gallium scanning was often combined with technetium scanning to improve both the sensitivity and specificity, and this combination can still be used but rarely needs to be.

The imaging modality of choice is MRI. MRI has a sensitivity greater than scintigraphy (around 95%) and much higher specificity (greater than 90%), while additionally providing detailed imaging of the extent of pathologic involvement and the specific structures involved. Because a positive or even equivocal bone scan will almost always lead to ordering an MRI, our practice is to utilize this test initially when infection of the spine is suspected.

A characteristic MRI picture is seen in vertebral osteomyelitis (Fig. 12.33). We rely most heavily on the T2-weighted images, wherein increased signal is seen in the disk space as well as involved areas of the vertebral bodies. This is more striking following the administration of gadolinium, which should be ordered with the study when infection is suspected. The most significant finding is the increased signal in the disk space, which clearly differentiates infection from degenerative change. MRI distinctly defines disk and end plate destruction, enabling distinction between infection and tumor of the spine. Neoplasms, as previously explained, do not involve the disk space while infections do.

Finally, CT scanning is not typically used in the initial evaluation for infection. However, many times CT can be very helpful in preoperative planning to better define the amount of bony destruction.

Before treatment is initiated, laboratory confirmation of the presence of infection and the causative organism should be sought. Confirmation by a positive culture from the spine or blood is preferable to beginning empiric antibiotic therapy unless systemic sepsis is present. Biopsy of the spine can usually be performed via a percutaneous approach. Fluoroscopy and, when needed, CT guidance allow for minimally invasive access to the entire spine and have been reported to lead to accurate diagnosis in 68% to 86% of cases of vertebral osteomyelitis. When initial percutaneous aspiration does not result in positive culture or histopathologic findings, the decision must then be made about the next step in evaluation and treatment. In our practice, only rarely is empiric medical management

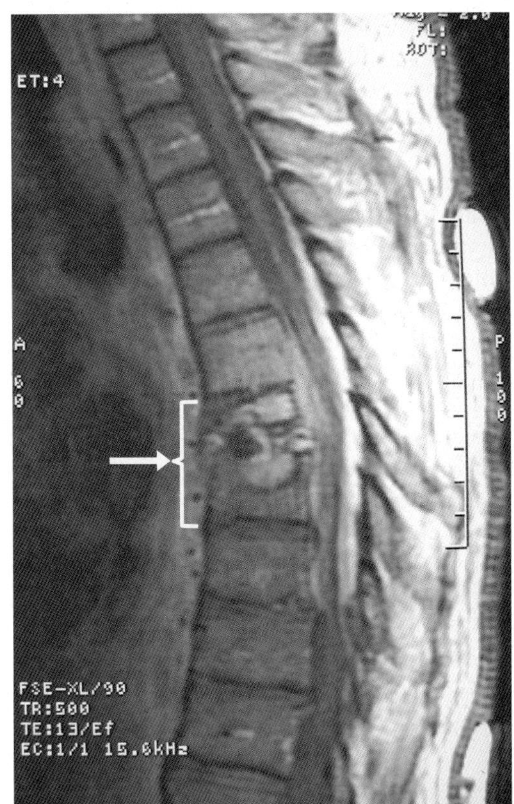

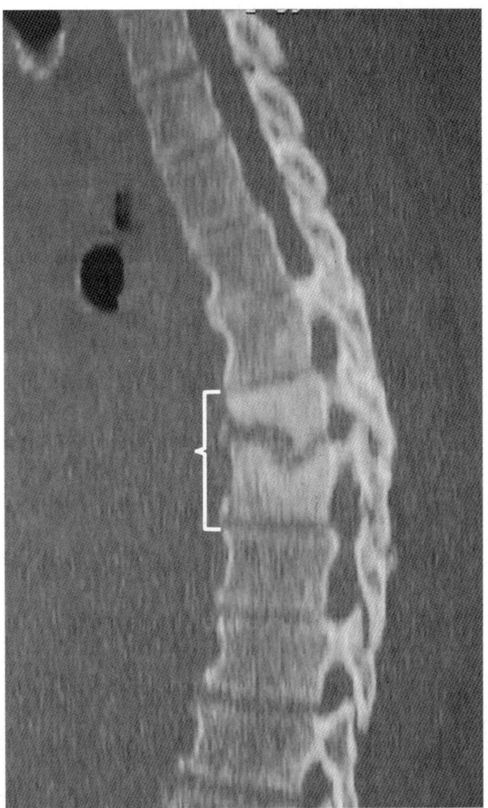

Figure 12.33 Vertebral osteomyelitis. A 78-year-old male on hemodialysis presented with back pain, fevers, and progressive paraplegia, though incomplete. **(A)** Sagittal T1 gadolinium MRI demonstrating enhanced signal within T7 and part of T8 and an anterior epidural mass compressing the cord. **(B)** Sagittal reconstruction CT scan shows advanced destruction of T7 and part of T8. Sclerotic changes in the infected vertebrae are noted. (*Reproduced with permission from* Frymoyer JW, Wiesel SW, An HS, et al. *The Adult and Pediatric Spine*, 3rd ed. Philadelphia: Lippincott Williams & Wilkins, 2003.)

undertaken at this stage. We find it helpful to consult with our interventional radiologists to see if they believe that another attempt at biopsy is likely to be more rewarding; if not, we typically proceed with open biopsy and definitive debridement.

Treatment of pyogenic vertebral osteomyelitis can be medical or surgical, but, regardless of the method, the goals remain the same. The goals of treatment are identification of the pathogen, eradication of the pathogen, and maintenance of stability and neurologic function. The type and duration of medical treatment are dictated by the causative organism cultured. Because of the continuous evolution in available antibiotics, we routinely utilize infectious disease consultation to select the agent used. It should be noted that cephalosporin penetration into the nucleus pulposus is less effective than that of bone and, in most cases, the use of an aminoglycoside should be considered. We favor the use of parenteral antibiotics for 6 weeks followed by the use of oral antibiotics, when available, for another 6 weeks. When medical management of vertebral osteomyelitis is undertaken, it should be appreciated that a protracted course of treatment is necessary before symptomatic resolution can be expected, and we have found that extending treatment for a total of 3 months leads to increased success. Response to treatment can be monitored by response of the ESR and CRP. The CRP is a better indicator as a response can be seen in 48 to 72 hours, while the ESR takes around 1 to 2 weeks. The CRP can be monitored over the first few days following treatment and then extending ESR and CRP monitoring to weekly checks for 3 to 4 weeks followed by monthly testing until a return to normal is seen.

Medical treatment of spinal infections is accompanied by immobilization. The hospitalized patient is usually placed on bed rest for several days and then mobilized, as symptoms allow, in a custom-molded or custom-made orthosis. Ambulatory patients diagnosed in the outpatient setting, now seen with increasing frequency, are not placed on bed rest but are placed into a custom-molded TLSO or a cervical orthosis depending on the level of involvement.

The indications for surgery include the need for tissue for diagnosis, the presence of significant destruction or deformity, failure of medical management, neurologic deficit caused by spinal cord compression by either abscess, disk, or bone, and the presence of a clinically significant paraspinal or epidural abscess. Each of these indications is somewhat subjective and open to interpretation.

As noted, we believe strongly in the need for a bacteriologic diagnosis whenever possible, and when minimally invasive techniques fail, we prefer definitive surgical treatment as a means of obtaining tissue rather than a limited open technique.

The extent of bony destruction or deformity leading to the need for surgical treatment has not been clearly defined; it is important when evaluating the patient with a possible neurologic deficit to recognize the extent to which kyphosis can contribute to compression of the spinal cord and cauda equina. Progressive kyphosis with retropulsion of disk or bone will not respond to bracing or antibiotics and should be promptly recognized and treated surgically. Failure of medical management requires the correlation of a number of factors. In the patient with minimal anterior column destruction who is neurologically intact without evidence of abscess formation, we favor a minimum of 4 weeks of antibiotic treatment along with rest and bracing. At that time, the absence of a significant decrease in the patient's pain as well as the absence of a significant decline in the ESR/CRP would lead to consideration of either repeat biopsy to ensure that the proper organism is being treated, or definitive surgical treatment.

The significance of the radiographic appearance of abscess formation should be mentioned. The presence of a soft-tissue mass in the paraspinal or epidural space is usually not, in our experience, evidence of pus under pressure. Although frequently a large paraspinal or epidural mass is present in a patient with significant destruction or neurologic compromise, in the absence of these more concrete surgical indications we typically prefer to undertake nonoperative management and closely follow the patient. Awareness of the previously described risk factors for neurologic injury, including increasing age, immunosuppression, and involvement of the cervical spine facilitates appropriate decision making in this setting.

Vertebral osteomyelitis is primarily a disease of the anterior column, and being such, it is axiomatic that surgical treatment should approach this disease directly from an anterior approach. The anterior approach to the spine was pioneered by Hodgson for the treatment of tuberculous spondylitis and is still favored in the vast majority of cases. With the exception of limited posterior or posterolateral approaches for biopsy, there is little advantage of an isolated posterior approach as thorough debridement is rarely possible and laminectomy for decompression has been demonstrated to destabilize an infected spine.

The anterior approach lends itself ideally to thorough surgical debridement, decompression of the spine or cauda equina, and stabilization of the spine. Once debridement of the infection is carried out, and bleeding bone above and below the involved area is seen, autogenous strut grafting has been demonstrated to be safe and effective. As an alternative, in recent years, the use of titanium surgical mesh with autogenous bone graft has been used with success as well, though long-term follow-up is lacking.

Anterior stabilization alone followed by casting or bracing is usually sufficient for single-level involvement in which the kyphotic deformity can be mostly corrected. A combined approach with posterior stabilization is generally reserved for cases of multilevel disease or cases with residual kyphosis of 20 degrees or greater. This most typically occurs in long-standing infections at the thoracolumbar junction. When posterior stabilization is undertaken, most authors believe that the risk of secondary infection of the orthopedic implants posteriorly is acceptable, and this has certainly been our experience.

The improvement in outcomes seen following medical and surgical management of pyogenic vertebral osteomyelitis is striking. Nonoperative treatment is successful in the majority of patients particularly in those that are not immunocompromised, and surgical treatment has a success rate of over 90% to 95% in terms of obtaining solid bony fusion and pain relief. In short, modern surgical and medical techniques have almost completely eliminated the risk of death, in the absence of failure of other organ systems, lead to predictably good rates of healing of the spine with good relief of pain, and lead to predictable improvement in neurologic function when impaired.

Epidural Abscess

Abscess formation in the epidural space occurs almost exclusively in adults and, with increasing numbers of elderly and immunosuppressed patients, appears to be increasing in frequency. Although epidural abscess can occur secondary to spread from a focus of vertebral osteomyelitis, a distinct entity of epidural abscess arising from hematogenous spread from a remote source of infection or from direct inoculation is also seen. It is important to distinguish primary epidural abscess from a secondary abscess associated with vertebral osteomyelitis; primary infection of the epidural space is not associated with destruction or instability of the spine, is frequently seen posterior to the cord and cauda equina, and therefore has significantly different treatment implications. It is by all accounts a medical and surgical emergency.

A high index of suspicion is mandatory when approaching the patient with a potential epidural abscess. The initial diagnosis is missed in approximately 50% of cases, and there are various modes of presentation. Therefore, one must keep in mind the risk factors that are the same as for pyogenic infection. Symptoms may be short lived, of less than 1 to 2 weeks duration, or chronic extending over several months. The most common findings with acute epidural abscess are fever, back pain, and localized tenderness, but one or all of these may be absent with a more chronic presentation. An ominous progression of the disease has been described. Pain in the midline of the back or neck persists for a variable period of time, followed by radicular pain, possibly weakness, and finally paraparesis and paralysis. The timing of this progression varies, and deterioration to the next neurologic stage may be gradual or sudden.

Diagnosis requires bacteriologic confirmation. Laboratory findings suggestive of epidural abscess include elevation of the ESR, which is almost always elevated, averaging 86.3 mm/hr in a study by Gardner. The WBC count is more variable (less sensitive), at times with no elevation, but is generally elevated as well. In the same study by Gardner, the average WBC count was 22,000 cells/mm^3. Patients with more long-standing disease typically have less dramatic leukocytosis. The CRP is also generally elevated, though less research has focused on the CRP as it is a relatively new laboratory value in comparison to the ESR. Radiographic evaluation is undertaken, but plain radiographic findings are frequently minimal. Historically, myelography has been used to evaluate for epidural abscess, but as with vertebral osteomyelitis, MRI has evolved as the imaging modality of choice. Ideally with the addition of gadolinium to improve sensitivity, MRI provides visualization of the abscess and the extent of neural element compression while giving the added benefit of identifying concurrent vertebral osteomyelitis when present. T1 images typically appear hypointense (may be isointense), T2 images appear hyperintense, and the addition of gadolinium often shows peripheral enhancement typically seen with abscesses.

Prompt intervention is required once an epidural abscess is diagnosed. Most authors consider epidural abscess a surgical emergency and we concur. Certainly all patients, once a bacteriologic diagnosis is achieved, should be started on high-dose IV antibiotics. Surgery is indicated unless the patient is such a poor surgical candidate that the risks outweigh the benefits. There are some advocates for initial nonoperative management for those patients who are neurologically intact, though this is controversial.

Unlike epidural abscess secondary to vertebral osteomyelitis, primary epidural abscess is routinely treated surgically by laminectomy. Spinal stability can usually be preserved while still thoroughly unroofing and debriding the epidural space. It is imperative to prove intraoperatively that the cephalocaudad extent of decompression is adequate.

Aggressive medical and surgical management of epidural abscesses has radically improved the historically bleak results of treatment. Perioperative death is exceedingly rare, and depending on the extent of neurologic deficit, significant improvement is frequently seen. Poor prognostic factors include dense or long-standing neurologic deficit, diabetes, and advanced age.

Tuberculosis of the Spine

TB and tuberculous spondylitis are both diseases that have a historical significance and are still very common in developing countries. However, in industrialized countries, they are not nearly as widespread as they once were, but they are still present. In 1980s and 1990s, the frequency of TB in the Western World was on the rise secondary to chronic immunosuppressive disorders, mainly HIV, but it has subsequently been on the decline again in recent years. Although it is not as prevalent in our society as it once was, a basic understanding of the disease process and treatment insomuch as it relates to the spine is necessary for all orthopedic surgeons.

In the United States, TB is primarily a disease of adults, while in Asia and Africa significant numbers of children are affected. Approximately 5% of patients with TB develop it in the spine with a neurologic deficit reported in 10% to 45% of these patients. The possibility of tuberculous spondylitis should be considered in any individual with persistent unexplained back pain, particularly in patients who have emigrated from or recently traveled to underdeveloped areas of the world, or patients with chronic immunosuppressive disorders such as IV drug abuse or HIV infection.

Tuberculous spondylitis usually develops from hematogenous spread, most commonly from the pulmonary system. Initial inoculation of the spongiosa of the vertebral body leads to local spread of the disease. This spread has been described in several patterns including peridiscal, central, and anterior. Peridiscal spread involves infection of one vertebral body extending out of the anterior cortex and under the ALL to involve the adjacent body. A distinguishing characteristic of tuberculous spondylitis is the relative resistance of the disk to infection, unlike pyogenic vertebral osteomyelitis. Central and anterior spread occur much less commonly than peridiscal. Central involvement occurs with significant destruction of the vertebral body without extension anteriorly or into either disk space, giving the appearance of metastasis. Anterior "skip" lesions may also be seen where spread underneath the ALL extends over several segments, seen radiographically as anterior scalloping.

Patients typically present with back pain, weight loss, and intermittent fevers. On physical examination, one sees muscle spasm, local tenderness, and restricted range of motion, though kyphosis, abscess formation, and draining sinuses can be seen in severe cases. Neurologic involvement is more common with more cephalad levels and occurs anywhere from 10% to 45% of the time.

Patients generally have been previously diagnosed with TB, though spinal involvement can be the presenting symptom that leads to the diagnosis. Typically, the PPD will be positive, though it can be negative. With tuberculous spondylitis, laboratory values typically show an extremely elevated ESR (typically over 100 mm/min), with a variable increase in WBC count. Once suspected, a systemic workup for TB should be undertaken.

Concerning the spine, plain films are gathered followed by MRI, the imaging modality of choice. The earliest finding on plain film is vertebral body osteopenia, while the disk space is preserved. MRI findings mirror the previously described pathologic picture, and the differences between

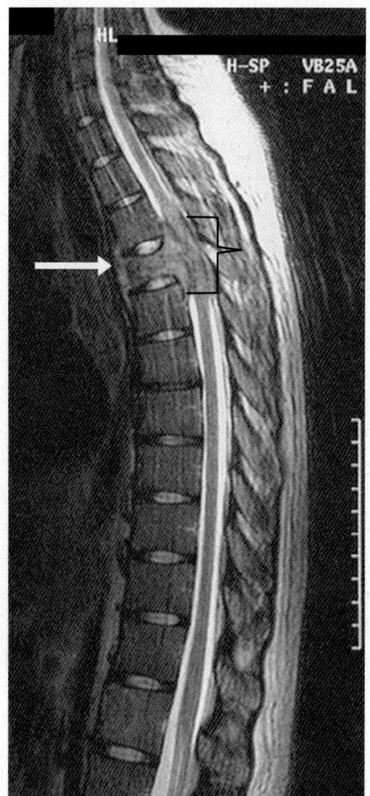

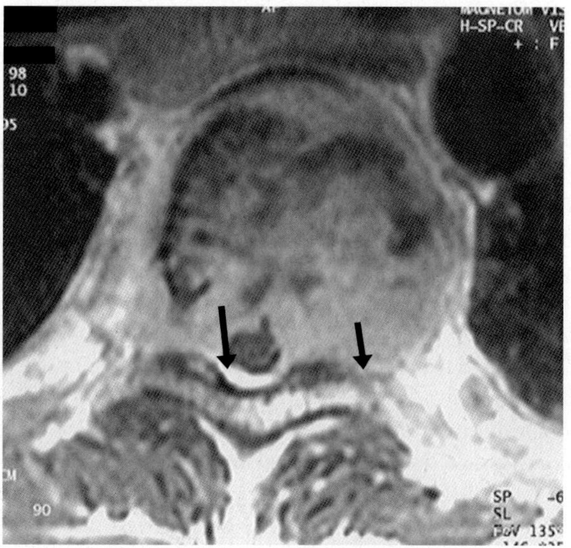

Figure 12.34 Tuberculosis of the spine. **(A)** Sagittal T2 MRI scan demonstrates involvement of upper thoracic vertebral body with soft-tissue mass extending anteriorly and posteriorly into the spinal canal, causing cord compression. Note relative preservation of disks at this stage of disease, which is frequently the case with tuberculous versus pyogenic spondylitis. **(B)** T1 axial MRI of same patient shows extensive soft-tissue mass in the left foraminal and extraforaminal regions. (*Reproduced with permission from* Frymoyer JW, Wiesel SW, An HS, et al. *The Adult and Pediatric Spine*, 3rd ed. Philadelphia: Lippincott Williams & Wilkins, 2003.)

pyogenic and tuberculous infection on MRI (Fig. 12.34) will reflect the potential for extensive bony destruction before significant disk involvement, multilevel spread under the ALL, or central involvement mimicking tumor. Additionally, tuberculous spondylitis is more likely to result in extensive abscess formation, either in the paraspinal region or in the psoas.

The treatment for spinal TB has evolved over the years and has made significant strides with medical management sufficing in most cases. We favor a 9-month course of medical management for the majority of cases consisting of a four-drug combination, per recent CDC recommendations, of isoniazid, rifampin, pyrazinamide, ethambutol, and streptomycin with isoniazid and rifampin always taken throughout the entire treatment period. Surgery is reserved for patients with a neurologic deficit who have failed to respond to 3 months of nonoperative therapy as medical management has proven to be beneficial even in the face of neurologic involvement. The details of surgical intervention are beyond the scope of this article, but an anterior approach is typically utilized followed by radical debridement of infected bone and soft tissue and debridement of any abscesses. Following adequate debridement, reconstruction of the spine is undertaken, typically with strut grafting and immobilization following surgery in a fiberglass body jacket to protect the strut. With multilevel involvement or the potential for instability, posterior stabilization is performed as well.

Outcomes have improved significantly over the past 30 years with modern medical and modern surgical techniques. Prognosis for these patients is now good. The mortality following surgery is only approximately 5%, which is significantly decreased from the 30%, which it was not too long ago.

CONCLUSIONS

Disorders of the spine encompass a wide spectrum from minor problems such as neck strain to disabling conditions such as severe degenerative spinal stenosis. Most conditions can be treated successfully with conservative management following the algorithms outlined in the article. The success of treatment revolves around a good doctor–patient relationship centered on patient education and informed decision making. When operative intervention is necessary, fairly predictable results can be obtained when surgery is performed for the proper indications and when patients are well informed about the realistic goals and risks of surgery. While much progress has been achieved in the realm of spine surgery over the past 20 years, newer technologies such as disk replacements may continue to improve operative results in the years to come.

RECOMMENDED READINGS

Cousins JP, Haughton VM. Magnetic resonance imaging of the spine. *J Am Acad Orthop Surg.* 2009;17:22–30.

Daniels AH, et al. Adverse events associated with anterior cervical spine surgery. *J Am Acad Orthop Surg.* 2008;16:729–738.

Heck AH, et al. Venous thromboembolism in spine surgery. *J Am Acad Orthop Surg.* 2008;16:656–664.

Reilly CW. Pediatric spine trauma. *J Bone Joint Surg.* 2007;89:98–107.

Rihn JA, et al. The use of bone morphogenic protein in lumbar spine surgery. *J Bone Joint Surg.* 2008;90:2014–2025.

The Shoulder

13

Brent B. Wiesel **Benjamin Shaffer** **Gerald R. Williams**

The primary purpose of the shoulder is to position the upper extremity in space and provide a stable platform for hand and elbow function. It is also the major power generator of the upper extremity. Often thought of as a single joint, it is more appropriately described as the *shoulder complex*, consisting of multiple bones, articulations, and muscle–tendon units. When all of these elements are working correctly, the complex is able to obtain a remarkable range of motion (ROM) and generate significant power. Unfortunately, the complexity of the interaction makes the shoulder complex susceptible to a number to traumatic and atraumatic conditions that can lead to dysfunction and pain. Several of these conditions have quite similar presentations, and a thorough understanding of each disorder is essential in making the correct diagnosis and rendering effective treatment. This chapter reviews the shoulder's functional anatomy, outlines a basic approach to the evaluation of shoulder problems, and describes the evaluation and management of several of the common pathologic conditions affecting the shoulder complex.

FUNCTIONAL ANATOMY

The shoulder complex consists of five articulations working in synchrony to obtain a tremendous ROM. The primary articulation is the glenohumeral (GH) joint, in which the round humeral head articulates with the oval glenoid. The remaining articulations are the sternoclavicular (SC) joint, the acromioclavicular (AC) joint, the scapulothoracic articulation, and the subacromial space (Fig. 13.1). Of these five articulations, only the GH, SC, and AC joints are true diarthrodial joints with a joint capsule containing synovial fluid separating opposing articular surfaces. The remaining two articulations are contact areas between two mobile surfaces with an intervening bursa to facilitate motion.

When considering motion about the shoulder it is important to realize that almost any activity represents a complex pattern of coordinated movement at each of the five articulations. For example, elevation of the arm generally consists of two-thirds movement at the GH joint and one-third at the scapulothoracic articulation, accompanied by rotation and translation at the SC and AC joints. Furthermore, when pathology affects one of the articulations it will often induce secondary pathology at the other articulations. If movement at the GH joint is limited by adhesive capsulitis, patients will often attempt to compensate by increasing motion at the scapulothoracic articulation, leading to fatigue in the muscles responsible for scapular motion and periscapular pain.

Osteology

The clavicle is an S-shaped bone that serves as a strut to maintain the normal relationship of the shoulder girdle to the body (Fig. 13.2). On the medial side, the strut is attached to the sternum and the first rib at the SC joint, whereas on the lateral end, the clavicle articulates with the acromion via the AC joint. Fractures of the clavicle most commonly occur through the midportion, which is the thinnest and narrowest portion of the bone and therefore mechanically weakest.

The proximal humerus consists of the nearly round humeral head, which is approximately one third to one half of a sphere, and the greater and lesser tuberosities (Fig. 13.3). The junction between the articular surface and the tuberosities forms the anatomic neck of the humerus, whereas the junction of the tuberosities to the shaft is referred to as the *surgical neck*. The articular surface is angled superiorly, with a neck shaft angle of 135 degrees (angle between the humeral shaft and a line drawn perpendicular to the anatomic neck) and in 30 degrees of retroversion when compared to the transepicondylar axis of the elbow. The

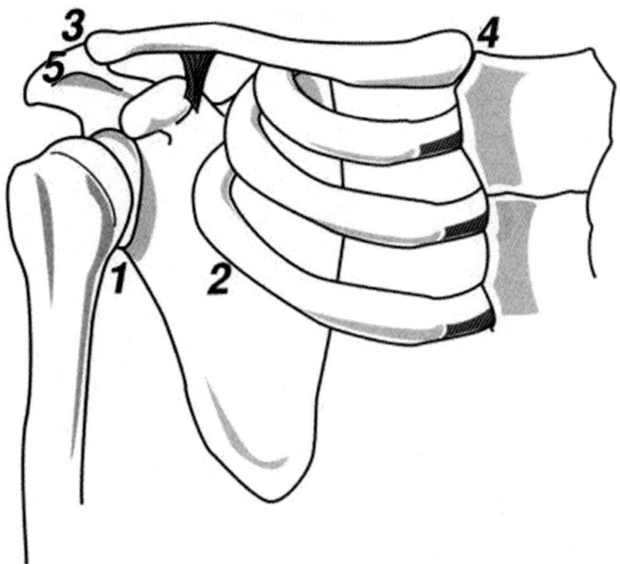

Figure 13.1 The five articulations of the shoulder complex: (1) glenohumeral, (2) scapulothoracic, (3) acromioclavicular, (4) sternoclavicular, and (5) subacromial. (*From* Chapman MW, Szabo RM, Marder RA, et al. *Chapman's orthopaedic surgery*. Philadelphia, Lippincott Williams & Wilkins, 2001, with permission.)

greater tuberosity serves as the insertion point for the three superior and posterior rotator cuff muscles (supraspinatus, infraspinatus, and teres minor), while the lesser tuberosity is the insertion for the anterior cuff muscle, the subscapularis. The tuberosities are separated by the bicipital groove, which contains the tendon of the long head of the biceps. When considering arthroplasty, whether for reconstruction after a four-part proximal humerus fracture or the sequela of arthritis, it is important to remember that the tip of the articular surface is 5 to 10 mm superior to the tip of the greater tuberosity. The blood supply to the proximal humerus is primarily via the arcuate artery, which is a terminal branch of the anterior humeral circumflex artery (Fig. 13.4). This vessel can be disrupted following proximal humerus fractures, leading to avascular necrosis.

The third bone of the shoulder girdle is the scapula, which has two primary purposes (Fig. 13.5). First, the scapula is the attachment site for the majority of muscles involved in shoulder motion (Table 13.1). Second, the bone provides a mobile base for the glenoid portion of the GH articulation. In addition to the glenoid, the lateral aspect of the scapula contains two boney projections: the coracoid and the acromion. The coracoid serves as the point of origin for three muscles (the short head of the biceps, the coracobrachialis, and the pectoralis minor) as well as the attachment point for two ligaments that stabilize the AC joint and the coracoacromial (CA) ligament. The acromion is an extension of the scapular spine and provides the point of origin for a portion of the deltoid muscle as well as the scapular side of the AC joint. The supraspinatus and anterior portion of the infraspinatus run underneath the inferior portion of the acromion as they

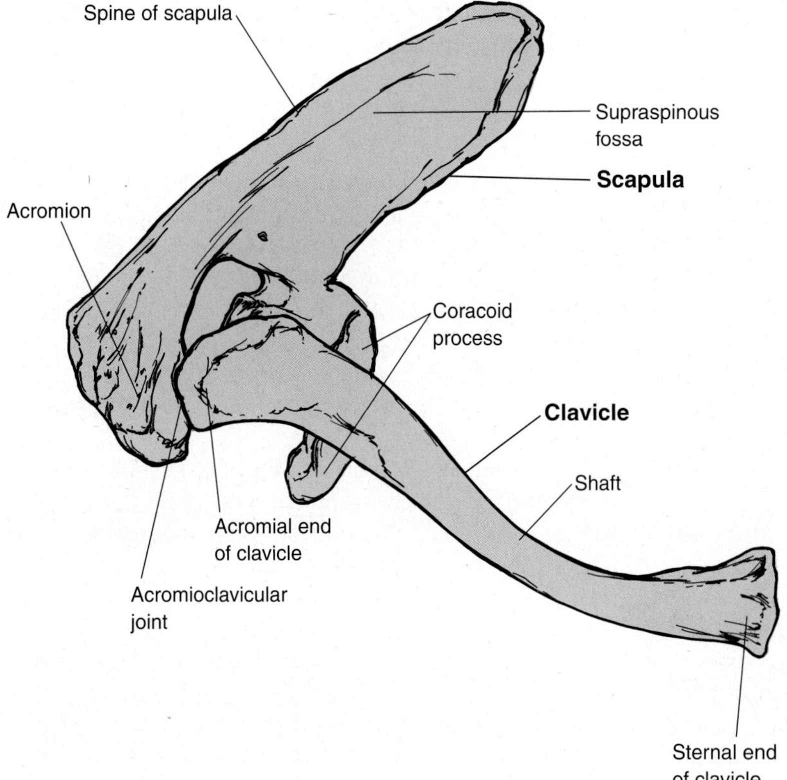

Figure 13.2 The clavicle is an S-shaped bone that serves as a strut to maintain the normal relationship of the shoulder girdle to the body. (*From* Oatis CA. *Kinesiology. The mechanics and pathomechanics of human movement*. Baltimore: Lippincott Williams & Wilkins, 2003, with permission.)

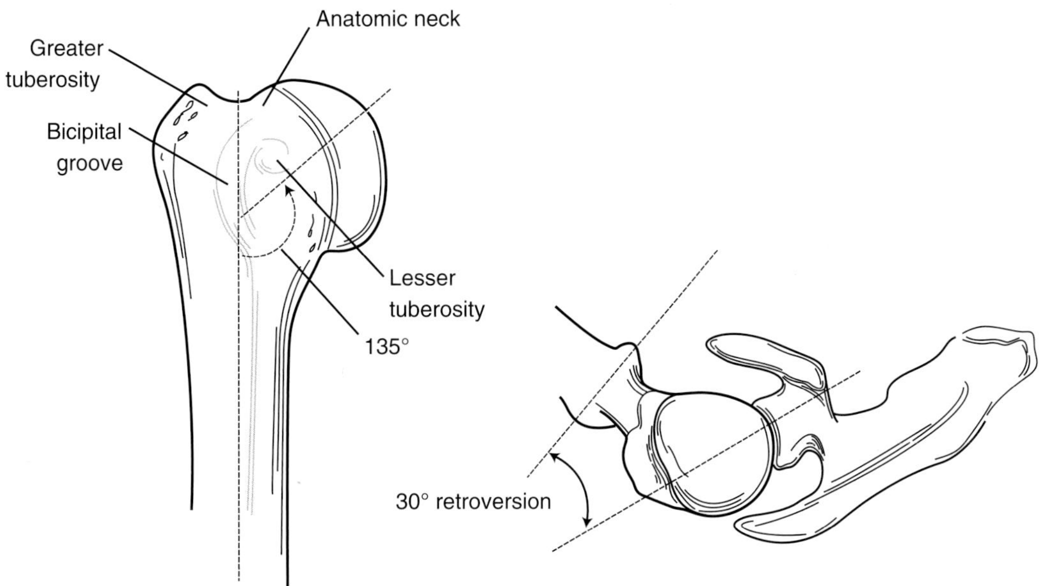

Figure 13.3 The proximal humerus consist of the humeral head and the greater and lesser tuberosities. The highest point of the humeral head is 5–10 mm above the top of the greater tuberosity. The articular surface is angled superiorly 135 degrees and is in 30 degrees of retroversion when compared to the transepicondylar axis of the elbow.

transverse laterally toward their insertion on the proximal humerus.

Glenohumeral Joint

The GH joint has the largest ROM of any joint in the body. This extreme ROM comes at the cost of stability, and the GH joint is therefore the most frequently dislocated major joint. Only 20% to 30% of the articular surface of the humeral head is in contact with the shallow glenoid at any given time. This relationship has very little inherent stability and has been compared to a golf ball sitting on a tee (Fig. 13.6). The stability of the articulation is enhanced by the labrum, a triangularly shaped fibrous ring attached to periphery of the glenoid that enhances the glenoid depth by up to 50% (Fig. 13.7). Although similar in appearance to the meniscus of the knee, the labrum is made of fibrous tissue rather than fibrocartilage. The remaining stability of the GH joint is provided by the capsular structures, which provide primarily static restraint at the extremes of the ROM, and the rotator cuff muscles, which are dynamic stabilizers through the functional arch of motion.

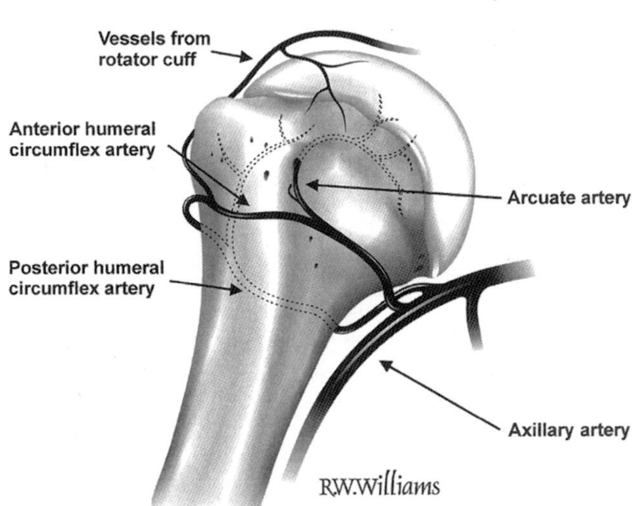

Figure 13.4 The primary blood supply of the humeral head is the arcuate artery, which is a branch of the anterior humeral circumflex artery. (*From* Craig EV. *Master Techniques in Orthopaedic Surgery: The Shoulder*, 2nd ed. Philadelphia: Lippincott Williams & Wilkins, 2004, with permission.)

When viewed from its external surface (as in open surgery), the GH joint capsule appears to be a bland fibrous structure; however, when seen internally (as in arthroscopy or histologic section) the capsule is found to contain several discrete ligaments, each with a specific function (Figs. 13.8 and 13.9). The GH ligaments originate from various locations on the glenoid rim and labrum, for which they are named, and attach to the proximal humerus distal to the articular surface.

The superior glenohumeral ligament (SGHL) is the primary restraint to inferior translation and external rotation with the arm in adduction. The middle glenohumeral ligament (MGHL) is not present in all individuals but, when it is, it resists anterior translation with the arm at 45 degrees of abduction. The inferior glenohumeral ligament is divided into anterior (AIGHL) and posterior (PIGHL) bands, with

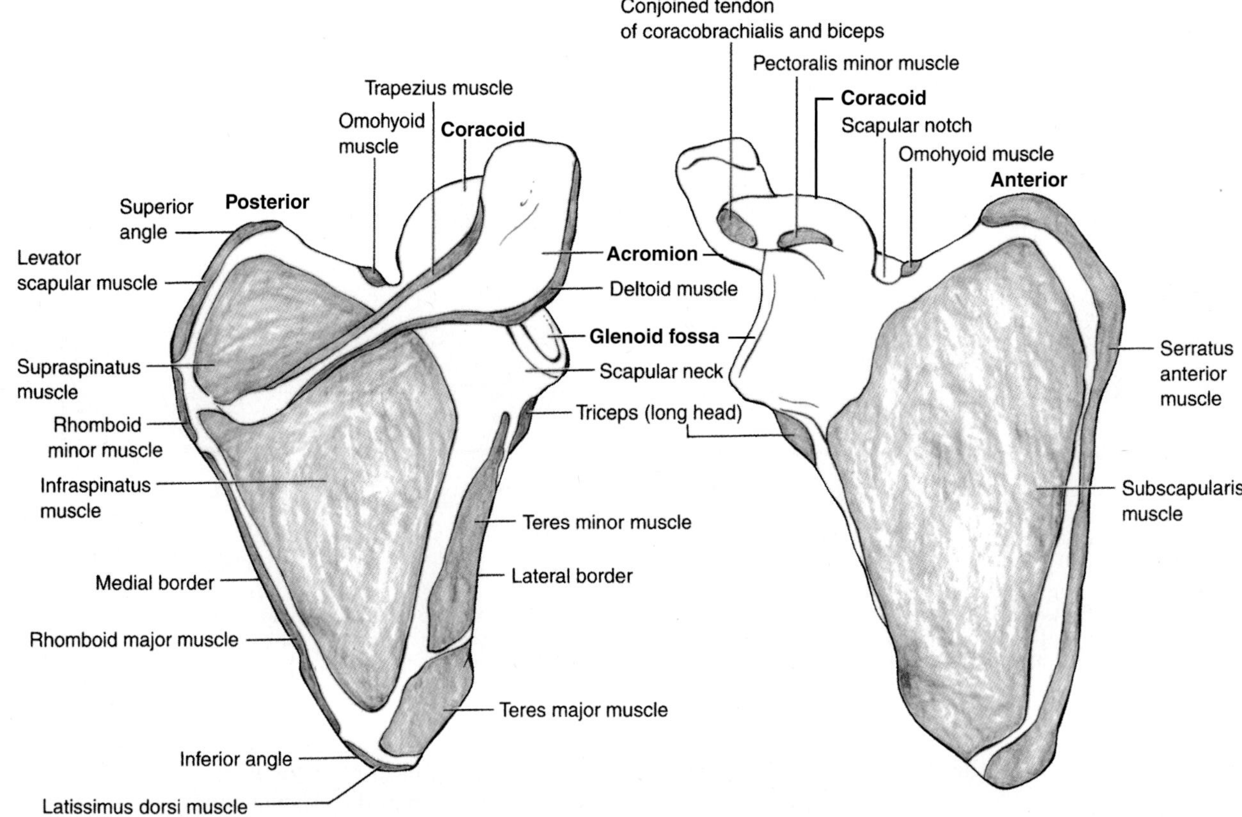

Figure 13.5 Anterior and posterior view of the scapula demonstrating the multiple muscle attachments as well as the glenoid, coracoid, and acromion. (*From* Iannotti JP, Williams GR. *Disorders of the Shoulder: Diagnosis and Management*, 2nd ed. Philadelphia: Lippincott Williams & Wilkins, 2007, with permission.)

TABLE 13.1
MUSCULAR ATTACHMENTS TO THE SCAPULA

Scapulohumeral Muscles
Long head of biceps
Short head of biceps
Deltoid
Coracobrachialis
Teres major
Long head of triceps
Scapulothoracic Muscles
Levator scapulae
Omohyoid
Rhomboid major
Rhomboid minor
Serratus anterior
Trapezius
Pectoralis minor
Rotator Cuff Muscles
Supraspinatus
Infraspinatus
Subscapularis
Teres Minor

Seventeen muscles attach the scapula to the neck, thorax, and humerus, making it the control tower for coordinated upper-extremity activity. *From* Iannotti JP, Williams GR. *Disorders of the shoulder: Diagnosis and management*, 2nd ed. Philadelphia: Lippincott Williams & Wilkins, 2007, with permission.

an intervening pouch. These inferior ligaments become taut at 90 degrees of abduction. In this position, the AIGHL is the primary restraint against anterior translation and the PIGHL resists posterior translation. The inferior capsular pouch also cradles the humeral head in abduction, further enhancing stability.

Acromioclavicular Joint

The AC joint consists of a fibrocartilaginous disk interposed between the distal clavicle and the acromion. With aging, natural degeneration of this disk occurs, often leading to arthritis of the AC joint. Fortunately, this arthritis is often asymptomatic. Stability is provided by the joint capsule, which surrounds the joint circumferentially. The superior and posterior aspects of the capsule are the most important horizontal stabilizers of the AC joint, whereas the coracoclavicular (CC) ligaments are the most important vertical stabilizers. These ligaments run between the coracoid process and the distal clavicle and consist of the medial conoid and lateral trapezoid ligament (Fig. 13.10).

Sternoclavicular Joint

The SC joint is the medial articulation between the clavicle and the manubrium of the sternum. This joint is supported

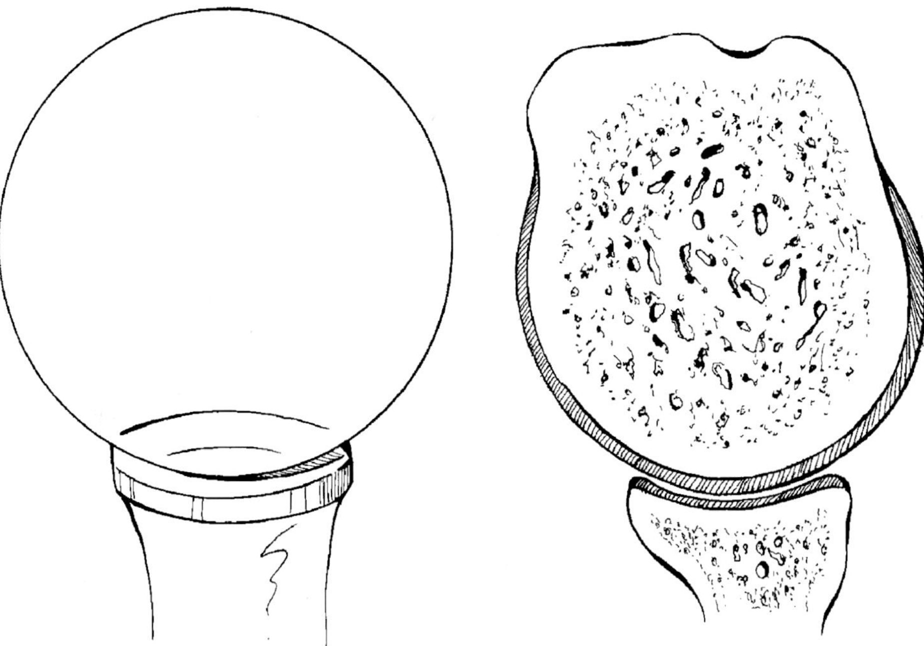

Figure 13.6 The glenohumeral joint has been compared to a golf ball sitting on a tee. (*From* Boardman ND III, Fu FH. Shoulder biomechanics. In: McGinty JB, Cas-pari RB, Jackson RW, Poehling GG, eds. *Operative Arthroscopy*. Philadelphia: Lippincott-Raven, 1996:627, with permission.)

by a strong capsular ligament (SC ligament) as well as by the costoclavicular ligament, which is a robust structure linking the medial clavicle to the first rib (Fig. 13.10). The posterior SC ligament has been shown to be the most important structure in preventing both anterior and posterior instability of this joint.

Disorders of the SC joint are much less common than pathology of the other four articulations within the shoulder girdle; however, the joint is susceptible to a number of conditions including degenerative arthritis, spontaneous subluxation, and septic arthritis. Of particular importance, posterior dislocation of this joint can lead to compression of the underlying trachea and great vessels. These dislocations generally require reduction in the operating room, with a thoracic surgeon immediately available.

Scapulothoracic Articulation

The anterior aspect of the scapula is covered by the subscapularis muscles, whose anterior side articulates with

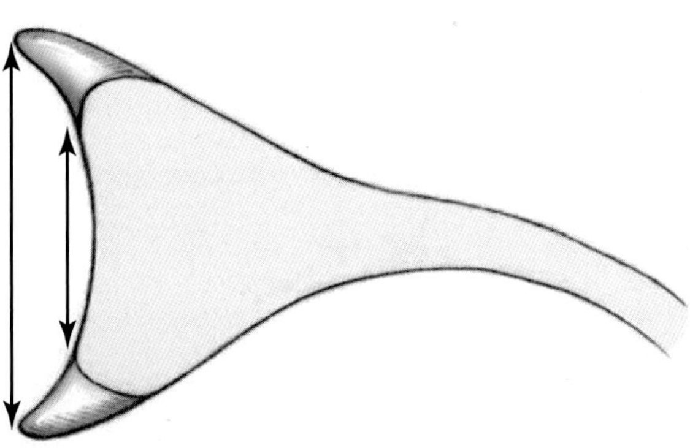

Figure 13.7 The glenoid labrum increases the depth and surface area of the glenoid socket, which improves stability of the glenohumeral joint. (*From* Iannotti JP, Williams GR. *Disorders of the Shoulder: Diagnosis and Management*, 2nd ed. Philadelphia: Lippincott Williams & Wilkins, 2007, with permission.)

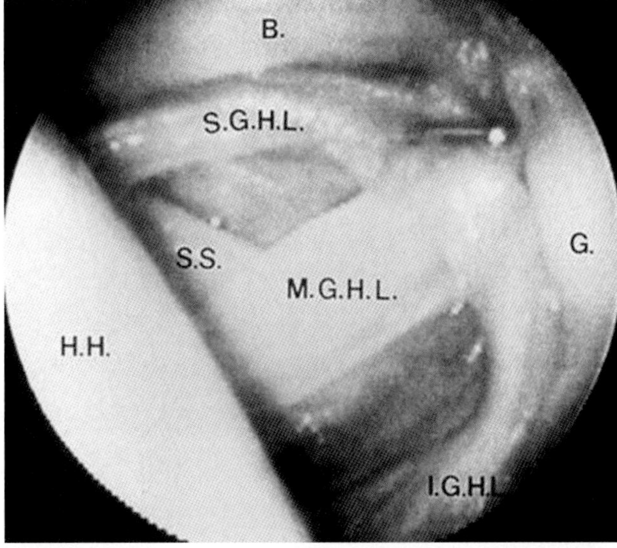

Figure 13.8 Arthroscopic view from the posterior portal of the anterior capsular structures of a left shoulder. HH, humeral head; G, glenoid; B, biceps tendon; SGHL, superior glenohumeral ligament; SS, subscapularis tendon; MGHL, middle glenohumeral ligament; IGHL, inferior glenohumeral ligament. (*From* Chapman MW, Szabo RM, Marder RA, et al. *Chapman's orthopaedic surgery*. Philadelphia, Lippincott Williams & Wilkins, 2001, with permission.)

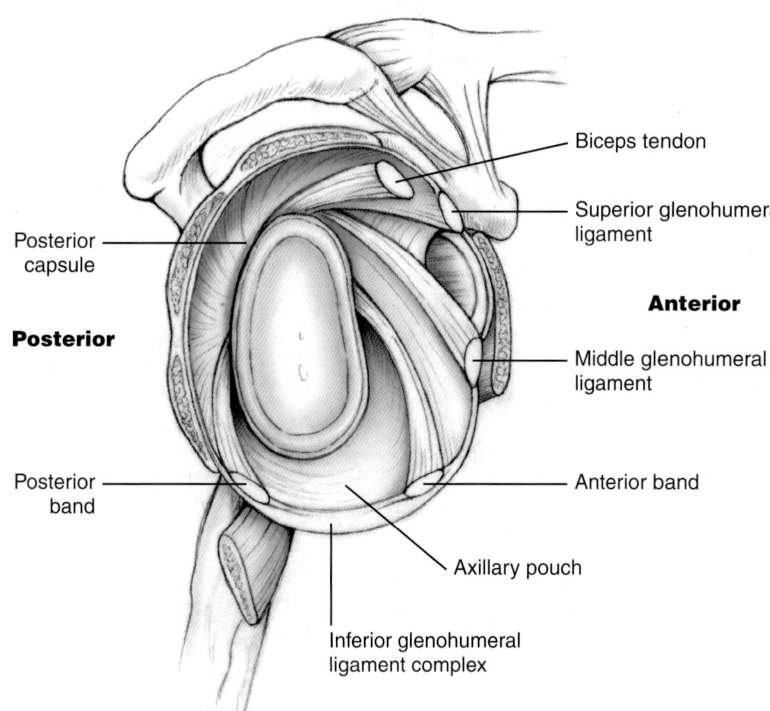

Figure 13.9 Capsuloligamentous anatomy viewed from the side with the anterior aspect to the right and the posterior aspect to the left. The humeral head has been removed, leaving the glenoid. The superior glenohumeral ligament and middle glenohumeral ligament are labeled. The inferior glenohumeral ligament complex consists of an anterior band, posterior band, and interposed axillary pouch. The posterior capsule is the area above the posterior band. The biceps is also labeled. (*Adapted from* O'Brien SJ, Neves MC, Arnoczky SP, et al. The anatomy and histology of the inferior glenohumeral ligament complex of the shoulder. *Am J Sports Med* 1990;18:449–456, with permission.)

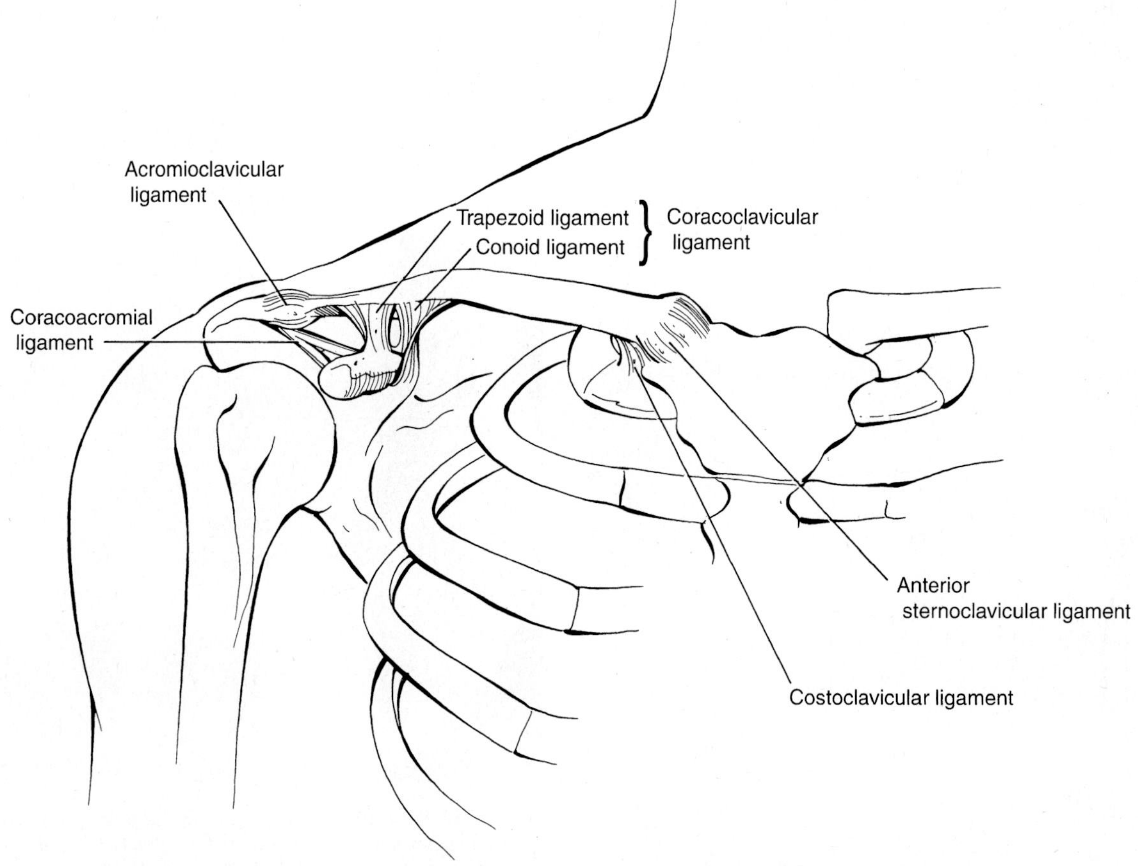

Figure 13.10 The acromioclavicular joint is stabilized by the joint capsule and the coracoclavicular ligaments, while the sternoclavicular joint is stabilized by the costoclavicular and sternoclavicular ligaments. (*From* Iannotti JP, Williams GR. *Disorders of the Shoulder: Diagnosis and Management*, 2nd ed. Philadelphia: Lippincott Williams & Wilkins, 2007, with permission.)

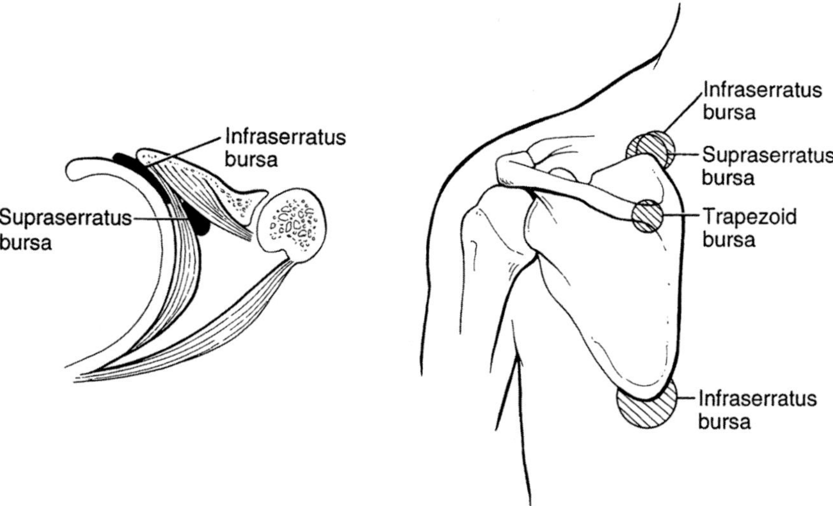

Figure 13.11 Location of the scapulothoracic bursa. (*From* Iannotti JP, Williams GR. *Disorders of the Shoulder: Diagnosis and Management*, 2nd ed. Philadelphia: Lippincott Williams & Wilkins, 2007.)

the posterior thoracic cage. These surfaces are separated by several scapulothoracic bursa that aid in motion at this interface (Fig. 13.11). Occasionally, these bursa can become inflamed and lead to posterior shoulder pain. When this inflammation is due to abnormal mechanics used to compensate for other deficits within the shoulder complex, the pain normally resolves with correction of the underlying problem. When the inflammation is the primary pathology, it often responds to conservative treatment using physical therapy and occasionally steroid injections.

Subacromial Space

The subacromial space is located between the superior aspect of the superior rotator cuff tendons and the inferior aspect of the acromion. Within this space, the subacromial bursa helps to facilitate motion between the two opposing surfaces (Fig. 13.12). Inflammation of this bursa, narrowing of the space, or degeneration of the rotator cuff tendons within the space is a common source of shoulder pain, as discussed in the section on rotator pathology.

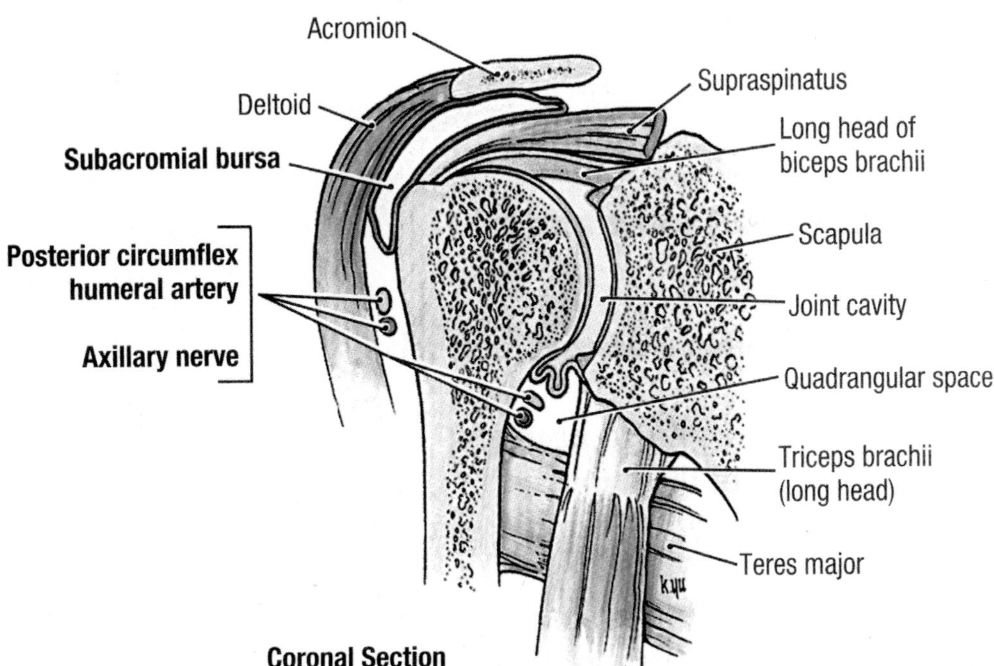

Figure 13.12 The subacromial bursa is between the rotator cuff and the overlying acromion. When a full-thickness rotator cuff tear is present, this bursa communicates with the glenohumeral joint. (*From* Agur AMR, Dalley AF. *Grant's Atlas of Anatomy*, 11th ed. Philadelphia: Lippincott Williams & Wilkins, 2005.)

Rotator Cuff Muscles

A large number of muscle groups contribute to normal movement of the shoulder. These muscles can be divided into groups that primarily function to stabilize the shoulder, move the shoulder, or move the scapula.

Immediately superficial to the GH joint capsule is a set of four muscles called the *rotator cuff*. Although these muscles contribute to rotation and elevation about the GH joint, their primary purpose is to keep the humeral head centered within glenoid cavity while the larger, more powerful muscles of the shoulder complex move the arm. All four muscles originate on the scapula and coalesce as a tendinous cuff to insert onto the greater and lesser tuberosities of the proximal humerus (Fig. 13.13). The supraspinatus cuff muscle is most frequently involved in rotator cuff pathology. It originates from the suprascapular fossa and inserts on the anterior portion of the greater tuberosity. As the supraspinatus tendon passes laterally, it runs underneath the CA arch that is formed by the anterior acromion and the CA ligament. The infraspinatus muscle originates from the infraspinatus fossa of the scapula and inserts onto the greater tuberosity immediately posterior to the supraspinatus. The infraspinatus plays a major role in moving the arm, providing the majority of external rotation strength. Both the supra- and infraspinatus are innervated by the suprascapular nerve, which arises from the superior trunk of the brachial plexus and passes posteriorly through the suprascapular notch. After innervating the supraspinatus, the nerve then passes through the spinoglenoid notch before innervating the infraspinatus. Injury or compression of the nerve in the suprascapular notch will lead to atrophy

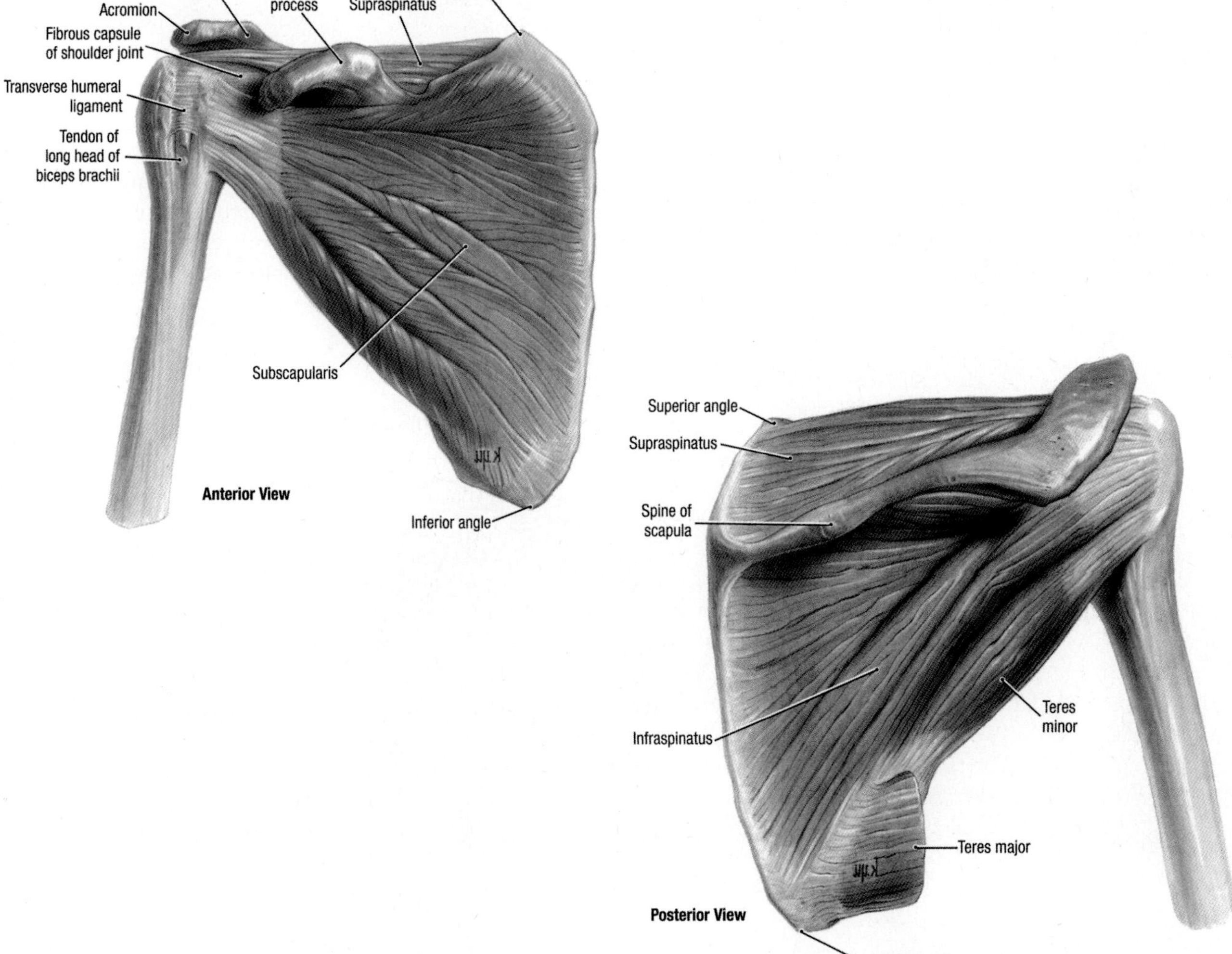

Figure 13.13 The four rotator cuff muscles originate on the scapula and insert on the greater and lesser tuberosities of the proximal humerus. The long head of the biceps tendon runs in a groove between the two tuberosities. (*From* Agur AMR. *Grant's Atlas of Anatomy*, 9th ed. Philadelphia: Williams and Wilkins, 1991.)

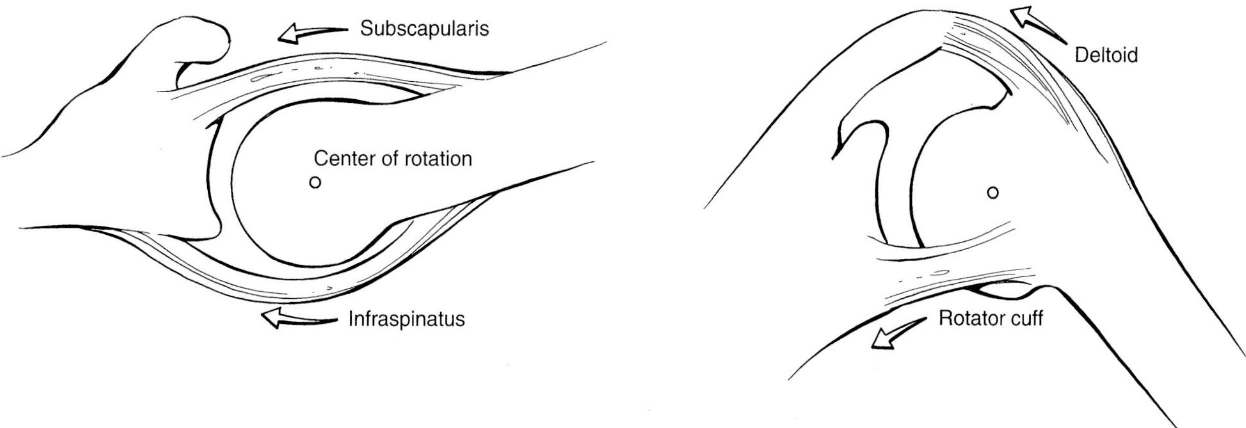

Figure 13.14 **A:** Contraction of the anterior and posterior rotator cuff muscles provides a compressive force that keeps the humeral head centered in the glenoid during rotation of the arm. **B:** During elevation of the arm, the inferior and medially directed force generated by the rotator cuff keeps the humeral head centered in the glenoid and allows the force generated by the deltoid to rotate humeral head. (*From* Iannotti JP, Williams GR. *Disorders of the Shoulder: Diagnosis and Management*, 2nd ed. Philadelphia: Lippincott Williams & Wilkins, 2007.)

of both muscles, whereas injury at the spinoglenoid notch will cause isolated atrophy of the infraspinatus.

The teres minor arises below the infraspinatus and attaches posteriorly on the greater tuberosity. The muscle is innervated by the axillary nerve as the nerve passes posteriorly just below the muscle through the quadrangular space (Fig. 13.12). Like the infraspinatus, it is an external rotator of the arm but is more effective with the arm at 90 degrees of elevation.

Anteriorly, originating from the subscapular fossa, lies the subscapularis muscle. It inserts onto the lesser tuberosity and is innervated by the upper and lower subscapular nerves. The subscapularis contributes to internal rotation of the arm.

Contraction of the rotator cuff muscles stabilizes the GH joint by providing a compressive force across the joint (Fig. 13.14). The cuff muscles also act as a *force couple* with the deltoid to allow for elevation of the arm. A force couple is a paired set of coordinated muscle contractions that together achieve a function not possible by either muscle group acting alone. If the deltoid were to contract without the rotator cuff, the humeral head would simply slide superiorly on the glenoid. When both the deltoid and rotator cuff muscles fire together, the overall medial and inferior vector generated by the cuff muscles keeps the humeral head centered on the glenoid, and the force generated by the deltoid leads to rotation of the humeral head and elevation of the arm.

Between the anterior border of the supraspinatus tendon and superior border of the subscapularis tendon lies a triangularly shaped area of uncovered capsule known as the *rotator interval*. This interval contains the SGHL, the coracohumeral ligament, and the long head of the biceps tendon (LHBT). The function of the LHBT remains controversial, with some authors believing it plays a major role in depressing the humeral head, especially when a deficiency of the rotator cuff is present. Others believe that its functional purpose is inconsequential and that it is a significant source of pain. The tendon originates from the supraglenoid tubercule and superior glenoid labrum and runs laterally through the GH joint to exit out the bicipital groove (Figs. 13.9 and 13.13). Tears of the subscapularis muscles are often associated with medial instability of the LHBT. Given its close anatomic proximity, pathology of the supraspinatus is often associated with tendinosis of the LHBT within the GH joint.

Glenohumeral Movers

The primary muscles responsible for generating motion and power about the GH joint are the deltoid, pectoralis major, latissimus dorsi, and teres major (Fig. 13.15). The deltoid is the largest muscle of the shoulder girdle, with an anterior head arising from the mid to lateral clavicle, a middle head arising from the lateral acromion, and a posterior head that arises from the scapular spine. All three heads coalesce to insert on the deltoid tuberosity of the proximal humerus. Innervation is via the axillary nerve, which passes posteriorly through the quadrangular space and then wraps back around the arm anteriorly on the deep surface of the deltoid muscle (Fig. 13.16). The nerve travels 5 cm below the tip of the lateral acromion as it passes in an anterior direction from the middle to the anterior deltoid. When splitting the deltoid between the anterior and lateral heads to access the rotator cuff, it is important that the split does not extend greater than 5 cm below the lateral acromion in order to avoid injuring the nerve and deinnervating the anterior deltoid. The primary action of the deltoid is elevation

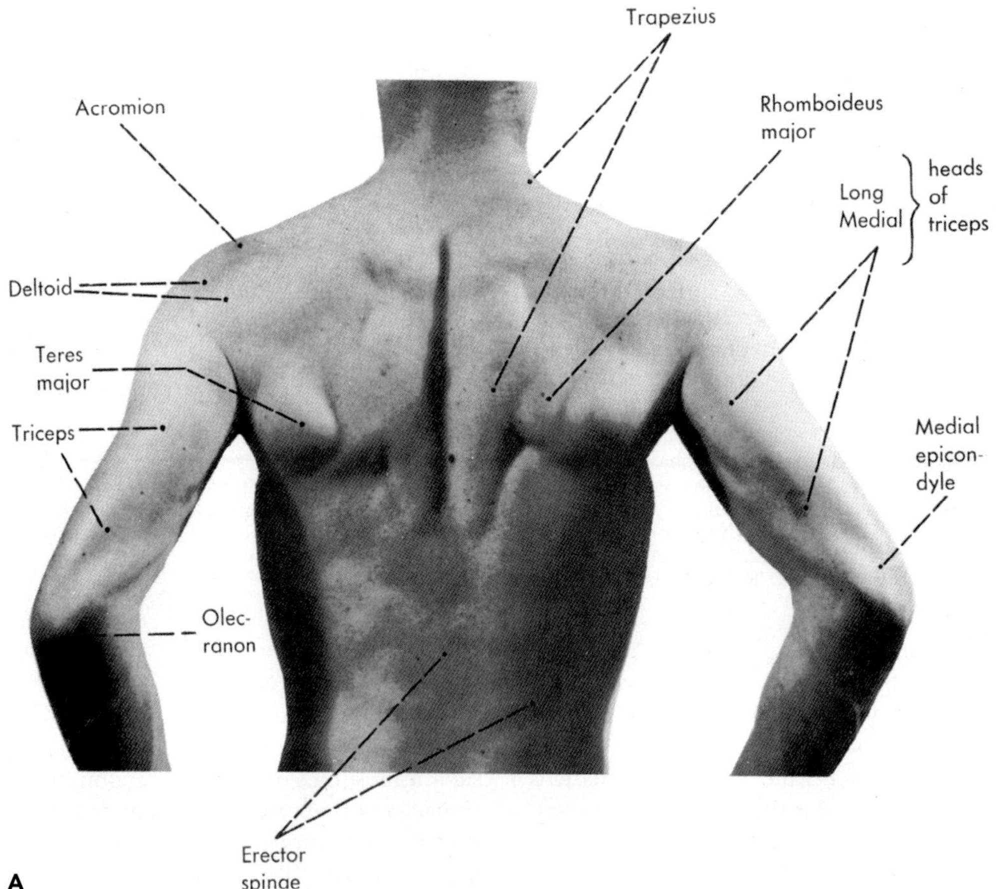

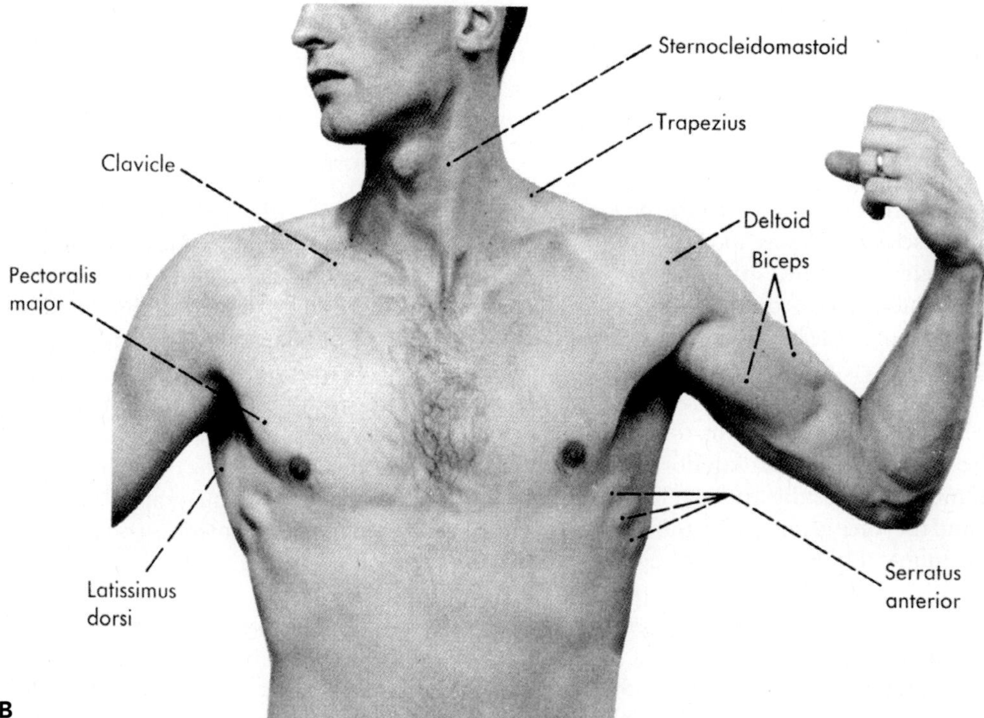

Figure 13.15 Anterior **(A)** and posterior **(B)** views of the primary movers of the glenohumeral joint, which are the deltoid, pectoralis major, latissimus dorsi, and teres major. (*From* Moore KL. *Clinically Oriented Anatomy*, 3rd ed. Baltimore: Williams & Wilkins, 1992, with permission.)

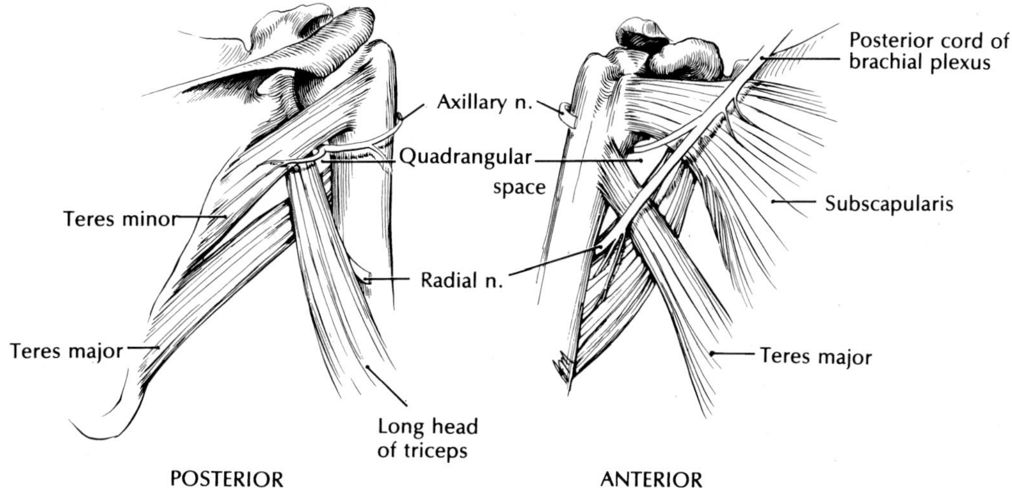

Figure 13.16 The axillary nerve passes posteriorly through the quadrangular space and then wraps back around the humerus anteriorly on the undersurface of the deltoid muscle. (*From* Moore KL. *Clinically Oriented Anatomy*, 3rd ed. Baltimore: Williams & Wilkins, 1992, with permission.)

of the arm, although the anterior and posterior heads also contribute to internal and external rotation of the arm.

The pectoralis major originates from the manubrium of the sternum, first six ribs, and medial two thirds of the clavicle. It inserts on the lateral lip of the bicipital groove and is innervated by the medial and lateral pectoral nerves. The muscle is important for forward flexion, adduction, and internal rotation of the arm. In cases of irreparable subscapularis tears, the pectoralis major can be transferred to the lesser tuberosity to substitute for the anterior rotator cuff.

The latissimus dorsi arises posteriorly from a large aponeurosis between T7 and L5 as well as the sacrum, ilium, and occasionally the lower three or four ribs and inferior scapular angle to insert on the medial lip of the bicipital groove. Innervation is via the thoracodorsal nerve. Activation of the muscle internally rotates, adducts, and extends the arm. The latissimus can be transferred to substitute for irreparable tears of the supra- and infraspinatus.

The teres major originates from the posterior scapula's inferior lateral border and attaches just medial to the latissimus on the medial aspect of the bicipital groove. It provides internal rotation, adduction, and extension of the arm and is innervated by the lower subscapular nerve.

Scapular Movers

In everyday life, the majority of movements about the shoulder complex consist of composite motion at both the GH and scapulothoracic articulation. Because the scapula's only boney articulation with the axial skeleton is via the AC joint, a group of large muscles is required not only to move the scapula but to stabilize it on the posterior aspect of the thorax. The muscles responsible for scapular movement and stability include the trapezius, levator scapulae, rhomboids, and serratus anterior (Fig. 13.17).

The trapezius is the largest of the scapulothoracic musculature and is innervated by the spinal accessory nerve. The muscle originates from the spinous processes of C7 through T12 and inserts along the scapular spine, acromion, and distal third of the clavicle. The trapezius is responsible for retraction and upward rotation of the scapula. Injury to the spinal accessory nerve, especially after the dissection of lymph nodes in the neck for the treatment of cancer, can lead to a palsy of the trapezius muscles and lateral winging of the scapula. In this condition, the medial border of the scapula will ride off or "wing" from the posterior chest wall (Fig. 13.18). The inferior tip of the scapula will also sit laterally compared with the opposite side. This deformity can be exaggerated by having the patient elevate his arm or perform a wall push-up.

The second major scapular rotator is the serratus anterior muscle, which originates as fleshy slips along the anterolateral first through ninth ribs and inserts along the anterior surface of the scapula's medial boarder. Innervated by the long thoracic nerve, the serratus protracts and upwardly rotates the scapula. Palsy of the serratus muscle will also lead to scapular winging, but the winging will be medial instead of lateral. The medial boarder of the scapula will continue to wing, but the inferior tip will ride medial and superior when compared with the opposite side. As with lateral winging, the deformity can be exaggerated with elevation of the arm or a wall push-up.

The levator scapula and rhomboids serve to retract and inferiorly rotate the scapula. The levator scapula lies deep to the trapezius and arises from the transverse processes of C1 to C3. It inserts on the superior border of the medial scapula and is innervated by deep branches of C3 and C4, as well as by the dorsal scapula nerve. The rhomboid minor and major originate from the spinous processes of C7 to

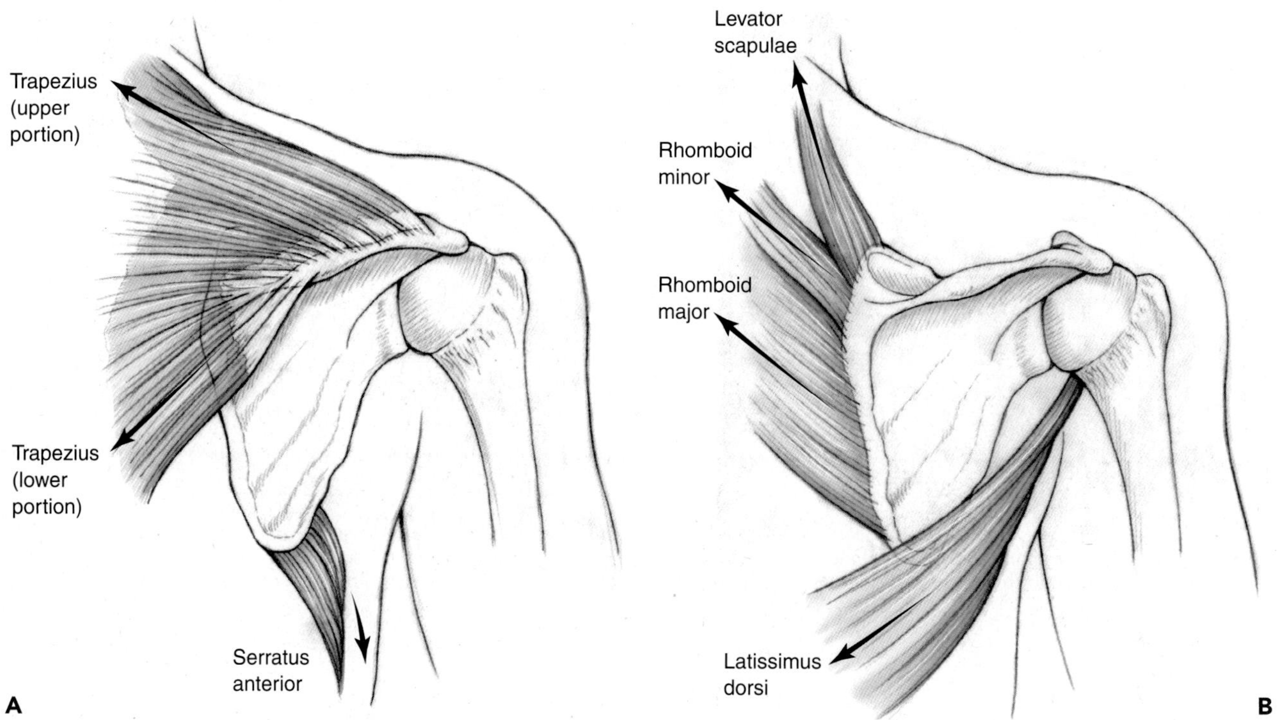

Figure 13.17 The scapular rotators. **A:** The trapezius and serratus anterior are the primary upward rotators of the scapula. **B:** The rhomboids, levator scapula, and latissimus dorsi are responsible for downward rotation. (*From* Iannotti JP, Williams GR. *Disorders of the Shoulder: Diagnosis and Management*, 2nd ed. Philadelphia: Lippincott Williams & Wilkins, 2007, with permission.)

T5 and insert along the medial border of the scapula. They are innervated by the dorsal scapular nerve.

Neurovascular Structures

Although the blood supply to the proximal humerus and innervation of the various muscles surrounding the shoulder has been previously discussed, it is extremely important to keep in mind the close proximity of the major neurovascular structures of the upper extremity to the shoulder girdle. The axillary artery and vein, surrounded by the brachial plexus, typically lie medially and distally to the coracoid process (Fig. 13.19). Damage to these vital structures following traumatic injuries to the shoulder region is uncommon but certainly can occur. Missing such damage, especially when it involves the vasculature, can have catastrophic consequences.

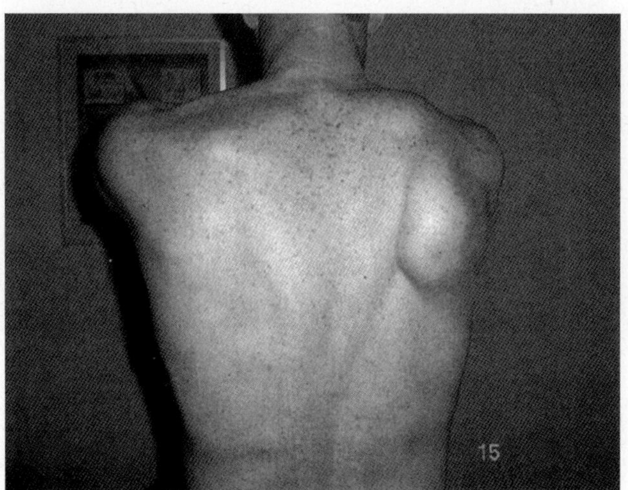

Figure 13.18 Weakness of the serratus anterior or trapezius muscles can lead to scapular winging. (*From* Krishnan SG, Hawkins RJ, Warren RF. *The Shoulder and the Overhead Athlete*. Philadelphia: Lippincott Williams & Wilkins, 2004, with permission.)

EVALUATION OF SHOULDER PROBLEMS

The most common shoulder complaints are pain, weakness, stiffness, and instability. Despite the widespread use of sophisticated imaging modalities, a thorough history and physical examination remain the most important tools in the evaluation of shoulder disorders.

History

For all patients presenting with upper extremity complaints, the history should begin with their age, dominant hand, and occupation. Age is particularly important when evaluating shoulder problems, because many of the common pathologies affecting the shoulder have a marked

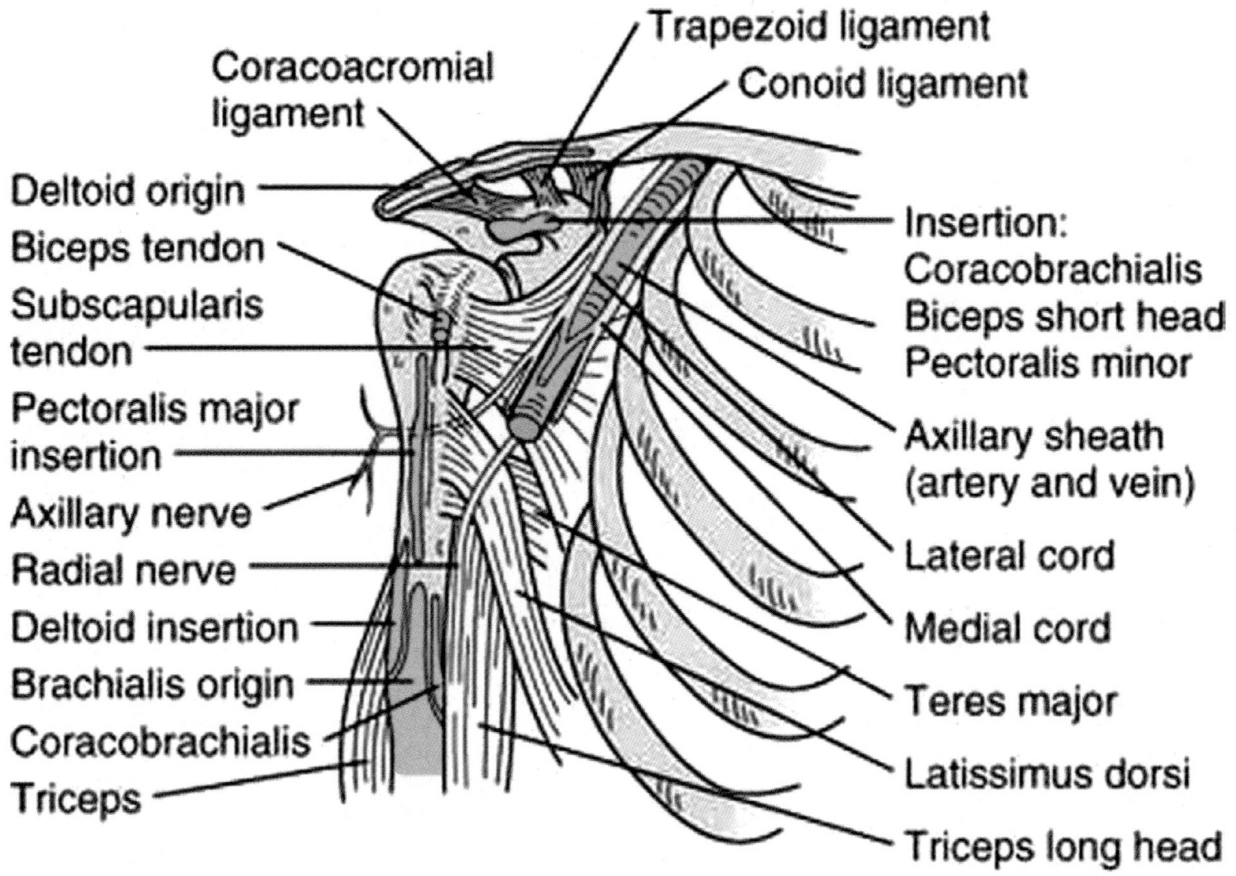

Figure 13.19 The axillary vessels and brachial plexus lie medial and distal to the coracoid process. (*From* Chapman MW, Szabo RM, Marder RA, et al. *Chapman's Orthopaedic Surgery*. Philadelphia: Lippincott Williams & Wilkins, 2001, with permission.)

predilection for certain age groups. Patients under the age of 30 are more likely to experience GH instability or labral lesions, whereas rotator cuff pathology and arthritis are more common in elderly patients.

Next, it is important to ask the patient to describe his problem. Patients will generally complain of pain, weakness, stiffness, instability, or a traumatic event. For each of these complaints, it is important to note the acuity of onset, duration, frequency, and severity of the symptoms. In patients who have experienced a traumatic injury, the exact nature of the injury and position of the extremity at the time of the injury are important. The function of the shoulder prior to the injury should also be noted, as this can influence decision making when evaluating the patient's physical examination and imaging findings. It is important to question the patient regarding litigation concerning any injury. Likewise, the examiner should inquire as to whether the patient began experiencing symptoms or was injured while working. Unfortunately, the literature has demonstrated that the outcomes for the treatment of pathology about the shoulder are significantly worse for patients who are involved in worker's compensation claims.

Pain is the most common shoulder problem. Its location about the joint is important. Pain over the superior shoulder is often due to disorders of the AC joint, whereas pain over the trapezius may be referred from the cervical spine or secondary to fatigue when the patient is attempting to compensate for GH or subacromial pathology through increased scapulothoracic motion. Rotator cuff pathology is almost always associated with pain over the lateral aspect of the upper arm, whereas GH arthritis leads to a dull ache within the shoulder joint that is exacerbated with motion.

Radiation of pain is an important consideration. In general, pain from shoulder problems does not radiate below the elbow. If the patient is complaining of pain that radiates to the forearm or hand, other sources of pathology, such as peripheral nerve compression or cervical spine disease, should be suspected.

The nature of the patient's pain and any exacerbating movements should be obtained. Burning pain suggests a neurologic cause. Pain from rotator cuff pathology and impingement syndrome is often described as a dull ache that is exacerbated by overhead activities and reaching behind the back. These patients will often complain that the pain wakes them from sleep, especially when they lie on the involved side. As in other areas of the body, severe night or rest pain should always raise concern for neoplasm or infection.

Patients with decreased motion of the shoulder may complain of stiffness. They may also complain of pain occurring primarily at the extremes of their ROM. Weakness is another common complaint. In these patients, it is important to attempt to determine whether they feel weak because of associated pain or whether they actually lack strength. When a patient complains of instability, the etiology, frequency, direction, and severity of the instability should be recorded.

Cervical spine pathology often leads to pain that is referred to the shoulder region; therefore, all patients with shoulder pain should be questioned regarding neck pain and neurologic symptoms radiating down the arm. Finally, the specifics and efficacy of any previous treatment that the patient may have already received for his shoulder complaint should be obtained. This includes the location (i.e., subacromial, GH, trigger point) and number of any injections, and the duration and nature of any physical therapy programs.

Physical Examination

The physical examination of the shoulder involves the same basic elements as examination of the other joints in the musculoskeletal system including inspection, palpation, ROM, strength testing, and neurovascular examination. Additionally, several special tests are useful in the evaluation of specific pathologic conditions (Table 13.2). Each of these tests need not be performed on every patient. Instead, only those maneuvers related to suspected pathology, as determined by the history and basic elements of the physical examination, should be performed. This section describes the basic elements of the physical examination; the specific tests are described in the physical examination sections of the conditions that they evaluate.

TABLE 13.2
SPECIAL TESTS FOR EXAMINATION OF THE SHOULDER

Test	Condition Examined
Neer impingement sign	Impingement
Hawkins impingement sign	Impingement
Jobe test	Rotator cuff weakness, impingement
External rotation lag sign	Infraspinatus weakness
Hornblower sign	Infraspinatus and teres minor weakness
Lift-off test	Subscapularis weakness
Belly-press test	Subscapularis weakness
Apprehension test	Glenohumeral instability
Relocation test	Glenohumeral instability
Load and shift test	Glenohumeral laxity
Sulcus sign	Inferior glenohumeral laxity
O'Brien test	SLAP tear
Mayo sheer test	SLAP tear

Given the close anatomic location and frequent overlap in presenting symptoms, it is important to begin the examination of all patients with shoulder pain with a brief examination of the cervical spine. Pain or stiffness with rotation or flexion/extension of the neck can be indicative of cervical disease and should prompt a more thorough workup.

Inspection

The patient must be appropriately gowned to allow inspection of both shoulders and the neck. Examination begins with inspection of the shoulders for asymmetry, masses, swelling, erythema, ecchymoses, and muscle atrophy. The location and condition of any previous surgical incisions should be noted. As with all elements of the shoulder examination, comparison of the two sides is essential. Ecchymoses may be present in a number of traumatic shoulder conditions including fractures, dislocations, muscle ruptures, and large, acute rotator cuff tears. Prominence of the distal clavicle at the AC joint is a common finding after AC separation or osteophyte formation with AC arthritis. Atrophy of the muscles about the shoulder can occur with disuse secondary to pain, tendon rupture, or following de-innervation. When longstanding rotator cuff tears lead to muscle atrophy, hollowing often occurs over the supraspinatus and infraspinatus fossa. Atrophy of the deltoid muscle, especially following traumatic injury or previous surgery, should raise concern for injury to the axillary nerve.

Inspection of the position of the scapula on the posterior chest wall is important. Winging of the scapula can indicate weakness of the serratus anterior or trapezius (Fig. 13.18). While viewed posteriorly, the patient should be asked to raise both hands overhead while the examiner inspects for scapulothoracic rhythm, which should be smooth and symmetric. Abnormalities can be due to scapulothoracic bursitis or scapular winging. They may also be secondary as the patient attempts to compensate for stiffness or pain in other aspects of the shoulder complex.

Palpation

Palpation begins medially at the SC joints and continues laterally along the clavicle, AC joint, coracoid, acromion, and scapular spine. Patients with SC or AC joint pathology will generally be tender directly over those joints. The insertion of the rotator cuff tendons on the greater tuberosity can be palpated through the deltoid muscle lateral to the acromion and is often tender in patients with impingement or rotator cuff tears. Tenderness to palpation over the trapezius is often seen with cervical spine pathology or with muscle spasm during scapulothoracic compensation for GH abnormalities.

Range of Motion

In the traumatized or obviously fractured or dislocated shoulder, ROM assessment should be considered only after

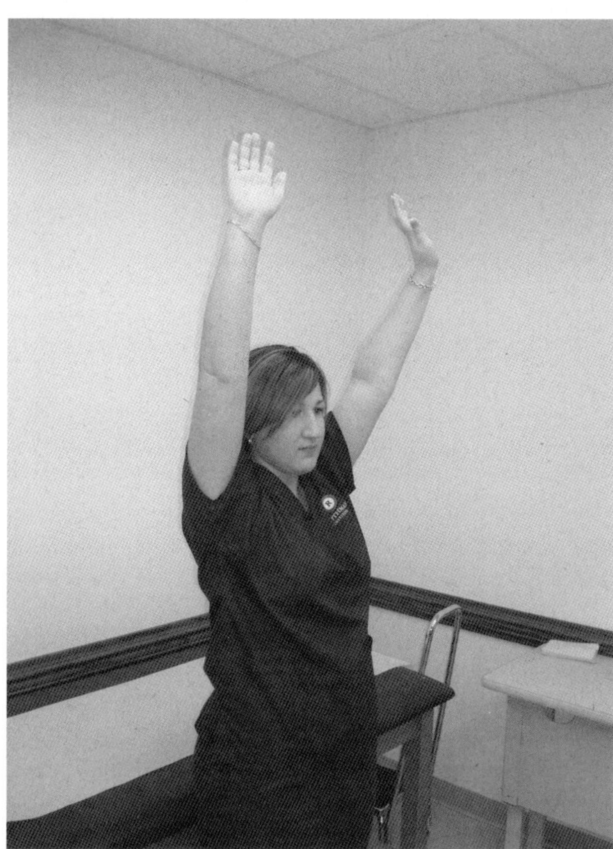

Figure 13.20 Forward elevation is assessed by asking the patient to raise her hands directly overhead.

review of radiographs. In all other patients, both active and passive ROM should be evaluated for forward elevation and internal and external rotation.

Forward elevation is a composite of GH and scapulothoracic motion and is assessed by asking the patient to raise his hands directly overhead (Fig. 13.20). Internal and external rotation are evaluated with the arm both at the side and at 90 degrees of abduction. For external rotation with the arm at the side, the patient's elbow is placed at the side of the body and flexed 90 degrees. Glenohumeral rotation is then measured by rotating the forearm laterally while the elbow is stabilized at the side (Fig. 13.21). Zero degrees is achieved when the forearm points straight ahead, whereas 90 degrees is achieved when the forearm is positioned in line with the shoulders. Internal rotation is assessed by having the patient put the hand behind the back to touch as high as possible, noting the relationship of the thumb to the tip of the spinal column (Fig. 13.22). As a reference, the spine of the scapula is considered approximately at the T2 level and the tip at T7.

For rotation with the arm at 90 degrees of abduction, the arm is abducted 90 degrees in the plane of the scapula with the elbow in 90 degrees of flexion (Fig. 13.23). The examiner then uses one hand to externally rotate the patient's arm while steadying the patient's elbow with the

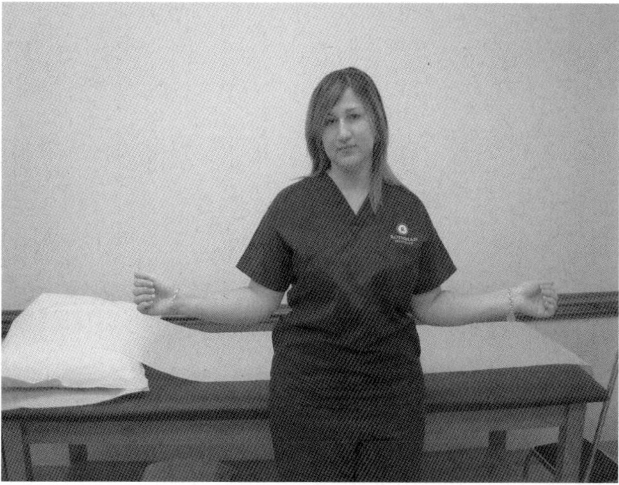

Figure 13.21 External rotation with the arm at the side is assessed by asking the patient to place her elbow at the side of the body and flex it 90 degrees. The patient is then asked to externally rotate the forearm while maintaining the elbow at her side.

opposite hand. At neutral rotation, the forearm is parallel to the floor; at 90 degrees of external rotation, the forearm is parallel to the body with the hand pointing toward the ceiling. This is followed by internal rotation, which is

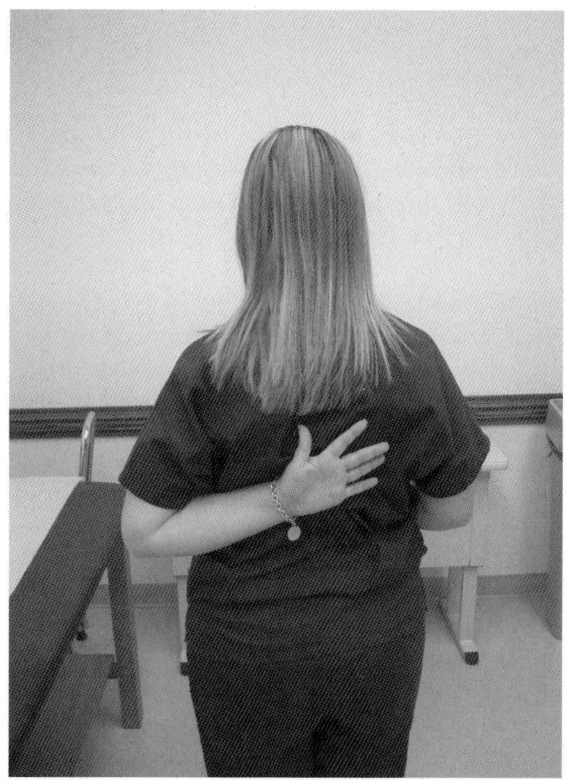

Figure 13.22 Internal rotation is assessed by asking the patient to put her hand behind her back and touch as high as possible. The relationship of the thumb to the spinous processes of the vertebral bodies is used as a reference for measurement. This patient has internal rotation to the T5 level.

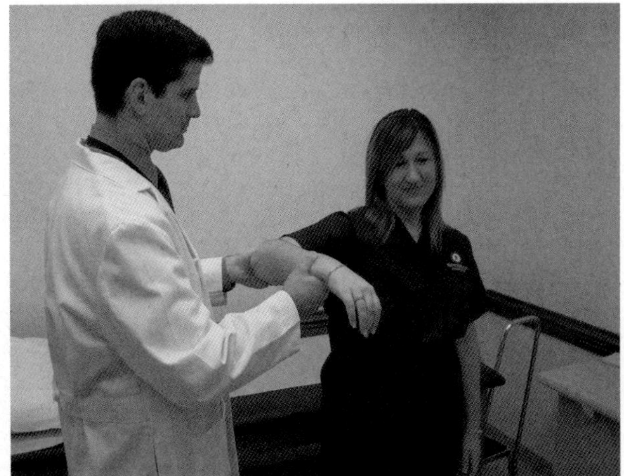

A

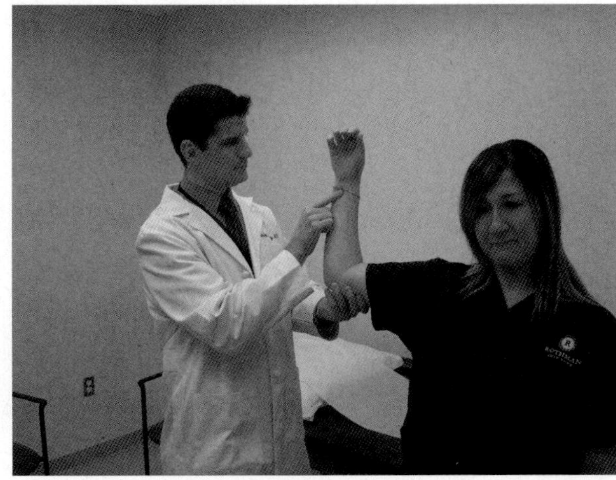

B

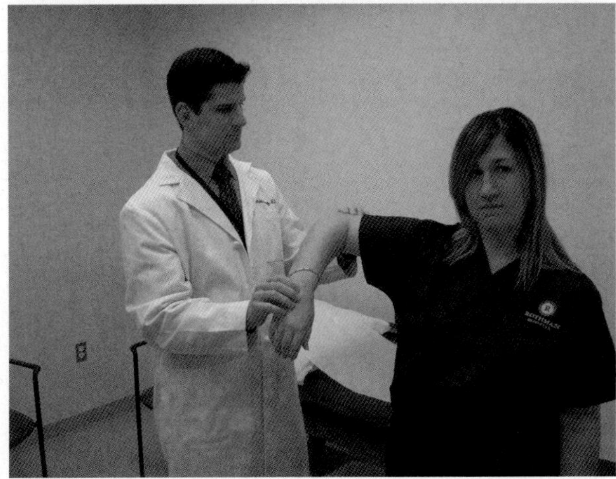

C

Figure 13.23 **A–C:** For rotation with the arm at 90 degrees of abduction, the arm is abducted 90 degrees in the plane of the scapula with the elbow in 90 degrees of flexion (A). The arm is then maximally externally (B) and then internally (C) rotated.

measured by rotating the hand toward the floor and noting the degrees of downward rotation from the neutral position.

Strength Testing

Strength testing about the shoulder focuses on evaluation of the rotator cuff. The supraspinatus is best evaluated by testing resisted abduction in the plane of the scapula of the extended, internally rotated arm. This is known as the Jobe test or the "empty can" sign. The patient is asked to resist downward pressure from the examiner with the shoulder abducted 90 degrees, the elbow extended, and the thumb pointing downward toward the floor (Fig. 13.24). Weakness with this maneuver can be indicative of supraspinatus dysfunction, although it can be difficult to distinguish true weakness from weakness secondary to pain. Furthermore, some patients with full-thickness tears of the supraspinatus tendon will exhibit minimal strength deficits with this test.

The posterior rotator cuff muscles (infraspinatus and teres minor) are evaluated by testing external rotation strength of the arm with the elbow at the side (Fig. 13.25). Significant weakness in external rotation should be evaluated with lag signs. With the elbow flexed 90 degrees and at

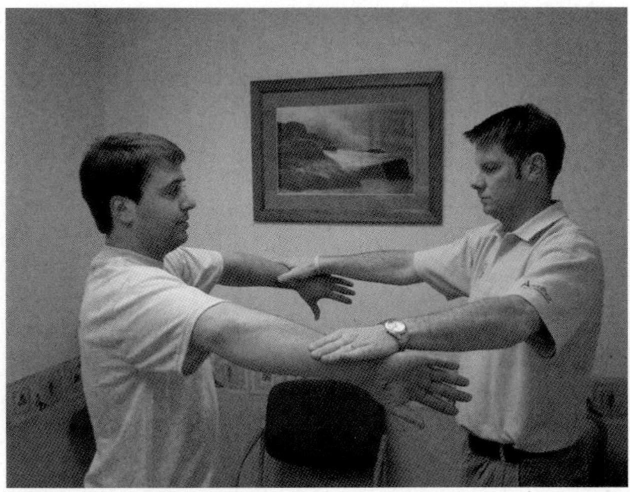

Figure 13.24 Jobe test is performed by having the patient abduct the shoulder 90 degrees in the plain of the scapula and internally rotate the arm (thumb pointing toward the floor). The patient is then asked to resist a downward force applied by the examiner. The test can be performed separately on each side, or both shoulders can be tested simultaneously. (*From* Schepsis AA, Busconi BD. *Orthopaedic Surgery Essentials: Sports Medicine*. Philadelphia: Lippincott Williams & Wilkins, 2006, with permission.)

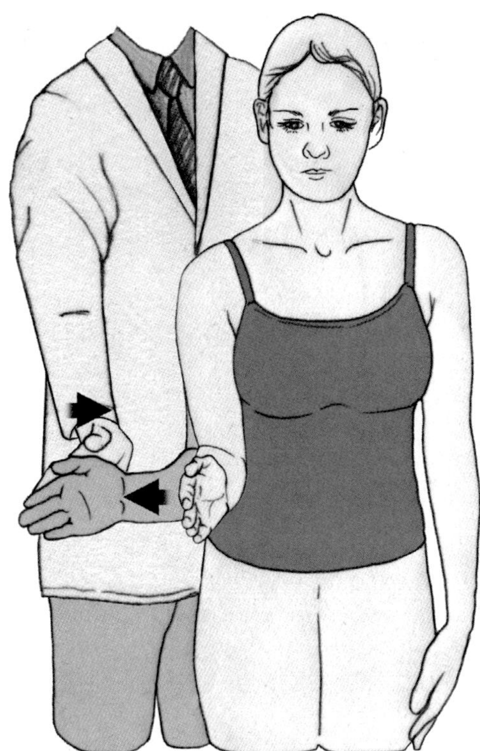

Figure 13.25 The posterior rotator cuff is evaluated by testing external rotation strength with the elbow at the side. (*From* Johnson DH, Pedowitz RA. *Practical Orthopaedic Sports Medicine and Arthroscopy*. Philadelphia: Lippincott Williams & Wilkins, 2007, with permission.)

the side, the forearm is placed in maximal external rotation by the examiner. As the examiner releases the forearm, the patient is asked to maintain it in maximal external rotation (Fig. 13.26). If the patient is unable to do so, the sign is considered positive, and a tear or dysfunction of the infraspinatus should be suspected. An inability to maintain the 90-degree abducted arm in maximal external rotation is known as the Hornblower sign and is indicative of pathology of the lower half of the infraspinatus and teres minor (Fig. 13.27).

Two maneuvers have been described to evaluate subscapularis strength. For the lift-off test, the patient is asked to lift his hand away from the lower back (Fig. 13.28). Inability to lift and maintain the hand off the back is considered a positive test and indicates subscapularis weakness. The belly press test can also be used to evaluate subscapularis strength. The patient is asked to place his hand on his abdomen and internally rotate the shoulder so that the elbow is in front of the trunk. The patient is then asked to press down on his abdomen while maintaining the elbow in front of the plane of the body. With subscapularis weakness, the elbow will fall posteriorly when the patient attempts to push on his abdomen (Fig. 13.29).

The strength of the scapular stabilizers can be evaluated by asking the patient to perform a wall push-up when there is a suggestion of scapular winging. For patients with significant weakness or atrophy about the shoulder, the larger GH movers can be evaluated for integrity and function by testing resistance against their primary direction of motion. For example, the deltoid is evaluated by resisted abduction and the pectoralis major is tested by resisted adduction of the arm in 90 degrees of forward flexion.

Neurovascular Assessment

The majority of the neurologic examination has already been completed by evaluation of the strength of the muscles about the shoulder. Motor function of the remaining major nerves to the arm can be tested by resisted elbow flexion (musculocutaneous), elbow extension (radial), finger flexion (median), finger abduction (ulnar), and thumb abduction (posterior interosseous). Sensation is evaluated by assessing light touch over the lateral deltoid (axillary),

A

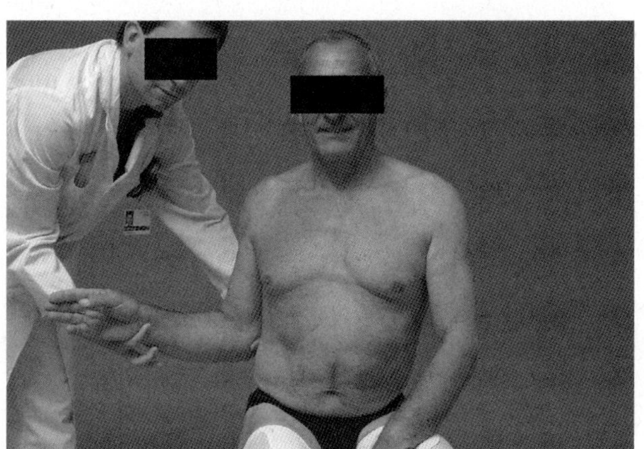

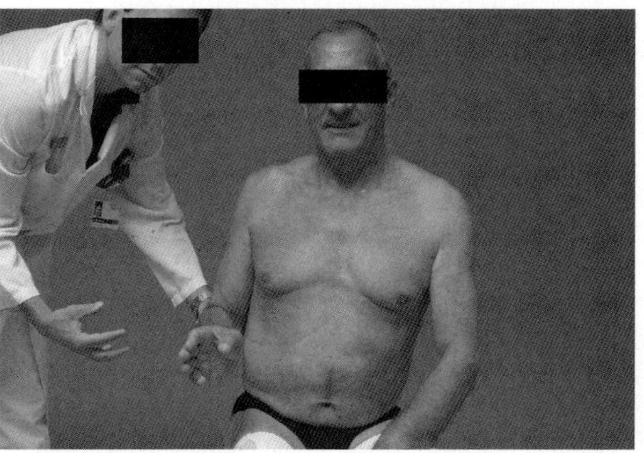

B

Figure 13.26 A lag between maximal passive and active external rotation with the arm at the side constitutes a positive external rotation lag signs and is associated with infraspinatus weakness. (*From* Iannotti JP, Williams GR. *Disorders of the Shoulder: Diagnosis and Management*, 2nd ed. Philadelphia: Lippincott Williams & Wilkins, 2007, with permission.)

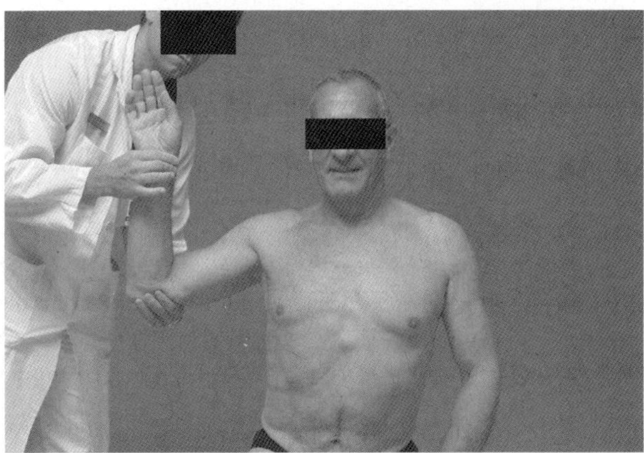
A

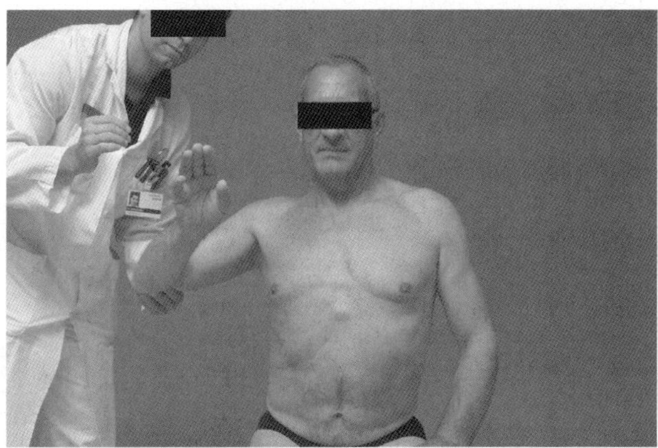
B

Figure 13.27 An inability to keep the arm in maximal external rotation at 90 degrees of abduction constitutes a positive Hornblower sign and is associated with weakness of the infraspinatus and teres minor. (*From* Iannotti JP, Williams GR. *Disorders of the Shoulder: Diagnosis and Management*, 2nd ed. Philadelphia: Lippincott Williams & Wilkins, 2007, with permission.)

lateral forearm (musculocutaneous), thumb web space (radial), radial aspect of the index finger (median), and lateral aspect of the little finger (ulnar). For patients with suspected neurologic pathology, a more detailed neurologic exam including reflex evaluation is necessary. Vascular integrity should be evaluated by palpating the radial pulse and measuring the capillary refill time for the fingers.

Imaging

Multiple imaging modalities are available for the evaluation of disorders of the shoulder complex. A standard set of plain radiographs should be obtained in all patients presenting with shoulder complaints. Additional views and more advanced imaging techniques are then ordered based on the patient's history, physical examination, and initial radiographic findings.

Radiographs

The standard radiographic examination of the shoulder includes the anterior–posterior (AP), scapular Y, and axillary lateral views. To evaluate the GH joint, it is important to obtain a true AP view of the shoulder, not of the chest. Because the scapula is angled anteriorly on the thorax, the x-ray beam must angled 30 to 45 degrees laterally, so that the beam is perpendicular to the GH joint (Figs. 13.30–32). The Zanca view, described below under the evaluation of AC sprains, is used to evaluate the AC joint. A variety of

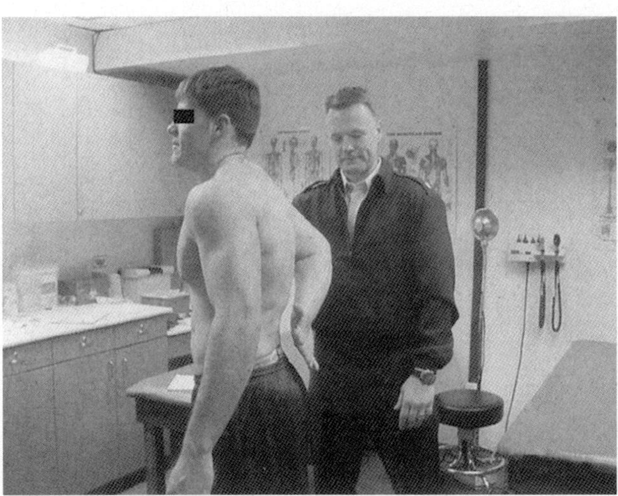

Figure 13.28 The lift-off test is used to evaluated subscapularis strength. (*From* Krishnan SG, Hawkins RJ, Warren RF. *The Shoulder and the Overhead Athlete*. Philadelphia: Lippincott Williams & Wilkins, 2004, with permission.)

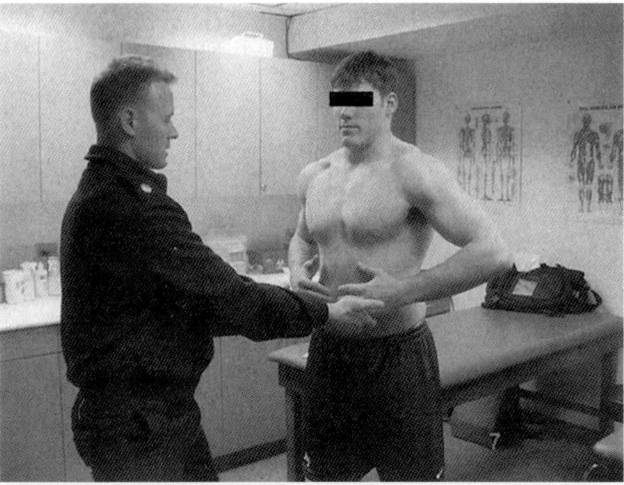

Figure 13.29 A patient with subscapularis weakness will be unable to keep his elbow in front of the plane of the body when asked to press down on his belly. This patient's elbow remains forward on the normal left side, whereas on the right side, the elbow falls posterior making the belly-press test positive. (*From* Krishnan SG, Hawkins RJ, Warren RF. *The Shoulder and the Overhead Athlete*. Philadelphia: Lippincott Williams & Wilkins, 2004, with permission.)

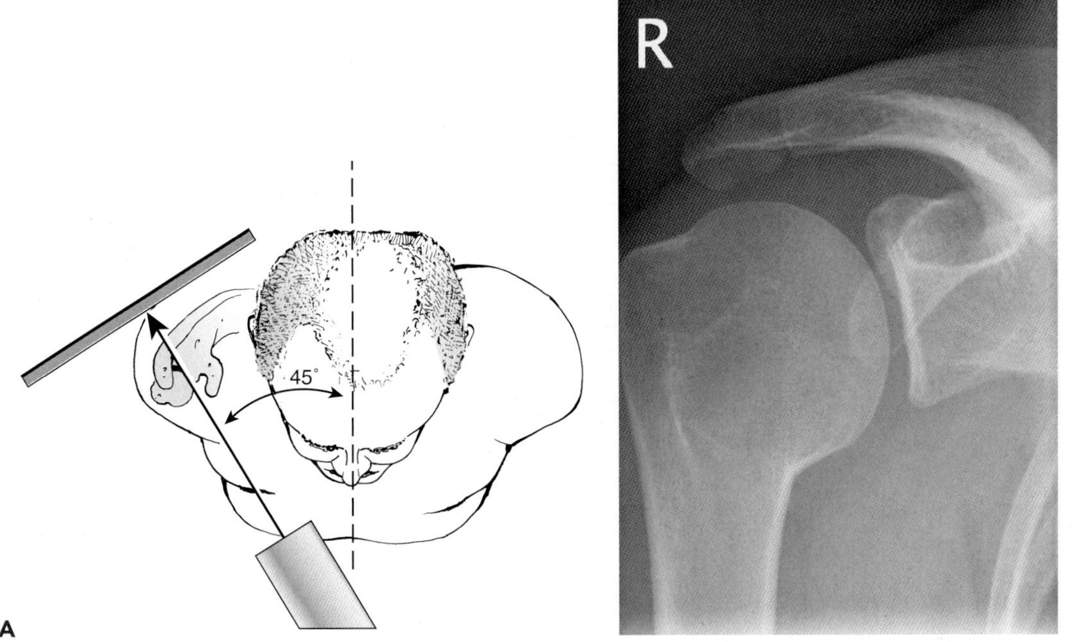

A B

Figure 13.30 **A:** The true anterior–posterior (AP) view of the glenohumeral joint is obtained by angling the beam 30 to 45 degrees from the sagittal plane. **B:** The true AP shows the glenohumeral joint without overlap of the proximal humerus on the glenoid, as occurs on an AP of the chest. (*From* (A) Buholz RW, Heckman JD, Court-Brown CM. *Rockwood and Green's Fractures in Adults,* 6th ed. Philadelphia: Lippincott Williams & Wilkins, 2006; and (B) Iannotti JP, Williams GR. *Disorders of the Shoulder: Diagnosis and Management*, 2nd ed. Philadelphia: Lippincott Williams & Wilkins, 2007, with permission.)

additional radiographic views have been described to better visualize specific areas of injury associated with GH instability, although these techniques are utilized less frequently owing to the widespread use of computed tomograph (CT) and magnetic resonance imaging (MRI) scans.

Computed Tomography Scans

Computed tomography scans provide a more detailed three-dimensional evaluation of the boney anatomy about the shoulder. They are the imaging modality of choice for the evaluation of complex fractures of the proximal humerus or scapula. They are also useful for the evaluation of posterior glenoid bone stock in patients being considered for total shoulder arthroplasty.

Magnetic Resonance Imaging Scans

Magnetic resonance imaging scans are the imaging modality of choice for the evaluation of the soft tissue structures about the shoulder. They are especially useful for evaluation of disorders of the rotator cuff. As in other areas of the body, T1 weighted images are best suited for evaluating anatomic structures, whereas T2 weighted images highlight areas of pathology. Standard MRI examination of the shoulder includes axial, coronal oblique, and sagittal oblique cuts. The coronal and sagittal oblique views are termed "oblique," because they are oriented parallel and perpendicular to the plane of the scapula which, because of the scapula's orientation on the chest wall, is oblique to the plane of the body. When using MRI for the evaluation of rotator cuff tears, it is important to correlate the patient's clinical findings with the pathology seen only in the imaging study. Over 50% of asymptomatic patients older than 60 years of age will have complete or partial rotator cuff tears on MRI scans.

Magnetic resonance imaging is less accurate in the evaluation of disorders of the glenoid labrum, such as superior labrum anterior to posterior (SLAP) tears and Bankart lesions. Although the sensitivity and specificity can be increased with injection of intra-articular contrast prior to the study, MRI findings continue to be less accurate than history and physical examination for these disorders.

Ultrasound

Ultrasound evaluation is rapidly gaining popularity for the evaluation of soft tissue pathology about the shoulder, especially disorders of the rotator cuff. Compared to MRI scans, ultrasound has the advantage of being quicker, less expensive, and better tolerated by patients, and it allows for dynamic as well as static examinations. On the downside, the accuracy is highly operator-dependent and associated muscle atrophy and intra-articular pathology is not well visualized. For these reasons, MRI remains the imaging

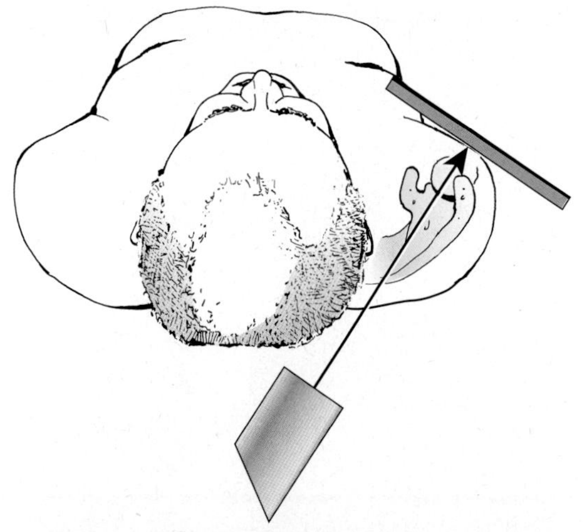

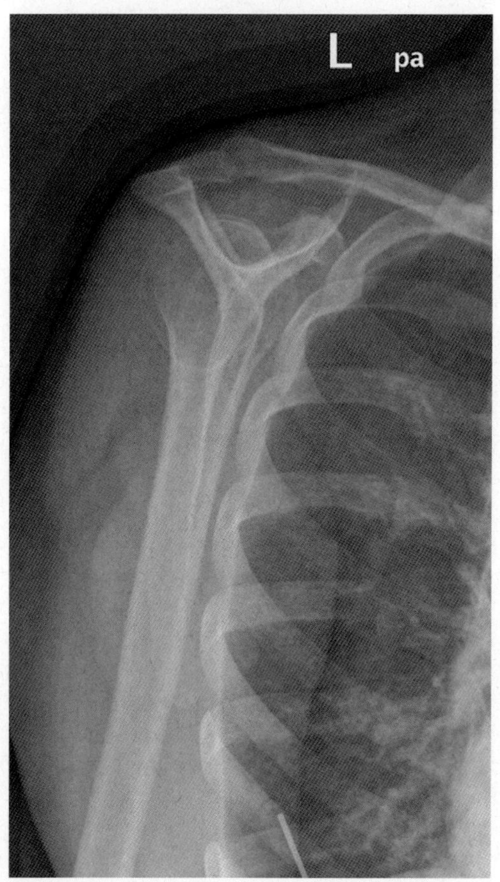

Figure 13.31 **A:** The Y view is obtained by shooting the x-ray beam parallel to the scapular spine. **B:** This view visualizes the shape of the acromion and the subacromial space. (*From* (A) Buholz RW, Heckman JD, Court-Brown CM. *Rockwood and Green's Fractures in Adults*, 6th ed. Philadelphia: Lippincott Williams & Wilkins, 2006, with permission.)

modality of choice at most centers except for those patients who are unable to undergo MRI scans. Ultrasound is especially useful following previous rotator cuff surgery, in which postsurgical artifact often makes MRI scans difficult to interpret.

Arthrography

Arthrography involves the injection of radiopaque contrast material into the GH joint followed by radiographic evaluation of the shoulder to determine the distribution pattern of the dye. In patients with full-thickness tears of the rotator cuff, the dye will leak through the cuff defect into the subacromial space. Although extremely accurate in the detection of full-thickness rotator cuff tears, the use of arthrography has been supplanted by MRI and ultrasound examination due to their less invasive nature and ability to better detect partial-thickness cuff tears and tendonitis. This study is now reserved for patients unable to undergo an MRI scan in locations where ultrasound is not available.

TRAUMATIC INJURIES TO THE SHOULDER COMPLEX

Clavicle Fractures

The clavicle is the most frequently fractured bone in the shoulder complex. Although the majority of these fractures heal uneventfully with nonoperative treatment, recent evidence suggests that the incidence of nonunion and the disability associated with malunion is more significant than was previously thought.

Classification

Fractures are classified according to their anatomic location into medial, middle, and lateral thirds. The majority of fractures (80%) occur in the middle third, where the bone is biomechanically weakest and less soft tissue protection is present. Fractures of the lateral third are further divided according to the relationship of the fracture pattern to the CC ligaments and the AC joint (Fig. 13.33). Medial fractures are much less common, accounting for only 5% of all clavicle fractures.

Mechanism of Injury

The most common cause of clavicle fractures is a fall on the involved shoulder. Direct impact to the clavicle and a fall on an outstretched hand are other, less common, mechanisms of injury.

Presentation

Patients usually present with localized pain, swelling, and deformity over the clavicle following a traumatic injury. The affected arm is often adducted across the body and supported by the opposite hand in an effort to decrease the deforming forces across the fracture site.

Physical Findings

Visible deformity and ecchymosis at the fracture site are common. The medial fragment can "tent" the skin, occasionally leading to a complete puncture and an open fracture. It is important to look for, and document, any open wounds, as their presence could have a significant impact on treatment. A thorough neurovascular examination is

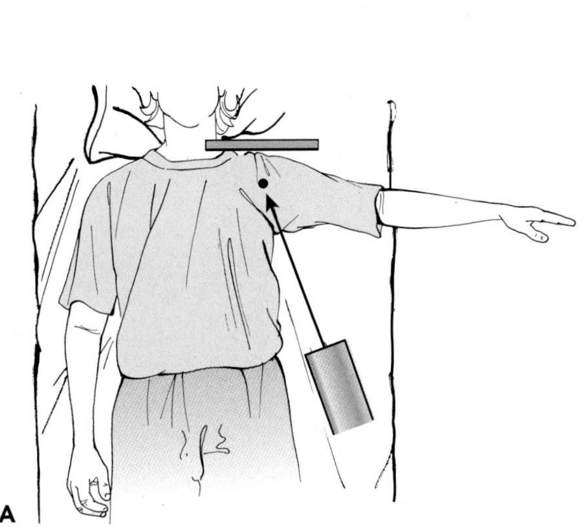

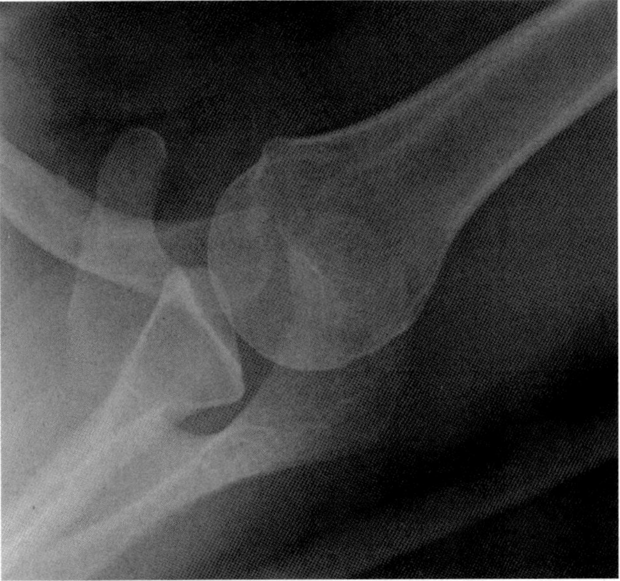

Figure 13.32 **A:** The axillary lateral is obtained by aiming the x-ray beam into the axilla with the plate on the superior shoulder. **B:** The axillary view demonstrates the relation of the humeral head to the glenoid articular surface in the anterior and posterior plane. (*From* (A) Buholz RW, Heckman JD, Court-Brown CM. *Rockwood and Green's Fractures in Adults*, 6th ed. Philadelphia: Lippincott Williams & Wilkins, 2006; and (B) Iannotti JP, Williams GR. *Disorders of the Shoulder: Diagnosis and Management*, 2nd ed. Philadelphia: Lippincott Williams & Wilkins, 2007, with permission.)

necessary, especially in patients with a high-energy mechanism of injury. The brachial plexus and axillary artery lie in close proximity to the inferior surface of the bone and are vulnerable to injury, especially with fractures of the medial third. The chest should be auscultated for bilateral breath sounds to rule out a pneumothorax.

Radiographic Evaluation

Two views of the clavicle are needed. For medial clavicle fractures, an AP and an AP with 40 degrees of cephalic tilt are used. Lateral fractures are better evaluated with an AP, a Zanca view (Fig. 13.34), and an axillary lateral of the shoulder.

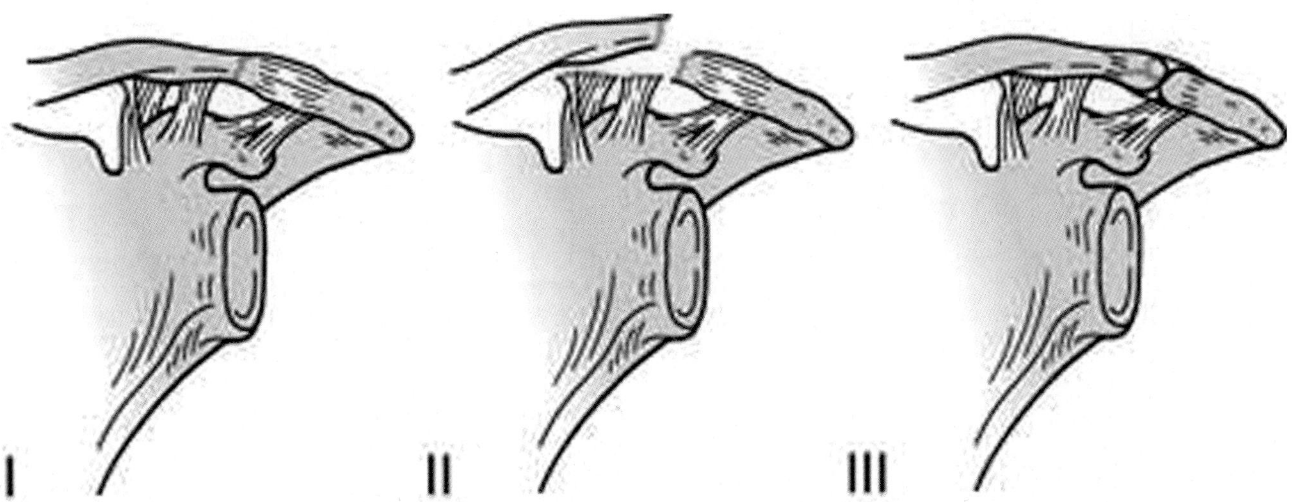

Figure 13.33 Fractures of the distal clavicle are divided into three types. Type I fractures are lateral to the cricoclavicular (CC) ligaments. Type II fractures are medial to the CC ligaments or lead to rupture of the ligaments from the medial clavicle. Type III fractures are lateral to the CC ligaments with extension into the acromioclavicular joint. (*From* Chapman MW, Szabo RM, Marder RA, et al. *Chapman's Orthopaedic Surgery*. Philadelphia: Lippincott Williams & Wilkins, 2001, with permission.)

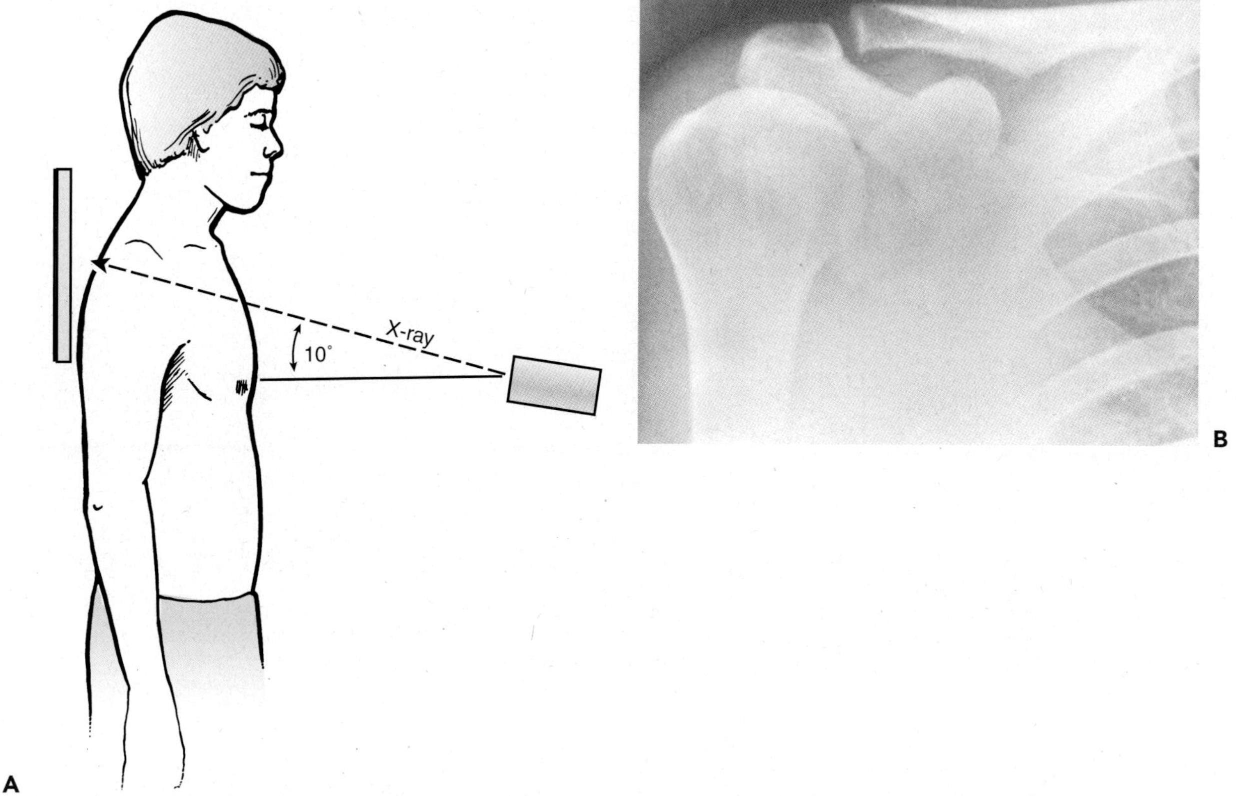

Figure 13.34 **A:** The Zanca view is obtained by shooting an anterior-posterior view with 10 degrees of cephalic tilt and half of the normal kV. **B:** The view provides excellent visualization of the acromioclavicular joint and the cricoclavicular space. (*From* (A) Rockwood CA, Young DC. Disorders of the acromioclavicular joint. In: Rockwood CA, Matsen F III, eds. *The Shoulder*. Philadelphia: WB Saunders, 1990; and (B) Buholz RW, Heckman JD, Court-Brown CM. *Rockwood and Green's Fractures in Adults*, 6th ed. Philadelphia: Lippincott Williams & Wilkins, 2006, with permission.)

Special Tests

Special tests are rarely needed. If there is difficulty understanding the fracture pattern, CT scan can be helpful. This is especially true for medial third fractures. If, based on the physical examination, there is concern for vascular injury, an arteriogram is needed. For patients with a neurologic deficit, an electromyograph (EMG) is useful for diagnostic and prognostic purposes but not until 3 to 4 weeks after the injury.

Differential Diagnosis

Clavicle fractures must be differentiated from other traumatic injuries about the shoulder. This is easily accomplished by physical examination and radiograph. When evaluating injuries about the AC and SC joints in younger patients, it is important to remember that the medial and lateral physes often do not fuse until the late teens or early twenties. Suspected AC and SC dislocations in this patient population are often Salter Harris type I fractures of the clavicle through the physis. A CT scan is helpful in making this distinction.

Treatment

Historically, almost all midshaft clavicle fractures were treated nonoperatively and thought to heal with a very low incidence of nonunion and residual disability. Nonoperative management consists of sling immobilization for 4 to 6 weeks, followed by a gradual return to activity. Stiffness of the shoulder is generally not a problem because the injury does not involve the GH joint. Several recent studies have demonstrated that, in adults, the incidence of nonunion following displaced or comminuted fractures of the middle third may be as high as 20%. Furthermore, patients who heal with more than 1.5 to 2 cm of shortening often have some residual loss of shoulder function. These studies have led to an increased interest in operative fixation, either with plates and screws or intramedullary pins, for fractures with greater that 100% displacement, comminution, or greater than 2 cm of shortening (Fig. 13.35). The absolute indications for operative management of middle-third fractures continue to be open fractures, fractures associated with a neurovascular injury, and fractures in polytrauma patients who need rapid use of the upper extremity for weight bearing.

For lateral clavicle fractures, types I and III are stabilized by the intact CC ligaments, so they are generally treated nonoperatively. If symptoms persist, they can be treated with excision of the distal clavicle. Because the CC ligaments are either disrupted or attached to the lateral piece, type II factures are inherently unstable and associated

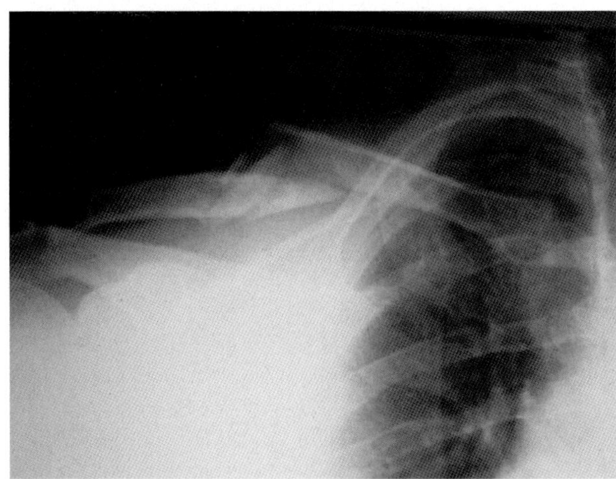
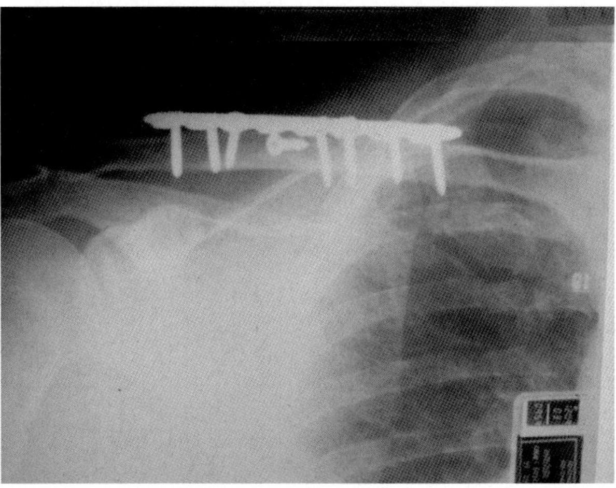

Figure 13.35 **A:** A comminuted fracture of the middle third of the clavicle. Recent evidence suggests that this type of fracture is more prone to nonunion than previously thought. **B:** The fracture was treated with open reduction and internal fixation using a plate and screws. (*From* Buholz RW, Heckman JD, Court-Brown CM. *Rockwood and Green's Fractures in Adults*, 6th ed. Philadelphia: Lippincott Williams & Wilkins, 2006, with permission.)

with a high rate of nonunion. This has led most authors to favor operative treatment of these fractures, although fixation can be technically challenging because of the small amount of bone lateral to the fracture site. Medial-third fractures generally respond well to nonoperative treatment.

Proximal Humerus Fractures

Proximal humerus fractures account for 4% to 7 % of all fractures and have a bimodal age distribution. In young patients, the fractures are a result of high-energy trauma and often require open reduction and internal fixation (ORIF). Proximal humerus fractures are also common in elderly patients, in whom they occur through osteoporotic bone, often after a fall. In this patient population, these fractures frequently do well with nonoperative treatment. If significant displacement is present, then ORIF or hemiarthroplasty may be necessary.

Classification

The most useful and commonly used classification of proximal humerus fractures is the Neer classification (Fig. 13.36). The scheme is based upon dividing the proximal humerus into four segments, as described by Codman (Fig. 13.37). In order for a segment to be considered a fracture part, it must be displaced at least 1 cm or angulated 45 degrees. Fractures are then described based on the number of parts. In a one-part fracture, none of the components is sufficiently displaced to qualify as a part, regardless of the number of fracture lines. Two-part fractures involve displacement of either the articular surface (through the anatomic neck), the entire head (through the surgical neck), the greater tuberosity, or the lesser tuberosity. In three-part fractures, there is displacement of either the lesser or greater tuberosity, as well as the head through the surgical neck. Four-part fractures involved displacement of all four segments of the bone. Proximal humerus fractures can also be associated with dislocations, in which case the direction of the dislocation and the number of parts to the fracture are described.

When using the Neer classification, it is important to remember that the system was not intended as a pure radiographic classification system. Instead, it was meant to provide a structured way to think about these complex fractures and place them into groups with defined natural history and treatment options. Several studies have criticized the reproducibility of this classification, but it remains the most commonly used method for describing these fractures. Adequate imaging, often involving CT scans, and increased rater experience have been shown to improve the accuracy of the classification.

Mechanism of Injury

In the elderly, the majority of proximal humerus fractures are the result of falls onto an outstretched hand. Younger patients are more frequently the victims of significant trauma, such as a motor vehicle collision or a fall from a significant height.

Presentation

The typical presentation is that of pain, swelling, and shoulder deformity following a traumatic injury. The patient typically holds the arm at the side and complains of significant pain with any movement of the shoulder. If the fracture is more than 6 to 12 hours old, ecchymoses extending from the axilla to below the elbow and swelling of the extremity all the way to the hand is not uncommon.

Physical Examination

As with all fractures, it is important to make sure that the overlying skin is intact, although open fractures of the proximal humerus are rare. Given the close proximity of the

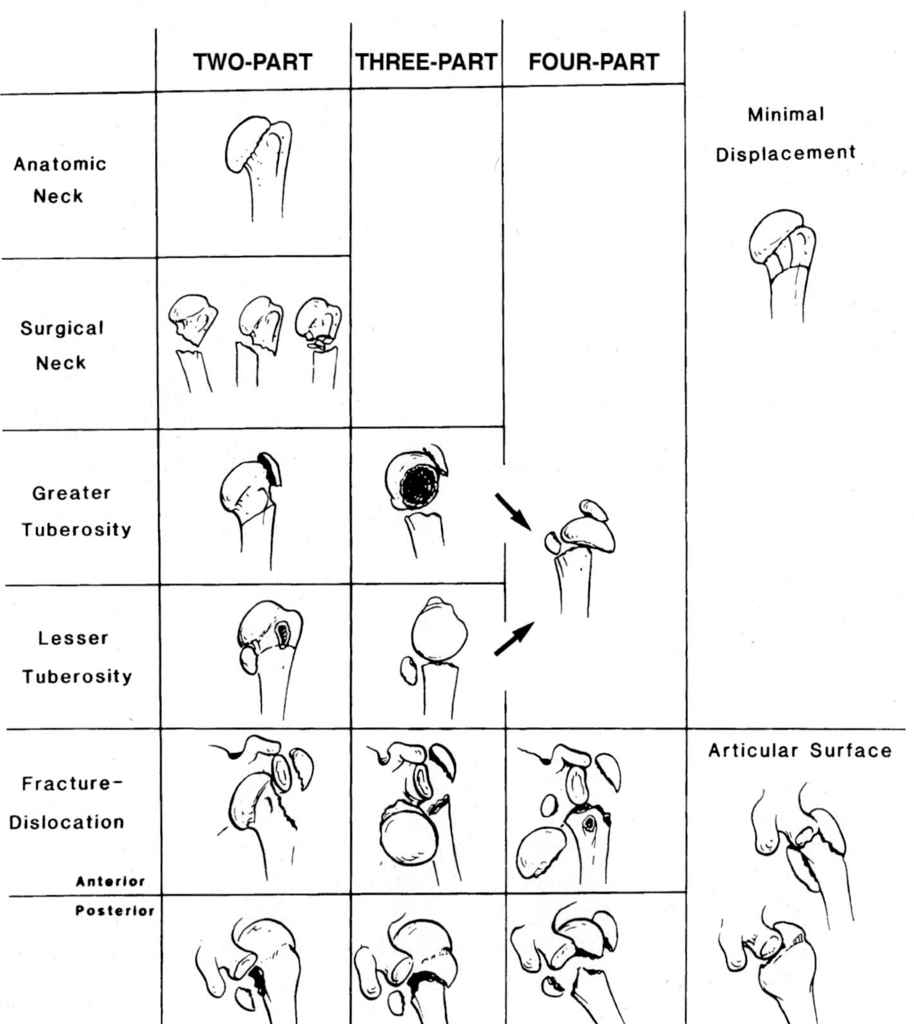

Figure 13.36 The Neer classification of proximal humerus fractures (see text for detailed explanation). (*From* Iannotti JP, Williams GR. *Disorders of the Shoulder: Diagnosis and Management*, 2nd ed. Philadelphia: Lippincott Williams & Wilkins, 2007, with permission.)

axillary artery to the proximal humerus, it is important to check distal pulses in the extremity. It is possible to have an intact radial pulse in the presence of a vascular injury, so any evidence of an expanding hematoma should be further investigated with an arteriogram. Neurologic injuries are not uncommon following these injuries, so it is important to perform and document a thorough neurologic examination. The axillary nerve is particularly at risk as it courses inferiorly below the subscapularis and through the quadrangular space (Fig. 13.16). Sensation over the lateral aspect of the upper arm is not an accurate indicator of axillary nerve function. Although pain will likely prevent the patient from actually abducting the arm, it is important to evaluate the axillary nerve by checking for deltoid muscle activation with attempted abduction of the arm.

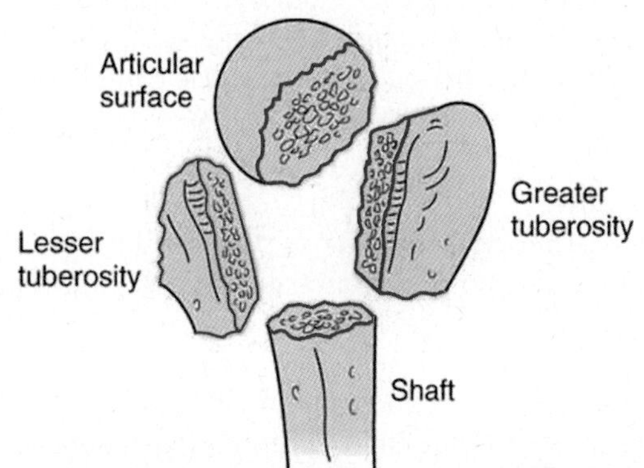

Figure 13.37 The Neer classification is based on dividing the proximal humerus into four segments, as described by Codman. (*From* Chapman MW, Szabo RM, Marder RA, et al. *Chapman's Orthopaedic Surgery*. Philadelphia: Lippincott Williams & Wilkins, 2001, with permission.)

Radiographic Examination

Radiographic evaluation must include an AP view of the GH joint, a scapular Y view, and an axillary lateral view. The axillary view is especially important in evaluating for the presence of a dislocation of the GH joint.

Special Tests

Even experienced clinicians can have difficulty describing the exact fracture pattern based on plain radiographs. In most displaced fractures, CT scans are useful to better

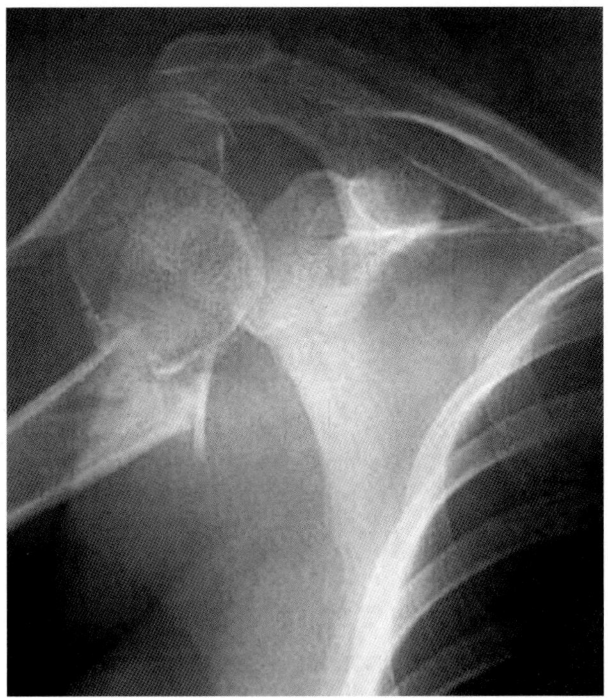

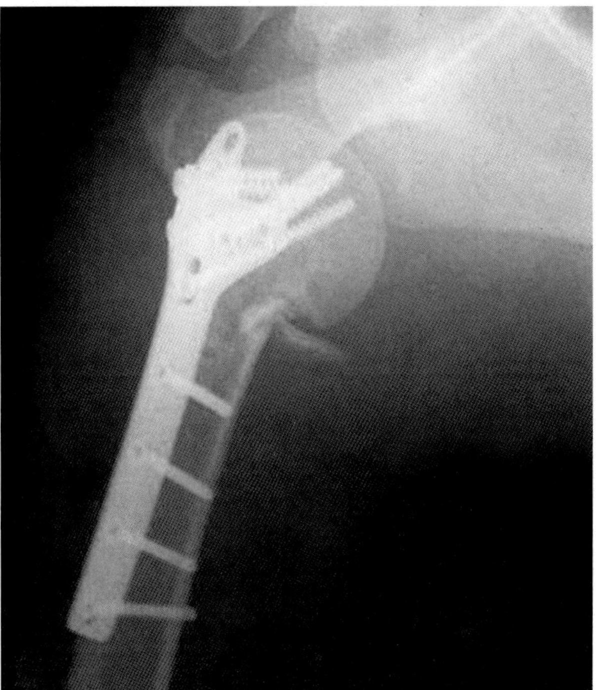

Figure 13.38 **A:** Anterior-posterior radiograph demonstrating a three-part fracture of the proximal humerus. The fracture lines separate the greater tuberosity, humeral shaft, and head fragment. The lesser tuberosity remains attached to the head fragment. **B:** Open reduction and internal fixation was obtained using a plate and screws. (*From* Chapman MW, Szabo RM, Marder RA, et al. *Chapman's Orthopaedic Surgery*. Philadelphia: Lippincott Williams & Wilkins, 2001, with permission.)

visualize and understand the injury pattern and aid in treatment decision making. For patients with neurologic deficits or those with an unexpectedly prolonged recovery, neurodiagnostic testing is valuable in detecting and classifying neurologic injury.

Differential Diagnosis

The differential diagnosis includes other traumatic injuries to the shoulder region. In the patient who presents with considerable shoulder pain following a fall, but has negative radiographs, consideration should be given to a nondisplaced proximal humeral fracture or acute rotator cuff tear. Both entities can be seen on an MRI scan.

Treatment

Greater than 70% of proximal humerus fractures are nondisplaced and do well with nonoperative treatment consisting of 4 to 6 weeks of immobilization in a sling. Given the intra-articular nature of the injury, stiffness is a significant concern. If the fracture pieces move as a single unit with motion of the arm, the patient is asked to remove his sling several times a day and perform gentle pendulum exercises. Unstable fractures should be reevaluated weekly and started on motion exercises as soon as the pieces move as a unit.

Two-part and some three-part fractures without significant displacement, especially in elderly patients, can be treated nonoperatively, as described earlier. For fractures with significant displacement, especially in younger, higher-demand patients, operative fixation using a variety of fixation techniques is preferred. Although several techniques have been described, the goal of surgery is always to achieve an anatomic reduction with enough stability to permit early motion (Fig. 13.38).

In four-part fractures, avascular necrosis is a particular concern because the fragment containing the articular surface is generally separated from its soft tissue attachments and blood supply. In younger patients, attempts at ORIF should be made when possible, whereas older individuals are generally treated with hemiarthroplasty. Although hemiarthroplasty for the treatment of proximal humerus fractures is often effective in relieving patients' pain, functional results are highly variable, with a significant number of patients failing to achieve more than 90 degrees of forward elevation.

Acromioclavicular Joint Sprains

Injury to the AC joint is a frequent cause of shoulder pain, especially in younger patients participating in athletic activities. Sprains of the AC joint result in varying disruption of the supporting structures between the distal clavicle and proximal acromion, leading to separation of the joint surfaces—which is why this entity is also referred to as a "shoulder separation."

Classification

Sprains of the AC joint are classified based on the degree of ligament disruption and the amount and direction of clavicular displacement, as described by Rockwood (Fig. 13.39). Type I injuries are a sprain of the AC ligament with no displacement of the joint. In type II injuries, the AC ligaments are torn and there is a sprain of the CC ligaments. Type III sprains involve disruption of both the AC and CC ligaments, with up to 100% superior displacement of the distal clavicle from the acromial joint surface. Separation types IV through VI involve complete disruption of the AC and CC ligaments and wide displacement of the clavicle.

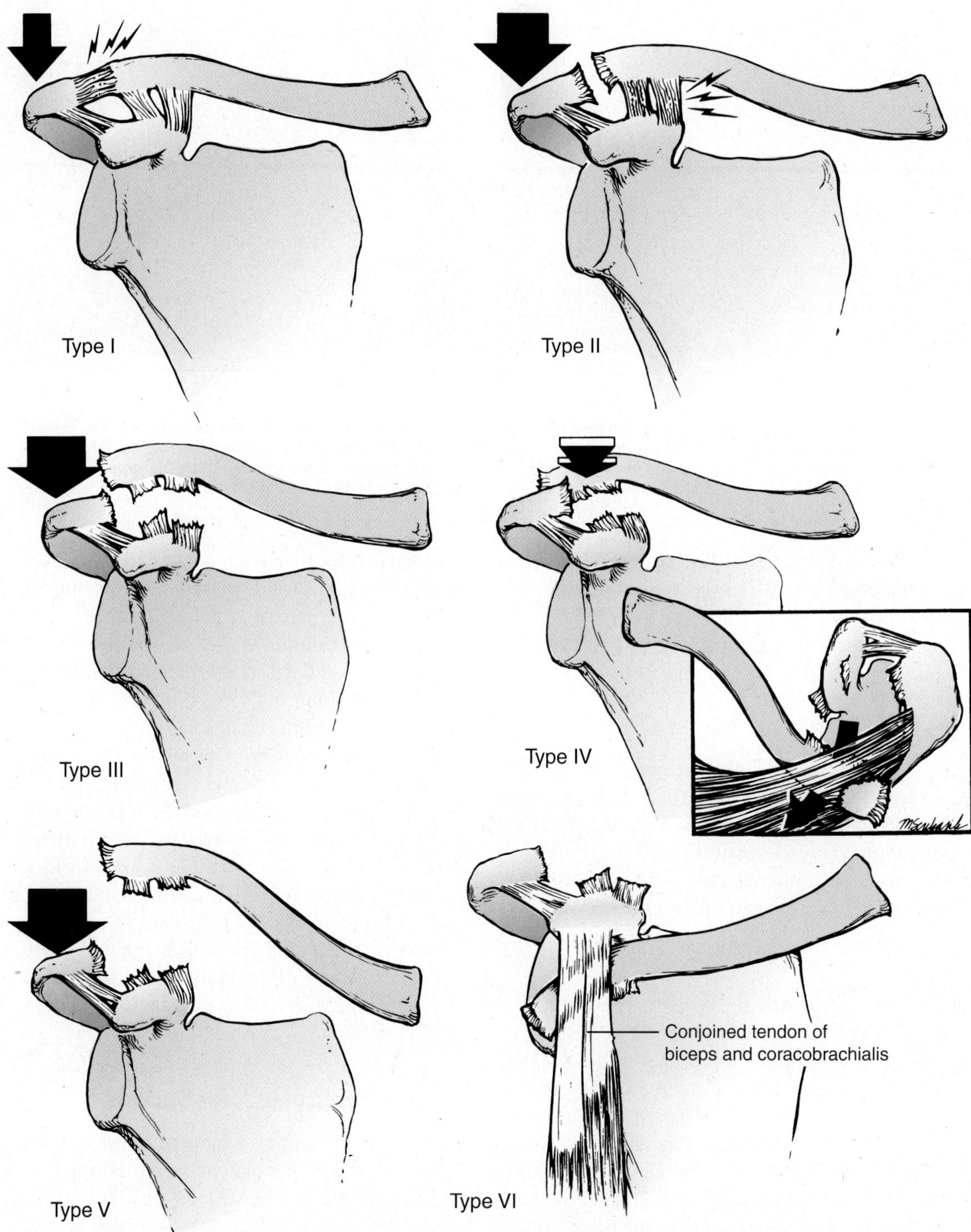

Figure 13.39 **A:** The Rockwood classification of injuries to the acromioclavicular joint (see text for detail explanation). (*From* Bucholz RW, Heckman JD, Court-Brown C, et al. *Rockwood and Green's Fractures in Adults*, 6th ed. Philadelphia: Lippincott Williams & Wilkins, 2006, with permission.)

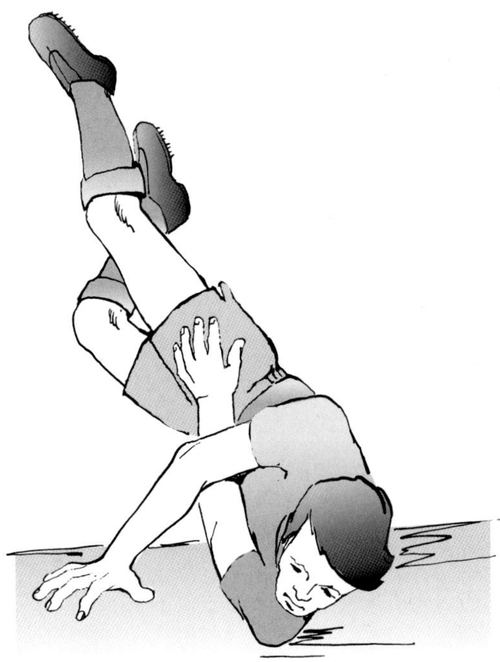

Figure 13.40 The most common mechanism of injury to the acromioclavicular joint is a direct force from a fall on the tip of the shoulder. (*From* Buholz RW, Heckman JD, Court-Brown CM. *Rock-wood and Green's Fractures in Adults*, 6th ed. Philadelphia: Lippincott Williams & Wilkins, 2006, with permission.)

In type IV, the displacement is posterior; in type V it is superior, and in type VI the clavicle is displaced inferior to the coracoid process.

Mechanism of Injury

Acromioclavicular injury is the result of direct trauma to the lateral aspect of shoulder. Most commonly, this occurs as a fall onto the tip of the shoulder during a sporting activity (Fig. 13.40). The traumatic load applies an inferiorly directed force on the acromion relative to the clavicle. Depending on the degree of the force, there is progressive disruption first of the AC ligaments and then of the CC ligaments.

Presentation

Patients with acute AC sprains present with pain localized to the AC joint following direct trauma to the shoulder. Occasionally, these patients will present in a delayed manner, in which case they may have milder symptoms over the AC joints accompanied by fatigue and cramping around the shoulder and scapula worsened by overhead activity.

Physical Examination

Patients with AC joint injuries will typically have pain and tenderness directly over the AC joint. With increased severity of injury, there will also be increased step-off and deformity across the joint. Although pain is often present with active motion of the shoulder, especially with higher-grade injuries, it should localize to the AC joint. Examination of the SC joint, clavicle, and GH joint is important to rule out any associated injuries.

Radiographic Examination

An AP view and axillary lateral are needed for evaluation of AC joint trauma. The Zanca view is preferred over a standard AP radiograph. This view is obtained by angling the x-ray beam 10 degrees toward the head and decreasing the kV by half in order to better visualize the AC joint (Fig. 13.34). Although this view will demonstrate step-off at the AC joint, the degree of superior displacement of the distal clavicle can best be described by comparing the CC distance in each shoulder. In type III sprains, this distance is typically increased 25% to 100%, whereas in type V injuries it is increased 100% to 300%. The axillary view is important for ruling out an associated GH dislocation and posterior displacement of the clavicle, as seen in type IV injuries.

Special Tests

No special tests are necessary for the evaluation of AC injuries. If there is question as to the degree of separation, stress views can be obtained by taking Zanca views of each shoulder with 5 to 10 pounds of weight suspended from each wrist. In type II separations, the CC distance should remain unchanged, whereas type III sprains will demonstrate an increase in the distance from the additional stress caused by the weights. Clinically, stress views are rarely needed because if a type III separation is not apparent on standard radiographs, it is likely to respond well to conservative treatment.

Differential Diagnosis

Acromioclavicular joint sprains must be distinguished from distal clavicle fractures, which can be accomplished with radiographs. Degenerative conditions of the distal clavicle, such as AC joint arthritis and distal clavicle osteolysis, can also cause pain over the AC joint. These conditions have a more insidious onset and lack both the characteristic isolated traumatic event to the lateral shoulder, as well as an increase in the CC distance on plain film.

Treatment

The initial treatment for all AC joint injuries is supportive care with the use of a sling, ice, and nonsteroidal anti-inflammatory drugs (NSAIDs). Type I and II injuries are treated conservatively, with a gradual return to activity as symptoms decrease. Athletes with type I injuries will generally be able to return to their sport within a few days, whereas type II injuries often require several weeks before a substantial improvement in symptoms occurs.

The treatment for type III injuries is controversial. The majority of patients do well with conservative treatment. It is important to advise patients that the step-off across the articular surface will result in a lasting cosmetic deformity but the pain generally resolves with a corresponding return in shoulder function. Return to athletic activity may take several months. Operative treatment is reserved for patients who fail conservative measures. These patients will often complain of fatigue of the shoulder and pain about the anterior trapezius. Manual laborers and overhead athletes with injury to their dominant arms are candidates for acute repair, although surgery will often result in a prolonged absence from work or athletic activity when compared to conservative treatment. A vast array of surgical techniques to repair the CC ligaments have been described; often the AC ligament is detached from the end of the acromion and transferred to the distal clavicle (Weaver-Dunn procedure) or an allograft hamstring tendon is used. Type IV to VI separations are treated with early surgical reconstruction.

Glenohumeral Instability

As previously mentioned, the shoulder has the largest ROM of any joint in the body. Unfortunately, this mobility comes at the expense of stability: The GH joint is also the most frequently dislocated major joint. When discussing instability of the GH joint, it is important to keep the definition of four key terms in mind. *Laxity* is asymptomatic translation of the humeral head on the glenoid. Laxity is required for normal GH motion, has a large variation between individuals, and tends to decrease with increasing age. *Instability* is a pathologic condition characterized by pain associated with excessive translation of the humeral head on the glenoid. If the instability leads to complete separation of the articular surfaces, it is referred to as a *dislocation*. Typically, a reduction maneuver performed by the patient or another individual is required to restore the alignment of the joint. When the increased translation of the humeral head results in partial separation of the articular surfaces, and the GH relationship spontaneously returns to normal following removal of the deforming force, the event is termed a *subluxation*.

Classification

Several factors must be considered when classifying GH instability, the most important of which is presence of a traumatic event leading to the initial episode of instability. Thomas and Matsen divided GH instability into two broad categories with the mnemonics TUBS and AMBRI. *Traumatic unidirectional Bankart surgery* (TUBS) refers to the fact that traumatic instability of the shoulder is generally unidirectional, associated with a Bankart lesions (see the section *Mechanism of Injury*), and responds well to surgical treatment. *Atraumatic multidirectional bilateral rehabilitation inferior capsular shift* (AMBRI) describes atraumatic instability that tends to occur bilaterally and responds to rehabilitation, or if that fails, an inferior capsular shift. Although these mnemonics oversimplify this complex condition, they provide an excellent framework for thinking about shoulder instability.

TABLE 13.3
SHOULDER INSTABILITY CLASSIFICATION

I. Degree
   A. Dislocation
   B. Subluxation
   C. Subtle

II. Frequency
   A. Acute (primary)
   B. Chronic
      1. Recurrent
      2. Fixed

III. Etiology
   A. Traumatic (macrotrauma)
   B. Atraumatic
      1. Voluntary (muscular)
      2. Involuntary (positional)
   C. Acquired (microtrauma)
   D. Congenital
   E. Neuromuscular (Erb palsy, cerebral palsy, seizures)

IV. Direction
   A. Unidirectional
      1. Anterior
      2. Posterior
      3. Inferior
   B. Bidirectional
      1. Anteroinferior
      2. Posteroinferior
   C. Multidirectional

Current classification of GH instability involves the description of the direction, etiology, frequency, degree, and volitional control of the instability (Table 13.3).

Unidirectional instability can be either anterior, posterior, or inferior, with anterior being the most common. *Multidirectional instability* always includes inferior instability combined with either anterior, posterior, or anterior and posterior instability. The etiology of the instability is traumatic, atraumatic, or congenital. Frequency is important in determining the impact of the instability on the patient's life. Degree of instability is described using the terms *dislocation, subluxation,* and *subtle* (meaning the patient experiences pain without instability, and the physician is able to reproduce the patient's symptoms by translating the humeral head on physical examination). Finally, any voluntary component to the instability must be described. A subset of patients will voluntarily dislocate or sublux their shoulders because of emotional disorders associated with secondary gain. These patients do extremely poorly with orthopaedic intervention and are better addressed by psychiatric evaluation. It is important to distinguish these patients from a second group of patients who are able to recreate their instability by selective muscle contraction and position of the arm but attempt not do so except when being examined by a physician.

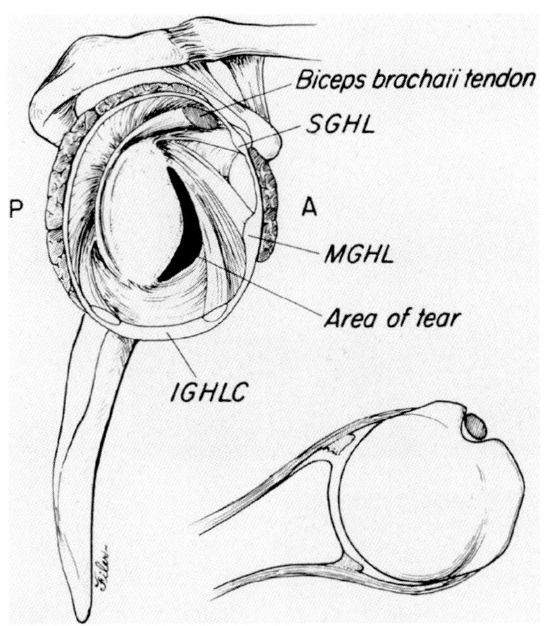

Figure 13.41 Illustration of a Bankart lesion involving a tear of the anterior inferior labrum off the glenoid rim. (From Johnson DH, Pedowitz RA. *Practical Orthopaedic Sports Medicine and Arthroscopy*. Philadelphia: Lippincott Williams & Wilkins, 2007, with permission.)

Mechanism of Injury

A traumatic blow to a maximally abducted, externally rotated arm is the most common mechanism of injury for an acute anterior shoulder dislocation. With the arm in this provocative position, GH stability is provided primarily by the anterior band of the inferior glenohumeral ligament (AIGHL). Further external rotation of the arm, an anterior directed force applied to the posterior shoulder, or a posterior force directed toward the hand or elbow levers the humeral head away from the glenoid and results in an anterior dislocation. These injuries frequently occur during a wide variety of athletic activities and are more common in males than females.

The anterior dislocation of the humeral head results in the disruption of the anterior stabilizing structures, especially the AIGHL and anterior inferior glenoid labrum. This was classically described as an avulsion of these structures from the anterior inferior glenoid rim and termed the *Bankart lesion* (Fig. 13.41). It is now clear that these restraining structures can fail anywhere along their length, including at the glenoid rim (Bankart lesion), as a midsubstance rupture or stretch, and at their humeral attachment (referred to as a humeral avulsion of the glenohumeral ligament or HAGL lesion). Contraction of the shoulder girdle musculature once the humeral head has slipped forward over the glenoid rim can lead to an impaction fracture of the posterior lateral humeral head, called a *Hill-Sachs lesion* (Fig. 13.42).

Acute posterior instability typically occurs following a posteriorly directed force transmitted through a flexed, adducted, and internally rotated arm. Posterior dislocations can also occur following sudden muscle contractions associated with seizures and electrical shocks. As the name implies, atraumatic instability occurs without antecedent trauma. It is more commonly multidirectional and often occurs in patients with hyperlaxity of their joints.

A second group of patients who are prone to atraumatic instability are those involved in sports that place significant stress on the capsular restraints that limit shoulder mobility, such as overhead throwers, gymnasts, and swimmers. The instability in these athletes is not truly atraumatic; instead, it develops as a result of microtrauma that occurs with the repetitive stretching of the capsule and ligaments during participation in these sports.

Presentation

Patients with acute dislocations will present with a sudden onset of pain and deformity of the shoulder following a traumatic event. The patient will keep the arm splinted at the side, often supporting the wrist with the opposite hand. Any rotation through the GH joint will lead to severe pain.

When recurrent, the shoulder may dislocate with little or no trauma and, especially as the capsular structures are stretched with an increasing number of dislocations, the patient is often able to relocate the joint without assistance. In these patients, it is important to determine the nature of the injury at the time of the first dislocation, how it was initially treated, the number of recurrences, and the specific activities or positions that now cause instability.

Patients with subluxation or multidirectional instability will present with complaints of pain when the joint shifts out of place with provocative positioning of the arm. In athletes with subtle instability, the presenting complaint is often shoulder pain and a decrease in athletic performance. This pain often occurs only when they are participating in athletics and may or may not be associated with a sensation of instability or loss of strength in the arm.

Physical Examination

With an acute anterior dislocation, prominence of the humeral head anteriorly will be present, with noticeable flattening of the normal rounded contour of the posterior shoulder. The shoulder is globally painful and prereduction examination is generally limited to the assessment of the neurovascular status. As with proximal humerus fractures, the axillary nerve is at particular risk for injury with shoulder dislocation, as it passes along the inferior shoulder capsule to transverse the quadrangular space (Fig. 13.16). Assessment and documentation of deltoid muscle motor function is important prior to attempting any reduction maneuvers.

With posterior dislocations, the arm will be held internally rotated at the side, and any attempts at external rotation will cause significant pain. There may be some anterior flattening and posterior prominence although this is often difficult to appreciate because of the increased

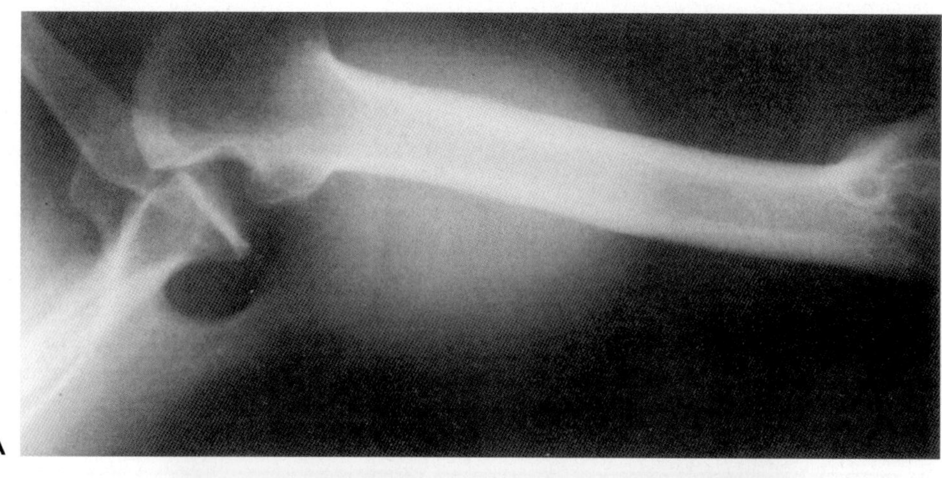

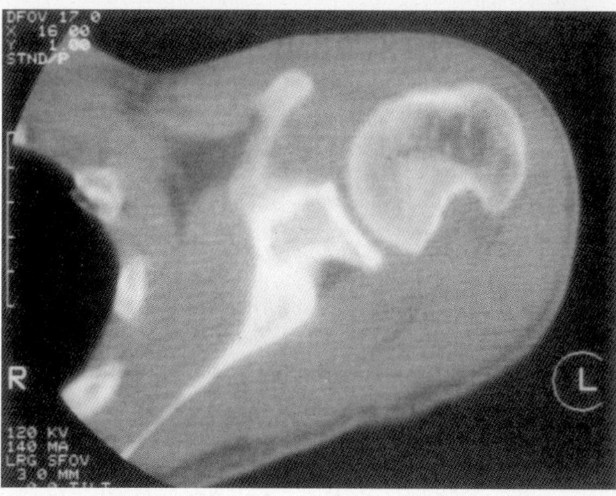

Figure 13.42 Impaction of the posterior superior humeral head on the glenoid rim leads to a Hill-Sachs lesion of the humeral head. **A:** An axillary radiograph demonstrating an anterior dislocation with a Hill-Sachs lesion. **B:** A post-reduction computed tomography scan further demonstrating the impaction fracture. (*From* Iannotti JP, Williams GR. *Disorders of the Shoulder: Diagnosis and Management*, 2nd ed. Philadelphia: Lippincott Williams & Wilkins, 2007, with permission.)

bulk of the posterior shoulder. There is a high incidence of missed posterior dislocation of the shoulder, often with disastrous consequences. For this reason, any patient experiencing trauma to the upper extremity, a seizure, or an electrical shock and decreased external rotation of the GH joint should be suspected of having a posterior dislocation until proven otherwise by axillary radiographs.

Patients presenting for evaluation of recurrent or atraumatic instability should undergo a standard physical examination of the shoulder including ROM and strength testing. Several specific tests have been developed to assess GH laxity and instability by assessing pain and apprehension with provocative positioning of the arm. Anterior instability is evaluated via the apprehension test. The patient is placed in the supine position to stabilize the scapula, and the elbow is flexed 90 degree while the shoulder is abducted 90 degrees (Fig. 13.43). The examiner then slowly externally rotates the arm. A positive test occurs when the patient experiences apprehension of impending instability. This is followed by the relocation test, in which the examiner uses his opposite hand to place a posteriorly directed force on the humeral head. For a positive test, the patient's apprehension is relieved by the posteriorly directed force. Posterior instability is assessed by applying a posteriorly directed force to the arm with the shoulder adducted, internally rotated, and flexed 90 degrees. A positive test is indicated by pain with posterior subluxation of the humeral head. These maneuvers should be carried out with great care or skipped altogether in patients with a recent dislocation. In a patient with a clear history of dislocation, there is no need to confirm instability by dislocating the patient's joint during the office examination, as this will lead to an extremely uncomfortable experience for both patient and physician.

Anterior/posterior laxity of the GH joint is evaluated with the load and shift test, which can be done in both the upright and supine positions. For the supine test, the examiner positions the patient's arm in the plane of the scapula, at 45 to 60 degrees of abduction and neutral rotation. The examiner the places his opposite hand around

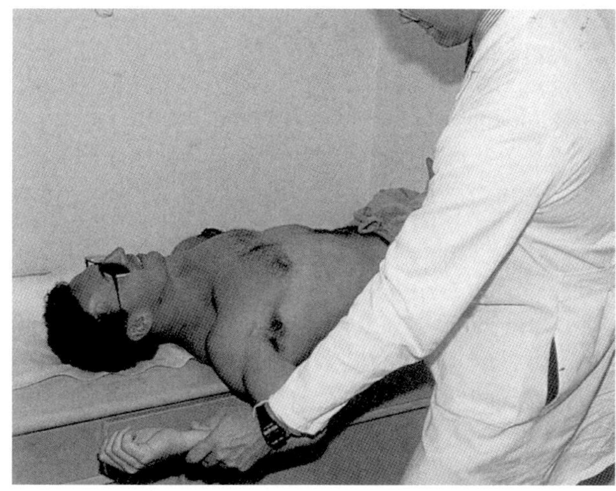

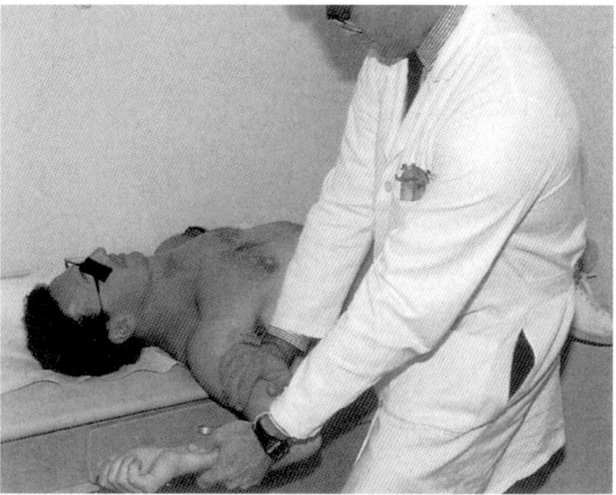

Figure 13.43 The apprehension **(A)** and relocation **(B)** tests for anterior instability. (*From* Iannotti JP, Williams GR. *Disorders of the Shoulder: Diagnosis and Management*, 2nd ed. Philadelphia: Lippincott Williams & Wilkins, 2007, with permission.)

the arm at the level of the deltoid tuberosity and applies an anterior and then posterior force to the arm while compressing the GH joint. Laxity is graded based on direction and the amount of translation of the humeral head from grade 0 (minimal movement) to grade 3 (dislocation of the humeral head) (Fig. 13.44).

Inferior laxity is evaluated by the sulcus sign. With the elbow flexed 90 degrees and adducted to the side, an inferior force is applied to the arm. The distance between the acromion and humeral head is then observed and measured in centimeters (Fig. 13.45). Greater than 2 cm of inferior translation is indicative of inferior laxity.

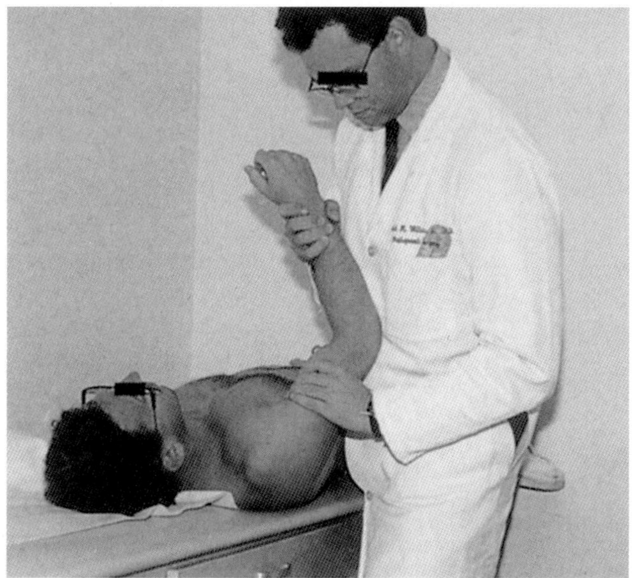

Figure 13.44 Laxity of the glenohumeral joint is evaluated with the load and shift test. (*From* Iannotti JP, Williams GR. *Disorders of the Shoulder: Diagnosis and Management*, 2nd ed. Philadelphia: Lippincott Williams & Wilkins, 2007, with permission.)

Radiographs

Any patient with a possible shoulder dislocation should be evaluated with AP, scapular Y, and axillary radiographs. Of the three views, the axillary lateral is by far the most important. Radiology technologists will often shoot a three-view shoulder series consisting of an AP in internal and external

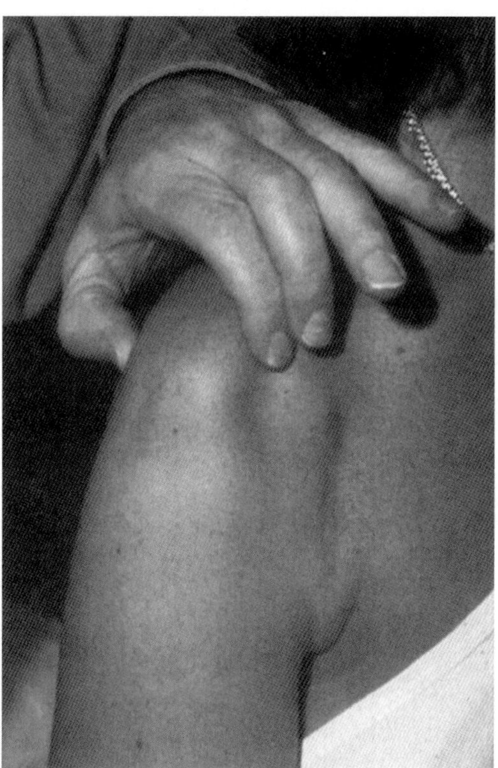

Figure 13.45 A positive sulcus sign indicating inferior laxity. (*From* Krishnan SG, Hawkins RJ, Warren RF. *The Shoulder and the Overhead Athlete*. Philadelphia: Lippincott Williams & Wilkins, 2004, with permission.)

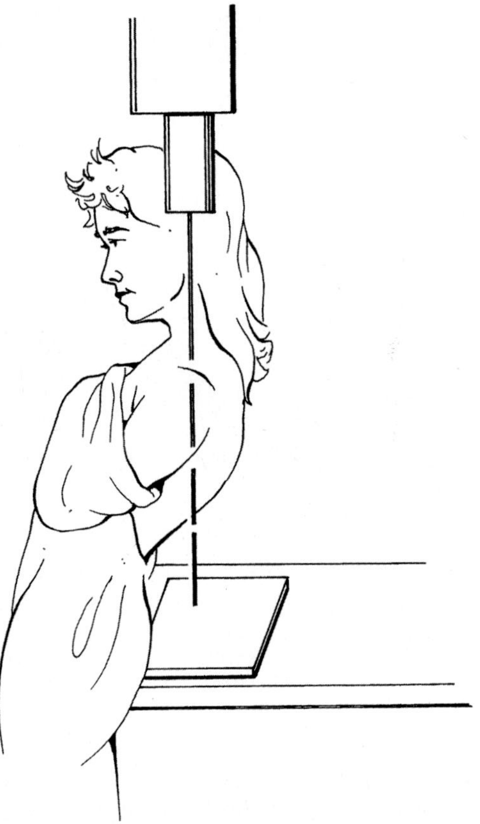

Figure 13.46 The Velpeau view is obtained by having the patient lean backward 30 degrees over the cassette with his arm in the sling. The beam is then directed superior to inferior through the shoulder. This view provides a magnified axillary view in patients who cannot tolerate abduction of the arm. (*From* Iannotti JP, Williams GR. *Disorders of the Shoulder: Diagnosis and Management*, 2nd ed. Philadelphia: Lippincott Williams & Wilkins, 2007, with permission.)

rotation and a scapular Y. Although it is often possible to detect a dislocation on the Y view, it is also easy to miss a dislocation, especially if the beam is not exactly parallel to the scapula. The axillary view will clearly demonstrate any anterior or posterior translation of the humeral head on the glenoid and is mandatory in these patients. If the patient cannot tolerate abduction of the arm for an axillary view, the Velpeau view can be obtained without removing the patient's arm from the sling (Fig. 13.46). A number of special x-ray views have been described to detect various pathologies that can accompany shoulder instability; however, these views have generally been replaced by the widespread use of CT and MRI scans.

Special Studies

Following a simple dislocation and reduction, no additional studies are needed if no boney abnormalities are suspected on the pre- and postreduction radiographs. If there is concern regarding the size of Hill-Sachs lesions or bone defects about the anterior glenoid rim, then a CT scan is useful. For patients with an unclear history of instability or pain and a physical examination suggestive of instability, MRI scanning is a useful tool. This study can be used to evaluate the soft tissue restraints to instability and also to rule out other pathologic conditions about the shoulder. The use of intra-articular contrast to obtain an MRI arthrogram increases the accuracy in evaluating in the labrum and capsular structures.

Differential Diagnosis

The differential diagnosis of acute shoulder dislocations in patients with severe pain after trauma injury includes AC separations and fractures about the shoulder complex. These can be easily distinguished by physical and radiographic examination.

For patients, especially athletes, with subtle instability presenting primarily as pain, the differential diagnosis includes several other shoulder disorders such as rotator cuff pathology, SLAP tears, AC joint arthritis, and scapulothoracic motion abnormalities.

Treatment

Following clinical and x-ray evaluation, the initial treatment for acute anterior dislocations involves closed reduction under conscious sedation. This can be accomplished by a variety of maneuvers that generally involve traction–counter traction across the joint (Fig. 13.47). Following reduction, the arm is placed in a sling, the neurovascular status is rechecked, and postmanipulation films are obtained to confirm the reduction.

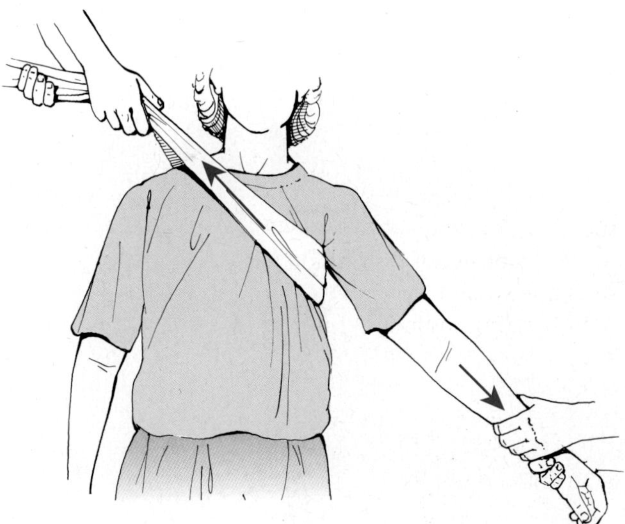

Figure 13.47 The most commonly used technique for reduction of an anterior shoulder dislocation uses a sheet around the axilla to provide a counter-traction force. A longitudinal force is then applied to the arm to disengage the humeral head from the anterior glenoid rim and allow it to return to the articular surface. (*From* Buholz RW, Heckman JD, Court-Brown CM. *Rockwood and Green's Fractures in Adults*, 6th ed. Philadelphia: Lippincott Williams & Wilkins, 2006, with permission.)

Traditionally, the arm has been maintained in a sling in internal rotation for a period ranging from several days to several weeks. This has led to a high recurrence rate in younger patients (between 50% and 90% in patients under the age of 20). Recent evidence suggests that immobilization in 10 degrees of external rotation for 3 weeks can significantly decrease the recurrence rate in patients under the age of 30. Following immobilization, the patient is started on a physical therapy program to regain motion and strengthen the dynamic stabilizers of the shoulder and is permitted a gradual return to activity.

Most surgeons reserve operative treatment for patients with recurrent instability. After the second dislocation, the patient is unlikely to remain stable unless he is willing to significantly modify his activity. Operative treatment consists of either open or arthroscopic repair of the injured structures, most commonly, the anterior inferior labrum and capsule. Although the early results of arthroscopic treatment were inferior to open repair, advances in arthroscopic techniques have led to success rates of greater than 90% in more recent series. The two exceptions to an initial trial of nonoperative treatment for first time dislocators are (a) high-level athletes for whom a second dislocation would result in the loss of an additional season of play and (b) individuals involved in activities in which a recurrent dislocation could compromise their overall safety.

In patients over the age of 40, the risk of recurrent instability is less than the risk of stiffness. Immobilization in this age group is for patient comfort only, and ROM exercises are begun as soon as the patient tolerates movement. These patients are at a much higher risk of rotator cuff tears or neurologic injuries following dislocation. Any weakness persisting more than a week or two after the dislocation should be further investigated with an MRI scan and possibly a nerve conduction study (NCS)/EMG.

Acute posterior dislocations should be reduced under conscious sedation. Following reduction, the GH joint may be unstable when placed in a sling. If this is the case, the arm should be held in neutral or external rotation using a specially designed sling or shoulder spica cast. If the diagnosis of a posterior dislocation has been delayed for more than a few days, reduction requires general anesthesia in the operating room and often must be done in an open manner. In the absence of boney injuries, recurrent posterior instability is less common than anterior instability. When surgery is required, posterior capsular repair or placation is more easily accomplished via arthroscopic rather than open techniques.

The first line of treatment for atraumatic and multidirectional instability is physical therapy to strengthen the rotator cuff muscles and scapulothoracic stabilizers. If the instability persists despite 3 to 12 months of therapy, then the patient may be a candidate for operative management. Surgical treatment involves either an open or arthroscopic procedure to reduce the capsular volume; however, the results of surgical treatment are not as predictable as they are for traumatic instability. Operative intervention in athletes with subtle instability is difficult because the procedure needs to decrease the patient's laxity enough to eliminate his instability while maintaining enough motion for the patient to continue participation in his sport.

Superior Labrum Anterior to Posterior (SLAP) Lesions

Since the increase in use of shoulder arthroscopy in the 1980s and 1990s, SLAP lesions have been recognized as a source of intra-articular shoulder pain in patients under the age of 40. These injuries involve the superior glenoid labrum and the insertion of the long head of the biceps tendon onto the supraglenoid tubercle.

Classification

Superior labrum anterior to posterior tears were originally described by Andrews in 1985, and further defined and classified into four types by Snyder in 1990 (Fig. 13.48). Type I tears involve fraying or degeneration of the superior labrum without detachment of the labrum or the biceps anchor. In type II tears, there is detachment of the superior labrum and biceps anchor from the glenoid rim. Type III tears are characterized by a "bucket-handle tear" of a portion of the superior labrum, with the remaining superior labrum and biceps anchor still firmly attached to the glenoid rim. The type IV SLAP involves a "bucket-handle tear" of the superior labrum that extends into the biceps tendon. Since Snyder's original classification, several additional types of SLAP tears have been described. These involve extension of the tear into varying portions of the anterior or posterior labrum and may be associated with shoulder instability.

Mechanism of Injury

Superior labrum anterior to posterior lesions are typically caused by traction or compression injuries to the shoulder. The most common mechanism is a fall on an abducted, forwardly flexed arm, which leads to a direct compressive force on the superior labrum. Reflex contraction of the biceps muscle may provide additional traction on the biceps anchor during the fall.

Superior labrum anterior to posterior tears are frequently found to occur in overhead athletes. In these patients, it is believed that the lesions are due to microtrauma from repeated traction transmitted through the biceps tendon during the throwing motion. This population also tends to have hypertrophy of their posterior inferior capsular structures, which causes a posterior superior shift of the contact point between the humeral head and glenoid when the arm is placed in abduction and external rotation (as in the late cocking phase of the throwing motion). This shift can lead to damaging sheer and compressive forces across the superior labrum.

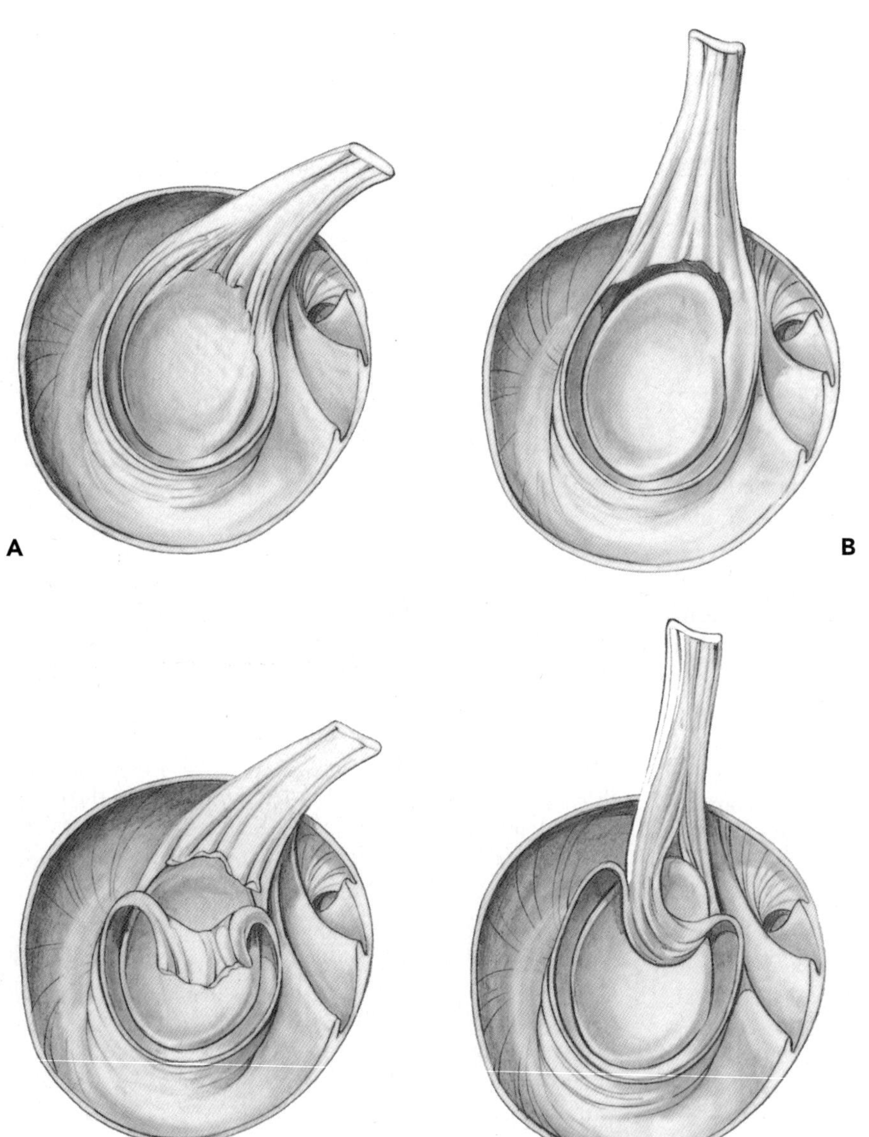

Figure 13.48 The classification of superior labrum anterior to posterior lesions. **(A)** Type I. **(B)** Type II. **(C)** Type III. **(D)** Type IV. (*From* Iannotti JP, Williams GR. *Disorders of the Shoulder: Diagnosis and Management*, 2nd ed. Philadelphia: Lippincott Williams & Wilkins, 2007, with permission.)

Presentation

The presentation of patients with SLAP lesions can be quite variable, and the diagnosis should be considered in all patients younger that 40 with pain coming from within the shoulder joint. The most common presentation is a young, active patient with activity-related pain deep within the shoulder following a traumatic event. The inciting injury typically involves a fall on an outstretched hand, weight lifting, automobile accidents, or traction on the extended arm. In overhead athletes, rarely is a single traumatic event the cause; rather, the player will complain of shoulder pain and a loss of strength and power with throwing or overhead activities.

Physical Examination

Patients with SLAP lesions will typically have full range of motion and good strength about the shoulder, especially of the rotator cuff muscles. The exception is overhead athletes with hypertrophy of the inferior capsule. They will have a decrease in internal rotation with the arm at 90 degrees of abduction.

A large array of special tests has been described to aid in the diagnosis of SLAP tears. Unfortunately, none of them of has been found to be particularly sensitive or specific. Three maneuvers that we have found useful are the O'Brien test, the Mayo sheer test, and the apprehension test. For the O'Brien test (Fig. 13.49), also known as the active biceps compression test, the patient places the arm in 90 degrees of forward flexion, 20 degrees of adduction, and active, full internal rotation (thumb points toward floor). The examiner then provides a downward force on the patient's forearm as the patient raises his arm toward the ceiling. If this reproduces the patient's pain, the patient is asked to full externally rotate the arm (thumb pointing toward the ceiling), and the downward force is reapplied. For a positive test, the pain experienced with the arm in internal rotation

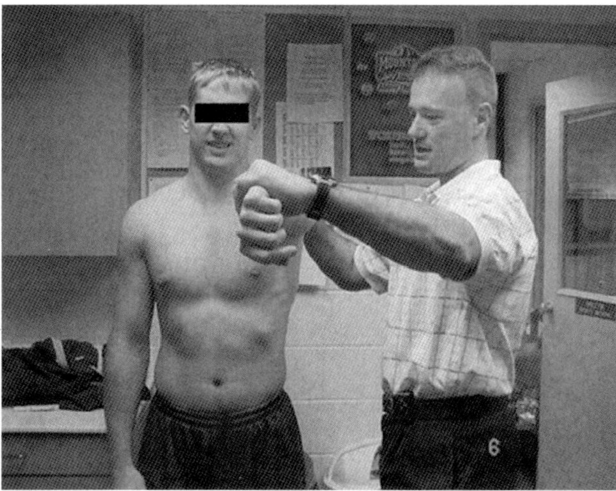

Figure 13.49 O'Brien test for the detection of superior labrum anterior to posterior tears. For a positive test, the patient will have pain when resistance is applied to the internally rotated arm that is not present when resistance is applied to the externally rotated arm. (*From* Krishnan SG, Hawkins RJ, Warren RF. *The Shoulder and the Overhead Athlete*. Philadelphia: Lippincott Williams & Wilkins, 2004, with permission.)

must be relieved or dramatically lessened with external rotation.

In the Mayo sheer test (also known as the dynamic labral sheer test), the patient's elbow is placed at his side and flexed 90 degrees. The examiner then puts the arm in maximal passive external rotation and gradually abducts the arm while stabilizing the patient's posterior scapula with the opposite hand. A patient with a positive test will experience pain with abduction between 60 and 120 degrees. A positive test may include pain, pain and a click, or simply a click.

Although apprehension testing is classically used to diagnose anterior shoulder instability, patients with SLAP tears will often have pain without a sensation of instability when the arm is placed in the abducted, externally rotated position. This test is most easily performed with the patient supine on the examination table to stabilize the scapula. For a positive test, the patient's pain should be relieved when a posteriorly directed force is applied to the proximal humerus.

Radiographic Findings

Standard radiographs are unremarkable in patients with a SLAP tear.

Special Studies

Magnetic resonance imaging is the most useful imaging modality for the diagnosis of labral pathology. The diagnosis is made when fluid is visualized between the superior glenoid rim and the labrum on the oblique coronal images (Fig. 13.50). The specificity and sensitivity of MRI in detecting SLAP tears can be markedly improved through the use of an MRI arthrogram, which involves the injection

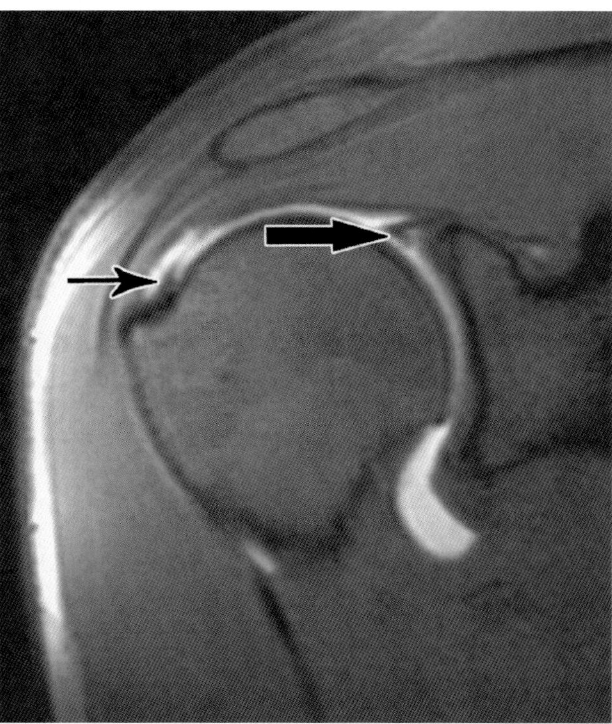

Figure 13.50 Coronal oblique magnetic resonance image arthrogram demonstrating a superior labrum anterior to posterior tear (*big arrow*). (*From* Magee T, Willams, D, Mani N, *Shoulder MR arthography: which patient group benefits most?* AM J Roentgol 2004:183:969–970, with permission.)

of contrast material into the GH joint prior to the MRI examination. Magnetic resonance imaging is also useful for identifying other pathology, such as partial articular-sided rotator cuff tears and Bankart lesions that can lead to shoulder pain in younger patients.

Differential Diagnosis

The differential diagnosis for SLAP tears includes any entity that can cause shoulder pain in young patients. For patients who have experienced a compression or traction injury to the shoulder, GH instability, AC joint injuries, rotator cuff tears, bursitis, and adhesive capsulitis must be excluded based on history, physical examination, and imaging studies. In overhead athletes, subtle anterior instability, articular-sided rotator cuff tears, and isolated deficits of GH internal rotation can lead to a loss of strength and performance and must be differentiated from SLAP tears. Patients over the age of 40 commonly have some degeneration or even frank tearing of their superior labrum that may be an asymptomatic part of normal aging. Therefore, in this population, other conditions, especially rotator cuff– related pathology, are much more likely to be responsible for that patient's symptoms.

Treatment

Superior labrum anterior to posterior tears generally do not respond well to conservative treatment. In young patients with a history, physical examination, and imaging studies consistent with a labral tear, surgical intervention is advised. For patients suspected of having a SLAP tear, but without the majority of characteristic finding on history and physical examination, a trial of physical therapy is warranted. Several of the conditions that can present in a similar manner will often respond well to therapy whereas those patients with superior labral pathology will not improve and may even have an exacerbation of their symptoms.

The surgical treatment of SLAP tears involves arthroscopic fixation or debridement. Type I and III tears are generally treated with debridement, whereas the treatment of type II and IV tears consists of repair of the labrum back to the glenoid rim using suture anchors. In patients over the age of 40, SLAP tears are often encountered at the time of arthroscopy for other shoulder pathology (especially rotator cuff pathology). If the biceps anchor is stable and the biceps tendon is in good condition, these tears should be ignored. If there is instability of the biceps anchor or degeneration of the tendon, a biceps tenotomy or tenodesis should be considered.

ATRAUMATIC SHOULDER CONDITIONS

Rotator Cuff Pathology

Rotator cuff pathology is the most common atraumatic condition responsible for shoulder pain. The spectrum of disease includes subacromial bursitis, rotator cuff tendinopathy, and partial or complete tears of the rotator cuff. The exact cause of the patient's symptoms is often unclear, leading the caregiver, especially the nonorthopaedist, to label any pain associated with the rotator cuff as impingement syndrome.

In degenerative disease of the rotator cuff, the supraspinatus tendon is the most commonly involved tendon, and the prevalence of tendon tears increases with increasing age. Interestingly, a large number of these tears, especially those that develop gradually, are asymptomatic. Traumatic injuries can occur in patients of any age, are often associated with significant weakness, and tend to require surgical treatment.

Pathophysiology and Classification

As the supraspinatus muscle passes laterally toward its insertion on the greater tuberosity, its tendon travels underneath the CA arch composed of the undersurface of the acromion, CA ligament, and AC joint (Fig. 13.51). The tendon is separated for the arch by the subacromial bursa, which allows frictionless gliding between the tendon and overlying structures. Even in the nonpathologic state there is a decrease in the subacromial space with abduction of the arm, leading to some impingement of the CA arch on the underlying tendon and bursa. Any process resulting in a decrease in this space can worsen this impingement and lead to inflammation of the bursa and disorders within the rotator cuff tendon. Dysfunction of the cuff muscles causing a decrease in their ability to keep the humeral head centered on the glenoid during motion of the arm can lead to superior translation of the humeral head and a decrease in the subacromial space. Likewise, the space can be reduced from above by abnormal tilt or shape of the overlying acromion or hypertrophy of the CA ligament or AC joint.

Two main theories attempt to explain the underlying cause of rotator cuff pathology. The *external theory* suggests that the initial pathologic change is caused by external compression of the rotator cuff by the overlying structures. This compression leads to inflammation within the subacromial bursa and degeneration and eventual tearing of the rotat or cufftendons. The *intrinsic model* suggests that the initiating event is degeneration within the rotator cuff tendons themselves. The degeneration may be due to several factors, including aging and decreased vascularity within the critical area of the tendon. The abnormal rotator cuff is no longer able to keep the humeral head centered on the glenoid, which can lead to superior translation of the head and worsening tendon destruction by subacromial impingement. In reality, in most patients, some element of

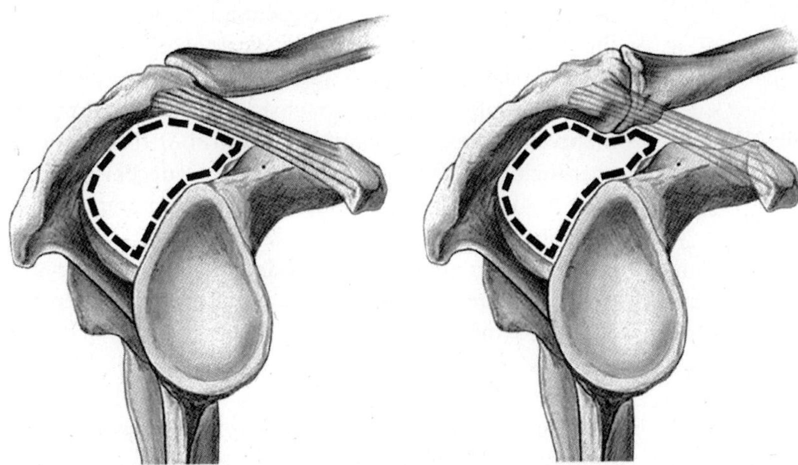

Figure 13.51 As the supraspinatus tendon passes laterally, it travels through an enclosed space covered by the coracoacromial arch. (*From* Johnson DH, Pedowitz RA. *Practical Orthopaedic Sports Medicine and Arthroscopy.* Philadelphia: Lippincott Williams & Wilkins, 2007, with permission.)

both intrinsic and extrinsic pathology probably occurs in rotator cuff disease. With either theory, once the process begins, increased impingement occurs between the cuff and the CA arch, which can lead to further degeneration of the cuff and hypertrophy of the overlying structures that worsens the impingement.

Presentation

The most common presentation of rotator cuff disease is a late middle-aged patient with the gradual onset of dull pain over the anterior lateral shoulder. The pain often radiates to deltoid insertion on the lateral arm, awakens the patient from sleep (especially when lying or rolling onto the affected side), and is exacerbated by overhead activities or reaching behind the back (as when putting a wallet in the back pocket of pants or hooking a bra). Alternately, the pain may begin following increased use of the arm, such as painting a room or playing several sets of tennis.

Occasionally, the pain may follow a traumatic event. This is more common in younger patients, and these patients are more likely to complain of weakness in addition to pain. As described in the section on GH instability, it is important to suspect a rotator cuff tear in any patient over the age of 40 with a dislocation of the GH joint.

Physical Examination

Patients with longstanding rotator cuff tears may have atrophy of the posterior shoulder over the supra- or infraspinatus fossa. They will often have tenderness to palpation about the cuff insertion on the greater tuberosity. With the exception of those with full-thickness tears, full active forward elevation is generally normal, although it is often accompanied with significant discomfort in the impingement zone between 70 and 120 degrees. It is not uncommon for patients with cuff pathology to lack several levels of internal rotation when measured with the arm behind the back. Placing the arm in this position increases the contact between the anterior superior rotator cuff and CA arch and is often provocative of the patient's pain.

The evaluation of rotator cuff strength is especially important in the examination of patients presenting with rotator cuff disease. In patients with inflammation of the subacromial bursa, it can be difficult to distinguish between true weakness and weakness secondary to pain, although with proper instruction, most patients with an intact cuff are able to maintain at least 4+/5 strength. Significant weakness on strength evaluation, especially positive lag signs, belly-press, or lift-off tests, is concerning for complete tears of the cuff tendons.

Several additional tests have been described for the evaluation of rotator cuff pathology. Best known for the name of the examiner who originally described them, these tests attempt to reproduce the patient's symptoms by manipulating the arm to increase impingement within the subacromial space. Unfortunately, although sensitive for the detection of cuff pathology, they are also positive in a number of other conditions causing pain about the shoulder.

In the Neer impingement sign, the involved extremity is passively elevated in the scapular plane with the scapula stabilized (Fig. 13.52A). The test is positive when the patient's pain is reproduced as the cuff and bursa are compressed against the CA arch. The Hawkins impingement sign is tested by passively internally rotating the arm while holding it in 90 degrees of forward flexion with the elbow also held in 90 degrees of flexion (Fig. 13.52B). Again, a positive test involves recreation of the patient's pain. In addition to evaluating supraspinatus strength, pain with the Jobe test is indicative of rotator cuff pathology.

Patients with subacromial bursitis, rotator cuff tendonitis, and partial-thickness cuff tears will have pain with strength testing of the involved portion of the rotator cuff and positive impingement maneuvers, but no strength deficits. Patients with small complete tears of the supraspinatus also generally present with pain but no or minimal strength deficits. In contrast, patients with larger tears of the rotator cuff will present with both pain and weakness on examination. Occasionally, a patient with a large tear will present with a chief complaint of weakness with no or minimal associated pain.

Radiographic Findings

The AP radiograph may demonstrate sclerosis of the undersurface of the acromion and cyst formation in the greater tuberosity. In elderly patients, it is important to carefully evaluate the films for GH and AC joint arthritis. With longstanding disease, the humeral head may be riding superiorly on the glenoid, with decrease in the acromiohumeral interval. This is an important finding as it indicates a large, and often irreparable, tear of the cuff (Fig. 13.53).

The axillary view is useful for demonstrating abnormal ossification centers within the acromion. These are known as *os acromiale* and, when present, may contribute to pain and impingement.

A modified scapular Y view, called the *outlet view*, is used to evaluate the morphology of the acromion and the space available under the CA arch. The radiograph is obtained by orienting the beam parallel to the spine of the scapula and then angling it 10 to 30 degrees caudally. Bigliani classified the acromion according to its shape on this view. Type I involves a straight, smooth acromion. In a type II acromion, there is a gentle inferior curve anteriorly, whereas a type III acromion involves an anterior hook (Fig. 13.54). Type III acromion are more common in patients with full-thickness tears, but the exact relationship between acromial morphology and rotator cuff disease remains unclear.

Special Tests

Magnetic resonance imaging scans are the imaging modality of choice in evaluating disorders of the rotator cuff. Full- and partial-thickness tears are best seen on the T2 weighted coronal oblique images (Fig. 13.55). Any associated

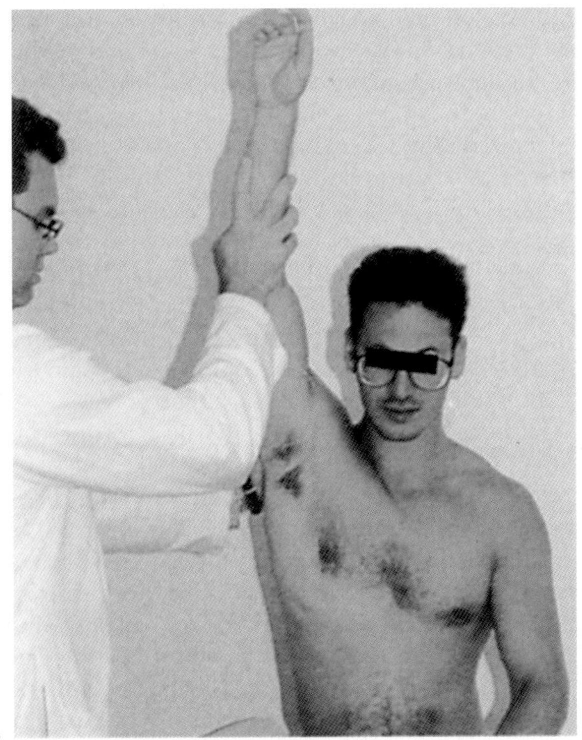

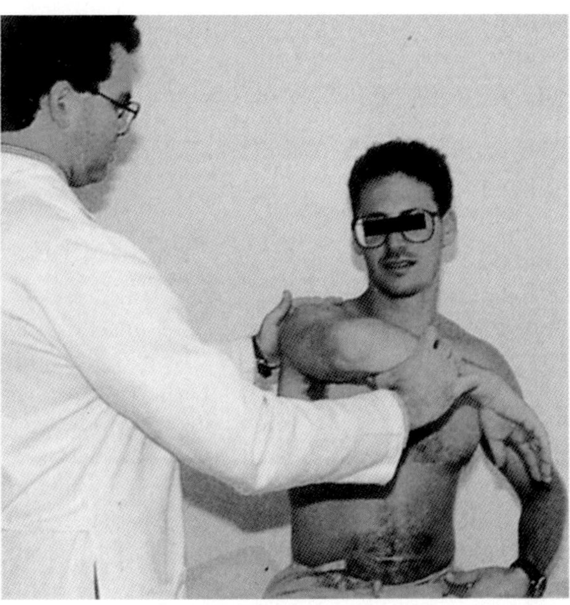

Figure 13.52 **A:** The Neer impingement sign. **B:** Hawkins impingement test. (*From* Iannotti JP, Williams GR. *Disorders of the Shoulder: Diagnosis and Management*, 2nd ed. Philadelphia: Lippincott Williams & Wilkins, 2007, with permission.)

tendon retraction and atrophy or fatty infiltration of the cuff muscles can be appreciated on MRI. Atrophy and fatty infiltration are best seen on the most medial sagittal oblique images and are important indicators of the chronicity of full-thickness cuff tears (Fig. 13.56). It is becoming increasingly clear that when these two processes are present, the chance of tendon healing following rotator cuff repair is significantly decreased.

Figure 13.53 Loss of the interval between the acromion and the humeral head indicates a large, full-thickness tear of the rotator cuff. (*From* Johnson DH, Pedowitz RA. *Practical Orthopaedic Sports Medicine and Arthroscopy*. Philadelphia: Lippincott Williams & Wilkins, 2007, with permission.)

Ultrasound is also gaining popularity in the evaluation of cuff disease. When compared to MRI, it has the advantage of being less expensive and better tolerated by patients, but it is highly operator-dependent and less suited to evaluating atrophy and fatty infiltration of the muscles. It is especially useful in postoperative patients, in whom artifact can make the interpretation of MRI scans difficult.

For patients with confusing historical and physical examination findings, the impingement injection test is useful for localizing pain to the subacromial space. Following examination, the patient is injected with 3 to 5 mL of 1% lidocaine into the subacromial space. If this results in the elimination of the patient's pain with provocative maneuvers, then it is likely that the pain is associated with pathology within the subacromial space. Strength examination following injection also allows for evaluation of muscle function without interference from pain.

Differential Diagnosis

The differential diagnosis of rotator cuff disease is age-dependent. In older patients, it includes cervical spine pathology, GH arthritis, metastatic disease and referred sources of shoulder pain such as cardiac disease. Impingement and cuff pathology is much less frequent in younger patients, and more common sources of shoulder pain

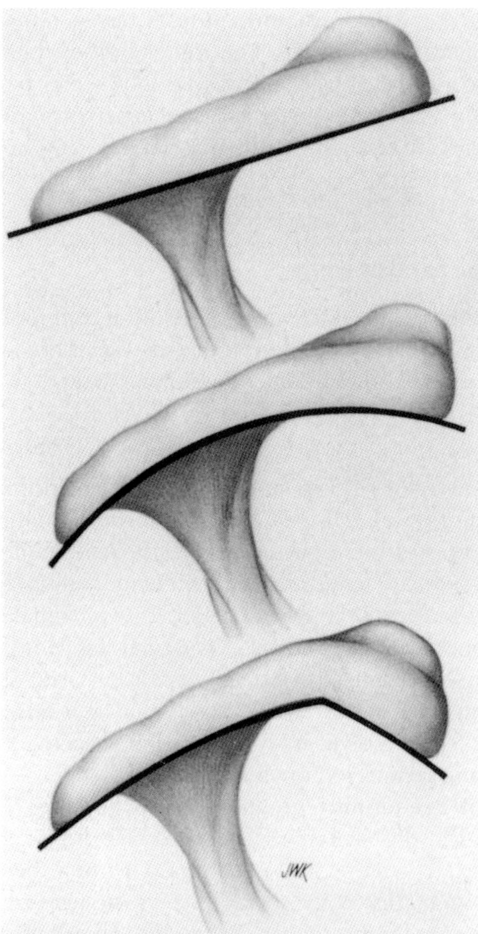

Figure 13.54 Acromial morphology as described by Bigliani: type I, flat; type II, curved; type III, hooked. This is evaluated on the supraspinatus outlet view. (*From* Iannotti JP, Williams GR. *Disorders of the Shoulder: Diagnosis and Management*, 2nd ed. Philadelphia: Lippincott Williams & Wilkins, 2007, with permission.)

in this population (such as instability and labral tears) should be considered. In any age group, adhesive capsulitis, calcific tendonitis, and AC joint arthritis should be considered.

Treatment

The treatment of rotator cuff disease depends on the pathology and the age of the patient. If there is no suggestion of a full-thickness cuff tear on the history, physical examination, and radiographs, then the presumptive diagnosis is cuff tendonitis or bursitis, and the initial treatment is nonoperative. At first, this consists of rest and education. This is followed by a progressive physical therapy program to regain motion, strengthen the cuff, and restore normal scapulothoracic strength and rhythm. Specific exercises to strengthen the cuff muscles help to keep the humeral head centered in the glenoid during motion, thereby creating more space for the tendons in the subacromial space. The speed of the patient's improvement can be enhanced through the use of subacromial corticosteroid injection. Although there are no absolute guidelines regarding these injections, concerns about tendon damage should limit their use to no more than three with at least 3 months in between injections in most patients. It is important to emphasize to patients that, while the injections

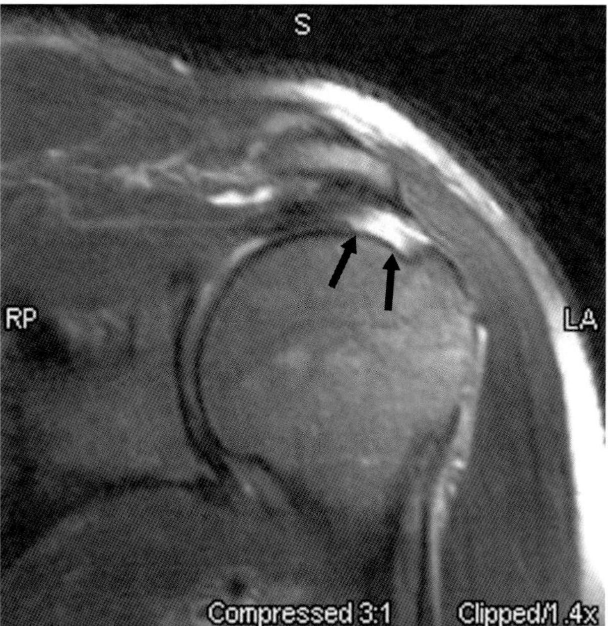

Figure 13.55 T2 weighted coronal oblique magnetic resonance image demonstrating a full thickness tear (*arrows*) of the supraspinatus tendon. (*From* Johnson DH, Pedowitz RA. *Practical Orthopaedic Sports Medicine and Arthroscopy*. Philadelphia: Lippincott Williams & Wilkins, 2007, with permission.)

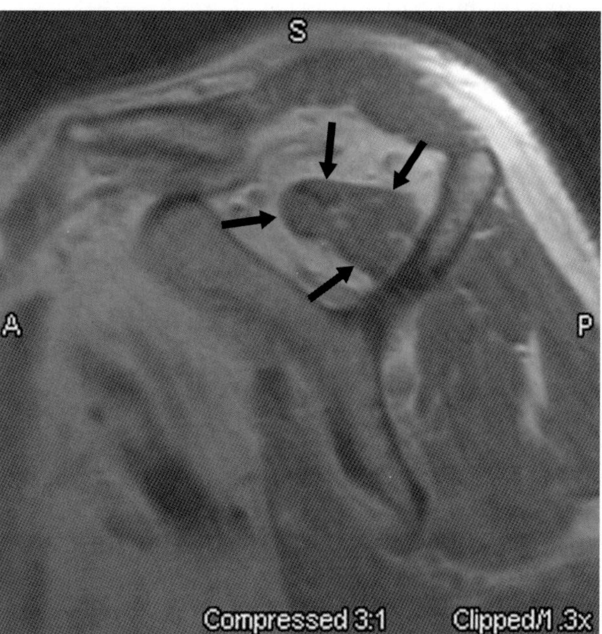

Figure 13.56 T1 weighted sagittal oblique magnetic resonance image depicting atrophy (*arrows*) of the supraspinatus muscle. (*From* Johnson DH, Pedowitz RA. *Practical Orthopaedic Sports Medicine and Arthroscopy*. Philadelphia: Lippincott Williams & Wilkins, 2007, with permission.)

will relieve their symptoms, the pain will return unless the patient complies with the therapy program.

Patients who fail to improve with 2 to 3 months of conservative treatment should undergo an MRI scan or ultrasound to evaluate the structural integrity of the cuff. Immediate imaging should also be considered in patients with significant weakness or following a traumatic injury. Patients with a structurally intact cuff should continue with another 2 to 3 months of conservative treatment. If they continue to be symptomatic then arthroscopic or open subacromial decompression is effective.

For patients with full-thickness rotator cuff tears, treatment depends on the age of the patient and the chronicity of the tear. If MRI demonstrates atrophy and fatty infiltration of the cuff muscles, surgical repair is unlikely to restore cuff integrity and function, so an extended course of physical therapy is indicated. Continued pain can be treated with arthroscopic debridement, partial cuff repair and, in selected cases, muscle transfers.

Patients who are physiologically older and less active with a full-thickness cuff tear but no atrophy and fatty infiltration will generally become asymptomatic with physical therapy. Decision making in these patients involves extensive counseling by the surgeon. If the patient opts for nonoperative treatment, it is important that he understands that the tear may progress and the muscles may atrophy; therefore if he becomes symptomatic again in the future, repair may no longer be an option. On the other hand, successful surgical treatment involves immobilization followed by an extended course of physical therapy that the patient may be unwilling or unable perform.

Younger, more active patients are less likely to be satisfied with nonoperative treatment and generally choose operative intervention. Controversy exists concerning asymptomatic patients under the age of 50 or 60 who present with full-thickness tears without muscle changes. These patients are at significant risk for progression of their tear and a return of symptoms in the future. It is important to discuss this with the patient when considering operative versus nonoperative treatment.

Acute tears of the rotator cuff that result from trauma are more likely to be associated with significant weakness, as the remaining cuff muscles do not have time to adapt and compensate. Because these patients are often younger and do not have degenerative changes of the tendon, these tears have the best healing rates following surgical repair. Consequently, that is the recommend treatment.

Partial-thickness cuff tears can be treated with an extended nonoperative course. The intact portion of the cuff continues to transmit force to the muscle, so there is less chance of atrophy or fatty infiltration. If symptoms persist, surgical management is an option. Surgery consists of subacromial decompression with debridement of the tear if it involves less than 50% of the tendon, and repair if more than 50% of the tendon is torn.

Surgical repair of rotator cuff tears can be done either open or arthroscopically. The initial healing rates with arthroscopic repair were inferior to open repair but, with improved techniques and increasing experience, more recent series are reporting comparable repair rates in all but the largest tears.

Calcific Tendonitis

Calcific tendonitis is a common disorder in middle-aged patients in whom calcification occurs within the tendons of the rotator cuff, especially the supraspinatus.

Pathophysiology and Classification

The etiology of calcific tendonitis is unknown but it involves multifocal, cell-mediated calcium deposition within the tendons of the rotator cuff. Calcific tendonitis differs from rotator cuff tendonitis in that it tends to occur in well-vascularized areas of the tendons 1 to 2 cm proximal to their insertion, rather than at the dysvascular tissue at the tendon's insertion into the tuberosity. Furthermore, the natural history of calcific tendonitis is that of a self-limited disorder that resolves with time rather than the gradual worsening seen in rotator cuff tendonitis.

Calcific tendonitis progresses through three distinct phases: the precalcifying stage, the calcifying stage, and the postcalcifying or resorptive phase. During the precalcifying stage, histologic metaplasia of the tenocytes into chondrocytes occurs within the tendon. This phase is generally asymptomatic. The calcifying stage involves the deposition and coalition of calcium within the tendon into well-delineated deposits. This stage is often asymptomatic, but when symptoms do occur they are generally similar to those characteristic of patients with mild to moderate subacromial impingement. Radiographs at this stage demonstrate a homogenous, well-demarcated calcium deposit within the tendon. The duration of this stage is variable, and it may last several years. The resorptive phase involves an inflammatory response by the body to the deposit resulting in break up and resorption of the calcification. Patients in this stage can experience severe pain secondary to the increased intratendinous pressure generated by the inflammatory response associated with resorption. Radiographs will demonstrate a fluffy, poorly delineated deposit.

Presentation

Calcific tendonitis is most common in patients between 40 and 50 and is more frequent in woman than men. The patient's symptoms depend on the stage of the disease. During the early stages, patients may be asymptomatic or complain of dull anterior lateral shoulder pain that is worse with activity, as is common in impingement syndrome. In the resorptive phase, patients may have severe, acute-onset shoulder pain that is extremely debilitating and can mimic a septic joint.

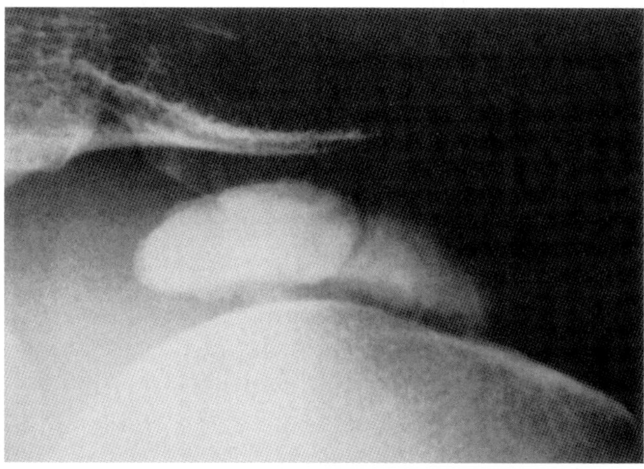

Figure 13.57 The characteristic calcification with the supraspinatus tendon seen in calcific tendonitis. (*From* Iannotti JP, Williams GR. *Disorders of the Shoulder: Diagnosis and Management*, 2nd ed. Philadelphia: Lippincott Williams & Wilkins, 2007, with permission.)

Physical Examination

In the precalcifying and calcifying stages, physical examination findings are similar to subacromial impingement, with a mild decrease in ROM and positive impingement signs. During the resorptive phase, the patient may have severely limited active and passive motion accompanied by intense pain.

Radiographic Findings

Radiographs are diagnostic for this disorder and will demonstrate calcification within the rotator cuff tendon (Fig. 13.57). A single AP view may miss the calcification if overlying bone is present, so additional AP radiographs in internal and external rotation can be helpful. The scapular Y and axillary views are useful for visualizing calcification with the subscapularis or posterior cuff muscles.

Special Tests

Radiographs are diagnostic of calcific tendonitis, so no further tests are necessary.

Differential Diagnosis

Calcific tendonitis is differentiated from other disorders of the rotator cuff by the presence of calcification within the tendon on plain radiographs. In patients presenting with acute pain characteristic of the resorptive phase, consideration must be given to septic arthritis. If the patient has any systemic signs of infection or underlying medical problems making him more prone to infection, the disorders can be distinguished by aspiration of the joint.

Treatment

The vast majority of patients with calcific tendonitis respond well to nonoperative treatment. Patients presenting with severe pain in the resorptive phase will benefit from subacromial injection of a mixture of local anesthetic and corticosteroid. Many authors have reported success with percutaneous needling of the deposits either alone or in combination with a steroid injection in these patients. For patients in the calcifying stage, nonoperative treatment with a rotator cuff–directed physical therapy program is generally successful in alleviating the impingement-type pain. If this fails, the deposits can be surgically excised.

Acromioclavicular Joint Arthritis

Arthritis of the AC joint is very common, and because of the joint's proximity to the subacromial space, often contributes to symptoms in patients with rotator cuff pathology.

Pathophysiology

Acromioclavicular joint arthritis can occur as a consequence of several disease processes. The three most common are primary osteoarthritis, posttraumatic arthritis, and osteolysis of the distal clavicle. As in other joints, primary osteoarthritis involves progressive cartilage loss resulting in joint space narrowing, sclerosis, and osteophyte formation. Osteoarthritis of the AC joint is ubiquitous, with intrinsic degeneration of the intra-articular disk in most individuals by age 40. Some radiographic evidence of arthritis is present in the majority of adults over the age of 50; however, the majority of these patients are asymptomatic.

Symptomatic posttraumatic arthritis is common, occurring in approximately 10% to 15% of those individuals with grade I or grade II AC separations. A history of trauma from a previous fall or injury during a contact sport is common. Identifying the subset of patients with a history of trauma is important because, in these individuals, an element of AC instability may contribute to their pain.

Patients with osteolysis of the distal clavicle are generally younger and typically involved in repetitive weight-lifting activities. The etiology of this condition is thought to be due to stress fractures of the subchondral bone and secondary joint breakdown. They complain of pain over the AC joint, particularly with bench pressing, dips, flies, and push-ups.

Presentation

Patients typically present with pain over the top of the shoulder, occasionally with radiation up into the trapezius or down the shoulder. The pain is often a mild ache, worsened with specific activities, especially reaching across the body. Symptoms can be worse at night, and lying or rolling onto the involved side may awaken the patient from sleep.

Physical Examination

Inspection may reveal prominence due to previous trauma with some residual separation or hypertrophy of the distal clavicle. Palpation yields tenderness directly over the AC joint. The joint is compressed by having the patient place the arm in adduction across the body at the level of the shoulder. In symptomatic patients, this maneuver will

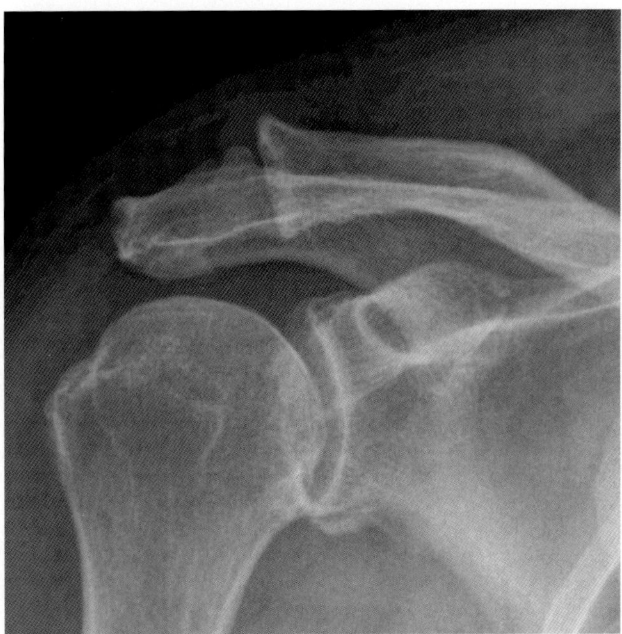

Figure 13.58 Anterior-posterior radiograph of the right shoulder demonstrating joint space narrowing, sclerosis and osteophyte formation typical of acromioclavicular joint arthritis.

reproduce their pain. Instability is examined by grasping the distal clavicle and attempting to translate it in an anterior–posterior or superior–inferior direction while the opposite hand stabilizes the acromion.

Radiographic Findings

As described in the section on AC sprains, the AC joint is best visualized in the AP plane using the Zanca view. With AC arthritis, there will be joint space narrowing, sclerosis, juxtacortical cysts, and osteophyte formation (Fig. 13.58). The axillary view provides further visualization of the joint space as well as any anterior or posterior translation of the distal clavicle. In osteolysis, the distal clavicle is enlarged and appears radiolucent. In this condition, the joint space may actually appear increased.

Special Tests

Additional studies are generally not necessary in the diagnosis of AC arthritis. Rarely, stress radiographs can be used to evaluate the contribution of instability to the patient's complaints. In complex cases, an injection of 1% lidocaine into the AC joint followed by repeat examination can be used to confirm the AC joint as the source of the patient's pain. Assuming the medication is correctly placed in the joint space, pain from AC arthritis should be temporarily eliminated by the injection.

Differential Diagnosis

Acromioclavicular joint pain may be due to a number of entities other than degenerative arthritis. These include acute AC joint separation, chronic pain or instability following AC separation, inflammatory arthritis, and septic arthritis. Many patients with rotator cuff pathology will present with symptoms similar to those seen in AC joint arthritis, and it is not uncommon for the two entities to coexist. Generally, pain with palpation directly over the AC joint is due to AC arthritis whereas pain associated with cuff pathology localizes over the anterolateral shoulder and deltoid.

Treatment

The treatment of primary osteoarthritis, posttraumatic arthritis, and osteolysis is similar. It is important to remember that AC arthritis is a common radiographic finding, and only those patients who are symptomatic warrant treatment. Initial treatment involves activity modification and NSAIDs. In mildly symptomatic patients, this is often effective in reducing their acute inflammation, and they can gradually return to their normal activities without a return of pain. In the weight-lifting athlete with osteolysis, changing the grip distance or eliminating bench presses and dips from the workout routine may eliminate symptoms. If pain persists, an injection of corticosteroid into the joint often provides dramatic if not permanent relief. Up to three injections can be performed for recurrent symptoms.

Surgical treatment with joint debridement and removal of the distal end of the clavicle is curative in most patients. This can be done with either an open or arthroscopic procedure. Care is taken to keep the resection lateral to the CC ligaments in order to avoid destabilizing the distal clavicle. In patients with symptomatic AC joints who are undergoing surgery for the treatment of rotator cuff pathology, conservative treatment is generally bypassed and excision of the distal clavicle is performed at the time of the cuff procedure.

Glenohumeral Arthritis

Although less common than arthritis of the hip and knee, degenerative arthritis of the GH joint is still relatively common. As in any joint in the body, the characteristic finding of GH arthritis is destruction of the articular cartilage, and a number of different pathologic entities can lead to this destruction. Given the importance of the periarticular soft tissues in shoulder function, the effect of arthritis on these structures is particularly important in determining the symptomatic effects and treatment of the disease.

Pathophysiology and Classification

Osteoarthritis is the most common form of GH arthritis. The exact etiology of this disease continues to remain an area of active research. As in other joints, the characteristic findings on radiographs include joint space narrowing, osteophyte formation, subchondral sclerosis, and juxtaarticular cysts. The pathognomic finding of osteoarthritis of the GH joint is the presence of osteophytes along the inferior margin of the humeral articular surface (Fig. 13.59). These osteophytes increase tension within the anterior joint

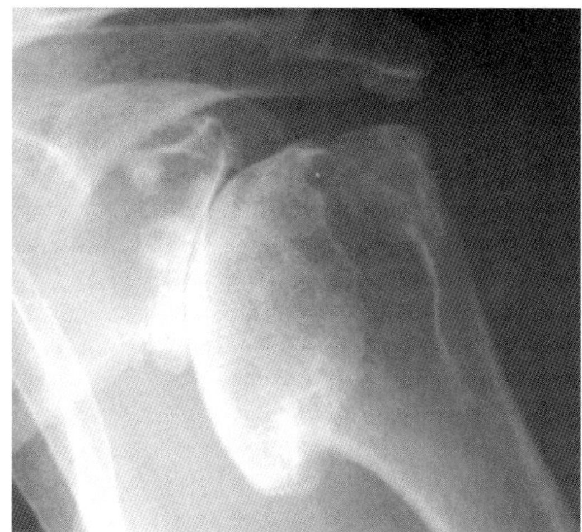
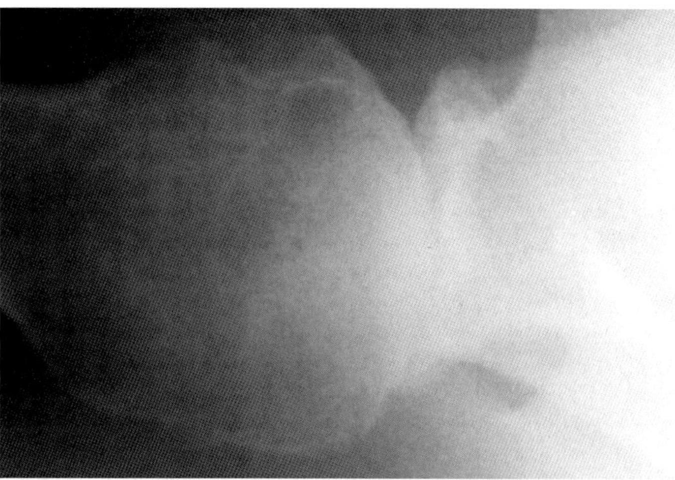

Figure 13.59 Anterior-posterior **(A)** and axillary **(B)** radiographs demonstrating moderately severe glenohumeral arthritis. Osteophytes along the inferior humeral neck are pathognomonic of osteoarthritis. (*From* Iannotti JP, Williams GR. *Disorders of the Shoulder: Diagnosis and Management*, 2nd ed. Philadelphia: Lippincott Williams & Wilkins, 2007, with permission.)

capsule, leading to hypertrophy of this structure and a characteristic decrease in external rotation. Disease progression leads to a preferential posterior wear of the glenoid eventually resulting in posterior subluxation of the humeral head. The disease process appears relatively protective of the rotator cuff, which is intact in 90% of these patients.

A second major cause of GH arthritis is inflammatory arthritis, especially rheumatoid arthritis. In these patients, the initiating event in cartilage destruction is a proliferative, inflammatory process of the synovium. Unfortunately, the destructive process is not limited to the articular cartilage but also involves the surrounding soft tissue, leading to attenuation and rupture of capsular restraints and rotator cuff. On radiographs, the osteophytes and sclerosis of osteoarthritis are absent, replaced by diffuse osteopenia and periarticular erosions in areas where the synovium has access to the bone (Fig. 13.60). Glenoid wear tends to be symmetrical, and patients do not have the dramatic loss of external rotation seen in osteoarthritis.

End-stage rotator cuff disease can lead to a unique form of arthritis termed *cuff tear arthropathy*. With massive, chronic rotator cuff tears, the humeral head can migrate superiorly, leading it to articulate with the superior margin of the glenoid and the undersurface of the acromion (Fig. 13.61). This leads to destruction of the articular surface and, if loss of the CA ligament occurs, can result in anterior–superior subluxation of the humeral head with attempted abduction of the arm. These patients often have significant pain and complete functional loss or pseudoparalysis of the shoulder.

A number of other disease processes, including osteonecrosis, GH dislocations, and posttraumatic articular incongruity, can lead to destruction of the GH articular surfaces. In most cases, this results in secondary osteoarthritis with joint destruction and symptoms similar to primary

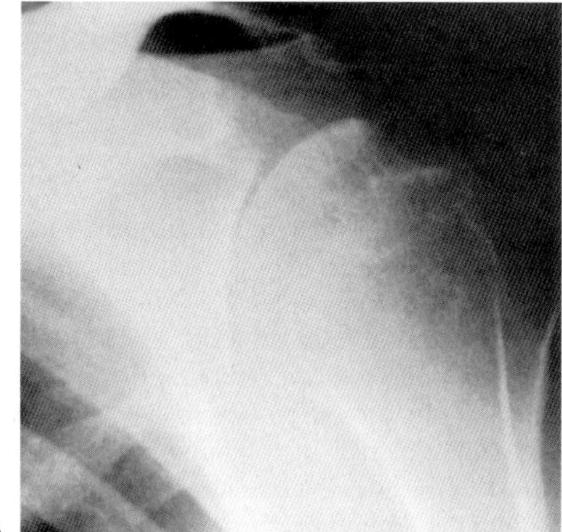
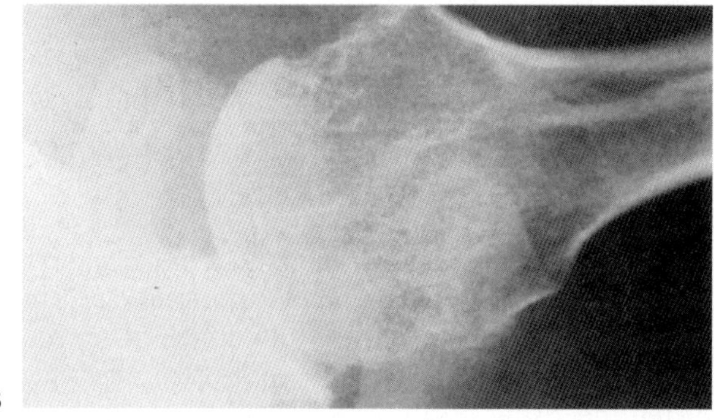

Figure 13.60 Anterior-posterior **(A)** and axillary **(B)** radiographs demonstrating rheumatoid orthritis of the glenohumeral joint. Note the periarticular osteopenia, symmetric cartilage loss, and lack of osteophytes. (*From* Iannotti JP, Williams GR. *Disorders of the Shoulder: Diagnosis and Management*, 2nd ed. Philadelphia: Lippincott Williams & Wilkins, 2007, with permission.)

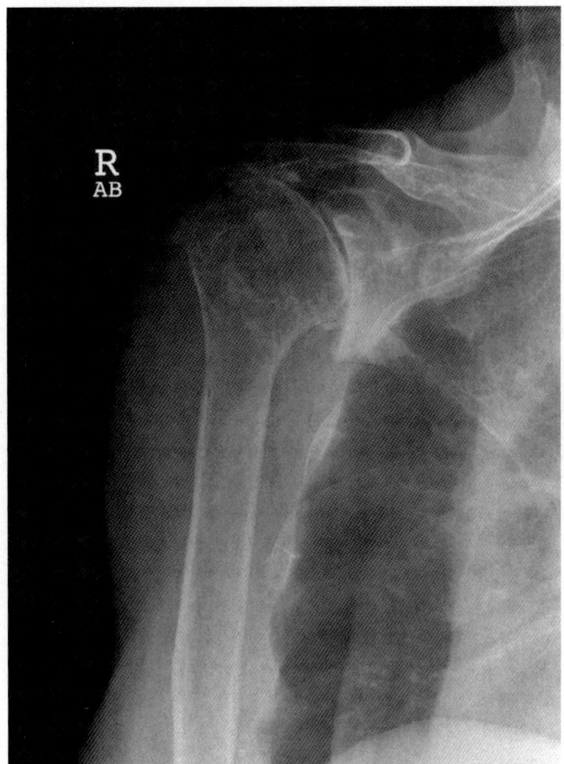

Figure 13.61 Anterior-posterior radiograph demonstrating the superior humeral translation seen in cuff tear arthropathy. (*From* Iannotti JP, Williams GR. *Disorders of the Shoulder: Diagnosis and Management*, 2nd ed. Philadelphia: Lippincott Williams & Wilkins, 2007, with permission.)

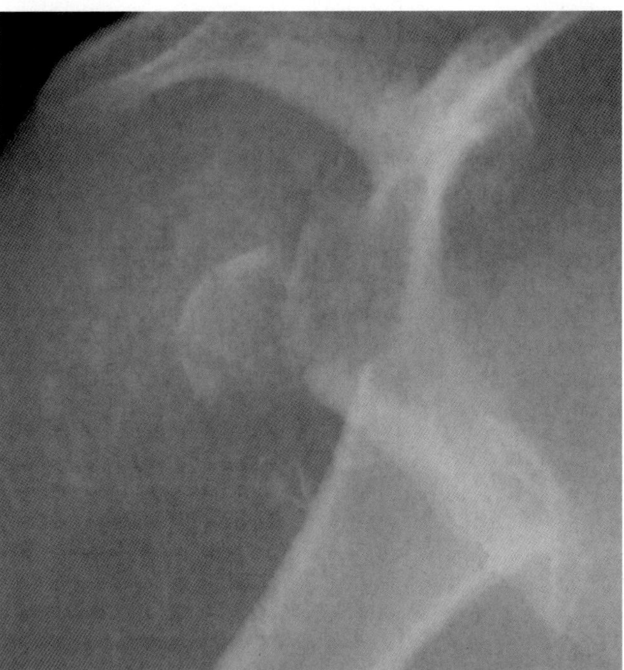

Figure 13.62 Radiograph demonstrating neuropathic arthropathy with complete destruction of the normal joint architecture. (*From* Iannotti JP, Williams GR. *Disorders of the Shoulder: Diagnosis and Management*, 2nd ed. Philadelphia: Lippincott Williams & Wilkins, 2007, with permission.)

osteoarthritis, although the specific patient presentation and clinical course may be altered by the initiating process.

Decreased proprioception can lead to a highly destructive neuropathic arthritis of the shoulder. These patients will have dramatic bone loss on radiographs and functional deficits, but often present with much less pain than one would expect given their radiographic findings (Fig. 13.62). The most common cause of neuropathic arthropathy in the shoulder is syringomyelia of the cervical spine. Recognition of a neuropathic shoulder should prompt detailed neurologic evaluation and MRI of the cervical spine.

Presentation

Patients with GH osteoarthritis generally present with a chief complaint of pain. Typically, the pain has an insidious onset, is progressive, and intensifies with use. Patients may also notice some limitation of motion, especially external rotation. The pain often interferes with sleep, especially if the patient rolls or lies on the involved side.

The presentation of other forms of GH arthritis depends on the underlying disease. Patients with rheumatoid arthritis may already know their diagnosis or present with pain and effusions in multiple joints. In cuff tear arthropathy, the pain is typically accompanied by the inability to raise the affected arm and weakness typical of massive rotator cuff tears.

Physical Examination

In primary osteoarthritis, atrophy about the shoulder girdle may be present secondary to disuse. Palpation of the joint often demonstrates crepitans with motion as the incongruous surfaces slide past each other. Posterior joint line tenderness may be present. Active motion is typically limited by pain, whereas passive motion is decreased secondary to capsular contracture. The most dramatic finding is often a significant loss of external rotation. With the arm at the side, these patients often have zero degrees of, or even negative, external rotation. They typically have significant pain with stretch of the anterior capsule, which can be demonstrated be placing the arm in maximal external rotation and then gently applying a mild external rotational force. Although the limited ROM can make the evaluation of the rotator cuff difficult, it is important to evaluate, as cuff integrity can have a significant impact on treatment if the decision is made to proceed with arthroplasty.

Patients with inflammatory arthritis are likely to have a relatively preserved ROM but may lack strength secondary to rotator cuff tears. In patients with cuff tear arthropathy, significant hollowing about the scapula is often present, secondary to atrophy of the cuff muscles. If the patient has anterior–superior subluxation, the humeral head will be visible anterior to the acromion.

Radiographic Findings

True AP and axillary radiographs will demonstrate joint space narrowing in all patients with arthritis. Once the presence of cartilage loss is observed, it is important to distinguish between the various types of arthritis, as this will have an impact on prognosis and treatment. The primary distinction is between osteoarthritis and inflammatory arthritis. This is easily accomplished given the characteristic osteophyte formation and sclerosis seen with osteoarthritis of the GH joint. In patients with osteoarthritis, the axillary radiograph is useful for evaluating the amount of posterior glenoid bone loss and any posterior subluxation of the humeral head.

Special Tests

In the straightforward presentation of osteoarthritis, no special studies are needed. In patients being considered for shoulder arthroplasty, CT scans are useful to further define posterior glenoid wear. When there are questions regarding the integrity of the rotator cuff, especially in patients with inflammatory arthritis, MRI continues to be the study of choice. Early in the course of some secondary causes of osteoarthritis, such as osteonecrosis, MRI is also useful in demonstrating changes that may not be apparent on plain radiographs. Patients with radiographic findings of inflammatory arthritis without a diagnosis of a systemic inflammatory process (rheumatoid arthritis, lupus, spondyloarthropathy) should be referred to a rheumatologist for further clinical and laboratory evaluation.

Differential Diagnosis

The differential diagnosis of GH arthritis consists of any condition that can present with a stiff, painful shoulder. The most common entities to present in a similar manner are adhesive capsulitis and rotator cuff disease. The distinction can generally be easily accomplished through history, physical examination, and radiographic studies. It is important to remember that more than one of these entities can exist in a given shoulder. Generally, if significant loss of the joint space has occurred, arthritis is responsible for the patient's symptoms.

Treatment

The treatment of arthritis depends on the patient's discomfort and ability to function. For patients with minor or moderate pain and preserved function, nonoperative treatment consisting of activity modification and anti-inflammatory medications is utilized. Physical therapy may be useful in maintaining the ROM, but it can also aggravate the patient's symptoms. For patients with more significant pain and a decreasing ability to perform the activities they want or need to do, shoulder replacement is an excellent treatment option.

Total shoulder arthroplasty (TSA) involves replacement of the humeral head with a metal sphere and replacement of the glenoid surface with an ultra-high-molecular-weight polyethylene disc (Fig. 13.63). In most current designs, the humeral component is placed in press-fit manner while the glenoid component is held in place by bone cement.

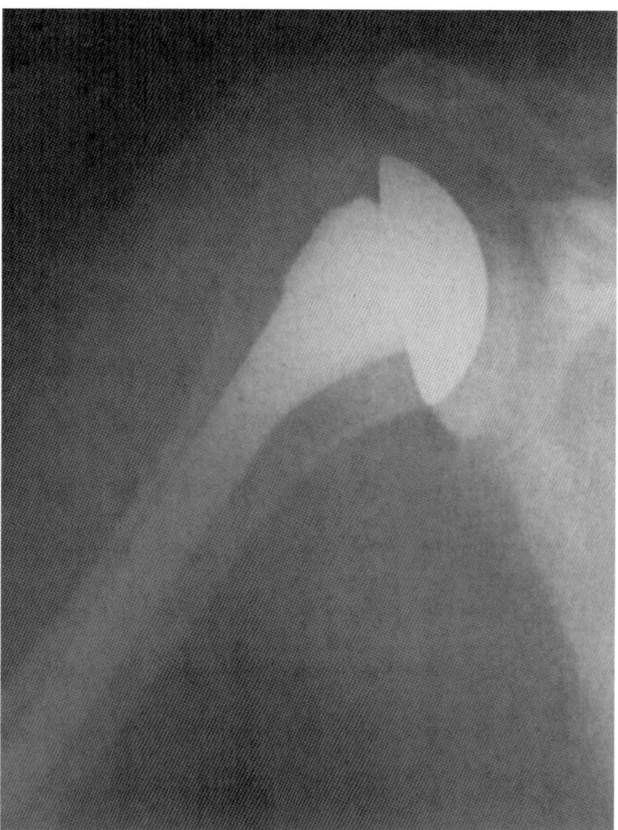

Figure 13.63 Anterior-posterior view demonstrating a total shoulder arthroplasty used to treat glenohumeral arthritis. (*From* Iannotti JP, Williams GR. *Disorders of the Shoulder: Diagnosis and Management*, 2nd ed. Philadelphia: Lippincott Williams & Wilkins, 2007, with permission.)

Patients often achieve dramatic, lasting pain relief and 85% to 90% good to excellent results have been reported at 10 to 15 year follow-up. Return to most activities, including golf, is permitted, although the patient is generally advised not to repetitively lift more than 25 pounds with the involved extremity. Controversy exists over the need to resurface the glenoid, but recent evidence suggests that, in patients with an intact rotator cuff, TSA provides superior function and pain relief when compared to hemiarthroplasty.

Total shoulder arthroplasty is a resurfacing procedure and relies on the integrity of surrounding soft tissue structures to provide stability and proper function of the joint. Improper positioning or sizing of the components or loss of integrity or function of the rotator cuff can lead to significant decreases in the postoperative function and early failure of the prosthesis.

Given the propensity for posterior glenoid wear with GH osteoarthritis, it is important to carefully evaluate the extent of glenoid bone loss on the preoperative axillary radiographs and CT scan. Occasionally, the amount of posterior bone loss will preclude the placement of a glenoid component, in which case the glenoid can be reamed to create a smooth surface with placement of a hemiarthroplasty

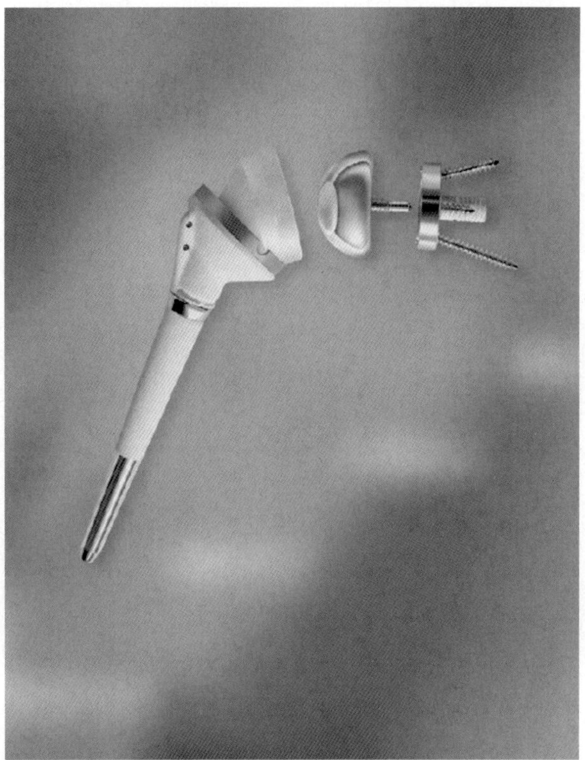

Figure 13.64 The reverse shoulder prosthesis is used to treat some patients with cuff tear arthropathy. The articular geometry is reverse, so that the convex component is placed on the glenoid and the concave component is on the humerus. (*From* Iannotti JP, Williams GR. *Disorders of the Shoulder: Diagnosis and Management*, 2nd ed. Philadelphia: Lippincott Williams & Wilkins, 2007, with permission.)

on the humeral side. Hemiarthroplasty is also favored in patients with osteoarthritis and an irreparable rotator cuff tear, as well as those under the age of 50.

Glenoid bone loss is an important consideration when advising the patient about continued conservative treatment for osteoarthritis. The patient needs to understand that once he begins to have significant posterior wear and subluxation, continuation of nonoperative treatment may lead to insufficient glenoid bone for placement of a glenoid component during future arthroplasty.

The functional results of TSA in patients with inflammatory arthritis are inferior to those of patients with osteoarthritis secondary to the attrition of their surrounding soft tissue envelope. In cuff tear arthropathy, glenoid replacement is contraindicated because the humeral head is no longer concentrically articulating with the glenoid. These patients can be managed with hemiarthroplasty or a new type of prosthesis known as a *reverse shoulder arthroplasty*. In this device, the geometry of the shoulder is reversed and the sphere is placed on the glenoid side of the articulation while the concave surface is placed on the humeral side (Fig. 13.64).

Adhesive Capsulitis

Adhesive capsulitis, or *frozen shoulder*, is a painful condition characterized by the loss of both active and passive motion of the GH joint. Given the paramount role of GH motion in proper shoulder girdle function, patients often find this disease remarkably debilitating. Primary adhesive capsulitis is an idiopathic process that tends to occur in middle-aged patients. Restricted ROM can also occur as a result of a traumatic injury, surgery, or other pathologic process of the shoulder, in which case it is referred to as *secondary adhesive capsulitis*.

Pathophysiology and Classification

Despite more than 100 years of familiarity with the condition, the underlying etiology of frozen shoulder remains unclear. Diabetes mellitus and thyroid disease are predisposing factors for the development of idiopathic adhesive capsulitis. The decrease in GH motion is associated with hypertrophy of the capsular and ligamentous restraints to shoulder motion as well as inflammation of the joint's synovial lining. In most patients, the process is self-limited, with the eventual return of near normal motion.

Idiopathic adhesive capsulitis has been divided into three distinct but overlapping clinical phases: freezing, frozen, and thawing. During the freezing phase there is an insidious, progressive loss of shoulder motion, often associated with significant pain with both rest and activity. In the frozen phase, the loss of motion stabilizes. Pain is generally limited to activities that place the joint near its end ROM. The thawing phase is characterized by a gradual return of the GH motion. The duration of each phase is highly variable, with the overall course of the disease generally ranging for 9 months to 3 years.

Presentation

The presentation of adhesive capsulitis depends on the stage of the disease. The majority of patients will present in the freezing phase complaining of pain over the anterior lateral aspect of the shoulder and arm. This pain is generally described as a dull ache and is often worse at night, leading to nocturnal awakening. The discomfort is often accompanied by a sharp pain with movements that stretch the inflamed capsular structures such as fastening a bra, putting on a coat, or reaching into the back seat of a car. As the disease progresses, patients will note decrease in the functional ROM of their shoulder. They may also have pain and muscle cramping about the scapula as they attempt to compensate for decreased GH motion with increased scapulothoracic motion.

Physical Examination

The hallmark of frozen shoulder on physical examination is the loss of both active and passive ROM. Restriction is present in several planes but is often most pronounced in external rotation and abduction. It is not uncommon for patients to lack sufficient abduction to examine rotation at 90 degrees of abduction. When examining patients with adhesive capsulitis, it is particularly important to identify and control compensatory motions in order to get a true measurement of GH motion. Patients will often have sharp pain when a stretch is applied to the capsule at the extreme ranges of passive motion.

Radiographic Findings

Radiographs of patients with adhesive capsulitis are generally unremarkable. They are important to rule out other conditions that can lead to restricted ROM, especially GH arthritis.

Special Tests

Frozen shoulder is diagnosed on the basis of history and physical examination findings, and no special tests are needed. In rare circumstances, arthrography can be used to confirm the diagnosis. The normal shoulder will accommodate 15 to 30 mL of contrast fluid, whereas the contracted capsule of the typical frozen shoulder will hold less than 10 mL. Postcontrast radiographs will also demonstrate a small, blunted axillary fold. Occasionally, MRI examination is warranted to rule out other soft tissue disorders about the shoulder that can lead to pain and secondary adhesive capsulitis.

Differential Diagnosis

During the early phases of adhesive capsulitis, it can be extremely difficult to differentiate the condition from rotator cuff disease. Both groups of patients will present with pain that is very similar in nature. It is not uncommon for patients with adhesive capsulitis to present having self-diagnosed themselves with impingement syndrome. Patients with cuff pathology will often have small decreases in the range of active motion, especially internal rotation. Further complicating the issue, patients with frozen shoulder will often experience some degree of secondary impingement syndrome as their tight posterior inferior capsule leads to anterior superior translation of the humeral head toward the acromion with elevation of the arm. The distinction is best accomplished over time. Both sets of patients can be started on an initial therapy program that emphasizes capsular stretching and strengthening of the rotator cuff muscles outside of the impingement zone. In the compliant patient, reexamination in 1 month will generally reveal an improvement in the ROM in patients with cuff disease. In patients in the early stages of adhesive capsulitis, further decrease in the ROM will often occur despite the stretching program.

Glenohumeral arthritis and missed traumatic injuries to the shoulder, especially posterior GH dislocations, can lead to decreased ROM. These disorders can be easily differentiated on plain radiographs.

Treatment

The most important aspect of treatment of the patient with adhesive capsulitis is educating the patient regarding the self-limited nature of the disease. The variable time course and generally slow restoration of motion can make the treatment of this condition extremely frustrating for both patient and physician. During the freezing phase, the patient is started on a passive stretching program in an attempt to maintain as much motion as possible. Although supervision of the program by a therapist is often helpful, in order to be effective, the stretching must be performed by the patient at home, a minimum of four to five times a day. For patients with significant pain, NSAIDs or an intra-articular cortisone injection are helpful in relieving the patients' symptoms, so that they can participate in the therapy program. The stretching is continued during the frozen and thawing phases in an attempt to restore motion as quickly as possible. The majority of patients are left with some small limitations in GH motion following adhesive capsulitis; however, these deficits rarely result in any functional limitations.

For patients with no improvement or a decrease in their ROM despite 3 to 6 months of aggressive therapy, operative intervention is a consideration. Traditionally, manipulation under anesthesia has been the procedure of choice, although fractures of the proximal humerus are a significant risk. More recently, an arthroscopic capsular release has been favored. Although more invasive, this procedure allows controlled sectioning of the contracted capsular structures. Regardless of which surgical option is utilized, aggressive postoperative therapy is crucial to maintaining the increased ROM achieved in the operating room.

CONCLUSION

When healthy, the shoulder complex is able to achieve a remarkable ROM while generating significant power for the functional activities of the upper extremity. In order to achieve these functions, it relies on a complex interaction between multiple bones, joints, and muscles, making it susceptible to a wide range of pathologic processes. Significant advances in our understanding of the function of the various elements of the complex, as well as advances in open and arthroscopic surgical techniques, have led to an enhanced ability to diagnose and treat dysfunction about the shoulder. Disorders of the shoulder complex remain an area of active orthopaedic research, and future findings will continue to advance our understanding of these conditions and our ability to diagnose and treat them.

RECOMMENDED READINGS

Tennent DT, Beach WR, Meyers JF. A review of special test associated with shoulder examination. Part I: The rotator cuff tests. *Am J Sports Med* 2003;31(1):154–160.

A detailed description of each of the various special tests used in the evaluation of rotator cuff disease.

Tennent DT, Beach WR, Meyers JF. A review of special tests associated with shoulder examination. Part II: Laxity, instability, and superior labral anterior and posterior (SLAP) lesions. *Am J Sports Med* 2003;31(2):301–307.

A detailed description of the many of the special tests used in the evaluation of several common disorders of the glenohumeral joint.

Iannotti JP, Ramsey ML, Williams GR, et al. Nonprosthetic management of proximal humeral fractures. *Am J Bone Joint Surg* 2003;85-A(8):1578–1593.
This reprint of an Instruction Course Lecture describes the multiple options available for the surgical treatment of proximal humerus factures.

Robinson CM, Dobson RJ. Anterior instability of the shoulder after trauma. *Br J Bone Joint Surg* 2004;86-B(4):469–479.
An excellent review of the epidemiology, pathoanatomy, and results of open and arthroscopic treatment of traumatic anterior shoulder instability.

Williams GR, Rockwood Jr. CA, Bigliani LU, et al. Rotator cuff tears: Why do we repair them? *Am J Bone Joint Surg* 2004;86-A(12):2764–2776.
This article provides a thorough review of both nonoperative and operative management of rotator cuff tears.

Boileau P, Sinnerton RJ, Chuinard C, et al. Arthroplasty of the shoulder. *Br J Bone Joint Surg* 2006;88-B(5):562–575.
A comprehensive discussion regarding the design rationale behind the current generation of implants available for shoulder replacement, as well as a review of factors influencing the success of shoulder arthroplasty.

The Elbow

14

Brian Magovern ***Matthew L. Ramsey***

INTRODUCTION

While the shoulder allows placement of the upper extremity throughout a large sphere of motion, the elbow allows fine-tuned motions within that sphere. Through its three articulations and a complex interplay of muscles and ligaments, the elbow is capable of both fine motions and great power. The elbow has a very unique anatomical and biomechanical profile, which adds to the complexity when evaluating and treating disorders of this region. Traumatic and atraumatic elbow conditions can have a dramatic influence on a patient's ability to function during work, recreation, or activities of daily living. This chapter describes the anatomy, biomechanics, evaluation, and management of the most common pathologic conditions of the elbow.

FUNCTIONAL ANATOMY

The elbow is a highly constrained hinge joint (trochoginglymoid) that is made up of three articulations. The three joint surfaces consist of hyaline cartilage and are found within one shared joint capsule. The ulnohumeral joint is the primary articulation of the elbow. It allows flexion and extension and provides a large degree of elbow stability. The other two articulations are the radiocapitellar and proximal radioulnar joints, which allow for supination and pronation. Pathologic conditions that interfere with these important joint surfaces, such as rheumatoid arthritis (RA), will lead to painful loss of motion and poor function.

Several important structures are vital to the normal function of these articulations. They consist of bones, ligaments, and muscles, which provide static and dynamic stability as well as motion and power. Conditions that disrupt these structures lead to a breakdown in the complex chain necessary for fluid and powerful elbow motion.

Osteology

The distal humerus is a triangular-shaped long bone that flattens in the coronal plane as it nears the elbow joint (Fig. 14.1). Distally, it flares medially and laterally into two strong bony columns, leaving a very thin segment of intervening bone. The two columns end as the medial and lateral epicondyles, respectively, which serve as important attachment sites for the ligaments and muscles that cross the elbow. At the level of the joint, the humeral columns are separated by two main articular segments. Medially, the spool-shaped trochlea makes up the majority of the ulnohumeral articulation. Lateral to the trochlea lies the capitellum, a convex projection of the distal humeral joint surface, which articulates with the concave radial head to form the radiocapitellar joint. In the coronal plane, the trochlea has a 6 to 8 degree valgus alignment, which gives the elbow its carrying angle. Commonly, women have a larger carrying angle than do men. In the sagittal plane, the capitellum is angled 30 degrees relative to the humeral shaft, which may be helpful in the evaluation of fractures.

The proximal ulna is a saddle-shaped articulation that closely matches the shape of the trochlea on the humeral side of the joint. The elbow, unlike the shoulder, has an inherent bony stability primarily because of the congruity of these two irregular surfaces. The ulna is also made up of the anterior coronoid process and the posterior olecranon process, which act as important tendon, ligament, and capsular attachment sites. The coronoid is an important buttress to prevent anterior dislocation of the elbow joint. The distal humerus has two corresponding concavities known as the coronoid and olecranon fossae. The coronoid process engages its fossa at greater than 120 degrees of flexion and the olecranon process at less than 20 degrees of flexion (Fig. 14.2). Bony stability is the most prevalent during these end ranges of motion. The proximal ulna also articulates with the proximal radius at the area known as the lesser sigmoid notch.

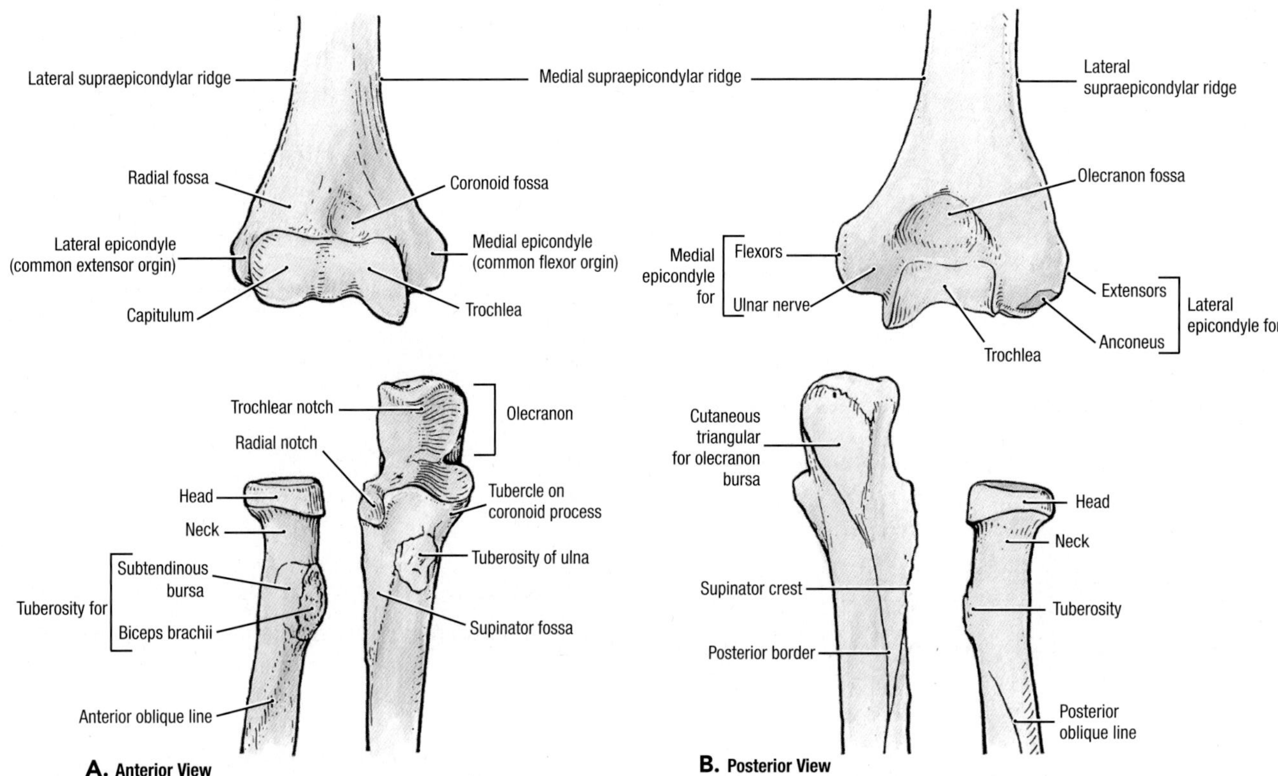

Figure 14.1 Osteology. (*Reproduced with permission from* Agur AMR, Dalley AF. *Grant's Atlas of Anatomy*. 11th ed. Philadelphia, PA: Lippincott Williams & Wilkins, 2004.)

The proximal end of the radius consists of the radial neck and head. The radial head is slightly elliptical and concave. It is an important secondary stabilizer to valgus stress of the elbow and a restraint to proximal migration of the radius. It articulates with both the capitellum and the proximal ulna to allow nearly 200 degrees of rotation. By necessity, most of the radial head is covered in articular cartilage. This is clinically important in the treatment of radial head fractures, as there is roughly a 90-degree "safe" arc for placement of internal fixation. The radial head is supported by the radial neck distally. Further distal, the radial tuberosity serves as the attachment site for the distal biceps tendon.

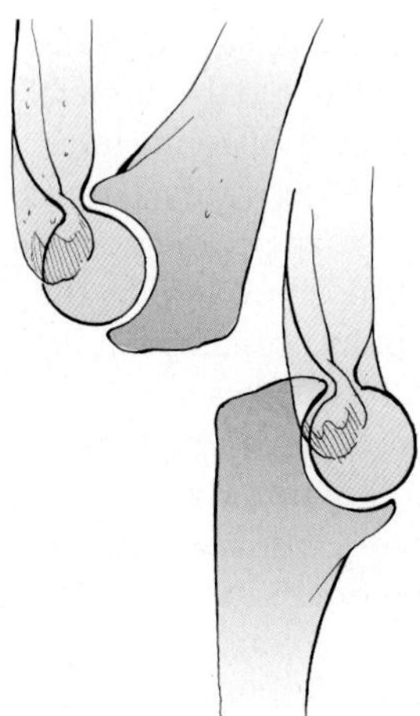

Figure 14.2 The coronoid and olecranon process engage at terminal flexion and extension so bony stability of the ulnohumeral joint is greatest at these end ranges of motion. (*Reproduced with permission from* Bucholz RW, Heckman JD, Court-Brown C, et al. *Rockwood and Green's Fractures in Adults*. 6th ed. Philadelphia, PA: Lippincott Williams & Wilkins, 2005.)

Ligaments

Two major ligament complexes offer stability to the elbow joint. They are most important in the arc of 20 to 120 degrees, where there is less bony stability. On the medial side, the medial ulnar collateral ligament (MUCL) complex is a triangular structure that acts as a major restraint to valgus stress (Fig. 14.3). It is made up of three components. The anterior bundle is the primary stabilizer to valgus stress and spans from the undersurface of the medial epicondyle to the sublime tubercle on the coronoid process of the ulna. The posterior bundle is found between the medial epicondyle and the olecranon and provides more stability in higher degrees of flexion. The transverse bundle is a smaller, less important structure that completes the triangle of the MUCL complex.

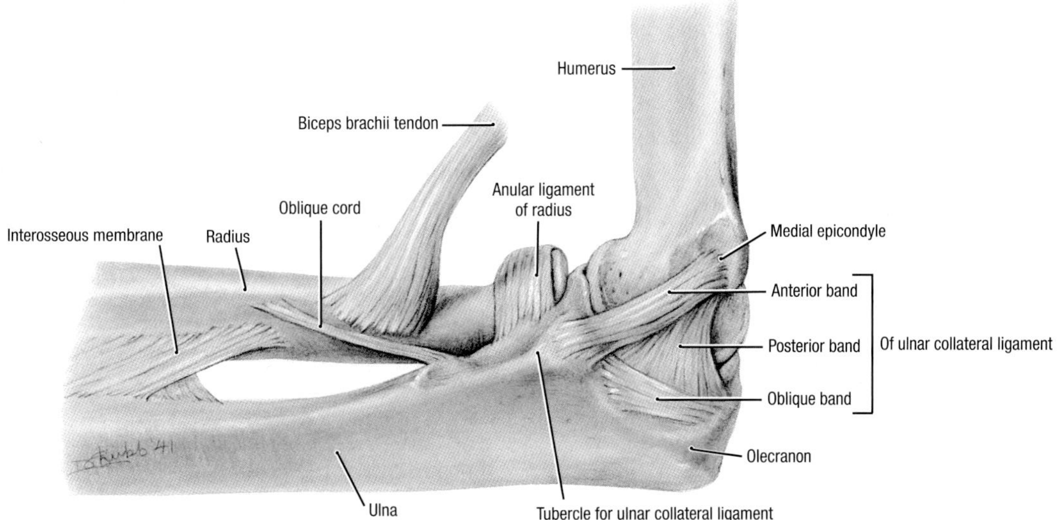

Figure 14.3 Medial ulnar collateral ligament complex. (*Reproduced with permission from* Agur AMR, Dalley AF. *Grant's Atlas of Anatomy*. 11th ed. Philadelphia, PA: Lippincott Williams & Wilkins, 2004.)

On the lateral side, the lateral ulnar collateral ligament (LUCL) is a thickening of the elbow capsule that spans from the lateral epicondyle to a process on the proximal ulna known as the *crista supinatoris* (Fig. 14.4). The LUCL is the primary restraint to posterolateral rotatory instability (PLRI) of the elbow. The annular ligament arises from the LUCL and encompasses the radial head, adding stability to the proximal radius.

Important capsular insertions make up the remainder of the static stabilizers to the elbow. The anterior capsule inserts on the slope of the coronoid process (not at the tip), offering restraint to anterior subluxation of the elbow. The posterior capsule lies deep to the triceps. It does not offer significant stability, but when diseased, it can play a major role in elbow stiffness and contracture.

Muscles

The elbow joint is powered by several major muscles. These muscles can be divided into groups based on the elbow motion that they perform. There are also many important muscles that cross the elbow joint providing motor function to the wrist and hand.

Elbow extension is primarily performed by the triceps muscle (Fig. 14.5). It is made up of three heads proximally that form one tendon that attaches to the olecranon process distally. It is innervated by the radial nerve. Flexion of the elbow is driven by the structures of the anterior arm compartment (Fig. 14.6). The brachialis originates from the anterior humerus and inserts just distal to the tip of the coronoid process along the anterior slope. It is the primary flexor of the elbow and has a dual innervation. The lateral fibers are innervated by the radial nerve, whereas its medial fibers are innervated by the musculocutaneous nerve. This allows longitudinal splitting of the brachialis during the anterior approach to the humerus. The brachioradialis, also innervated by the radial nerve, is a weak flexor of the elbow. It originates on the lateral aspect of the distal humerus and inserts on the radial styloid of the wrist. The biceps muscle adds additional flexion strength but is more important as the primary supinator of the forearm. It originates from two heads proximally and inserts on the bicipital tuberosity of the proximal radius. It is innervated by the musculocutaneous nerve. A fascial reflection known as the *bicipital aponeurosis* or *lacertus fibrosis* extends medially from the biceps tendon onto the forearm fascia covering the median nerve and brachial artery. In some cases of distal biceps tendon rupture, the bicipital aponeurosis remains intact, preventing proximal retraction of the muscle belly. The supinator provides secondary supination strength. Finally, pronation is mainly powered by the pronator teres (PT) with some contribution from the remaining flexor–pronator mass of muscles that originate from the medial epicondyle. The pronator teres (PT) inserts on the radial shaft and is innervated by the median nerve.

There are many other important muscle groups that originate or insert at the elbow but do not contribute significantly to elbow motion. The lateral epicondyle serves as the origination of the wrist and digital extensors, namely the extensor carpi radialis longus and extensor carpi radialis brevis (ECRB), extensor digitorum communis, and extensor carpi ulnaris (ECU). The anconeus is a small muscle posterior to the ECU, which may function as a weak stabilizer to the elbow, but its function is not entirely clear. The medial epicondyle serves as the attachment site for the PT,

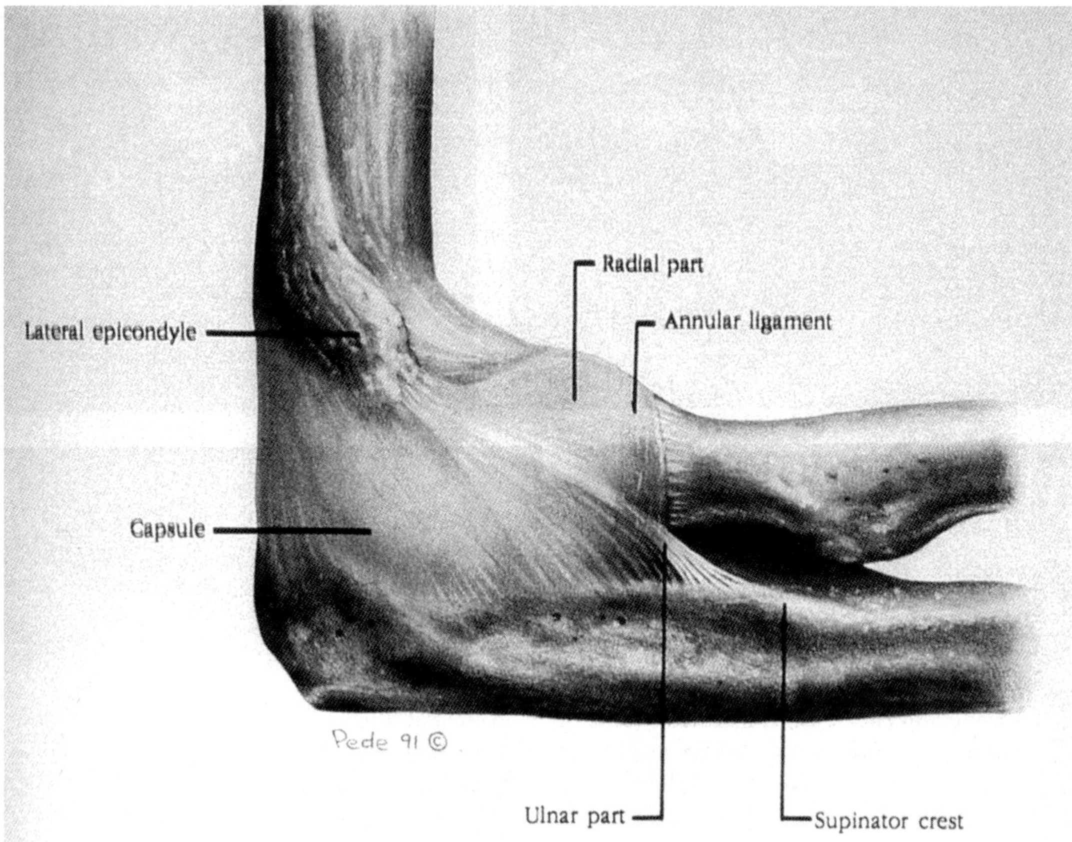

Figure 14.4 Lateral ulnar collateral ligament complex. (*Reprinted with permission from* O'Driscoll SW, Horii E, Morrey BF, et al. Anatomy of the ulnar part of the lateral collateral ligament of the elbow. *Clin Anat*. 1992;5:296–303.)

flexor carpi ulnaris, flexor digitorum superficialis (FDS), and flexor carpi radialis (FCR).

Neurovascular Structures

The elbow is surrounded by major neurovascular structures all within close proximity to one another. Knowledge of the relationship between structures in the elbow is crucial during surgical dissection as there is little room for error.

The brachial artery runs along the medial arm and crosses anterior to the elbow joint as it bifurcates into the radial and ulnar arteries underneath the bicipital aponeurosis (Fig. 14.7). The radial artery runs along the medial aspect of the biceps tendon and into the radial forearm. The ulnar artery continues along the ulnar side of the forearm.

The median nerve courses along with the brachial artery, passing under the bicipital aponeurosis medial to the artery. It then continues between the FDS and FDP into the forearm. It supplies the PT and the remainder of the flexor–pronator mass. The ulnar nerve also travels along the medial arm, passing into the posterior compartment through the intermuscular septum proximal to the elbow joint. It then runs under the medial epicondyle into the cubital tunnel. The posterior bundle of the ulnar collateral ligament makes up the floor of the cubital tunnel while the anterior bundle lies anterior to the nerve running parallel to it. The nerve passes between the two heads of the PT and runs along the ulnar aspect of the forearm into the hand. The musculocutaneous nerve enters the anterior arm from underneath the coracoid process where it supplies the coracobrachialis, the biceps, and the medial two-thirds of the brachialis. It then exits the arm between the biceps and brachialis muscles proximal to the elbow joint, forming the lateral antebrachial cutaneous nerve. It pierces the anterior fascia of the forearm, becoming subcutaneous and is in danger during surgical approaches to the anterior forearm, such as those used for distal biceps tendon repair. The radial nerve enters the arm from the posterior cord of the brachial plexus and passes posterior to the humerus in the spiral groove. The nerve then enters the anterior compartment of the arm between the brachialis and the brachioradialis muscles. It travels in close proximity to the anterior elbow capsule and bifurcates distal to the elbow joint. The superficial branch runs on the

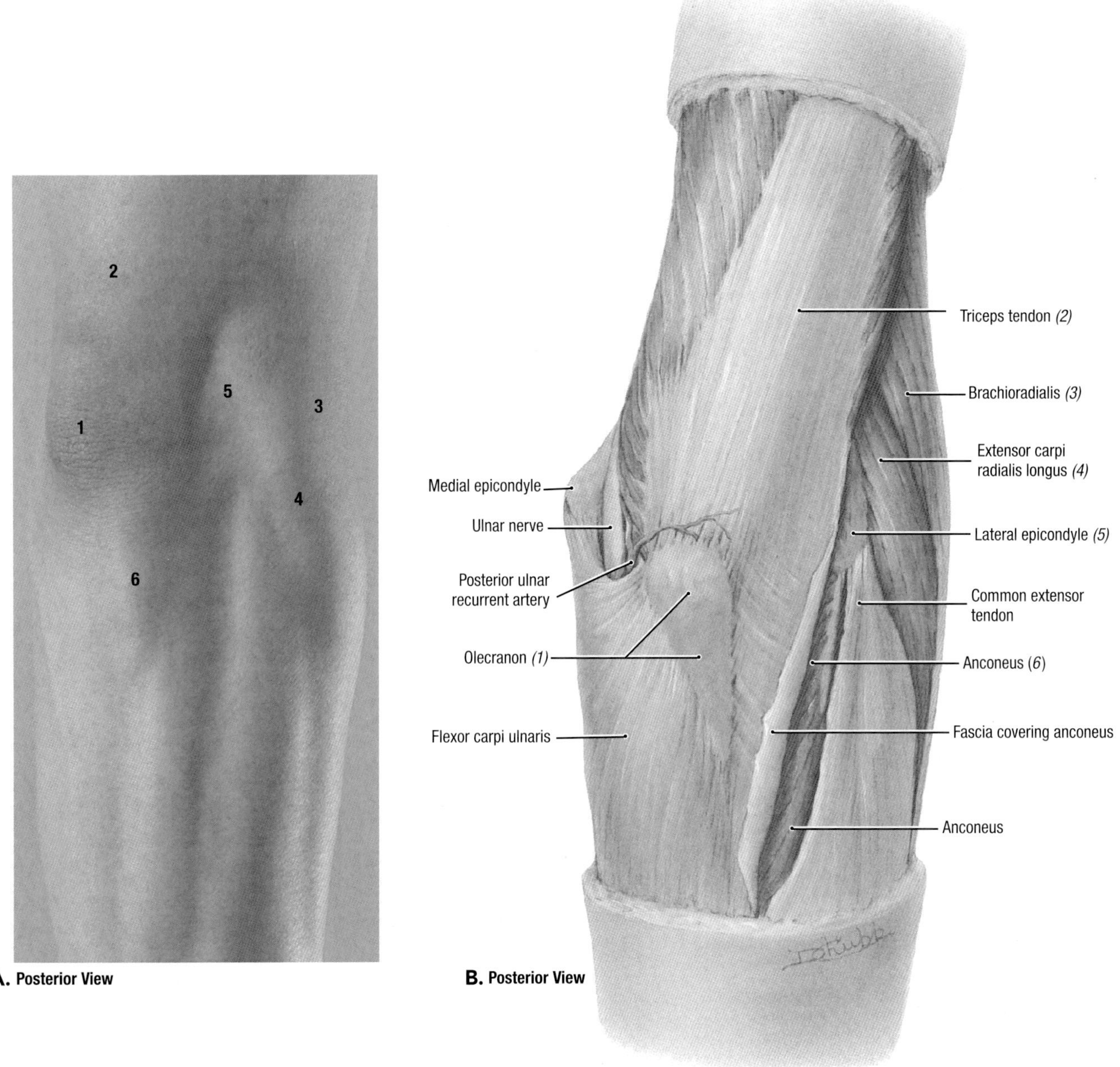

Figure 14.5 Posterior elbow muscles. (*Reproduced with permission from* Agur AMR, Dalley AF. *Grant's Atlas of Anatomy*. 11th ed. Philadelphia, PA: Lippincott Williams & Wilkins, 2004.)

undersurface of the brachioradialis and provides sensation to the radial forearm and first dorsal webspace of the hand. The deep branch becomes the posterior interosseous nerve (PIN) as it passes under the arcade of Struthers and into the supinator muscle. The PIN then travels along the radius and along the interosseous membrane, giving important branches to the wrist and digital extensors. It should be noted that the PIN runs on the opposite side of the bicipital tuberosity, which should be remembered during surgical approaches to the proximal radius. Pronation tends to bring the nerve medially, while supination tends to put the nerve in a more lateral position. Therefore, during the lateral approach to the elbow, the forearm should be pronated to move the PIN away from the field of dissection (Fig. 14.8).

EVALUATION OF ELBOW DISORDERS

History

In the evaluation of elbow disorders, the history remains the most crucial component of the diagnosis. An initial determination of the age of the patient, location of the

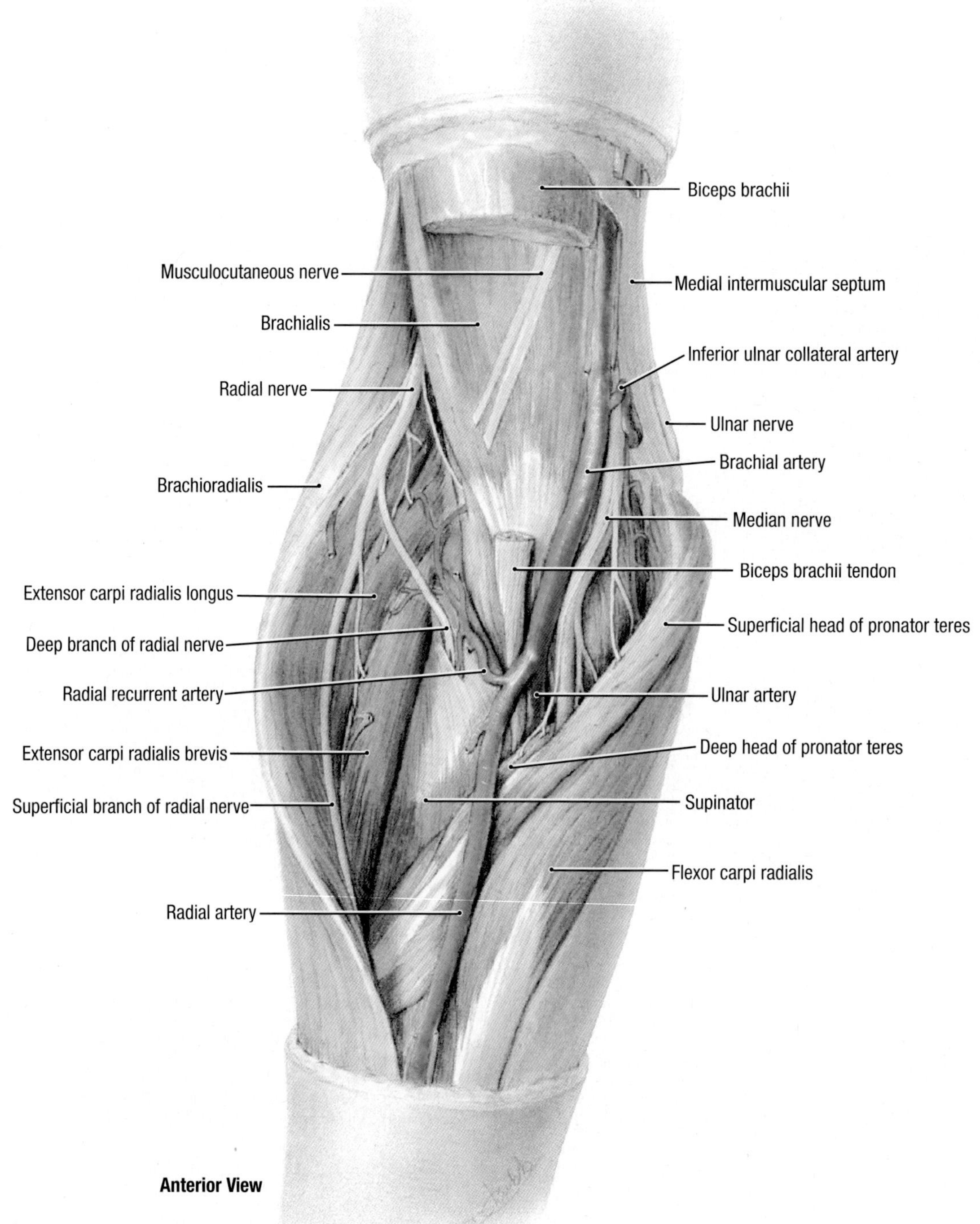

Figure 14.6 Anterior elbow muscles. (*Reproduced with permission from* Agur AMR, Dalley AF. *Grant's Atlas of Anatomy*. 11th ed. Philadelphia, PA: Lippincott Williams & Wilkins, 2004.)

symptoms, and mechanism of injury will significantly narrow the differential diagnosis. An overhead throwing athlete with medial elbow pain, for example, has a very different set of possible diagnoses compared with an elderly woman with chronic elbow pain. Further investigation can then be tailored for each patient. If the mechanism of injury is traumatic, make note of the type of trauma and the position of the arm at the time of injury. Ask the patient whether there was a sense of subluxation or whether any reduction maneuver was required. If the patient presents

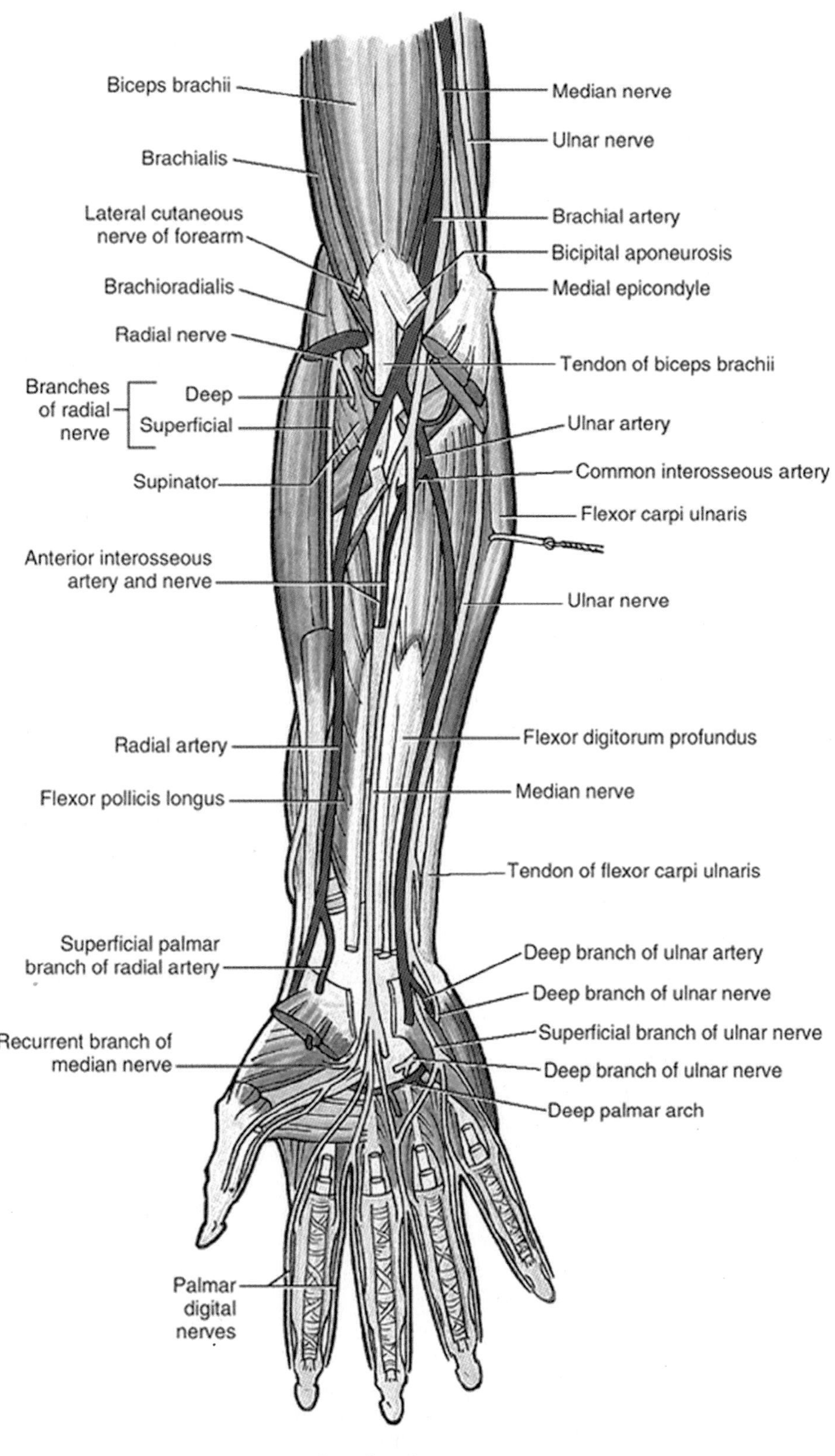

Figure 14.7 Elbow arteries and nerves. (*Reproduced with permission from* Moore KL, Agur AM. *Essential Clinical Anatomy*. 3rd ed. Philadelphia, PA: Lippincott Williams & Wilkins, 2006.)

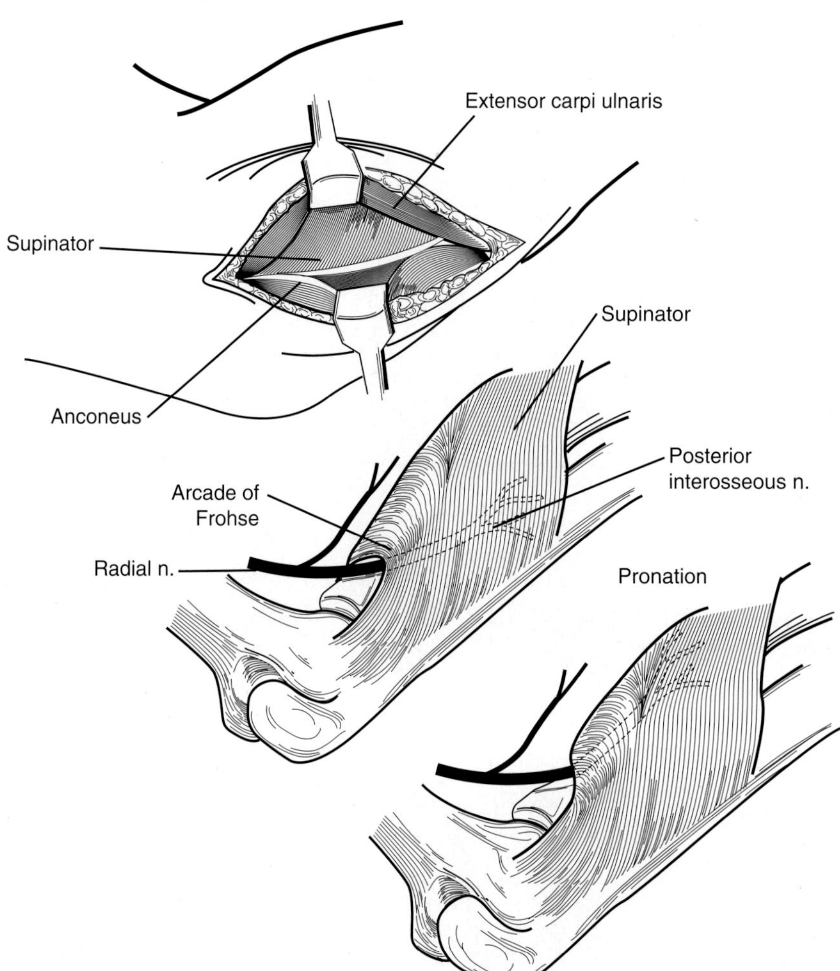

Figure 14.8 Posterior interosseous nerve during lateral approach. (*Adapted from* Hoppenfeld S, deBoer P. *Surgical Exposures in Orthopaedics: The Anatomic Approach.* 2nd ed. Philadelphia, PA: Lippincott Williams & Wilkins, 1984.)

with an overuse injury, determine the length of time since the onset of symptoms, aggravating or alleviating factors, and the effect of any prior treatments, particularly surgical interventions. The location of the symptoms will often be localized to the medial, lateral, or posterior aspects of the elbow, helping to greatly limit the differential diagnosis. If pain is the main complaint, note the character of the pain. Constant burning and radiating pain is classically more neurogenic, whereas activity-related pain is more typical of musculoskeletal pathology. It is important to remember that symptoms may overlap in patients with cervical spine pathology. Questioning the patient for any neck injury or cervical spine complaints is, therefore, mandatory. While pain is the most common presenting complaint, it is important to note other symptoms as well. Patients with unstable elbows may report feeling a "clunk" with certain activities and arm positions. Patients with loose bodies will often complain of locking and catching.

Physical Examination

The physical examination of the elbow will often confirm the diagnosis after the history has narrowed down the differential. A systematic approach will ensure that a complete examination is performed and no pathology is overlooked. The basic components of the physical examination include inspection, palpation, range-of-motion, stability, and a neurovascular evaluation. The contralateral limb may be used as a normal comparison if it is asymptomatic. Further testing for specific disorders is added to the examination depending on clinical suspicion. These tests will be further discussed in the sections on the pathologic entities that they detect.

As previously stated, there is significant overlap between cervical spine and upper extremity disorders, and they can frequently occur simultaneously. Prior to examination of the extremity, a complete cervical spine examination is necessary. Range of motion, tenderness, and the presence of a Spurling or Lehrmite sign are noted. In addition, a complete shoulder examination will help identify coexisting pathology.

Inspection

The physical examination begins with a thorough circumferential inspection. The location and character of traumatic wounds, such as bruising or lacerations, are recorded.

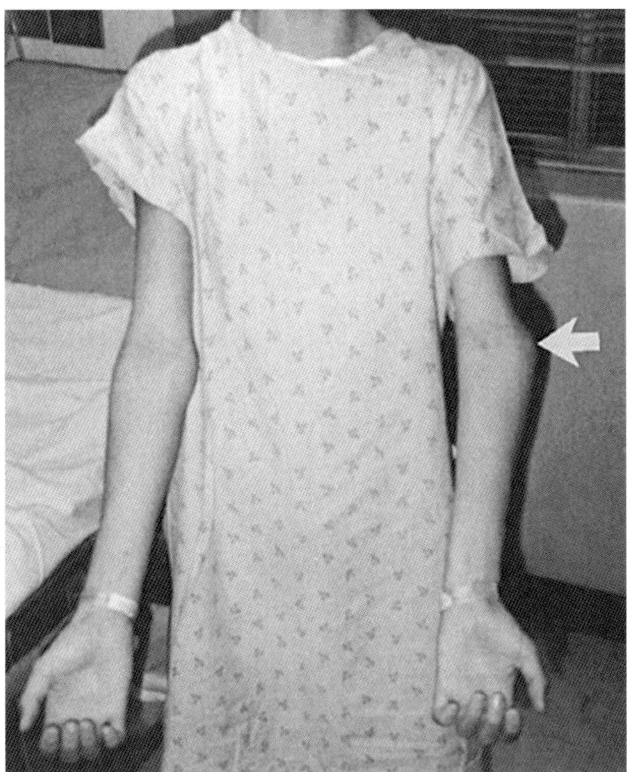

Figure 14.9 Cubitus varus. (*Reproduced with permission from* Beaty JH, Kasser JR. *Rockwood and Wilkins' Fractures in Children.* 6th ed. Philadelphia, PA: Lippincott Williams & Wilkins, 2006.)

An elbow joint effusion, indicative of intraarticular pathology, may be seen on the lateral side of the elbow between the radial head and the olecranon. Any asymmetric muscle atrophy should raise the concern of chronic denervation. The presence and location of any prior surgical incisions is also important. Open wounds, draining sinuses, and warmth and erythema should be considered as possible evidence of infection. Elbow alignment is also evaluated. The carrying angle, formed between the humerus and forearm, should be 5 to 7 degrees of valgus. Asymmetry is most commonly seen following pediatric trauma to the supracondylar humerus (Fig. 14.9).

Palpation

Careful palpation of all structures is performed. The elbow offers an advantage during physical examination in that many structures are subcutaneous and readily palpable even in obese patients. This is a diagnostic examination and should be conducted circumferentially so as not to miss any potential problem areas. Beginning on the lateral side, palpate the lateral epicondyle. Tenderness is indicative of lateral epicondylitis. The radial head is palpated and can be felt rotating underneath the skin with forearm pronation and supination. An effusion may be palpated in the triangular area between the lateral epicondyle, radial head, and proximal tip of the ulna. The lateral collateral ligament is palpated along the posterior half of the radial head. Moving posteriorly, the olecranon bursa is examined for tenderness, fluid, and evidence of infection. The insertion of the triceps is also examined for tenderness. On the medial aspect of the elbow, the ulnar nerve is examined for tenderness, subluxation, or a Tinel sign. The medial epicondyle and flexor pronator mass are palpated for tenderness, indicative of medial epicondylitis. Last, palpate the anterior elbow, including the biceps tendon and radial tunnel.

Range of Motion

The elbow is capable of flexion, extension, pronation, and supination. The functional range of motion has been determined to be a flexion–extension arc of 30 to 130 degrees and pronation and supination of 50 degrees each. The passive and active range of all four motions is examined and recorded. The contralateral elbow, if uninvolved, can be used as a comparison. Any crepitus, clicking, or grinding during range of motion should be noted. If limitations in motion exist, the firmness of the endpoint should be noted. A soft endpoint may be more indicative of soft tissue contracture that may improve with stretching, whereas a more firm endpoint may indicate a process less likely to resolve with nonoperative treatment, such as a synostosis. The presence of pain during range-of-motion examination can also be informative. Pain during the midrange as opposed to the end range of motion may indicate abnormality of the joint surface instead of surrounding soft tissue pathology.

Stability

Assessment of stability of the elbow is often difficult for two reasons. One, instability is often very painful and patients will guard against attempts at recreating the unstable scenario. Second, shoulder motion must be controlled so that varus and valgus stressing of the elbow is not falsely positive simply because the humerus is rotating. There are specific tests for different types of instability, which will be discussed in their respective sections later.

Neurovascular Assessment

A thorough neurovascular examination is undertaken. The radial, median, ulnar, and several cutaneous nerves cross the elbow and may be subject to traumatic or surgical injury or atraumatic neuropathy from compression. Neural examination should include muscle strength testing and sensory examination. Strength testing should be conducted methodically and should include all four motions of the elbow. Sensory testing should include light touch and two-point discrimination for greater accuracy. Knowledge of cervical root innervation and peripheral nerve innervation is crucial for delineating the location of potential lesions. For example, elbow extension by the triceps in innervated by the radial nerve peripherally and the seventh cervical root centrally. This must be taken into account so that a weak triceps is not misdiagnosed as a radial nerve injury when it is in fact a cervical lesion. Comparison of motor testing with any sensory deficits can help narrow the location of the lesion. The vascular examination should start above the elbow with palpation of the brachial artery and followed down the arm into the wrist with palpation of the radial and potentially the ulnar artery. Comparison with the contralateral side and pulse differences with elevation or positioning may be evidence of vascular compression such as thoracic outlet syndrome.

Imaging

Imaging makes up the third step in the evaluation of elbow disorders. The most common imaging modalities in use are plain radiographs, magnetic resonance imaging (MRI), computed tomography (CT), and ultrasound (US). After a thorough history and physical examination, imaging studies can often help confirm a diagnosis either through a positive finding or by eliminating an item from the differential diagnosis. Imaging studies can be misleading, however, if viewed without considering the history and physical examination. Imaging studies are most effective when used to confirm a suspected diagnosis from the history and physical examination. For example, a CT scan may be used to identify the exact size and location of a coronoid fracture, which will potentially alter management. Imaging studies are less effective when used as a "shot in the dark," such as obtaining an MRI, looking for any pathology to explain vague symptoms.

Radiography

Plain radiographs remain the initial imaging study for virtually all disorders of the elbow. A standard series includes anteroposterior (AP), lateral, and oblique views (Fig. 14.10). Additional radiographs such as radiocapitellar, traction, or stress views are obtained, depending on the condition under investigation. Radiographs are relatively inexpensive and noninvasive and can provide a large amount of information. A standard radiographic series will often give more information about conditions such as fractures, arthritis, and angular deformities than any advanced imaging modality. Radiographs must be scrutinized for the presence of osseous lesions or soft tissue swelling consistent with a neoplastic process. They also must be scrutinized for multiple injuries. It is easy to make the mistake of identifying the primary abnormality on the radiograph and then missing an additional injury that may not be as obvious.

Additional Imaging

Additional imaging may be added to the diagnostic arsenal depending on the pathology in question. CT scan will delineate osseous structures, and it offers multiplanar imaging that plain radiographs do not. It is an excellent modality for evaluating the three-dimensional configuration of fractures. MRI with or without an arthrogram can evaluate distinct soft tissues such as collateral ligaments and the biceps tendon. Soft tissue neoplastic processes are best evaluated with MRI. A combination of MRI and CT is typically used for diagnosis and evaluation of osseous tumors. US is a constantly improving imaging modality that is being used more commonly in the evaluation of a great deal of elbow pathology. It is a relatively inexpensive and noninvasive study with the downside that it is highly operator dependent.

Synovial Fluid/Laboratory Studies

Depending on the pathology in question, laboratory work and synovial fluid analysis can be very beneficial. The workup for infection often includes a complete blood cell count, erythrocyte sedimentation rate (ESR), and C-reactive protein (CRP). Synovial fluid is examined for the white blood cell (WBC) count, Gram stain, and culture. If concern exists, fungal and viral cultures and acid-fast bacillus (AFB) testing may also be added. Laboratory and synovial fluid analysis are also useful in the workup of inflammatory arthritis and crystalline arthropathies.

TRAUMATIC INJURIES TO THE ELBOW

Fractures

Fractures of the Humeral Shaft

Fractures of the humeral shaft come in many varieties. They are seen in all age groups following both low- and high-energy mechanisms of injury. Most humeral shaft fractures will heal with nonoperative treatment. There are, however, certain absolute and relative indications for operative fixation.

Classification

Fractures of the humeral shaft are generally classified by location and fracture type. The location is described as midshaft, junction of the middle and distal third, or junction of the proximal and middle third. The fracture type is described as transverse, oblique, spiral, or comminuted. The presence of a butterfly fragment or a segmental component is also noted.

Mechanism of Injury

The mechanism of injury of humeral shaft fractures may vary widely. A young patient with good bone stock will often present following high-velocity trauma. Alternatively, activities that place high torsional force on the arm, such as

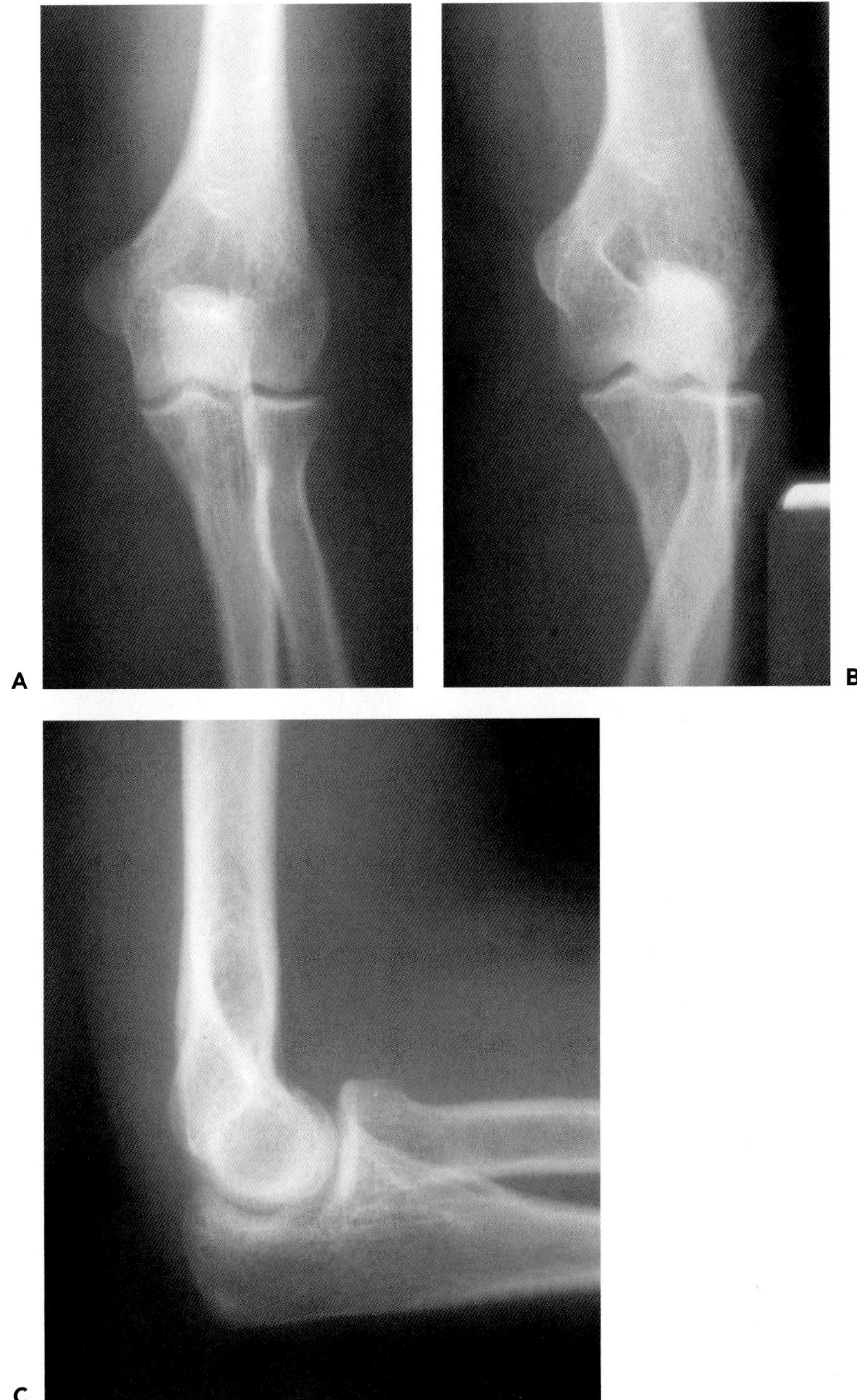

Figure 14.10 Anteroposterior **(A)**, oblique **(B)**, and lateral **(C)** radiographs of elbow.

arm wrestling, may also lead to fracture. An elderly patient may only have had a ground-level fall. Last, a direct blow, such as following an assault, may lead to a humeral shaft fracture. The fracture pattern will often give clues to the mechanism of injury. Spiral fractures, for example, are common from torsional injuries, whereas comminuted, transverse fractures are caused by higher energy trauma. Unusually low-energy injuries and patients with preexisting arm pain or constitutional symptoms should raise concern for the presence of a pathologic fracture.

Presentation

Patients will present with pain, swelling, and varying degrees of deformity. They will have pain with attempts at elbow or shoulder motion and will be comforted with support under the arm or sling immobilization.

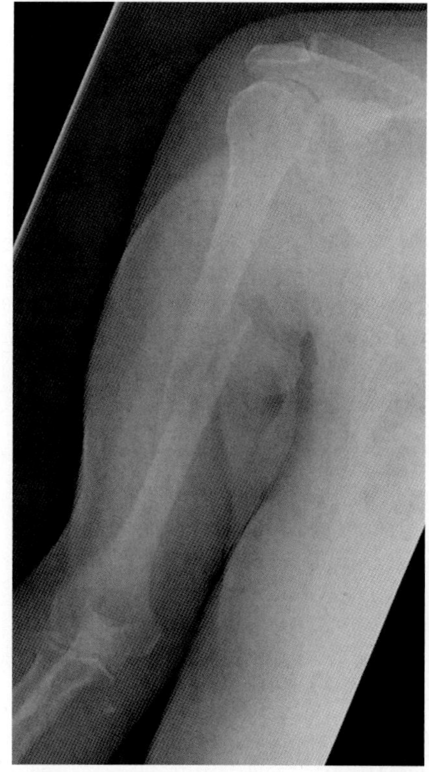

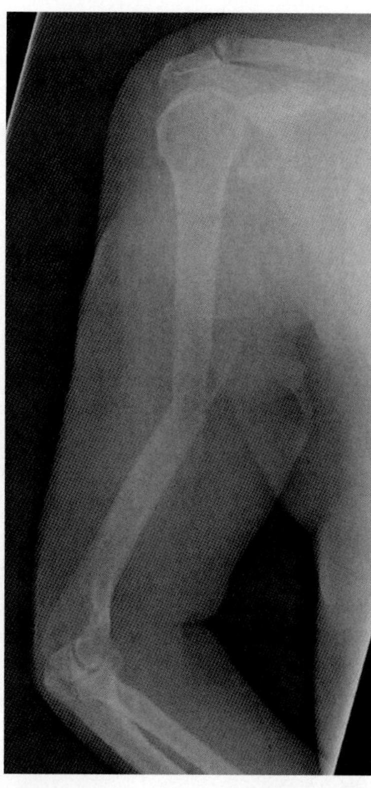

Figure 14.11 Internal rotation and external rotation views of the humerus attempting to obtain two orthogonal views. Rotation occurs through the fracture site leading to patient discomfort and inadequate radiographs.

Physical Findings

The skin will often display evidence of trauma, such as bruising and ecchymoses, particularly in higher energy injuries. Open humeral shaft fractures are relatively uncommon, secondary to the large soft tissue envelope, but the skin must be thoroughly examined such that an open injury is not missed. A careful neurovascular examination should be performed and documented, with specific attention placed on distal examination of the radial nerve. The nerve runs along the posterior humeral shaft in the spiral groove and may be injured during or after fracture.

Radiographic Evaluation

Radiographs of the humeral shaft must include two orthogonal views that are taken 90 degrees to one another. The radiological technologist will often attempt to take two orthogonal views by taking two AP views, one with the humerus internally rotated and one externally rotated (Fig. 14.11). This will only lead to motion through the fracture site and inadequate radiographs. A transthoracic lateral is an alternative method to obtain a view that is orthogonal to the AP. It is also crucial that the radiographs include the elbow and shoulder to identify the presence of any articular extension or additional injury to these adjacent structures.

Special Studies

Further studies are rarely required for the evaluation of humeral shaft fractures. A CT scan may help determine the presence and degree of involvement of the shoulder or elbow joint if there is a concern for articular extension. Irregularity at the fracture site that suggests pathologic fracture should be further evaluated with advanced imaging such as MRI or bone scan. An electromyogram (EMG)/nerve conduction velocity (NCV) may be ordered if there is a neurologic deficit but is rarely helpful until several weeks following the injury.

Differential Diagnosis

The diagnosis of a humeral shaft fracture is rarely in question after the history, physical examination, and radiographs. Adjacent joint involvement and pathologic lesions should be carefully eliminated from the differential diagnosis.

Treatment

The vast majority of humeral shaft fractures can be treated nonoperatively with predictably high rates of healing and little residual deformity. Initially, a coaptation splint is applied from the axilla to the base of the neck, with a gentle valgus mold (Fig. 14.12). When patient comfort allows, the splint is converted to a clamshell orthosis and shoulder and elbow motion is initiated. At 6 to 8 weeks, the orthosis may be discontinued if the physical examination and radiographs demonstrate healing. Up to 30 degrees of varus angulation and 3 cm of shortening is acceptable. Relative indications for surgical treatment include an inability to maintain a closed reduction secondary to body habitus or the presence of polytrauma with the need for immediate use of the extremity. Absolute indications for operative fixation include open fractures and those with vascular

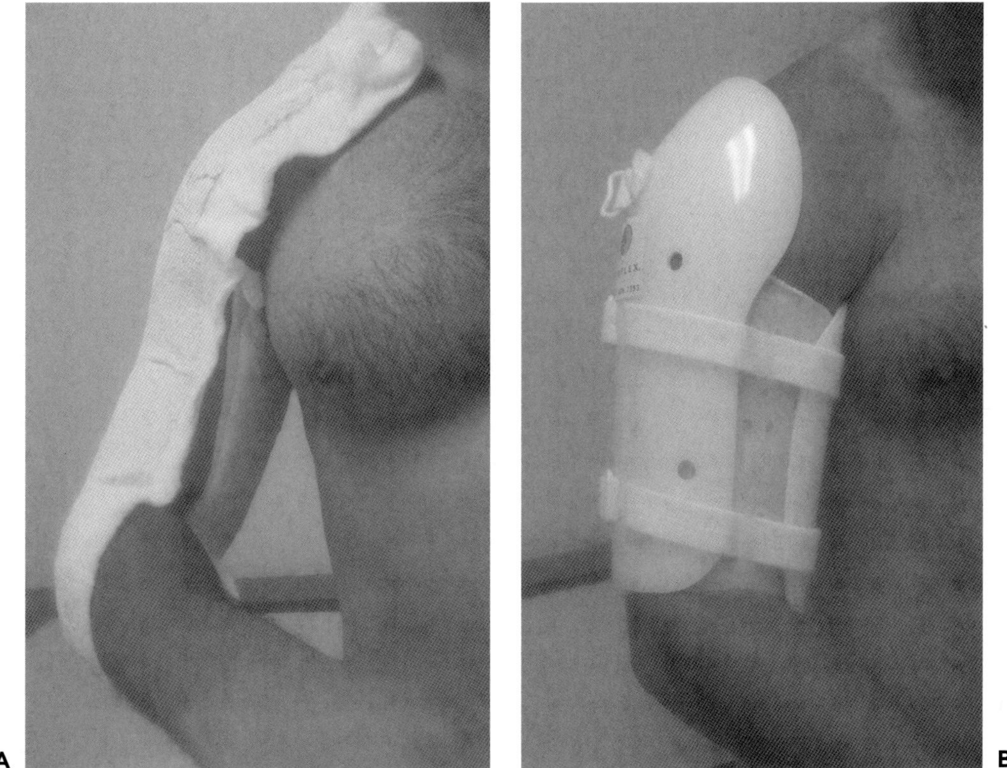

Figure 14.12 The majority of humeral shaft fractures are initially treated with a coaptation splint. This is converted to a clamshell orthosis once the discomfort for the initial injury subsides.

injuries. Plate fixation and intramedullary (IM) nailing have both been used successfully (Fig. 14.13). Plate fixation is more likely to cause radial nerve injury and elbow stiffness, whereas IM nailing is more likely to cause shoulder pain from entry through the rotator cuff and is associated with a higher incidence of nonunion. The presence of a radial nerve palsy at the time of injury does not necessitate operative fixation. In the absence of sharp, penetrating trauma, the nerve injury may be observed, as most injuries are neuropraxia with predictable recovery. Failure of recovery by 3 to 4 months mandates further investigation with possible surgical exploration.

Fractures of the Distal Humerus

Fractures of the distal humerus represent a large spectrum of injuries varying widely in complexity, treatment, and prognosis. They occur in all ages, and treatment is dependent on factors such as fracture pattern, activity level, and bone quality.

Classification

The Orthopaedic Trauma Association system is currently the most comprehensive and reproducible classification scheme for fractures of the distal humerus. Extraarticular fractures are labeled as type A, partial articular fractures (medial, lateral, anterior) as type B, and complete articular fractures as type C. Further breakdown of the classification is based on the presence of metaphyseal and articular comminution (Fig. 14.14).

Mechanism of Injury

Fractures of the distal humerus occur in a bimodal distribution. Younger patients usually require a large force to fracture the bone, such as a high-speed motor vehicle collision, whereas older patients may sustain a fracture simply from a fall from standing height. In both groups, the mechanism of injury is usually a direct axial load on a flexed elbow.

Presentation

Patients will present with pain, swelling, and deformity at the elbow following trauma. The elbow will be held at the side, and any attempted elbow motion will be painful. Often a splint will have been placed by paramedics or another physician prior to orthopaedic evaluation.

Physical Findings

As with any fracture, the skin must be examined carefully for any wound that may be evidence of an open fracture. Any splint or dressing must be completely removed such that a thorough examination may be undertaken. A careful neurovascular examination is performed next. The ulnar nerve is near the medial epicondyle and requires special attention. Interosseous muscle motor strength and sensation to the small and ulnar side of the ring finger must be

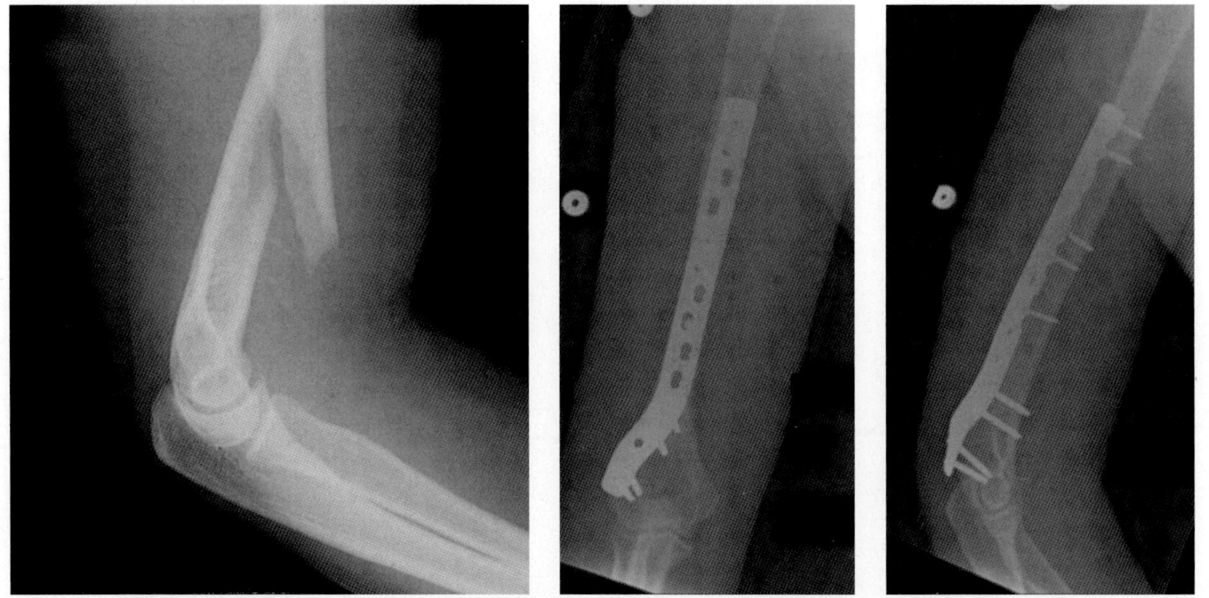

Figure 14.13 **(A)** Preoperative radiograph of a displaced humeral shaft fracture. **(B** and **C)** Postoperative radiographs demonstrating open reduction and internal fixation with a plate and screws.

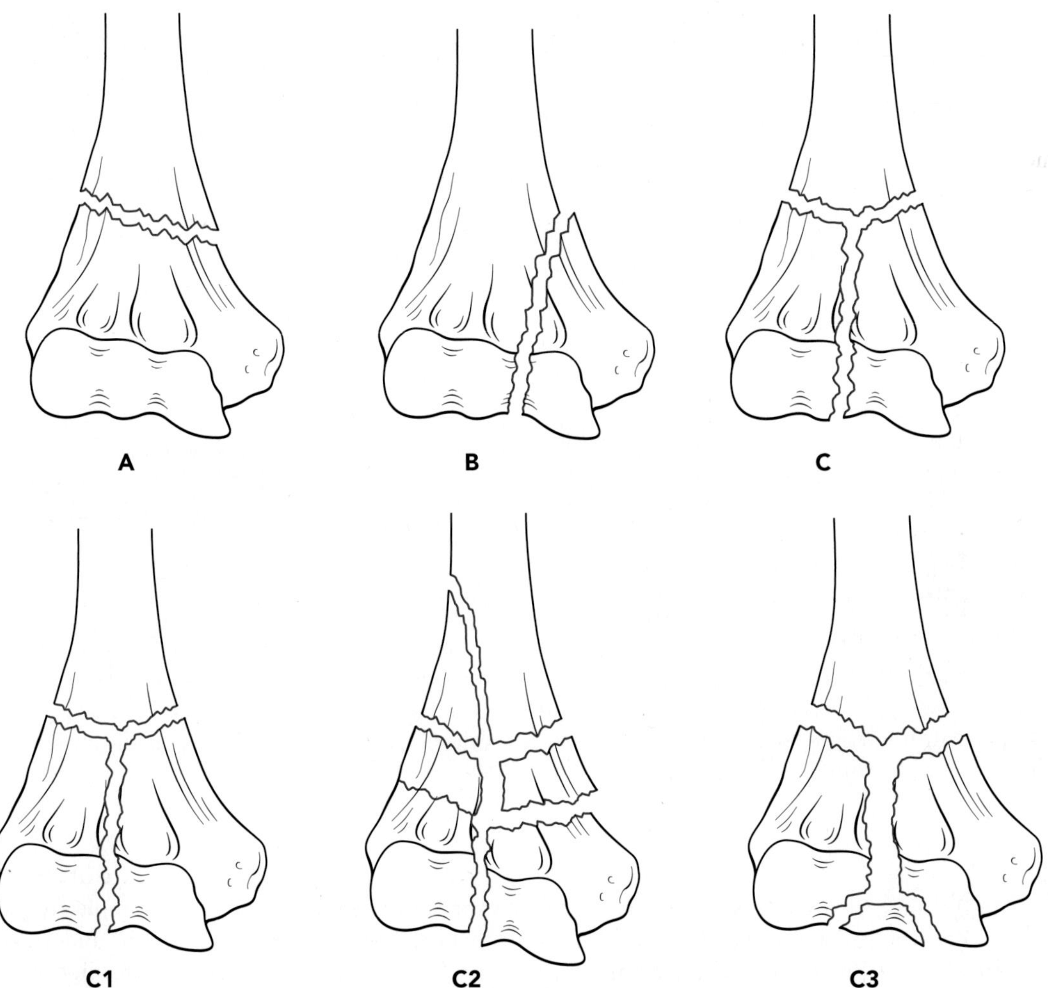

Figure 14.14 Orthopaedic Trauma Association classification of distal humerus fractures. (*Reproduced with permission from* Bucholz RW, Heckman JD, Court-Brown C, et al. *Rockwood and Green's Fractures in Adults*. 6th ed. Philadelphia, PA; Lippincott Williams & Wilkins, 2005.)

documented. A secondary survey for undiagnosed injuries should be performed, particularly in high-velocity trauma or unconscious patients.

Radiographic Evaluation

The standard series of plain radiographs includes AP, lateral, and oblique views of the elbow. If there is shortening of the bones with overlapping segments, gentle traction can be applied to the elbow while radiographs are taken.

Special Studies

In a simple fracture pattern, plain radiographs may be sufficient for diagnosis, classification, and treatment. A CT scan is a very useful additional study and should be obtained if there is any question as to the location of the fracture fragments or degree of complexity (Fig. 14.15).

Differential Diagnosis

The diagnosis of distal humeral fractures is typically obvious on plain radiographs. In the absence of fracture on radiograph, soft tissue injuries such as an elbow dislocation or ligament rupture must be considered. Fractures in other areas of the elbow, such as the olecranon, should also be considered in the differential diagnosis.

Treatment

The treatment of distal humerus fractures depends on many factors. The elbow joint is prone to stiffness and immobilization must be kept to a minimum. Nonsurgical treatment, therefore, is indicated only for patients with essentially nondisplaced fractures who can withstand gentle early motion and those with medical comorbidities that place them at excessive surgical risk. Operative treatment is favored in most patients. In younger patients, open reduction and internal fixation (ORIF) is recommended (Fig. 14.16). The goals of surgery are to restore the articular congruity and obtain stable internal fixation that will allow early motion. Failure to restore the joint surface may lead to posttraumatic arthrosis, which is difficult to treat in the younger population. Osteotomy of the olecranon may be necessary for improved exposure of the joint surface, in the presence of comminution. Stiffness and heterotopic ossification (HO) formation are common complications following ORIF. Elderly patients with osteoporosis will often have significant fracture comminution and a low-demand lifestyle. Obtaining stable internal fixation may not be possible. Whenever possible, ORIF is the preferred treatment for distal humerus fractures in the elderly. However, if poor bone quality prevents primary ORIF, acute total elbow arthroplasty (TEA) is the preferred treatment. The most concerning complication of TEA is the development of infection. Because of the limited soft tissue envelope around the elbow, infection rates reach as high as 5%, substantially higher than other joint arthroplasties.

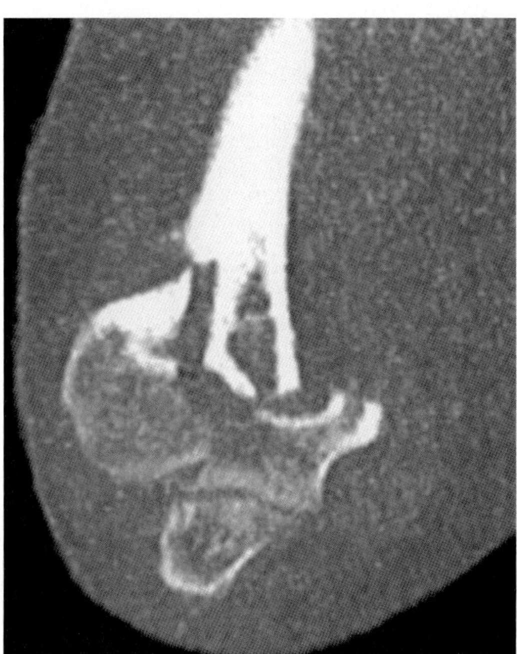

Figure 14.15 A coronal computed tomography reconstruction demonstrating a distal humerus fracture with articular displacement.

Fractures of the Radial Head

Fractures of the radial head are relatively common injuries about the elbow. They may occur in isolation or in association with other bony or soft tissue injuries. There are multiple treatment options depending on the fracture type.

Classification

Radial head fractures are classified according to Mason (Fig. 14.17). Type I fractures are nondisplaced. Type II fractures have a marginal fracture or impaction but have a portion of the head that is not fractured. Type III fractures are comminuted and involve the entire radial head. A type IV fracture was later added to the classification to include radial head fractures with an associated elbow dislocation.

Mechanism of Injury

Fractures of the radial head usually occur following a fall onto the outstretched hand. The force is transmitted through the forearm into the elbow. When an elbow dislocation has occurred, the radial head may be fractured by the distal humerus as it exits the joint.

Presentation

Patients present with variable degrees of pain depending on the extent of injury. Minimally displaced fractures may cause little pain with range of motion and present much like a bruise or sprain. More displaced fractures will cause significant pain, and the patient will be reluctant to move the elbow.

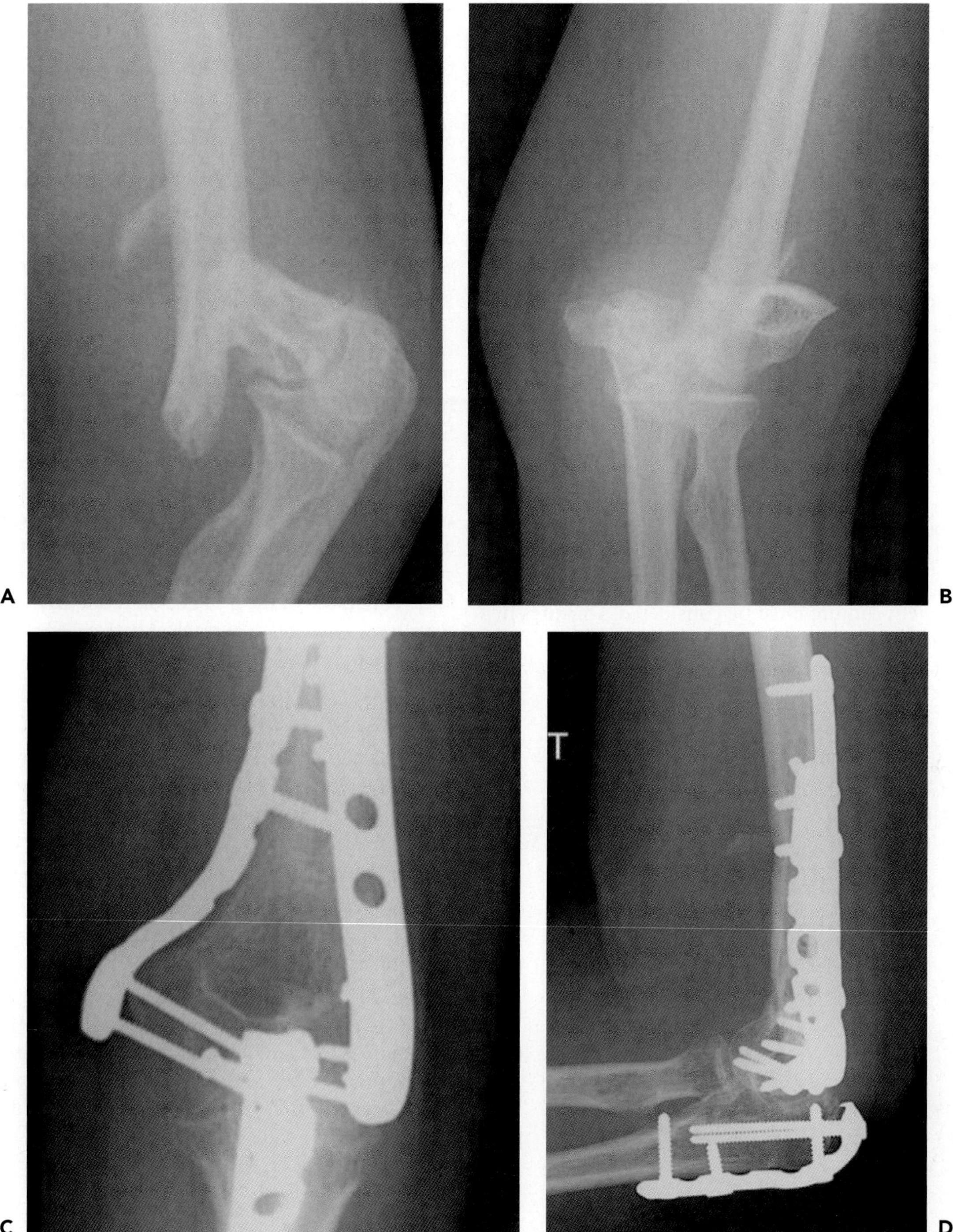

Figure 14.16 Pre- **(A** and **B)** and postoperative **(C** and **D)** radiographs of a distal humerus fracture treated with open reduction and internal fixation. An olecranon osteotomy was performed to improve visualization of the articular surface during reduction. This was repaired with a precontoured proximal ulna plate.

Physical Findings

The radial head is consistently palpable along the lateral aspect of the elbow, even in obese patients. The examiner can feel for tenderness over the radial head as it is rotated with forearm pronation and supination. An effusion may be palpable in this area as well. Range of motion is a crucial component of the physical examination, as any block to motion that is not secondary to pain is an indication for surgery. Aspiration of the hemarthrosis followed by injection of local anesthetic into the joint will provide pain relief so that the range of motion can be assessed (Fig. 14.18). A careful wrist examination is performed to determine the

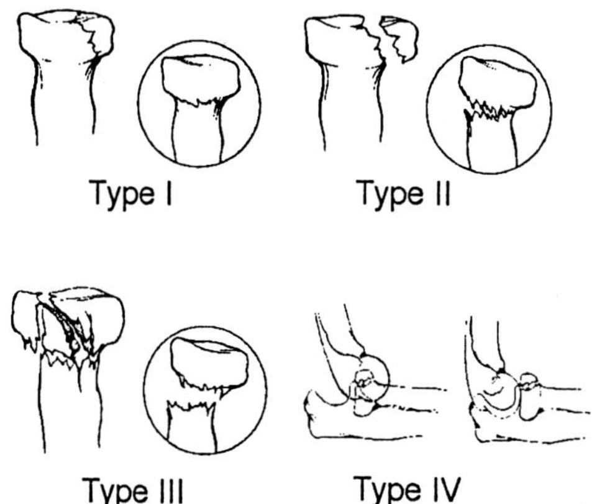

Figure 14.17 The Mason classification of radial head fractures. (*Reproduced with permission from* Koval KJ, Zuckerman JD. *Handbook of Fractures*. 3rd ed. Philadelphia, PA: Lippincott Williams & Wilkins, 2006.)

presence or absence of an Essex–Lopresti lesion. This is a longitudinal injury that begins at the distal radioulnar joint and propagates along the interosseous membrane, finally ending at the radial head. This is a more complex injury than an isolated radial head fracture and its presence may significantly alter management.

Radiographic Evaluation

The diagnosis is typically made from plain radiographs. A plain radiographic series includes AP, lateral, and oblique views. A radiocapitellar view is a lateral view of the elbow with an oblique angle to minimize overlap between the radial head and the proximal ulna. This can give a more complete view of the proximal radius.

Special Studies

If further definition of the fracture is necessary, a CT scan is obtained. It can give valuable information regarding the number and location of fragments. It may also help diagnose other pathology, such as coronoid fractures, not seen on plain radiograph.

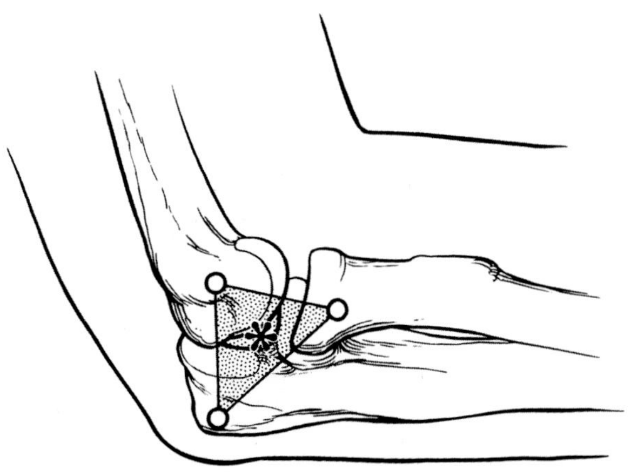

Figure 14.18 The elbow can be aspirated via the lateral soft spot, which is located at the center of a triangle formed by the lateral epicondyle, radial head, and olecranon. (*Reproduced with permission from* Bucholz RW, Heckman JD, Court-Brown C, et al. *Rockwood and Green's Fractures in Adults*. 6th ed. Philadelphia, PA: Lippincott Williams & Wilkins, 2005.)

Differential Diagnosis

Displaced radial head fractures will be seen on plain radiograph. Nondisplaced fractures, however, may demonstrate only a posterior fat pad sign, or an effusion, on radiographs. Other causes of intraarticular pathology, such as occult fracture or ligamentous injury, must be ruled out in this instance. A careful physical examination is performed and radiographs and advanced imaging are scrutinized for the presence of these other injuries.

Treatment

Fractures with less than 2 mm of displacement are treated nonoperatively. The elbow is immobilized briefly in a sling for comfort, and early motion is begun when the patient is able to tolerate it. The elbow should not be used for strenuous activities until 6 weeks after injury when a gradual increase in weight-bearing is allowed. Fractures with more significant articular displacement or an osseous block to motion are treated with ORIF or radial head replacement. Younger patients with simpler fracture patterns are treated with ORIF (Fig. 14.19). Older, sedentary patients or those with comminuted fractures are treated with radial head replacement. Postoperative early motion is again critical to reduce stiffness. Associated injuries must be assessed such that early motion is limited to a safe and stable zone. Partial or complete radial head excision may be considered in rare circumstances but must not be performed if an Essex–Lopresti lesion is present. In general, a radial head replacement is favored to prevent proximal migration of the radius.

Fractures of the Olecranon

Fractures of the olecranon present following several different injury mechanisms and with several different fracture patterns. The olecranon makes up the ulnar side of the ulnohumeral joint and fractures through the area are intraarticular, which affects management. The olecranon also serves as the attachment site for the triceps tendon and fractures will usually disrupt the extensor mechanism of the elbow.

Classification

Fractures of the olecranon are classified according to the amount of displacement and the presence or absence of comminution. Fractures are undisplaced, displaced with a stable ulnohumeral joint, and displaced with an unstable ulnohumeral joint. For each fracture type there are noncomminuted and comminuted subgroups (Fig. 14.20).

Mechanism of Injury

Fractures of the olecranon typically occur through two different mechanisms. One type of fracture is an avulsion of the triceps mechanism, which is typically a transverse

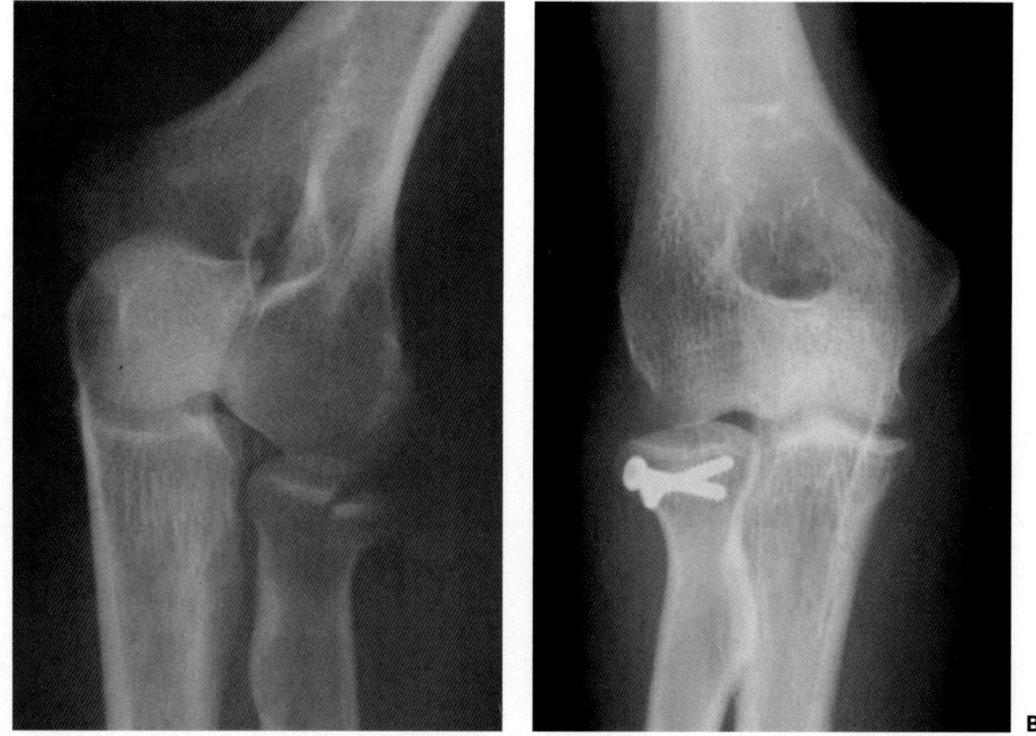

Figure 14.19 **(A)** Pre- and **(B)** postoperative radiographs of open reduction and internal fixation of a radial head fracture.

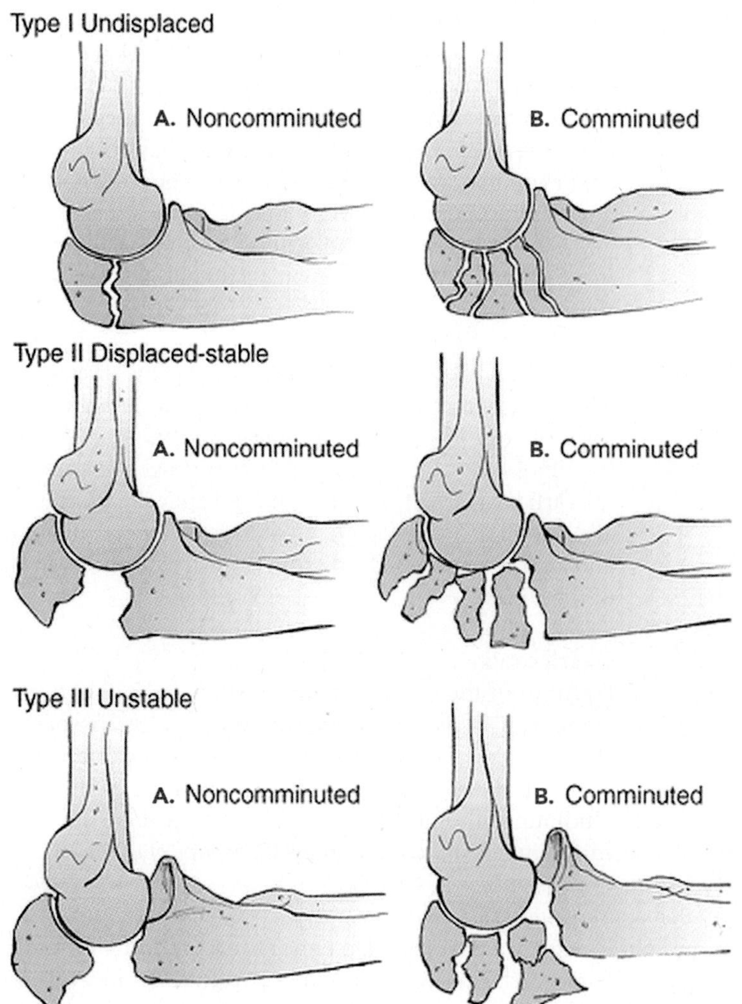

Figure 14.20 Mayo classification of olecranon fractures. (*Reproduced with permission from* Bucholz RW, Heckman JD, Court-Brown C, et al. *Rockwood and Green's Fractures in Adults*. 6th ed. Philadelphia, PA: Lippincott Williams & Wilkins, 2005.)

fracture with minimal comminution. The second type of fracture occurs from a direct axial load onto the flexed elbow. Varying degrees of comminution and articular impaction may be present.

Presentation
Presentation will vary depending on the mechanism of injury and severity of the fracture. Patients will have pain, tenderness, and swelling about the proximal ulna. They will have pain with attempted range of motion.

Physical Findings
The status of the extensor mechanism of the elbow must be evaluated. Inability to fully extend the elbow against gravity is an indication for operative treatment. The skin overlying the proximal ulna must be carefully examined for open wounds, as the majority of the bone is subcutaneous and an open fracture cannot be overlooked. As always, a careful neurovascular examination is undertaken with particular attention to the ulnar nerve because of its close proximity to the olecranon.

Radiographic Evaluation
Plain radiographs are typically sufficient for diagnosis. The three standard views of the elbow are obtained. The lateral view will demonstrate the degree of displacement, the stability of the ulnohumeral joint, and the presence of comminution.

Special Studies
CT scan can be useful if concern for articular comminution or impaction exists. It may also be helpful to determine whether there is extension of the fracture into the coronoid process.

Differential Diagnosis
If plain radiographs do not reveal any osseous abnormality, other soft tissue injuries must be considered. Rupture of the distal triceps will have a similar presentation as olecranon fractures, with loss of elbow extension. Injury to the medial or lateral ligaments must also be evaluated.

Treatment
The treatment of olecranon fractures depends on the fracture pattern and patient factors. With fracture displacement of less than 2 mm and full-elbow extension against gravity, nonoperative treatment is indicated. A short period of immobilization followed by early motion is instituted. Exercises should be limited to active flexion and passive extension to reduce the pull of the triceps against the fracture. If significant displacement exists or triceps function is compromised, operative treatment is favored. Simple fracture patterns may be treated with tension band wiring (Fig. 14.21), whereas plate fixation is required if significant comminution or impaction is present. In elderly patients with comminuted fractures, resection of the fracture with reattachment of the triceps can be performed. At least 50% of the olecranon may be excised without compromising elbow stability, provided the medial and lateral collateral ligaments are intact.

Fractures of the Coronoid

The coronoid process acts to buttress against posterior translation of the ulna on the humerus. It also serves as the attachment site for the anterior elbow capsule, the

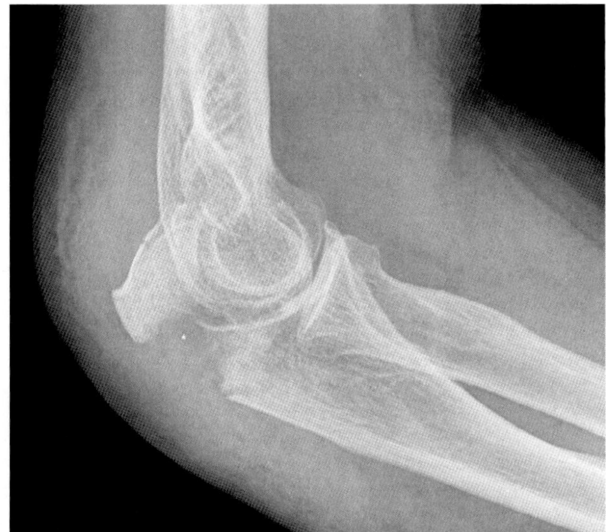

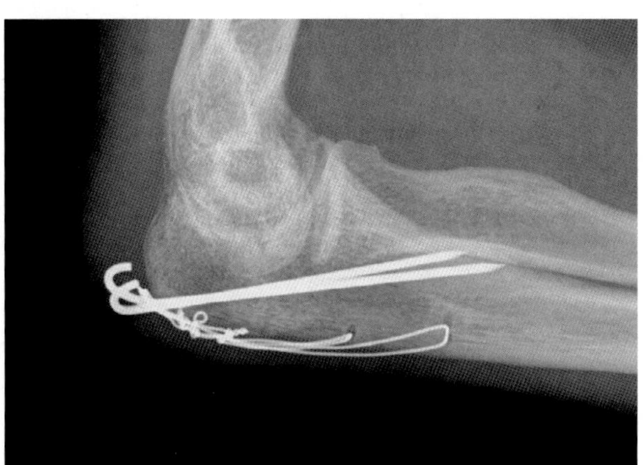

Figure 14.21 Tension band wiring of an olecranon fracture. (*Reproduced with permission from* Bucholz RW, Heckman JD, Court-Brown C, et al. *Rockwood and Green's Fractures in Adults.* 6th ed. Philadelphia, PA: Lippincott Williams & Wilkins, 2005.)

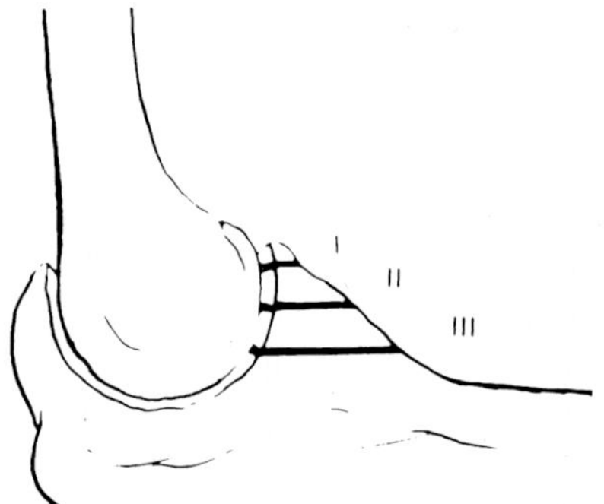

Figure 14.22 Regan and Morrey classification of coronoid fractures. (*Reprinted with permission from* Regan W, Morrey BF. Fractures of coronoid process of the ulna. *J Bone Joint Surg Am.* 1989;71:1348–1354.)

brachialis, and the medial collateral ligament. Fractures of the coronoid are often seen in conjunction with other injuries to the elbow, such as dislocations.

Classification

Fractures of the coronoid are classified according to Regan and Morrey (Fig. 14.22). A type I fracture involves just the tip of the coronoid. Type II and type III fractures involve less than 50% or greater than 50% of the coronoid, respectively. Recently, more focus has been placed on the importance of the location of the fracture. The anteromedial facet plays a key role in elbow stability and is the basis for the O'Driscoll classification (Fig. 14.23).

Mechanism of Injury

Coronoid fractures are frequently seen in the setting of acute elbow instability, most commonly a posterior elbow dislocation. Coronoid fractures are frequently associated with radial head fractures. As the distal humerus subluxes anteriorly, the coronoid is subjected to shearing forces that can lead to fracture. Coronoid fractures are also seen as the extension of a complex proximal ulna fracture, such as the transolecranon fracture dislocation.

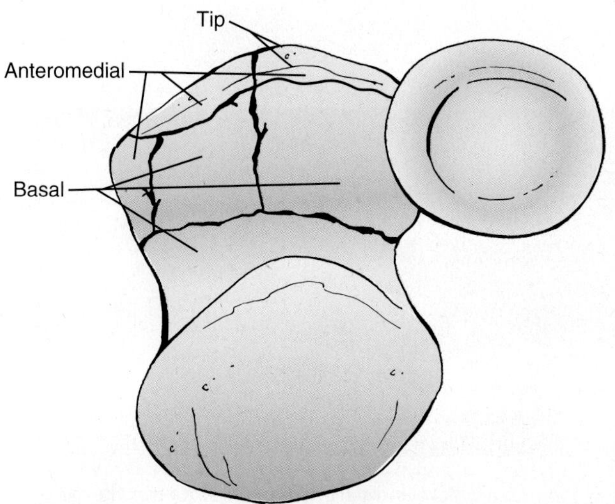

Figure 14.23 O'Driscoll classification of coronoid fractures. (*Reproduced with permission from* Bucholz RW, Heckman JD, Court-Brown C, et al. *Rockwood and Green's Fractures in Adults.* 6th ed. Philadelphia, PA: Lippincott Williams & Wilkins, 2005.)

Presentation

The patient's history will often give clues to the diagnosis. Patients may describe a subluxation of the elbow that self-reduced. If the patient reports that a closed reduction was required, a coronoid fracture should be considered. Patients will have diffuse pain and swelling and be reluctant to move the elbow.

Physical Findings

After a careful neurovascular examination and close evaluation of the skin integrity, a range-of-motion and stability examination is performed. Stability is often difficult to evaluate secondary to pain and guarding. An examination under anesthesia is considered if further information is needed.

Radiographic Evaluation

Plain radiographs consisting of three views of the elbow are obtained initially (Fig. 14.24). Fractures of the coronoid may be very small and the radiographs must be closely scrutinized. While frank dislocations will be obvious, subtle subluxation must not be overlooked.

Special Studies

Coronoid fractures may be difficult to appreciate on plain radiographs secondary to overlap of the radial head and other bony structures. CT scans are very helpful in these cases where the size and configuration of the fracture remains in question (Fig. 14.25).

Differential Diagnosis

The differential diagnosis of coronoid fractures includes other osseous and soft tissue injuries of the elbow. Dislocation of the elbow, radial head fracture, and olecranon fracture must be considered.

Treatment

The management of coronoid fractures depends on multiple factors. Fractures of the tip of the coronoid have traditionally been considered capsular avulsions from an elbow dislocation. In reality, the tip of the coronoid is intraarticular and the capsule inserts more distal so these likely represent sheer injuries. These isolated fractures can be managed nonoperatively as long as a concentric reduction of the elbow can be maintained during early controlled motion and associated injury to the radial head does not require surgical management. If repair is required, the fragment is often too small for ORIF and suture repair of the overlying capsule down to the ulna is performed. Larger fractures will contribute more to elbow stability and may require ORIF.

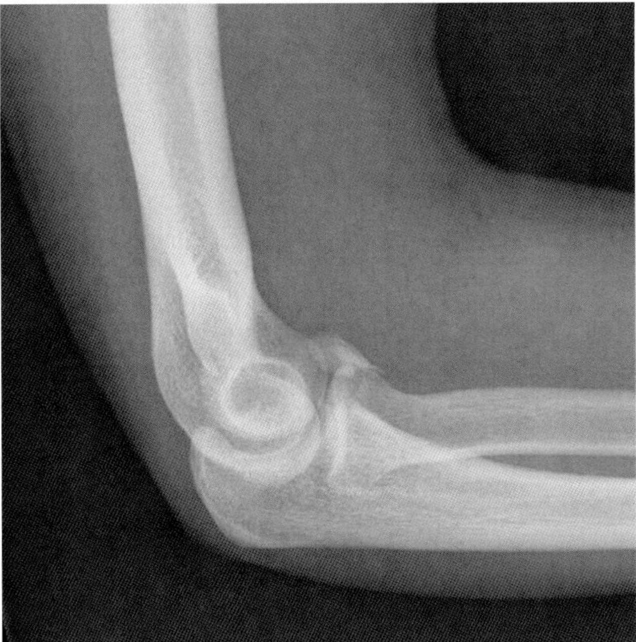
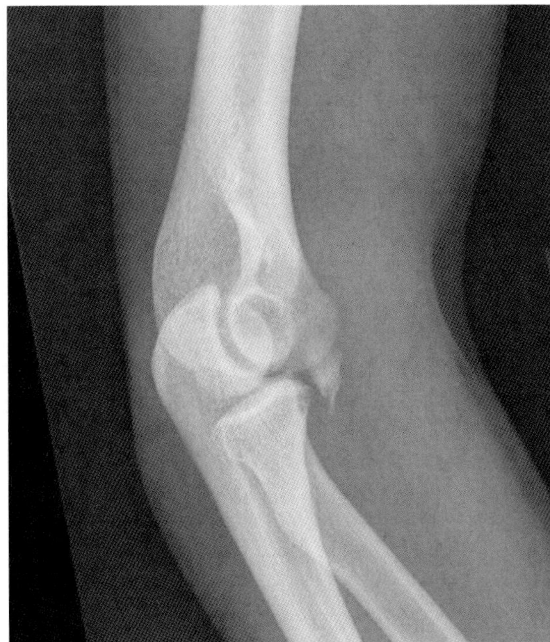

Figure 14.24 Plain lateral **(A)** and oblique **(B)** radiographs of a Type II coronoid fracture.

Fractures of the anteromedial facet, in particular, lead to varus posteromedial instability. Restoration of the coronoid buttress with screw or plate fixation is often necessary to achieve stability of the elbow (Fig. 14.26). Often times, the lateral soft tissues of the elbow will be disrupted as well. The treatment of other injuries associated with elbow instability is discussed later.

Instability

Elbow Dislocation

Dislocation of the elbow is a relatively common injury, making up as many as 25% of all elbow injuries. They typically occur in younger patients, often during contact sports or activities. Associated injuries are common and play a major role in the management of elbow dislocations.

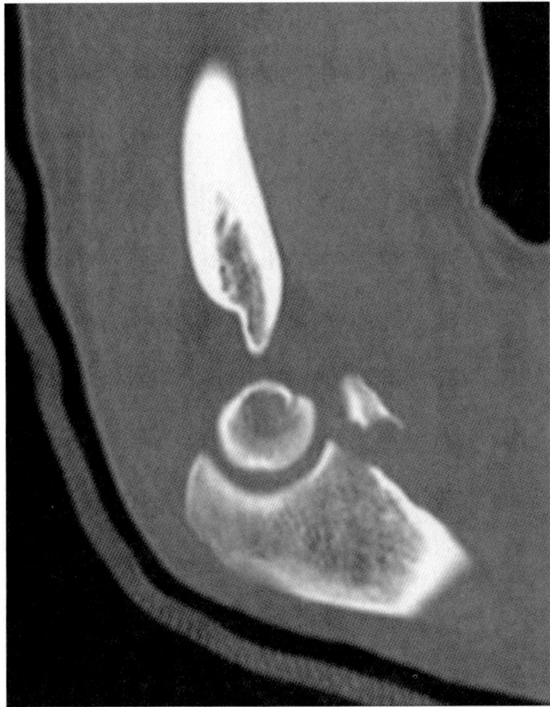
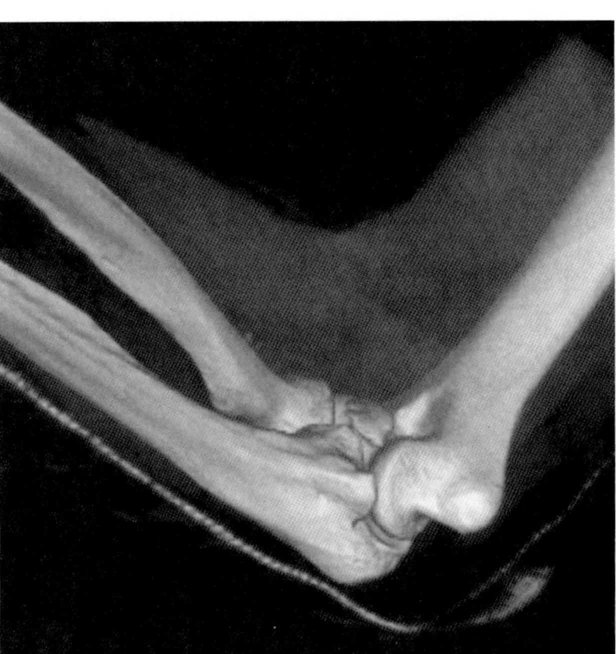

Figure 14.25 Lateral **(A)** and three-dimensional **(B)** computed tomography scan reconstructions of a coronoid fracture.

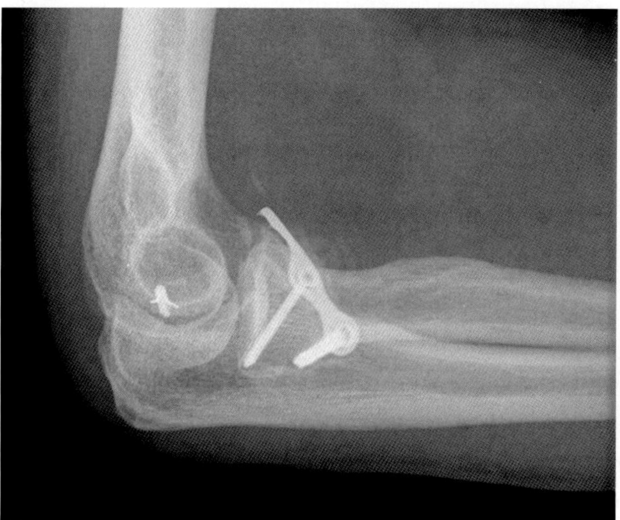

Figure 14.26 Open reduction and internal fixation coronoid. (*Reproduced with permission from* Bucholz RW, Heckman JD, Court-Brown C, et al. *Rockwood and Green's Fractures in Adults.* 6th ed. Philadelphia, PA: Lippincott Williams & Wilkins, 2005.)

Classification

Elbow dislocations are classified first according to the direction of the dislocation (Fig. 14.27). Standard orthopaedic nomenclature describes a dislocation based on the location of the distal segment in relation to the proximal segment. A posterior elbow dislocation, for example, implies that the forearm lies posterior to the humerus. They are further classified on the basis of the presence of associated injuries. Simple elbow dislocations do not have any associated fractures, whereas complex elbow dislocations will have associated fractures of the radial head, coronoid process, or distal humerus.

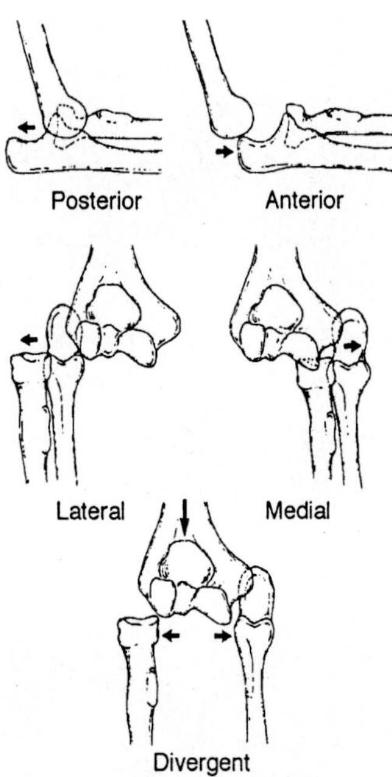

Figure 14.27 Classification of elbow dislocations. (*Reproduced with permission from* Browner BD, Jupiter JB, Levine AM, eds. *Skeletal Trauma.* Philadelphia, PA: WB Saunders, 1992:1142.)

Mechanism of Injury

The vast majority of elbow dislocations are posterior. They typically occur from a fall onto an outstretched arm. O'Driscoll has proposed that elbow dislocations begin with failure of the lateral tissues, specifically the LUCL. As the force dissipates, the capsule continues to tear anteriorly and posteriorly and ultimately the medial ligamentous structures are disrupted.

Presentation

Patients will present with acute pain, deformity, and inability to range the elbow. They will typically hold the arm at the side with the elbow partially flexed.

Physical Findings

A careful neurovascular examination prior to any reduction maneuver is critical in the initial evaluation. The examination must be repeated following reduction, as nerve entrapment within the joint has been reported. Although rare, compartment syndrome does occur and must be diagnosed and emergently treated.

Radiographic Evaluation

Plain radiographs will clearly demonstrate a dislocated elbow. The presence of associated fractures may not be as obvious. Postreduction radiographs may be more helpful in the diagnosis of other injuries. They should be evaluated to ensure that there is not an incarcerated fragment of bone within the joint. Any residual subluxation must be identified and treated accordingly.

Special Studies

As stated earlier, a CT scan is obtained if a coronoid or radial head fracture requires further evaluation. Rarely, an MRI may be useful in determining the extent of ligamentous injury.

Differential Diagnosis

The differential diagnosis of elbow dislocations includes fractures of the distal humerus, olecranon, and radial head. Plain radiographs will rule out these other injuries.

Treatment

Simple Elbow Dislocation. The initial management of an elbow dislocation is a gentle reduction maneuver. After the induction of appropriate sedation, gentle traction and countertraction are applied. The elbow is slightly extended to allow the coronoid to be brought back anterior to the humerus. The elbow is examined to determine stability while the patient is still anesthetized. Postreduction radiographs are obtained to ensure a concentric reduction. A short period of immobilization is followed by controlled early motion. If the elbow is unstable moving into the extended position, a hinged brace is utilized. The brace is set to limit extension within stable limits for the first few weeks. It is gradually opened and discontinued between 3 and 6 weeks, depending on the stability examination. In elbows that are more unstable and cannot be treated closed, open repair is indicated. Operative treatment begins with repair of the LUCL. Stability is reevaluated and if instability persists, repair of the MUCL is considered. Last, a hinged external fixator may be placed if residual instability exists.

Complex Elbow Dislocation. Associated fractures with an elbow dislocation suggest that the elbow may be unstable following reduction, making closed treatment more unpredictable. An elbow dislocation with a radial head and coronoid fracture, known as the *terrible triad,* is best treated surgically. The lateral side of the elbow is addressed first. The radial head is fixed or replaced depending on the fracture. The coronoid fracture can often be approached through a lateral incision once the radial head has been resected prior to replacement. However, a separate medial approach is necessary for larger and more medial fragments or if the radial head fracture does not permit adequate exposure. The LUCL is repaired as part of the closure. If residual instability is present, the MUCL is repaired. A hinged external fixator is placed if the elbow is still unstable.

Ligament and Tendon Injury

Medial Collateral Ligament

The anterior band of the MUCL is the primary restraint to valgus stress on the elbow. High valgus loads are placed across the elbow during overhead throwing. For overhead athletes, injury to the MUCL is a very disabling and potentially career ending injury. Many professional athletes have had their careers cut short by this injury, which may explain the attention it receives in the media.

Classification

Injuries to the MUCL are classified as acute versus chronic ruptures. They are further classified into midsubstance tears and bony avulsions.

Mechanism of Injury

There are two primary mechanisms of injury to the MUCL. A single event such as an elbow dislocation or acute valgus load may rupture the ligament. The force across the elbow during a pitch far exceeds the strength of the ligament. More commonly, repetitive trauma from overhead activities will lead to attenuation and ligament insufficiency.

Presentation

The history will often reveal the mechanism of injury. Patients present with medial-sided elbow pain following an injury or with certain activities. Some patients will also complain of pain, numbness, and weakness in the ulnar nerve distribution. Ulnar nerve symptoms are typically transient occurring with throwing and improve once throwing is discontinued.

Physical Findings

The MUCL is examined for tenderness to palpation. The milking maneuver places a valgus stress across the elbow (Fig. 14.28). The moving valgus stress test is a dynamic test

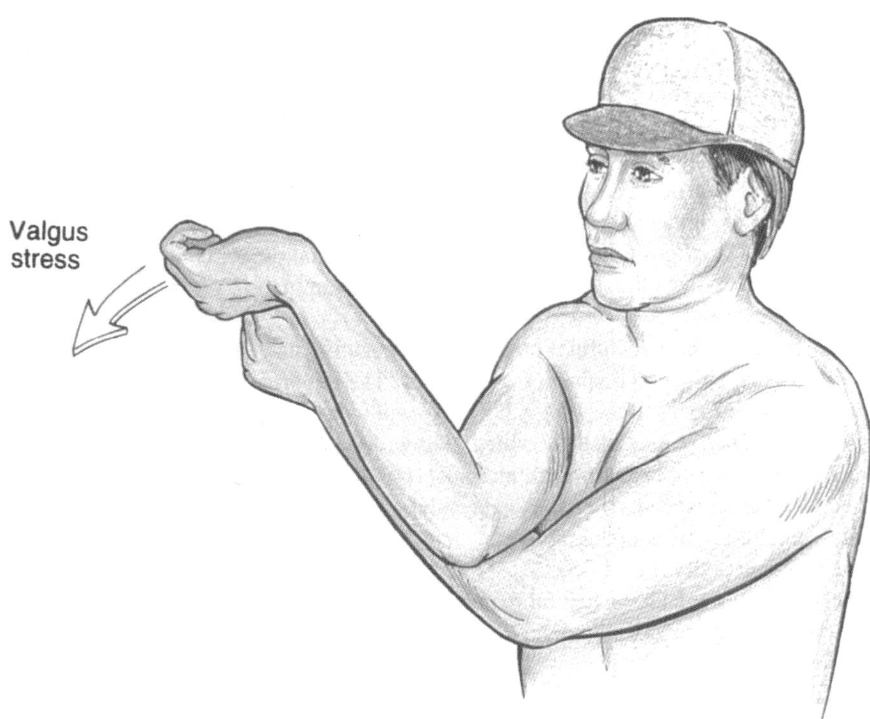

Figure 14.28 The milking maneuver for evaluation of the medial ulnar collateral ligament. (*Reproduced with permission from* Morrey BF. *Master Techniques in Orthopaedic Surgery: The Elbow.* 2nd ed. Philadelphia, PA: Lippincott Williams & Wilkins, 2002.)

that places a valgus stress across the elbow while simulating a throwing motion. Pain with either test is evidence of MUCL insufficiency. The ulnar nerve must be closely examined for subluxation and any sign of nerve dysfunction. The lateral side of the elbow must be examined closely as well, as attenuation of the MUCL may lead to higher compressive forces across the radiocapitellar joint and diseases such as osteochondritis dissecans.

Radiographic Evaluation

A standard elbow series is obtained initially and may reveal a bony avulsion of the ligament. Valgus stress radiographs may demonstrate widening of the medial joint space.

Special Studies

An MRI arthrogram is the most sensitive and specific test for MUCL rupture. Concomitant pathology can also be diagnosed by MRI. Ultrasonography has recently shown promise in the diagnosis of MUCL injury, through noninvasive means.

Differential Diagnosis

MUCL insufficiency must be distinguished from other causes of medial-sided elbow pain. Medial epicondylitis, cubital tunnel syndrome, and medial epicondyle fractures can present with symptoms similar to MUCL injury. In skeletally immature athletes, Little League elbow should be considered. Radiographs and a careful physical examination are usually sufficient to make the diagnosis.

Treatment

Initial treatment is typically conservative. Rest from inciting activities for up to 3 months is appropriate. Elbow range of motion and strengthening of the flexor–pronator musculature are also initiated. Once symptoms subside, the patient is gradually allowed to return to throwing. If the patient does not respond to conservative treatment, surgical reconstruction is indicated. Multiple reconstructive techniques using different grafts and fixation methods have been described. Classically, autograft tendon is woven through bone tunnels in the humerus and ulna (Fig. 14.29). Use of allograft tissue and fixation with interference screws

A

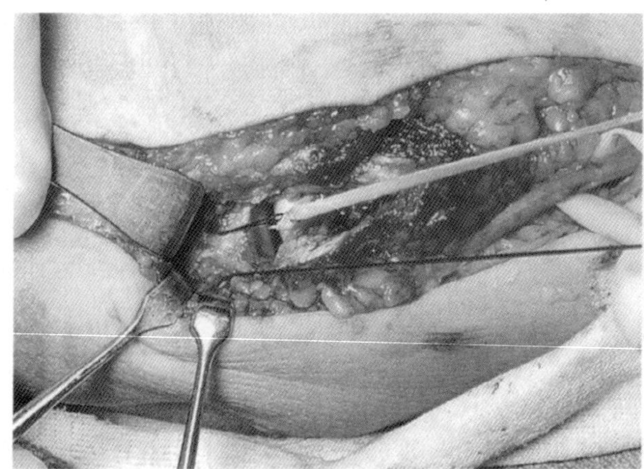

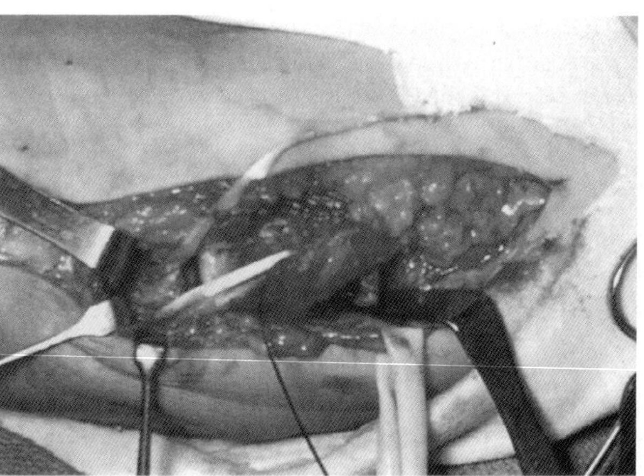

B

MAYO ©2000

C Three-ply reconstruction

Figure 14.29 Medial ulnar collateral ligament reconstruction. (*Reproduced with permission from* Morrey BF. *Master Techniques in Orthopaedic Surgery: The Elbow*. 2nd ed. Philadelphia, PA: Lippincott Williams & Wilkins, 2002.)

has been described more recently. An ulnar nerve transposition is not typically required when the nerve symptoms are transient with activity. However, when the ulnar neuropathy is more profound, transposition may be required. Postoperatively, valgus stresses must be avoided. Early range of motion is initiated in a hinged brace. At 3 months, early strengthening is begun. Light pitching from flat ground begins at 6 months and off the mound pitching begins at 9 to 12 months.

Lateral Ulnar Collateral Ligament

Injury to the lateral ligamentous structures of the elbow has received increasing focus in the recent literature. Insufficiency of the LUCL can lead to PLRI of the elbow. Rupture of the LUCL is now considered the essential lesion in the majority of elbow dislocations.

Classification

LUCL injuries are classified primarily on the basis of chronicity of the injury. Associated injuries, such as radial head and coronoid fractures, are also documented.

Mechanism of Injury

The majority of LUCL injuries occur following subluxation or dislocation of the elbow. After a fall on the outstretched arm, the lateral ligaments fail first. As the injury progresses and the forearm rotates, the force is carried across the joint. The capsule tears and eventually the medial ligaments fail (Fig. 14.30). Iatrogenic injury is another cause of ligament compromise during procedures such as tennis elbow release. The LUCL is avoided during the lateral approach to the elbow by staying anterior to the midline of the radial head. Overuse injuries are less likely to cause LUCL injury but have been reported.

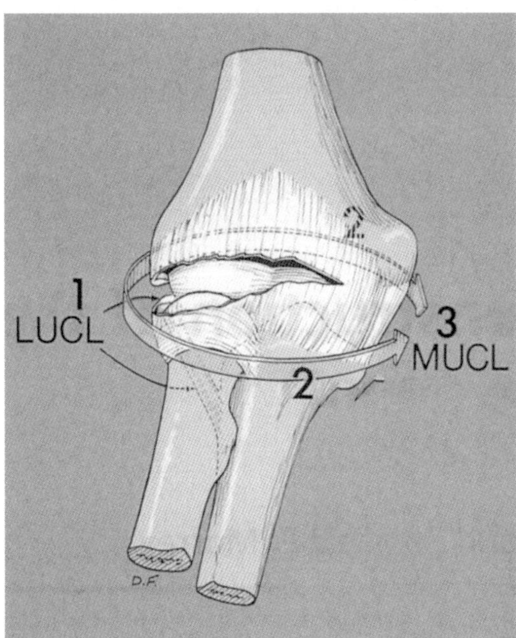

Figure 14.30 Progressive failure of the elbow ligaments with dislocation of the elbow. (*Reproduced with permission from* Morrey BF. *Master Techniques in Orthopaedic Surgery: The Elbow.* 2nd ed. Philadelphia, PA: Lippincott Williams & Wilkins, 2002.)

Presentation

Patients will present with lateral-sided elbow pain and varying degrees of instability. They will often give a history of a dislocation. Activities that classically cause pain are those that place a valgus load across a supinated forearm as it moves in to extension, such as rising from a chair using the armrests.

Physical Findings

On physical examination, patients will have tenderness over the lateral aspect of the elbow. The pivot shift maneuver stresses the incompetent ligament complex (Fig. 14.31). With the patient supine, the arm is elevated overhead. The elbow is slightly flexed, the forearm supinated, and a valgus and axial load is placed across the elbow. This results in supination of the ulna away from the humerus. The radial head follows the ulna posteriorly. The elbow is slowly brought into flexion, and there will be a palpable reduction of the radial head. The maneuver is reversed, and the radial head is subluxed. A dimple in the skin may be present over the radial head. If prior surgery has been performed, the location of any previous incisions should be noted as evidence of a possible iatrogenic injury. A subcutaneous fluid-filled cyst or a chronic draining sinus following surgical treatment of lateral epicondylitis is evidence of insufficiency of the lateral capsule and LUCL

Radiographic Evaluation

Plain radiographs will reveal a dislocation or subluxation but are usually normal in cases of ligament insufficiency. The radial head should point directly toward the capitellum on all radiographic views. Fluoroscopic examination under anesthesia will often reveal subluxation or dislocation in the provocative positions. US has been successfully reported as a diagnostic test as well but is highly operator dependent.

Differential Diagnosis

Other causes of lateral-sided elbow pain are lateral epicondylitis, radiocapitellar arthritis, synovial plica, and lateral epicondylar fracture. Physical examination and imaging will help narrow the differential.

Treatment

Acute elbow dislocation may be initially treated nonoperatively, as stated earlier. In the case of continued instability, acute ligament repair is usually sufficient to stabilize the elbow. However, chronically unstable elbows require ligament reconstruction, not repair. The LUCL is reconstructed with autograft or allograft tendon. It is placed between the

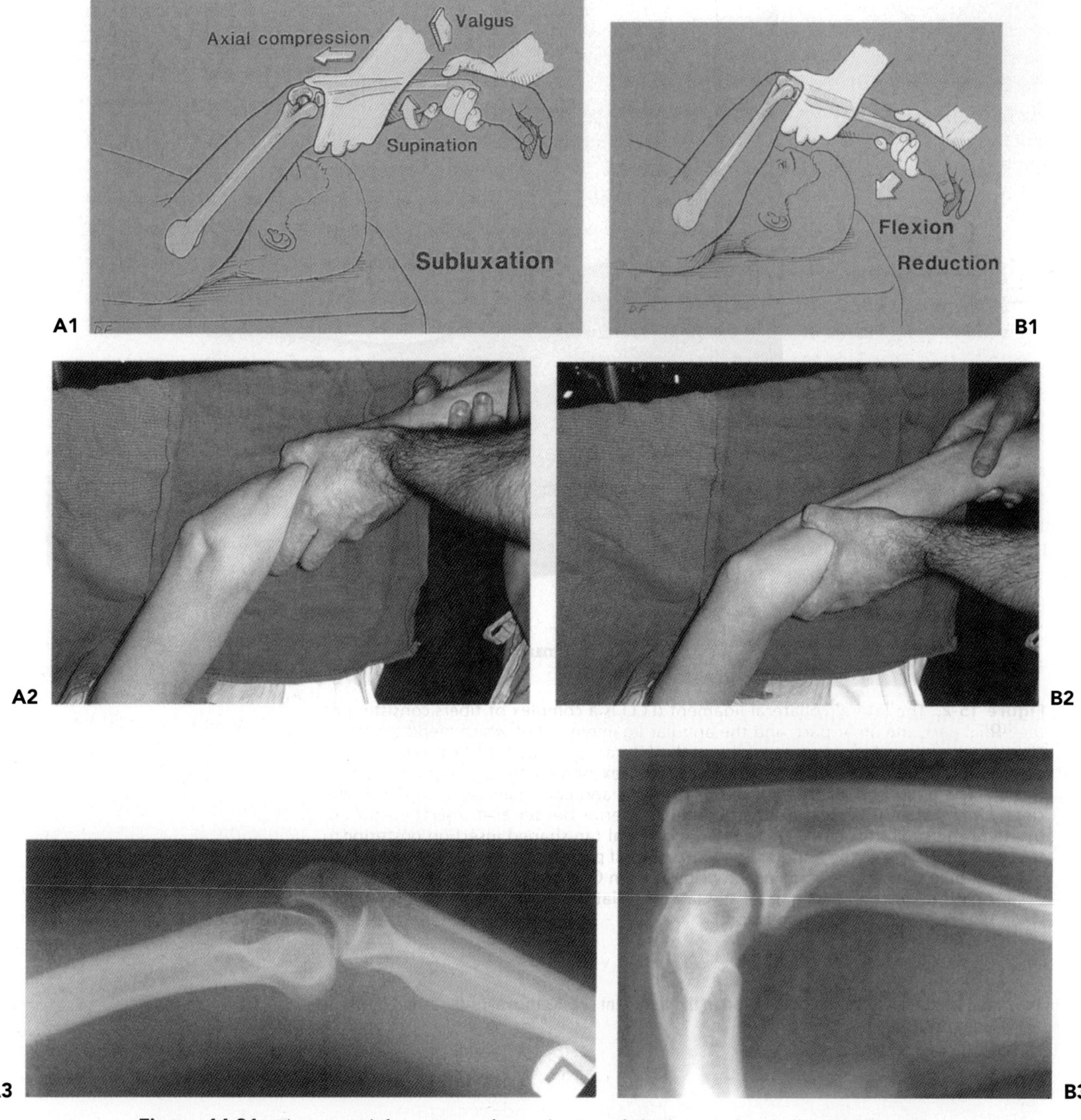

Figure 14.31 The pivot shift maneuver for evaluation of the lateral ulnar collateral ligament. (*Reproduced with permission from* Morrey BF. *Master Techniques in Orthopaedic Surgery: The Elbow.* 2nd ed. Philadelphia, PA: Lippincott Williams & Wilkins, 2002.)

lateral epicondyle and the supinator crest on the ulna. Various fixation techniques have been described. Postoperative care includes early motion in a safe range determined at surgery. Extension and supination are avoided. Varus stress across the repair is also avoided, most commonly by keeping the arm at the side. By 6 weeks, full motion is allowed and stretching is employed. Gradual increased use of the arm is permitted over the next 12 weeks and strengthening is added to the postoperative regimen. Patients are allowed full activity at 6 months after surgery.

Distal Biceps Tendon Rupture

Rupture of the distal biceps is a relatively uncommon injury. Only 3% of biceps injuries involve the distal tendon insertion. The biceps muscle is the primary supinator of the forearm and inserts on the bicipital tuberosity of the radius. The distal tendon fibers undergo degeneration with age, which likely predisposes patients to injury. Rupture of the tendon leads to loss of supination strength and endurance. Flexion strength is also lost, but to a lesser degree given that the brachialis remains intact.

Classification

Distal biceps tendon ruptures may be partial or complete. Complete ruptures are broadly classified into acute and chronic injuries. The definition of an acute rupture is arbitrary and varies from less than 2 to 6 weeks after injury but generally is considered acute if the injury is less than 4 weeks old.

Mechanism of Injury

The mechanism of injury is typically an eccentric load forcefully extending an actively flexing elbow.

Presentation

Ruptures of the distal biceps tendon primarily occur in men in their 50s. There have been a few reports of women sustaining this injury. Other risk factors include weightlifting, steroid use, and smoking. Patients may describe a tearing sensation and pain in the anterior elbow following an injury. Some patients note a second distinct tear that represents failure of the bicipital aponeurosis.

Physical Findings

Patients with an acute rupture will have swelling, tenderness, and ecchymoses around the proximal medial forearm. The biceps tendon will not be palpable along the anterior elbow. Proximal migration of the muscle belly with supination may help confirm the diagnosis but may not occur if the lacertus fibrosis remains intact (Fig. 14.32).

Radiographic Evaluation

Plain radiographs are usually normal but should be scrutinized for any abnormalities of the bicipital tuberosity.

Special Studies

MRI and US have been used for confirmation of the rupture and may demonstrate the degree of proximal migration (Fig. 14.33). A special MRI view of the biceps is obtained with the patient placed prone with the elbow flexed to 90 degrees, the shoulder abducted, and the forearm supinated (FABS view). This view provides a longitudinal view of the biceps tendon

Differential Diagnosis

Although rare, muscle–tendon junction tears may occur and will have a similar presentation. Other sources of pathology to consider are partial tendon ruptures, cubital bursitis, and lateral antebrachial nerve compression.

Treatment

Direct tendon repair to the bicipital tuberosity is indicated in active individuals to restore supination and flexion strength and endurance. Nonoperative treatment is reserved for low-demand patients or those who are medically unfit for surgery. Multiple fixation methods using either a one-incision or a two-incision approach have been described. Historically, the one-incision technique had a high rate of radial nerve injury, leading to the development of the two-incision repair. Recent advances in fixation using suture anchors and fixation buttons have led to a renewed

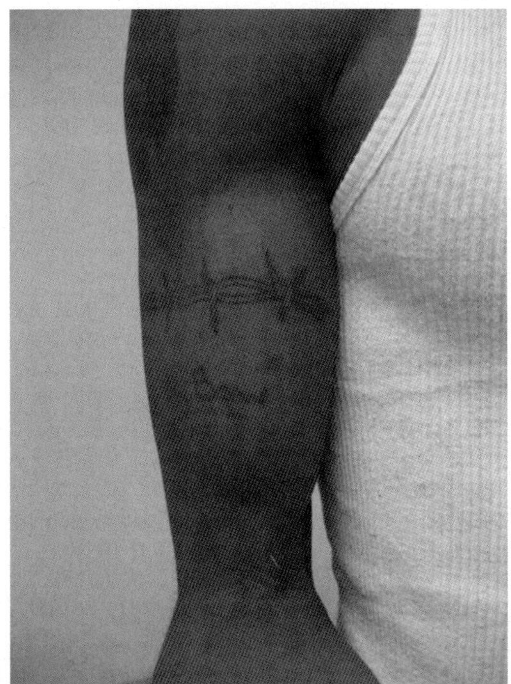
A

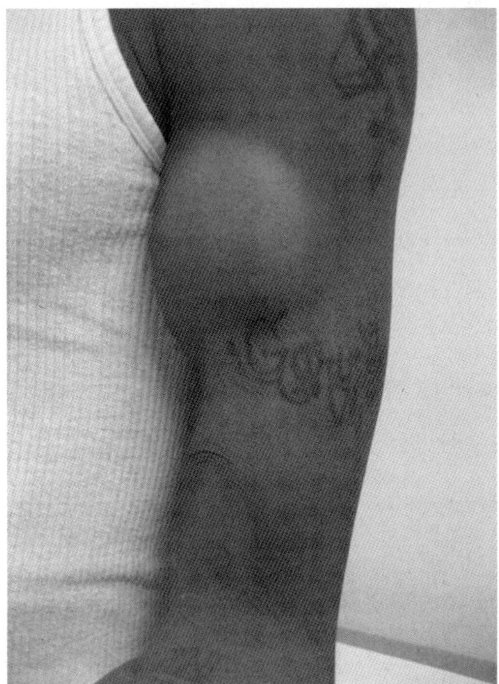
B

Figure 14.32 Clinical photographs demonstrating the right biceps with an intact tendon **(A)** and the left biceps where there is a distal biceps rupture **(B)**.

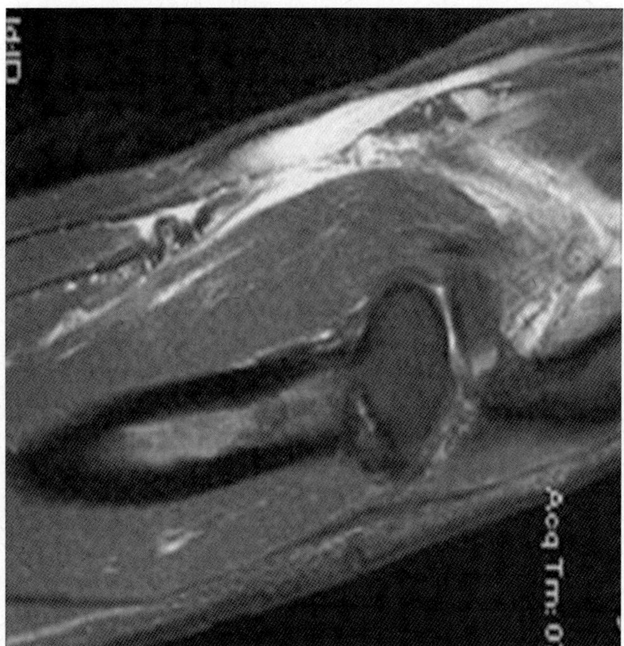

Figure 14.33 Sagittal magnetic resonance image demonstrating a distal biceps rupture.

interest in the one-incision approach. Complications with both approaches, including heterotopic bone formation and nerve damage, remain a potential problem. Partial tendon ruptures are initially treated conservatively. Failure to achieve relief of symptoms is an indication for surgical treatment. Results have been promising with the completion of the partial tear and tendon reattachment. Chronic ruptures are a much more difficult problem to treat. Because of proximal migration of the biceps tendon, tendon graft if often required and results are much less predictable.

ATRAUMATIC CONDITIONS OF THE ELBOW

Degenerative Joint Disease

Similar to other joints in the body, degenerative joint disease (DJD) of the elbow occurs in several forms. It is typically classified into osteoarthritis (OA), posttraumatic arthritis, and inflammatory arthritis such as rheumatoid disease. Each has its own different characteristics, but all can lead to substantial disability.

Rheumatoid Arthritis

With the recent advent of disease-modifying antirheumatic drugs, severe destructive elbow arthritis is becoming less common. RA, however, remains the most common cause of elbow joint arthritis and can be severely debilitating.

Pathophysiology and Classification

Autoimmune complexes form and incite a painful inflammatory response in the synovial lining of the joint. This leads to synovial hypertrophy and pannus formation, which is responsible for the ultimate destruction of the joint. The hyaline cartilage surfaces are eroded initially. Bone resorption and soft tissue attenuation follow, leading to loss of the joint stability and architecture. The Mayo classification is based on radiographs and consists of four grades that closely mirror the pathophysiology. Grade I represents synovitis, and radiographs are normal or may show osteopenia. Grade II demonstrates joint space narrowing consistent with loss of the joint cartilage. Grade III disease demonstrates loss of joint architecture and is further subdivided into A or B, on the basis of severity. Grade IV represents end-stage disease with gross joint instability, severe incongruity, and extensive bone loss.

Presentation

Patients with early-stage disease will present with a painful range of motion and joint effusion. In later stages, they will complain of increasing loss of motion and varying degrees of joint deformity. Patients have usually been diagnosed with RA prior to orthopaedic consultation and will often have adjacent joint or cervical spine involvement. Occasionally, however, patients will present prior to diagnosis, and a proper workup or referral is imperative.

Physical Examination

An initial inspection should note any soft tissue swelling, joint effusion, and deformity. The elbow is then taken through a range of motion, noting any crepitus, grinding, or instability. The cervical spine, shoulder and wrist are examined, as well, for the presence of any dysfunction or deformity.

Radiographic Findings

The radiographic findings in rheumatoid disease demonstrate the classic changes of inflammatory arthritis. Periarticular osteopenia is seen in early stages. Symmetric joint space narrowing and periarticular bone erosion follow. Ultimately, bone loss and soft tissue attenuation lead to loss of joint stability and architecture. In contrast to OA, very few osteophytes are typically present.

Special Tests

Generally, the plain radiographs are sufficient for diagnosis. CT scans or MRI may be helpful if the degree of bone loss or soft tissue attenuation is in question. Laboratory workup for RA, such as rheumatoid factor and other inflammatory markers, is considered if a diagnosis has not yet been made.

Differential Diagnosis

RA is a form of inflammatory arthritis, which can typically be distinguished from other forms of DJD by radiographs. Other causes of inflammatory arthritis should be considered, such as hemophilic arthropathy and psoriatic

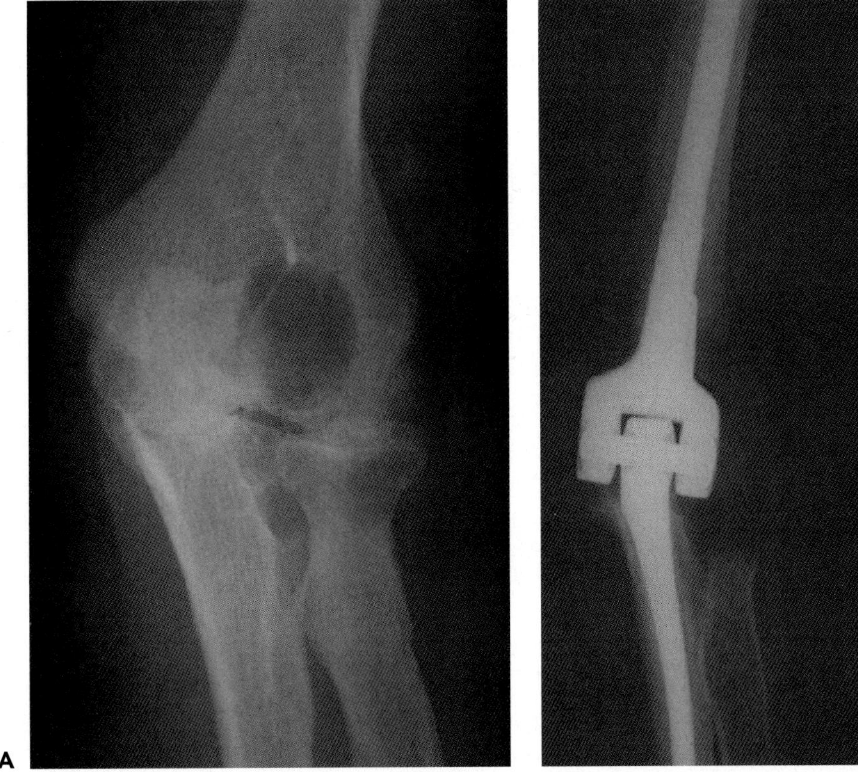

Figure 14.34 **(A)** Preoperative radiograph of an elbow with advanced rheumatoid arthritis. **(B)** Postoperative image following treatment with a total elbow arthroplasty.

arthritis. Patient history and laboratory workup will help distinguish the different causes of inflammatory arthritis. Earlier stages of the disease may be more difficult to diagnose, especially if the presentation is monoarticular. In these cases, septic arthritis must be considered and one must have a low threshold for aspiration of the joint.

Treatment

Early stages of RA can often be treated with medications, selective steroid injections, and activity modification. Synovectomy, either open or arthroscopic, is considered if painful synovitis exists in a relatively well-preserved joint. Once joint destruction has reached end stages, TEA becomes the most viable option (Fig. 14.34). Elbow replacement designs fall into two main categories. Linked implants offer immediate stability through a coupled articulation but have higher rates of loosening and bushing wear. Unlinked implants have no physical linkage between the components and rely on the native soft tissues for stability. They typically have a lower rate of loosening but have a higher incidence of instability. Patients with RA typically have attenuated soft tissues, and a linked implant offers a more stability. Infection is a major concern following TEA and can be as high as 5%. Any wound complication must be taken seriously, and prompt irrigation and debridement should be undertaken in attempt to salvage the prosthesis.

Osteoarthritis

OA is relatively uncommon in the elbow joint. Nonetheless, the pain and stiffness that occur can greatly affect a patient's livelihood.

Pathophysiology and Classification

OA is a poorly understood disease despite being the most common cause of DJD throughout the body. It is likely that multiple factors, including genetics and lifestyle, contribute to the formation of OA. Patients whose jobs require high-impact or repetitive trauma, such as using a jackhammer, seem to be at higher risk for the development of elbow OA. Unlike other joints in the body, the cartilage surface is initially spared in the elbow with OA. Abundant osteophytes form in the periarticular region, which limit motion. Eventually, the joint surface becomes involved and joint space narrowing occurs.

Presentation

The classic presentation of elbow OA is loss of motion with pain at terminal extension before terminal flexion. As the elbow enters the end range of motion, osteophytes cause a painful impingement. Midrange motion, on the other hand, will typically not be painful, as the joint surface is initially preserved. In later stages, however, as the joint surface becomes affected, midrange motion will become more painful.

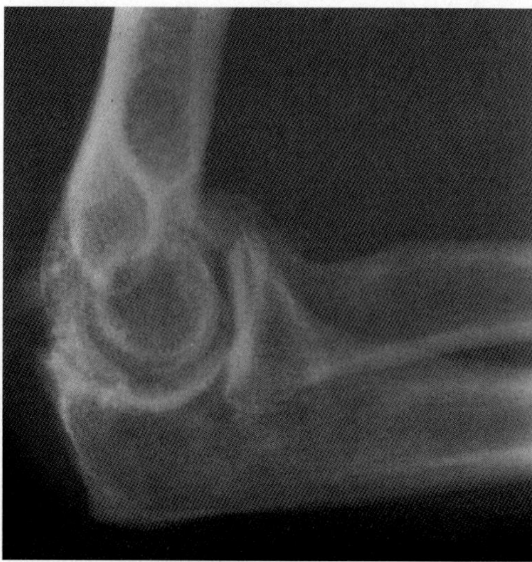

Figure 14.35 Lateral radiograph of elbow osteoarthritis demonstrating significant periarticular osteophytes with preservation of the chondral surfaces.

Physical Examination

Range of motion is the most important component of the examination of the osteoarthritic elbow. The overall range is recorded first. Next, the presence of pain during the examination is carefully evaluated. As stated earlier, the presence of midrange pain implies involvement of the joint surface which may significantly affect treatment.

Radiographic Findings

Plain radiographs will reveal the changes of OA. In particular, periarticular osteophytes are often very impressive and explain the lack of motion seen on physical examination (Fig. 14.35). Joint space narrowing is typically not seen initially. The deformity and instability seen with inflammatory arthritis is usually not seen with OA.

Special Tests

The plain radiographs may be difficult to interpret in two dimensions. A three-dimensional study, such as a CT scan, will better define the size and location of the osteophytes and may be useful for preoperative planning.

Differential Diagnosis

OA of the elbow is typically diagnosed by plain radiographs. It must be distinguished from other forms of elbow DJD. In the presence of normal radiographs, soft tissue contracture may cause similar pain and loss of motion.

Treatment

Initial treatment is conservative, consisting of anti-inflammatory medications and activity modification. Later stages may respond to arthroscopic debridement, capsular release, and removal of osteophytes. Care must be taken not to destabilize the elbow joint with overaggressive resection. Total elbow replacement is rarely required in patients with OA.

Posttraumatic Arthritis

Posttraumatic arthritis is an extremely difficult condition to treat. Because patients tend to be younger, arthroplasty with lifelong activity restrictions is an unrealistic treatment option. Patients typically have a high-demand lifestyle and require a functioning elbow for their livelihood.

Pathophysiology and Classification

The articular cartilage of the elbow, particularly of the distal humerus, is among the thinnest in the body. Failure to anatomically restore the joint surface can lead to uneven wear of the remaining cartilage, followed by rapid degeneration of the joint. However, even after an anatomic reduction, there may be cartilage loss. A direct impact to the joint surface has been shown to cause apoptosis of the chondrocytes with subsequent loss of articular cartilage. Patients are typically classified on a descriptive basis. The original injury pattern, presence or absence of hardware, and degree of soft tissue or bony contracture are noted.

Presentation

While posttraumatic arthritis will occur in many different forms, the common thread is the history of trauma. Patients will usually complain of pain and loss of motion. They often will have had multiple prior procedures. Any operative reports, radiographs, or office notes are helpful. It is important to determine whether the original injury was open or closed and whether any wound complications occurred following surgery.

Physical Examination

A thorough inspection of the skin is the initial step in the physical examination. Many patients will exhibit compromise of the soft tissue envelope. Any open wounds or draining sinuses should be noted. Prior surgical incisions are examined for evidence of infection and for future surgical planning. Range of motion is recorded along with the presence of crepitus or grinding. Any deformity or instability is also noted.

Radiographic Findings

The radiographic findings of posttraumatic arthritis will show a similar loss of joint space as seen in other forms of DJD. Usually, however, there will also be hardware present, which can obscure the images. The hardware should be evaluated for loosening, breakage, or penetration into the joint. Varying degrees of bone loss and evidence of ununited segments may also be present. HO is a common finding after elbow trauma, and its presence and location should be noted.

Special Tests

A major concern in the posttraumatic elbow is the possibility of infection. Laboratory workup including WBC, ESR, and CRP will offer evidence for or against the presence of infection. Joint aspiration can also aid in the diagnosis. CT scan is helpful in determining such factors as the location of HO, the presence of nonunited segments, and areas of bone loss.

Differential Diagnosis

The main difficulty is the diagnosis of posttraumatic arthritis is the evaluation of the joint surface. In the presence of trauma, many other factors besides cartilage loss can cause symptoms. HO, soft tissue contracture, infection, and nonunion may all contribute to painful loss of motion in the elbow. Treated separately, these conditions may relieve a great deal of the patient's complaints, without requiring intervention at the joint surface.

Treatment

The treatment of posttraumatic arthritis varies on the basis of the presenting complaints and must be tailored to each individual. Conservative measures include anti-inflammatory medications and activity restriction. Any suspicion for infection should be diagnosed and treated accordingly. Operative treatment is chosen on the basis of the patient's needs. Hardware removal, contracture release, and repair of nonunited segments can relieve many symptoms. Addressing articular surface degeneration is more challenging. Arthrodesis of the elbow is less successful than it is in other joints, leaving patients very disabled. TEA requires lifelong activity restriction and conversion to a low-demand lifestyle. This is often not possible for a young, active patient who must use the elbow for work. Interposition arthroplasty, using fascial tissue, has been used with success but is a technically demanding procedure with results that may be unpredictable.

Lateral and Medial Epicondylitis

Lateral and medial epicondylitis, also known as *tennis* and *golfer's elbow*, respectively, are among the most common conditions causing elbow pain. Simple activities of daily living are painful to impossible, leading to a great deal of disability with lost time from work and recreation.

Pathophysiology and Classification

The term *epicondylitis* is actually a misnomer. The suffix -*itis* implies that an inflammatory process is taking place. Histologic analysis, however, has revealed that the process is an age-related degeneration of the tendon fibers. In tennis elbow, the fibers of the ECRB are most often involved, whereas the PT and FCR are involved in golfer's elbow. The conditions are broadly classified into medial or lateral epicondylitis on the basis of location of the symptoms. They are further subdivided into acute and chronic processes, with 6 weeks being an arbitrary cutoff for an acute epicondylitis.

Presentation

Because the condition is a degenerative process, patients typically present during their middle age. They usually have a history of overuse or repetitive trauma, but some patients will describe an acute inciting event. Patients with lateral epicondylitis present with lateral elbow pain, which is exacerbated by activities involving resisted wrist extension. Tight grasping will also cause pain, as wrist extension is component of a power grip. Patients with medial epicondylitis complain of medial elbow pain with activities involving resisted wrist flexion and pronation.

Physical Examination

When medial or lateral epicondylitis is suspected by history, a complete elbow examination must still be performed such that concomitant pathology is not missed. This should include a complete range of motion and stability examination. A careful neurovascular examination is also important to rule out compressive neuropathies, such as radial or cubital tunnel syndrome. For lateral epicondylitis, palpation over the lateral epicondyle will reproduce the patient's symptoms. Pain with resisted wrist extension (Fig. 14.36), known as *Mill test,* or pain with passive wrist flexion and elbow extension are two specific maneuvers that will cause pain in lateral epicondylitis. The radiocapitellar joint and radial tunnel should be palpated for tenderness. Pain with resisted supination is more likely secondary to a partial biceps rupture or radial tunnel syndrome. A pivot shift is performed to identify PLRI.

For medial epicondylitis, the medial epicondyle is palpated for tenderness. Pain with resisted flexion and pronation will reproduce the symptoms. The ulnar nerve is examined for subluxation, tenderness, or a Tinel sign to rule out ulnar nerve involvement. Valgus stress testing will

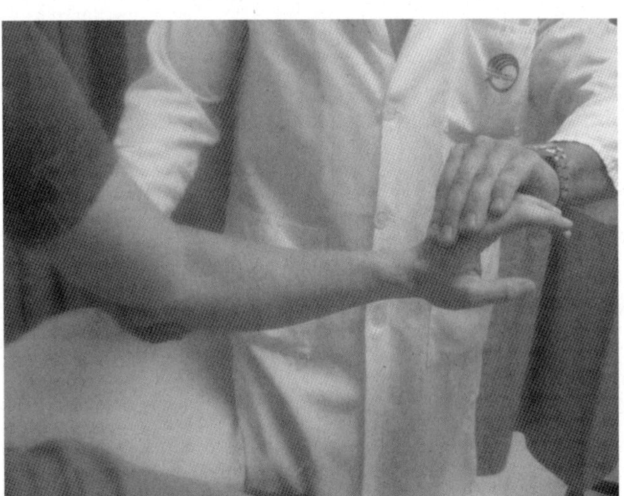

Figure 14.36 Mill test for lateral epicondylitis.

cause pain if the pathology is secondary to MUCL insufficiency.

Radiographic Findings

Imaging studies are rarely helpful in medial and lateral epicondylitis as the diagnosis is generally a clinical one. Plain radiographs may demonstrate calcifications around the involved epicondyle, but this has no known prognostic or treatment value.

Special Studies

Advanced imaging does not typically add any information as the diagnosis is based on clinical findings. EMG studies are obtained if suspicion for ulnar or PIN involvement exists. Unfortunately, EMG studies are oftentimes normal in these conditions.

Differential Diagnosis

The differential diagnosis for lateral epicondylitis includes radial tunnel syndrome, radiocapitellar DJD, PLRI, and intraarticular plical folds. The differential diagnosis on the medial side includes cubital tunnel syndrome and MUCL insufficiency. Again, it must be remembered that more than one condition may occur simultaneously.

Treatment

Initial treatment is conservative and aimed at relieving symptoms. A period of rest from 2 to 6 weeks is advocated, particularly in acute cases, with avoidance of aggravating activities. Braces are designed to transfer the force from the origin of the tendon to the muscle belly. An injection of corticosteroid may help to relieve symptoms. Therapy may offer an additional resource in the treatment armamentarium, with techniques such as cross-friction massage and US. The vast majority of patients will respond to a nonoperative program.

Those patients who fail 6 months of conservative management, however, are candidates for surgical treatment. For lateral epicondylitis, the procedure can be performed either open or arthroscopically. In the open approach, the fibers of the ECRB are identified, the degenerative tissue is excised, and the footprint of the ECRB is drilled or decorticated. The LUCL must be avoided to prevent iatrogenic PLRI. The arthroscopic approach offers the advantage of removal of any concomitant intraarticular plicae and a faster return to work; however, there is a greater risk of complications, especially nerve injury. Similar to lateral epicondylitis, the approach to medial epicondylitis involves excision of the degenerated portion of the flexor–pronator tendon. Care must be taken not to injure the MUCL.

Olecranon Bursitis

The olecranon bursa lies on the dorsal aspect of the proximal ulna as a protective tissue between the skin and bone. It is a frequent area of inflammation and a common cause of elbow pain.

Pathophysiology and Classification

The bursa is a potential space that normally has only a thin layer of fluid but may become significantly larger when inflamed. Olecranon bursitis can begin from overuse or a direct trauma. Septic bursitis occurs when the bursa is seeded or inoculated with bacteria.

Presentation

Patients will present with pain along the posterior elbow and will report varying degrees of swelling. Often, they will not recall a specific trauma but will report a history of pressure on the area, such as resting it on a car door while driving. Septic bursitis must be considered in patients who present with fevers, erythema, or history of penetrating trauma to the area.

Physical Examination

Some cases of olecranon bursitis are obvious and present with a massive fluid-filled bursa. Other cases are less dramatic with tenderness to palpation and only mild or no swelling. Chronic cases may have tender, palpable nodules within the bursa. Inspection for open wounds, purulent drainage, erythema, or warmth should raise the suspicion for a septic process.

Radiographic Findings

Plain radiographs may show the fluid within the bursa. Many patients will have an olecranon spur.

Special Studies

Advanced imaging is rarely necessary for the diagnosis of olecranon bursitis. US may confirm the presence of fluid within the bursa. MRI can also confirm the presence of fluid and help identify characteristics of the fluid, such as the presence of loculations. MRI can also yield information regarding other tissues, such as the integrity of the triceps tendon, if it is in question. Laboratory values are obtained if infection is a possibility. Aspiration of the bursa is sent for culture in cases of septic bursitis if identification of an organism is necessary.

Differential Diagnosis

A partial or complete triceps tendon rupture must be considered in a patient with posterior elbow pain. Pain with resisted elbow extension will help distinguish a triceps tear from olecranon bursitis.

Treatment

Treatment of the inflamed bursa begins conservatively with unloading of the area. Avoiding aggravating activities or using elbow padding is effective in most cases. Aspiration of the bursa is controversial in that it relieves much of the swelling, but concerns exist regarding recurrence and formation of a draining sinus. In chronic cases that fail to respond to nonoperative treatment, bursal excision may be considered; however, recurrence and wound failure remain common complications. Septic bursitis can be empirically treated with antibiotics in a stable patient. Failure to respond to appropriate antibiotics, however, necessitates irrigation and debridement with bursal excision.

Cubital Tunnel Syndrome

Ulnar nerve compression at the elbow, or cubital tunnel syndrome, is the second most common compressive neuropathy after carpal tunnel syndrome. There are many causes of cubital tunnel syndrome and many other disease processes with similar symptoms, making diagnosis challenging.

Pathophysiology and Classification

As the ulnar nerve crosses the elbow, it passes beneath the medial epicondyle of the humerus. When the elbow is flexed and pronated, maximum traction is placed across the nerve, with some patients experiencing nerve subluxation. Repetitive use of the elbow in these positions is the cause of symptoms in most patients. Other causes include direct trauma, delayed trauma in the form of tardy ulnar nerve palsy, and space-occupying lesions, such as gouty tophi or ganglion cysts.

Presentation

Patients will present with vague pain along the medial elbow. Classically, they will have paresthesias and dysesthesias along the ulnar forearm into the ring and small finger. Patients will often complain of weakness of the hand, as the intrinsic muscles are innervated by the ulnar nerve. Symptoms commonly occur with the elbow in the flexed position.

Physical Examination

The physical examination is crucial in the evaluation of cubital tunnel syndrome, as many other conditions have similar symptoms. The ulnar nerve is made up of the lower roots of the brachial plexus, specifically C8 and T1. The roots become the medial cord of the plexus and ultimately the ulnar nerve. Compression anywhere along the pathway can cause the symptoms of cubital tunnel syndrome. The examination begins with testing for cervical nerve root compression by evaluating the range of motion and performing a Spurling maneuver. The axilla is then examined for any palpable masses, and an Adson or Wright maneuver is performed for the presence of thoracic outlet syndrome. The elbow examination begins with palpation of the medial elbow. Tenderness, nerve subluxation, or Tinel sign are all noted. Reproduction of symptoms with the elbow held in a flexed position helps confirm the diagnosis. The carrying angle should also be evaluated for the possibility of tardy ulnar nerve palsy from posttraumatic deformity. A complete elbow examination for range of motion and stability is performed. The wrist is examined for presence of nerve compression at Guyon canal. A Tinel sign is elicited and the hook of the hamate examined for tenderness or a pulsatile mass. Weakness may exist when testing intrinsic muscles. Patients may compensate for the loss of finger abduction with finger hyperextension. The first dorsal interosseous muscle is easily palpated in the first webspace, with attempted index finger abduction. Decreased sensation may be present along the little finger and ulnar side of the ring finger.

Radiographic Findings

Plain radiographs of the elbow are obtained and are usually normal. They may demonstrate posttraumatic deformity or callus within the area of the cubital tunnel. An epicondylar view may be added to obtain a clear image of the groove and evaluate for the presence of osteophytes or other lesions. Radiographs of other areas of the body, such as the cervical spine, chest, and wrist are taken, depending on clinical suspicion following the physical examination.

Special Tests

Advanced imaging is rarely helpful in the diagnosis of cubital tunnel syndrome. MRI can be obtained if concern exists for a space-occupying lesion. Electrodiagnostic studies, such as EMG and NCV, help to confirm the diagnosis and localize the compression in equivocal situations. False negatives do occur and treatment for cubital tunnel syndrome should proceed accordingly if the clinical examination is clear, despite a normal EMG/NCV.

Differential Diagnosis

As stated earlier, the differential diagnosis is extensive. Many conditions have overlapping symptoms, and different conditions may occur simultaneously. The differential diagnosis begins with cervical nerve root compression. Traveling down the arm, brachial plexus compression from thoracic outlet syndrome or a Pancoast tumor is considered. At the elbow, MUCL insufficiency and medial epicondylitis are evaluated. At the wrist, ulnar nerve compression at Guyon canal, around the hook of the hamate, or secondary to ulnar artery aneurysm is also considered. Last, systemic abnormalities that may produce peripheral neuropathy, such as vitamin deficiency, heavy metal intoxication, and alcoholism, are all included in the differential diagnosis.

Treatment

Initial treatment is conservative. Splinting is effective in reducing the amount of elbow flexion, particularly at night. Nighttime 45-degree splints relieve a significant portion of involuntary compression. Daytime flexion is avoided, and full-time splinting may be considered in severe cases. Anti-inflammatory medications and therapy modalities may also be added. In refractory cases, surgical treatment is indicated. There is controversy in the various treatment measures available. In all cases, however, all areas of compression or potential compression must be addressed. Surgical techniques vary from simple decompression to nerve

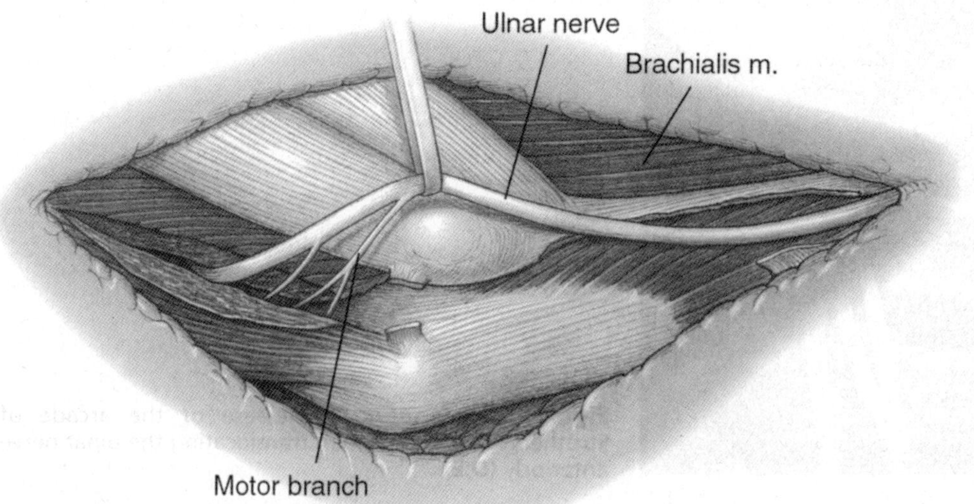

Figure 14.37 Ulnar nerve transposition. (*Reproduced with permission from* Morrey BF. *Master Techniques in Orthopaedic Surgery: The Elbow.* 2nd ed. Philadelphia, PA: Lippincott Williams & Wilkins, 2002.)

transposition (Fig. 14.37). If transposition is performed, multiple methods have been described placing the nerve in a subcutaneous or a submuscular position. Head-to-head trials demonstrating a significant benefit of one treatment compared with another are lacking. The possible complications from surgical treatment are nerve dysfunction or damage, incomplete release, and damage to the medial antebrachial cutaneous nerve.

CONCLUSION

For normal elbow function, a delicate interplay of bones, ligaments, and muscles must exist. Traumatic and atraumatic disorders disrupt this delicate interplay in multiple different ways. They all lead to a common endpoint, which is disability, often limiting the patient's ability to perform daily activities. Advances in the understanding of elbow biomechanics and pathology have led to improved diagnostic and treatment options for patients with elbow disorders. Further research will continue to advance our knowledge and expand our ability treat these devastating conditions.

RECOMMENDED READINGS

Cheung EV, Steinmann SP. Surgical approaches to the elbow. *J Am Acad Orthop Surg*. 2009;17:325–333.

Cheung EV, Adams R, Morrey BF. Primary osteoarthritis of the elbow: current treatment options. *J Am Acad Orthop Surg*. 2008;16:77–87.

Mathew PK, Athwal GS, King GJW. Terrible triad injury of the elbow: current concepts. *J Am Acad Orthop Surg*. 2009;17:137–151.

Sarmiento A, Waddell JP, Latta LL. Diaphyseal humeral fractures: treatment options. *J Bone Joint Surg Am*. 2001;83:1566–1579.

Hand and Wrist

15

Nick Pappas *Jonas L. Matzon* *Pedro K. Beredjiklian*

HAND AND WRIST SURGERY

Our hands serve as our gateway to the outside world. They enable us to touch, eat, communicate, and perform countless other tasks of daily living. Without them, we are limited in our ability to interact in society. Perhaps one can only truly appreciate their importance when an injury or disease process limits their use. In this chapter, the diagnosis and treatment of several basic hand injuries and conditions will be explored.

ANATOMY

Anatomy of the hand is more intricate than perhaps any other area of the musculoskeletal system. Knowing the anatomy is fundamental to understanding the basic hand function and to diagnosing dysfunction when evaluating a patient with a hand injury in the clinic or emergency department setting.

BONE AND LIGAMENT

Carpus

The carpus is composed of eight bones that are organized in two rows of four. The proximal row includes the scaphoid (navicular), lunate, triquetrum, and pisiform (Fig. 15.1). Each of these bones has characteristic features that assist in its radiographic identification. The scaphoid is boat-shaped and has a prominent tubercle distally. The lunate is moon-shaped and has been classified into two types. A type I lunate (30% of patients) does not articulate with the hamate, whereas a type II lunate (70% of patients) has a medial facet that articulates with the proximal hamate and increases the risk of potential hamate arthrosis. The triquetrum is pyramidal in shape. Last, the pisiform is a small round sesamoid bone that sits on the volar surface of the triquetrum and is contained within the flexor carpi ulnaris (FCU) tendon. Collectively, the proximal row is referred to as the *intercalary* segment because it connects the forearm to the distal carpal row and is not controlled by any musculotendinous structures.

The distal carpal row is made up by the trapezium, trapezoid, capitate, and hamate. The trapezium is four-sided and sits at the base of the thumb metacarpal (TM). The trapezoid is wedge-shaped and is the smallest bone of the distal row. The capitate is the largest carpal bone and has a rounded portion that articulates with the scaphoid and lunate. The hamate is also wedge-shaped and has a hook-like process on its volar surface known as the *hamulus* or *hook of the hamate.*

The carpal bones are stabilized by numerous ligaments, which can be divided into intrinsic and extrinsic. In the proximal row, the two most important intrinsic ligaments are the scapholunate and the lunotriquetral. They stabilize their respective bony structures but also allow for small amounts of rotational motion between them.

The most important of the extrinsic ligaments of the proximal row are the volar ligaments and include the radio–scaphoid–capitate, long radiolunate, and short radiolunate (Fig. 15.2A). These ligaments are thickenings of the joint capsule and serve to anchor the proximal row to the distal radius and ulna. While these ligaments stabilize the radiocarpal joint radially, the ulnocarpal ligaments (including the ulnolunate, ulnotriquetral, and ulnocapitate) provide support ulnarly.

The most important dorsal ligaments are the dorsal transverse intercarpal, which runs from the scaphoid to the triquetrum, and the dorsal radiocarpal ligament, which connects the radius to the triquetrum. These two ligaments form a "V" with the apex of the "V" directed ulnarly (Fig. 15.2B).

The radiocarpal joint is composed of the distal radius and proximal carpal row. The distal radius has a separate

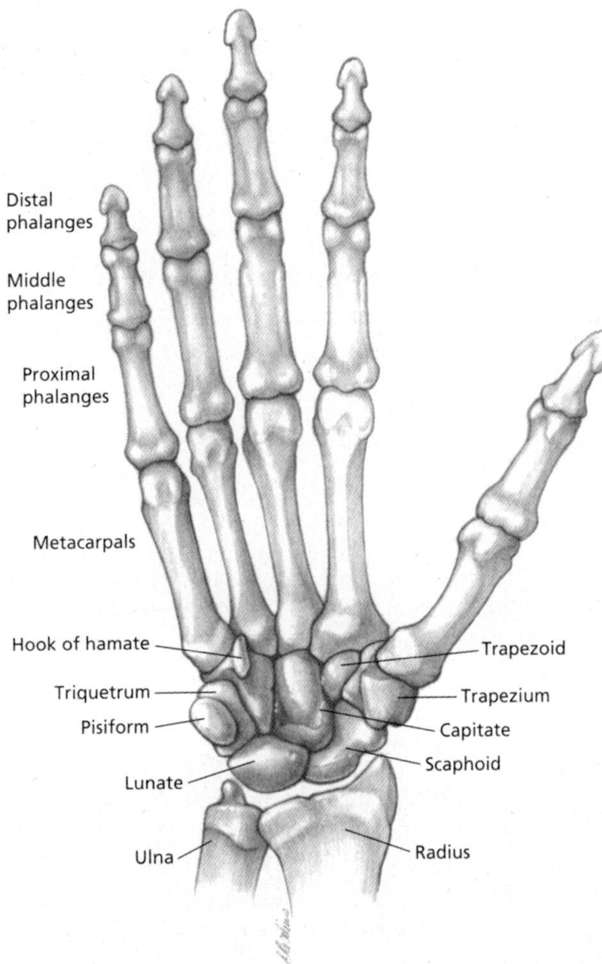

Figure 15.1 Bony anatomy of the hand and wrist. (*Reprinted with permission from* Doyle JR, Botte MJ. *Surgical Anatomy of the Hand and Upper Extremity.* Philadelphia, PA: Lippincott Williams & Wilkins, 2003.)

facet for articulation with both the scaphoid and lunate. The distal radius is tilted volarly at an angle of approximately 11 degrees (Fig. 15.3). Its angle of inclination is roughly 22 degrees, whereas its height is approximately 11 mm relative to its most ulnar surface. The mnemonic "11–22–11" can be useful for remembering these relationships, which are important in evaluating distal radius fractures.

The distal radioulnar joint (DRUJ) is the last articulation in the radiocarpal region that merits attention. The distal ulna is divided into two separate articular surfaces: the *ulnar seat,* which abuts the sigmoid notch, and the *ulnar pole,* which faces the carpus. The ulnar seat is surrounded by a 105-degree arc of articular cartilage, which corresponds to a 10 mm radius of curvature. This radius of curvature of the ulnar seat is substantially less than that of the sigmoid notch, which is 15 mm and corresponds to an arc of curvature of approximately 60 degrees. Therefore, the DRUJ is not congruent. This incongruency enables translational motion (in addition to the rotational motion) of the ulna on the radius during pronation and supination.

The ulnar pole and DRUJ are surrounded by a structure called the *triangular fibrocartilage complex* (TFCC) (Fig. 15.4). The TFCC serves to stabilize the DRUJ and absorb force directed from the carpus to the ulnar pole. It is composed of the ulnotriquetral and ulnolunate ligaments, the volar and dorsal radioulnar ligaments, the ulnar collateral ligament, the subsheath of the extensor carpi ulnaris (ECU), a meniscus homolog, and an articular disk (triangular fibrocartilage).

METACARPAL AND PHALANGEAL STRUCTURES

The metacarpus is the skeletal region of the hand, bordered by the distal carpal row proximally and the phalanges distally. It consists of five elongated bones with a head, neck, body, and base area. The TM differs slightly from the others in that its epiphysis is located proximally instead of distally, and its base is saddle-shaped, which increases overall mobility. All the MC heads are cam-shaped, meaning that their diameter from palmar to dorsal is larger than from the distal head to neck junction. The metacarpophalangeal (MCP) joints are stabilized medially and laterally by radial and ulnar collateral ligaments. These ligaments start dorsally on the MC head and attach volarly on the proximal phalanx. Because of the cam shape of the MC heads, the collateral ligaments are taut in flexion and lax in extension (Fig. 15.5). In addition, the volar surface of the MCP joint contains fibrous thickenings of the joint capsule, collectively referred to as *volar plates,* which add stability to the joint and serve as restraints to hyperextension.

The phalanges articulate directly with the MC heads. Each digit is composed of three phalanges (proximal, middle, and distal) with the exception of the thumb, which has only a proximal and distal phalanx. The phalanges decrease in size as one moves from proximal to distal. Their heads are bicondylar in shape, unlike those of the aforementioned MCs. They are stabilized laterally and medially by collateral ligaments, which share the same orientation as those in the MCs.

MUSCLES AND TENDONS

Extrinsic Flexors

The flexors of the hand and wrist include the flexor carpi radialis (FCR), palmaris longus (PL), FCU, flexor pollicis longus (FPL), flexor digitorum superficialis or sublimis (FDS), and flexor digitorum profundus (FDP). The FCR originates on the medial epicondyle of the humerus and

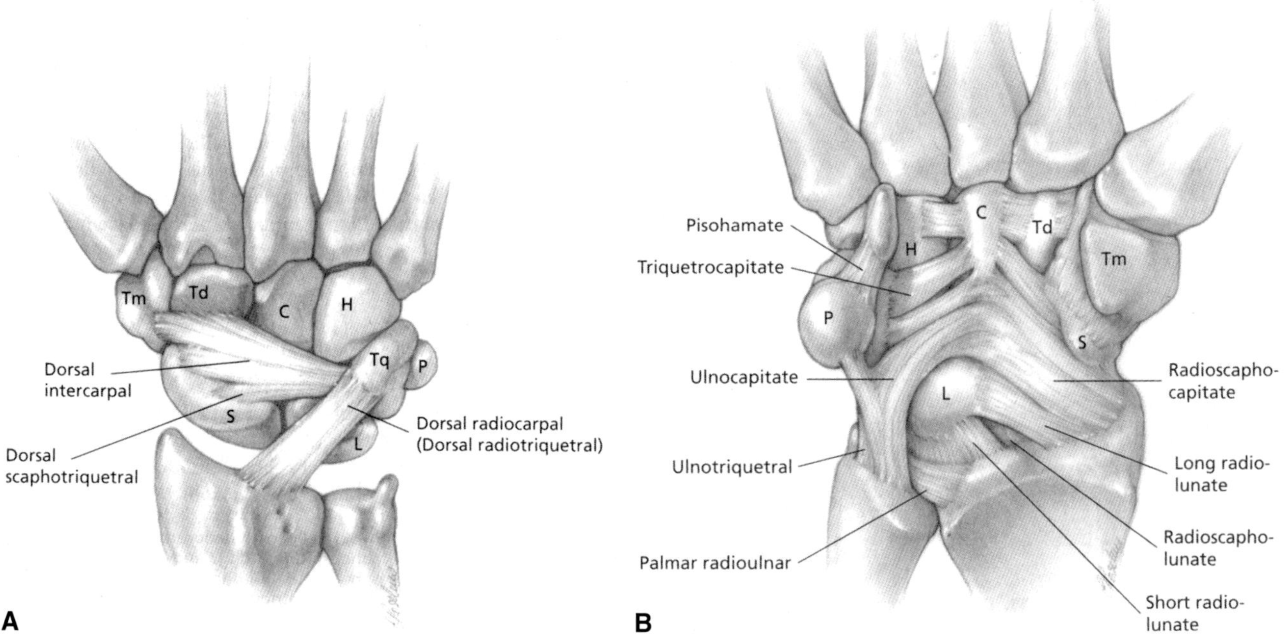

Figure 15.2 **(A)** Volar radiocarpal ligaments. **(B)** Dorsal radiocarpal ligaments. (*Reprinted with permission from* Doyle JR and Botte MJ. *Surgical Anatomy of the Hand and Upper Extremity.* Philadelphia: Lippincott Williams & Wilkins, 2003.)

inserts at the base of the second and third MCs. It helps to flex and radial deviate the wrist. Of note, it runs outside the carpal tunnel at the wrist, just superficial and radial to the median nerve. The PL originates on the medial epicondyle and inserts at the palmar aponeurosis. It is a weak wrist flexor and is absent in approximately 10% of patients. One can readily identify the PL on his or her own wrist by touching the thumb to the small finger and flexing the wrist. If present, the tendon can be visualized. The FCU originates from the medial epicondyle and posterior ulna to insert on the hook of the hamate and fifth MC base. It is the most powerful wrist flexor and helps to flex and ulnar deviate the wrist. Of note, its muscle belly extends farther distally as compared with other wrist flexors.

Regarding the finger flexors, the FPL originates on the anterior aspect of the radius and the coronoid process to insert on the distal phalanx of the thumb. It passes through the carpal tunnel and lies just radial to the median nerve. It assists in thumb flexion at the interphalangeal joint. The FDS originates on the medial epicondyle, coronoid process, and anteroproximal radius and passes through the carpal tunnel to insert on the middle phalanges of the index through small fingers. It assists in flexion of the proximal interphalangeal (PIP) joints of those digits. Of note,

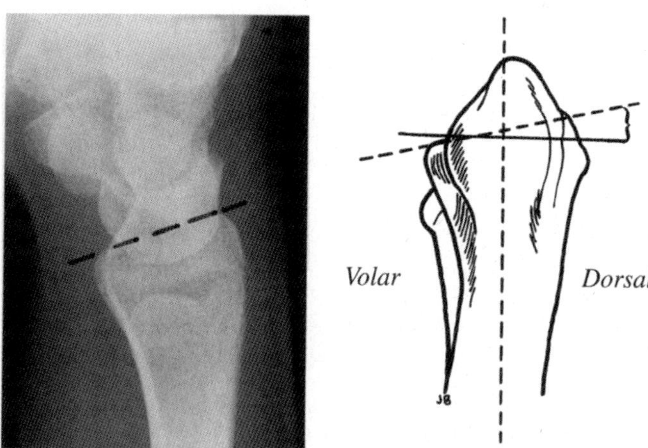

Figure 15.3 The normal volar tilt of the distal radius averages 11 degrees. (*Reprinted with permission from* Harris JH, Harris WH. *Radiology of Emergency Medicine.* 4th ed. Philadelphia, PA: Lippincott Williams & Wilkins, 2000.)

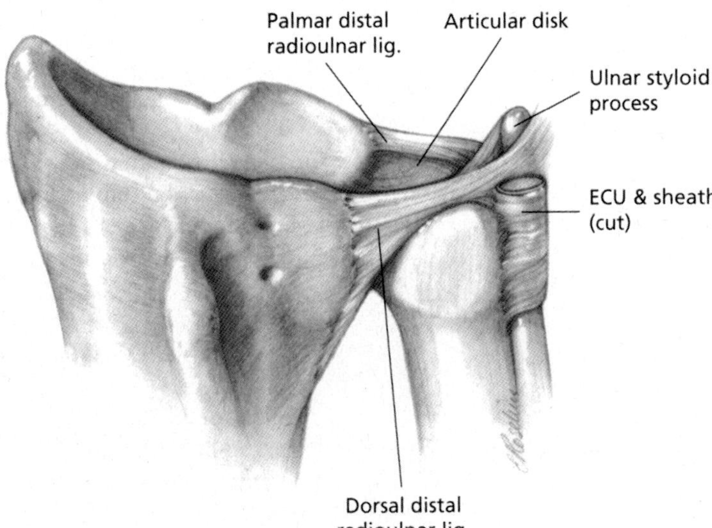

Figure 15.4 Components of the distal radioulnar joint. ECU, extensor carpi ulnaris. (*Reprinted with permission from* Doyle JR, Botte MJ. *Surgical Anatomy of the Hand and Upper Extremity.* Philadelphia, PA: Lippincott Williams & Wilkins, 2003.)

the tendons to the long and ring fingers are more superficial than those to the index and small at the level of the carpal tunnel. The FDP originates off the anterior ulna and interosseous membrane and runs through the carpal tunnel on its way to inserting on the distal phalanges of the index through small finger. It allows flexion of the distal interphalangeal (DIP) joints of all but the thumb (Fig. 15.6). The FDS and FDP tendons share a unique relationship at the level of the MP joints. In this region, which is known as *Camper chiasma,* the FDS splits into a radial and ulnar slip and inserts dorsal to the FDP on the proximal one-third of the middle phalanx. The FDP tendon runs through this

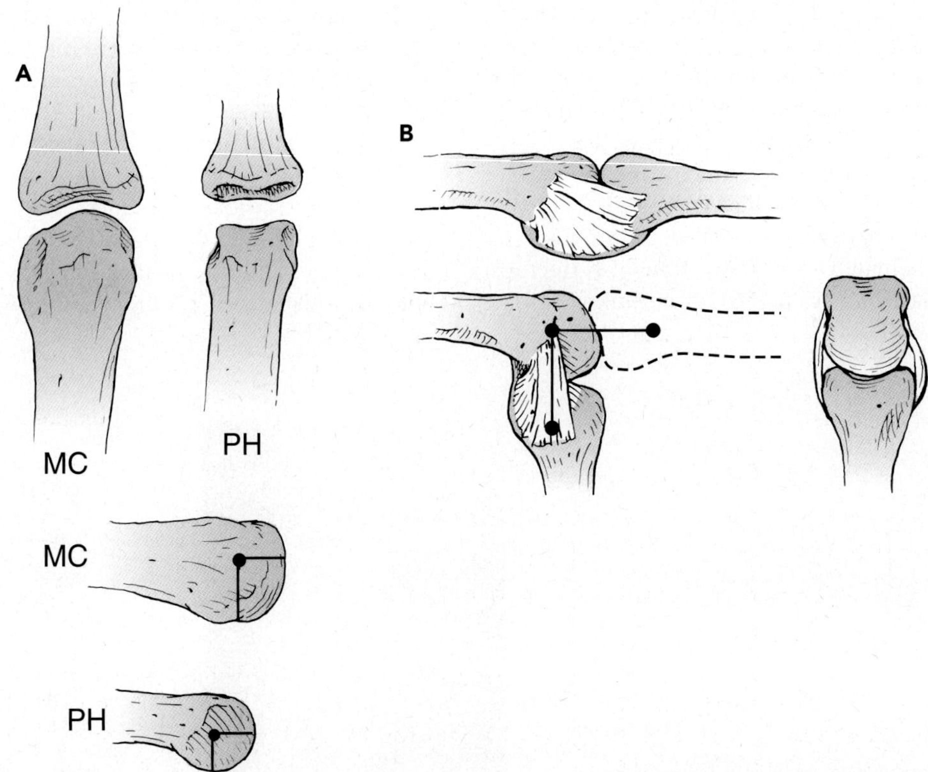

Figure 15.5 The cam shape of the metacarpal heads causes the collateral ligaments to be more taut in flexion than extension. MC, metacarpal; PH phalanx. (*Reprinted with permission from* Bucholz RW, Heckman JD, Court-Brown CM, et al. *Rockwood and Green's Fractures in Adults.* 6th ed. Philadelphia, PA: Lippincott Williams & Wilkins, 2006.)

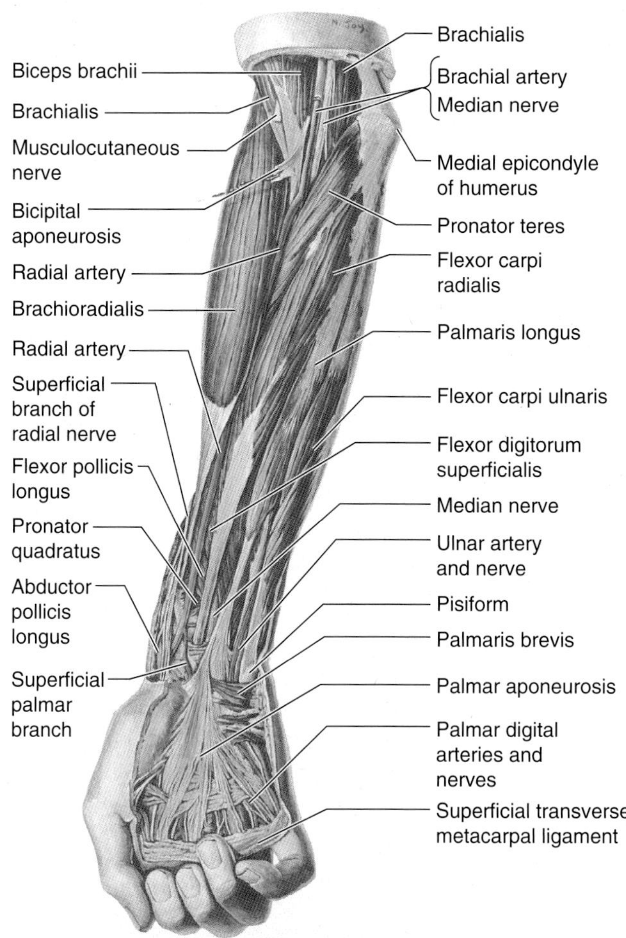

Flexor pollicis longus
Pronator quadratus
Pronator quadratus
Dorsal (cutaneous) branch
Palmar carpal branch
Dorsal carpal branch
Flexor digitorum profundus
Palmar radiocarpal branch
Persisting median artery
Median nerve
Superficial palmar branch
Palmaris longus
(B)
Flexor carpi radialis

Figure 15.6 Two views of the volar forearm, showing the relationships of the volar forearm flexors to one another and the surrounding neurovascular structures. (*Reprinted with permission from* Moore KL, Dalley AF. *Clinically Oriented Anatomy*. 4th ed. Philadelphia, PA: Lippincott Williams & Wilkins, 1999.)

split and inserts on the distal phalanx, as mentioned previously.

The flexor tendons enter fibro-osseous tunnels known as *flexor sheaths* at the level of the MCP joints. These sheaths are lined with synovium and enable the flexor tendons to glide smoothly as the finger flexes. Surrounding these sheaths are bandlike thickenings known as the *annular* and *cruciate pulleys*. There are five annular pulleys and three cruciate. The A-1 pulley is attached to a volar plate at the level of the MP joint and is often responsible for digit triggering. The A-2 and A-4 pulleys are located at the base of the proximal and middle phalanx, respectively, and are the most important mechanically due in part to their direct attachment to bone. They are essential in preventing bowstringing of the tendons. The A-3 and A-5 pulleys are found at the level of the PIP and DIP joints, respectively, and also attach to volar plates (Fig. 15.7). The three cruciate pulleys—C-1, C-2, and C-3—run between the annular pullies, providing an additional tether of the flexor sheath to the phalangeal bones. Proximal to the A-1 pulley, the flexor tendons receive their nutrition from the surrounding *paratenon*. Distal to the A-1 pulley, the flexor tendons receive their blood supply dorsally via *vinculae*, which are folds of mesotenon that run from the tendons to the bone.

The pulley system of the thumb is slightly modified due in part to its having only one flexor tendon, the FPL. In addition to the A-1 pulley at the MCP joint, there is an *oblique* pulley that lies over the proximal phalanx. Last, an A-2 pulley can be found over the IP joint. Both the A-1 and A-2 pulleys attach to volar plates as opposed to the oblique pulley, which attaches to bone.

Extrinsic Extensors

The extensors of the wrist and hand include the extensor carpi radialis longus (ECRL), extensor carpi radialis brevis (ECRB), ECU, extensor digitorum communis (EDC), extensor indicis proprius (EIP), and extensor digiti minimi (EDM) (Fig. 15.8). The extensor tendons run in six separate dorsal compartments, which are formed by the extensor retinaculum. The contents of the individual compartments are listed in Table 15.1.

The ECRL originates on the lateral aspect of the supracondylar humerus and inserts at the base of the second MC.

TABLE 15.1
EXTENSOR COMPARTMENTS OF THE WRIST

1. Abductor pollicis longus, extensor pollicis brevis
2. Extensor carpi radialis longus, extensor carpi radialis brevis
3. Extensor pollicis longus
4. Extensor digitorum communis, extensor indicis proprius
5. Extensor digiti minimi
6. Extensor carpi ulnaris

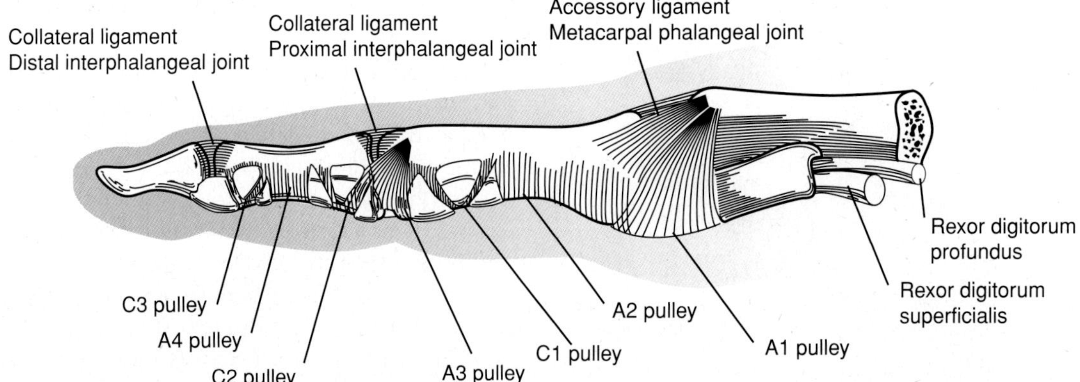

Figure 15.7 The pulley system of the finger. *(Adapted with permission from* Hoppenfeld S, deBoer P. *Surgical Exposures in Orthopaedics: The Anatomic Approach.* 3rd ed. Philadelphia, PA: Lippincott Williams & Wilkins, 2003.)

It enters the wrist as part of the second dorsal compartment along with the ECRB. It functions to extend the wrist. The ECRB originates on the lateral epicondyle of the humerus and inserts more centrally than the ECRL at the base of the third MC. In a manner similar to the ECRL, it functions to extend the wrist. The ECRB is often implicated in *lateral epicondylitis* (i.e., tennis elbow). The ECU originates on the lateral epicondyle and inserts at the base of the fifth MC. It assists in extending the hand in an ulnar direction.

The extensor mechanism of the fingers is more complex than that of the wrist. The EDC originates from the lateral epicondyle to insert on the *sagittal bands* of the extensor hood of the index through small fingers. The EIP and EDM also insert on the sagittal bands but only on the index and small fingers, respectively. These tendons lay ulnar to their respective common extensor tendon on the dorsum of the hand. The EIP originates from the posterior aspect of the ulna while the EDM originates from the lateral epicondyle. The sagittal bands are localized to the MP joint and help to centralize the extensor tendons over this region, which is collectively known as the *extensor hood*. Distal to the sagittal bands at the level of proximal phalanx, the tendons of the lumbricals and interossei insert and become part of the *lateral bands*. The extensor tendon trifurcates just distal to the MCP joint, forming a *central slip*, which inserts on the middle phalanx and two other slips, which join the lateral bands to insert on the distal phalanx. The *oblique retinacular ligament* (ligament of Landsmeer) originates volarly on the flexor sheath and attaches dorsally on the lateral terminal extensor tendon. It links motion of the DIP and PIP joints. The *transverse retinacular ligament* originates on the flexor sheath at the PIP and inserts on the lateral bands. This ligament stabilizes the lateral bands, preventing excessive dorsal migration during PIP extension and volar migration during flexion (Fig. 15.9).

The extensors of the thumb include the extensor pollicis longus (EPL), extensor pollicis brevis (EPB), and the abductor pollicis longus (APL) (Fig. 15.10). The EPL originates on the posterior ulna and inserts at the base of the distal phalanx of the thumb. If serves to extend the thumb IP joint. The EPL makes a 45-degree turn at Lister tubercle on the dorsum of the radius just after passing through the third dorsal extensor compartment of the wrist. It is the most common tendon rupture associated with a distal radius fracture. The EPB originates on the posterior radius and inserts at the base of the proximal phalanx of the thumb. It extends the thumb at the carpometacarpal (CMC) joint. The APL originates on the posterior aspect of the radius and ulna, and together with the EPB, courses through the first dorsal extensor compartment before inserting at the base of the first MC. It abducts and extends the thumb at the CMC joint.

INTRINSIC HAND MUSCLES

The intrinsic muscles in the hand are termed *intrinsic* because they both originate and insert on the hand (Fig. 15.11). They can be divided into four groups: lumbricals, interossei, thenar, and hypothenar. The lumbricals originate on the FDP tendons and insert on the *radial aspect of the lateral bands*, which are part of the extensor hood. The muscle bellies of the lumbricals of the index, and long finger are *unipennate*, whereas those of the ring and small fingers are *bipennate*. They function to extend the PIP joints and flex the MCP joints. Lumbricals are unique in that they insert on their own antagonist (i.e., the termination of the extensor tendons, which extend the MCP joints). The two most radial lumbricals are innervated by the median nerve, whereas the two ulnar lumbricals are innervated by the ulnar nerve.

There are seven interosseus muscles: three volar and four dorsal. The volar interossei originate on the ulnar side of the index finger MC and the radial side of the ring and small finger MC to insert at the base of the proximal phalanx and extensor hood. They are unipennate and assist in digit adduction. The dorsal interossei originate from the thumb to small finger MC to insert in the same location

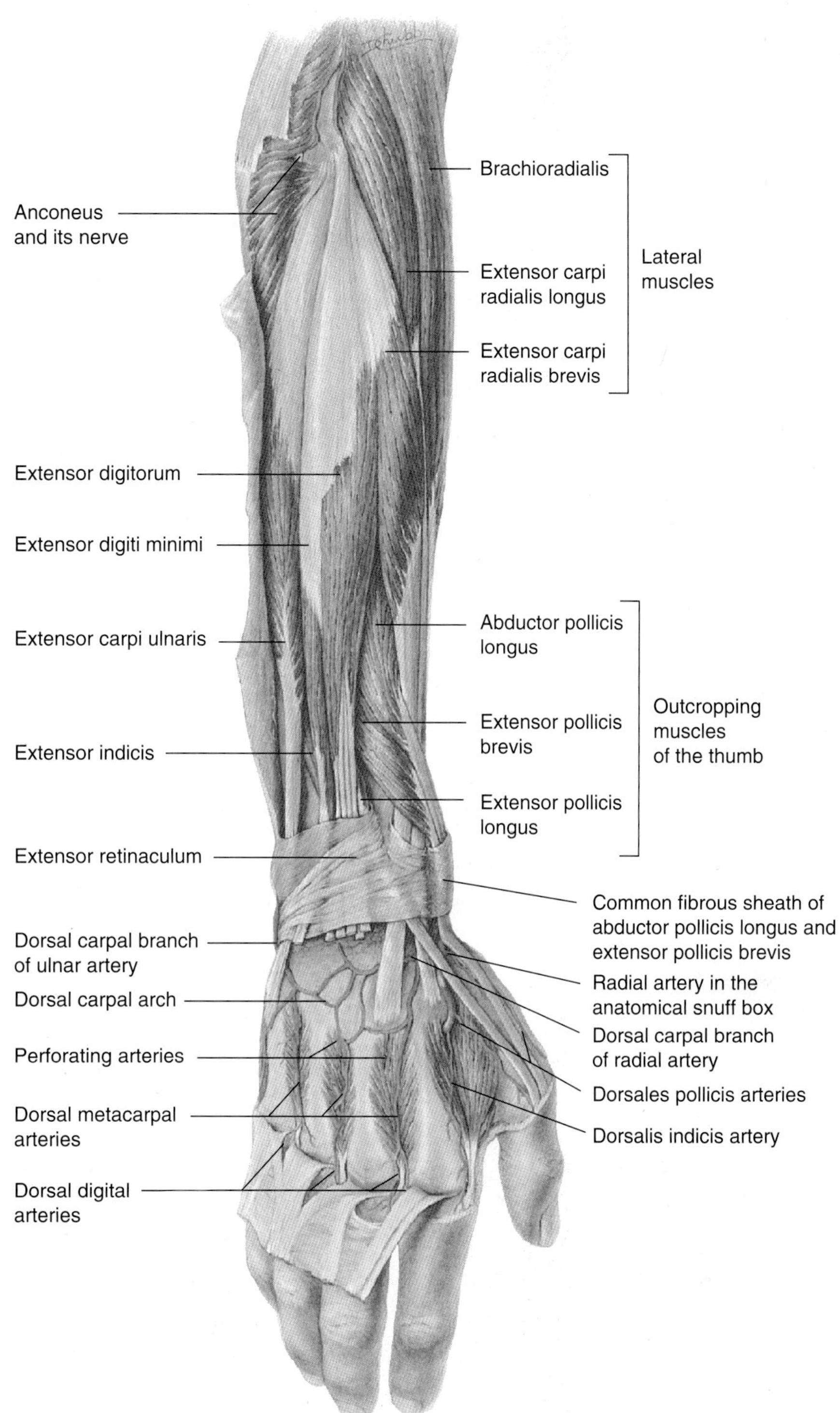

Figure 15.8 Illustration demonstrating the muscles of the extensor compartment of the forearm and hand. (*Reprinted with permission from* Moore KL, Dalley AF. *Clinically Oriented Anatomy*. 4th ed. Philadelphia, PA: Lippincott Williams & Wilkins, 1999.)

as their volar counterparts. However, they are all bipennate muscles and assist in digit abduction. Both groups of interossei are innervated by the ulnar nerve. In addition, they both help the lumbricals with MCP flexion and IP extension.

The thenar muscles are composed of the abductor pollicis brevis (APB), flexor pollicis brevis (FPB), and opponens pollicis (OP). The APB originates on the scaphoid and trapezium to insert at the lateral aspect of the proximal phalanx of the thumb. It is innervated by the *recurrent branch of the median nerve* and serves to abduct the thumb. The FPB originates on the trapezium to insert at the base of the proximal phalanx of the thumb. It has two heads: superficial and deep. The superficial head is innervated by the recurrent branch of the median, whereas the deep head is innervated by the ulnar nerve. It aids thumb MCP flexion.

Deep to these muscles, the OP originates on the trapezium to insert on the lateral aspect of the thumb MC. It is innervated by the recurrent branch of the median nerve and serves to flex and medially rotate the TM.

The adductor pollicis (AP) muscle is composed of an oblique and transverse head. The oblique head originates from the capitate and base of the index and middle MC, whereas the transverse head originates from the distal third of the index MC. Both heads insert on the base of the proximal phalanx of the thumb. The AP assists in thumb adduction and is ulnarly innervated.

The hypothenar muscles include the palmaris brevis (PB), abductor digiti minimi (ADM), flexor digiti minimi brevis (FDMB), and opponens digiti minimi (ODM). The PB originates on the transverse carpal ligament (TCL) and inserts on the undersurface of the medial palm epidermis. It is innervated by the superficial branch of the ulnar nerve and wrinkles the skin on the medial palm. The ADM originates on the pisiform to insert on the base of the small finger proximal phalanx. It assists with small finger abduction. The FDMB originates on the hamate and TCL to insert at the base of the small finger proximal phalanx. It assists with small finger MCP flexion. Deep to these muscles, the ODM originates on the hamate and TCL to insert on the medial side of the small finger MC. It flexes the small finger MC and rotates it laterally. All of the hypothenar muscles, except for the PB, are innervated by the deep branch of the ulnar nerve.

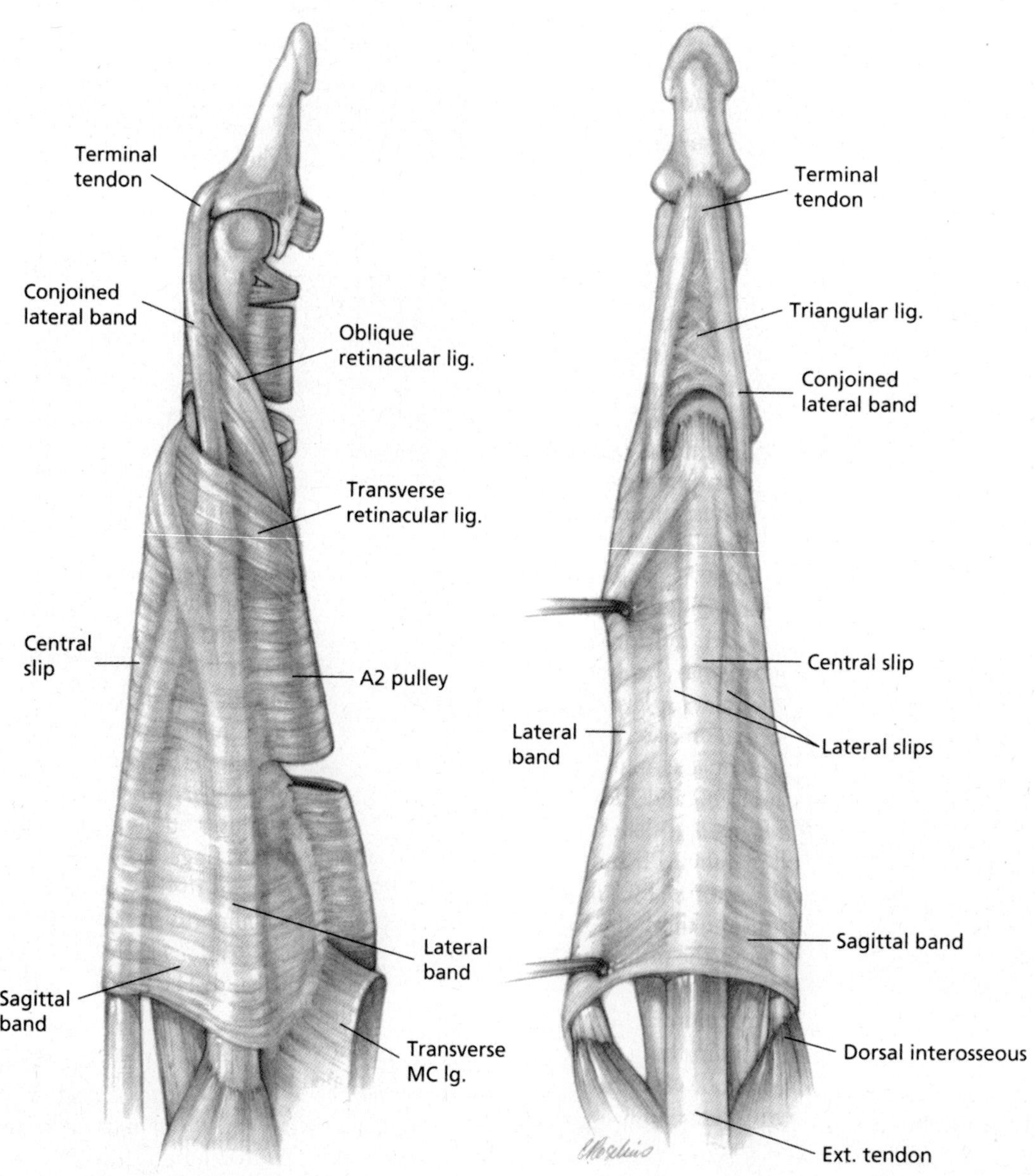

Figure 15.9 The extensor mechanism of the finger. (*Reprinted with permission from* Doyle JR and Botte MJ: *Surgical Anatomy of the Hand and Upper Extremity.* Philadelphia: Lippincott Williams & Wilkins, 2003.)

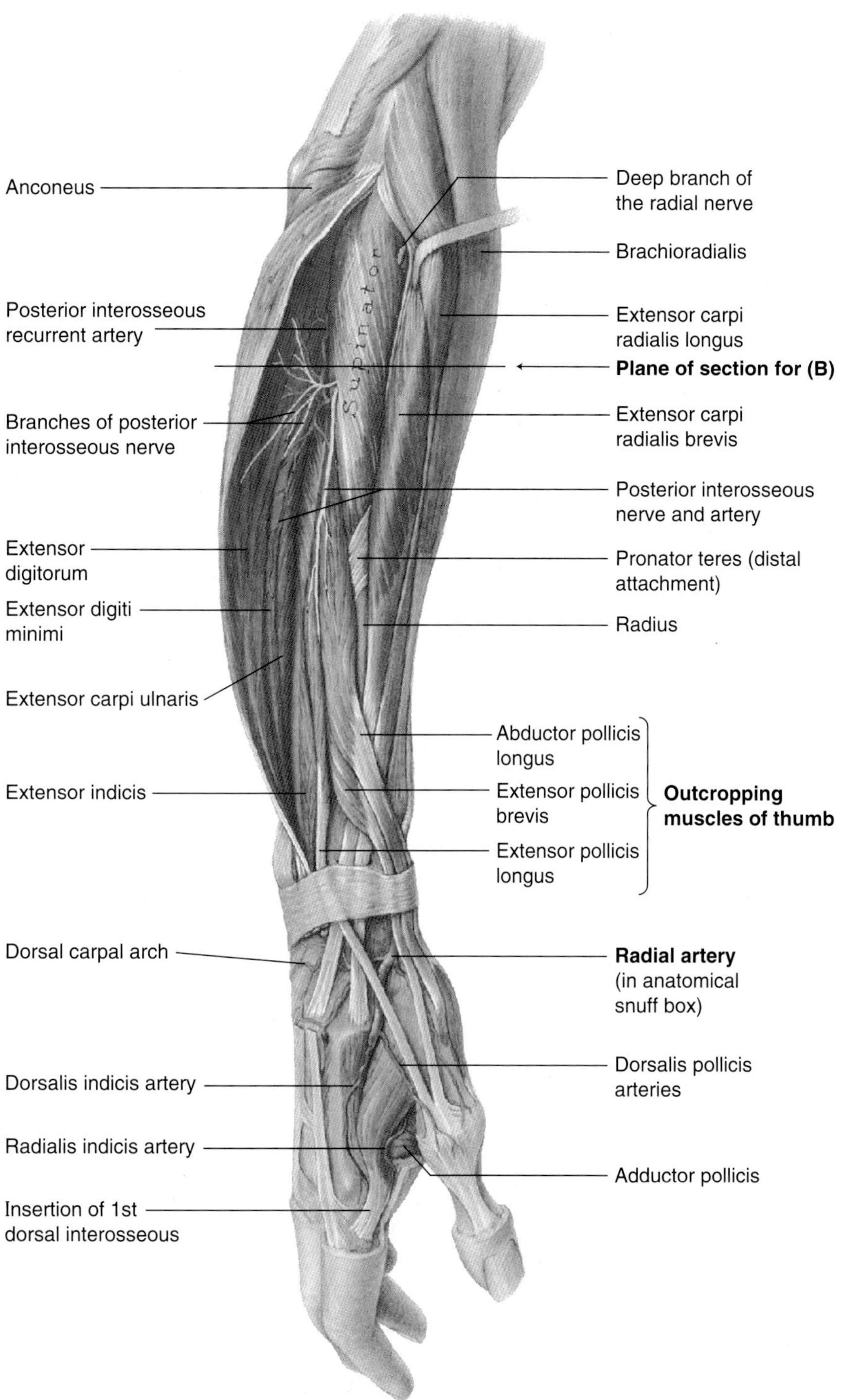

Figure 15.10 Deep musculature of the extensor compartment of the forearm. (*Reprinted with permission from* Moore KL, Dalley AF. *Clinically Oriented Anatomy*. 4th ed. Philadelphia, PA: Lippincott Williams & Wilkins, 1999.)

VASCULAR

The main blood supply to wrist and hand is via the radial and ulnar arteries, which are terminal branches of the brachial artery (Fig. 15.12). The ulnar artery, which is slightly larger than its radial counterpart, starts in proximal forearm, running on top of FDP and beneath both FDS and FCU. As it travels more distal, the ulnar artery is located just radial to ulnar nerve. After traversing the TCL, it enters the Guyon canal. At this point, it gives off three branches—the palmar carpal branch, dorsal carpal branch, and deep palmar branch—before terminating in the hand as the superficial palmar arch. The deep palmar branch anastomoses with the radial artery to complete the deep palmar arch (see Fig. 15.12).

The radial artery is located just lateral to the FCR tendon from the proximal forearm to the radiocarpal joint, where it gives off three branches—palmar carpal branch, dorsal

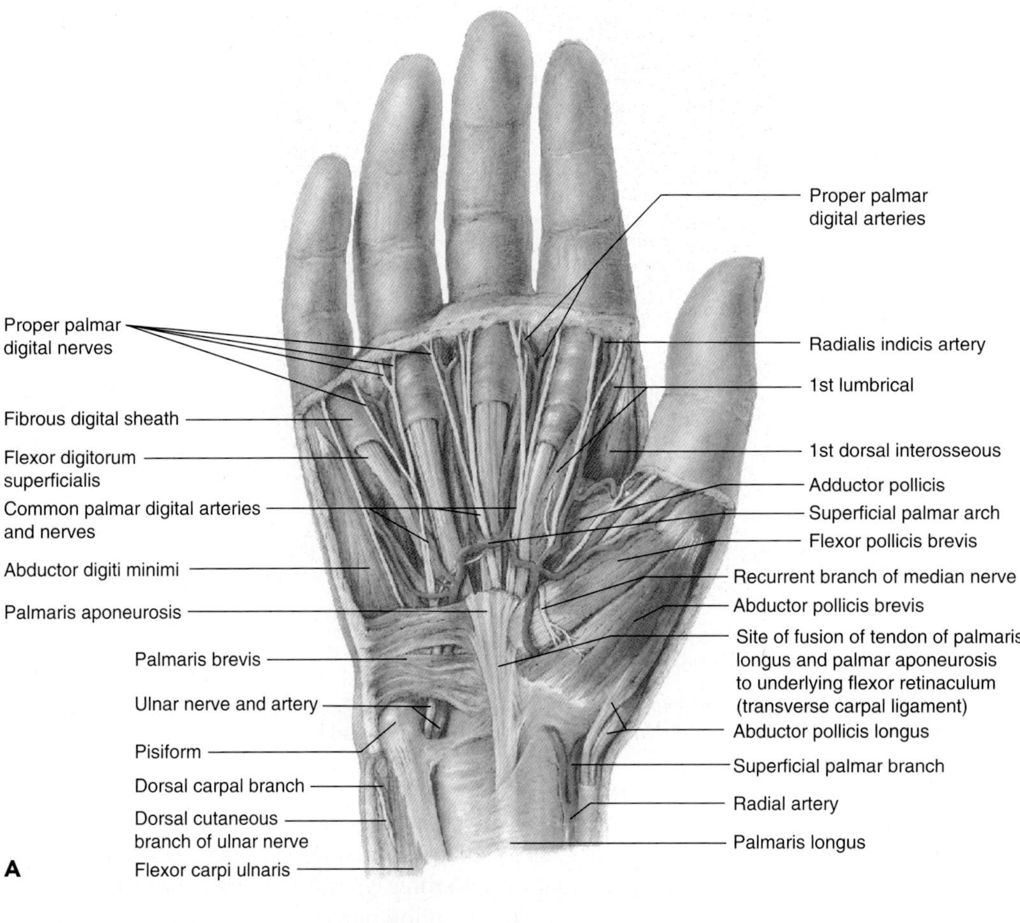

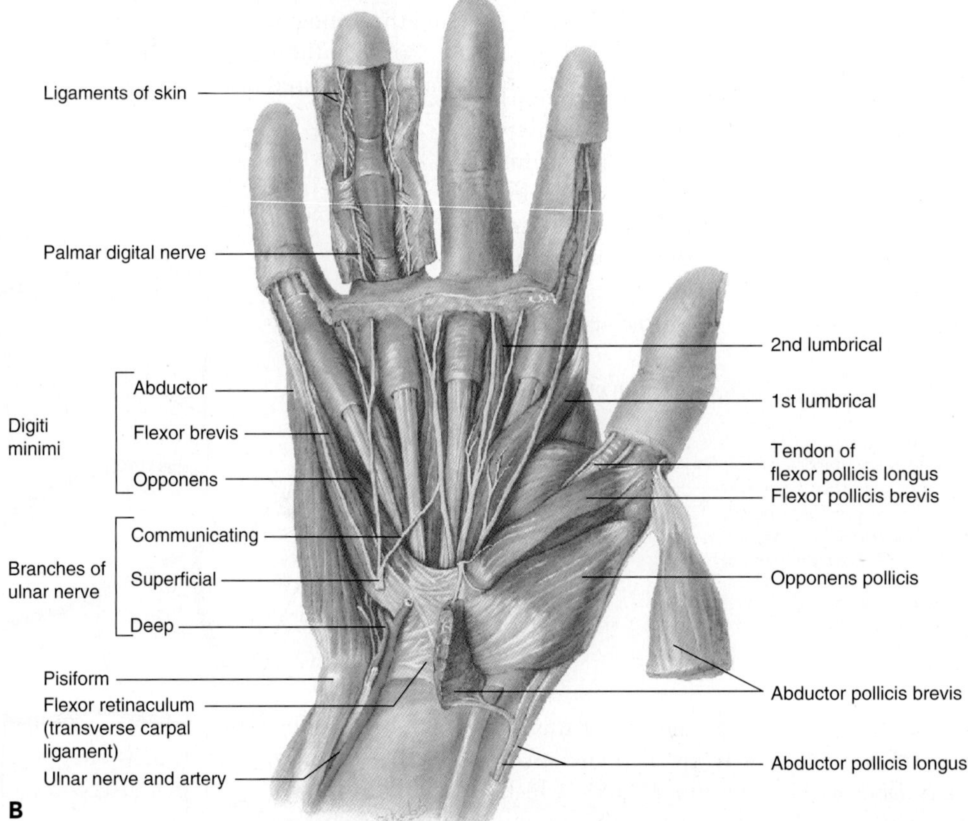

Figure 15.11 The superficial **(A)** and deep **(B)** intrinsic hand muscles. (*Reprinted with permission from* Moore KL, Dalley AF. *Clinically Oriented Anatomy*. 4th ed. Philadelphia, PA: Lippincott Williams & Wilkins, 1999.)

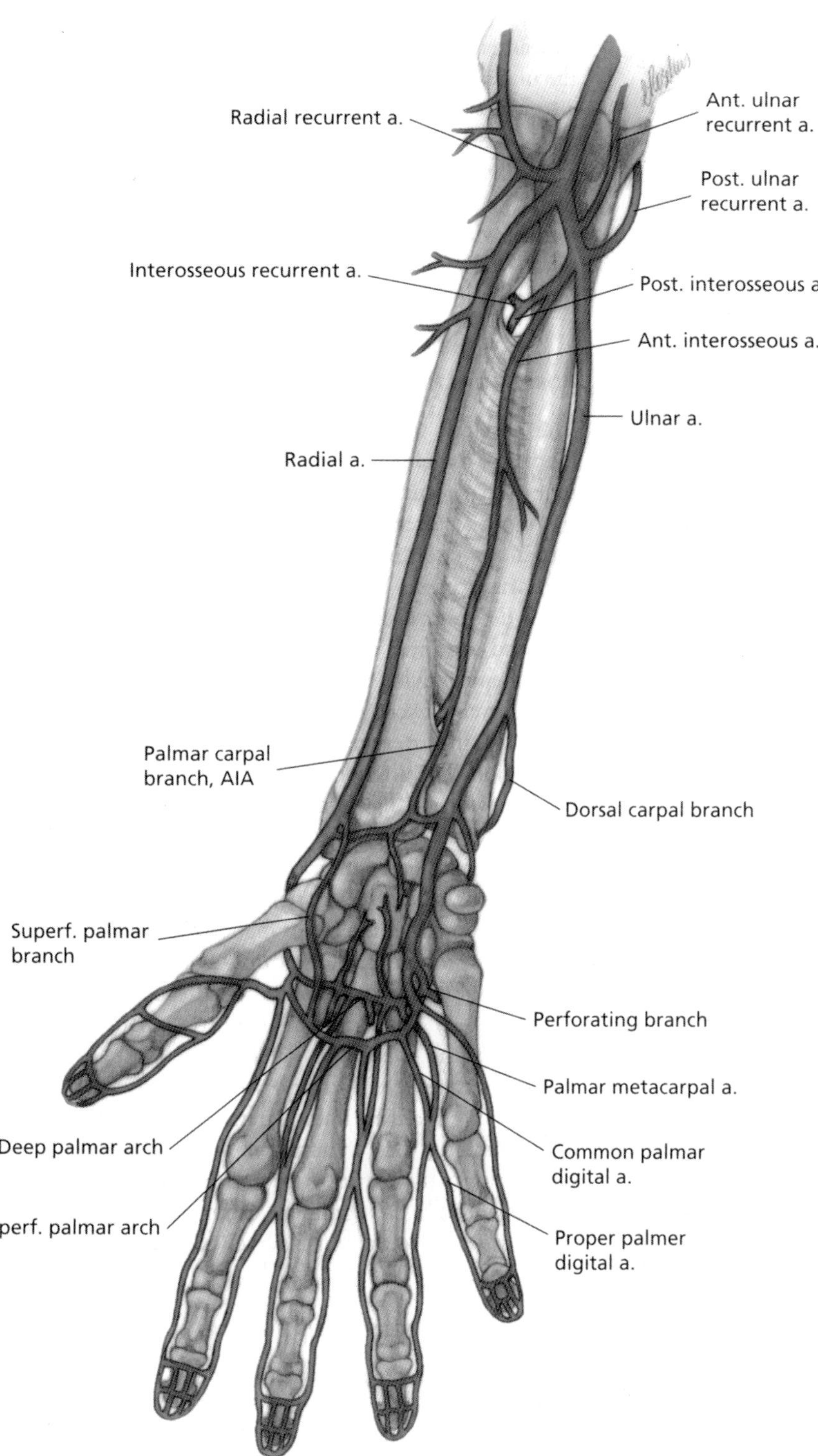

Figure 15.12 Blood supply to palmar forearm and hand. (*Reprinted with permission from* Doyle JR, Botte MJ. *Surgical Anatomy of the Hand and Upper Extremity.* Philadelphia, PA: Lippincott Williams & Wilkins, 2003.)

carpal branch, and a superficial palmar branch. The superficial palmar branch anastomoses with the ulnar artery to complete the superficial palmar arch. The radial artery continues dorsally under the APL and EPB tendons as it enters the anatomic snuffbox. After passing through the snuffbox, it dives between the heads of the first dorsal interosseus muscle and gives off two additional branches: the princeps pollicis, which supplies the thumb, and the radialis indicis artery, which supplies the radial index finger. The remainder of the radial artery terminates into the deep palmar arch.

The deep arch gives off three palmar MC arteries and the superficial arch gives off three common palmar digital arteries. The palmar MC arteries join the common palmar

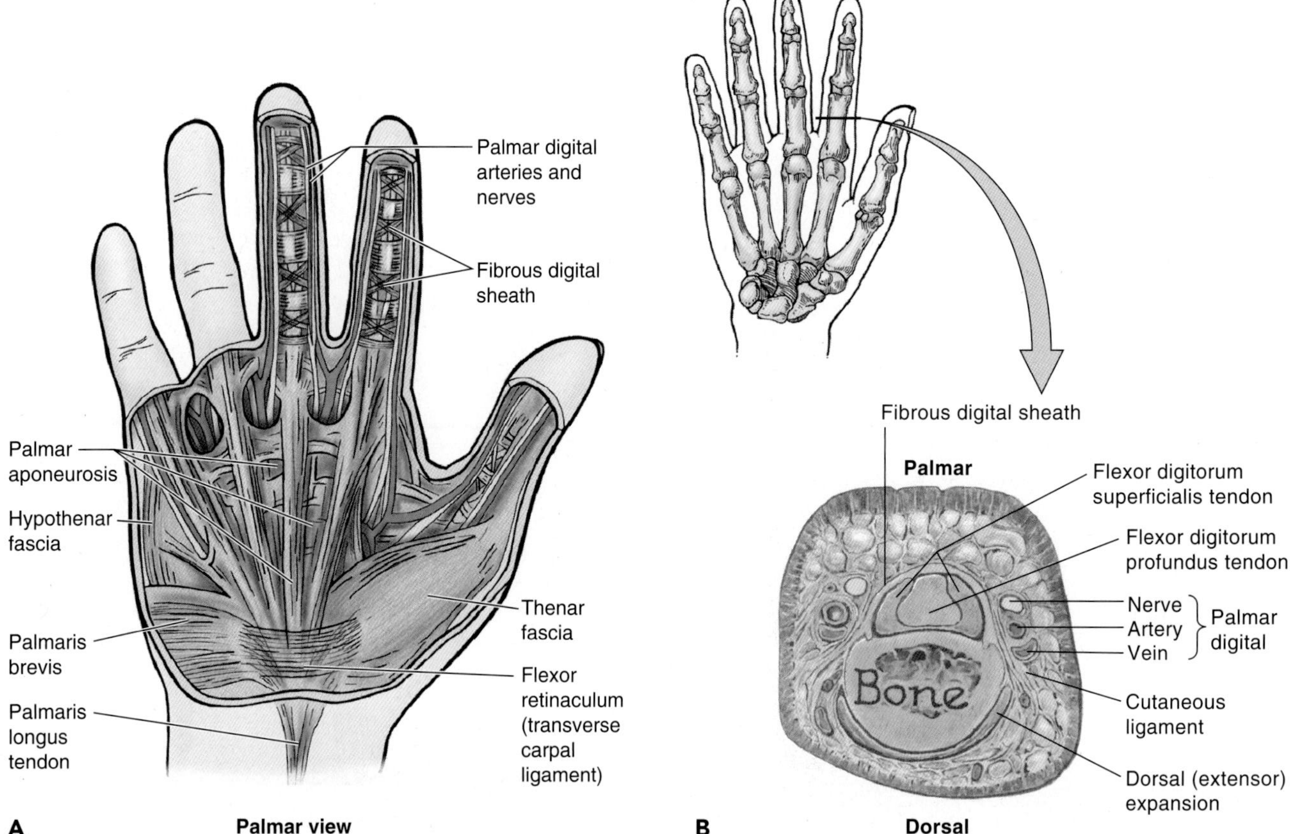

Figure 15.13 Cross section of a finger showing the relationships between the tendons and surrounding neurovascular structures. (*Reprinted with permission from* Moore KL, Dalley AF. *Clinically Oriented Anatomy*. 4th ed. Philadelphia, PA: Lippincott Williams & Wilkins, 1999.)

digital arteries, which subsequently bifurcate to form the proper palmar digital arteries. It is important to note that the proper palmar digital arteries lies at the periphery, not the center, of the fingers.

One last take-home point regarding the vasculature of the fingers is that, unlike in the palm, the arteries lie deep to the nerves. The latter has implications for identifying nerve injuries in patients with finger lacerations, for if one determines an artery has been severed, then nerve injury should be suspected (Fig. 15.13).

NERVE ANATOMY

The three main nerves that supply the hand are the ulnar, median, and radial. The ulnar nerve enters the forearm after emerging from the medial epicondylar groove and piercing the two heads of the FCU. It runs down the length of the forearm, just radial to the ulnar artery. Before reaching the radiocarpal joint, it gives off dorsal and palmar sensory branches. After entering the Guyon canal, it divides into a superficial and deep branch. The superficial branch turns into the proper digital nerves to the small finger and ulnar aspect of the ring finger, while the deep branch provides motor innervation to all intrinsic muscles not innervated by the median nerve.

The median nerve enters the forearm between the two heads of the pronator teres and quickly dives beneath the FDS throughout the length of the forearm. Just before entering the carpal tunnel at the wrist crease, it gives off a *palmar cutaneous branch,* which supplies sensation to the thenar eminence. The rest of the median nerve courses through the carpal tunnel and forms a *recurrent branch,* which supplies motor to the thenar muscles. It is important to note that the recurrent motor branch is formed *before* entering the carpal tunnel in some individuals and that there can be some anatomic variability. The remainder of the median nerve terminates in digital sensory nerves, which supply the dorsal distal phalanges of the thumb, index, long, and radial half of the ring finger and the palmar thumb through radial half of the ring finger.

The radial nerve divides into the superficial and deep radial nerve, which becomes the posterior interosseus nerve, just proximal to the lateral epicondyle of the humerus. The superficial radial nerve runs just beneath the brachioradialis throughout the length of the forearm before emerging

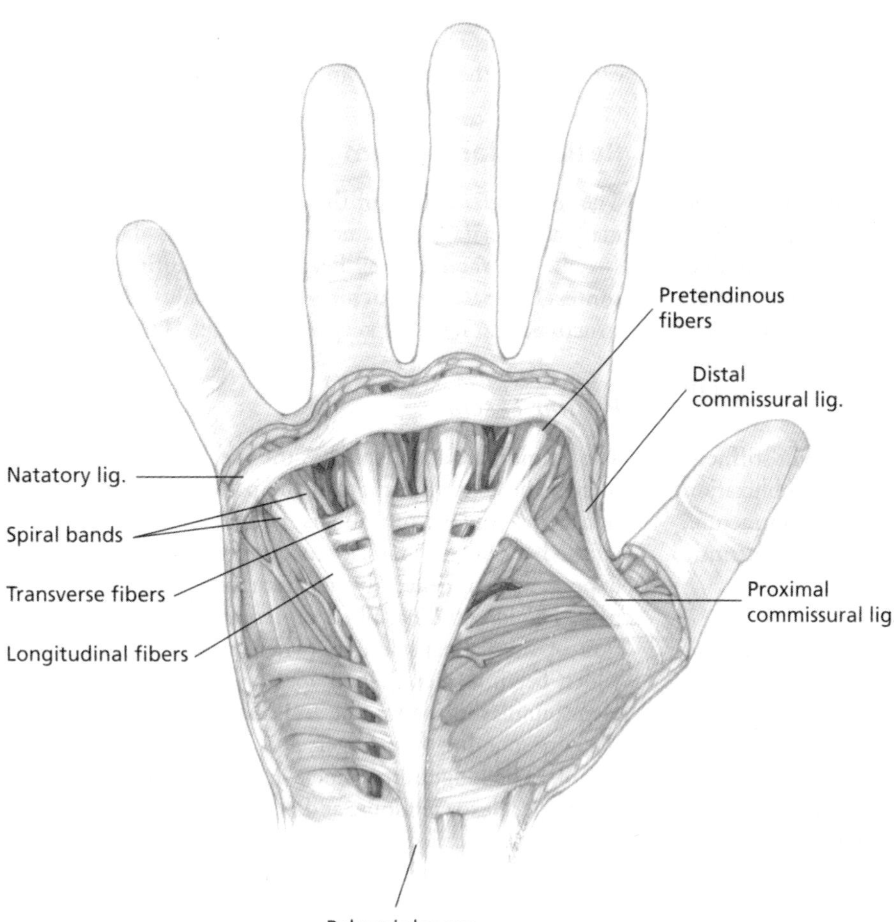

Figure 15.14 The relationship of Grayson and Cleland ligaments to the neurovascular bundle. NV, neurovascular; MC, metacarpal; PA, palmar aponeurosis. (*Reprinted with permission from* Doyle JR, Botte MJ. *Surgical Anatomy of the Hand and Upper Extremity.* Philadelphia, PA: Lippincott Williams & Wilkins, 2003.)

more superficially a few centimeters proximal to the extensor retinaculum. The superficial radial nerve is purely sensory in function and provides sensation to the dorsum of both the wrist and the proximal half of the following digits: thumb, index, long finger, and radial half of the ring finger.

The digital nerves lie volarly and at the periphery of the digits. As mentioned previously, they are superficial to the digital arteries. The neurovascular bundle is protected by two thickened ligaments—*Grayson and Cleland ligaments*—which are located volarly and dorsally, respectively. The digital arteries and nerves are protected by these ligaments (see Figs. 15.13 and 15.14).

PATIENT EVALUATION

History

The key to diagnosing any hand pathology begins with a well-taken history. One should begin by obtaining the patient's age, handedness, mode of employment, and exploring his or her chief complaint. Typically, a patient will complain of pain in a specific area of the hand. A good strategy is to have the patient localize the pain by having him or her point with one finger to the area of maximal tenderness. The examiner should then ask the typical pain evaluation questions, which include the following: When did the pain start? Was there an initial trauma? What aggravates it? What makes it better? One should inquire about a recent travel history or exposures and any relevant medical history such as rheumatoid arthritis (RA) or diabetes. The answers to these questions can steer the physician toward the correct diagnosis. For instance, golfers and baseball players are prone to hook of the hamate fractures so knowing that a patient has had ulnar-sided pain in the palm region since a golf outing a few days prior can assist one in making this diagnosis. One should also inquire whether the patient is involved in worker's compensation for this injury, as this patient population has been shown to have unique outcomes.

Physical Examination

As in any medical field, the physical examination of the hand should begin with inspection. Once inspection is complete, one should proceed with palpation and range of motion of all joints of the hand, especially the area of maximal tenderness. Radial pulse and capillary refill time should be explored. Motor and sensory function of the median, ulnar, and radial nerve should be tested. Grip and pinch strength can also be quantified.

Radiographic Evaluation

Radiographically, the initial investigation begins with plain radiographs showing three views of the hand and/or finger (anteroposterior or posteroanterior [PA], lateral, oblique) depending on the circumstances. Occasionally, a special view may be requested depending on the patient's symptomatology and the suspected diagnosis. For example, if the clinician is worried about a hook of the hamate fracture, he or she might request a *carpal tunnel view*, which provides a better view of the hook itself. Another important additional view is the *scaphoid view*, which is shot with the wrist in ulnar deviation. Ulnar deviation causes scaphoid to extend, which places it in the plane of the radius, making it easier to evaluate for fracture.

More sophisticated imaging may be necessary for certain types of suspected injuries. For example, a patient with unexplained anatomic snuffbox tenderness 2 weeks after a fall onto an outstretched hand might merit a magnetic resonance imaging (MRI) scan to rule out a scaphoid fracture. MRI can also be useful for evaluation of TFCC tears, scapholunate ligament disruption, or suspected avascular necrosis of a carpal bone. CT scan can be useful for evaluating bone injuries such as intraarticular distal radius fractures or hook of the hamate fractures.

TRAUMATIC INJURIES TO THE HAND AND WRIST

The hand is a frequent recipient of trauma. Fractures of the bones in the hand are among the most common in the body. Because our hands are essential to many of our everyday activities, deformity or loss of function is not well tolerated.

FRACTURES AND DISLOCATIONS

Distal Phalangeal Fractures

The distal phalanx is one of the most frequently fractured bones in the body.

Classification

Distal phalanx fractures are classified on the basis of location, into three types: tuft, shaft, and intraarticular.

Mechanism of Injury

Fractures of the distal phalanx are generally the result of a crush injury.

Presentation and Physical Examination

Patients typically complain of pain and swelling over the distal phalanx after trauma to the finger. On examination, the patient will have tenderness over the distal phalanx and may have a concomitant nail bed injury. If the fracture is intraarticular, the patient may not be able to actively flex or extend the DIP.

Radiographic Findings/Special Studies

Plain anteroposterior, lateral, and oblique radiographs of the finger will demonstrate a visible fracture line.

Treatment

Treatment varies depending on the type of distal phalanx fracture. Because of their surrounding soft tissue envelope, tuft fractures are usually stable and can be treated nonoperatively with an aluminum finger splint. However, soft tissue injury can often be a concern with these injuries, especially damage to the underlying nail bed. Classically, the teaching is that if there is a subungual hematoma involving greater than 50% of the nail bed, the physician should remove the nail plate and repair the sterile matrix, although this issue remains controversial.

Distal phalangeal shaft fractures can usually be treated nonoperatively with aluminum splinting unless they are significantly displaced or unstable, in which case they may require percutaneous pinning (Fig. 15.15). Beware of distal phalangeal shaft fractures in children who go through the physis (Salter I fractures), known as *Seymour fractures*. These are often associated with open nail bed injuries and are susceptible to infection if missed.

Distal phalanx intraarticular fractures are more difficult to treat and may require operative fixation if the fracture fragment is large or if it is attached to either the FDP or terminal extensor tendon. When the terminal extensor

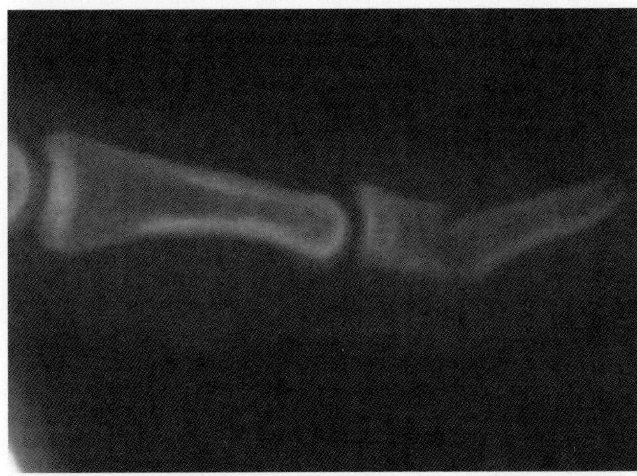

Figure 15.15 Distal phalanx fracture. (*Reprinted with permission from* Bucholz RW, Heckman JD, Court-Brown CM, et al. *Rockwood and Green's Fractures in Adults*. 6th ed. Philadelphia, PA: Lippincott Williams & Wilkins, 2006.)

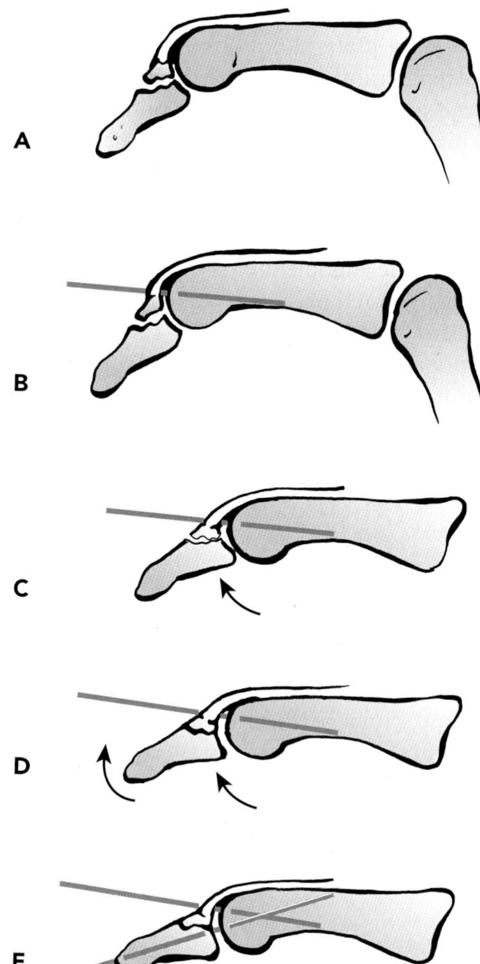

Figure 15.16 **(A–E)** Technique of extension block pinning. (*Reprinted with permission from* Bucholz RW, Heckman JD, Court-Brown CM, et al. *Rockwood and Green's Fractures in Adults.* 6th ed. Philadelphia, PA: Lippincott Williams & Wilkins, 2006.)

tendon is attached to the avulsed fragment, the injury is often referred to as a *bony mallet finger*. This injury frequently requires closed reduction and percutaneous pinning, especially if greater than 50% of the joint surface is involved or there is DIP joint subluxation (Fig. 15.16). The majority of injuries that involve an FDP avulsion fracture have to be repaired surgically to restore the flexion mechanism of the finger.

Proximal and Middle Phalangeal Fractures

Fractures of the proximal and middle phalanx are also common.

Classification

Fractures of the proximal and middle phalanx can be divided into the following types based on anatomic location: base, shaft, neck, and condylar (Fig. 15.17)

Mechanism of Injury

The typical mechanisms are crush injury and axial load.

Presentation and Physical Examination

The patient typically complains of pain and swelling over the affected phalanx after a traumatic event. On examination, the patient will have tenderness and swelling over the affected phalanx with decreased range of motion.

Radiographic Findings/Special Studies

Plain PA, lateral, and oblique radiographs of the hand will demonstrate a visible fracture line.

Treatment

Nondisplaced or even minimally displaced fractures can be treated nonoperatively with buddy tape, aluminum splinting, or even casting. If a cast or splint is applied, one must keep the wrist in 20 degrees of extension with fingers in intrinsic plus position (i.e., MCP joints flexed with IP joints in full extension). This position prevents the MCP collateral ligaments (due to the CAM effect of the MC heads) and IP volar plates from shortening. Fractures that are more severely displaced, rotated, comminuted, or display more than 10 to 20 angulation in any plane often require operative fixation. They can be stabilized with screws, Kirshner wires, plates, or external fixation.

Phalangeal Dislocations

Classification

Phalangeal dislocations are classified as dorsal, volar, rotatory, or lateral.

Mechanism of Injury

These injuries are commonly the result of an axial load to an extended digit.

Presentation and Physical Examination

The patient will often complain of pain and difficulty moving the involved joint.

The patient will have tenderness over affected joint, an obvious deformity, and reduced active and passive motion of the joint.

Radiographic Findings/Special Studies

Plain anteroposterior, lateral, and oblique radiographs of the involved finger will demonstrate dorsal, volar, or lateral dislocation of the more distal phalanx relative to the more proximal phalanx (or MC).

Treatment

DIP dislocations are commonly dorsal and easily reduced. PIP dislocations can be volar, dorsal, or lateral and are also easily reduced, usually with a maneuver consisting of gentle traction and volar or dorsal pressure on the middle phalanx (Fig. 15.18). Rotational PIP dislocations can be irreducible by closed methods and may require surgical intervention.

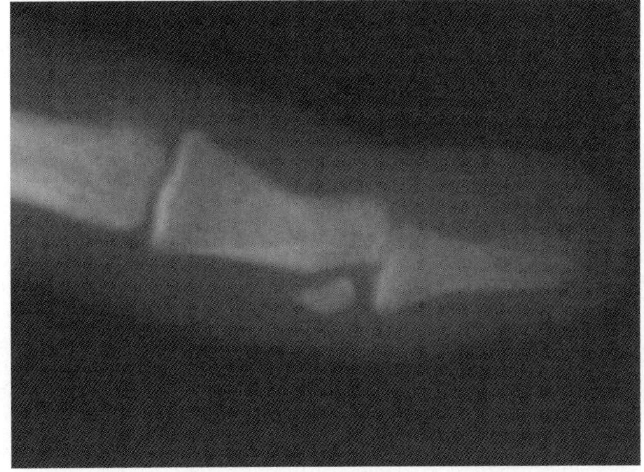

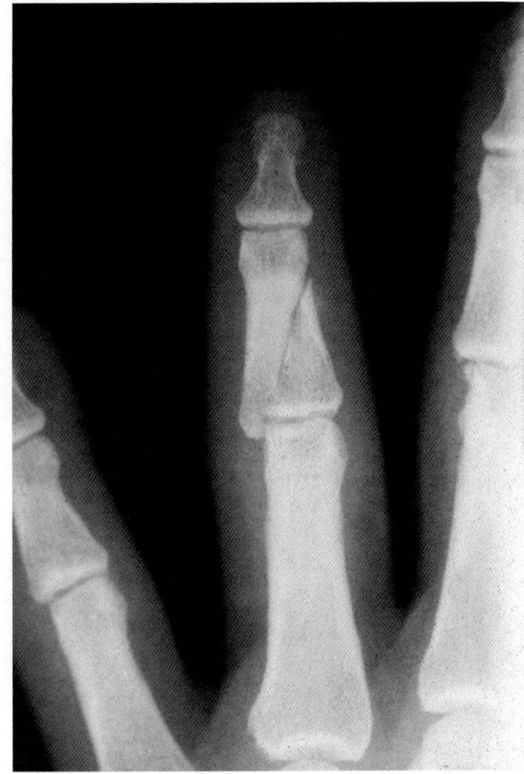

Figure 15.17 **(A)** Intraarticular fracture of the head and **(B)** an oblique shaft fracture. (*Reprinted with permission from* Bucholz RW, Heckman JD, Court-Brown CM, et al. *Rockwood and Green's Fractures in Adults.* 6th ed. Philadelphia, PA: Lippincott Williams & Wilkins, 2006.)

MCP dislocations are less common but often more difficult to treat. With a dorsal MCP dislocation, a noose can be formed around the MC head by the flexor tendon ulnarly and the lumbrical radially. In this scenario, longitudinal traction can cause the volar plate to become entrapped in the joint, making closed reduction impossible. Reduction is best achieved with application of force from dorsal to volar over the base of the proximal phalanx. When reduction cannot be afforded by this maneuver, open reduction via a dorsal approach is often required to remove the interposed volar plate.

Metacarpal Fractures

The MCs are common sites of injury in the hand. They are often injured during physical altercations when one individual attempts to punch another person or object with a closed fist.

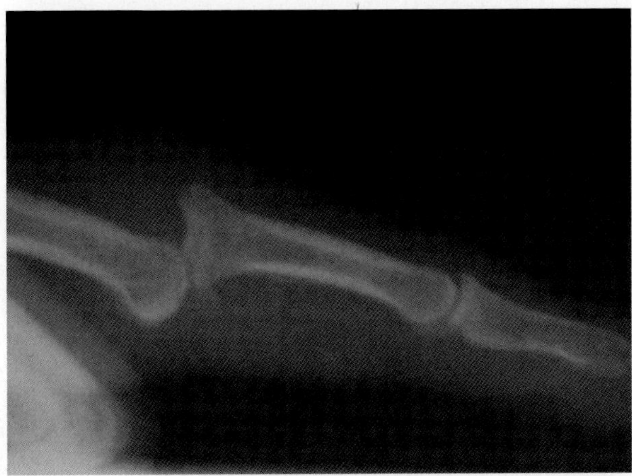

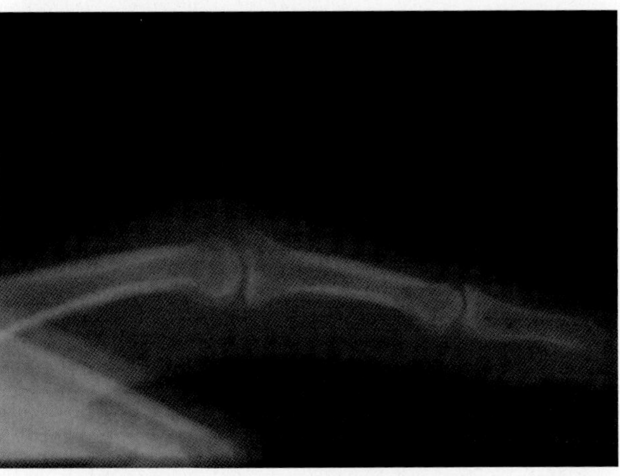

Figure 15.18 **(A)** Dorsal proximal interphalangeal dislocation and **(B)** subsequent reduction. (*Reprinted with permission from* Bucholz RW, Heckman JD, Court-Brown CM, et al. *Rockwood and Green's Fractures in Adults.* 6th ed. Philadelphia, PA: Lippincott Williams & Wilkins, 2006.)

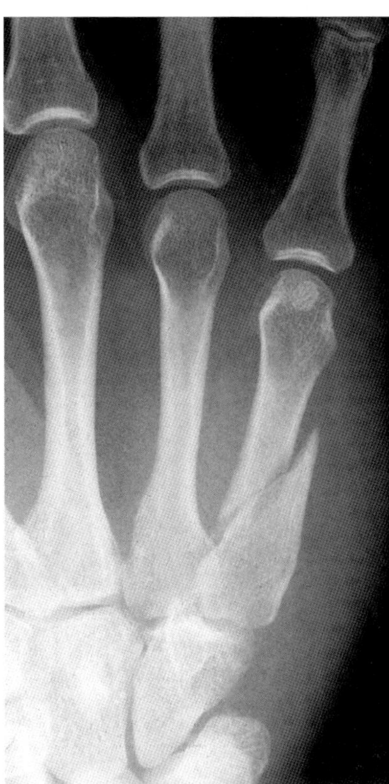

Figure 15.19 Oblique fracture of metacarpal shaft with shortening. (*Reprinted with permission from* Bucholz RW, Heckman JD, Court-Brown CM, et al. *Rockwood and Green's Fractures in Adults.* 6th ed. Philadelphia, PA: Lippincott Williams & Wilkins, 2006.)

Classification

MC fractures are classified on the basis of anatomic location as head, neck, shaft, and base (Fig. 15.19).

Mechanism of Injury

The fractures are typically the result of either a crush injury or an axial load to the MC (e.g., when punching an object with a clenched fist).

Presentation and Physical Examination

Patients typically complain of pain and swelling over the affected MC after an injury. Patients typically demonstrate tenderness and swelling over the affected MC. The MC head may be depressed, giving the appearance of a "missing knuckle."

Radiographic Findings/Special Studies

Plain PA, lateral, and oblique radiographs of the hand will demonstrate a visible fracture line. A Brewerton view can be helpful to evaluate for collateral ligament avulsion fractures. It is taken with the MP joints flexed 60 to 70 degrees, the dorsal surfaces of the digits placed flat on the x-ray cassette, and the beam angled 15 degrees radial.

Treatment

MC head fractures are relatively uncommon but when they occur, they are often difficult to treat and generally require operative stabilization. A simple fracture pattern can be managed effectively with either closed reduction and percutaneous pinning or open reduction internal fixation (ORIF). Comminuted fractures can be managed similarly but have poorer outcomes and may require future arthroplasty.

Fractures of the MC neck are relatively frequent. They carry the eponym "boxer's fractures" because of their mechanism, which is an axial load across a clenched fist. MC neck fractures generally assume an apex dorsal angulation deformity. They may also exhibit rotational deformity, which is important to note as it may merit reduction even if angulation is minimal. Criteria for acceptable angulation varies depending on the source, but many surgeons use the *10–20–30–40 rule* in which 10 degrees is acceptable for the index finger, 20 for the long, 30 for the ring, and 40 for the small. There is little evidence in the literature regarding what "acceptable" angulation is, and there are some biomechanical data for the small finger MC that suggest that angulation of more than 30 degrees leads to significant dysfunction of the flexor system. If displacement is greater than the accepted degree for a particular finger, a closed reduction is warranted. A commonly applied technique is the *Jahss maneuver,* in which the affected digit is volar flexed to 90 degrees and a volar to dorsal force is applied through the proximal phalanx so as to restore the normal alignment of the MC neck (Fig. 15.20). Any rotational deformity can also be corrected while performing this maneuver. A plaster spint or cast should be applied to maintain this reduction with the affected digit in a 90 degree volar flexed position, which serves to maintain reduction and prevent the MC head collateral ligaments from shortening. As reduction is often difficult to maintain in a splint or cast, these fractures may require a repeat reduction with percutaneous pinning in the operating room setting.

As noted earlier, MC shaft fractures are typically the result of either an axial load or a crush injury. They generally create an apex dorsal angulation deformity due to the vector of pull of the interosseus muscles, which is volar (Fig. 15.21). Most clinicians consider nonoperative treatment in a spint or cast if sagittal plane deformity is less than 30 degrees and there is no significant rotational malalignment. In general, unstable MC shaft fractures require operative fixation, which consists of percutaneous pinning versus ORIF with plates and/or screws. It is important to be aware that multiple MC shaft fractures in the same hand can result in a compartment syndrome, in which the patient will present with a very swollen painful hand held in the *intrinsic minus* (MP joint extension and IP joint flexion) position.

Fractures of the MC base are less common than in the neck but can be more problematic, particularly when intraarticular. The often involve the thumb and small finger.

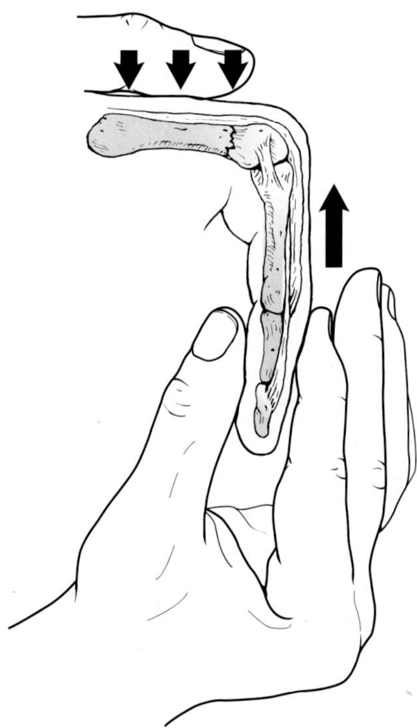

Figure 15.20 Jahss maneuver for reducing metacarpal neck fractures. (*Reprinted with permission from* Bucholz RW, Heckman JD, Court-Brown CM, et al. *Rockwood and Green's Fractures in Adults.* 6th ed. Philadelphia, PA: Lippincott Williams & Wilkins, 2006.)

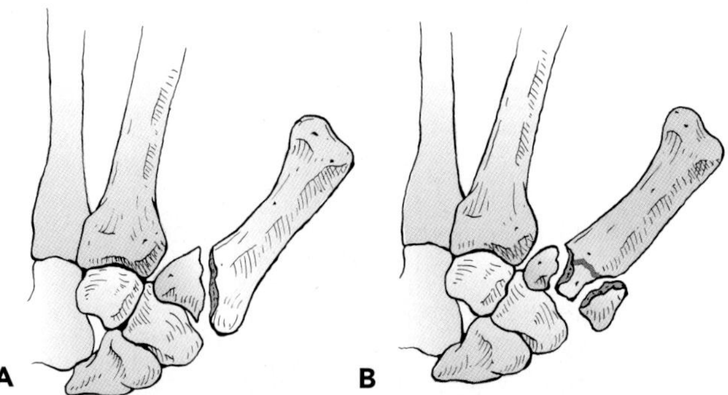

Figure 15.22 Bennett fracture **(A)** and Rolando fracture **(B)**. (*Reprinted with permission from* Bucholz RW, Heckman JD, Court-Brown CM, et al. *Rockwood and Green's Fractures in Adults.* 6th ed. Philadelphia, PA: Lippincott Williams & Wilkins, 2006.)

An intraarticular fracture at the base of the thumb MC is often referred to as a *Bennett fracture* (Fig. 15.22). This injury is typically caused by axial load to flexed thumb. Deformity and difficulty with healing is the result of the fact that the APL pulls the thumb MC shaft radially and dorsally while the deep volar oblique (*beak ligament*) remains attached to the ulnar-sided fragment. Of note, the eponym "Rolando fracture" is used when there is comminution at the thumb MC base and both an ulnar and radial fragment are visible. Last, a "baby Bennett" is the term used for an intraarticular fracture at the base of the small finger MC. In this scenario,

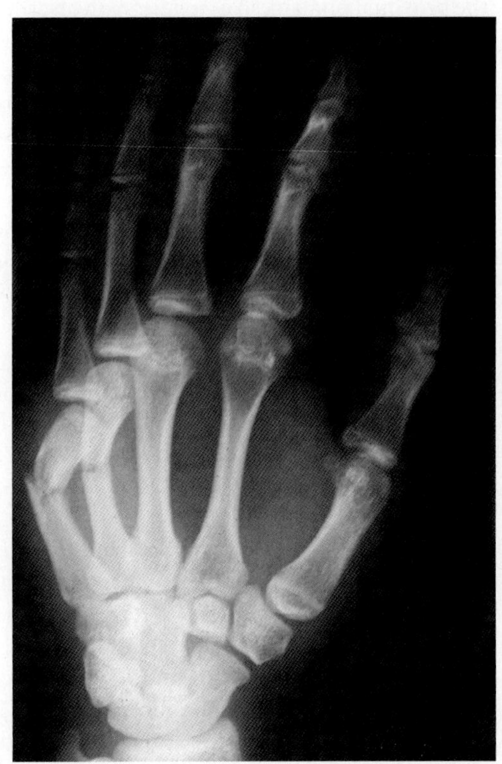

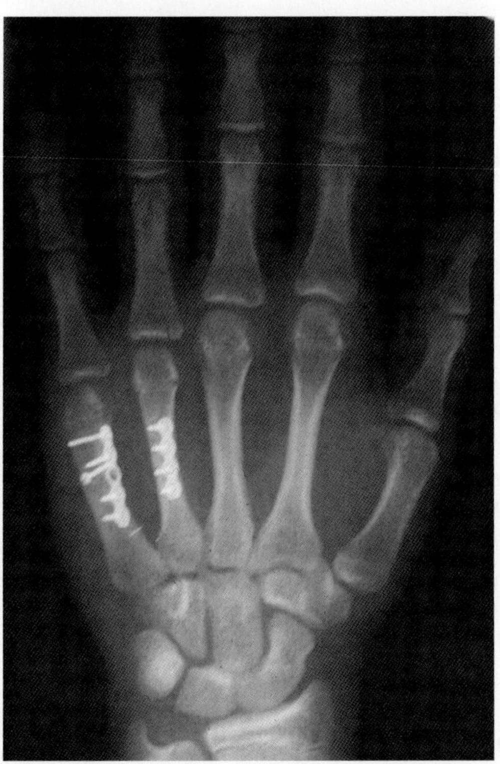

Figure 15.21 Ring and small finger metacarpal fracture **(A)** status post open reduction internal fixation **(B)**. (*Reprinted with permission from* Bucholz RW, Heckman JD, Court-Brown CM, et al. *Rockwood and Green's Fractures in Adults.* 6th ed. Philadelphia, PA: Lippincott Williams & Wilkins, 2006.)

the ECU pulls the small finger MC shaft ulnarly, making healing difficult. Each of these intraarticular MC base fractures generally require percutaneous pinning versus ORIF.

Gamekeeper's Thumb

Ligamentous injury involving the MCs occurs quite frequently, with the MCP joint of the thumb being the most vulnerable due to its hypermobility. Classically, *gamekeeper's thumb* refers to chronic attenuation of the ulnar collateral ligament, while *skier's thumb* refers to acute rupture of the ligament.

Mechanism of Injury

Radial-directed stress on the thumb MCP joint can damage the ulnar collateral ligament, resulting in a gamekeeper's thumb.

Presentation and Physical Examination

The patient typically complains of pain and instability at the thumb MCP joint.

On examination, the patient will have tenderness to palpation at the ulnar aspect of the thumb MCP joint and will have gapping at the joint with radial stress. The joint should be stressed in full extension and in 30 degrees of flexion. Compared with the contralateral side, greater than 35 degrees of increased angulation in extension or greater than 15 degrees of increased angulation in flexion is diagnostic.

Radiographic Findings

Standard anteroposterior, lateral, and oblique radiographs of the thumb may demonstrate a bony fleck in the region of the thumb MCP representing the avulsion of the ulnar collateral ligament.

Special Studies

Stress radiographs of the thumb with a radial-directed force may reveal gapping at the MCP joint. Ultrasonography and MRI can also help in establishing the diagnosis.

Treatment

Patients who demonstrate minimal gapping with radial stress are likely to have only a partial ulnar collateral ligament rupture, which can be treated with thumb spica casting for 6 weeks. However, gapping with radial stress greater than 35 degrees in extension or greater than 15 degrees in 30 degrees of flexion suggests a complete rupture. In complete tears, the ligament can become lodged behind AP aponeurosis, which prevents healing (known as a *Stener lesion*) (Fig. 15.23). Therefore, early surgery is advocated for complete tears.

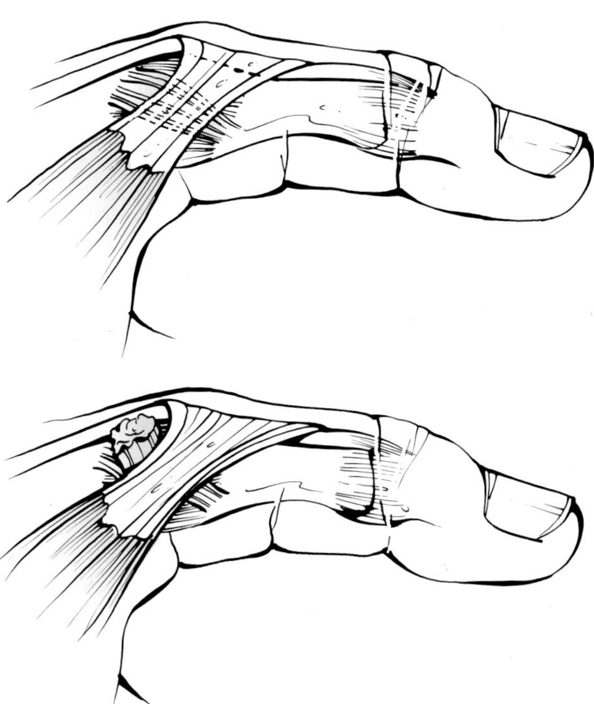

Figure 15.23 Stener lesion in gamekeeper's thumb. (*Reprinted with permission from* Bucholz RW, Heckman JD, Court-Brown CM, et al. *Rockwood and Green's Fractures in Adults.* 6th ed. Philadelphia, PA: Lippincott Williams & Wilkins, 2006.)

CARPUS

Scaphoid Fractures

The scaphoid is the most frequently fractured bone in the carpus and the slowest to heal. Scaphoid fractures are frequently missed since they often cannot be visualized on initial radiographs and require close follow-up for detection. All scaphoid fractures can be problematic but fractures of the proximal pole are the most worrisome. Since the scaphoid has a retrograde blood supply from the radial artery, which enters mainly on its dorsal ridge, the proximal pole is particularly susceptible to avascular necrosis when fractured.

Classification

Fractures of scaphoid are often described on the basis of anatomic location as tubercle, proximal pole, waist, or distal pole (Fig. 15.24).

Mechanism of Injury

The scaphoid is typically injured by a fall onto an outstretched hand.

Presentation and Physical Examination

The patient will typically complain of pain over the region of the anatomical snuffbox after a fall. The patient often has radial-sided swelling and pain with movement. Frequently, there is tenderness to palpation dorsally over the anatomical snuffbox or volarly over the scaphoid tubercle.

Radiographic Findings

Standard radiographic evaluation of the scaphoid begins with three plain radiograph views of the wrist, which include a PA, lateral, and oblique.

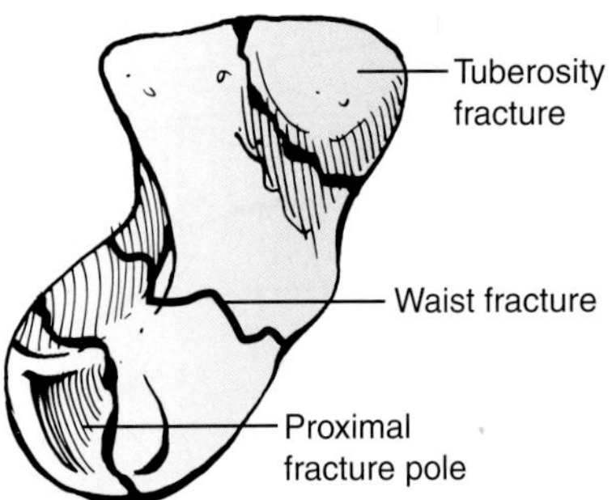

Figure 15.24 The classification of scaphoid fractures based on anatomical location. (*Reprinted with permission from* Bucholz RW, Heckman JD, Court-Brown CM, et al. *Rockwood and Green's Fractures in Adults.* 6th ed. Philadelphia, PA: Lippincott Williams & Wilkins, 2006.)

Special Studies

To better visualize the scaphoid, one can request a "scaphoid view" of the wrist, which is a PA shot with approximately 20 degrees of ulnar deviation. Ulnar deviation rotates the scaphoid into the same axis as the radius and minimizes overlap between the waist and tubercle, allowing one to visualize the scaphoid along its entire length (Fig. 15.25).

Since scaphoid fractures may not show up on initial radiographs, any patient who complains of anatomic snuffbox pain after trauma to the hand/wrist should be placed in thumb spica splint and should be followed up for repeat radiographs in 2 to 3 weeks (Fig. 15.26). At that time, bone

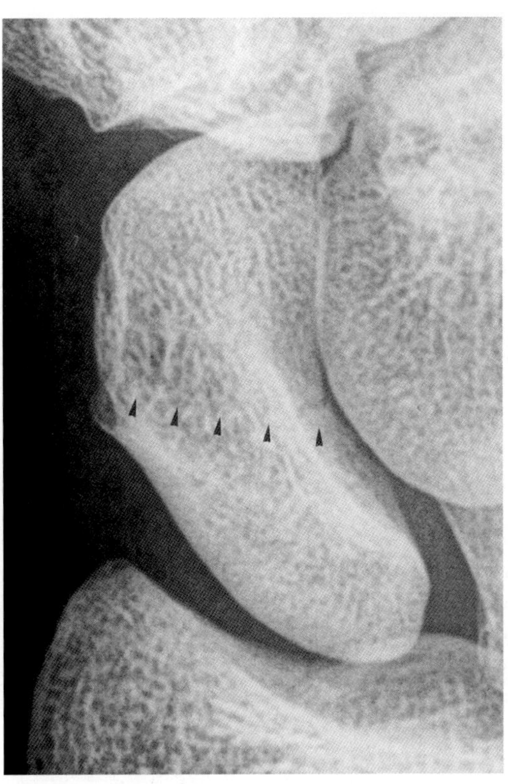

Figure 15.26 Radiograph of a very subtle scaphoid fracture that could easily be missed. (*Reprinted with permission from* Bucholz RW, Heckman JD, Court-Brown CM, et al. *Rockwood and Green's Fractures in Adults.* 6th ed. Philadelphia, PA: Lippincott Williams & Wilkins, 2006.)

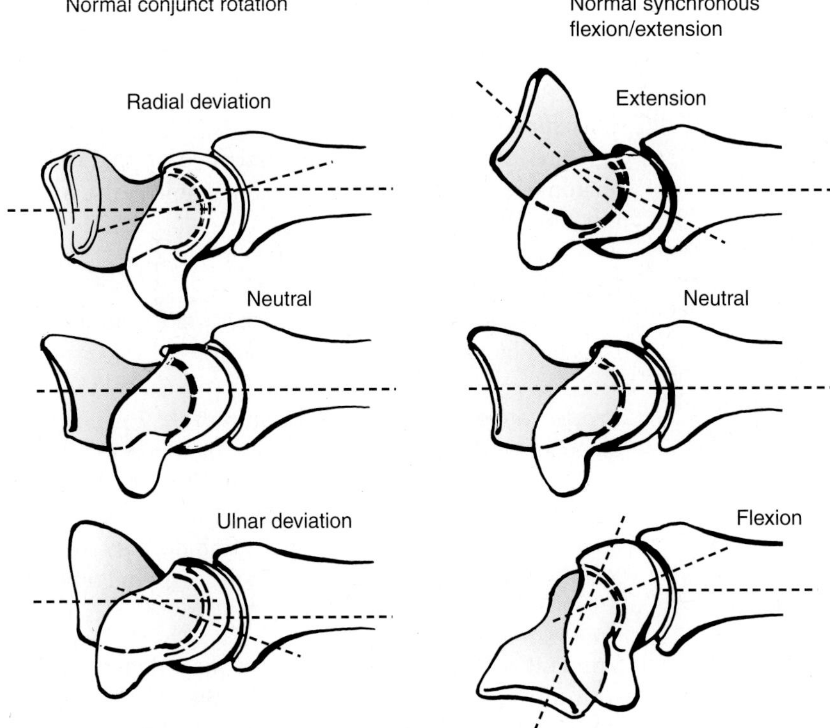

Figure 15.25 The kinematics of the proximal carpal row during radial/ulnar deviation and flexion/extension. (*Reprinted with permission from* Bucholz RW, Heckman JD, Court-Brown CM, et al. *Rockwood and Green's Fractures in Adults.* 6th ed. Philadelphia, PA: Lippincott Williams & Wilkins, 2006.)

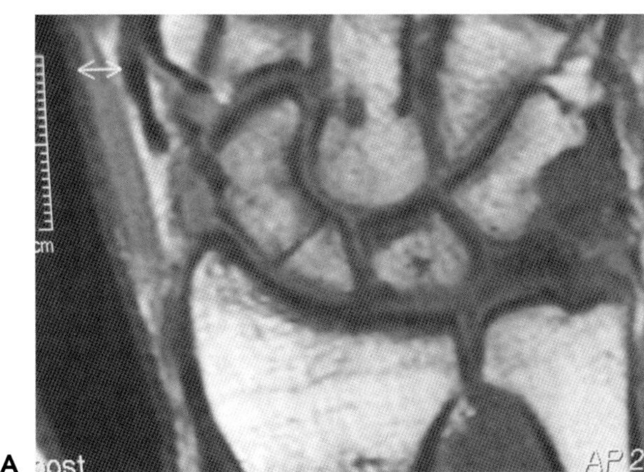

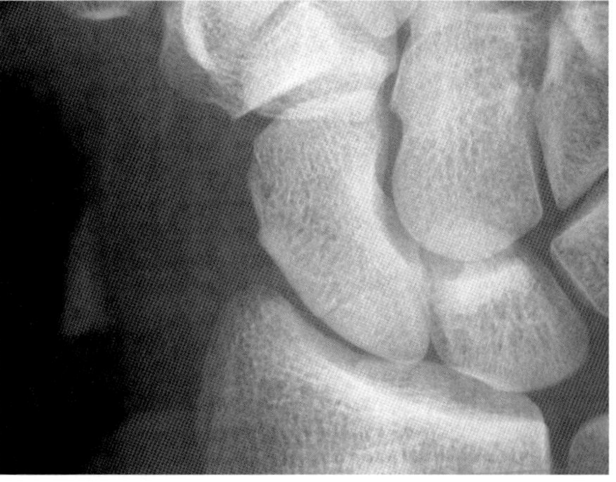

Figure 15.27 A clear scaphoid fracture on magnetic resonance imaging (A), which is difficult to see on plain radiograph (B). (*Reprinted with permission from* Bucholz RW, Heckman JD, Court-Brown CM, et al. *Rockwood and Green's Fractures in Adults.* 6th ed. Philadelphia, PA: Lippincott Williams & Wilkins, 2006.)

resorption may be evident if there was indeed a fracture. One radiographic clue suggesting a possible scaphoid fracture is alteration of the *navicular fat stripe,* which is a thin radiolucent line just radial to the scaphoid. It is present in normal individuals and may become displaced or obliterated secondary to a scaphoid fracture. Ultimately, one may need either MRI or CT scan of the wrist with 1 mm cuts through plane of scaphoid to diagnose an occult scaphoid fracture (Fig. 15.27). Bone scan is another useful diagnostic test but is used less frequently than MRI or CT.

Treatment

As note earlier, scaphoid fractures come in four varieties: tubercle, proximal pole, waist, and distal pole. In general, scaphoid fractures are treated on the basis of displacement; however, some surgeons choose to surgically fix all proximal pole fractures to minimize the chances of avascular necrosis. Nondisplaced fractures can be treated with a thumb spica cast. Some surgeons place patients in a long arm thumb spica for 6 weeks, after which they are placed in a short arm thumb spica until the fracture has healed. These fractures can take from 3 to 6 months to heal. Waist fractures average approximately 12 weeks to heal, whereas proximal pole fractures generally take approximately 20 to 25 weeks. Because of these prolonged healing times, patients may be given a choice of surgical fixation even for nondisplaced injuries.

Displaced scaphoid fractures require operative fixation, usually with a headless compression screw. Other criteria for fixation include scapholunate angle of greater than 60 degrees and radiolunate angle of greater than 15 degrees. The procedure can be done either percutaneously or open. If done open, most surgeons advocate a volar approach for waist to distal pole fractures and dorsal approach for waist to proximal pole (Fig. 15.28).

Delayed union and nonunion are of particular concern in scaphoid fractures. Some support the use of electrical bone stimulator for nondisplaced fractures. The standard of care for a displaced nonunion is bone grafting and screw fixation. Bone grafting options include cancellous, corticocancellous, and vascularized. Cancellous bone grafting is usually used for nondisplaced nonunions. However, in many scaphoid fractures, volar comminution in the area of the waist can cause an apex dorsal or "humpback" deformity. In cases like these, a corticocancellous wedge of bone graft must be placed volarly to correct the deformity.

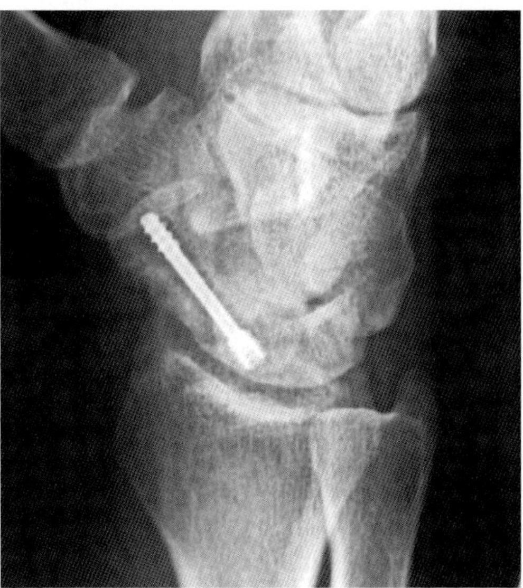

Figure 15.28 Proximal pole fracture of the scaphoid treated with open reduction and internal fixation via a dorsal approach. (*Reprinted with permission from* Bucholz RW, Heckman JD, Court-Brown CM, et al. *Rockwood and Green's Fractures in Adults.* 6th ed. Philadelphia, PA: Lippincott Williams & Wilkins, 2006.)

Finally, fractures of the proximal pole or those demonstrating avascular necrosis may require vascularized bone grafts. The most commonly used is the distal radius vascularized bone graft based on the 1,2 intercompartmental supraretinacular artery, which has demonstrated union rates of approximately 70%. More recently, some centers have attempted free vascularized grafts from the medial femoral condyle.

Lunate Fractures

The lunate is the fourth most commonly fractured bone in the carpus. Similar to the scaphoid, it has a tenuous blood supply that can be disrupted when a fracture occurs.

Classification

There are five types of lunate fractures: palmar pole, osteochondral chip, dorsal pole, sagittal oblique, and coronal split.

Mechanism of Injury

The typical mechanism is a fall onto an outstretched, hyperextended wrist.

Presentation and Physical Examination

Patients often complains of central wrist pain and/or pain with wrist movement after a fall. Physical findings include tenderness to palpation in the center of the wrist and pain with wrist range of motion.

Radiographic Findings

Standard PA, lateral, and oblique radiographs of the hand may be negative.

Special Studies

CT of the wrist may help to delineate a lunate fracture if plain radiographs are negative. MRI is indicated if Kienbock disease (osteonecrosis of the lunate) is suspected.

Treatment

In general, minimally displaced lunate fractures can be treated with 4 to 6 weeks of immobilization in a short or long arm cast. Fractures associated with intraarticular incongruity or instability are generally treated with ORIF.

Complications

Of note, one of the potential and more devastating complications of lunate trauma is Kienbock disease. It is believed that trauma, which can be acute or chronic from repetitive stress (e.g., as in patients with negative ulnar variance, which causes increased stress on the lunate), disrupts the tenuous blood supply of the lunate, leading to avascular necrosis. MRI or bone scan should be obtained if there is any suspicion. This disease and its severity can be characterized by the *Lichtman classification system*. This system is based on plain radiograph appearance and divides Kienbock disease into four stages. Stage I represents no visible changes in the lunate on plain film, only MRI. Stage II is sclerosis of the lunate. Stage III involves sclerosis and fragmentation of the lunate and is divided into A and B based on either the absence (A) or presence (B) of fixed scaphoid rotation. Stage IV is degenerative arthritis of the adjacent intercarpal joints.

In terms of treatment, Stage I can be treated with immobilization, whereas stages II through IIIA may require revascularization and joint leveling procedures (e.g., ulnar lengthening, radial shortening) or even carpal fusions, which help to unload the lunate. With fixed rotation of the scaphoid, a proximal row carpectomy (PRC) or intercarpal fusion may be indicated. Finally, with stage IV disease, a total wrist fusion or PRC is recommended.

Triquetral Fractures

Triquetral fractures are the second most common type of carpal fracture behind fractures of the scaphoid.

Classification

There are two types of triquetral fractures: dorsal rim chip fractures, which are the most common, and body fractures.

Mechanism of Injury

Wrist hyperflexion with radial deviation is a common cause of dorsal chip fractures, whereas triquetral body fractures are often caused by direct trauma.

Presentation and Physical Examination

The patient complains of pain and swelling about the ulnar wrist after trauma.

The patient typically has ulnar-sided wrist tenderness and pain with wrist range of motion.

Radiographic Findings/Special Studies

Standard PA, lateral, and oblique radiographs of the hand should be obtained. Dorsal chip fractures can best be seen on the lateral radiograph.

Treatment

Small dorsal chip triquetral fractures and minimally displaced body fractures can typically be treated with 4 to 6 weeks of cast immobilization. If the fragment is sizable, it results in instability, or if it is significantly displaced, ORIF may be indicated.

Trapezium Fractures

Trapezial fractures are the third most common carpal fracture.

Classification

There are five types of trapezium fractures: vertical transarticular, horizontal, dorsoradial tuberosity, anteromedial ridge, and comminuted.

Mechanism of Injury

The most common mechanism is an axial load to the TM.

Presentation and Physical Examination

The patient typically complains of pain and swelling at the base of the thumb after trauma. On examination, the patient will have tenderness over the base of the thumb and pain with thumb range of motion.

Radiographic Findings/Special Studies

Standard PA, lateral, and oblique radiographs of the hand should demonstrate the fracture.

Treatment

Minimally displaced trapezial fractures can be treated with cast immobilization for 3 to 6 weeks. Displaced, intraarticular fracture may require ORIF. Anteromedial ridge fractures often result in painful nonunion and frequently must be excised.

Capitate Fractures

Capitate fractures are rather rare but often have poor outcomes.

Classification

There are four types: transverse body, transverse proximal pole, coronal oblique, and parasagittal.

Mechanism of Injury

The most common mechanism of injury is an axial load on a hyperextended wrist.

Presentation and Physical Examination

The patient typically complains of central wrist pain after a fall. Tenderness can generally be elicited over the center of the carpus.

Radiographic Findings/Special Studies

Standard PA, lateral, and oblique radiographs of the hand should demonstrate the fracture; however, CT may be required to better visualize the fracture lines.

Treatment

Nondisplaced fractures can be treated with cast immobilization. Displaced or intraarticular fractures can be treated with K-wires or ORIF. Proximal pole fractures are particularly difficult to manage. Even if nondisplaced, they can result in avascular necrosis due to a tenuous blood supply, which, similar to that of the scaphoid, is retrograde. Capitate fractures can occur concomitantly with fractures of the scaphoid. *Scaphocapitate syndrome* is a term used to describe a scaphoid waist fracture and associated capitate neck fracture. This injury usually occurs via a wrist hyperdorsiflexion mechanism and requires ORIF to prevent migration of the proximal capitate.

Hamate Fractures

Hook of hamate fractures are most frequently seen in those who engage in stick or racquet sports, such as golfers and baseball players. These fractures can be difficult to heal and may result in painful nonunion. The resultant deformity of the hook can lead to rupture of adjacent ring and small finger flexor tendons over time (Fig. 15.29).

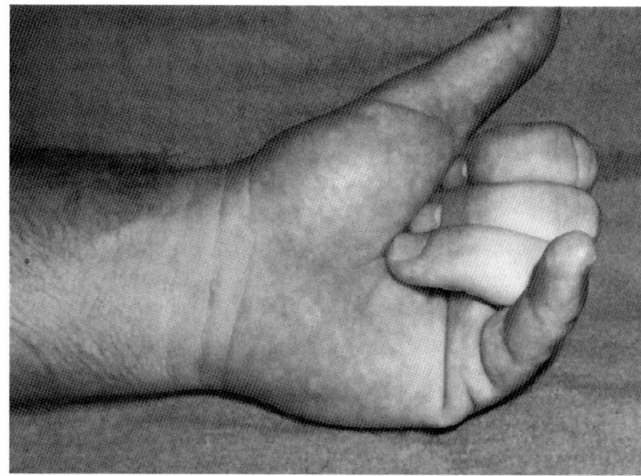

Figure 15.29 Small finger flexor rupture due to hook of hamate malunion. (*Reprinted with permission from* Doyle JR, Tornetta P, Einhorn TA. *Orthopaedic Surgery Essentials: Hand and Wrist.* Philadelphia, PA: Lippincott Williams & Wilkins, 2006.)

Classification

Hamate fractures can involve either the body or hook, the latter of which is exceedingly more common.

Mechanism of Injury

Hamate fractures can result from a direct blow to the hamate or from chronic repetitive impact (Fig. 15.30).

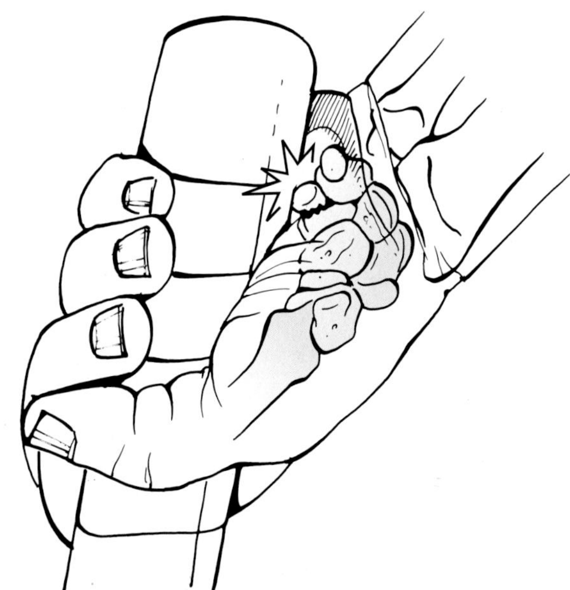

Figure 15.30 The mechanism for hook of the hamate fractures. (*Reprinted with permission from* Bucholz RW, Heckman JD, Court-Brown CM, et al. *Rockwood and Green's Fractures in Adults.* 6th ed. Philadelphia, PA: Lippincott Williams & Wilkins, 2006.)

Presentation and Physical Examination

The patient complains of ulnar-sided pain distal and radial to the pisiform after sustaining acute or repetitive trauma. Patients demonstrate tenderness over the ulnar side of the wrist, diminished grip strength, and possibly paresthesias in the ulnar nerve distribution. The hook of the hamate can be palpated by the examiner by placing his/her own thumb IP joint on the patient's pisiform and then palpating 45 degrees radial and distal. This is usually the point of maximal tenderness.

Radiographic Findings/Special Studies

The hook of the hamate can be visualized by a *carpal tunnel view*, which is an axial view of the wrist at maximal dorsiflexion, or by CT scan, which is more accurate.

Treatment

Nondisplaced hamate body fractures can be treated with cast immobilization, whereas displaced or unstable fractures may require excision of the fractured hook, or rarely ORIF. It is generally recommended that displaced fractures or nonunions of the hook be excised.

Pisiform Fractures

Pisiform fractures are rather uncommon injuries seen in the carpus.

Classification

There are four types: transverse (most common), parasagittal, comminuted, and pisotriquetral impaction.

Mechanism of Injury

The typical mechanism is direct trauma to the pisiform.

Presentation and Physical Examination

The patient typically complains of ulnar-sided wrist pain and will exhibit tenderness to palpation directly over the pisiform.

Radiographic Findings/Special Studies

Standard PA, lateral, and oblique radiographs of the hand should demonstrate the fracture adequately. If not, a CT scan can be considered.

Treatment

These fractures can generally be treated in a short arm cast but may require excision if a painful nonunion develops.

Distal Radius Fractures

Distal radius fractures are common, representing up to 15% of all fractures in the upper extremity. They are seen frequently in young, active patients as a result of a high-energy trauma or elderly, osteoporotic patients as a fragility fracture. In both groups of patients, restoration of normal wrist function is the guiding principle for treatment. Internal fixation with plating of these fractures has become increasingly popular over the past decade.

Classification

A variety of classification systems exist, including the Frykman and Melone, but there is no general consensus as to which one should be used (Fig. 15.31). In general, distal radius fractures are referred to by certain eponyms, which include Colles (dorsal displacement), Smith (volar displacement), Barton (radial rim fracture with either volar or dorsal displacement of the carpus), or Chauffeur fractures

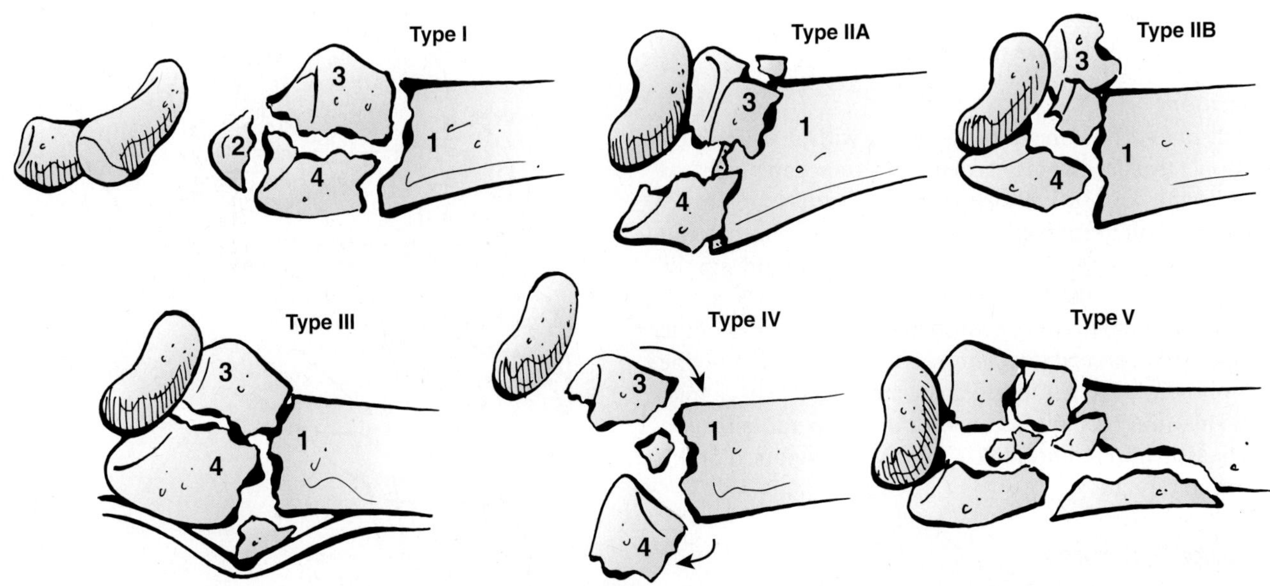

Figure 15.31 The Melone classification for distal radius fractures. (*Reprinted with permission from* Bucholz RW, Heckman JD, Court-Brown CM, et al. *Rockwood and Green's Fractures in Adults*. 6th ed. Philadelphia, PA: Lippincott Williams & Wilkins, 2006.)

(radial styloid). Distal radius fractures are also classified on the basis of whether they are intra- or extraarticular.

Mechanism of Injury

These generally occur by a fall onto an outstretched hand.

Presentation and Physical Examination

The patient complains of pain and swelling over the wrist after a fall. On examination, the patient will exhibit tenderness over the wrist with limited range of motion. A detailed neurovascular examination must be performed, with special attention given to the median nerve. Patients who present with numbness in the median nerve distribution often have improved symptoms after fracture reduction. However, on occasion, patients develop progressive deterioration of median nerve function, which is suggestive of acute carpal tunnel syndrome (CTS). In these situations, any restrictive dressings, splints, and/or casts should be removed, and the wrist should be placed in a neutral position. If the symptoms do not improve, the patient should be taken to the operating room for an emergent carpal tunnel release.

Radiographic Findings/Special Studies

Standard anteroposterior, lateral, and oblique views of the wrist are initially obtained. In cases in which the fracture is comminuted or intraarticular, a CT scan can be obtained to assist with preoperative planning.

Treatment

Treatment options for distal radius fractures differ depending on several variables, such as a patient's age, activity level, and occupation. However, the degree of displacement is the most important factor that influences managment. Recall from the anatomy section that the distal radius is tilted volarly at an angle of approximately 11 degrees. Its angle of radial inclination is roughly 22 degrees while its height radially is approximately 11 mm relative to its most ulnar surface. These numbers are important in determining whether a reduction, open or closed, is necessary. However, even after reduction, fractures have a tendency to return to their initial displacement. Although no consensus exists, most would consider acceptable alignment in a healthy, active patient to be up to 10 degrees of dorsal tilt (20 degrees from normal), less than 2 mm of intraarticular step-off at radiocarpal joint, less than 5 mm of radial shortening, a congruent DRUJ, and more than 15 degrees of radial inclination.

If closed reduction is warranted, the reduction maneuver may vary depending on the nature of the fracture. The general principle is to recreate the mechanism that caused the deformity. For example, a Colles fracture occurs via a wrist hyperextension mechanism; therefore, when reducing these fractures, one should not simply pull longitudinal traction on the wrist but hyperextend it so as to lever the dorsally displaced fragment back into position. Conversely, for a Smith fracture, a wrist hyperflexion reduction maneuver might be employed. Once reduction is achieved, the patient should be immobilized in sugar tong plaster splint.

A few notable complications can occur after a distal radius fracture, both in the short and long term. In the short term, one can develop an *acute CTS*, especially after repeated closed reduction attempts. In acute CTS, the patient typically develops a sudden numbness in the median nerve distribution several hours after the injury and this numbness gets progressively worse. When this occurs, immediate carpal tunnel release is indicated. Of note, acute CTS should be distinguished from median nerve contusion. Unlike acute CTS, median nerve contusion causes numbness in the median nerve distribution at the time of injury that does not get progressively worse.

A long-term complication that can occur, particularly with nondisplaced distal radius fractures, is *rupture of the EPL tendon*. This is attributed to ischemia of the tendon secondary to the pressure exerted by the fracture hematoma.

When closed reduction techniques fail to hold the distal radius in acceptable alignment, surgery is indicated. The use of percutaneous pinning to augment closed reduction is a method more appropriate for younger patients with extraarticular fractures. Advances in low profile and locked plating have made either volar or dorsal plating a more commonly used option for distal radius fractures in adults (Fig. 15.32). The decision of whether to approach the fracture from volar or dorsal is dependent on fractures pattern and surgeon preference. External fixation may be indicated for highly comminuted distal radius fractures in which there is significant bony or soft tissue loss.

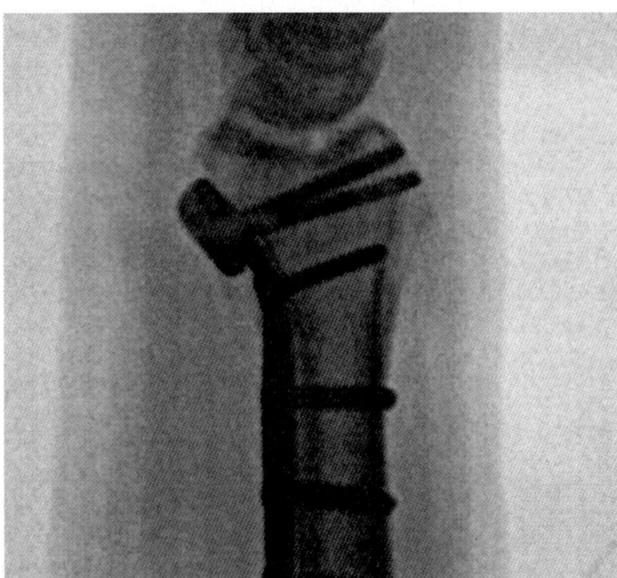

Figure 15.32 A volar distal radius plate. Note that the more distal the plate placement, the more likely a screw will penetrate the articular surface. (*Reprinted with permission from* Bucholz RW, Heckman JD, Court-Brown CM, et al. *Rockwood and Green's Fractures in Adults*. 6th ed. Philadelphia, PA: Lippincott Williams & Wilkins, 2006.)

Of note, a related fracture pattern seen in the distal forearm is the *Galeazzi fracture,* in which a distal radial shaft fracture occurs in combination with a DRUJ dislocation. This injury requires ORIF of radial shaft with possible percutaneous pinning of the DRUJ, depending on the stability of the DRUJ after closed reduction.

Distal Forearm Fractures

Ulnar Shaft Fractures

Isolated ulnar shaft fractures, also known as *nightstick fractures,* are commonly seen fractures of the distal forearm.

Classification

There is no universal classification system for ulnar shaft fractures. The fracture is described on the basis of its location and characteristics.

Mechanism of Injury

Ulnar shaft fractures typically occur by a direct trauma to the ulna, such as when one is struck by a nightstick while raising his or her arm in defense (hence the eponym "nightstick fracture").

Presentation and Physical Examination

Patients complain of pain over the ulnar aspect of the forearm after trauma.

Tenderness usually is found over the ulna and pain is worsened with supination/pronation.

Radiographic Findings/Special Studies

Standard anteroposterior and lateral radiographs of the forearm will demonstrate a visible fracture line.

Treatment

If nondisplaced, ulnar shaft fractures can be treated with a long arm cast for 6 to 8 weeks. If angulated greater than 10 degrees or displaced greater than 50% of the shaft, most surgeons would advocate ORIF by using a 3.5 mm dynamic compression plate.

Radial Shaft Fractures

The radial shaft is less commonly fractured in isolation than the ulnar shaft.

Classification

The classification of radial shaft fractures is largely descriptive.

Mechanism of Injury

The typical mechanism is a high-energy direct trauma to forearm.

Presentation and Physical Examination

The patient complains of severe forearm pain after trauma. The patient will exhibit considerable tenderness over the forearm, accompanied by swelling. A comprehensive neurovascular examination should be performed, and the forearm should be examined carefully for signs of compartment syndrome. The DRUJ should be examined for stability by pronating and supinating the forearm and directly stressing the distal radioulnar articulation.

Radiographic Findings/Special Studies

Standard anteroposterior and lateral radiographs of the forearm and the wrist are essential to both identify the fracture and rule out DRUJ instability.

Treatment

This injury usually occurs as a result of a high-energy mechanism and can cause significant soft tissue trauma. In the pediatric population, these fractures can be treated with closed reduction and long arm casting. In adults, ORIF is typically required. Of note, if the radial shaft fracture occurs in combination with a DRUJ dislocation, which is known as a *Galeazzi fracture,* ORIF of radial shaft with possible percutaneous pinning of the DRUJ is necessary, depending on the stability of the DRUJ after treatment of the radial shaft.

Ulnar and Radial Shaft Fractures

Fractures of both the ulnar and radial shafts, known as *both bone forearm fractures,* are more common than isolated fractures of either the radius or ulna.

Classification

The classification of both bone forearm fractures is largely descriptive.

Mechanism of Injury

The typical mechanism is a high-energy direct trauma to forearm.

Presentation and Physical Examination

The patient complains of severe forearm pain after trauma. The patient will exhibit considerable swelling and tenderness over the forearm and may have an obvious deformity. A comprehensive neurovascular examination should be performed and compartments of the forearm should be examined carefully for signs of increased pressure.

Radiographic Findings/Special Studies

Standard anteroposterior and lateral radiographs of the forearm are generally sufficient to make the diagnosis.

Treatment

This injury usually occurs as a result of a high-energy mechanism and can cause significant soft tissue trauma (Fig. 15.33). In the pediatric population, both bone forearm

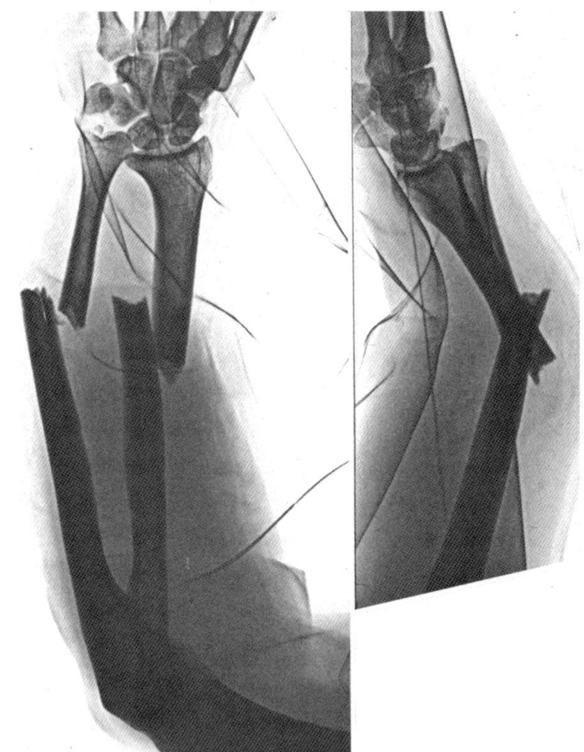

Figure 15.33 Both bone forearm fracture. (*Reprinted with permission from* Bucholz RW, Heckman JD, Court-Brown CM, et al. *Rockwood and Green's Fractures in Adults.* 6th ed. Philadelphia, PA: Lippincott Williams & Wilkins, 2006.)

fractures can typically be treated with closed reduction and long arm casting. In adults, ORIF is required, generally through two separate incisions.

Tears of the TFCC

Injury to the TFCC is a common cause of ulnar-sided wrist pain. It is more likely to occur in patients with ulnar-positive variance.

Classification

TFCC tears have been divided by Palmer into two classes: traumatic (Class I) and degenerative (class II). Class IA tears are central perforations of the articular disc. Class IB lesions are ulnar-sided avulsions that may or may not be associated with an ulnar styloid fracture. These lesions can destabilize the DRUJ. Class IC lesions are distal avulsions of either the ulnolunate or ulnotriquetral ligaments. Class ID lesions involve radial-sided avulsions of either the dorsal or volar radiocarpal ligaments.

Class II lesions are degenerative and are often the result of ulnocarpal abutment syndrome—excessive loading of the ulnocarpal joint secondary to positive ulnar variance. Class IIA lesions involve TFCC thinning, while class IIB involves thinning plus lunate and/or ulnar chondromalacia. Class IIC is the addition of perforation to the TFCC while class IID is perforation plus a lunotriqetral ligament tear. Last, class IIE is identical to class IID with the addition of ulnocarpal arthritis.

Mechanism of Injury

The TFCC is susceptible to injury, either from general wrist overuse or from acute trauma. The specific mechanism is an extension or pronation force to an axially loaded wrist.

Presentation and Physical Examination

Patients with TFCC tears typically present with ulnar-sided wrist pain and may complain of a clicking sensation in their wrist with certain movements. Patients usually experience tenderness to palpation over the fovea, which is the area between the FCU and ECU. Also, the TFCC compression test, which involves axial loading and ulnar-deviating the wrist, can often exacerbate pain.

Radiographic Findings/Special Studies

Plain radiographs of the wrist are usually unremarkable. The gold standard for diagnosing a TFCC tear was once wrist arthrography; however, MRI has proven more accurate and is considered the current study of choice. Wrist arthroscopy is another diagnostic modality and is most useful for staging these lesions.

Differential Diagnosis

Other causes of ulnar-sided wrist pain should be included in the differential diagnosis for a TFCC tear, including both ECU and FCU tendonitis, ulnocarpal abutment, lunotriquetral instability, ulnar styloid fracture, triquetrum fracture, and pisiform fracture.

Treatment

Although certain types of TFCC tears may require surgical treatment, all TFCC tears warrant an initial trial of conservative therapy, which includes splinting, anti-inflammatory medication, and activity modification for 6 weeks. Only if symptoms persist should arthroscopic or open surgery be considered.

Class IA tears involve a relatively avascular zone and, therefore, cannot be repaired. Instead, arthroscopic debridement is the treatment of choice. Class IB lesions can destabilize the DRUJ. Since they occur in the more vascular periphery of the articular disc, they are amenable to repair. Associated ulnar styloid fractures should undergo ORIF or closed reduction and pinning. Class IC lesions often require open repair. For class ID lesions, direct repair (either open or arthroscopic) is advocated.

Class IIA through IID can be managed with ulnar shortening, either at the head (wafer procedure) or diaphysis. The goal is to make the ulnar variance negative. Class IIE lesions should be managed with either a *Suave–Kapandji* (DRUJ arthrodesis with ulnar neck resection) or *Darrach procedure* (distal ulna resection).

Carpal Instability

Carpal instability is a commonly encountered problem in hand surgery; however, it remains difficult to both diagnose and treat.

Classification

Although many systems pervade the literature, the Mayo clinic classification system appears the most widely used. It divides carpal instability into *four* major categories: carpal instability dissociative (CID), carpal instability nondissociative (CIND), complex instabilities (dissociative and nondissociative), and longitudinal or axial loading instabilities.

CID involves disruption of *intrinsic* interosseous ligaments of the proximal carpal row, in contrast to nondissociative instability, which results from disruption of the *extrinsic* radiocarpal ligaments with intact intrinsic ligaments. Within the CID category are two important subgroups of instability: dorsal intercalated segment instability (DISI) and volar intercalated segment instability (VISI). The DISI deformity, which describes a palmar-flexed scaphoid in combination with a dorsiflexed lunate–triquetram, is a result from either a scapholunate ligament disruption or unstable scaphoid fracture. The VISI deformity, which describes a palmar-flexed scaphoid–lunate in combination with a dorsiflexed triquetram, usually results from lunotriquetral ligament disruption. The reason for these deformities relates to the biomechanics of the wrist, which are such that the scaphoid generally wants to assume a palmar-flexed position while the triquetrum wants to extend dorsally. When the lunate loses its tether to the scaphoid from a SL ligament disruption or scaphoid fracture, the lunate moves with the triquetrum, assuming a dorsiflexed position. Conversely, when the lunate loses its tether to the triquetram from a LT ligament disruption, the lunate moves with the scaphoid, assuming a volar-flexed position. In DISI, PA radiographs of the wrist may demonstrate the *Terry-Thomas sign*, which is SL widening greater than 3 mm, and/or the *cortical ring sign*, which represents the appearance of tubercle of the scaphoid when palmar-flexed (Fig. 15.34). In VISI, PA radiographs of the wrist may show widening of the LT interval. Lateral radiographs of the wrist will show SL angle greater than 60 degrees in DISI or less than 30 degrees in VISI.

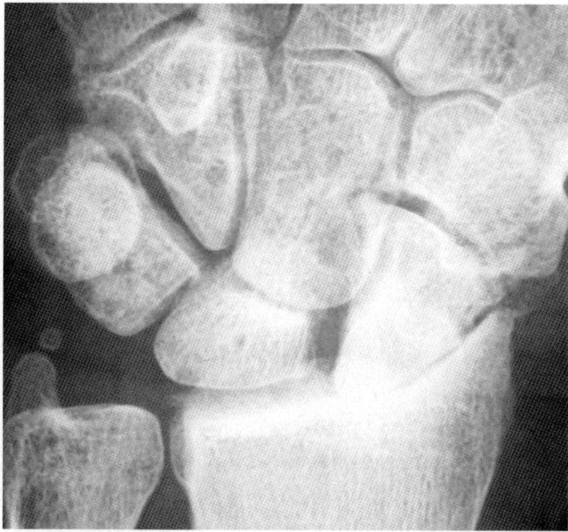

Figure 15.34 The Terry-Thomas sign for SL ligament disruption. (*Reprinted with permission from* Bucholz RW, Heckman JD, Court-Brown CM, et al. *Rockwood and Green's Fractures in Adults.* 6th ed. Philadelphia, PA: Lippincott Williams & Wilkins, 2006.)

The second category is CIND, which involves disruption of the *extrinsic* radiocarpal ligaments with intact intrinsic ligaments and results in instability at the radiocarpal joint and midcarpal rows. This category is further subdivided into three types: radiocarpal instability, midcarpal instability, and ulnar translation. In radiocarpal instability, disruption of either the dorsal or volar radiocarpal ligaments results in carpal drift. Midcarpal instability, the second subtype, involves instability between the proximal and distal carpal row. A capitolunate angle of greater than 15 degrees or less than 0 degrees on a true lateral radiograph is characteristic. The third subtype, ulnar translation, occurs after global ligamentous injury to the radiocarpal joint. It describes ulnar migration of the lunate relative to its normal position in the lunate facet of the distal radius. Radiographically, when less than 50% of the lunate remains in contact with the distal radius, the diagnosis of ulnar translation can be made. Ulnar translocation is traditionally seen in patients with inflammatory arthropathy such as RA.

The third category of carpal instability is complex instabilities, known as *carpal instability combined* (CIC). CIC involves disruption of ligaments between and within the carpal rows. It is helpful to divide the perilunate region into two arcs: the greater and lesser arcs. The *greater arc* consists of the bony structures surrounding the lunate, including the scaphoid, trapezium, capitate, hamate, and triquetrum. An example of a greater arc injury is the transscaphoid perilunate dislocation. The *lesser arc* is the ligamentous region surrounding the lunate. Injuries to the lesser arc are less common than those to the greater. An example of a lesser arc injury is a pure lunate dislocation, which is usually volar. According to Mayfield, there are four stages of perilunar instability proceeding from radial to ulnar around the lunate (Fig. 15.35). Stage I involves disruption of the scapholunate joint, whereas stage II violates both the scapholunate and capitolunate articulations. In stage III the scapholunate, capitolunate, and lunotriquetral ligaments are disrupted, and the result is a perilunate dislocation. Finally, in stage IV, all the ligaments surrounding the lunate are disrupted and the lunate dislocates volarly.

The fourth category of carpal instability is longitudinal or axial loading instabilities. These injuries are essentially fracture-dislocations in which the attached MCs travel with the involved carpal bone. They are caused almost exclusively by high-energy trauma to the carpus. They are further

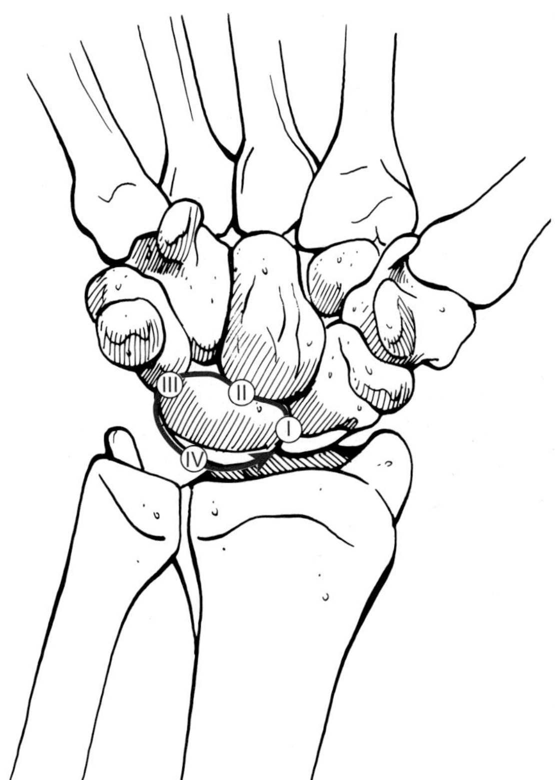

Figure 15.35 The Mayfield stages of perilunar instability. (*Reprinted with permission from* Bucholz RW, Heckman JD, Court-Brown CM, et al. *Rockwood and Green's Fractures in Adults.* 6th ed. Philadelphia, PA: Lippincott Williams & Wilkins, 2006.)

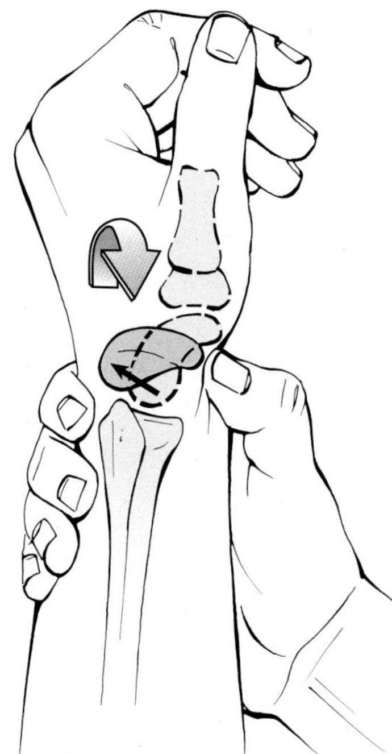

Figure 15.36 The scaphoid shift test. (*Reprinted with permission from* Bucholz RW, Heckman JD, Court-Brown CM, et al. *Rockwood and Green's Fractures in Adults.* 6th ed. Philadelphia, PA: Lippincott Williams & Wilkins, 2006.)

subdivided into axial ulnar, axial radial, and combined on the basis of the location of the injury.

Mechanism of Injury

Mechanisms of injury range from a fall onto an outstretched hand to a high-energy axial load to the wrist, as may occur during a motor vehicle accident.

Presentation

The patient may present with vague symptoms of wrist pain anywhere in the carpal region depending on where the disruption has occurred. They may also report a clunking sensation with certain movements of the wrist.

Physical Examination

Physical examination for carpal instability include the *scaphoid shift* and *lunatotriquetral shear* tests. The scaphoid shift test was designed to evaluate the competency of the scapholunate ligament (Fig. 15.36). During this test, the examiner ranges the wrist from ulnar to radial deviation while maintaining constant pressure on the scaphoid tubercle. Under normal conditions, the scaphoid should palmar-flex; however, if the scapholunate ligament is disrupted, the direct pressure on the scaphoid tubercle can subluxate the scaphoid, causing the patient considerable pain. A clunking sensation may also be noted as the scaphoid proximal pole subluxes dorsally with respect to the radius. The lunatotriquetral shear test is used to evaluate lunatotriquetral instability. The thumb and index finger of one of the examiner's hands are used to stabilize the lunate and the other, to stabilize the triquetrum. Shear forces are introduced across the joint. An increase in translation versus the contralateral side indicates pathology at the lunatotriquetral interval.

Radiographic Findings/Special Studies

Standard radiographic evaluation for carpal instability includes PA, lateral, and oblique views of the hand. Additional views that are more specific for carpal instability include *clenched-fist* anteroposterior (accentuates SL interval widening), *scaphoid view*, and *flexion-extension lateral views* (for dynamic instability). On the PA view, three smooth curved lines that run across the proximal and distal cortices of the proximal carpal row and proximal cortices of the capitate and hamate, known as *Gilula lines*, can be drawn (Fig. 15.37). Any step-off in these lines indicates possible ligamentous disruption. In addition, the SL interval can be measured, with a gap greater than 3 mm indicating disruption of the scapholunate ligament (Terry-Thomas sign). On the lateral, angles that should be appreciated include radiolunate (RL, normal <15 degrees), capitolunate (CL, normal 0–15 degrees), and scapholunate (SL, normal <60 degrees). Arthrograms are still very useful for detecting

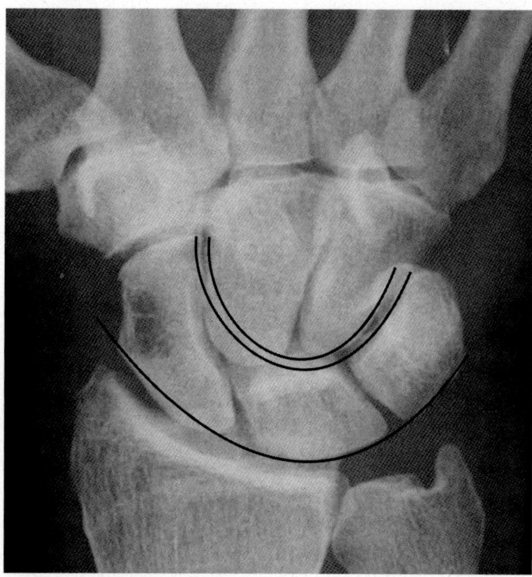

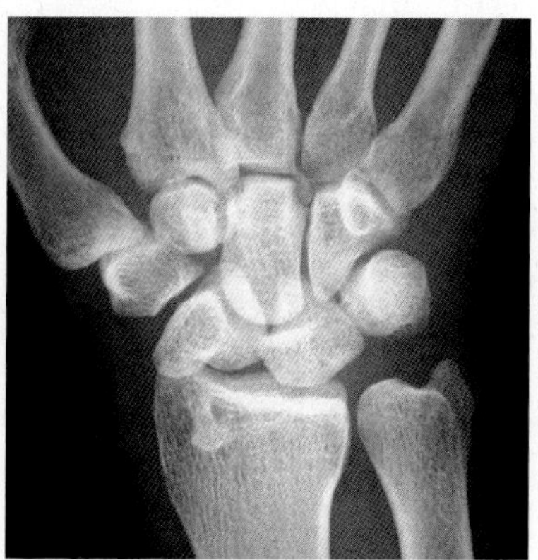

Figure 15.37 **(A, B)** Gilula lines. (*Reprinted with permission from* Bucholz RW, Heckman JD, Court-Brown CM, et al. *Rockwood and Green's Fractures in Adults.* 6th ed. Philadelphia, PA: Lippincott Williams & Wilkins, 2006.)

ligament tears in the carpus, but the improved resolution of MRI has rendered it the study of choice for detecting these injuries.

Treatment

Treatment for SL instability with DISI deformity is varied and depends on the reconstructability of the SL ligament. For acute SL ligament tears treated within the first 6 months, many advocate open reduction and primary ligament repair. The repair may be augmented by a Blatt dorsal capsulodesis. If the ligament is not repairable but the instability is reducible, reconstruction of the ligament with tendon or bone–ligament–bone autograft or capsulodesis is recommended. If the instability is not reducible, a scapho-trapezial–trapezoidal (STT) or scaphocapitate (SC) fusion may be indicated. When chronic instability is present, a pattern of arthritis known as *scapholunate advanced collapse* (SLAC) can result. This pattern is discussed in detail in the arthritis portion of the chapter. The second subgroup of CID is the VISI deformity, in which the lunate assumes a palmar-flexed position while the triquetrum remains in extension. Acute instability can be treated with pin fixation while fusion of the LT interval is need for chronic instability.

For CIND with midcarpal instability, nonoperative management with immobilization should be attempted initially. If that treatment fails, a midcarpal fusion may be indicated. Treatment for CIND with ulnar translation includes immediate open repair, reduction, and pin fixation.

CIC injuries are typically treated with ORIF, with focus on restoring the normal SL gap. A prolonged period of casting (8–12 weeks) typically follows. Last, for longitudinal or axial loading instabilities, ORIF is the mainstay of treatment.

SOFT TISSUE INJURIES

Skin and Nail Trauma

Trauma to the skin and nail region is extremely common, especially in children and young adults. Most injuries are simple lacerations and generally have a good prognosis.

Classification

There is no specific classification system for isolated skin and nail trauma. These injuries can be characterized by the extent of nail bed involvement, location of the injury, and the type of laceration (linear, stellate, etc.).

Presentation and Physical Examination

Patients usually present with the injured region wrapped. Because each injury to the skin and/or nail is different, there is no unifying presentation. The patient should be examined closely. Much information regarding associated injuries can be obtained by simply inspecting the hand. A subungual hematoma often indicates a nail bed disruption with an intact nail plate. Flexor and extensor tendon injuries can often be diagnosed by the posture of the hand. If the hand is not in the usual resting cascade, a tendon injury must be excluded (Fig. 15.38). Vascular injuries can be diagnosed by the color of the distal digits. Following inspection, a full neurovascular examination should be performed, and the function of all tendons should be tested.

Radiographic Findings/Special Studies

Radiographs are useful in diagnosing associated fractures and/or identifying foreign bodies. Orthogonal views are

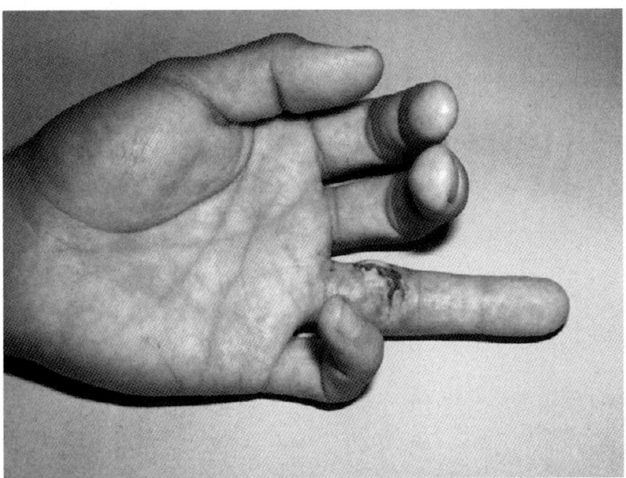

Figure 15.38 Loss of the normal resting cascade suggests underlying tendon injury. (*Reprinted with permission from* Doyle JR, Tornetta P, Einhorn TA. *Orthopaedic Surgery Essentials: Hand and Wrist*. Philadelphia, PA: Lippincott Williams & Wilkins, 2006.)

necessary to avoid missing any injuries. Typically, special studies are not indicated or necessary.

Treatment

On presentation, it is imperative that the patient's tetanus status is up to date. If not, a booster shot should be given. The appropriate treatment of nail trauma is dependent on the size of the injury. If a subungual hematoma occupies less than 25% of the nail, then treatment consists of symptomatic care. If a subungual hematoma involves 25% to 50% of the nail, then a small perforation can be made in the nail to relieve the fluid pressure, which decreases pain. If greater than 50% of the nail is involved, some hand surgeons recommend removing the nail and exploring the nail bed, although this remains controversial. Lacerations can be repaired by using fine absorbable sutures (6–0 chromic), although skin glue can be used for simpler injuries. After the repair, the removed nail or another type of stent should be replaced under the nail fold to prevent it from scarring down on the nail bed.

While wounds should be closely examined, they should not be extensively explored in the emergency department setting. Bleeding should be stopped by direct pressure, and one should avoid blindly clamping any bleeding vessels, given the proximity of the digital nerves to the digital vessels. If evaluation indicates no injuries to the deeper structures, the laceration should be copiously irrigated and then loosely closed with simple 4–0 or 5–0 nylon sutures. In children, absorbable sutures, such as chromic gut, may be preferred to avoid the need for removing the sutures in the office. Antibiotics should be given depending on the size and contamination of the wound.

If there is an amputation of the distal part of the finger, treatment is dependent on location. Distal injuries can often be treated with isolated debridement and composite grafting by using the amputated part. Even if this graft

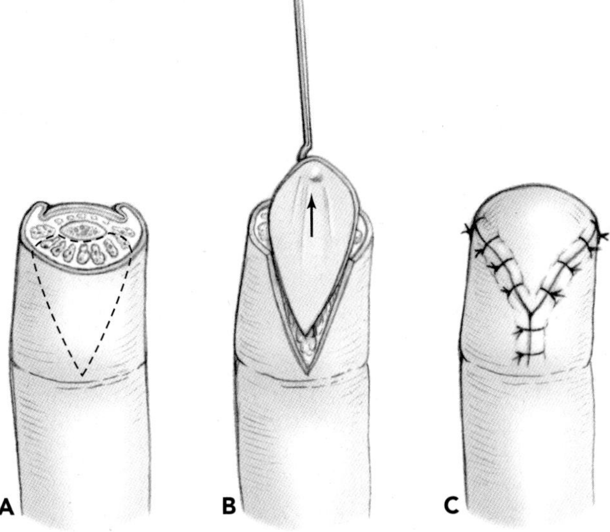

Figure 15.39 The Atasoy–Kleinert V-Y advancement flap. (*Reprinted with permission from* Moran SL, Cooney WP. *Master Techniques in Orthopaedic Surgery: Soft Tissue Surgery*. Philadelphia, PA: Lippincott Williams & Wilkins, 2009.)

fails, the finger tip can frequently heal by secondary intention in small wounds (<1 cm). If bone is exposed, it can be debrided back proximal to the skin defect to allow for primary closure. When this is done, it is important not to advance the nail bed distally as this will lead to a *hooked nail deformity*. More significant soft tissue defects can be treated in a variety of ways. Skin grafts are used for areas with skin loss but adequate deep soft tissue coverage. Split thickness skin grafts can cover large areas and are primarily used for the *dorsal* surface of the hand. Full-thickness skin grafts are more cosmetic and are preferred for *palmar* defects. When bone is exposed, local advancement flaps are ideal for obtaining coverage. Distal finger amputations can often be treated by either a *volar* or *lateral VY flaps* (Fig. 15.39). For amputations through the tip of the thumb, the *Moberg* advancement flap is preferred (Fig. 15.40). This flap can cover defects up to 2.5 cm, but it risks a thumb IP flexion contracture. These local flaps provide sensate soft tissue coverage for the fingertip in small central defects. Larger defects require regional flaps. The *cross-finger flap* is useful for volar finger defects and is based on the dorsal aspect of the middle phalanx (Fig. 15.41). The donor site requires skin grafting. The *thenar flap* is indicated for loss of skin and pulp of the long or ring fingers (Fig. 15.42). This flap can cause PIP joint contractures but remains useful in young patients. Other flaps, such as the neurovascular island flap and the first dorsal MC artery flap, are available for more proximal coverage, but these are more technically demanding.

Flexor Tendon Injuries

Flexor tendon injuries are relatively common but can have a detrimental effect on hand function. Historically, the out-

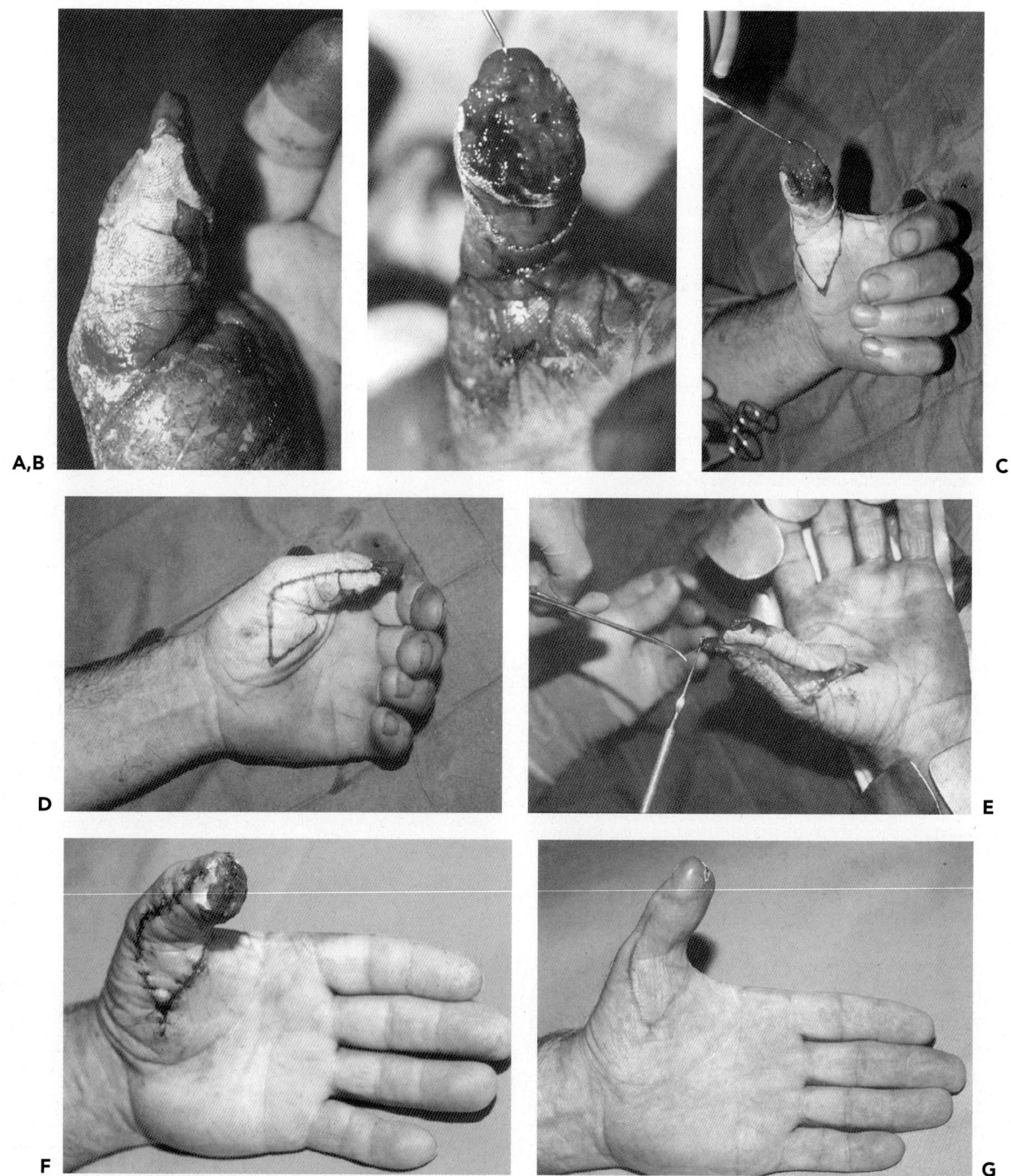

Figure 15.40 **(A–G)** The Moberg advancement flap. (*Reprinted with permission from* Moran SL, Cooney WP. *Master Techniques in Orthopaedic Surgery: Soft Tissue Surgery.* Philadelphia, PA: Lippincott Williams & Wilkins, 2009.)

comes from this injury were extremely poor secondary to tendon adhesions, but advances in basic science, surgical technique, and postoperative rehabilitation have improved results.

Pathophysiology

Tendon healing occurs by a combination of intrinsic and extrinsic mechanisms. The initial inflammatory phase begins immediately after the injury when the defect is filled with blood clot and inflammatory cells. As these cells proliferate, they promote migration of more fibroblasts into the repair site and begin the healing process. The next stage is fibroblastic. At approximately 1 to 2 weeks from injury, the fibroblasts begin secreting collagen, a process that continues for approximately 4 more weeks. At approximately 6 weeks, the remodeling stage begins and the fibroblasts

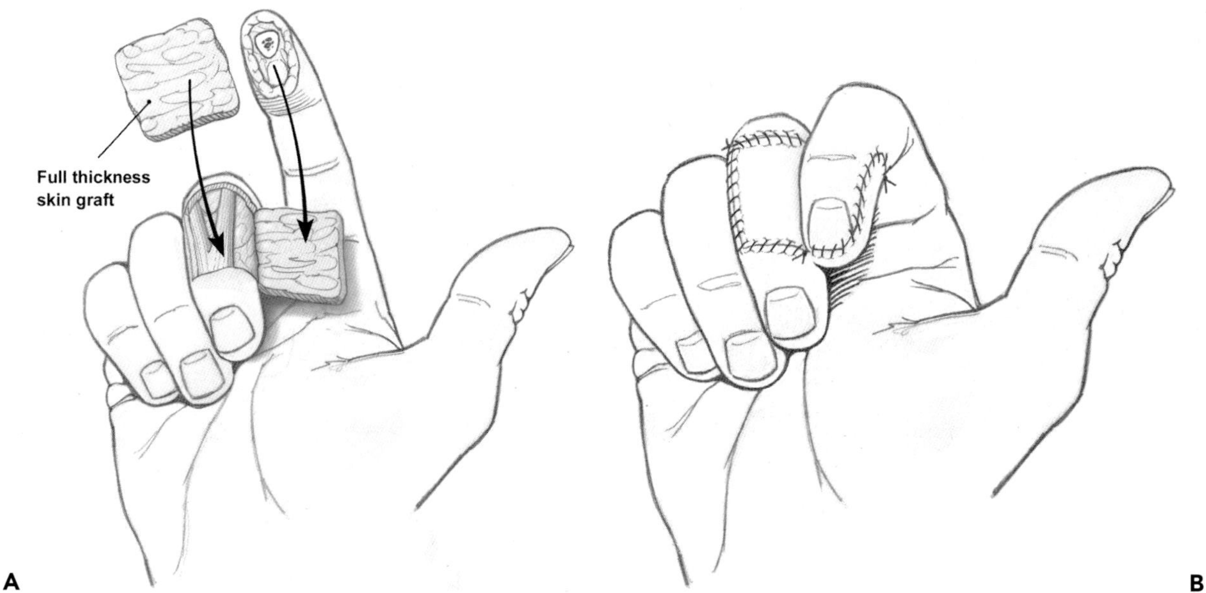

Figure 15.41 **(A, B)** The cross-finger flap. (*Reprinted with permission from* Moran SL, Cooney WP. *Master Techniques in Orthopaedic Surgery: Soft Tissue Surgery*. Philadelphia, PA: Lippincott Williams & Wilkins, 2009.)

begin to reorient themselves in line with the tendon; the collagen fibrils realign with them. At 8 weeks, the repair gap is completely filled with collagen. As physiologic loading begins, the tensile strength of the repair increases steadily.

Classification and Mechanism of Injury

Flexor tendon injuries are classified by the zone (location) of injury (Fig. 15.43). Zone I is distal to the FDS insertion and contains only one tendon (FDP or FPL). In this zone, the tendon can be lacerated or avulsed from its insertion. FDP avulsions occur secondary to forced extension of the digit during maximal contraction of the tendon and is referred to as a *jersey finger* (Fig. 15.44). This injury often occurs in athletes and is commonly misdiagnosed as a sprained or jammed finger. Leddy classified these injuries into three types, and the prognosis is based on the amount of tendon retraction, the remaining tendon blood supply, and the timing of repair.

Zone II is the region from the MC neck (A1 pulley) to the middle of the middle phalanx (FDS insertion) and contains

Figure 15.42 The thenar flap. (*Reprinted with permission from* Strickland JW, Graham TJ. *Master Techniques in Orthopaedic Surgery: The Hand*. Philadelphia, PA: Lippincott Williams & Wilkins, 2005.)

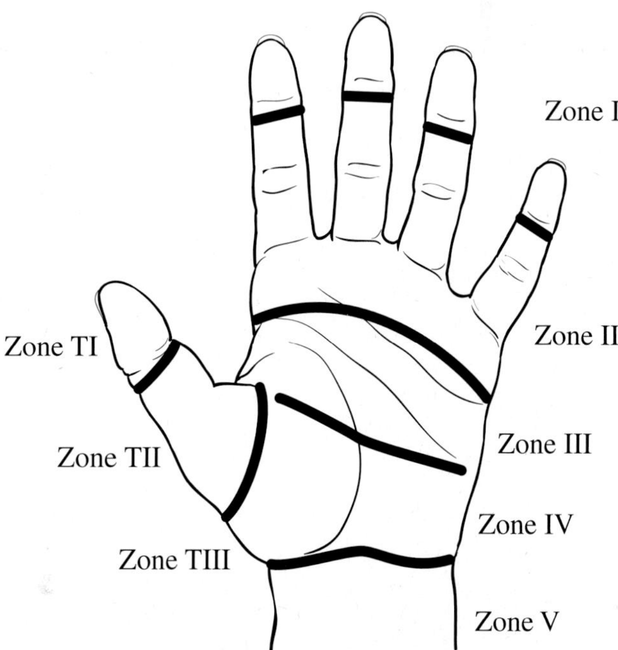

Figure 15.43 The flexor zones of the hand. (*Reprinted with permission from* Doyle JR, Tornetta P, Einhorn TA. *Orthopaedic Surgery Essentials: Hand and Wrist*. Philadelphia, PA: Lippincott Williams & Wilkins, 2006.)

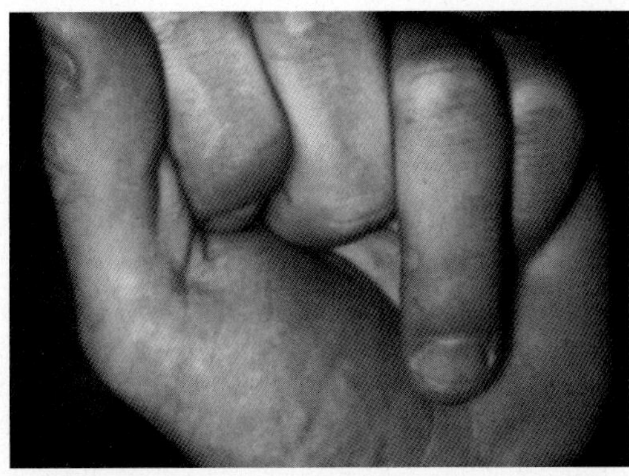

Figure 15.44 Avulsion of the flexor digitorum profundus of the ring finger. (*Reprinted with permission from* Strickland JW, Graham TJ. *Master Techniques in Orthopaedic Surgery: The Hand*. Philadelphia, PA: Lippincott Williams & Wilkins, 2005.)

both the FDS and FDP tendons. This zone is otherwise known as *no man's land* because it has poor results with direct repair secondary to adhesion formation. Zone III is in the palm where the lumbrical muscles originate and is defined by the area between the distal edge of the TCL and the distal palmar crease. Isolated injuries in this zone have a relatively good prognosis but are often complicated by associated nerve and/or vessel injury. Zone IV is the carpal tunnel. The TCL can protect tendon injuries in this area, but when they occur, they are usually associated with nerve (median and/or ulnar nerve) injuries. Zone V is in the forearm from the musculotendinous junction of the flexors to the proximal edge of the TCL. Concomitant nerve or vessel injuries in this zone result in the classic "spaghetti wrist." Overall, the prognosis for tendon reconstruction is best in this zone.

Presentation and Physical Examination

Flexor tendons are usually injured after a sharp laceration or significant blunt trauma. Patients present with the inability to flex the affected finger, and the normal finger cascade is usually disrupted (Fig. 15.45). The FDS and FDP tendons of each digit should be manually tested in isolation. It must be remembered that one-third of all normal individuals are missing the FDS to their small finger. Also, it is important to remember that the site of skin laceration does not always correlate with the zone of tendon laceration because the latter is dependent on the position of the fingers at the time of injury. Of course, the presence or absence of concomitant nerve and vessel injuries should also be determined.

Radiographic Findings

Radiographs are unnecessary in diagnosing flexor tendon ruptures. However, they provide some utility if there is concern regarding concomitant fractures.

Special Studies

Flexor tendon rupture can usually be diagnosed on the basis of history and physical examination. If the diagnosis is unclear, MRI or ultrasound can be used to confirm the diagnosis. These modalities also help to identify partial flexor tendon ruptures.

Differential Diagnosis

The differential of flexor tendon injuries include nerve injuries that cause muscle paralysis and underlying neurological conditions, such as polio or spinal muscular atrophy. A history of trauma generally distinguishes flexor tendon injuries from these other conditions.

Treatment

Complete flexor tendon ruptures should be repaired surgically. Partial tendon lacerations are difficult to diagnose, but lacerations greater than 60% should be repaired to prevent triggering or subsequent rupture.

In flexor tendon repair, several factors affect outcome. First, primary tendon repair should be performed early. No difference in results has been found between emergent and delayed early repairs, but worse outcomes may occur if

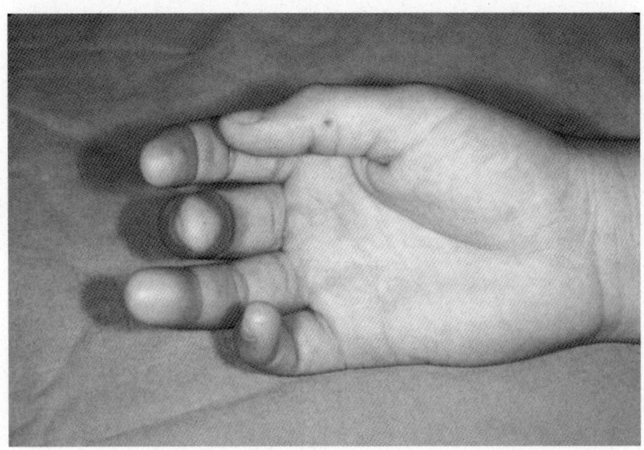

A

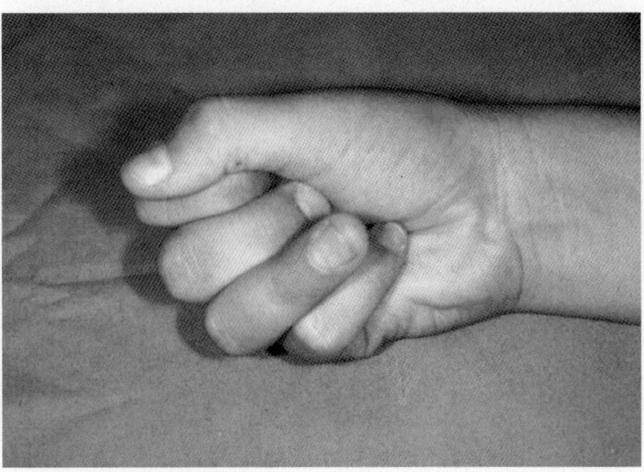

B

Figure 15.45 Note the loss of the normal cascade **(A)** and inability to flex the distal interphalangeal joint **(B)**. (*Reprinted with permission from* Doyle JR, Tornetta P, Einhorn TA. *Orthopaedic Surgery Essentials: Hand and Wrist*. Philadelphia, PA: Lippincott Williams & Wilkins, 2006.)

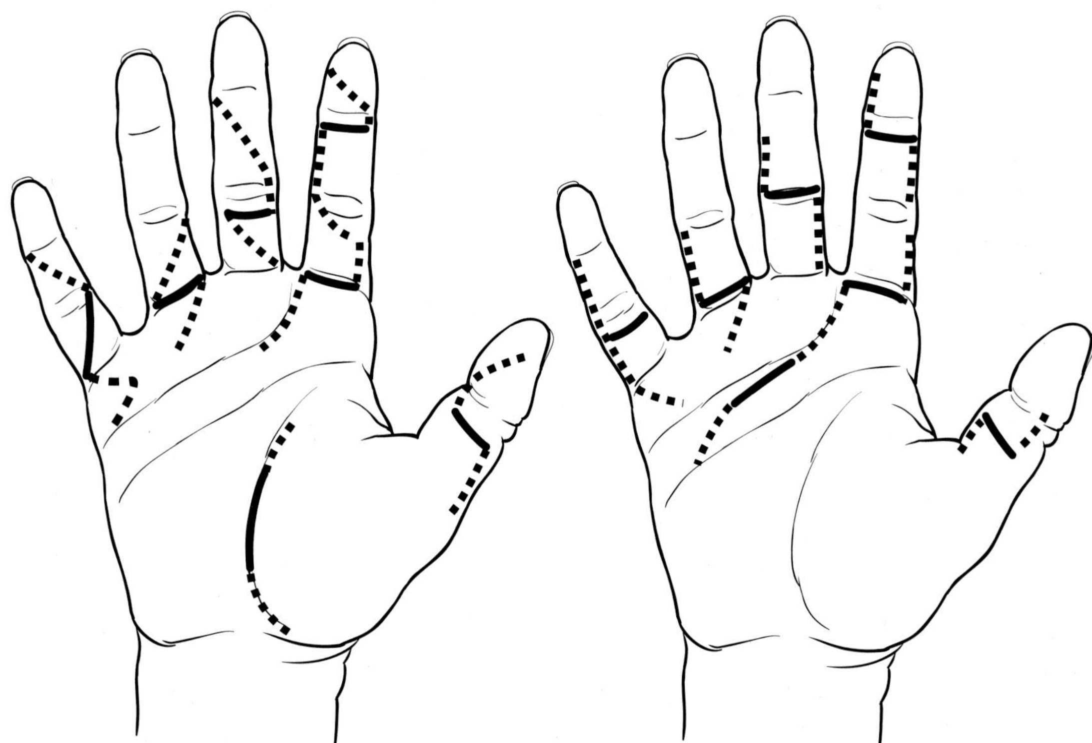

Figure 15.46 Recommended skin incisions for extension of traumatic hand wounds. *Dotted lines* represent the safe extensions of these wounds. (*Reprinted with permission from* Doyle JR, Tornetta P, Einhorn TA. *Orthopaedic Surgery Essentials: Hand and Wrist*. Philadelphia, PA: Lippincott Williams & Wilkins, 2006.)

surgery is done after several weeks due to tendon retraction. If diagnosis or treatment is delayed, the patient may require a two-stage reconstruction, using silicon rods. The rod is used to create a synovial sheath for eventual placement of tendon graft.

In addition to early timing, the repair must be strong enough to allow early motion. Many studies have examined different suture techniques. While several have been shown to be effective, including those advocated by Strickland (Fig. 15.46) and Tajima (Fig. 15.47), the general conclusion is that strength is directly proportional to the number suture strands crossing the repair site. Currently, most surgeons recommend at least four core stands of 3–0 nonabsorbable suture supplemented with a running epitenon stitch (usually 5–0 nylon). Ideally, core sutures are placed dorsally to provide additional strength.

For zone I injuries, treatment involves attachment of the proximal stump to the bone by using suture anchors or pull-out sutures over a button (Fig. 15.48). Tendon advancement greater than 1 cm must be avoided to prevent the *quadregia effect*, which is functional shortening of one of the profundus tendons. Primary end-to-end repair is the treatment of choice for zone I tendon lacerations, but occasionally the quality of the distal stump is so poor that these lacerations are treated as avulsions.

Postoperative rehabilitation is essential to achieve a good result. Early motion gives repaired tendons greater tensile strength, excursion, and function than seen with immobilization. The most common protocols are active extension with rubber band flexion (modified Kleinert), controlled passive motion (modified Duran) (Fig. 15.49), and controlled active motion. Unlike adults, children are immobilized for 4 weeks because they cannot comply with these protocols, and they are less likely to become as stiff.

Extensor Tendon Injuries

Although extensor tendon injuries are discussed less frequently than flexor tendon injuries, they can be quite complex with similar detrimental effects on hand function.

Classification

Similar to flexor tendon injuries, zones can be used to define the location of extensor tendon injuries. Nine zones have been defined anatomically, with the odd zones occurring over joints and the even zones occurring over bones (Fig. 15.50). Zone I is over the DIP joint and involves the disruption of the terminal tendon, which leads to DIP flexion. These injuries are commonly referred to as *mallet fingers* (Fig. 15.51). Zone II injuries occur over the middle phalanx. Zone III injuries are directly over the PIP joint and involve disruption of the central slip of the extensor mechanism. The PIP joint goes into flexion, and chronic injuries

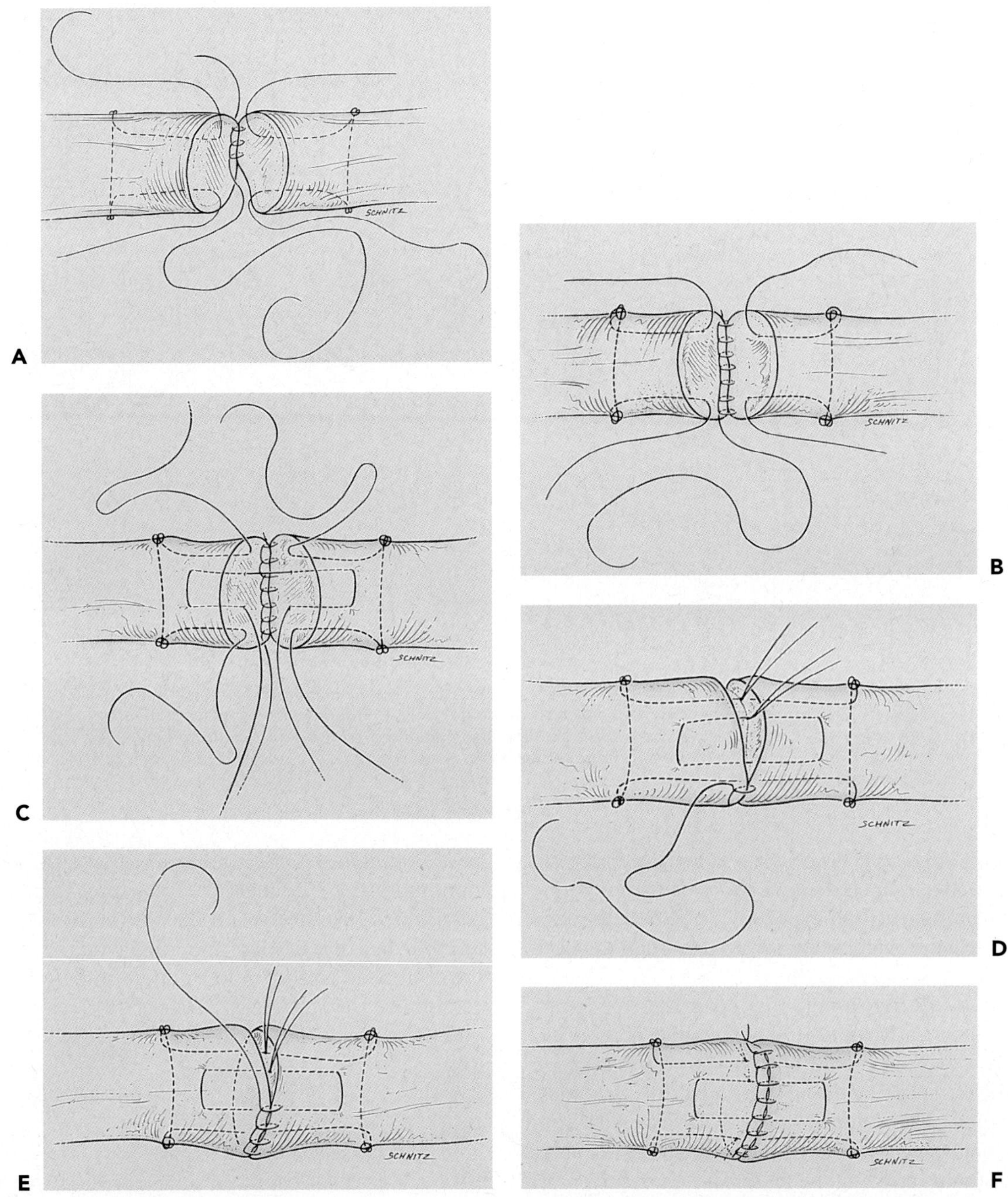

Figure 15.47 **(A–F)** Flexor tendon repair. (*Reprinted with permission from* Strickland JW, Graham TJ. *Master Techniques in Orthopaedic Surgery: The Hand.* Philadelphia, PA: Lippincott Williams & Wilkins, 2005.)

can develop a boutonniere deformity characterized by PIP flexion and DIP hyperextension secondary to volar migration of the lateral bands (Fig. 15.52). Zone V injuries occur over the MP joint and are extremely common. These injuries usually occur during altercations when a fist impacts the tooth of an opponent ("fight bites").

Presentation/Mechanism of Injury

Extensor tendon injuries usually occur via trauma. Common mechanisms are altercations, sharp lacerations, or "jamming" of a finger. Presentation and deformity is dependent on the location of the extensor tendon disruption (Fig. 15.53).

Physical Examination

As with the flexor tendons, extensor tendon injury is relatively straightforward to diagnose. Inspection will often reveal extensor lag, and examination reveals the inability to actively extend the finger. Each finger should be tested in isolation with the adjacent fingers flexed at the MP joints.

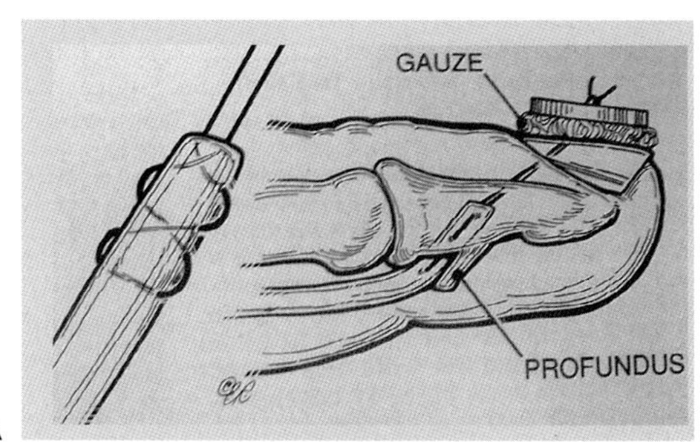

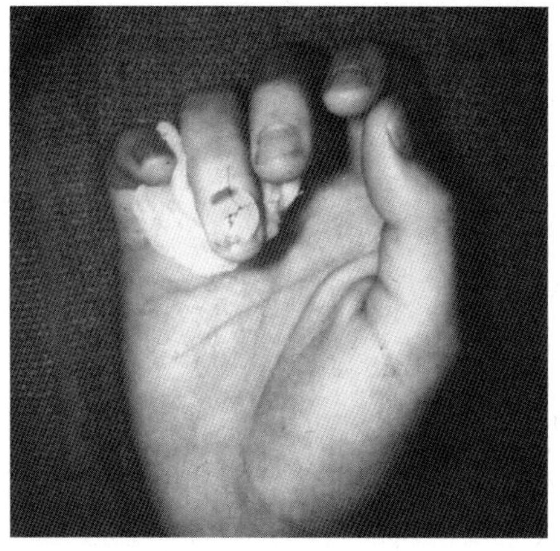

Figure 15.48 **(A, B)** Repair of the flexor digitorum profundus tendon. (*Reprinted with permission from* Strickland JW, Graham TJ. *Master Techniques in Orthopaedic Surgery: The Hand*. Philadelphia, PA: Lippincott Williams & Wilkins, 2005.)

This position eliminates the pull of the juncturae tendinae (fibrous connections between the tendons), which can mask isolated extensor tendon disruption. Also, active extensor strength should be tested at each joint or zone. The Elson test is a specific test for diagnosing an acute boutonniere deformity in a patient with a central slip injury (Fig. 15.54). It is performed with the finger flexed 90 degrees over a table at the PIP joint. In this position, the patient attempts to extend the PIP joint. With an intact central slip, there should be extension pressure through the middle phalanx while the distal phalanx is flail. With a disrupted central slip, the middle phalanx is lax, whereas the distal phalanx is rigid through the DIP joint.

Again, it is important to remember that the site of skin laceration does not always correlate with the zone of tendon laceration because it is dependent on the position of fingers at the time of injury. Of course, one should also evaluate the patient for concomitant nerve or vessel injuries.

Radiographic Findings

Radiographs are mandatory during evaluation to rule out fractures and foreign bodies such as teeth.

Special Studies

It is rare that advanced imaging is necessary in the diagnosis or treatment of extensor tendon injuries.

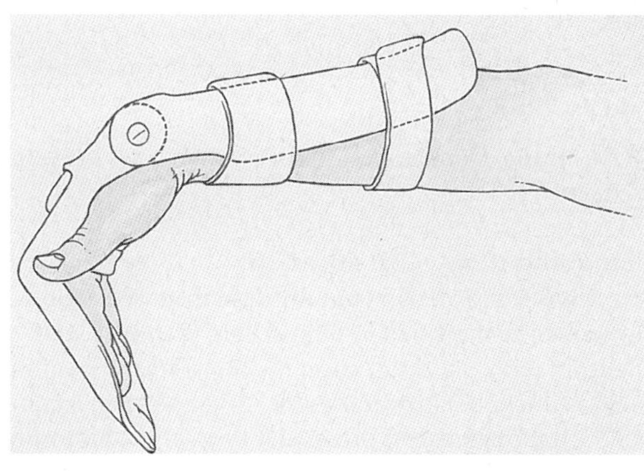

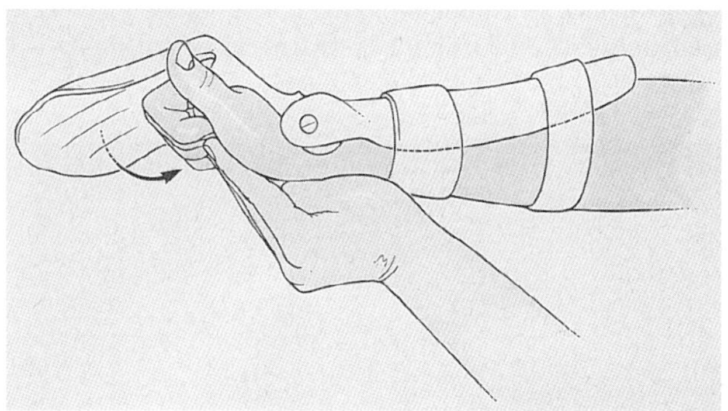

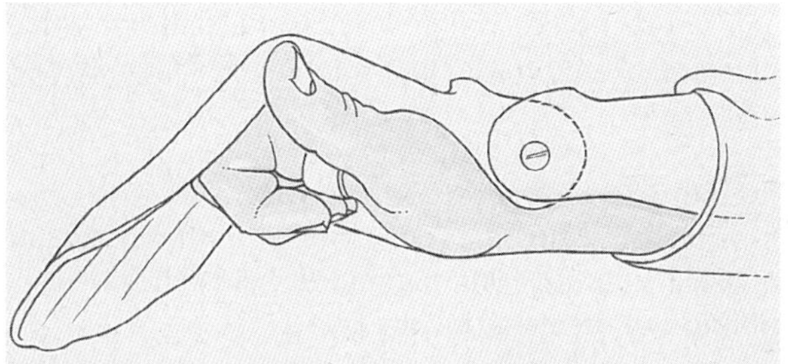

Figure 15.49 **(A–C)** Post flexor tendon repair motion protocol. (*Reprinted with permission from* Strickland JW, Graham TJ. *Master Techniques in Orthopaedic Surgery: The Hand*. Philadelphia, PA: Lippincott Williams & Wilkins, 2005.)

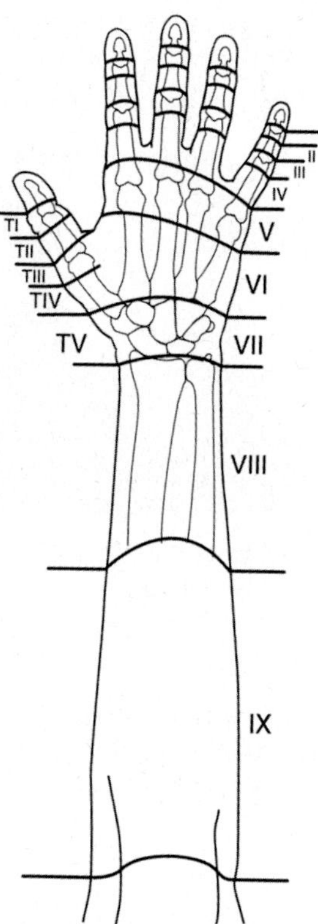

Figure 15.50 Zones of extensor tendon injury. (*Reprinted with permission from* Doyle JR, Botte MJ. *Surgical Anatomy of the Hand and Upper Extremity*. Philadelphia, PA: Lippincott Williams & Wilkins, 2003.)

Treatment

In managing these injuries, several general principles should be kept in mind. First, open injuries should generally be treated in an open manner with surgery, whereas closed injuries should be initially treated closed with splinting. Surgical repair should be performed with a nonabsorbable material and a core suture. Partial open tendon injuries should be repaired if greater than 50% of the tendon width is lacerated.

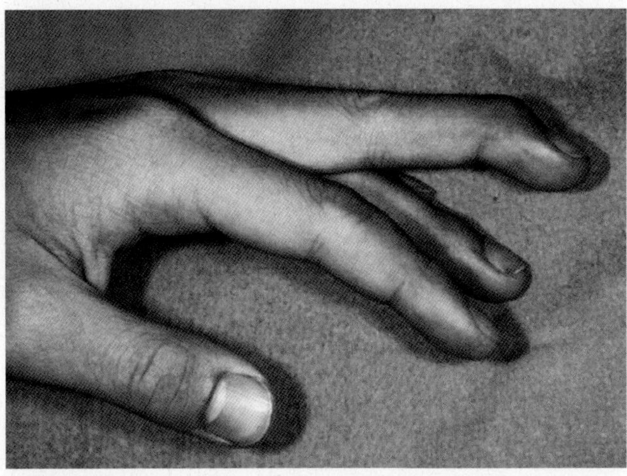

Figure 15.51 Mallet finger. (*Reprinted with permission from* Doyle JR, Tornetta P, Einhorn TA. *Orthopaedic Surgery Essentials: Hand and Wrist*. Philadelphia, PA: Lippincott Williams & Wilkins, 2006.)

Zone I injuries can be treated with extension splinting for 6 weeks with a Stack splint and then subsequent nighttime splinting for an additional 6 weeks (Fig. 15.55). Splinting is the primary treatment also in fingers presenting up to 6 months after injury. Untreated zone I injuries will lead to a swan-neck deformity with DIP flexion and PIP hyperextension secondary to dorsal migration of the lateral bands. This deformity requires significant surgical reconstruction to be corrected. Mallet fingers can also occur with an avulsion fracture of the distal phalanx. Treatment remains the same unless there is DIP subluxation or the fracture fragment is greater than 50% of the articular surface.

Zone II injuries require suture repair if greater than 50% of the tendon is disrupted. Again, nonabsorbable suture is preferred and core sutures should be used.

Similar to mallet fingers, zone III injuries are usually treated nonoperatively with extension splinting of the PIP joint for 6 weeks. Patient compliance is important because reconstruction of chronic boutonniere deformities (i.e., the Fowler procedure) is difficult.

Zones IV through IX injuries all require primary repair. In zone V injuries, urgent surgical irrigation and debridement is necessary if the joint capsule has been violated. A commonly associated injury is sagittal band rupture. Most often, the radial sagittal band of the long finger is ruptured, which leads to ulnar subluxation of the extensor mechanism. Closed injuries can be treated with extension splinting for 4 to 6 weeks, but open injuries should be repaired.

Nerve Injury

Nerve injuries from lacerations or crush injuries to the hand are relatively common.

Pathophysiology/Classification

The classification was originally described by Seddon and subsequently modified by Sunderland (Table 15.2). Type I (neuropraxia) is a conduction block with axon continuity preserved. Type II (axonotomesis) involves axonal damage but the endoneurium is preserved. Type III (axonotomesis) describes axonal damage but the perineurium is preserved. Type IV (axonotomesis) involves axonal damage with only the epineurium intact. Finally, type V is a complete nerve transection.

Presentation/Physical Examination

Presentation varies and is dependent on the specific nerve involved. Physical examination will yield deficits in the distribution of the nerve involved.

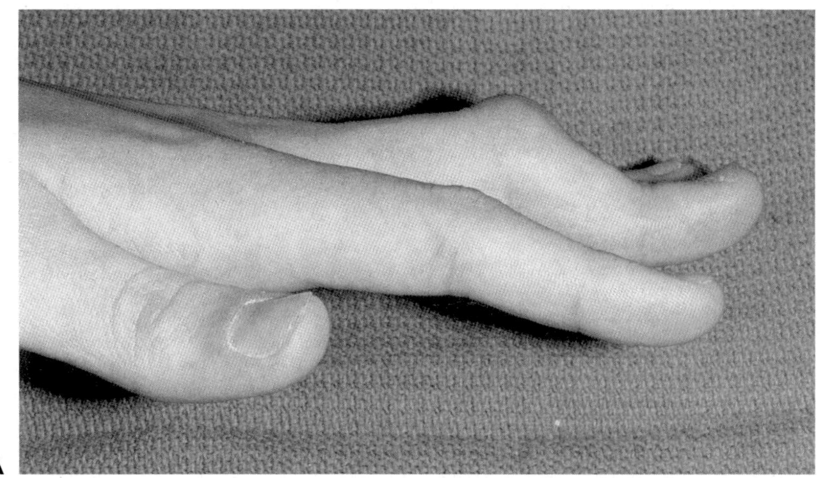

Figure 15.52 **(A, B)** Chronic boutonniere deformity. EDC, extensor digitorum communis; MP; PIP, proximal interphalangeal; DIP, distal interphalangeal. (*Reprinted with permission from* Strickland JW, Graham TJ. *Master Techniques in Orthopaedic Surgery: The Hand.* Philadelphia, PA: Lippincott Williams & Wilkins, 2005.)

TABLE 15.2
COMPARISON OF SUNDERLAND AND SEDDON CLASSIFICATION OF NERVE INJURIES

Author	Descriptive Term	Nature of Injury/Neuropathology
Sunderland	First-degree injury	Demyelinating injury with a temporary conduction block
Seddon	Neurapraxia	
Seddon Sunderland	Second-degree injury (axonotmesis)	Distal degeneration of the injured axon but with almost always complete regeneration due to intact endoneurium
Sunderland Seddon	Third-degree injury (neurotmesis)	Sunderland third-degree injury is less severe than the neurotmesis category of Seddon since the perineurial layer is intact. Regeneration occurs but is incomplete due to endoneurial scarring and loss of end-organ specificity within the fascicle
Sunderland	Fourth-degree injury	Axon, endoneurium, and perineurium are disrupted with extensive scarring that blocks axonal regeneration and often results in a neuroma-in-continuity
Sunderland	Fifth-degree injury	Severed nerve trunk without possibility of spontaneous regeneration

(*Reprinted with permission from* Doyle JR, Tornetta P, Einhorn TA. *Orthopaedic Surgery Essentials: Hand and Wrist.* Philadelphia, PA: Lippincott Williams & Wilkins, 2006.)

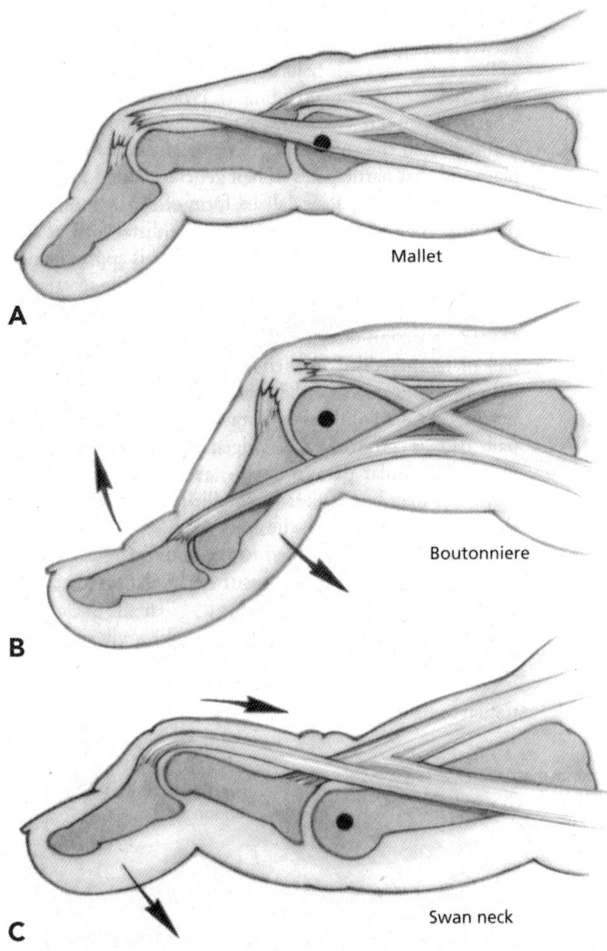

Figure 15.53 Deformities secondary to extensor mechanism injury. (*Reprinted with permission from* Doyle JR, Botte MJ. *Surgical Anatomy of the Hand and Upper Extremity.* Philadelphia, PA: Lippincott Williams & Wilkins, 2003.)

Radiographic Findings

Radiographs are unnecessary in nerve injuries unless associated bone injury is suspected.

Differential Diagnosis

The differential diagnosis includes tendon disruptions that may mimic nerve injuries. These two diagnoses can be distinguished by the use of the tenodesis effect, which should be present only in patients with nerve injuries but absent if there is a tendon injury. The *tenodesis effect* refers to spontaneous flexion of the digits when the wrist is passively extended and implies continuity of the extrinsic tendons. Also, underlying neurological conditions, such as polio or spinal muscular atrophy, must be excluded.

Treatment

When a lacerated nerve is found, microsurgical repair should be performed to facilitate nerve regeneration and to prevent neuroma formation. Primary nerve repair is favored, but nerve grafts should be considered if a tension-free nerve repair cannot be achieved. Common nerve grafts include the sural nerve, the anterior branch of the medial antebrachial cutaneous nerve, the lateral antebrachial cutaneous nerve, and the terminal branch of the posterior interosseous nerve. Recently, autogenous vein conduits and synthetic nerve grafts have been used with some success. After appropriate alignment of the nerve, epineurial repair is currently preferred because grouped fasicular repair has not been shown to be superior (Fig. 15.56). Suture size is dependent on the size of the nerve being repaired. In children, fibrin glue has been used successfully in place of a suture. After nerve repair, occupational therapy is important to provide motor and sensory reeducation.

Replantation

Advances in microsurgical techniques and instrumentation in the late 1950s and the early 1960s led to the ability to replant detached limbs. Malt and McKhann performed the first successful arm replantation in Boston in 1962, and Komatsu and Tamai performed the first successful digital replantation in 1968. Today, the survival rates for digital replants are greater than 90% if performed for appropriate indications.

Classification

No specific classification scheme exists. Injuries are described by location of amputation and the quality of soft tissue.

Mechanism of Injury

There are many different mechanisms that cause upper extremity amputations. Common causes include lawn mowers, snowblowers, industrial machines, and motor vehicle collisions.

Physical Examination

The most important aspect of the physical examination is inspection of the amputated site and residual part. It is vital to assess the quality of the soft tissues and to determine whether replantation has a chance to be successful. Most often, this is dependent on whether the amputation was a sharp or a crush injury.

Radiographic Findings

Radiographs of both the amputated part and the residual limb are necessary to assess the bone stock and to determine the best mode of bone fixation.

Treatment

Whenever a part of the hand or upper extremity is amputated, the part should be wrapped in saline-soaked gauze

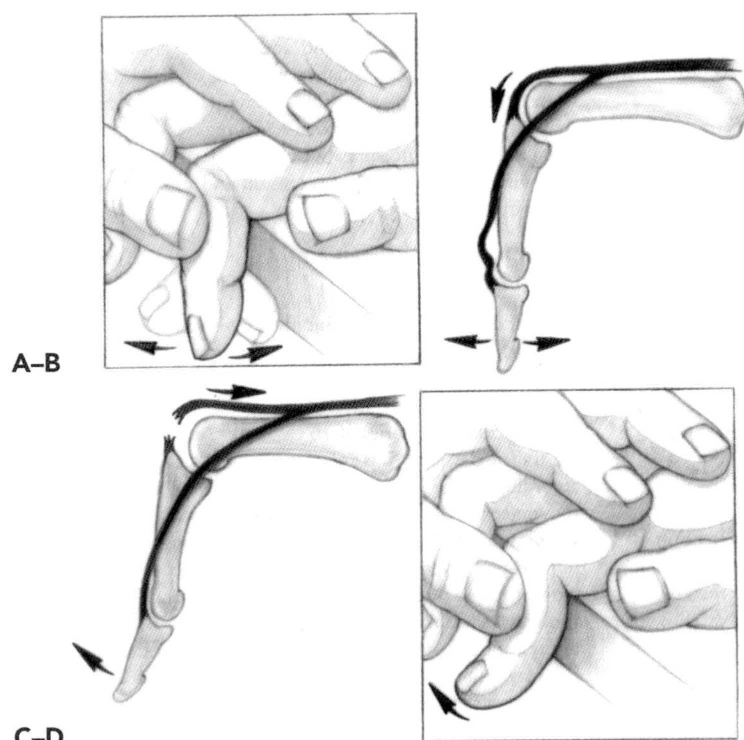

Figure 15.54 Elson test for detection of boutonierre deformity. (*Reprinted with permission from* Doyle JR, Botte MJ. *Surgical Anatomy of the Hand and Upper Extremity*. Philadelphia, PA: Lippincott Williams & Wilkins, 2003.)

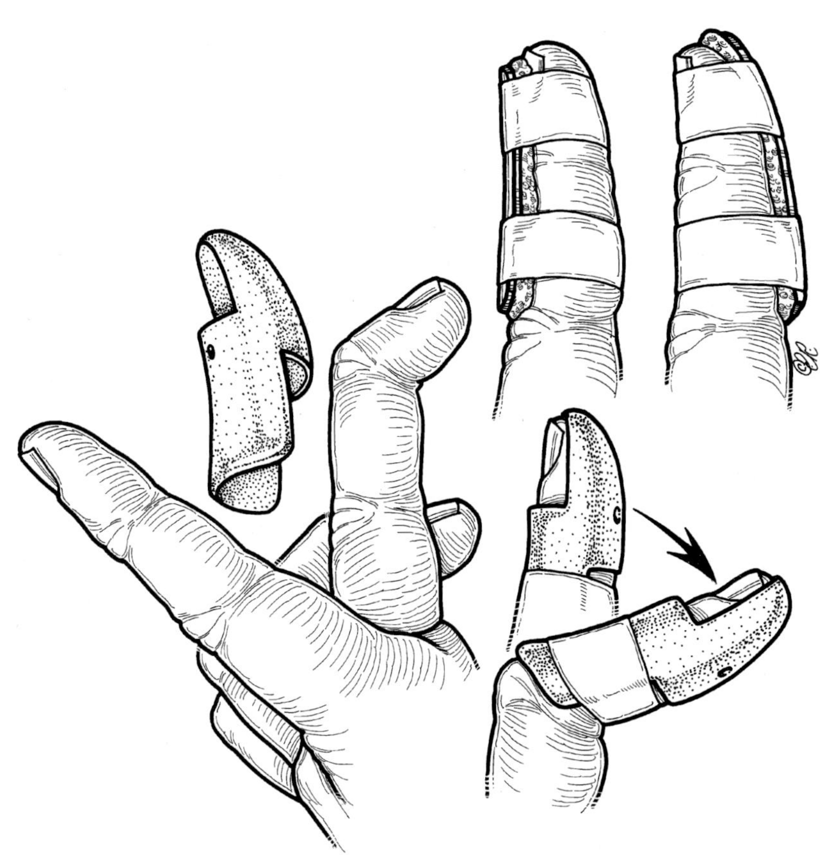

Figure 15.55 Splints used to treat mallet finger deformity. (*Reprinted with permission from* Doyle JR, Tornetta P, Einhorn TA. *Orthopaedic Surgery Essentials: Hand and Wrist*. Philadelphia, PA: Lippincott Williams & Wilkins, 2006.)

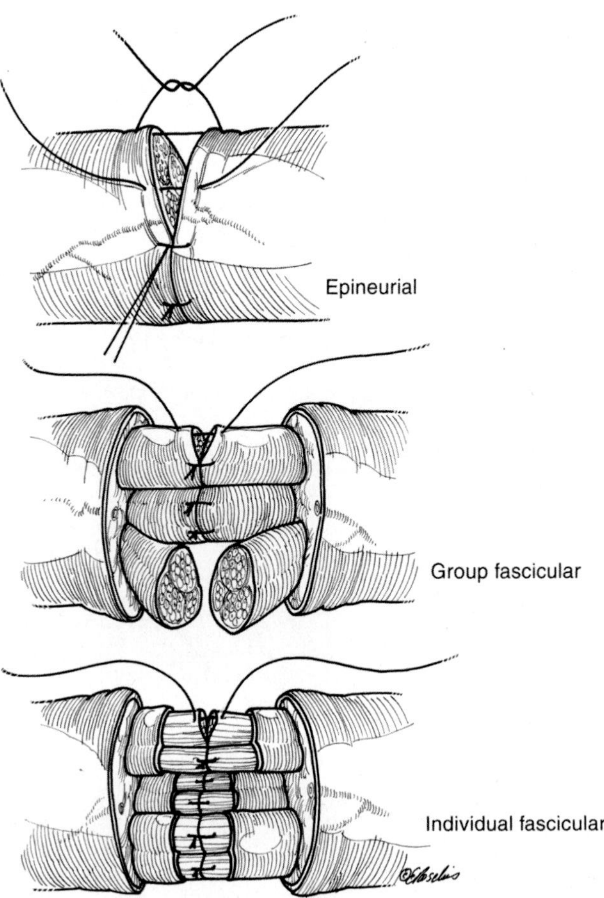

Figure 15.56 Techniques of peripheral nerve repair. (*Reprinted with permission from* Doyle JR, Tornetta P, and Einhorn TA: *Orthopaedic Surgery Essentials: Hand and Wrist.* Philadelphia: Lippincott Williams & Wilkins, 2006.)

and placed inside a plastic bag or sterile container. This should subsequently be placed on ice for transport to the definitive treatment center with the patient. Upon arrival, the patient should be given antibiotics and tetanus prophylaxis. The amputation site and part should then be evaluated to determine whether replantation is possible.

The currently accepted indications for replantation are any thumb amputation, multiple digit amputations, any amputation in a child, and partial hand amputations through the palm, wrist, or forearm (Table 15.3). The duration of ischemia time is also extremely important. Warm ischemia time of more than 12 hours for digital amputation or more than 6 hours for amputations proximal to the carpus leads to poor outcomes Cooling of parts gives an additional ischemia time of 24 hours for digits and 12 hours for major limbs. Acceptable ischemia time is less for more proximal amputation because muscle can tolerate less ischemia than tendon. The type of injury is also extremely important. Sharp amputations do significantly better than crush or degloving injuries. Finally, patient factors play a role in deciding whether replantation should be attempted. Younger patients have better outcomes. Preexisting conditions such as diabetes, peripheral vascular disease, hypercoagulopathy, nicotine dependence, and severe psychiatric conditions decrease success rates. Patients must also be able and willing to comply with the long postoperative rehabilitation program.

When replantation is attempted, a standard operative sequence is used. After identification of structures and debridement of necrotic tissues, the bone is shortened and fixed to allow decreased tension on the neurovascular structures. Next, the extensor tendons, the flexor tendons, the arteries, the nerves, and the veins are repaired in that order. All repairs must be performed using careful microvascular technique. In multiple digital amputations, repair of the same anatomic structure in each digit improves operative efficiency. In major limb replantation, arterial shunting is the first step to limit ischemic time.

Postoperatively, patients must be monitored closely to prevent unnecessary failure. Dressings and protective splints should be applied carefully to avoid compression. The extremity should be elevated high enough to prevent

TABLE 15.3
INDICATIONS AND CONTRAINDICATIONS FOR FINGER REPLANTATION

Indications	Controversial Indications
Amputation of the thumb at any level	Single-digit amputation at a level proximal to the insertion of the flexor digitorum superficialis tendon
Amputation of multiple digits	Ring avulsion injuries
Any amputation in children	Severe contamination
Single-digit injury in zone I	
Contraindications	
Amputated parts that are severely crushed or damaged	
Multiple-level amputations	
Significant associated trauma and/or medical conditions	

(Reprinted with permission from Moran SL, Cooney WP. *Master Techniques in Orthopaedic Surgery: Soft Tissue Surgery.* Philadelphia, PA: Lippincott Williams & Wilkins, 2009.)

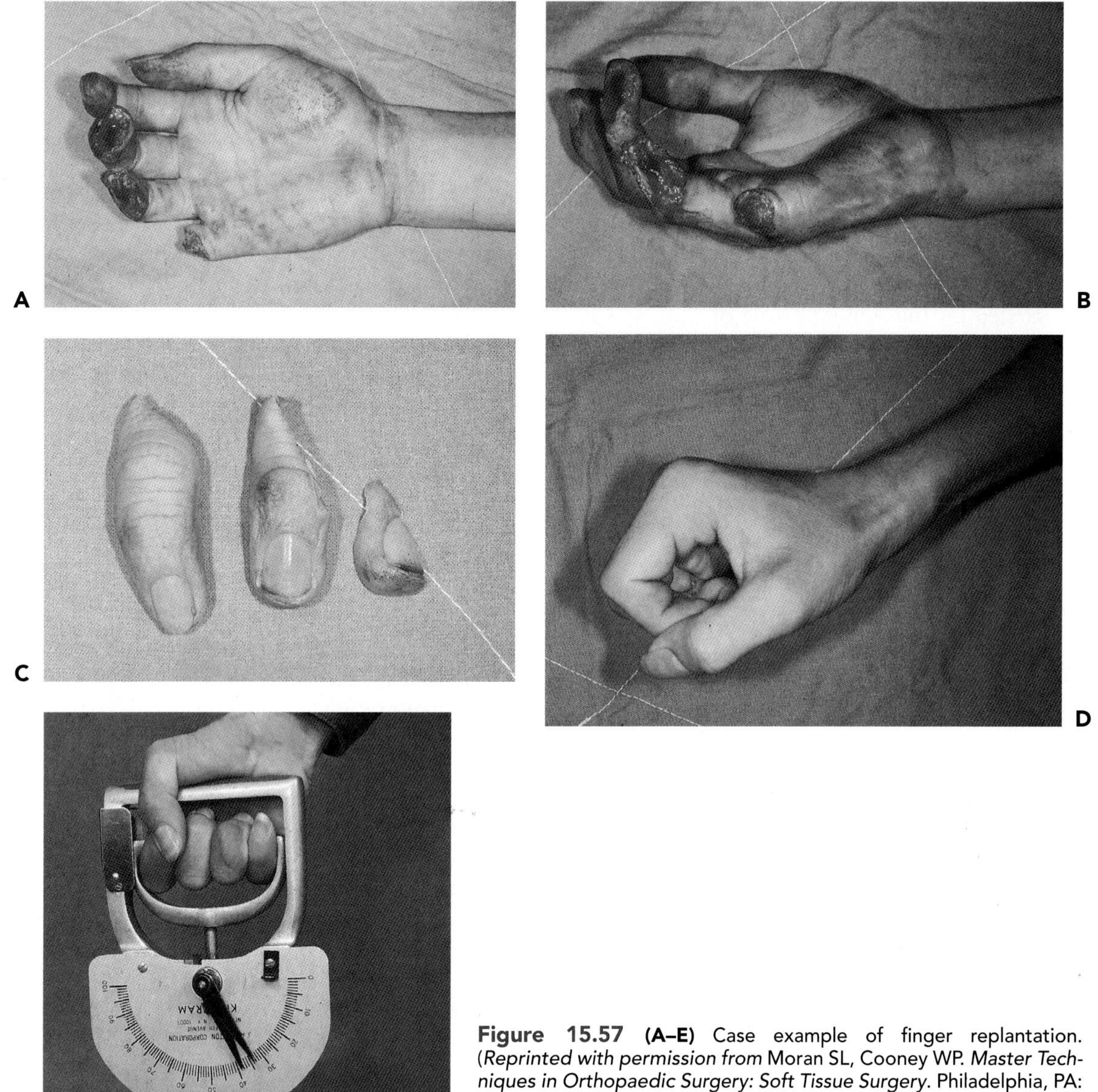

Figure 15.57 **(A–E)** Case example of finger replantation. (*Reprinted with permission from* Moran SL, Cooney WP. *Master Techniques in Orthopaedic Surgery: Soft Tissue Surgery*. Philadelphia, PA: Lippincott Williams & Wilkins, 2009.)

venous pooling but low enough to allow arterial inflow. The patients should avoid any vascoconstrictors such as nicotine, caffeine, and chocolate, and the room should be kept warm and quiet. Anticoagulation is dependent on the preference of the surgeon, but multiple agents such as aspirin, heparin, dextran, and dipyridamole have been used. Replants should be checked hourly for adequate perfusion. Leeches are occasionally used to relieve venous congestion if venous outflow is inadequate.

As stated earlier, the survival rates for replantation of clean amputations in appropriate patients is 90%. However, functional results vary significantly (Fig. 15.57). Stiffness, cold sensitivity, and chronic pain can be significant problems. Return to the operating room is often necessary. In summary, replantation is a powerful but technically demanding tool, which is associated with a high complication rate; correct patient selection is therefore imperative.

NONTRAUMATIC INJURIES TO THE HAND AND WRIST

Compressive Neuropathies

Compressive neuropathies result from mechanical compression that causes local nerve ischemia and dysfunction. Traction is also thought to play a role in this disease process. When diagnosed and released early, nerve recovery is predictably good. However, after a long-standing injury, decompression may only halt the progression of disease rather than reverse the symptoms.

The general assessment of a patient in whom a compressive neuropathy is suspected should involve a careful history and physical examination. The history should evaluate predisposing factors such as systemic or inflammatory conditions including diabetes, hyperthyroidism, RA, and infection. Also, the history should draw out conditions that alter fluid balance, such as pregnancy and hemodialysis. On examination, one should focus on finding objective signs of motor or sensory changes and trying to isolate the exact level at which the compression is present. Motor strength is graded on the standard scale of 1 to 5. Sensory examination consists of both threshold (light touch) and innervation density (2-point discrimination) testing. Semmes–Weinstein testing with monofilaments is helpful in diagnosing early sensory change. The concept of a double crush phenomenon, with entrapment at two levels, must always be considered because both sites of compression may require release.

Carpal Tunnel Syndrome

CTS is the most common upper extremity compressive neuropathy.

Pathophysiology

CTS is compression of the median nerve as it passes underneath the TCL in the wrist (Fig. 15.58). Potential causes include anatomic abnormalities (such as proximal lumbrical muscles), fluid imbalances (pregnancy, hemodialysis), trauma (hematoma, distal radius fractures), and positional factors.

Presentation/Mechanism of Injury

CTS usually presents with decreased sensation over the palmar aspect of radial three fingers and the radial side of the ring finger. The numbness is typically worse at night. As the syndrome progresses, patients complain of weakness and pain that can radiate into the volar forearm. If left untreated, CTS can lead to thenar atrophy.

Physical Examination

Physical examination includes Tinel test (tapping over the TCL, which elicits electric-like shocks that radiate into the fingers), Phalen test (manual volar flexion of the wrist, which reproduces the patient's symptoms), and the carpal tunnel compression test (reproduction of the patient's symptoms from direct compression over the volar aspect of the carpal tunnel) (Table 15.4). Each of these tests has varying degrees of sensitivity and specificity, but combined with a history and electromyography (EMG), a reliable diagnosis can usually be obtained.

Special Studies

EMG and nerve conduction studies (NCSs) are useful tests to help confirm the diagnosis of CTS. Changes consistent with a diagnosis of CTS include distal motor latency greater than 4.0 ms or asymmetry of 1.0 ms between the involved and uninvolved hands. In addition, a distal sensory latency greater than 3.5 ms or asymmetry of 0.5 ms between hands is highly suggestive of CTS.

Treatment

Once diagnosed, CTS can be treated nonoperatively or operatively. Initial treatment usually focuses on nighttime wrist splinting in a neutral position, oral anti-inflammatory medications to decrease synovitis and edema, and management of underlying medical problems. Corticosteroid injections can be performed directly into the carpal tunnel. Although injections provide transient relief to 80% of patients, only 22% of patients have continued symptomatic relief at 1 year. Although relief may be only transient, it is a good prognostic sign for surgical release.

Surgical treatment can be done either open or endoscopically. Although debate still exists over which is the optimal procedure, data continue to show minimal differences between the two procedures. Endoscopic carpal tunnel release may result in less pillar pain and earlier return to work, but there is a slightly increased risk of incomplete release. Success after either procedure results in improved pain and decreased numbness, which is proportional to the amount of preoperative EMG dysfunction.

Pronator Syndrome

Pathophysiology

Pronator syndrome involves proximal compression of the median nerve. Potential compression sites include a supracondylar process of the humerus with an associated ligament of Struthers, the lacertus fibrosis or bicipital aponeurosis, the pronator teres origin, and the origin of the FDS (Fig. 15.59).

Presentation

The primary presenting symptoms are numbness in the radial three fingers and the radial side of the ring finger, as well as forearm pain. Pronator syndrome rarely presents with motor weakness.

Physical Examination

Pronator syndrome is clinically differentiated from CTS by numbness in the palmar cutaneous branch distribution, pain with resisted wrist flexion and forearm pronation, and a negative Phalen and carpal compression tests.

Special Studies

EMG is usually necessary to definitively distinguish pronator syndrome from CTS, although the accuracy of the study for this condition can be variable.

Differential Diagnosis

Pronator syndrome must be differentiated from the more common CTS.

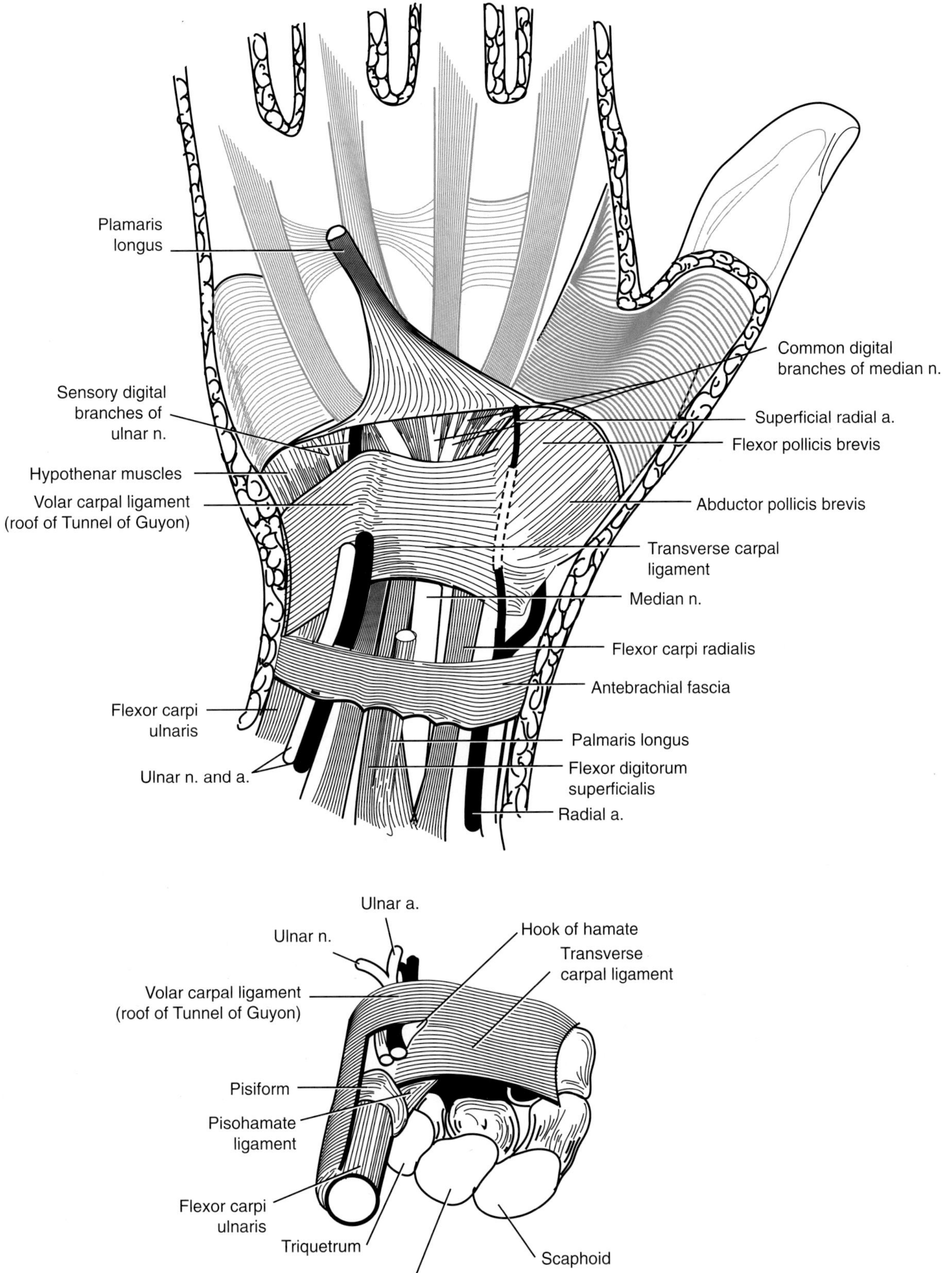

Figure 15.58 The carpal and ulnar tunnels. (*Adapted with permission from* Hoppenfeld S, deBoer P. *Surgical Exposures in Orthopaedics: The Anatomic Approach.* 3rd ed. Philadelphia, PA: Lippincott Williams & Wilkins, 2003.)

TABLE 15.4
TESTS FOR CARPAL TUNNEL SYNDROME (CTS)

Test	How to Perform	Condition Tested	Interpretation of Positive Result	Positive Result
Phalen test	Elbows on table, forearms vertical, wrists flexed	Paresthesia in response to position	Numbness or tingling on radial digits within 60 s	Probable CTS (sens 0.75, spec 0.47)
Percussion test (Tinel sign)	Lightly tap along median nerve from proximal to distal	Site of nerve lesion	"Electric" tingling response in fingers	Probable CTS if positive at the wrist (sens 0.60, spec 0.67)
Carpal tunnel compression test (Durkan)	Direct compression of median nerve at carpal tunnel	Paresthesia in response to compression	Paresthesia within 30 s	Probable CTS (sens 0.87, spec 0.90)
Hand diagram	Patient marks site of pain or altered sensation on outlined hand diagram	Patient's perception of symptoms	Markings on palmar side of radial digits, without markings in palm	Probable CTS (sens 0.96, spec 0.73, negative predictive value 0.91)
Hand volume stress test	Hand volume measured by displacement, repeat after 7-minute stress test and a rest of 10 minutes	Hand volume	Hand volume increased by 10 mL or greater	Probable dynamic CTS
Direct measurement of carpal tunnel pressure	Wick or infusion catheter placed in carpal tunnel	Hydrostatic pressure in resting and provocative positioning	Resting pressure 25 mm Hg or more (variable and technique related)	Hydrostatic compression is felt to be probable cause of CTS
Static two-point discrimination	Determine minimum separation of two distinct points when applied to palmar fingertip	Innervation density of slow-adapting fibers	Failure to determine separation of at least 5 mm	Advanced nerve dysfunction
Moving two-point discrimination	As mentioned earlier, with movement of the points	Innervation density of fast-adapting fibers	Failure to determine separation of at least 4 mm	Advanced nerve dysfunction
Vibrometry	Vibrometer placed on palmar side of digit, amplitude set to 120 Hz, and increase to threshold of perception; compare median and ulnar bilaterally	Threshold of fast-adapting fibers	Asymmetry compared with contralateral hand or median to ulnar in ipsilateral hand	Probable CTS (sens 0.87)
Semmes–Weinstein monofilaments	Monofilaments of increasing diameter touched to palmar side of digit until patient can determine which digit is touched	Threshold of slowly adapting fibers	Value greater than 2.83	Median nerve impairment (sens 0.83)
Distal sensory latency and conduction velocity	Orthodromic stimulus and recording across wrist	Latency, conduction of sensory fibers	Latency greater than 3.5 ms, or asymmetry of conduction velocity of greater than 0.5 m/s vs. opposite hand	Probable CTS
Distal motor latency and conduction velocity	Orthodromic stimulus and recording across wrist	Latency, conduction velocity of motor fibers of median nerve	Latency greater than 4.5 ms, or asymmetry of conduction velocity of greater than 1.0 m/s	Probable CTS
Electromyography	Needle electrodes placed in muscle	Denervation of thenar muscles	Fibrillation potentials, sharp waves, increased insertional activity	Advanced motor median nerve compression

Sens, sensitivity; spec, specificity.
(*From* Abrams R, Meunier, M. Carpal tunnel syndrome. In: Trumble TE, ed. *Hand Surgery Update 3, Hand, Elbow, Shoulder.* Rosemont, IL: American Society for Surgery of the Hand, 2003:299–312.)
(*Reprinted with permission from* Doyle JR, Tornetta P, Einhorn TA: *Orthopaedic Surgery Essentials: Hand and Wrist.* Philadelphia, PA: Lippincott Williams & Wilkins, 2006.)

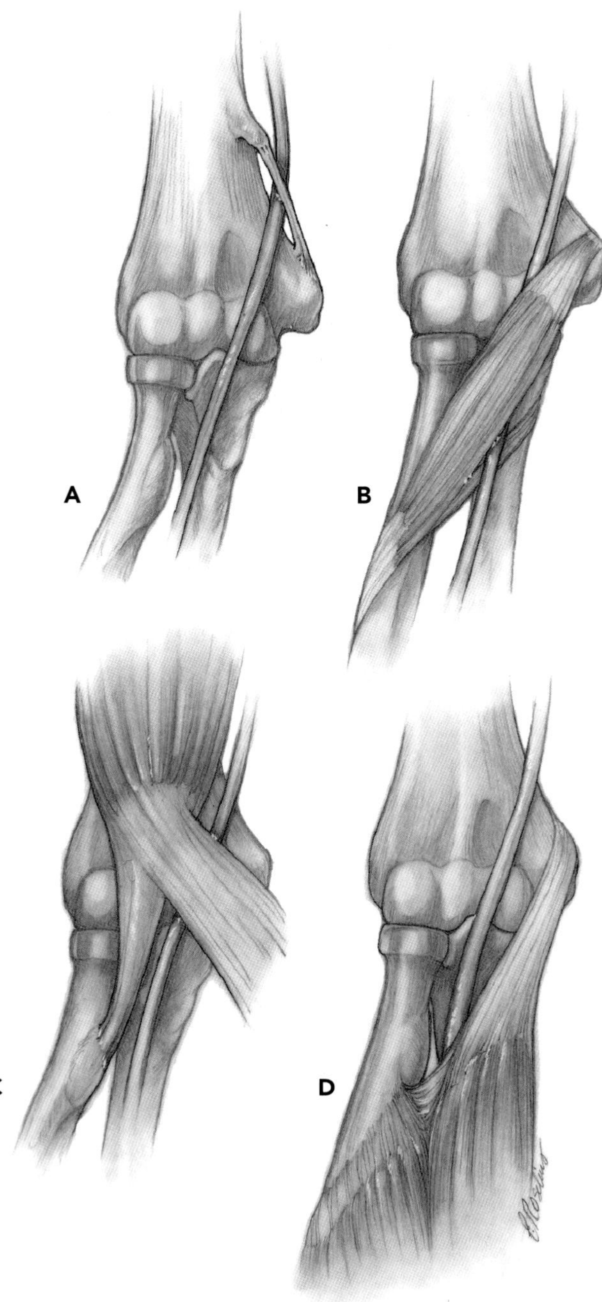

Figure 15.59 Sites of median nerve compression include **(A)** ligament of Struthers from supracondylar process, **(B)** pronator teres, **(C)** lacertus fibrosis, and **(D)** fibrous arch of flexor digitorum superficialis. (*Reprinted with permission from* Doyle JR, Tornetta P, Einhorn TA. *Orthopaedic Surgery Essentials: Hand and Wrist.* Philadelphia, PA: Lippincott Williams & Wilkins, 2006.)

Treatment

If the diagnosis is made, initial management is nonoperative with activity modification to decrease repetitive flexion and pronation. Splinting and nonsteroidal anti-inflammatory drugs (NSAIDs) are occasionally helpful. Operative treatment, which involves releasing all four potential compression sites, is considered only after a minimum of 6 months of conservative treatment.

Anterior Interosseous Syndrome

Pathophysiology

Anterior interosseous syndrome involves the compression of the anterior interosseous nerve (AIN) after it branches from the median nerve 4 to 6 cm below the elbow. Sites of compression include the deep head of the pronator teres, the FDS origin, the FCR origin, and accessory muscles such as Gantzer muscle, which is an accessory head to the FPL.

Presentation

Since the AIN is a motor nerve that innervates the FPL, the pronator quadratus, and the FDS to the index and little fingers, symptoms involve weakness to these muscles and forearm pain.

Physical Examination

Physical examination can demonstrate the inability to make an "O" sign with the index finger and the thumb. No sensory deficit should be evident.

Special Studies

EMG is necessary to make the diagnosis. Delayed conduction should be seen across the site of compression.

Differential Diagnosis

The differential diagnosis of this rare condition includes tendon ruptures and Parsonage–Turner syndrome (viral brachial neuritis).

Treatment

Initial treatment involves 3 to 6 months of observation. If symptoms do not resolve, surgical decompression or tendon transfers can be considered.

Cubital Tunnel Syndrome

Cubital tunnel syndrome is the second most common upper extremity compressive neuropathy.

Pathophysiology/Classification

Cubital tunnel syndrome involves ulnar nerve compression around the elbow, and there are five common sites of compression. The arcade of Struthers is a band of fascia that connects the medial intermuscular septum to the medial head of the triceps and is located approximately 8 cm proximal to the medial epicondyle (Fig. 15.60). This fascia, along with the intermuscular septum and a hypertrophied medial head of the triceps, can compress the ulnar nerve. Moving distally, the medial epicondyle can compress the ulnar nerve, especially during elbow flexion. Beyond the medial epicondyle, the nerve is at risk as it passes under the arcuate ligament, which connects the medial epicondyle to the olecranon and serves as the roof of the cubital tunnel. Osborne fascia, which is a fascial band between the two heads of the FCU, is another site of potential compression. Finally,

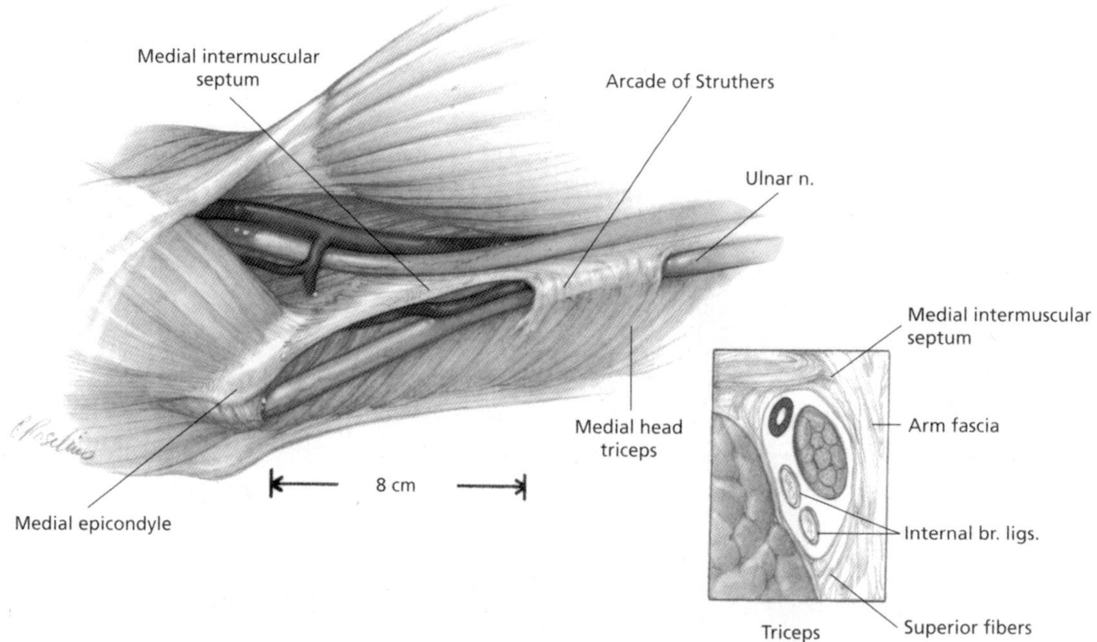

Figure 15.60 **(A)** The arcade of Struthers. (*Reprinted with permission from* Doyle JR, Botte MJ. *Surgical Anatomy of the Hand and Upper Extremity*. Philadelphia, PA: Lippincott Williams & Wilkins, 2003.)

as it exits from underneath the FCU, the ulnar nerve can be compressed by the deep flexor pronator aponeurosis. Less common causes of compression include anomalous muscles such as an anconeus epitrochlearis.

McGowan has categorized cubital tunnel syndrome into three grades. Grade I represents mild lesions of the ulnar nerve causing paresthesias and clumsiness in the affected hand, without intrinsic muscle weakness. Grade II describes intermediate lesions causing weakness in the interossei and muscle wasting. Grade III denotes severe lesions that cause interossei paralysis with substantial hand weakness.

Presentation

Cubital tunnel syndrome usually presents with numbness or paresthesias in the ulnar one and a half fingers. Other signs and symptoms include elbow pain, intrinsic weakness, and hand clumsiness. Symptoms are usually exacerbated by elbow flexion because this alters the shape of the cubital tunnel from an oval to a slit, thereby decreasing its volume by 50%.

Physical Examination

Beyond standard motor and sensory testing, several provocative physical examination signs may help in the diagnosis. Often, tapping over the cubital tunnel (Tinel sign) and full-elbow flexion will reproduce the patients' symptoms. A Froment sign is weakness during pinch. Patients are asked to pinch a sheet of paper between their thumb and index finger. Patients with cubital tunnel syndrome have weakness in thumb adduction (ulnar nerve) and compensate by flexing their FPL (AIN). Wartenberg sign is abduction of the small finger during repetitive flexion and extension of the fingers secondary to weakness of the third palmar interosseous muscle.

Special Studies

EMG and NCS are helpful in confirming the diagnosis. A nerve conduction velocity of less than 50 m/s or a drop in conduction velocity of greater than 10 m/s around the elbow is considered abnormal.

Differential Diagnosis

Differential diagnosis includes radiculopathy of C8–T1, Pancoast tumor, and thoracic outlet syndrome.

Treatment

Initial treatment involves NSAIDs and nighttime extension splinting. If nonoperative treatment fails or intrinsic atrophy occurs, surgery is indicated. In situ decompression is the least invasive option but does not address the potential traction phenomenon that the nerve experiences as the elbow flexes. In general, anterior transposition of the ulnar nerve is the most commonly used surgical technique for treating cubital tunnel syndrome. Although dissection of the nerve risks devascularization, the entire length of the nerve can be freed from compression. By moving the nerve anterior to the axis of motion at the elbow, traction on the nerve is also reduced. Two different techniques have been described for the transposition: submuscular and subcutaneous. Subcutaneous transpositions are technically easier and preserve the integrity of the flexor–pronator muscle mass. However, the superficial position of the nerve risks future injury in thin patients. Submuscular transpositions provide a safer haven for the ulnar nerve and are useful in revision cases but do violate the integrity of the flexor–pronator muscles. In general, this technique should be avoided in throwing athletes.

Ulnar Tunnel Syndrome

Pathophysiology

Ulnar tunnel syndrome is compression of the ulnar nerve at the Guyon canal in the wrist. The borders of the Guyon canal are defined by the flexor retinaculum (floor), the pisiform (ulnar border), the hook of the hamate (radial border), and the volar carpal ligament (roof). In this area, the ulnar nerve bifurcates into the deep motor branch and the superficial sensory branch. Compression is most usually secondary to ganglion cysts but can be associated with hook of the hamate fractures, ulnar artery thrombosis, and repetitive trauma.

Presentation/Physical Examination

Ulnar tunnel syndrome can be differentiated from cubital tunnel syndrome by intact sensation over the dorsal ulnar aspect of the hand, which is innervated by the dorsal sensory nerve.

Special Studies

EMG and NCS are important in confirming the location of compression.

Differential Diagnosis

The primary diagnoses that need to be excluded are compression of the ulnar nerve at the elbow or more proximal nerve compression, especially in the cervical spine.

Treatment

Treatment is based on etiology. Similar to other compression neuropathies, splinting, NSAIDs, and activity modification are attempted prior to surgical decompression.

Posterior Interosseous Syndrome

Pathophysiology

Posterior interosseous syndrome refers to compression of the posterior interosseous nerve by one of the following structures: fibrous bands anterior to the radiocapitellar joint, the leash of Henry (recurrent radial vessels), the arcade of Frohse (proximal edge of the supinator), the distal edge of the supinator, or the fibrous edge of the ECRB (Fig. 15.61).

Presentation/Physical Examination

Because the posterior interosseus nerve is primarily a motor nerve, symptoms do not include pain. Instead, patients have difficulty extending their fingers at the MP joints and the thumb at the IP joint. Wrist extension remains intact because the ECRL is innervated by the radial nerve.

Special Studies

EMG and NCS are useful for diagnosing posterior interosseous syndrome.

Differential Diagnosis

Intact wrist extension is important in differentiating posterior interosseous syndrome from a more proximal radial nerve palsy. The other differential diagnosis is extensor tendon rupture, which can be differentiated from posterior interosseus syndrome by the presence of the tenodesis effect (passive finger extension with wrist flexion).

Treatment

Once the diagnosis has been made, initial treatment involves activity modification and splinting. If this fails, surgical release or tendon transfers may be indicated.

Radial Tunnel Syndrome

Pathophysiology

Radial tunnel syndrome is a pain syndrome that is not associated with motor or sensory deficits.

Presentation

The chief complaint is pain in the proximal radial forearm, and it is usually related to repetitive work activities.

Physical Examination

On physical examination, tenderness over the radial nerve distal to the lateral epicondyle is one of the hallmark findings, and provocative maneuvers include pain with resisted middle finger extension. However, both of these findings lack sensitivity and specificity.

Special Studies

EMG and NCS usually have normal results.

Differential Diagnosis

The other major diagnosis in the differential is lateral epicondylitis. One method to differentiate these two conditions is selective injection of local anesthetic into the region of the posterior interosseous nerve. If this leads to pain relief while also causing a temporary, complete radial nerve palsy, it is considered diagnostic for radial tunnel syndrome. Unfortunately, lateral epicondylitis and radial tunnel syndrome can coexist in up to 5% to 10% of patients.

Treatment

Treatment is based on extended nonoperative modalities, such as splinting, activity modification, and NSAIDs. If symptoms persist despite 6 to 9 months of conservative treatment, surgical decompression can be considered.

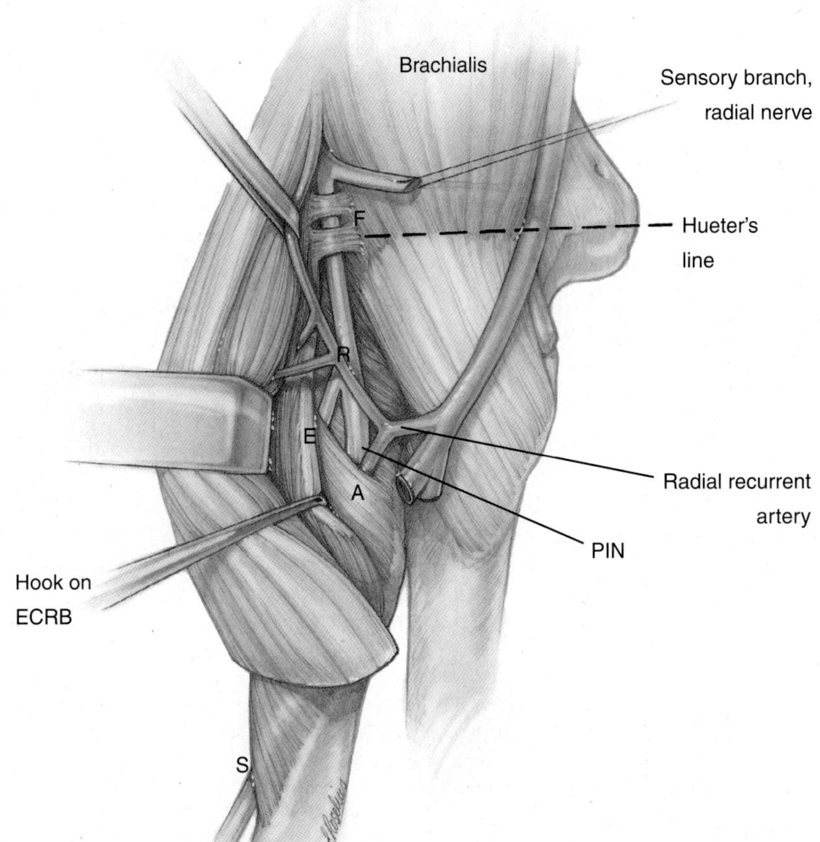

Figure 15.61 Sites of radial nerve compression in radial tunnel syndrome include (*F*) fibrous tissue bands, (*R*) radial recurrent vessels, (*E*) fibrous edge of ECRB, (*A*) arcade of Frohse, and (*S*) supinator. ECRB, extensor carpi radialis brevis; PIN, posterior interosseus nerve. (*Reprinted with permission from* Doyle JR, Tornetta P, Einhorn TA. *Orthopaedic Surgery Essentials: Hand and Wrist*. Philadelphia, PA: Lippincott Williams & Wilkins, 2006.)

Wartenberg Syndrome

Pathophysiology

Wartenberg syndrome (also known as *cheiralgia paresthetica*) is compression of the superficial radial nerve, which is a purely sensory nerve that runs in the forearm underneath the brachioradialis and exits dorsally between the tendons of the brachioradialis and ECRL. Compression occurs secondary to scissoring of the brachioradialis and the ECRL. Handcuffs, tight casts, tight watch bands, and direct blows have been implicated in its etiology.

Presentation

Symptoms are paresthesias on the dorsal radial aspect of the hand; wrist flexion, ulnar deviation, and pronation may exacerbate symptoms.

Physical Examination

A positive Tinel sign over the superficial radial nerve is diagnostic.

Special Studies

EMG and NCS are not indicated.

Treatment

Treatment is almost always nonoperative and is based on the removal of the inciting agent.

Thoracic Outlet Syndrome

Pathophysiology/Classification

There are two types of thoracic outlet syndrome: vascular and neurogenic. The vascular type is more common and usually involves compression of the subclavian artery. The neurogenic type is relatively rare, and the diagnosis is generally a clinical one. Compression is due to structures such as cervical ribs, the scalene muscles, abnormal fibrous bands, or a hypertrophic head of the sternocleidomastoid muscle compromising the space available for the brachial plexus.

Presentation/Mechanism of Injury

The condition is found most commonly in young or middle-aged female population. Symptoms are variable. Classically, it presents in a pattern similar to ulnar nerve compression at the elbow combined with neck pain and neurologic symptoms that are worse with overhead activity.

Physical Examination
Adson test is specific for thoracic outlet syndrome and involves obliteration of the radial pulse with slight abduction of the shoulder in the coronal plane and rotation of the neck to the affected side. Roos test is another useful physical examination for making the diagnosis. The test is positive when there is numbness or tingling of the ulnar-sided digits with 90 degrees of abduction of the shoulder, 90 degrees of external rotation, and opening and closing the hands rapidly for up to 3 minutes.

Radiographic Findings
Radiographs of the neck and chest should be obtained to check for cervical ribs, Pancost tumors, and other chest diseases or anomalies.

Special Studies
EMG and NCS can be helpful in making a diagnosis if a proximal site of compression can be identified.

Differential Diagnosis
Cervical radiculopathy and cubital tunnel syndrome are among the chief conditions in the differential diagnosis.

Treatment
This condition should be treated nonoperatively for an extended period unless there is an underlying structural abnormality, such as a cervical rib, that is found during the initial evaluation. Initial management includes strengthening of the upper extremity, trapezius, and neck muscles as well as stretching of the neck and shoulder. Weight loss and other physical therapy modalities can be helpful. If these fail, surgical options include anterior scalenotomy, exploration and resection of any anomalous fibrous bands, or first rib resection through an axillary approach.

Degenerative Arthritis

Pathophysiology
In the hand, degenerative arthritis occurs in diarthrodial joints that are subjected to abnormal loading conditions or that have abnormal cartilage. It tends to be a progressive condition and is classified as either primary, when there is no underlying cause, or secondary, when it is attributed to underlying factors, such as trauma, avascular necrosis, developmental dysplasia, or other disease.

Presentation/Physical Examination
Commonly, patients present with pain localized to the involved joint, decreased range of motion, and a progressive deformity.

Radiographic Findings
The diagnosis can usually be made with radiographs, which demonstrate four characteristic changes: joint space narrowing secondary to cartilage destruction, peripheral osteophyte formation, subchondral sclerosis, and subchondral cyst formation.

Special Studies
Radiographs are usually sufficient to make the diagnosis of degenerative arthritis. Occasionally, an MRI scan is useful for the diagnosis of early arthritis, and CT scans can potentially be helpful in surgical planning.

Differential Diagnosis
The primary differential diagnosis is inflammatory arthritis.

Treatment
Initial treatment is nonoperative and includes activity modification, splinting, and NSAIDs. The second line of nonoperative treatment often includes intraarticular corticosteroid injections that can provide excellent symptomatic relief. Surgical intervention is considered only when the patient has deformity or instability that interferes with function or pain that is refractory to nonoperative treatment.

Any joint in the hand and wrist can be involved, but arthritis most commonly affects the IP joints, the first CMC joint, and the STT joint. Specific surgical management is dependent on the patient and joint involved.

DIP Joint

The DIP joint is one of the most frequently involved joints. Presenting symptoms include pain, swelling, decreased range of motion, and deformity. Heberden nodes are the characteristic enlargements of the joint secondary to the underlying osteoarthritis. Mucous cysts, which are ganglion cysts associated with a joint osteophyte, can commonly be seen. Surgical treatment is dependent on the stage of the disease. Mucous cysts can often be managed by cyst excision with removal of the underlying osteophyte. More extensive arthritis is typically treated with DIP arthrodesis. Fusion is a simpler procedure and has been shown to have at least equal results to arthroplasty (Fig. 15.62). The joint is fused in a position of slight flexion (5 degrees to 10 degrees) to help with function. Multiple techniques, including the use of K-wires and compression screws, have been described.

PIP Joint

The PIP joint is also frequently involved in osteoarthritis. Arthritic disease presents similarly in the PIP joint, except that dorsal joint prominences are called *Bouchard nodes*. The primary difference between DIP and PIP arthritis is the preferred form of treatment. In the PIP joint, the primary surgical options are arthroplasty and arthrodesis. Arthroplasty with silicone or pyrocarbon implants can give an approximately 60-degree arc of motion, although implant durability and long-term results remain questionable. Arthrodesis in approximately 40 degrees of flexion

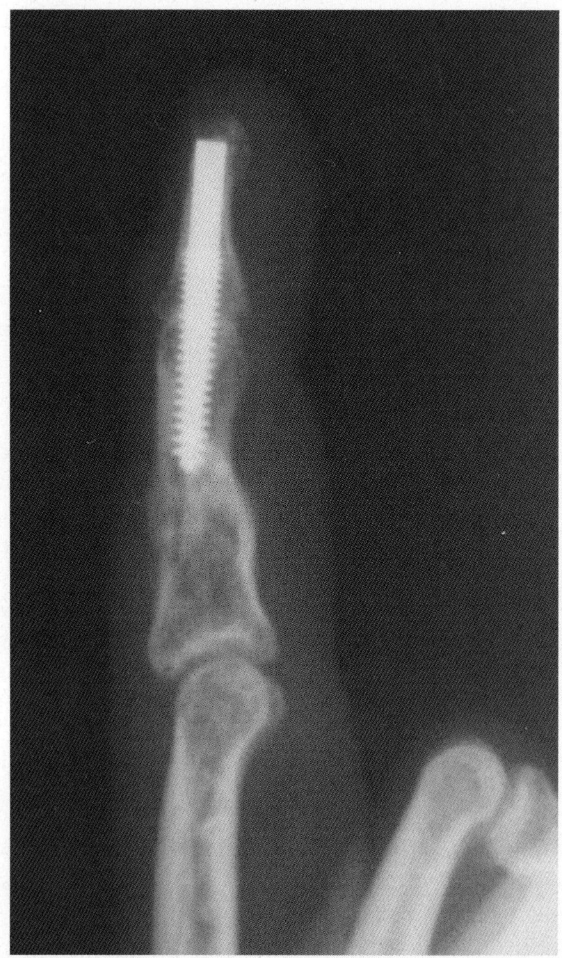

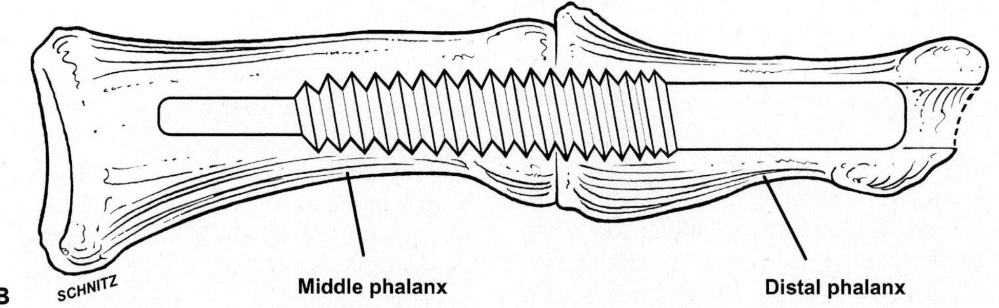

Figure 15.62 **(A)** Radiograph and **(B)** schematic of DIP fusion. DIP, distal interphalangeal. (*Reprinted with permission from* Strickland JW, Graham TJ. *Master Techniques in Orthopaedic Surgery: The Hand*. Philadelphia, PA: Lippincott Williams & Wilkins, 2005.)

has demonstrated better results in the index finger, which sees significant lateral stresses during pinch.

MP Joint

MP joint arthritis is significantly less common than either DIP or PIP arthritis. Disease at this location is usually secondary to trauma. Treatment is similar to that at the PIP joint, with arthroplasty being the preferred surgical option.

TM Joint (First CMC Joint)

The trapeziometacarpal joint is one of the most common sites of hand and wrist arthritis.

Classification

Eaton and Littler categorized TM arthritis into four stages (Fig. 15.63). Stage 1 involves a normal TM joint with possible joint widening secondary to synovitis. Stage 2 is

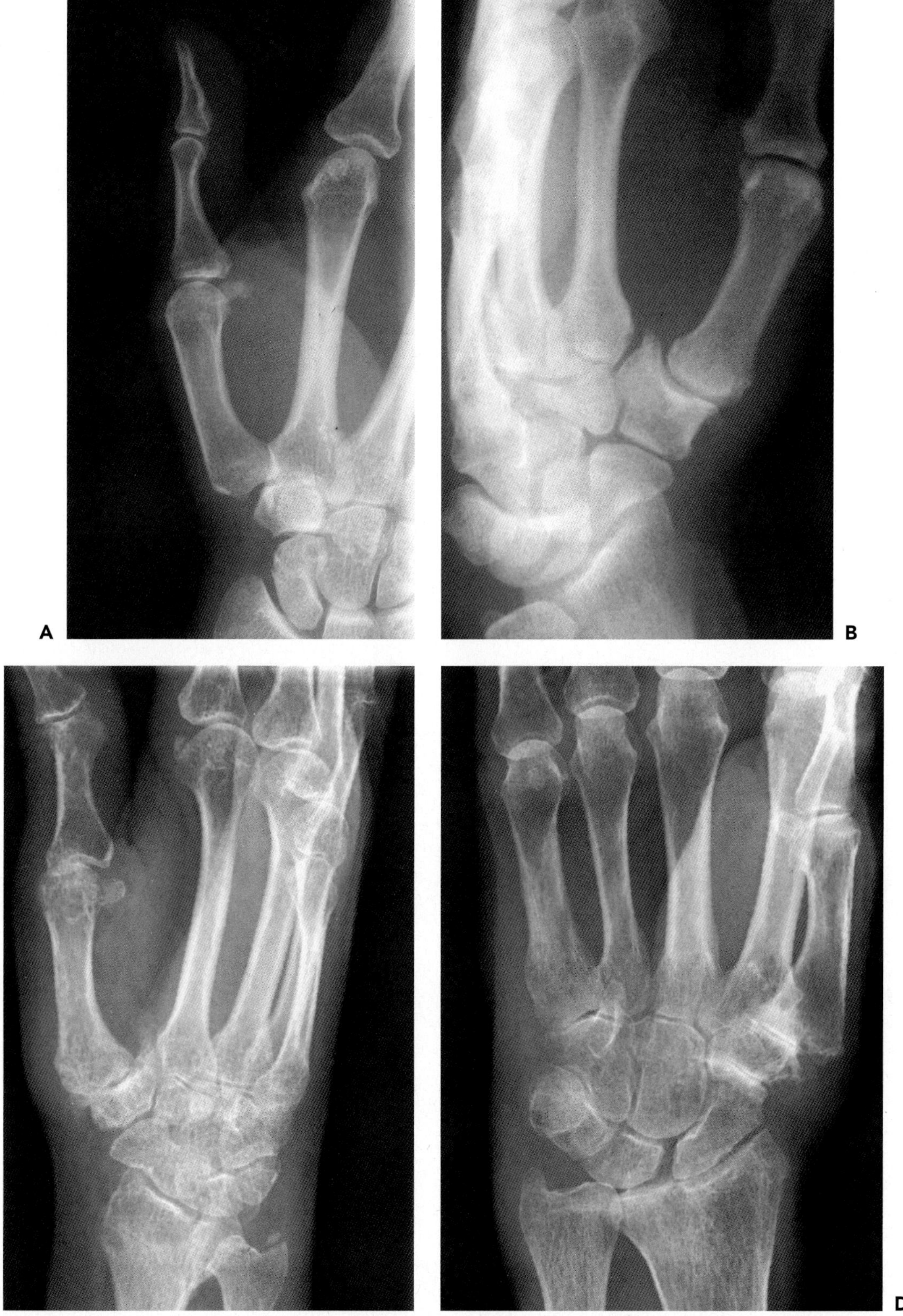

Figure 15.63 **(A–D)** Stages I–IV of thumb carpometacarpal arthritis. (*Reprinted with permission from* Lotke PA, Abboud JA, Ende J. *Lippincott's Primary Care Orthopaedics*. Philadelphia, PA: Lippincott Williams & Wilkins, 2008.)

characterized by mild joint space narrowing with osteophytes smaller than 2 mm. Stage 3 demonstrates joint space narrowing with osteophytes larger than 2 mm. Stage 4 involves pantrapezial arthrosis. These stages are important in determining treatment.

Presentation/Physical Examination

Patients usually present with pain at the base of the thumb. They commonly have a positive CMC grind test, which is axial load and rotation of the thumb. Careful evaluation of the thumb MP joint motion must be performed to assess for MP hyperextension.

Radiographic Findings

Radiographic evaluation includes a PA stress view, a lateral view, and a Robert view (a pronated anteroposterior view). One must keep in mind that the radiographic severity of the disease does not always correlate with clinical symptoms.

Differential Diagnosis

It is imperative to rule out other concomitant diagnoses, such as de Quervain tenosynovitis, stenosing tenosynovitis, CTS, MCP instability, or other wrist arthridities.

Treatment

As with arthritis at any other location in the hand and wrist, initial treatment is conservative with activity modification, thumb spica splinting, and NSAIDs. If nonoperative treatment is unsuccessful, surgical treatment can be considered. Stage 1 disease can be treated with arthroscopic debridement and synovectomy, MC extension osteotomy to redirect the MC force dorsally, and ligament reconstruction to improve joint laxity. The success of any of these treatments hinges on the correct staging of the TM arthritis. Stages 2 through 4 imply more advanced TM joint degeneration and usually require more extensive procedures. Ligament reconstruction tendon interposition (LTRI) arthroplasty was initially described by Burton and Pellegrini and remains the gold standard for end-stage pantrapezial arthritis (Fig. 15.64). This procedure involves trapezium excision, palmar (beak) ligament reconstruction using the FCR, and FCR interposition between the scaphoid and first MC. Long-term results have shown excellent pain relief and predictable increases in both grip and pinch strength. Hematoma or distraction arthroplasty is gaining popularity but risks include subsidence and loss of pinch strength. Arthroplasty has demonstrated high rates of loosening. Trapeziometacarpal arthrodesis in 30 degrees to 40 degrees of palmar abduction, 35 degrees of radial abduction, and 15 degrees of pronation is favored for young laborers. Synthetic spacers, such as Artelon, have recently been introduced and but lack long-term follow-up. Finally, with any of these procedures, it is important to address any thumb MCP deformity. Hyperextension of the thumb MP joint is a characteristic response to CMC arthritis and must be corrected to prevent early failure of a CMC reconstruction. Hyperextension of less than 30 degrees requires K-wire stabilization for 4 weeks, whereas hyperextension greater than 30 degrees requires volar capsulodesis or MP arthrodesis in 15 degrees of flexion and 10 degrees of pronation.

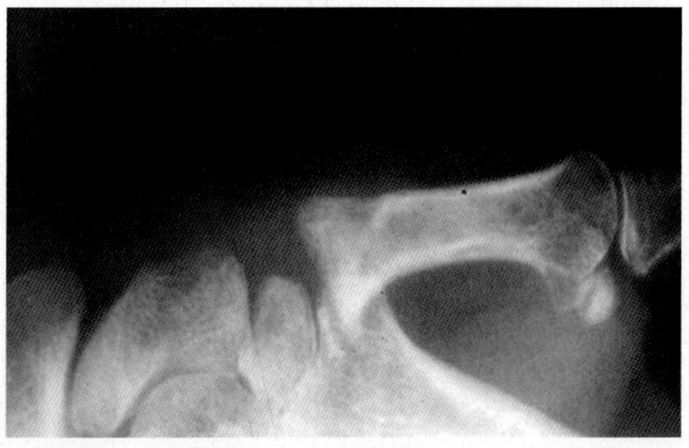

Figure 15.64 Postoperative radiograph of an LRTI. (*Reprinted with permission from* Lotke PA, Abboud JA, Ende J. *Lippincott's Primary Care Orthopaedics*. Philadelphia, PA: Lippincott Williams & Wilkins, 2008.)

STT Joint

While the scaphotrapezial–trapezoidal joint is a common site of arthritis, it rarely occurs in isolation. Usually this joint is involved in pantrapezial arthrosis, which is treated with ligament reconstruction with tendon interposition (LRTI) arthroplasty, or in SLAC wrist, where treatment is dependent on the stage of collapse. However, if the arthritis is limited to the STT joint, STT arthrodesis is a viable option.

SLAC/SNAC Wrist

Scapholunate advanced collapse (SLAC) and scaphoid nonunion advance collapse (SNAC) are two common forms of posttraumatic wrist arthritis.

Pathophysiology

SLAC occurs secondary to disruption of the scapholunate ligament and subsequent scaphoid flexion, whereas SNAC results from a scaphoid nonunion.

Classification

Watson was the first to describe the reproducible pattern of radiocarpal and intercarpal degeneration that occurs in a SLAC wrist. Stage I arthrosis is limited to the distal aspect of the scaphoid and the radial styloid. Stage II arthrosis involves the entire radioscaphoid joint. Stage III arthrosis affects the entire radioscaphoid joint and the capitolunate joint.

SNAC wrist is less common than SLAC wrist and has a different pattern of progression. Stage I arthrosis is limited to the distal scaphoid and radial styloid. Stage II arthrosis is stage I arthrosis plus scaphocapitate arthrosis. Stage III arthrosis is periscaphoid arthrosis.

Presentation

Patients usually present with a remote history of a fall on an outstretched hand. Initially, patients complain of wrist pain and swelling that resolves with time. Eventually, however, patients develop decreased wrist motion and decreased grip/pinch strength.

Physical Examination

Physical examination is dependent on the stage of disease, but patients usually have tenderness over the radioscaphoid articulation. Patients with an early SLAC wrist may have a positive Watson test, as described earlier.

Radiographic Findings

Radiographs are imperative in the diagnosis, staging, and treatment of these posttraumatic forms of arthritis.

Differential Diagnosis

The diagnosis of posttraumatic arthritis is generally straightforward, but SLAC and SNAC must be differentiated from each other.

Treatment

As with other forms of arthritis, conservative management in the form of activity restriction, simple splinting, and oral anti-inflammatory medications should be attempted first. For those patients who have recalcitrant symptoms, surgical management of symptomatic patients is based on the stage of disease. Stage I is best treated with radial styloidectomy and scaphoid stabilization. If the scaphoid can be reduced, it should be stabilized with a soft tissue procedure, such as a dorsal capsulodesis or scapholunate reconstruction. If it cannot be reduced, scaphoid stabilization requires a STT fusion. Stage II treatment is based on eliminating the radiocarpal joint, and this can be accomplished by performing a PRC, a scaphoid excision and four corner fusion of the lunate–capitate–hamate–triquetram (SLAC procedure) (Fig. 15.65), or a wrist arthrodesis (Fig. 15.66). In general, either a PRC or a SLAC procedure is preferred over a wrist fusion because there is preservation of approximately 50% to 60% of wrist motion. Stage III treatment requires either the SLAC procedure or a total wrist arthrodesis. PRC is contraindicated because capitate wear can lead to accelerated arthrosis between the capitate and the lunate fossa. Total

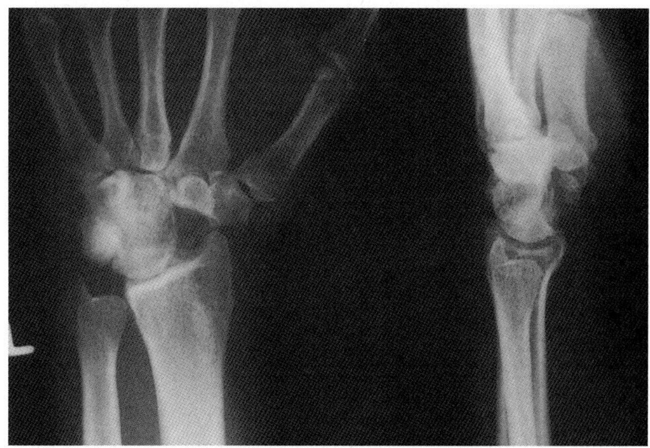

Figure 15.65 Radiographs of a healed scaphoid excision and four corner fusion of the lunate–capitate–hamate–triquetram (SLAC procedure). (*Reprinted with permission from* Gelberman RH. *Master Techniques in Orthopaedic Surgery: The Wrist.* Philadelphia, PA: Lippincott Williams & Wilkins, 2002.)

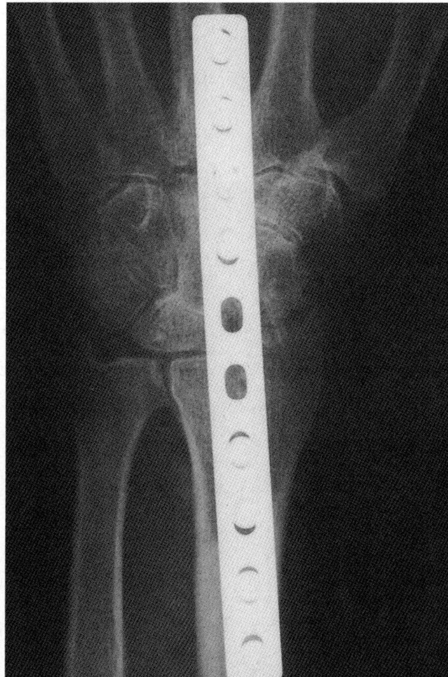

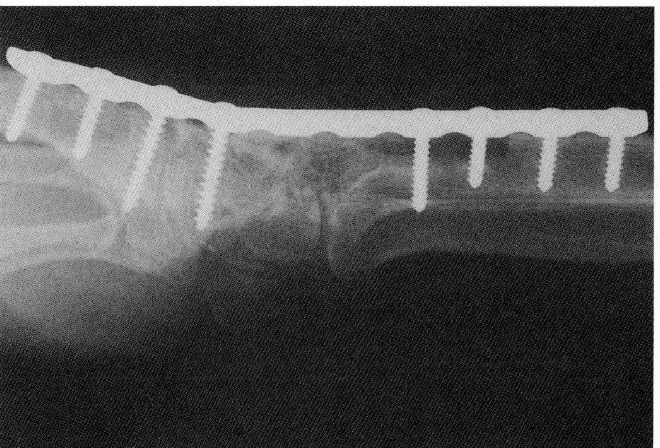

Figure 15.66 Radiographs of a healed wrist fusion. (*Reprinted with permission from* Gelberman RH. *Master Techniques in Orthopaedic Surgery: The Wrist.* Philadelphia, PA: Lippincott Williams & Wilkins, 2002.)

wrist arthrodesis is an excellent procedure in young laborers, in whom it reliably decreases pain and provides a rapid return of grip strength. Total wrist arthroplasty is gaining some popularity but does not have adequate long-term results to compare with total wrist arthrodesis.

Treatment of SNAC is similar to that of SLAC, except that surgery for stage I involves radial styloidectomy and fixation of scaphoid nonunion with some form of bone graft.

Distal Radioulnar Joint Arthritis

Pathophysiology/Classification

DRUJ arthritis can be posttraumatic or degenerative.

Presentation

Symptoms include pain, swelling, stiffness, and decreased grip strength.

Physical Examination

On physical examination, pain in located over the ulnar head and the DRUJ, and it is often exacerbated by forearm rotation.

Radiographic Findings/Special Studies

Radiographs will show standard degenerative changes of the DRUJ. MRI is sometimes helpful in evaluating the TFCC for potential tears and the lunate for ulnar impaction syndrome.

Differential Diagnosis

Differential diagnoses include ulnar impaction syndrome and TFCC tears.

Treatment

Surgical treatment is indicated only after conservative treatment has failed. For advanced arthritis, multiple procedures exist that eliminate the distal ulna and radius articulation, and each has its advantages and disadvantages. Bowers distal ulna hemiresection and tendon interposition preserves the TFCC insertion but is contraindicated in ulnar-positive individuals, who may have residual ulnocarpal impaction. Darrach distal ulnar resection and stabilization with ECU suspensionplasty has had good results in the low demand, elderly population, but has had problems with stump instability and subsequent weakness in younger patients. The Sauve–Kapandji procedure retains the distal ulna, fuses the ulnar head to the sigmoid notch, and creates a pseudoarthrosis of the ulnar neck. The procedure provides better support for the carpus than the distal ulna resection, but complications include proximal ulnar instability and ulnar regeneration with loss of motion. Finally, DRUJ arthroplasty is becoming increasingly popular, but few long-term studies exist to accurately assess its outcomes.

INFLAMMATORY ARTHRITIS

Rheumatoid Arthritis

RA is a systemic inflammatory autoimmune disease that initially affects the soft tissues and secondarily affects the bone. Approximately 1% of the population is affected, with a female:male ratio of 2.5:1. Onset is usually between ages 40 and 70, and the disease has a progressive course. Hand and wrist involvement is extremely common.

Pathophysiology

The true etiology of RA is unknown, but it is thought to be a combination of genetic and environmental factors. Over time, RA leads to synovial proliferation within joints and around tendons. Progressive destruction of these tissues results in secondary antibody reactions followed by lysozyme release from white blood cells, oxygen free radical formation, and collagenase release from the synovium. Cartilage, ligament, and tendons are eventually affected, leading to joint pain, instability, deformity, and tendon rupture.

Classification

RA can be classified by stage of joint involvement; accurate classification helps guide treatment. Stage 1 is synovitis without deformity and can be treated nonoperatively. Stage 2 is synovitis with passively correctable deformity. This stage is initially treated nonoperatively, but if symptoms persist, tenosynovectomy may be necessary. Stage 3 is fixed deformity without joint changes and is best treated with surgical reconstruction. Stage 4 is articular destruction; salvage surgery such as arthrodesis or arthroplasty is required.

Presentation/Physical Examination

The diagnosis of RA requires that at least four of the seven following criteria be present: periarticular morning stiffness lasting for at least 1 hour per day for at least 6 weeks, simultaneous arthritis and synovitis in three or more joints for at least 6 weeks, arthritis of the hand joints for at least 6 weeks, symmetric arthritis present for at least 6 weeks, presence of rheumatoid nodules, elevated rheumatoid factor titer, and radiographic evidence of subchondral erosions or osteopenia adjacent to involved joints.

Tendon ruptures are common in patients with RA. Etiologies include synovitis, attritional wear from osteophytes, and traumatic or iatrogenic causes. The Vaughn–Jackson lesion results from a subluxated, osteophytic, and sharp ulnar head that causes EDM and EDC tendon ruptures. A Mannerfelt lesion is a scaphotrapezial joint osteophyte that causes FPL rupture. The diagnosis of tendon rupture is relatively straightforward: patients will have normal passive motion but will be unable to actively move the joint. In addition, there is a loss of the tenodesis effect.

Deformity results when MP joints drift into ulnar deviation. This instability is secondary to synovitis, which attenuates the radial extensor hood sagittal fibers and causes

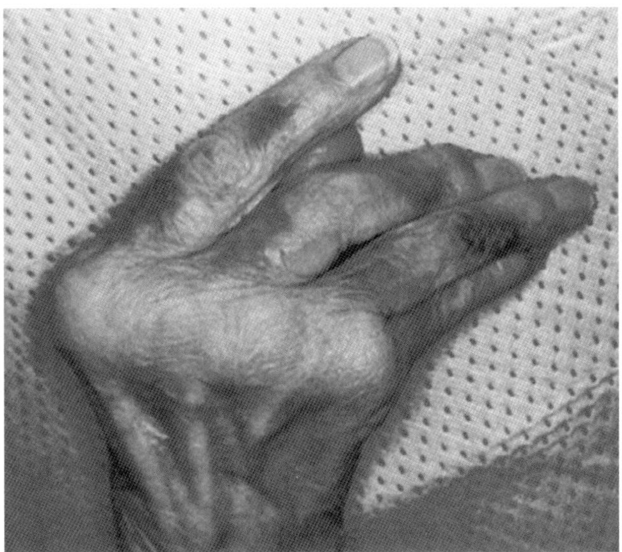

Figure 15.67 Typical ulnarly deviated hand of a patient with rheumatoid arthritis. (*Reprinted with permission from* Strickland JW, Graham TJ. *Master Techniques in Orthopaedic Surgery: The Hand.* Philadelphia, PA: Lippincott Williams & Wilkins, 2005.)

ulnar subluxation of the extensor tendon (Fig. 15.67). The PIP joints usually progress to a boutonniere deformity after PIP synovitis weakens the central slip.

Radiographic Findings/Special Studies

RA is characterized by severe deformity, periarticular erosions, and osteopenia, which distinguishes it from osteoarthritis.

Differential Diagnosis

Initially, RA must be distinguished from osteoarthritis and other forms of inflammatory arthritis. Once this is done, more specific clinical diagnoses have to be made. For instance, tendon ruptures must be differentiated from tendon subluxation and peripheral neuropathy.

Treatment

Initial treatment of acute flares is based on rest and activity modification. However, the current mainstay of treatment is early and aggressive use of disease-modifying antirheumatic drugs (DMARDs). These drugs, such as TNF-α inhibitors, have had a dramatic effect on symptoms and disease progression. By doing so, they have markedly reduced the need for surgical treatment of RA patients. However, surgical intervention is still necessary in managing certain aspects of the disease.

Persistent tenosynovitis is best managed by complete synovectomy. Tendon ruptures are treated by resection of the offending bony prominence, tenosynovectomy, and reconstruction via tendon transfers. Later stages of RA, which usually exhibit near-complete articular destruction, are best treated by arthrodesis or arthroplasty. The choice between the two options is dependent on the joint and is similar to the treatment of end-stage osteoarthritis.

Psoriatic Arthritis

Psoriatic arthritis is a relatively uncommon arthritis and presents only in 5% to 10% of patients with psoriasis.

Pathophysiology

Synovial disease in the hand leads to either osteolysis or ankylosis and autofusion. Osteolysis most commonly involves the DIP joint with erosion of the middle phalangeal condyles into a spike, creating the classic "pencil-in-cup" deformity. Spontaneous fusion occurs mainly at the DIP joint and occasionally at the PIP joints.

Presentation/Physical Examination

Patients usually have classic findings of psoriasis, such as the scaly erythematous rash, before developing joint symptoms. Early findings include nail pitting and sausage digits. However, once significant arthritis develops, it can affect all finger joints and cause severe deformity, which is often referred to as *arthritis mutilans*. Finger telescoping can also occur, which gives a characteristic appearance called "opera glass hand."

Radiographic Findings

As previously described, radiographs frequently show PIP fusions, MP erosions, and wrist autofusions. The classic deformity seen on radiographs is the DIP "pencil-in-cup" deformity.

Differential Diagnosis

Psoriatic arthritis must be differentiated from osteoarthritis, RA, and other inflammatory arthopathies. This usually can be accomplished with a thorough history and a search for the characteristic nonmusculoskeletal findings.

Treatment

Medical treatment is similar to that used for RA. Operative treatment primarily involves arthroplasty or arthodesis of arthritic joints.

Crystalline Arthropathy

Gout and pseudogout are the most common crystalline arthropathies.

Pathophysiology/Classification

Gout can be separated into primary gout, which is idiopathic, and secondary gout, which results from an imbalance in uric acid metabolism Pseudogout or calcium pyrophosphate deposition disease is thought to be due to increased level of calcium or pyrophosphate in cartilage.

Presentation/Physical Examination

Gouty attacks present with the sudden onset of a warm, swollen, erythematous, and painful joint. Pseudogout can present similarly, but usually the attack is less severe. Arthritis and tendon ruptures can occur secondary to chronic inflammatory changes.

Radiographic Findings/Special Studies

Radiograph in gout can demonstrate soft tissue densities (tophi) and articular erosion. Pseudogout appears as calcifications in the cartilage, most commonly seen in the TFCC. For both conditions, the diagnosis is made on the basis of joint fluid aspiration and analysis. Uric acid crystals in gout are negatively birefringent and needle-like under polarized microscopy, whereas calcium pyrophosphate crystals from pseudogout are weakly positively birefringent and rhomboid shaped.

Differential Diagnosis

Infection can often be confused with crystalline arthropathies since both present as hot, swollen joints. The diagnosis of infection can usually be excluded on the basis of analysis of the joint fluid cell count and of the Gram stain.

Treatment

Acute gout attacks are treated with colchicine and/or indomethacin. In between flares, allopurinol helps metabolize uric acid and prevent future attacks. Pseudogout is mainly treated symptomatically with NSAIDs and immobilization. For both diagnoses, surgery is limited to tophi excision, tenosynovectomies, and arthrodesis/arthroplasty of end-stage arthritic joints.

Hand Stiffness

Hand stiffness is a common problem that has many etiologies. To appropriately treat the stiffness, the correct diagnosis must first be made.

Classification

Stiffness can be due to either extrinsic or intrinsic causes. Extrinsic stiffness involves tendons that originate proximal to the wrist, whereas the source of intrinsic tightness originates at or distal to the wrist. Extrinsic extensor tightness manifests as limited IP joint flexion when the MP joint is held in flexion. When the MP joint is extended, motion is improved. Similarly, extrinsic flexor tightness manifests as limited IP joint extension when the MP joint is held in extension; this is improved with MP joint flexion. On the other hand, intrinsic tightness results in a positive Bunnell intrinsic tightness test (Fig. 15.68), which demonstrates less IP joint flexion with the MP joint in extension compared with when the MP joint is in flexion.

Presentation/Physical Examination

History should address the onset of symptoms, the progression of symptoms, and any associated trauma. Examination should include inspection for deformity and swelling, evaluation of active and passive range of motion, and testing

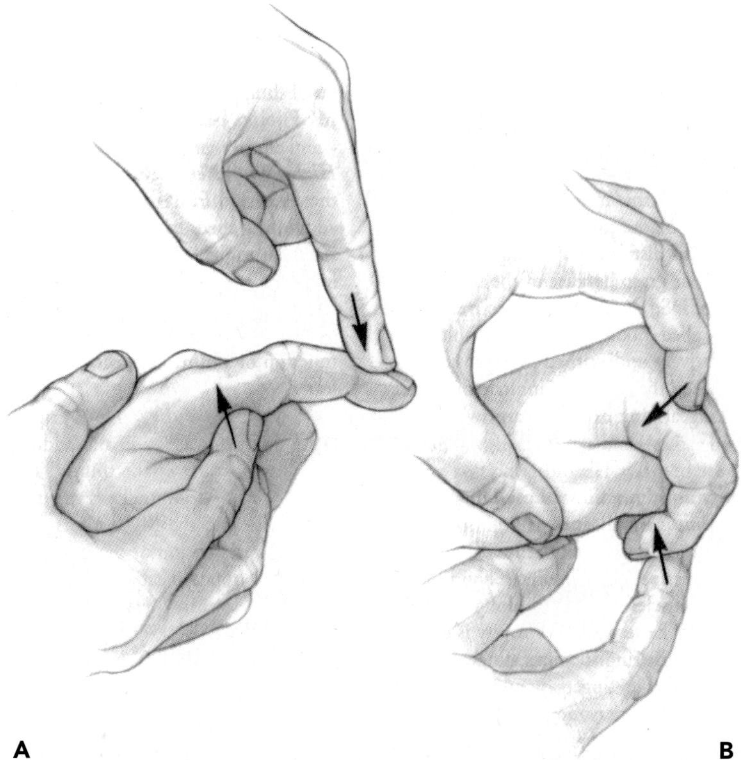

Figure 15.68 **(A, B)** Intrinsic tightness test. (*Reprinted with permission from* Doyle JR, Botte MJ. *Surgical Anatomy of the Hand and Upper Extremity.* Philadelphia, PA: Lippincott Williams & Wilkins, 2003.)

of neurologic function. The discrepancy between active and passive motion is particularly important. For example, joint contracture will have an equal decrease in passive and active ranges of motion, regardless of the position of the adjacent joints. This differs from stiffness secondary to tendon ruptures or adhesions, in which range of motion is affected by the type of movement and the position of adjacent joints.

Radiographic Findings/Special Studies

Radiographs are necessary only when stiffness is thought to be secondary to a bony process, such as a fracture, nonunion, joint dislocation, or arthritis.

Treatment

Initial treatment for hand stiffness involves splinting and aggressive range of motion exercises in an organized hand therapy program. If conservative management fails, surgery should be considered. The specifics of surgery are dependent on the structures that are contracted, but in general, all structures that are tight starting with the skin and ending with the joint capsule must be released until acceptable range of motion has been obtained. Postoperatively, early range of motion exercises are imperative for a successful result.

Complex Regional Pain Syndrome

Complex regional pain syndrome (CRPS) is the new nomenclature for the condition formerly known as *reflex sympathetic dystrophy (RSD)* or *causalgia*. CRPS is a diagnosis of exclusion, and its hallmark symptom is pain out of proportion to the inciting event. It is defined by the presence of pain, functional deficits, and objective sympathetic nervous system dysfunction.

Pathophysiology

The exact etiology or mechanism of CRPS is unknown. It has been hypothesized to occur from a positive feedback cycle in which peripheral nocicepter activation causes a spinal cord mediated reflex, which in turn activates the efferent sympathetic system. Another hypothesis is that CRPS is caused by exaggeration of the peripheral neural inflammatory response to tissue injury.

Classification

There are two types of CRPS. Type I, which corresponds to the classic RSD, is pain out of proportion to the initial noxious event that cannot be linked to any pathologic process. Type II, which corresponds to causalgia, is pain out of proportion to the initial noxious event that is associated with an identifiable nerve lesion.

Presentation/Physical Examination

CRPS develops after an initial painful or noxious event, and often is associated with trauma. Subsequently, patients complain of pain with light tough (allodynia), increased sensitivity to touch (hyperesthesia), pain at rest (hyperpathia), burning pain, and various extremity changes corresponding to the stage of disease. Specifically, three stages have been described. Stage I involves significant extremity swelling and edema, with hyperhidrosis. Stage II is the dystrophic phase characterized by marked stiffness. In this stage, skin changes such as loss of creases, loss of hair, and decreased moisture are evident. Stage III is the atrophic stage, during which the limb becomes hardly usable.

Radiographic Findings/Special Studies

No imaging study is diagnostic. Radiographs may demonstrate patchy osteopenia, and bone scans may show diffuse uptake in the involved joints.

Differential Diagnosis

As previously mentioned, CRPS is a diagnosis of exclusion. Therefore, any and all diagnoses that could potentially lead to similar symptoms must be ruled out before making the diagnosis.

Treatment

Treatment is based on early diagnosis and aggressive multidisciplinary treatment. Occupational and physical therapy are helpful in decreasing pain, reducing edema, and limiting stiffness. Many medications, including calcium channel blockers, antidepressants, and anticonvulsants, have demonstrated some success. Other modes of treatment such as transcutaneous electrical nerve stimulators (TENSs), autonomic blocks, and surgical sympathectomies have proven beneficial in some patients. These modalities are usually best prescribed and coordinated by pain specialists.

Dupuytren Disease

Dupuytren disease is a condition that is characterized by nodule and cord formation in previously normal fascial tissues of the hand, with progressive flexion contractures of the MP and/or PIP joints. It primarily affects 40- to 60-year-old men of Northern European ancestry. Although it can be inherited as an autosomal dominant condition with variable penetrance, it is most frequently sporadic. It has been linked to alcohol, diabetes, HIV, and smoking.

Pathophysiology

The exact etiology of Dupuytren disease is unknown, but many factors have been proposed. These include oxygen free radical formation secondary to hypoxia and dysfunction of multiple growth factors including PDGF and TGF-B1. The cell responsible for the disease has been identified as the myofibroblast, which has features of both smooth muscle cells and fibroblasts. These cells are responsible for the three stages of the disease. The proliferative stage is a vascular stage when the number of myofibroblasts increases. The involutional stage involves aligning of the myofibroblasts and the increasing ratio of type III to type I collagen. The residual stage demonstrates disappearance of the myofibroblasts and replacement with fibrous tissue.

The specific fascial tissues involved in the disease are the pretendinous bands, the ligaments of Legueu and Juvara, the spiral bands, the natatory ligament, the lateral digital sheet, and Grayson ligament (Fig. 15.69). Cleland ligaments are not affected by the disease. When the bands become thickened and contracted, they become cords. The common cords are the central cord, the ADM cord, the spiral cord, the retrovascular cord, the lateral cord, the natatory cord, and the first web's intercommissural cord (Fig. 15.70). The central cord has no fascial precursor but is a continuation of the pretendinous band. The spiral cord arises from four structures: the pretendinous band, the spiral bands, the lateral digital sheaths, and Grayson ligament. This cord passes beneath the neurovascular bundle and brings it more superficial.

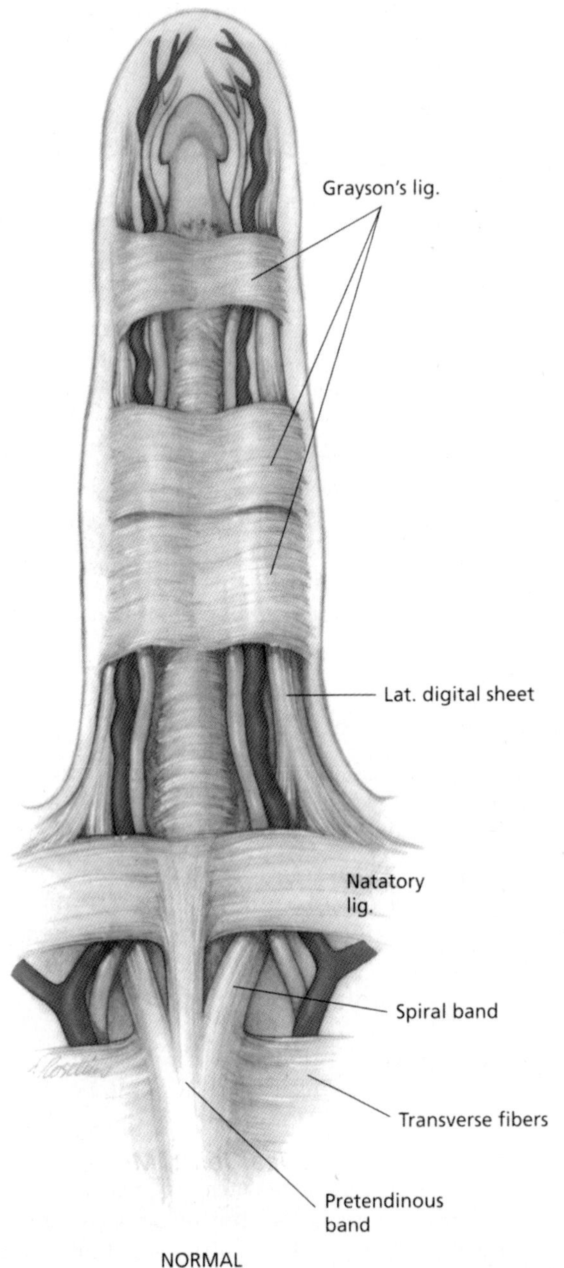

Figure 15.69 Normal components of palmar and digital fascia. (*Reprinted with permission from* Doyle JR, Botte MJ. *Surgical Anatomy of the Hand and Upper Extremity*. Philadelphia, PA: Lippincott Williams & Wilkins, 2003.)

Presentation

Patients usually present with single or multiple nodules and/or cords in the palmar fascia of the hand (Fig. 15.71). Although these nodules are often painless, they can cause skin dimpling, flexion contractures of the MP and PIP joints, and web space contractures. These contractures often limit function and usually progress over time. Eventually, patients complain of difficulty with fine motor movement.

Physical Examination

Physical examination varies depending on the severity of the disease. Range of motion of the involved joints should be accurately assessed. Distal neurovascular function must be confirmed, especially if operative intervention is being considered.

Radiographic Findings

Radiographs are usually unnecessary to make the diagnosis.

Treatment

Treatment is based on the severity of the disease. Nonoperative treatment is useful in the early stages of the disease when the patient has no pain and no functional limitations. However, as the disease progresses, surgical treatment is indicated for MP joint contractures greater than 30 degrees and any PIP joint contracture. Surgical options include palmar fasciotomies, partial palmar fasciectomies, and complete palmar fasciectomies. Fasciotomies allow joint contracture release but have higher rates of recurrence and increased incidence of neurovascular injuries. Complete fasciectomies have fallen out of favor due to the increased risk of complications such as neurovascular injury and infection. Partial fasciectomies are a compromise between the other two procedures. With any procedure, careful dissection must be performed to prevent injury to the neurovascular bundle. The skin is often left open to prevent hematoma formation, which has been implicated in flair reaction and RSD. Overall, the results of the procedures are relatively good, but the recurrence rate remains approximately 10% per year.

Recently, enzymatic fasciotomy with clostridial collagenase injections has shown some promising results. One randomized controlled trial showed a 90% success rate, with low recurrence rate. However, long-term results are pending.

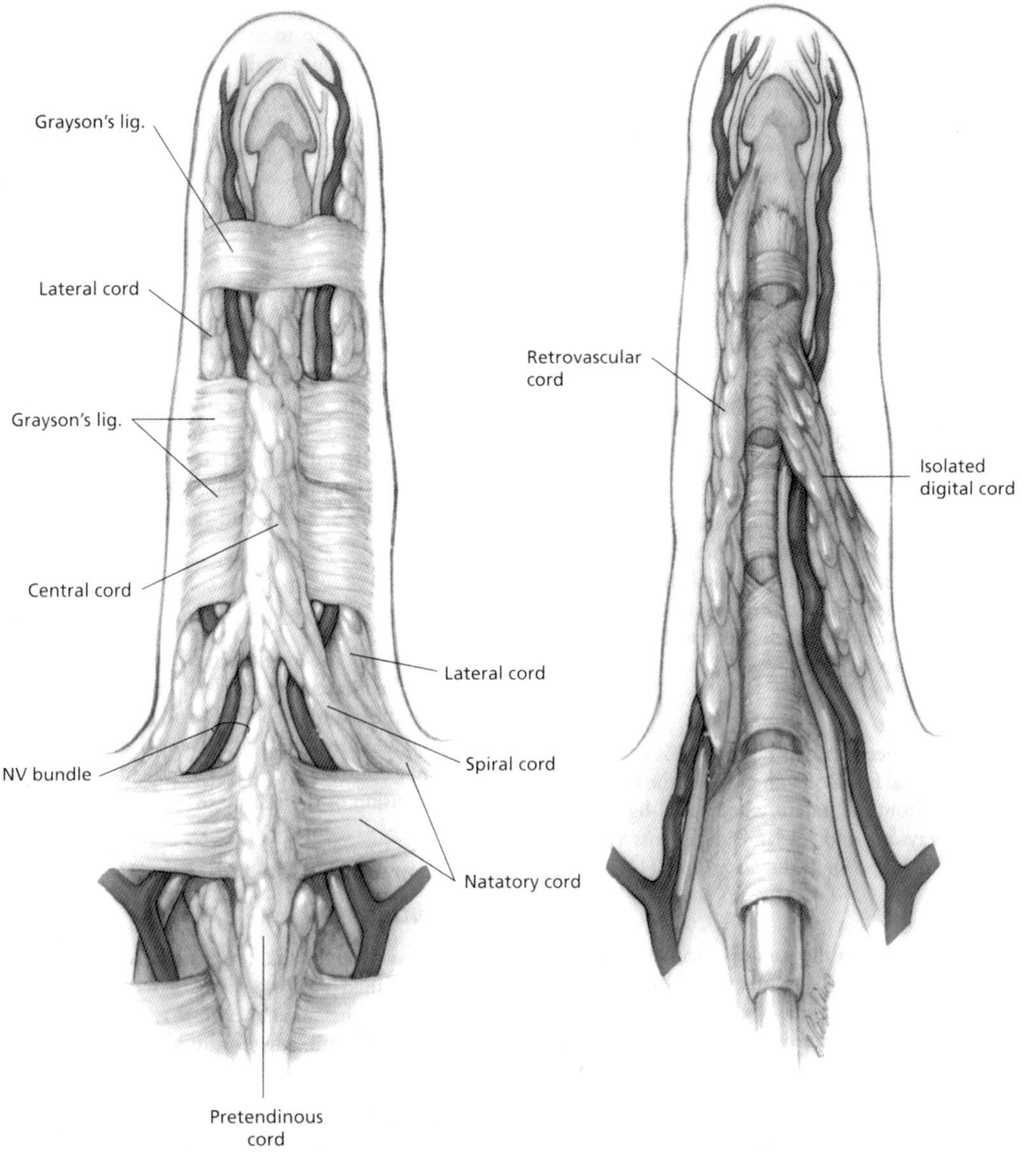

Figure 15.70 Changes in palmar and digital fascia seen in Dupuytren disease. (*Reprinted with permission from* Doyle JR, Botte MJ. *Surgical Anatomy of the Hand and Upper Extremity*. Philadelphia, PA: Lippincott Williams & Wilkins, 2003.)

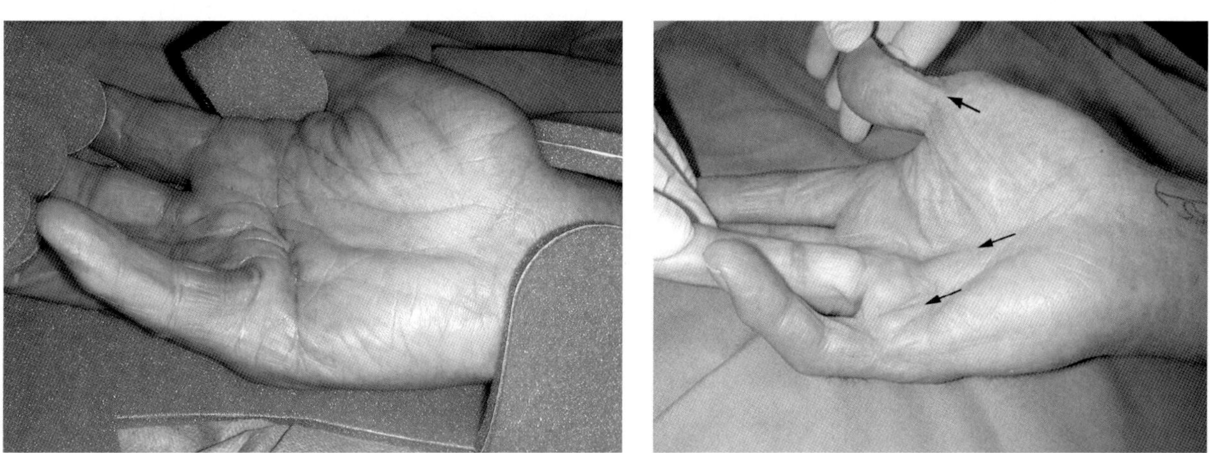

Figure 15.71 **(A, B)** Dupuytren cords. (*Reprinted with permission from* Lotke PA, Abboud JA, Ende J. *Lippincott's Primary Care Orthopaedics*. Philadelphia, PA: Lippincott Williams & Wilkins, 2008.)

TENDINOPATHIES

Tendinopathies are common conditions of the hand and wrist. The flexor/extensor tendons are restrained from displacing forces by the flexor retinaculum, the extensor retinaculum, and the digital fibro-osseous pulleys. If there is thickening of these restraints or of their contents, the tendons become compressed and the tenosynovium can become inflamed. Motion of the tendon is altered, and a vicious cycle of worsening pain and decreased range of motion results.

Trigger Finger

Trigger finger or stenosing tenosynovitis is a common problem that is characterized by the inability to flex or extend a digit. Normally, the flexor tendons can glide smoothly through the fibro-osseous flexor pulley system. However, in trigger digits, a discrepancy exists between the size of the flexor tendon and of the tendon sheath, and this leads to mechanical impingement.

Pathophysiology/Classification

Trigger finger exists in two forms. Nodular tenosynovitis is caused by thickening of the flexor tendon on the distal edge of the A1 pulley and has a distinct nodule. Diffuse tenosynovitis is caused by diffuse thickening of the flexor tenosynovium.

Presentation

Idiopathic trigger finger often occurs in middle-aged women, whereas secondary trigger finger is commonly seen in patients with diabetes, hypothyroidism, RA, chronic renal disease, or other inflammatory disease. All of these patients usually complain of palmar pain and stiffness of the involved finger. Depending on the severity, patients may also sense crepitus, catching, or locking of the finger.

Physical Examination

On examination, a palpable nodule can often be felt over the A1 pulley. Patients are tender to palpation over the nodule. Visible catching or locking can usually be seen with active range of motion.

Radiographic Findings

Radiographs are usually unnecessary to make the diagnosis.

Differential Diagnosis

Differential diagnoses include locking secondary to impingement of the collateral ligaments on a prominent MC head condyle, FDP avulsion or rupture, MP dislocation, and extensor tendon rupture.

Treatment

Treatment is based on the severity of disease. Initially, most patients are treated nonoperatively. This usually involves NSAIDs to decrease inflammation, extension splinting at night, and activity modification. The next step in treatment is a corticosteroid injection, which is indicated early in the disease process (Fig. 15.72). A single injection has been shown to effectively relieve symptoms in 47% to 87% of patients. A higher rate of failure has been seen in patients with diabetes, a long history of triggering, and multiple involved digits. If nonoperative treatment fails or if a patient has a locked digit, surgery is indicated. The procedure of choice is release of the A1 pulley (Fig. 15.73). The gold standard is an open surgical release, but recently some surgeons have been performing the release percutaneously. The primary risk of either procedure is injury to the digital nerve. Overall, the surgery has a greater than 90% success rate.

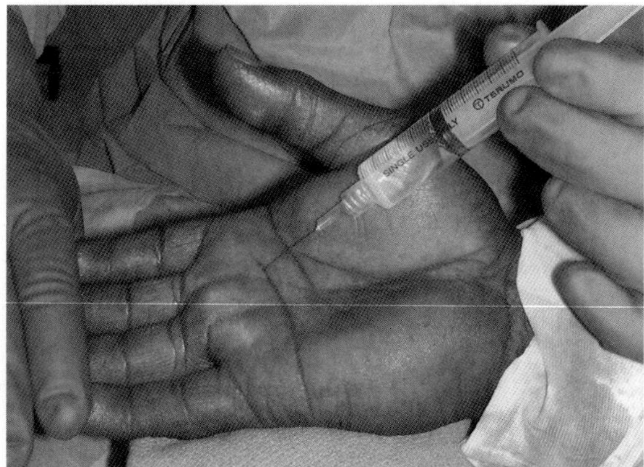

Figure 15.72 Trigger finger injection. (*Reprinted with permission from* Lotke PA, Abboud JA, Ende J. *Lippincott's Primary Care Orthopaedics*. Philadelphia, PA: Lippincott Williams & Wilkins, 2008.)

de Quervain Tenosynovitis

Pathophysiology

de Quervain tenosynovitis is tenosynovitis of the first dorsal compartment of the wrist. Common causes include repetitive use, inflammatory arthritis, and trauma. New mothers often are diagnosed with de Quervain tenosynovitis as a result of lifting their children with radial/ulnar deviation of the wrists.

Presentation

de Quervain tenosynovitis occurs primarily in middle-aged patients and presents with radial-sided wrist pain. The pain is exacerbated by thumb movements and may radiate distally or proximally.

Physical Examination

On examination, patients are tender over the first dorsal compartment of the wrist. Most patients have a positive Finkelstein test, which is pain with forced ulnar deviation of the wrist with the thumb inside a clenched fist.

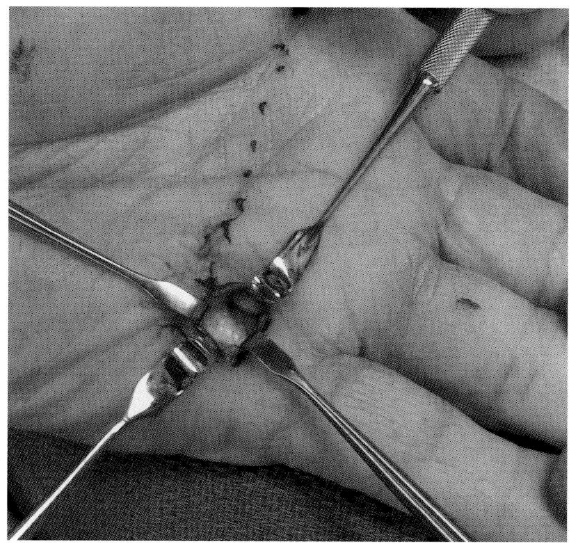

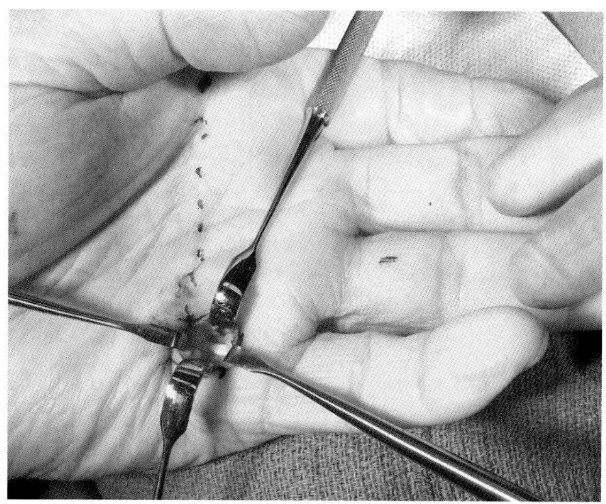

Figure 15.73 **(A, B)** Operative pictures of a trigger finger release. (*Reprinted with permission from* Lotke PA, Abboud JA, Ende J. *Lippincott's Primary Care Orthopaedics*. Philadelphia, PA: Lippincott Williams & Wilkins, 2008.)

Radiographic Findings

Radiographs are unnecessary in making the diagnosis but may be helpful to rule out other conditions.

Differential Diagnosis

It is important to exclude other causes of radial-sided wrist pain, such as CMC arthritis, intersection syndrome, Wartenberg syndrome, and scaphoid fracture.

Treatment

Initial treatment is nonoperative with thumb spica splinting and oral NSAIDs. A corticosteroid injection can also be performed to decrease inflammation and is successful approximately 60% of the time. If conservative treatment fails, surgery consisting of release of the first dorsal compartment is indicated. Given that the APL often has several slips, great care must be taken to release all tendon sheaths of both the APL and EPB. The tendon sheaths should be released on their ulnar aspect to prevent radial subluxation of the compartment. The sensory branches of the radial nerve have to be protected to avoid neuroma formation (Fig. 15.74).

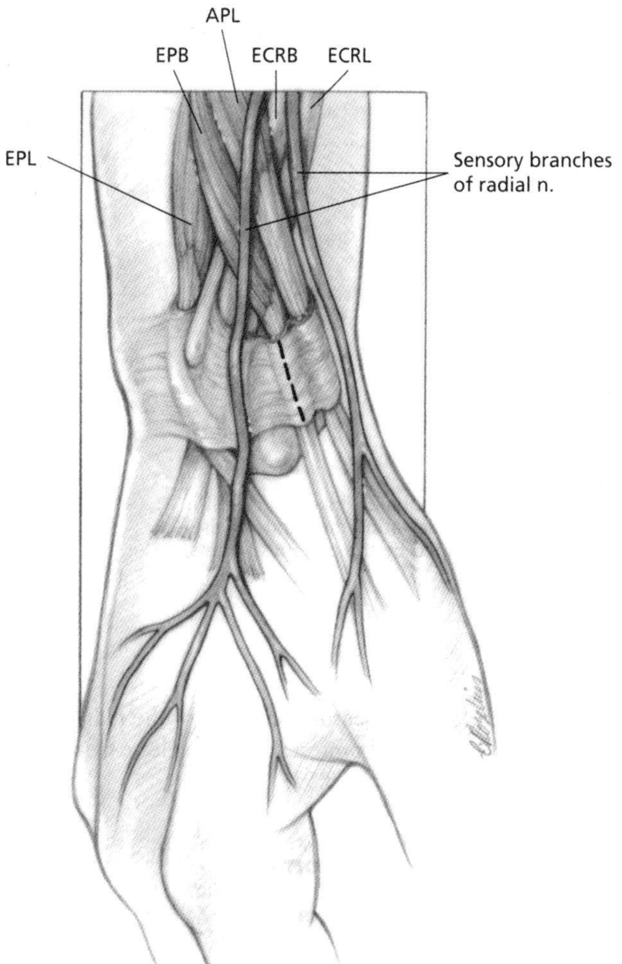

Figure 15.74 Anatomy pertinent to deQuervain's tenosynovitis. (*Reprinted with permission from* Doyle JR and Botte MJ: *Surgical Anatomy of the Hand and Upper Extremity*. Philadelphia: Lippincott Williams & Wilkins, 2003.)

Intersection Syndrome

Pathophysiology

Intersection syndrome is inflammation of the second dorsal extensor compartment secondary to overuse. It is characteristically seen in rowers.

Presentation/Physical Examination

Patients usually present with pain approximately 4 cm proximal to the wrist (Fig. 15.75). On examination, the second dorsal compartment is boggy and crepitation can be felt.

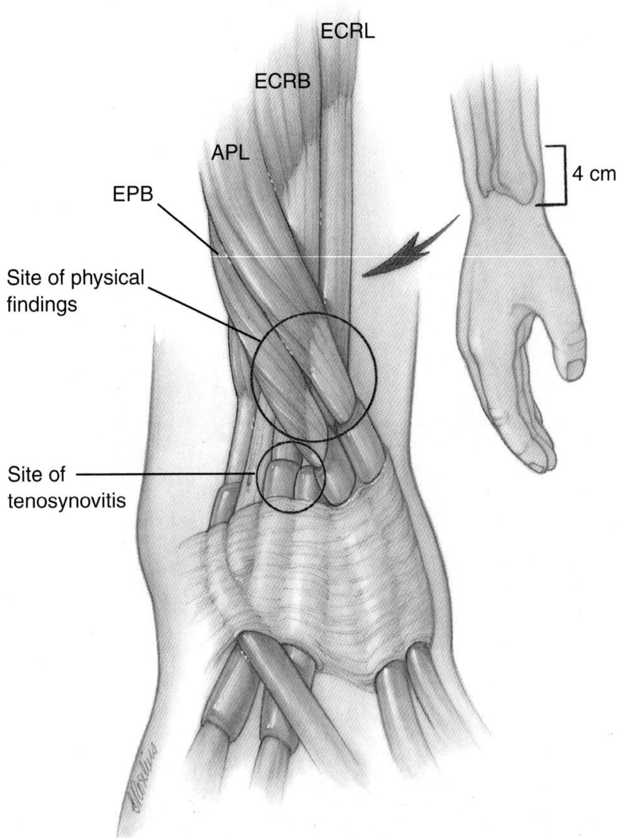

Figure 15.75 Intersection syndrome. ECRL, extensor carpi radialis longus; ECRB, extensor carpi radialis brevis; APL, abductor pollicis longus; EPB, extensor pollicis brevis. (*Reprinted with permission from* Doyle JR, Tornetta P, Einhorn TA. *Orthopaedic Surgery Essentials: Hand and Wrist*. Philadelphia, PA: Lippincott Williams & Wilkins, 2006.)

Radiographic Findings

Radiographs are unnecessary to diagnose intersection syndrome.

Differential Diagnosis

The differential diagnosis is similar to that of de Quervain syndrome.

Treatment

The mainstays of treatment are activity modification, wrist splinting, and oral NSAIDs. Corticosteroid injections are used if these modalities fail. Surgery, which involves complete release of the second compartment, is indicated after failure of nonoperative management.

HAND INFECTIONS

Although the hand is well perfused, frequent breaks in the skin and exposure to outside pathogens makes it a frequent site of infection.

Pathophysiology

The hand is constantly exposed to both minor and major trauma, which can disrupt the skin and allow inoculation of bacteria. Once bacteria have penetrated the skin, the progression of infection is dependent on several factors, including the location, the virulence of the organism, and the immune status of the host. The most common organisms involved in hand infections are *Staphylococcus aureus* and *Streptococcus*, but others are encountered.

Presentation

As with other locations in the body, hand infections present with pain, warmth, erythema, and swelling. Infections that become systemic can cause fevers, chills, and night sweats. Often, inflammatory markers, such as C-reactive protein (CRP), erythrocyte sedimentation rate (ESR), and white blood cell (WBC) count are elevated.

History/Physical Examination

A complete history is vital to appropriately treating infections. Key components of the history are mode of inoculation, duration of symptoms, change in symptoms, previous treatments, environmental exposures, occupation travel history, and immune status. On examination, it is important to determine the exact location of the infection. For instance, cellulitis is a superficial tissue infection and does not involve any deep loculated areas of purulence. On the other hand, septic arthritis affects joints cause micromotion pain and can lead to deep, fluctuant abscesses.

Radiographic Findings

Radiographic findings in osteomyelitis include osteopenia, bony erosions, lytic lesions. For other soft tissue infections, radiographs are less helpful but can sometimes demonstrate soft tissue swelling or subcutaneous air.

Special Studies

MRIs and ultrasounds are the best modalities for accurately localizing and diagnosing deep infections. For septic joints, aspiration and fluid analysis is diagnostic. Nuclear medicine testing may be beneficial in diagnosing osteomyelitis.

Differential Diagnosis

Tumors and crystalline arthropathies can often present similar to infection. Another common condition that can present like infection is pyogenic granuloma. These lesions form secondary to penetrating trauma and present as a red, friable mass; treatment consists of cauterization.

Treatment

In general, all infections of the hand are treated similarly with immobilization, elevation, antibiotics, and operative debridement if necessary. The specifics of treatment are based on the severity of the pathogen and the location of the infection. Empiric antibiotics, which should be used until culture results are available, have historically covered gram-positive cocci. With the recent increased incidence of community-acquired methicillin-resistant *S. aureus*, one must be sure that this pathogen is also covered. Mild infections can be treated with oral antibiotics, whereas severe infections require intravenous antibiotics.

Paronychia

Pathophysiology

Paronychia is an infection under the eponychial fold, and it usually occurs secondary to manicures, hang nails, or nail biting. The most common pathogen responsible is *S. aureus*.

Presentation/Physical Examination

Paronychia usually present with pain, swelling, and redness along the nail fold. Spontaneous drainage of purulent material can also be seen.

Radiographic Findings

Radiographs can evaluate the distal phalanx for osteomyelitis.

Differential Diagnosis

Severe paronychias can progress to felons.

Treatment

The treatment of paronychia is based on the stage of the infection. Early stages can be treated with warm water soaks and oral antibiotics. As the infection progresses, an irrigation and debridement (I&D) must be performed to decompress the pus. This can usually be performed in the emergency department setting, under digital block. The eponychial fold is separated from the nail, and often the involved portion of the nail is removed. After irrigation, the fold should be stented open with gauze to allow continued drainage. Chronic paronychia is usually caused by *Candida albicans*, is more resistant to treatment, and may require marsupialization for complete eradication (Fig. 15.76).

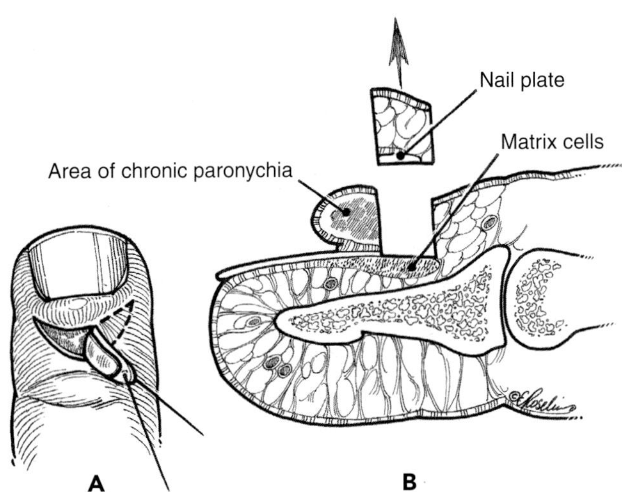

Figure 15.76 Surgical management of chronic paronychia with marsupialization technique. (*Reprinted with permission from* Doyle JR, Tornetta P, Einhorn TA. *Orthopaedic Surgery Essentials: Hand and Wrist*. Philadelphia, PA: Lippincott Williams & Wilkins, 2006.)

Felon

Pathophysiology

A felon is an abscess of the finger pulp overlying the distal phalanx, and it usually occurs secondary to minor trauma or extension of a paronychia. Similar to paronychia, felons are most frequently caused by *S. aureus*.

Presentation/Physical Examination

These infections present with tense swelling, warmth, redness, and pain localized to the finger pulp.

Radiographic Findings

Radiographs are beneficial in excluding osteomyelitis of the underlying distal phalanx in severe infections.

Differential Diagnosis

Severe infection can progress to adjacent structures. Therefore, osteomyelitis of the distal phalanx, septic arthritis of the PIP joint, and pyogenic flexor tenosynovitis must be excluded.

Treatment

Early cases can be treated with elevation, warm soaks, and antibiotics. However, the majority of felons require surgical decompression of all the pulp's multiple compartments. The procedure can usually be performed in the emergency department setting, under digital block. While many incisions have been described, the most common approach is through a midaxial, longitudinal incision. To avoid scar sensitivity, the incision should be placed on the ulnar side of the index finger, long finger, and ring finger, but on the radial sides of the thumb and small finger. The digital neurovascular bundle must be avoided, and then scissors or clamps are used to decompress all the small compartments. The wound is packed, and twice-a-day soaks are started after 24 hours. Empiric antibiotics covering gram-positive cocci are started until culture results are finalized.

Herpetic Whitlow

Pathophysiology

Herpetic whitlow is a finger infection caused by the herpes simplex virus. Most commonly, it is transmitted by oral secretions; and therefore, children and health care workers are at risk.

Presentation/Physical Examination

The infection presents as a single or a group of painful vesicles over the fingertips or other regions of the hand (Fig. 15.77). The pain may precede the appearance of the vesicles.

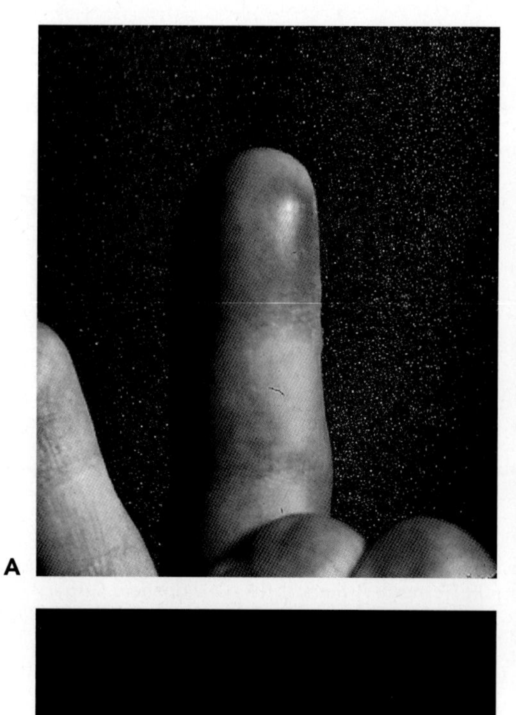

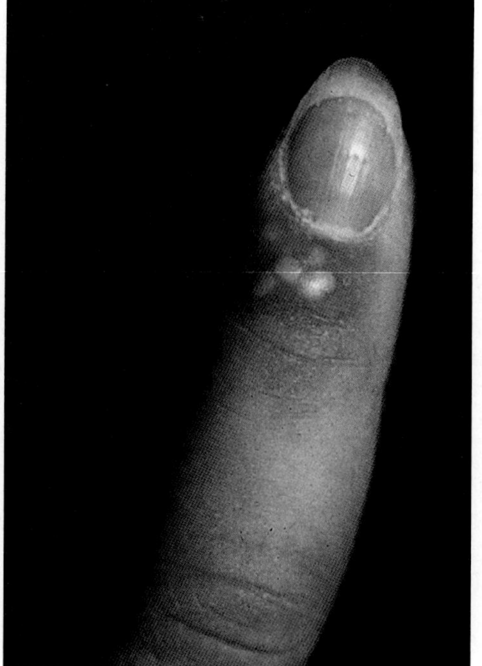

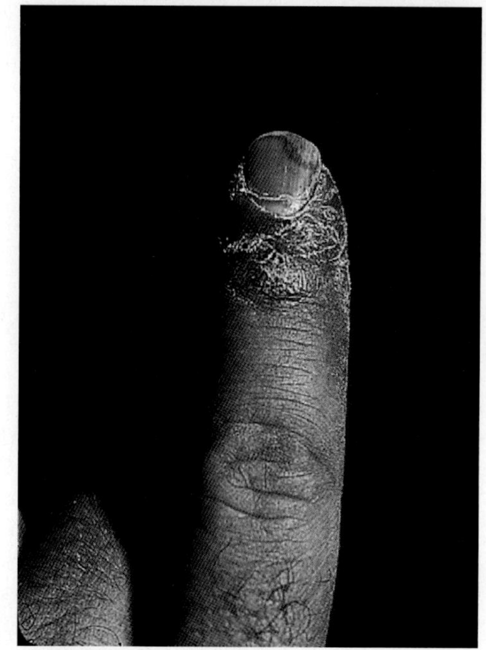

Figure 15.77 Three phases of herpes simplex infection: **(A)** erythematous, **(B)** pustular, and **(C)** desquamation. (*Reprinted with permission from* Doyle JR, Tornetta P, Einhorn TA. *Orthopaedic Surgery Essentials: Hand and Wrist*. Philadelphia, PA: Lippincott Williams & Wilkins, 2006.)

Radiographic Findings/Special Studies

Since the diagnosis is made by history and physical examination, no imaging modalities are necessary. Tzanck smear and viral culture can be used to confirm the diagnosis.

Differential Diagnosis

Bacterial infection must be excluded.

Treatment

Herpetic whitlows are usually self-limited with a 7- to 14-day course, during which the vesicles coalesce, unroof, form ulcers, and then epithelialize. Until epithelialization, the patient is considered contagious. Surgical incision and drainage must be avoided at all costs because this can lead to disseminated infection or superinfection.

Pyogenic Flexor Tenosynovitis

Pyogenic flexor tenosynovitis is purulent infection of the flexor tendon sheath. It causes scarring and adhesions of the flexor tendons and leads to significantly impaired motion.

Pathophysiology

Infection of the tendon sheath usually results from direct inoculation or from the spread from adjacent infection. If treatment is inadequate or delayed, infection can spread to adjacent tendon sheaths or to the radial/ulna bursa. The radial and ulna bursa can theoretically communicate through Parona space in the wrist, forming what is known as a *horseshoe abscess*.

Presentation/Physical Examination

Diagnosis is usually based on the Kanavel four cardinal signs, which are severe pain to passive extension, fusiform swelling of the involved digit (sausage digit), tenderness along the flexor tendon sheath, and partial flexed resting posture of the finger

Differential Diagnosis

The differential diagnosis for pyogenic tenosynovitis includes gout, other deep infections of the hand, and inflammatory arthropathy.

Treatment

Treatment is based on time to presentation. Early stages of the disease (<24 hours) can sometimes be managed with elevation, immobilization, intravenous antibiotics, and close observation. However, if the infection worsens or if the patient presents beyond 24 hours, irrigation and debridement of the flexor tendon sheath is mandatory. This can be accomplished via an open Brunner zigzag incision or a midaxial incision. Alternatively, it can be performed closed via a proximal and a distal incision into the tendon sheath, followed by irrigation of the sheath using an angiocatheter (Fig. 15.78).

Abscesses

The hand contains many deep spaces where abscesses can occur. These include the subcutaneous space, the dorsal subaponeurotic space, the thenar space, the hypothenar space, and the interdigital web spaces.

Pathophysiology

Most abscesses occur from a penetrating trauma or from contiguous infection of an adjacent area. However, a collar button abscess is an abscess of the web space that assumes a volar to dorsal hourglass configuration due to the superficial transverse MC ligament. This abscess often forms in laborers from a palmar blister, callus, or fissure.

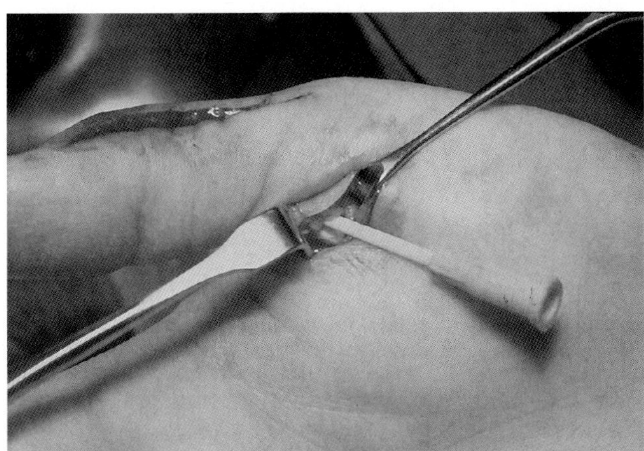

Figure 15.78 Flexor tendon sheath I&D. (*Reprinted with permission from* Strickland JW, Graham TJ. *Master Techniques in Orthopaedic Surgery: The Hand.* Philadelphia, PA: Lippincott Williams & Wilkins, 2005.)

Presentation/Physical Examination

Patients usually present with pain, erythema, warmth, and swelling. The swelling may be diffuse or localized. For example, mid palmar abscesses have a loss of the normal palmar concavity. Also, patients may have limited, painful finger motion depending on the location of the abscess.

Radiographic Findings/Special Studies

If a patient presents with diffuse swelling, an MRI is useful in differentiating cellulitis from an abscess.

Differential Diagnosis

Abscesses can mimic any adjacent infection. Tumor must also be excluded.

Treatment

All abscesses are treated with irrigation and debridement, but specific techniques are dependent on the exact location of the infection. Certain infections, such as a collar button abscess or a thenar space abscess, may require two incisions. The wounds should be packed open, and soaks should be initiated 1 to 2 days after surgery. Following surgery, appropriate intravenous antibiotics, elevation, and immobilization are critical for a successful outcome.

Septic Arthritis

Pathophysiology

Septic arthritis is infection of the joint, and it can be caused by direct inoculation from trauma or by secondary spread. Once there is infection in the joint, cartilage destruction will occur from the inflammatory process. The most commonly involved pathogens are *S. aureus* and *Streptococcus*.

Presentation/Physical Examination

Patients with septic arthritis complain of erythema, swelling, and significant joint pain that causes pain even with micromotion of the joint.

Radiographic Finding/Special Studies

Radiographs are mandatory to evaluate the joint for fractures or foreign bodies. For instance, fight bites often lead to septic arthritis of the MP joint, and chipped teeth can occasionally be seen in the joint. Although radiographs are helpful in excluding fractures and foreign bodies, the specific diagnosis of septic arthritis is made via joint aspiration. WBC count greater than 75,000, with neutrophils more than 75% is indicative of a septic arthritis.

Differential Diagnosis

Inflammatory arthritis can mimic septic arthritis but generally demonstrates lower WBC counts and lower percentages of neutrophils.

Treatment

Once the diagnosis of septic arthritis is made, the treatment is irrigation and debridement of the joint, followed by long-term oral or intravenous antibiotics. The one exception is septic arthritis caused by *Neisseria gonorrhoeae*, which can usually be treated nonoperatively by intravenous ceftriaxone.

Osteomyelitis

Pathophysiology

Osteomyelitis, or an infection of the bone, is typically caused by an open fracture or by spread of infection from adjacent sites. The risk of osteomyelitis is increased in immunocompromised patients, especially those who have diabetes.

Presentation/Physical Examination

Patients usually present with pain, swelling, erythema, and possible drainage. Inflammatory markers, such as CRP level and ESR, are elevated.

Radiographic Findings/Special Studies

Initial radiographs are often negative. However, after several weeks of osteomyelitis, radiographs will demonstrate osteopenia and periosteal reaction. Sequestra, which is dead bone with surrounding granulation tissue, and involucrum, which is periosteal new bone, can also be seen. When radiographs are negative, MRI and nuclear medicine studies are invaluable in making the diagnosis.

Differential Diagnosis

The differential diagnosis for osteomyelitis includes septic arthritis, crystalline arthropathy, trauma, and deep soft tissue infection.

Treatment

Antibiotics are the first line of treatment and are continued for 4 to 6 weeks. If conservative treatment fails, an associated abscess is present, or necrotic bone is seen, then surgical debridement is required.

Bite Wounds

Pathophysiology

Both human and animal bite wounds are a common source of infection in the hand. Human bites usually occur during an altercation when one person strikes another person in the mouth. The resulting wound over the MP joint is termed a *fight bite*. The most common organisms found in these wounds are *S. aureus* and *Eikenella corrodens*. Animal bite infections are usually secondary to *Streptococcus*, *Pasteurella multocida*, or *S. aureus*, but they can also be polymicrobial. Cat bites become infected more often than dog bites because cat teeth are sharper and therefore able to inoculate bacteria deeper within the tissue.

Presentation/Physical Examination

Patients usually present with a wound on the hand. If the patient presents with a dorsal wound over the MP joint after an altercation, careful physical examination is warranted to be sure that this fight bite does not communicate with the joint.

Radiographic Findings/ Special Studies

Radiographs are necessary to screen for fractures and foreign bodies, especially with fight bites.

Treatment

Most inoculated wounds should be copiously irrigated, left open, and treated with broad-spectrum antibiotics, such as ampicillin–sulbactam (Unasyn) or amoxicillin–clavulanate (Augmentin). If a wound is grossly infected or if the joint is infected, formal irrigation and debridement should be performed in the operating room. Rabies prophylaxis should be considered if the involved animal was a bat, fox, skunk, raccoon, unknown domestic animal, or a domestic animal demonstrating features of rabies.

Necrotizing Fasciitis

Pathophysiology

Necrotizing fasciitis is a rapidly progressive and potentially life-threatening infection of the soft tissues. It usually stems from relatively minor trauma to the extremity. The most common organism responsible is group A β-hemolytic streptococcus, but *S. aureus* and anaerobes may be present. It is seen more commonly in diabetic patients.

Presentation/Physical Examination

Patients present with rapidly spreading, painful erythema that is accompanied by induration and swelling. Inflammatory markers, such as CRP and ESR, and WBC count are usually extremely elevated. As the infection progresses, the patient may become hemodynamically unstable.

Radiographic Findings/Special Studies

Radiographs will show significant soft tissue swelling and potentially subcutaneous air. If the patient is stable and the diagnosis is unclear, an MRI can be performed, which will show edema and swelling of the fascial planes.

Differential Diagnosis

The primary differential diagnosis is cellulitis, which presents with less severe symptoms, stable vitals signs, slower disease course.

Treatment

Mortality rates of been described between 10% and 30%. Therefore, early and aggressive surgical debridement along with empiric, broad-spectrum antibiotics is warranted. Antibiotics must include coverage for gram-positive organisms (cephalosporins), gram-negative organisms (gentamicin), and anaerobes (penicillin). In the operating room, watery, foul-smelling fluid ("dishwasher pus") is usually found along the fascial planes. Multiple debridements are usually required, and amputation is occasionally necessary. If the limb can be salvaged, soft tissue coverage is often eventually required.

Atypical Infections

Besides common bacterial infections, atypical infections from mycobacterial species and fungi can be seen in the hand.

CONGENITAL HAND DISORDERS

Fortunately, congenital hand deformities are relatively rare occurrences. However, when they do arise, they can have devastating consequences, both for children and their families.

Embryology

The embryonic development of the upper limb occurs in a surprisingly consistent and reproducible pattern. On roughly day 26, the upper limb buds appear. At this time, limb growth is controlled by the *apical epidermal ridge*. All growth in the limbs proceeds from proximal to distal. By day 33, primitive arms and hands have formed. At 6 weeks, chondrification of the bones has begun. By 8 weeks, apoptosis (programmed cell death) has separated out the individual fingers.

Incidence and Etiology

Upper extremity anomalies are present in approximately 1 out of every 626 live births. However, only 10% of these anomalies cause any significant functional or cosmetic deficit. The root cause of half of these congenital defects is unknown, whereas the rest are believed to be either genetic or environmental in etiology. When an upper extremity congenital anomaly is encountered, it is important to evaluate the child for anomalies of other organ systems, such as cardiac, gastrointestinal, or renal.

Classification

Swanson has divided anomalies of the upper limb into 7 major categories, which are outlined below:

I. Failure of formation (e.g., amputations)
II. Failure of differentiation (e.g., syndactyly)
III. Duplication (e.g., polydactyly)
IV. Undergrowth
V. Overgrowth
VI. Congenital constriction ring syndrome
VII. Generalized skeletal abnormalities

Goals and Timing of Treatment

The ultimate goal of treatment for upper extremity congenital anomalies is to maximize function. Creation of a satisfactory grasp is tantamount to achieving this goal. The secondary aim is to restore normal aesthetic appearance. The parents of children with these anomalies simply desire that their children be "normal" and hope the hand surgeon can achieve this surgically. However, this is not always possible, and it is important to be honest with parents about this reality from the beginning. If possible, planned surgical correction of any congenital upper extremity anomaly should be undertaken before age 4 to 5, which is when school typically begins.

A complete discussion of all congenital hand conditions is beyond the scope of this text. Some of the Swanson major categories are discussed later, and several specific conditions are mentioned in Chapter 11 ("General and Regional Problems in Children").

Failure of Formation

Failures of formation can be either transverse or longitudinal. Transverse failures of formation typically present as amputations. They are seen most often in the proximal forearm but can occur anywhere in the upper extremity. The incidence is roughly 1 in every 20,000 live births. Treatment is rarely surgical and often includes fitting children for prostheses at an age as young as 6 months to encourage use of the limb. Otherwise, they may ignore the limb due to lack of function.

Longitudinal failure of formation is also known as *phocomelia* (derived from the Greek word for "seal"), a term used to denote limbs with a flipper-like appearance due to absence of either the forearm or the humerus. Patients with longitudinal deficiencies differ from those with transverse ones in that the former have digital structures. Longitudinal deficiencies come in three types: complete, proximal, and distal. In complete deficiencies, the hand is attached directly to shoulder. In proximal deficiencies, the hand is attached to an abnormal humerus. Last, in distal deficiencies, the hand is attached to the humerus with no intervening forearm. Of historical note, phocomelia was seen in the 1960s in children whose mothers ingested thalidomide during pregnancy. The mainstay of treatment for longitudinal deficiencies is nonoperative. Limb training should begin at an early age.

Failure of Differentiation

Failure of differentiation occurs when the normal mechanisms of apoptosis are disrupted and structures that normally are separate remain joined. Syndactyly is the most representative condition in which digits fail to separate. Syndactyly is discussed further in Chapter 11.

Duplication

Duplication refers to the presence of an extra structure in the hand, usually a finger or a thumb. *Preaxial duplication*, or *polydactyly*, refers to duplications of the thumb or the radial side of the hand. *Postaxial polydactyly* refers to duplication of the small finger.

RECOMMENDED READINGS

Barron OA, Glickel S, Eaton R. Basal joint arthritis of the thumb. *J Am Acad Orthop Surg*. 2000;8:314–323.

Cranford CS, Ho JY, Kalainov DM, et al. Hartigan carpal tunnel syndrome. *J Am Acad Orthop Surg*. 2007;15:537–548.

Freeland AE, Geissler WB, Weiss APC. Operative treatment of common displaced and unstable fractures of the hand. *J Bone Joint Surg Am*. 2001;83:928–945.

Gupta R, Bozentka D, Osterman AL. Wrist arthroscopy: principles and clinical applications. *J Am Acad Orthop Surg*. 2001;9:200–209.

Nana A, Joshi A, Lichtman DM. Plating of the distal radius. *J Am Acad Orthop Surg*. 2005;13:159–171.

Saldana MJ. Trigger digits: diagnosis and treatment. *J Am Acad Orthop Surg*. 2001;9:246–252.

The Hip and Femur

16

Neil P. Sheth J. Stuart Melvin Charles L. Nelson R. Bruce Heppenstall

INTRODUCTION

The hip joint is the most proximal joint of the lower extremity and plays an integral role in gait and balanced locomotion. The hip is designed for strength and mobility, and thus the bony architecture, soft-tissue structures, and surrounding musculature are geared toward conferring constraint and joint stability while allowing for a multitude of maneuvers and range of motion (ROM). Pathologic processes affecting the hip are common and include soft-tissue injuries such as labrum and cartilage defects, bony injuries such as fractures about the acetabulum and femur, vascular insults such osteonecrosis of the femoral head, and degeneration of the joint as seen in post-traumatic arthritis and osteoarthritis (OA). Hip pathology has a significant impact on a patient's mobility and thus may result in a significant degree of morbidity and dysfunction without adequate treatment.

This chapter will focus on a brief overview of the embryology and development of the hip, the osteology and musculature surrounding the hip joint, contribution of the hip to lower extremity gait and biomechanics, as well as a series of soft-tissue and bony pathologies with an emphasis on clinical diagnosis, radiographic diagnosis, and indications for surgical treatment.

ANATOMY

Embryology of the Hip

The hip is defined as a ball and socket-type joint. The femoral head is situated within the confines of the acetabulum that confers bony stability to the joint. The structural acetabulum is a result of a fusion between three separate pelvic bones: the ilium, ischium, and pubis (Fig. 16.1). These three bones are confluent at the tri-irradiate cartilage (Fig. 16.2), the medial acetabular growth plate, and eventually fuse together during skeletal maturity to comprise the innominate bone. Two innominate bones along with the intervening sacrum constitute the pelvis (Fig. 16.3).

Normal development of the acetabulum is dependent upon adequate articulation with the femoral head. In scenarios where the femoral head is subluxated or dislocated, the acetabulum is unable to properly develop and a condition known as developmental dysplasia of the hip (DDH) results. Depending upon the severity of the dysplasia, the patient may be predisposed to early onset osteoarthritis (OA) of the hip. Early diagnosis is paramount and may be treated with closed reduction and casting or open acetabular and/or femoral osteotomy, depending on patient's age (please see Chapter 11 on Pediatric Orthopaedics).

Osteology of the Pelvis and Proximal Femur

As mentioned earlier, the pelvis is composed of two innominate bones and the intervening sacrum. When evaluating each hemipelvis, the ilium has two important anterior prominences: the anterior superior iliac spine (ASIS) and the anterior inferior iliac spine (AIIS). The ASIS is the origin of the inguinal ligament, sartorius muscle and is the insertion of the transverse and internal oblique abdominal muscles. The AIIS is the origin of the direct head of the rectus femoris muscle and the Y ligament of Bigelow (iliofemoral ligament). The fusion of the ilium and the pubis results in another anterior prominence known as the iliopectineal eminence. The iliopsoas muscle traverses the groove between this eminence and the AIIS. Posteriorly, the posterior superior iliac spine (PSIS) is a prominence that has clinical significance as the point of referred lumbosacral pain. Just posterior and superior to the acetabulum is the greater sciatic notch (Fig. 16.1).

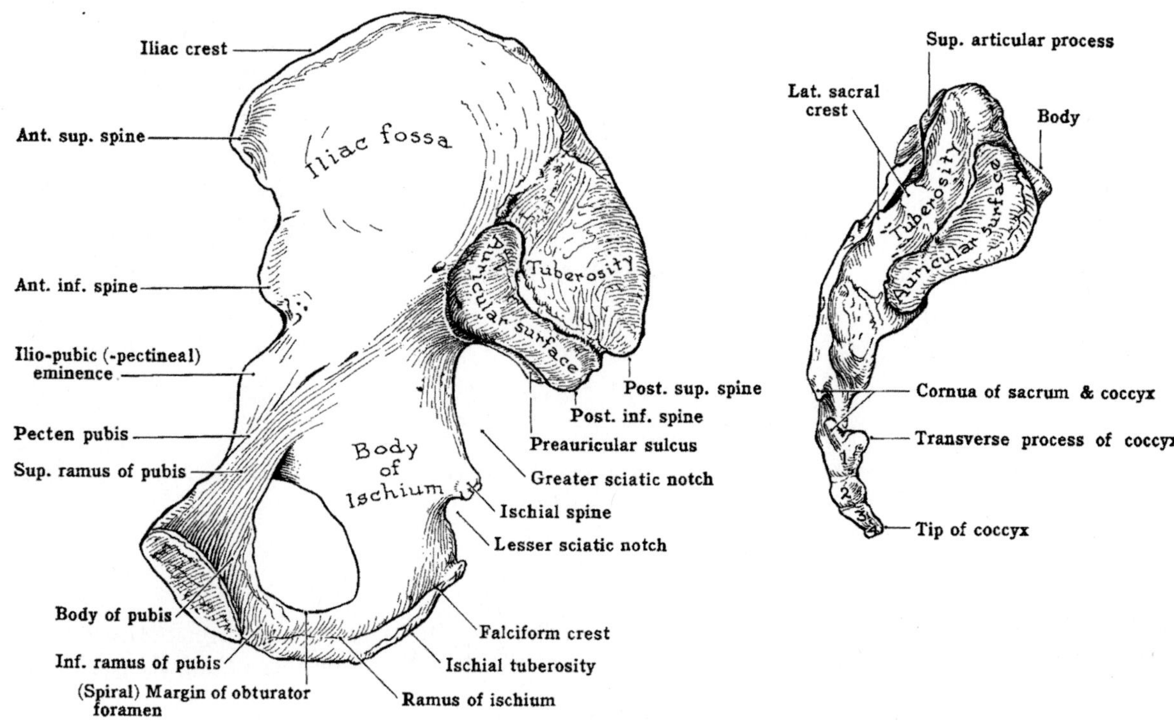

Figure 16.1 Hemipelvis depicting the three components of the innominate bone. (*Reprinted with permission from* Tile M, Helfet DL, Kellam JF. *Fractures of the Pelvis and Acetabulum*. 3rd ed. Philadelphia, PA: Lippincott Williams & Wilkins, 2003.)

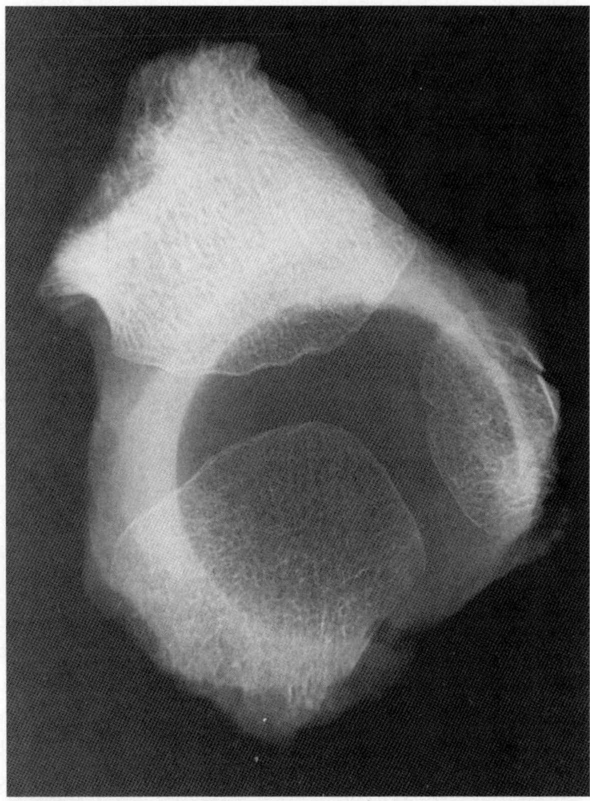

Figure 16.2 Image of the tri-irradiate cartilage in a 4-year-old patient. (*Reprinted with permission from* Callaghan JJ, Rosenberg AG, Rubash HE. *The Adult Hip*. 2nd ed. Philadelphia, PA: Lippincott Williams & Wilkins, 2007.)

In general, the acetabulum is oriented in 20 to 25 degrees of anteversion and 45 degrees of abduction or inclination. The central inferior surface is devoid of cartilage and comprises the cotyloid fossa bound by the transverse acetabular ligament. These landmarks are typically used for retractor placement and as reference points for acetabular reaming during total hip arthroplasty. In addition, a cartilaginous ring called the labrum surrounds the inner lining of the acetabulum like a horseshoe (Fig. 16.4). The purpose of the labrum is to deepen the acetabulum and enhance the stability conferred by the bony architecture of the acetabulum.

The proximal femur is composed of the femoral head, the femoral neck, the greater and lesser trochanters, and the femoral shaft. The femoral neck is further subdivided into regions, namely the subcapital, transverse cervical, and basicervical regions. The area between the two trochanters is named the intertrochanteric region and is composed primarily of cancellous bone. The named regions and the bony architecture become important considerations for the appropriate treatment of various hip fractures on the basis of location of the fracture line. Structurally, the femoral neck is anteverted approximately 12 to 15 degrees compared with the epicondylar axis between the medial and lateral femoral condyles, and the average neck shaft angle is 127 degrees (Fig. 16.5).

The proximal femur extending from just distal to the intertrochanteric region to 5-cm distal to the lesser trochanter is named the subtrochanteric region of the femur. The

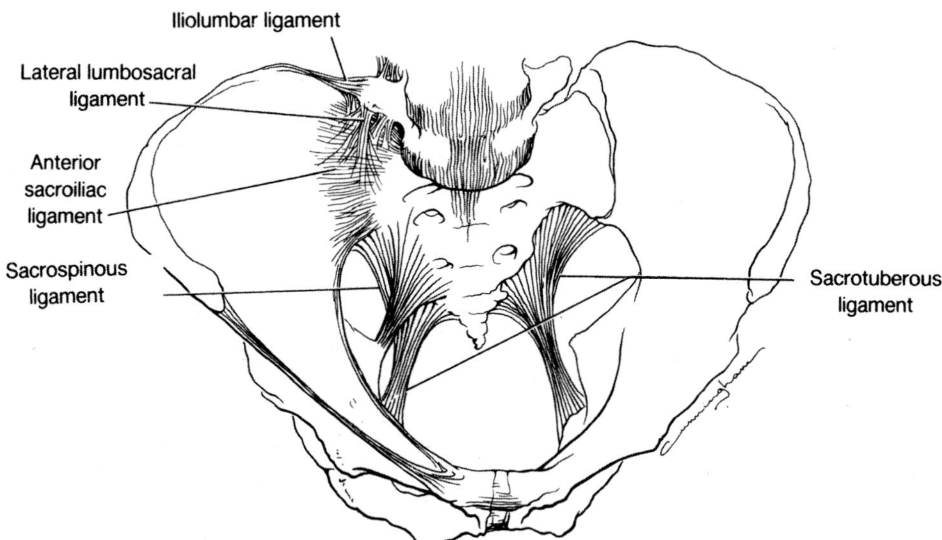

Figure 16.3 Anteroposterior view of the pelvis demonstrating two innominate bones along with the sacrum comprising the pelvis. (*Reprinted with permission from* Tile M, Helfet DL, Kellam JF. *Fractures of the Pelvis and Acetabulum*. 3rd ed. Philadelphia, PA: Lippincott Williams & Wilkins, 2003.)

subtrochanteric region contains the calcar femorale that extends from the femoral neck to the subtrochanteric region. This bony column is the strongest part of the proximal femur and is responsible for resisting varus rotational moments. Additionally, its integrity defines whether a subtrochanteric fracture is considered stable or unstable (see details in section on traumatic injuries to the hip and femur).

Soft-Tissue and Musculature Surrounding the Hip Joint

Soft-tissue structures surrounding the hip play a key role in its stability. These include capsular thickenings surrounding the hip: (a) iliofemoral ligament (strongest), (b) ischiofemoral ligament, and (c) pubofemoral ligament as well as the labrum (Fig. 16.6). These soft-tissue structures,

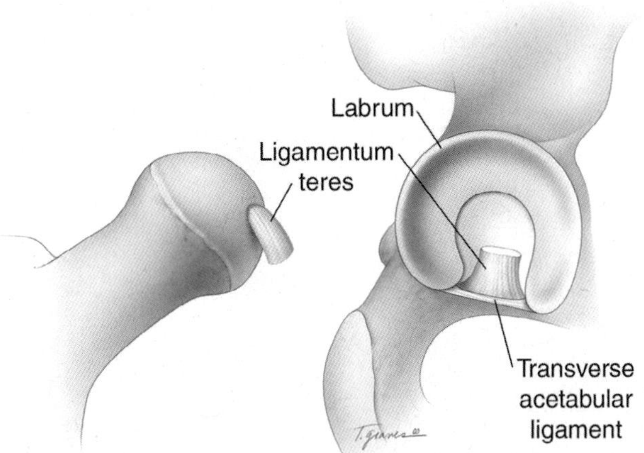

Figure 16.4 The labrum and transverse acetabular ligament within the acetabulum. (*Reprinted with permission from* Callaghan JJ, Rosenberg AG, Rubash HE. *The Adult Hip*. 2nd ed. Philadelphia, PA: Lippincott Williams & Wilkins, 2007.)

in addition to the bony anatomy of the acetabulum, make the hip a very stable joint when compared with other ball and socket joints such as the glenohumeral joint.

The muscular sleeve surrounding the hip adds additional dynamic stability to the joint. The gluteus medius and minimus are considered the abductor complex that plays an important role in both function and stability after total hip arthroplasty. A series of short external hip rotators insert onto the posterior aspect of the greater trochanter. The piriformis muscle insertion is typically used as a landmark during the posterior approach to the hip as well as a starting point for antegrade intramedullary nailing of femoral shaft fractures. The iliopsoas, the strongest hip flexor, inserts onto the lesser trochanter and may be involved in hip flexion contractures. The gluteus maximus, the main hip extensor, surrounds the posterolateral aspect of the hip. The gluteus maximus is just deep to the tensor fascia lata, which is also commonly used as a landmark during surgical exposure of the hip. The medial and posterior compartments of the thigh contain a series of adductor and hamstring muscles that originate from the pubic rami and the ischial tuberosity (Fig. 16.7).

APPLIED NEUROVASCULAR ANATOMY ABOUT THE HIP

Greater and Lesser Sciatic Foramen

Posteriorly, the sacrospinous (from the sacrum to the ischial spine) and sacrotuberous (from the sacrum to the ischial tuberosity) ligaments define the borders of the greater and lesser sciatic foramen or notches, respectively. The piriformis muscle is a key landmark with regards to all structures posterior to the hip joint. Using this muscle as a reference, the superior gluteal artery and nerve lie superior to the piriformis. The following structures lie deep to the

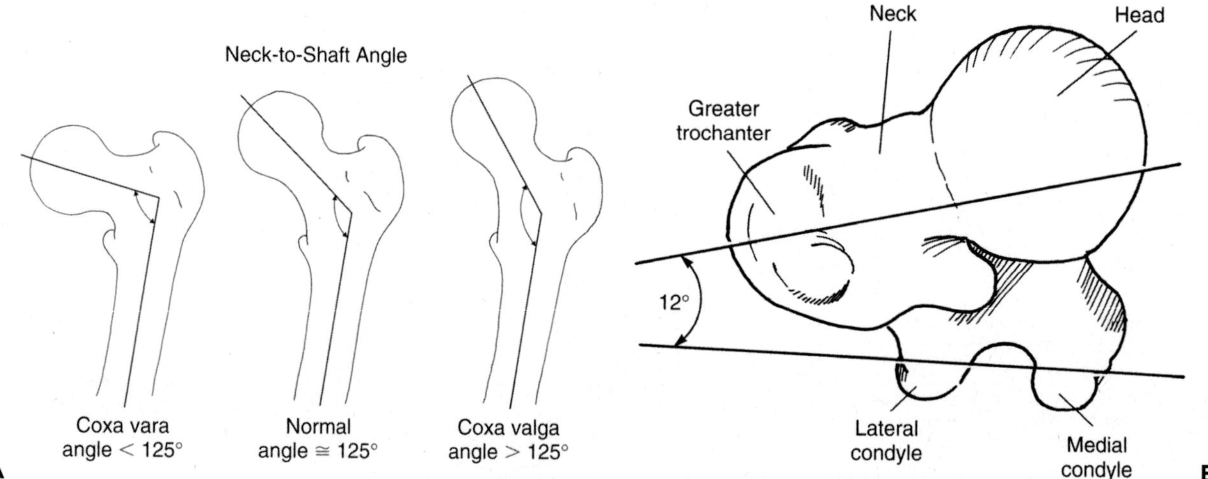

Figure 16.5 (**A**) The normal neck-to-shaft angle (angle of inclination of the femoral neck to the shaft in the frontal plane) is approximately 125 degrees. The condition in which this angle is less than 125 degrees is called coxa vara. If the angle is greater than 125 degrees, the condition is called coxa valga. (**B**) Top view of the left femur showing the angle of anteversion formed by the intersection of the long axis of the femoral head and the transverse axis of the femoral condyles. The angle averages approximately 12 degrees in adults. (*Reprinted with permission from* Nordin M, Frankel FH. *Basic Biomechanics of the Musculoskeletal System*. 3rd ed. Philadelphia, PA: Lippincott Williams & Wilkins, 2001.)

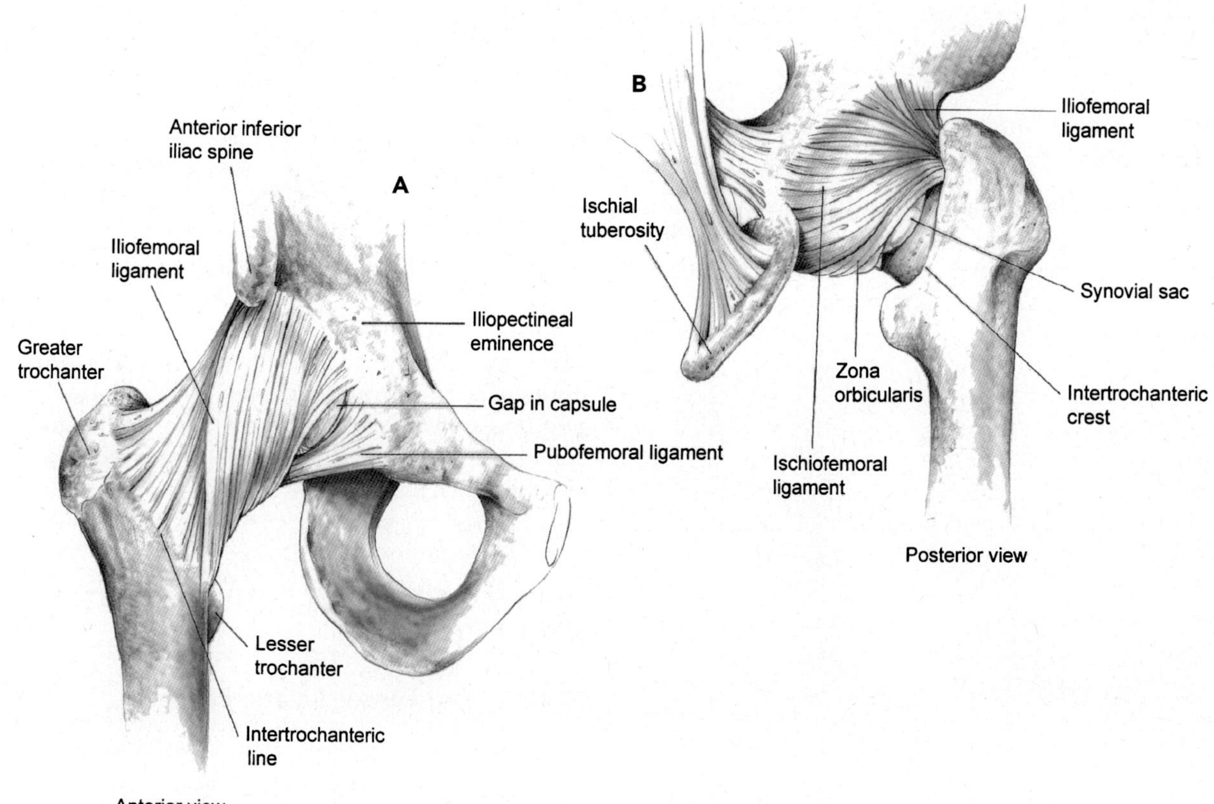

Figure 16.6 (**A**) Anterior and (**B**) Posterior views of the hip. Illustration of the three pericapsular hip ligaments. (*Reprinted with permission from* Callaghan JJ, Rosenberg AG, Rubash HE. *The Adult Hip*. 2nd ed. Philadelphia, PA: Lippincott Williams & Wilkins, 2007.)

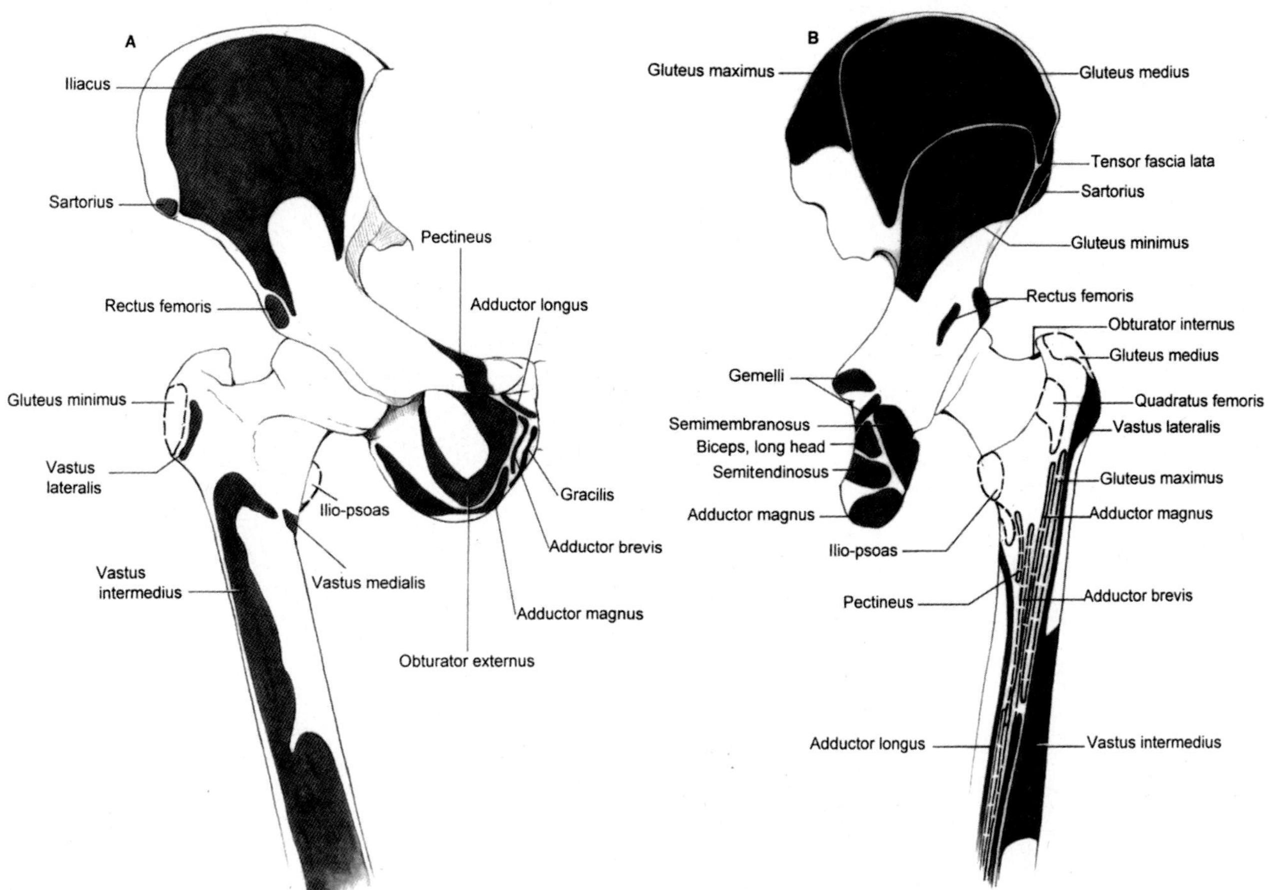

Figure 16.7 Origin and insertion of the major muscles surrounding the hip joint. (*Reprinted with permission from* Callaghan JJ, Rosenberg AG, Rubash HE. *The Adult Hip*. 2nd ed. Philadelphia, PA: Lippincott Williams & Wilkins, 2007.)

piriformis: (a) pudendal nerve, (b) nerve to obturator internus, (c) posterior femoral cutaneous nerve, (d) sciatic nerve, (e) inferior gluteal nerve, and (f) nerve to quadratus femoris. All of these structures, including the piriformis muscle, exit the pelvis through the greater sciatic foramen. However, both the pudendal nerve and the nerve to the obturator internus reenter the pelvis through the lesser sciatic foramen (Figs. 16.1 and 16.2). Clinically, the greater sciatic foramen or notch is a key landmark for identifying the location of the superior gluteal artery. Inadvertent injury to this artery in this location during surgery may result in significant bleeding and retraction of the damaged artery into the pelvis, making hemostasis difficult to achieve.

Sciatic Nerve

The sciatic nerve is the largest peripheral nerve in the body, and it is classified as a mixed nerve, containing both motor and sensory components. The nerve is composed of L4-S3 lumbosacral plexus nerve roots. The nerve is divided into a tibial and a peroneal nerve division, with the peroneal division positioned laterally, making it more susceptible to injury during posterior surgical approaches to the hip. Both divisions of the sciatic nerve travel down the posterior compartment of the thigh covered by the biceps femoris muscle. The tibial nerve division supplies innervation to the hamstring muscles (semimembranosus, semitendinosus, long head of the biceps femoris, and the hamstring portion of the adductor magnus), while the peroneal division only innervates the short head of the biceps in the posterior thigh compartment. The two divisions of the sciatic nerve formally separate posterior to the knee prior to traveling down the remainder of the lower leg.

Cruciate Anastomosis

There is a very rich vascular supply surrounding the hip joint. At the level of the L4 vertebral body, the aorta branches into the common iliac arteries, which in turn further divide into the internal and external iliac vessels at the level of the S1 sacral body. The internal iliac artery has several branches including the obturator, superior gluteal, inferior gluteal, and internal pudendal. An understanding of these named branches is important especially following traumatic pelvic fractures or when screws are needed for

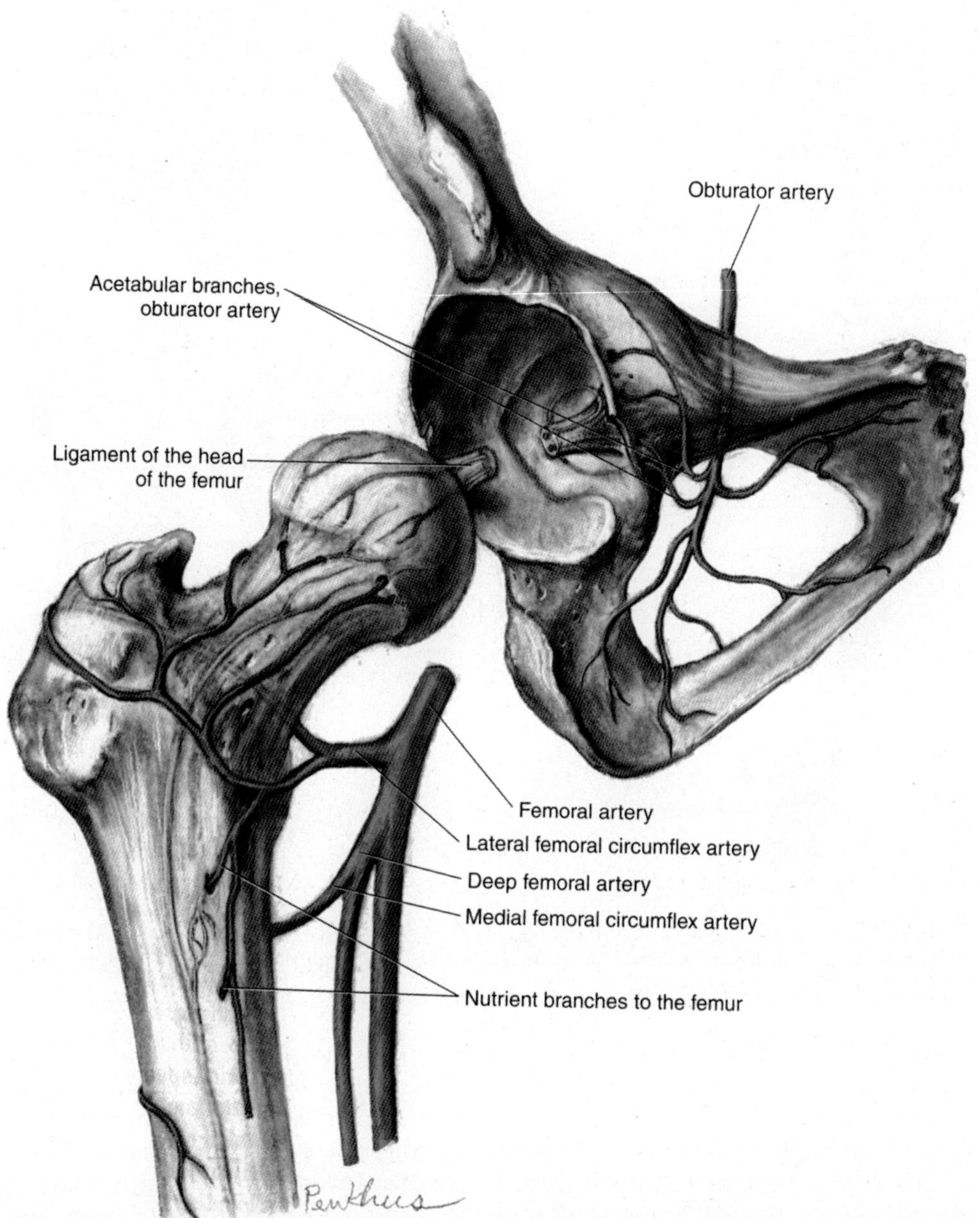

Figure 16.8 Illustration of arterial supply surrounding the hip joint. (*Reprinted with permission from* Clemente CD. *Clemente's. Anatomy Dissector*. 3rd ed. Philadelphia, PA: Lippincott Williams & Wilkins, 2011.)

fixation of the acetabular cup during total hip arthroplasty (see section on total hip arthroplasty).

The external iliac artery passes beneath the inguinal ligament to become the femoral artery. The femoral artery gives rise to the medial and lateral femoral circumflex arteries as well as the profunda femoris artery that branches into several perforating vessels. The cruciate anastomosis about the hip is a confluence of the descending branch of the inferior gluteal artery, the ascending branch of the first perforator, and the transverse branches of the medial and lateral femoral circumflex vessels. This anastomosis lies at the inferior margin of the quadratus femoris muscle and is often encountered during a posterior approach to the hip (Fig. 16.8).

Vascular Supply of the Femoral Head

The dominance of the blood supply to the femoral head changes according to patient's age. From birth to 4 years, the major vascular supply to the femoral head is derived from both the medial and lateral circumflex arteries. There is also a contribution from the artery of the ligamentum teres, a branch of the obturator artery that travels within a ligament that connects the femoral head to the cotyloid fossa (Fig. 16.9).

Beyond 4 years of age, the lateral femoral circumflex artery as well as the artery of the ligamentum teres contribute little to the blood supply of the femoral head. The medial femoral circumflex artery emerges as the dominant

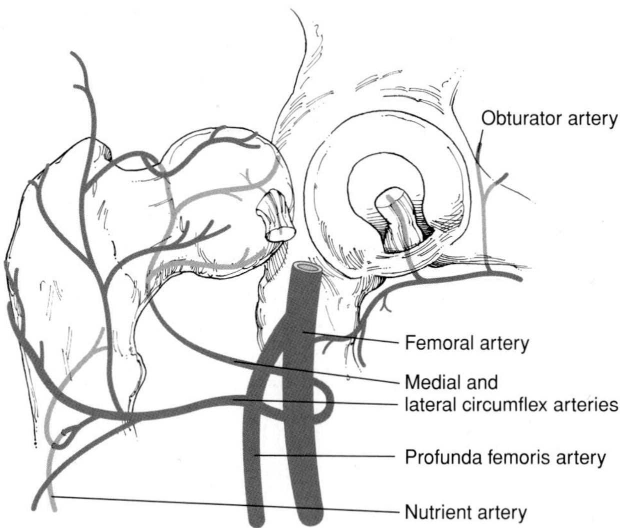

Figure 16.9 The vascular supply to the femoral head arises from the medial and lateral circumflex vessels, which create a ring giving rise to the cervical vessels. A minor contribution comes from the obturator artery via the ligamentum teres. From Bucholz RW, MD and Heckman JD, MD. *Rockwood & Green's Fractures in Adults*, 5th ed. Lippincott, Williams & Wilkins, 2001.

artery supplying the femoral head and does so through the posterosuperior and posteroinferior retinacular branches. In the adult, the medial femoral circumflex continues to be the major vascular supply to the femoral head via the lateral epiphyseal artery (Fig. 16.10). Disruption of this blood supply is of concern in displaced femoral neck fractures as well as piriformis entry femoral nails in pediatric patients due to the increase risk of femoral head osteonecrosis.

BIOMECHANICS OF THE HIP

Gait Analysis

The primary goal of the lower extremity is to allow for energy efficient ambulation. Gait analysis constitutes evaluation of the gait cycle that begins and ends with heel strike of the same limb. There are two components of the gait cycle: (a) stance and (b) swing. The foot is in contact with the ground during stance phase and is being propelled forward during the swing phase. The stance phase is approximately 60% of the gait cycle. Both feet are in contact (Fig. 16.11) with the ground during double-limb support that comprises 20% of the total gait cycle. Normal gait requires energy efficient locomotion. Efficiency is obtained through a level pelvis, which is maintained by hip abductor complex contraction. For normal ambulation to occur, the hip must be able to flex to 40 degrees and rotate 10 degrees, both internally and externally.

Joint Reaction Forces

The joint reaction force is defined as the sum of all forces that cross the hip joint. These forces are resolved into components from gravity, body weight, and muscle forces acting upon the joint. In the static phase of gait, during double-limb support, the joint reaction force is approximately 5/6 body weight. During single-limb stance, the joint reaction force across the hip can increase up to three times body weight. The increase seen during single-limb support is a result of an increased moment generated by the abductor complex, which helps to keep the pelvis level. During walking, the joint reaction force can reach four times body weight. In the postoperative recovery phase, non–weight-bearing status still results in joint reaction forces across the hip in the order of 1.5 to 1.8 times body weight, which is a result of hip flexion (via the iliopsoas muscle) used to avoid lower extremity contact with the floor. The lowest joint reaction forces seen with ambulation occur when patients use touch-down weight-bearing with the foot flat on the floor to steady the operative lower extremity.

PATIENT EVALUATION

Clinical History

The evaluation of a patient presenting with hip pain requires a thorough and detailed history. This history is complimented by physical examination and when necessary imaging studies, including plain radiographs, magnetic resonance imaging (MRI), and computed tomography (CT).

Several key elements are incorporated into obtaining a thorough patient history. The history should first focus on the exact location of the pain. It is important to determine whether the patient suffers from point tenderness versus diffuse pain encircling the hip. When possible, try to have the patient point with one finger to the location of maximal discomfort. Intra-articular hip pain typically manifests as groin pain with hip ROM, whereas referred pain to the hip from the lumbar spine presents as diffuse pain over the PSIS and buttock. Thigh pain typically is indicative of either hip or femoral pathology, especially when the patient has previously undergone total hip arthroplasty.

Next, the temporal nature of the pain should be determined. What has been the duration of this pain? Has the pain been there for 3 days, 2 weeks, or 1 year? Understanding the chronicity of the complaint is critical in assessing whether the patient is likely to need surgical intervention. Relating the onset of the pain to a specific event is also critical in determining the etiology. If the patients state that their hip pain started after a fall, it is important to obtain details surrounding the event to find a correlation between the mechanism of injury and the underlying pathology. After understanding the events leading up to the onset of hip pain, have the patient rate the pain on a scale of 1 to 10 to objectively document the degree of pain.

Ask the patient regarding remitting and exacerbating factors associated with their pain—what makes the pain worse and what makes it better? Are there specific motions that recreate the pain? Is the pain alleviated by the use of any

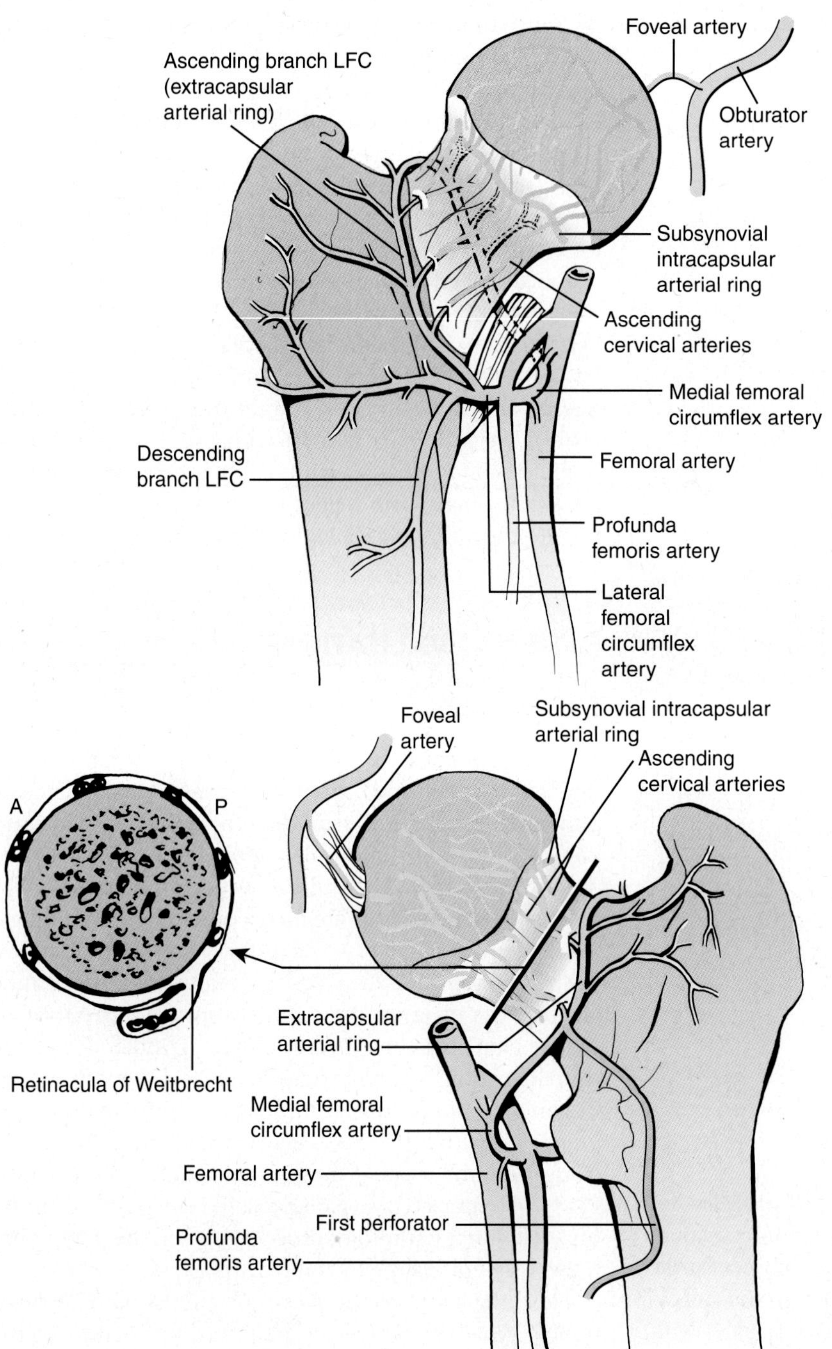

Figure 16.10 Vascular anatomy of the femoral head and neck. (**Top**) Anterior aspect. (**Bottom**) Posterior aspect. LFC: lateral femoral circumflex artery (*Reprinted with permission from* Bucholz RW, Heckman JD, Court-Brown CM, et al. *Rockwood and Green's Fractures in Adults.* 6th ed. Philadelphia, PA: Lippincott Williams & Wilkins, 2006.)

modalities? With long-standing pain from a degenerative process such as OA, patients may present with pain from prolonged sitting and pain with the first few steps of ambulation. Patients should be questioned regarding the requirement of pain medication, use of anti-inflammatory medications, previous interventions (e.g., aquatic therapy), as well as previous issues with the involved hip (e.g., delay in ambulation as a child, requirement of bracing as a child, or known history of developmental dysplasia). The use of an assistive device (e.g., cane or walker) for ambulation should be documented as well as a patient's inability to ambulate for any length of time. Has the patient been wheelchair-bound over the past 2 years? Information of this nature is important in determining the contribution of comorbidities (e.g., cerebrovascular accident) to the patient's condition and its effect on potential surgical treatment. Attention should also be given to the patient's history of medications (e.g., corticosteroids may lead to osteonecrosis) and social history (EtOH abuse is also associated with osteonecrosis).

It is imperative to question the patient regarding symptoms that may indicate concomitant lumbar spine involvement. Pain originating in the hip may radiate to the knee

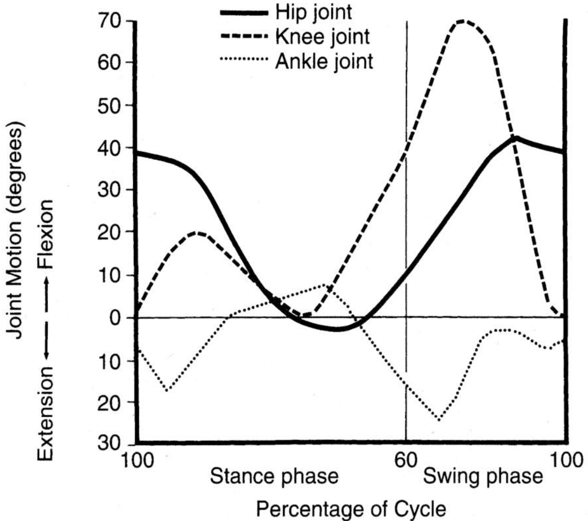

Figure 16.11 Range of hip joint motion in the sagittal plane for 30 normal men during level walking, 1 gait cycle. The ranges of motion for the knee and ankle joints are shown for comparison. (*Reprinted with permission from* Nordin M, Frankel FH. *Basic Biomechanics of the Musculoskeletal System.* 3rd ed. Philadelphia, PA: Lippincott Williams & Wilkins, 2001.)

via the obturator nerve; however, pain originating from the hip does not typically radiate below the tibial tubercle. Degenerative disc disease and spinal/foraminal stenosis may manifest as radicular pain extending beyond the knee into the lower leg and foot or as dull pain in the buttock and posterior thigh. Patients may also complain of subjective numbness, tingling and weakness in the lower extremity, inability to sit for long periods, or pain with valsalva maneuvers (sneezing or coughing). These signs and symptoms are crucial for differentiating lumbar spine pathology from hip pathology.

A detailed medical history should be obtained to determine a history of deep venous thrombosis (DVT), pulmonary embolus, pulmonary or cardiac disease, renal disease, immunocompromised, or recent/chronic infection. In addition, patients with arthritis are typically elderly and may be on medications such as blood thinners for other diagnoses. Use of these medications may be important in the timing of operative intervention.

Physical Examination

When conducting a physical examination of the painful hip, it is important to employ a thorough systematic approach. Gait analysis is the most important functional evaluation of the lower extremity. Observing a patient walking into the office can reveal a great deal about the patient's hip pathology and overall functional capacity. Typically, patients with a painful hip will spend a shorter time in stance phase on the involved lower extremity and lean over the affected hip when weight-bearing to reduce the joint reaction forces. This type of gait is termed as *Trendelenburg gait* and may also be seen with a weak abductor complex.

The method by which to conduct the physical examination of the hip follows the same principles used to examine any organ system. The examination should adhere to the following sequence: (a) inspection, (b) palpation, (c) active and passive ROM, (d) manual muscle/strength testing, (e) neurologic examination, (f) vascular examination, and (g) special tests based on the differential diagnosis developed from the history.

To inspect the hip properly, it is recommended to disrobe the patient. Inspect the hip for evidence of any skin discoloration, abrasions, ecchymosis, open wounds, draining sinus tracts, swelling, fluid collection (hematoma or abscess), as well as any previous incisions. Asymmetry existing between hips should be noted. In addition, use the positions of the ASIS to determine if pelvic obliquity exists and then assess for leg length discrepancy.

Bony palpation surrounding the hip should flow systematically from anterior to posterior. The anterior structures that should be palpated include the ASIS, iliac crests, and pubic tubercles. Next, attention should be focused on the greater trochanters. The posterior edge of the greater trochanter is relatively uncovered and is easily palpable in a thin patient. This is the region that is typically painful in patients with trochanteric bursitis. Continuing posteriorly, the PSIS and the ischial tuberosities should be palpated. Patients with referred pain from the lumbosacral spine typically are diffusely tender across the PSIS and sacrum.

The hip ROM should be documented. Normal hip flexion and extension are 130 and 20 degrees, respectively, while internal and external rotation of the hip is 30 and 70 degrees, respectively. These maneuvers are best tested with the patient in the supine position. In the lateral decubitus position (patient on their side), hip abduction and adduction can be tested and typically demonstrate 40 and 30 degrees, respectively. Passive ROM of the hip should be correlated to pain; patients with osteonecrosis of the hip typically maintain hip ROM but have painful internal rotation. In addition, all hip ROM maneuvers must be done with stabilization of the pelvis to avoid artificially inflated degrees of motion.

The neurovascular examination begins with manual muscle testing. Muscle strength is graded on a scale from 0 to 5: 0 is complete absence of muscle function; 1 demonstrates muscle fasciculations without any limb movement; 2 represents the ability to fire the muscle and move the limb, but not against gravity; 3 allows firing of the muscle and movement of the limb, but against gravity only; 4 is firing of the muscle against some resistance—this grade is subdivided into a 4− and 4+ on the basis of the degree of resistance that the patient can counter; and 5 is full muscle function. In general, the lower extremity muscles must not be able to be manually overcome to be given a grade of 5.

A detailed neurologic examination of the entire lower extremity as well as provocative spine maneuvers should be documented. Function of the major named nerves (e.g., femoral, tibial, deep, and superficial peroneal) should be tested. In addition, sensation to light touch should be determined in the dermatomal distribution of the lower extremity. A detailed sensory neurologic examination is more important in diabetic patients who may suffer from diabetic neuropathy.

Every patient should also undergo a vascular examination that starts with palpation of the dorsalis pedis and posterior tibial arteries. In patients who do not have palpable pulses, a formal vascular consultation should be ordered to determine the vascular status of the involved lower extremity. Vascular compromise may impede wound healing or may result in a vascular crisis in the early postoperative period following an elective hip procedure.

While obtaining a detailed history and performing a basic physical examination, the surgeon should formulate a differential diagnosis. On the basis of this differential diagnosis, special tests are performed to recreate patient symptomatology and confirm a diagnosis prior to employing imaging modalities.

Patients suffering from long standing hip pain, especially pain secondary to OA, may present with a hip flexion contracture due to contracture of soft-tissue structures surrounding the hip joint. The anterior capsule, hip capsule, is most frequently involved, resulting in decreased hip extension. The Thomas test aids in diagnosing the presence of a hip flexion contracture. The patient is placed supine on the examining table while maximally flexing the contralateral hip and knee by bringing the knee in toward the chest. As the examiner, make sure to place your hands on the ASIS to ensure that the pelvis is stable and flat against the examining table. If there is a flexion contracture about the hip, the involved extremity will not rest flat on the table (Fig. 16.12). If the pelvis is not flat on the table, patients may be able to reposition their pelvis and increase the degree of lumbar lordosis to compensate and demonstrate full extension of the involved hip.

Patients with a tight iliotibial (IT) band may also complain of lateral hip pain. The Ober's test demonstrates the presence of a tight IT band. The patient is placed in the lateral decubitus position with the uninvolved hip down on the table. The uninvolved extremity is flexed at the knee and hip. If the IT band is tight, the patient will be unable to adduct the involved extremity to contact the opposite extremity. Recently, the diagnosis of femoroacetabular impingement has been popularized due to its association with early OA of the hip in patients without developmental hip dysplasia. It is hypothesized that an abnormal anatomic relationship between the femoral head and neck may lead to impingement between the proximal femur and the acetabulum, resulting in early degenerative changes of the hip joint. Patients suspected to have femoroacetabular impingement typically present with limited hip ROM and often have a positive impingement test, depending on the location of the impingement. The anteroinferior impingement test is done with the patient in a supine position. The extremity is internally rotated while being passively flexed to 90 degrees and adducted. Contact between the femoral neck and the acetabular rim typically results in pain, especially if there is a cartilage lesion. This maneuver is sensitive but not specific for femoroacetabular impingement. Most intra-articular hip pathologic conditions will also illicit pain with this maneuver.

Less commonly, patients may suffer from posteroinferior impingement. The patient is supine and placed at the edge of the examining table. With full hip extension, the hip is externally rotated. A test is termed positive if the patient experiences groin pain due to impingement of the femoral neck on the posteroinferior acetabular rim.

Radiographic Evaluation

Standard radiographs used to evaluate a patient with hip pain include a standing AP pelvis (Fig. 16.13), and a standing AP of the involved hip with the hip internally rotated 15 degrees. A frog leg lateral or shoot-through lateral of the involved hip should also be obtained. These views provide

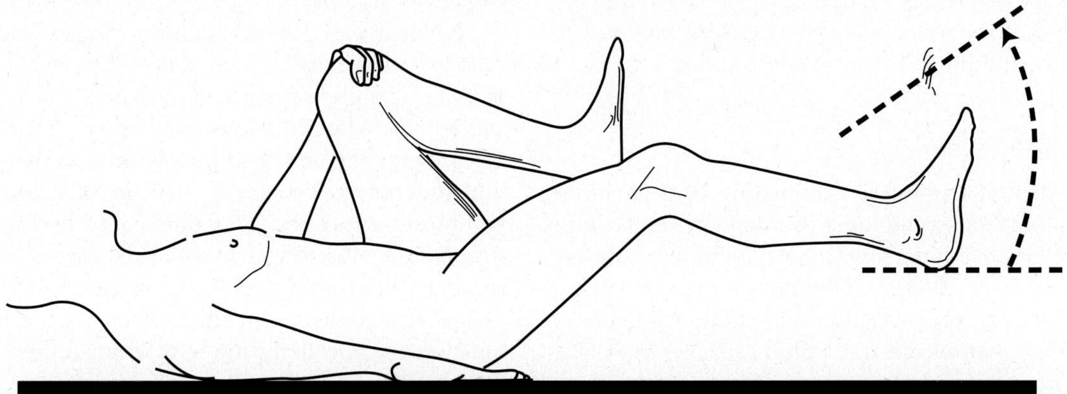

Figure 16.12 Thomas' test. After simultaneous flexion of both hips, each hip may be extended separately to record the arc from the horizontal to the femoral shaft. This indicated the degree of passive flexion contracture of the hip. (*Adapted from* Steinberg M. *The Hip and its Disorders.* Philadelphia, PA, WB Saunders, 1991.)

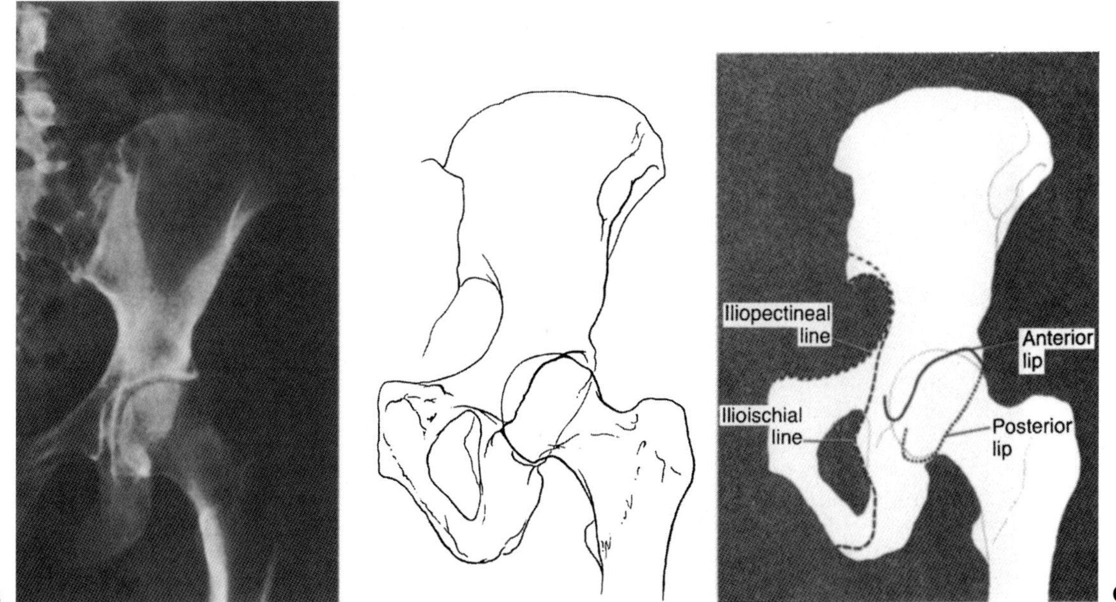

Figure 16.13 (**A**) AP radiograph of the left hemipelvis. (**B**) Diagram demonstrating the anatomic landmarks seen on the AP radiograph. (**C**) The major landmarks identified by various lines are as follows: diagonal dashes, the iliopectineal line (anterior column); straight dashes, the ilioischial line (posterior column); and solid line, the anterior lip of the acetabulum. The same identifying lines are used in Figures 16.14 and 16.15. (*Used with permission from* Tile M. *Fractures of the Pelvis and Acetabulum*. Baltimore, MD: Williams and Wilkins Co, 1984.)

information useful in defining disease and determining the location of a pathologic lesion.

Additional radiographic views can aid in trauma scenarios to define the extent of injury. The faux profile view is a weight-bearing, oblique AP radiograph with the patient's body rotated 60 degrees and the affected hip closest to the x-ray plate. This provides a weight-bearing lateral view and allows for assessment of anterior coverage and measurement of the anterior center-edge angle. Judet views are 45-degree angled hemipelvis radiographs that demonstrate injury to the pelvic ring. An obturator oblique view is obtained by tilting the involved hemipelvis 45 degrees upwards and making the obturator foramen perpendicular to the x-ray beam. This view highlights the anterior column of the pelvis and the posterior wall of the acetabulum (Figs. 16.14 and 16.15). The obturator oblique view on the involved side also renders an iliac oblique view of the opposite hemipelvis (tilting the uninvolved hemipelvis 45 degrees downwards). The iliac oblique view depicts the posterior column of the pelvis and the anterior wall of the acetabulum.

Additional inlet and outlet views of pelvis can be obtained, which provide information about sacral injuries and resulting translation of the hemipelvis. The inlet view is taken as an AP pelvis with the x-ray beam angled 45 degrees caudad and is beneficial for determining anterior and posterior translation of the hemipelvis. An outlet view is taken as an AP pelvis with the x-ray beam angled 45 degrees cephalad and is beneficial for determining superior and inferior translation of the hemipelvis. The outlet view renders a true AP view of the sacrum and allows the sacral foramina to be seen enface. (See detailed discussion of radiography and pelvic fractures in Chapter 10.)

In general, when enhanced bony detail of the pelvis and proximal femur is required, a CT scan is the imaging modality of choice. CT of the abdomen and pelvis typically extends down to the level of the lesser trochanters and when done with fine cuts (1 mm sections), provides great detail of the hip joint. CT scans are often used in the setting of acute trauma since most patients who sustain blunt abdominal injuries will have a CT of the abdomen and pelvis as part of their overall trauma evaluation. Images are obtained in the axial plane but can be reformatted to include reconstructed coronal and sagittal images or three-dimensional images. In the treatment of pelvic fractures, CT scan imaging can be very useful in fully understanding the fracture pattern and developing a sound preoperative plan.

In the outpatient setting, CT scans are a powerful adjunct to plain radiographs when diagnosing subtle subchondral collapse in patients with osteonecrosis of the hip, determining the degree of bony destruction by tumors about the hip, and evaluating an arthritic hip with minimal x-ray changes. In patients who have undergone total hip replacement and suffer from instability, CT scans can help determine the version of the acetabular component. CT often augments information derived from the radiographic evaluation and in certain circumstances can be invaluable in determining a treatment plan.

MRI in general is utilized for enhanced detail regarding the soft-tissue anatomy surrounding the hip joint,

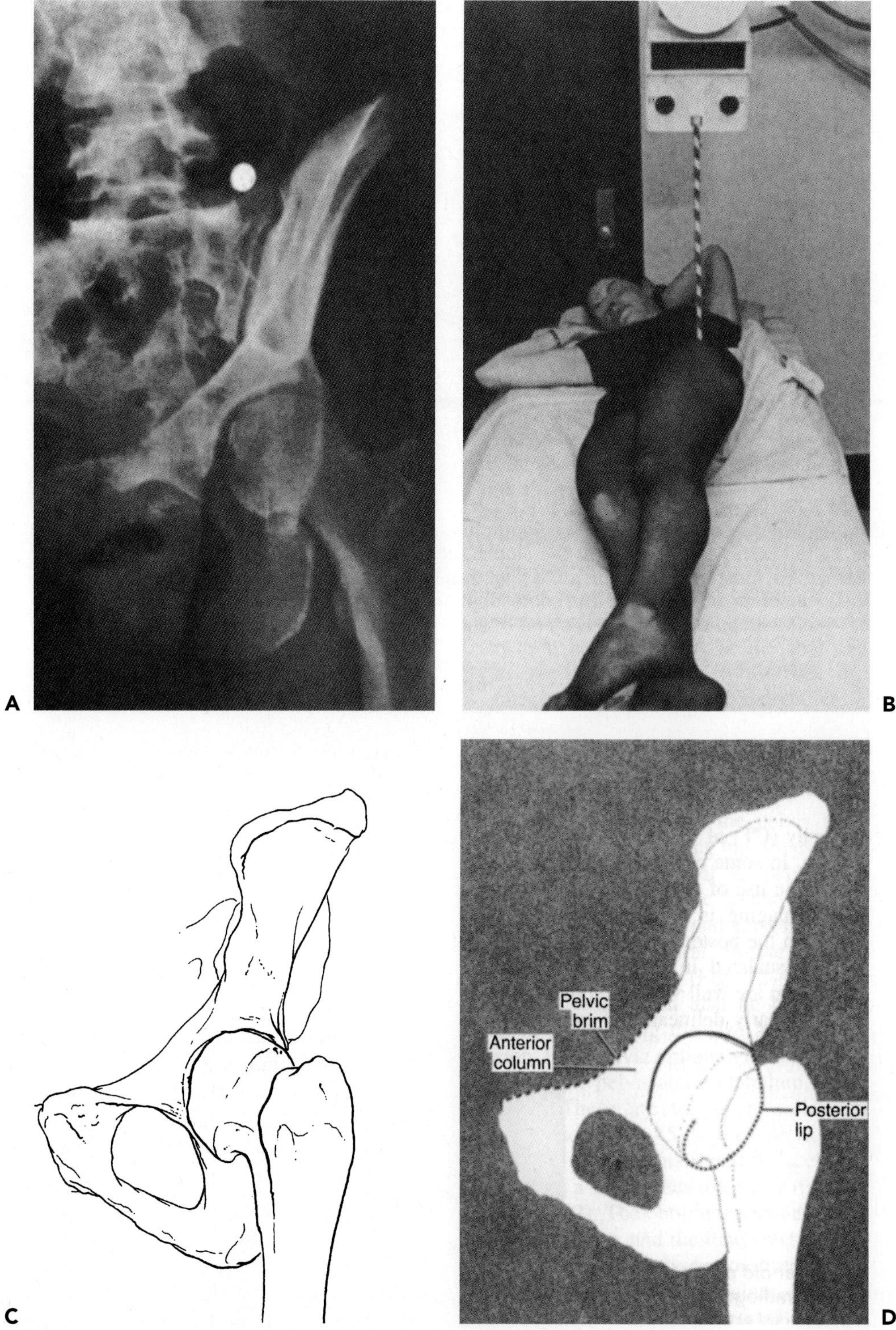

Figure 16.14 (**A**) Obturator oblique radiographic view of the left hemipelvis. (**B**) This view is taken by elevating the affected hip 45 degrees to the horizontal by means of a wedge and directing the beam through the hip joint with a 15-degree upward tilt. (**C**) Diagram demonstrating the anatomy of the pelvis on the obturators oblique view. (**D**) Diagram demonstrating the important anatomic landmarks by various lines (described in Fig. 16.13). In this view, note particularly the pelvic brim, indicating the border of the anterior column and the posterior lip of the acetabulum. (*Used with permission from* Tile M. *Fractures of the Pelvis and Acetabulum*. Baltimore, MD: Williams and Wilkins Co, 1984.)

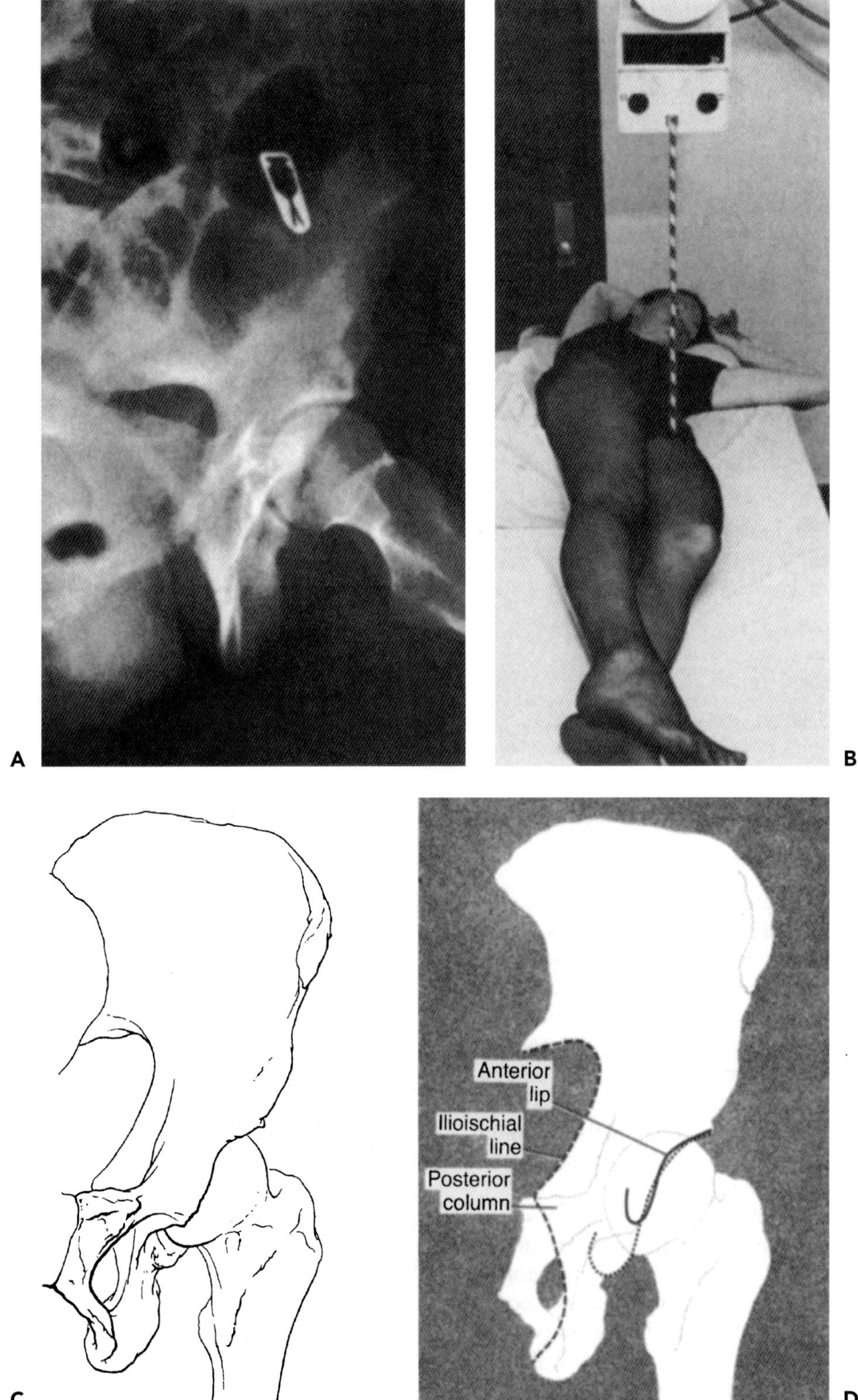

Figure 16.15 (**A**) Iliac oblique radiographic view of the left hemipelvis. This view is taken placing the patient in 45 degrees of external rotation by elevating the uninjured side on a wedge, as shown in (**B**). (**C**) Diagram demonstrating the anatomic landmarks of the left hemipelvis on the iliac oblique view, further clarified in (**D**) by the various lines described in Figure 16.13. This best demonstrated the posterior column of the acetabulum. (*Used with permission from* Tile M. *Fractures of the Pelvis and Acetabulum.* Baltimore, MD: Williams and Wilkins Co, 1984.)

especially the labrum. Often, an MRI arthrogram will be done to diagnose a labral tear. For this study, dye is injected into the hip prior to obtaining the MRI to distend the joint revealing soft-tissue structures that are normally apposed. MRI is also utilized for demonstrating the early stages of osteonecrosis of the hip where plain radiographs may not show any abnormalities. Rarely, MRI is indicated as an adjunct to plain radiographs in determining the etiology of hip pain that is unclear following radiographic evaluation.

Other modalities, such as bone scans and positron emission tomography, are helpful in determining the presence of metastatic lesions about the pelvis and proximal femur as well as osteonecrosis and osteomyelitis. In patients who are likely to have an infectious etiology as the source of their hip pain, hip aspiration under sterile conditions may be indicated. The fluid should be sent for gram stain, culture, and sensitivity. A single aspiration is approximately 50% accurate in identifying a microorganism. A second aspiration increases the accuracy to 80% in determining a bacterial source of infection.

TABLE 16.1
CLASSIFICATION SCHEMES FOR POSTERIOR HIP DISLOCATIONS

Thompson and Epstein

Type I	Dislocation with or without minor fracture
Type II	Dislocation with single large fracture of the posterior rim of the acetabulum
Type III	Dislocation with comminuted fracture of the rim, with or without a large major fragment
Type IV	Dislocation with fracture of the acetabular floor
Type V	Dislocation with fracture of the femoral head

Stewart and Milford

Type I	Simple dislocation without fracture
Type II	Dislocation with one or more rim fragments but with sufficient socket to ensure stability after reduction
Type III	Dislocation with fracture of the rim producing gross instability
Type IV	Dislocation with fracture of the head or neck of the femur

TRAUMATIC INJURIES TO THE HIP AND FEMUR

Hip Dislocations

The hip is a ball and socket joint with inherent bony stability that requires a tremendous amount force for dislocation. Thus, hip dislocations are typically the result of high-energy trauma with associated fractures and injuries being commonplace. Given the high-energy nature of these injuries, unsatisfactory outcomes may be anticipated in up to half of the patients. Factors such as damage to articular cartilage, nerves, and the vascular supply to the femoral head at the time of injury are beyond the control of the surgeon and contribute to the development of complications such as post-traumatic arthritis, neurologic deficit, and avascular necrosis (AVN). However, timely reduction along with appropriate treatment of associated femoral head and acetabular fractures often improves outcomes.

Classification

Hip dislocations are initially classified as anterior or posterior according to the relationship of the femoral head to the acetabulum. Thompson and Epstein first proposed a classification system for both anterior and posterior dislocations and incorporated associated fractures of the femoral head and acetabulum (Table 16.1). Stewart and Milford proposed a similar classification scheme that included postreduction stability. Both of these classifications have been commonly employed over the years and have been shown to predict outcome.

More recently, Levin introduced a comprehensive classification system that is useful for both anterior and posterior hip dislocations (Table 16.2). This classification system attempts to guide treatment on the basis of the pre- and postreduction physical findings, associated fractures, and diagnostic information gained from radiographs as well as CT scan.

Mechanism of Injury

The vast majority of hip dislocations are posterior and occur secondary to high-energy mechanisms such as motor vehicle accidents. They are due to a posteriorly directed force on a flexed knee. These injuries are commonly referred to as "dashboard" injuries. Other common mechanisms include falls, pedestrians struck by automobiles, and sports injuries.

The position of the hip, the direction of the force vector, and the patient's anatomy will determine the direction

TABLE 16.2
LEVIN'S CLASSIFICATION OF POSTERIOR AND ANTERIOR HIP DISLOCATIONS

Type I	No significant associated fractures; no clinical instability after concentric reduction
Type II	Irreducible dislocation without significant femoral head or acetabular fractures (reduction must be attempted under general anesthesia)
Type III	Unstable hip after reduction or incarcerated fragments of cartilage, labrum, or bone
Type IV	Associated acetabular fracture requiring reconstruction to restore hip stability or joint congruity
Type V	Associated femoral head or femoral neck injury (fractures or impactions)

Reprinted with permission from Browner BD, Levine AM, Jupiter JB, et al. *Skeletal Trauma: Expert Consult.* 4th ed. Saunders, 2008.

of the dislocation and whether an associated fracture occurs. More than 85% of hip dislocations are posterior. It has been shown that increasing degrees of adduction and flexion at the time of impact make pure dislocation more likely. Conversely, less hip adduction and flexion typically leads to fractures of the posterior wall of the acetabulum or shear fractures of the femoral head. Additionally, increased femoral anteversion has been shown to decrease the risk of posterior wall acetabular fracture in posterior dislocations.

Anterior dislocations occur much less frequently than posterior dislocations. The hip must be in a position of abduction and external rotation at the time of impact, as is often the case in motorcycle accidents, for an anterior dislocation to occur. The degree of flexion of the hip determines if the femoral head comes to rest in a suprapubic or obturator location. However, this anatomic distinction does not affect treatment or outcome. Associated femoral head fractures occur more commonly in anterior dislocations and typically are impaction-type fractures.

Presentation

Patients with hip dislocations typically present with severe pain and are unable to bear weight or move the affected hip. They may also complain of numbness in the sciatic or femoral nerve distributions. Often patients will have multiple injuries at presentation and may be obtunded or unconscious.

Physical Examination

Initially, the physical examination should be directed by the guidelines of the Advanced Trauma and Life Support System. Following a thorough trauma evaluation, examination of the patient should begin with observation of the position of the limb. Posterior hip dislocations cause the limb to be fixed in flexion, adduction, and internal rotation. On the contrary, marked abduction and external rotation are evidence of an anterior dislocation. However, associated fractures of the femoral neck or shaft will obscure these findings. Because of the typical dashboard mechanism causing most hip dislocations, associated injuries should be anticipated. Inspection and palpation must include the spine, pelvis, and the entire injured extremity. Close attention should be given to examination of the knee as knee injuries, such as patella fractures, ligamentous injuries, and dislocations, are especially common (Table 16.3).

Following careful inspection of the injured extremity, a detailed neurovascular examination should ensue. Sciatic nerve injury occurs in up to 20% of posterior dislocations, and it is important to make the diagnosis prior to reduction. Pulses should be palpated and compared with the contralateral extremity. Rarely, an anterior dislocation may lead to femoral vessel compromise, while posterior dislocations may have associated occult knee dislocations with injury to the popliteal artery. The neurovascular examination should be repeated immediately after reduction of the hip as the sciatic nerve can become incarcerated.

TABLE 16.3
ORTHOPEDIC INJURIES COMMONLY ASSOCIATED WITH HIP DISLOCATION

Pelvic ring injury
Acetabular fractures
Femoral head fractures
Femoral neck fractures
Femoral shaft fractures
Patella fractures
Ligamentous knee injuries
Knee dislocation
Foot and ankle fractures
Spine injuries
Sciatic and femoral nerve damage

Radiographic Examination

Radiographic evaluation begins with careful and systematic inspection of the AP pelvis radiograph. In a posterior dislocation, the affected femoral head will appear smaller than the unaffected hip, and there will be loss of congruence between the femoral head and acetabulum (Fig. 16.16). With anterior dislocations, the femoral head will appear larger than the contralateral femoral head. Rotation can be assessed through inspection of the relative positions of the lesser trochanters. It is very important to clearly visualize the femoral neck for evidence of fracture prior to attempted reduction. Femoral head fractures, pelvic ring injuries, and acetabular fractures should also be noted.

Following reduction, the five standard views of the pelvis (AP, inlet, outlet, obturator oblique, and iliac oblique) and a CT scan should be obtained. These studies

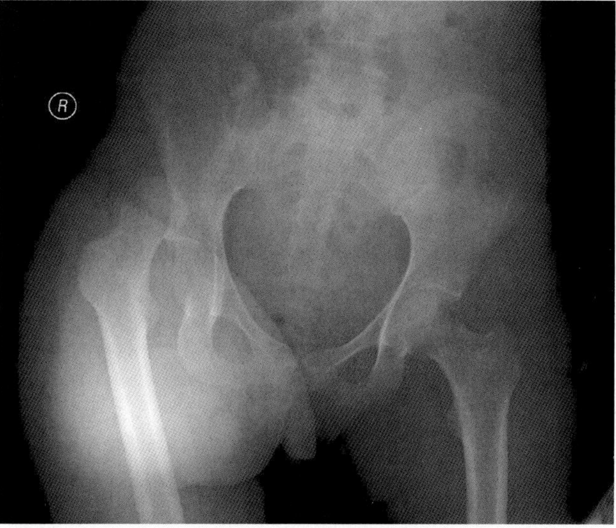

Figure 16.16 Anteroposterior radiograph of the pelvis depicting a right hip dislocation. Shenton's line on the right is disrupted, and there is a small posterior wall acetabulum fracture. Note that the right femoral head appears smaller than the left.

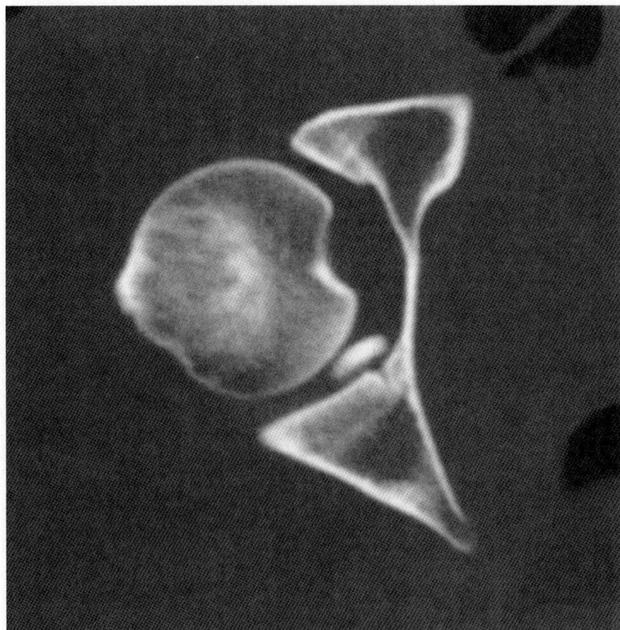

Figure 16.17 Computed tomography scan demonstrating a fragment of bone interposed between the femoral head and posterior articular surface that requires removal (*Reprinted with permission from* Bucholz RW, Heckman JD, Court-Brown CM, et al. *Rockwood and Green's Fractures in Adults.* 6th ed. Philadelphia, PA: Lippincott Williams & Wilkins, 2006.)

should be carefully scrutinized as to the congruency of the femoral head within the acetabulum and to identify associated fractures and loose bodies (Fig. 16.17). If the hip is unable to be reduced, a CT scan and Judet views should be emergently obtained prior to open reduction.

Special Tests

Bone scan or MRI may reveal vascular changes associated with AVN of the femoral head prior to evidence on plain radiographs. Additionally, MRI may be useful in the diagnosis of a labral tear. However, these studies have no current role in the acute management of hip dislocations.

Differential Diagnosis

The differential diagnosis is limited and includes fractures of the pelvis, acetabulum, and proximal femur.

Treatment

Hip dislocation constitutes an orthopedic emergency. The goal of initial treatment is to achieve reduction of the femoral head within in 6 hours of the injury. AVN of the femoral head has been reported to occur in up to 40% of dislocations; however, significantly lower rates of AVN occur for hips reduced within 6 hours of dislocation. Additionally, prompt reduction relieves pressure on the sciatic nerve.

In the absence of a concurrent fracture of the femur neck, closed reduction with conscious sedation or general anesthesia should be attempted. Closed reduction of a posterior dislocation is most often achieved with the Allis method (Fig. 16.18). With the patient supine, this method applies in-line traction to the femur while slowly flexing, adducting, and internally rotating the hip. An assistant applies downward pressure to the ASIS to stabilize the pelvis. Anterior dislocations may be reduced with the traction-countertraction method with lateral pressure applied to the medial thigh (Fig. 16.19). An audible and palpable clunk is often evident when the hip reduces.

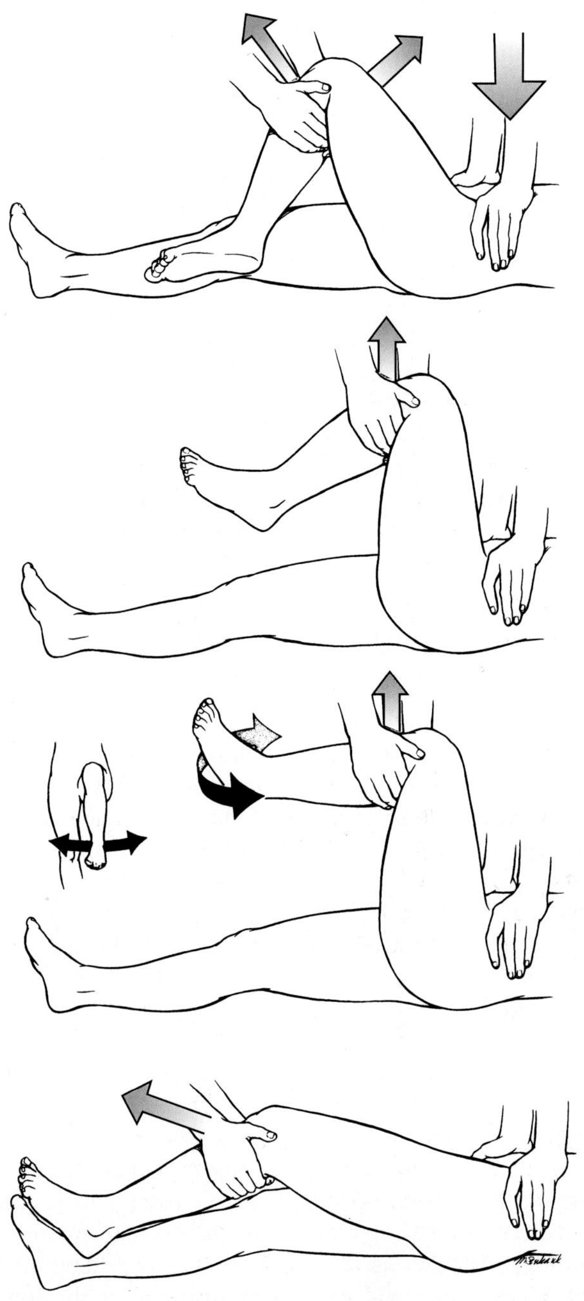

Figure 16.18 The Allis reduction technique for posterior hip dislocations. (*Reprinted with permission from* Bucholz RW, Heckman JD, Court-Brown CM, et al. *Rockwood and Green's Fractures in Adults.* 6th ed. Philadelphia, PA: Lippincott Williams & Wilkins, 2006.)

After reduction, it is important to assess the stability of the hip by taking the hip through a full ROM. In the absence

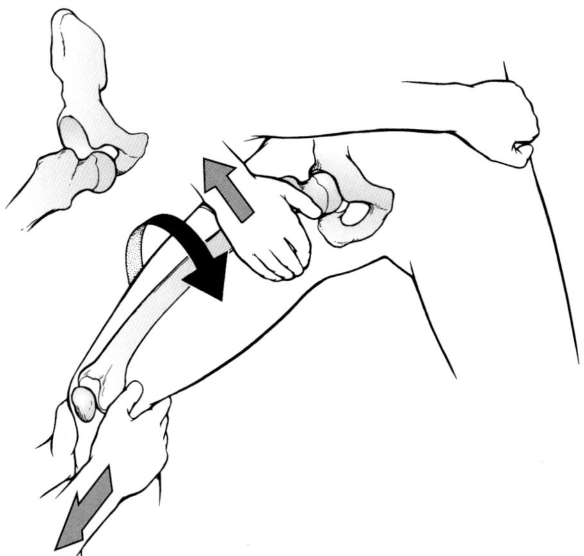

Figure 16.19 Reduction of an anterior dislocation with traction–countertraction and lateral pressure applied to the medial thigh. (*Reprinted with permission from* Bucholz RW, Heckman JD, Court-Brown CM, et al. *Rockwood and Green's Fractures in Adults.* 6th ed. Philadelphia, PA: Lippincott Williams & Wilkins, 2006.)

of an acetabular or femoral head fracture, the hip should be quite stable. As mentioned previously, the neurovascular examination should be repeated and a CT scan obtained to assess the congruency of reduction and identify associated fractures and loose bodies within the hip joint.

Open reduction is emergently indicated for irreducible hips and sciatic nerve injuries caused by closed reduction. An irreducible hip may be due to soft-tissue entrapment or blockage by a bony fragment. If excessive delay is not anticipated, Judet views and a CT scan should be obtained prior to open reduction in an effort to identify possible obstructions to reduction.

Once reduction of the femoral head is achieved, associated fractures of the acetabulum or femoral head, as well as incongruent reductions and loose bodies, may be addressed in a nonemergent fashion. However, for hips that continue to be unstable after reduction or contain intra-articular fragments, skeletal traction should be employed to decompress the acetabulum as the patient awaits joint debridement or definitive treatment of an acetabular or femoral head fracture.

Postreduction management of a patient suffering a pure hip dislocation who underwent reduction within 6 hours of dislocation should begin with partial weight-bearing. Full weight-bearing typically becomes tolerable within 2 to 4 weeks. For a hip that was reduced more than 6 hours after dislocation, 8 to 12 weeks of protected weight-bearing may be considered due to the significantly higher rate of AVN of the femoral head and potential for collapse. When there is dislocation with an associated fracture, the postreduction or postoperative regimen is variable and is determined by the associated fracture. Regardless of the time to reduction, early hip motion should be encouraged to minimize stiffness and adhesions. However, extremes in ROM should be avoided until the joint capsule has fully healed.

TABLE 16.4
COMPLICATIONS OF HIP DISLOCATION

Posttraumatic arthritis
Avascular necrosis of the femoral head
Sciatic nerve injury
Heterotopic ossification
Recurrent dislocation (rare)
Femoral nerve injury (rare)

Complications

The long-term outcome of a hip dislocation is variable and is often dependent on the complications encountered (Table 16.4). Posttraumatic arthritis is the most common complication, occurring in up to 70% of cases. Its development is likely multifactorial and may be related to cartilage damage at the time of injury, third body wear, or malreduction of associated fractures.

AVN of the femoral head is a dreaded complication whose incidence is diminished with emergent reduction. However, it may still occur in up to 10% of patients despite reduction within 6 hours of the injury. Its development is believed to be primarily related to ischemia induced by kinking and spasm of the ascending cervical and circumflex femoral vessels. Thus, reduction is thought to relieve vasospasm allowing for resumption of perfusion to the femoral head.

Sciatic nerve injury may complicate up to 20% of posterior dislocations and can lead to severe functional deficits. The injury is typically incomplete with the peroneal division of the nerve most commonly affected. Recovery of nerve function is often unpredictable and may be evaluated at 3 months with an electromyogram (EMG).

Heterotopic ossification is not uncommon after open reduction of a posterior hip dislocation and is more commonly associated with an anterior approach. Prophylaxis with indomethacin or radiation may reduce the development of clinically significant heterotopic ossification.

Femoral Head Fractures

Femoral head fractures are relatively rare injuries that are typically due to severe trauma to the hip joint. In fact, nearly all femoral head fractures are associated with a hip dislocation. The high-energy nature, as well as the frequency of associated injuries and complications, has historically led to relatively poor functional outcomes. More recently, improved surgical techniques and understanding of the relevant anatomy have improved our ability to treat these injuries.

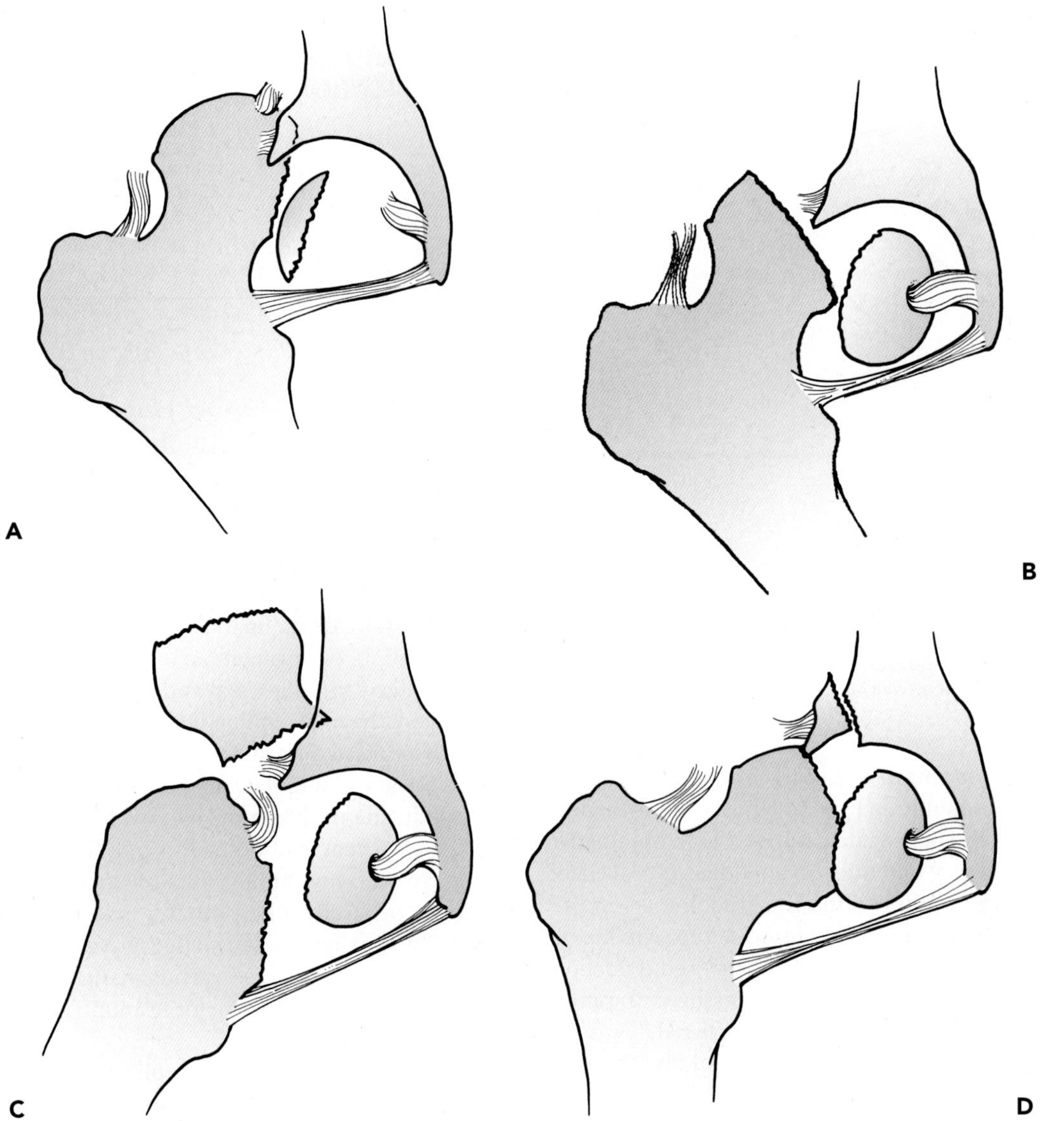

Figure 16.20 The Pipkin's classification of femoral head fractures. (**A**) Type I—fracture inferior to the fovea. (**B**) Type II—fracture superior to the fovea. (**C**) Type III—femoral head fracture with associated fracture of the femoral neck. (**D**) Type IV—femoral head fracture with associated fracture of the acetabular rim. (*Reprinted with permission from* Bucholz RW, Heckman JD, Court-Brown CM, et al. *Rockwood and Green's Fractures in Adults.* 6th ed. Philadelphia, PA: Lippincott Williams & Wilkins, 2006.)

Classification

The most commonly utilized classification scheme is proposed by Pipkin (Fig. 16.20). This relatively simple classification system is useful for communication and correlates with prognosis. Type I and Type II fractures are distinguished by the location of the fracture line in relation to the fovea. In Type I fractures, the fracture line is inferior to the fovea, while in Type II fractures, the fracture extends superior to the fovea into the weight-bearing portion of the femoral head. This important distinction often directs treatment and correlates with outcome as Type I fractures typically perform better than Type II fractures. As one might expect, femoral head fractures with an associated fracture of the femoral neck (Type III fracture) have the worst prognosis overall.

Brumbeck et al. and The Orthopaedic Trauma Association have each proposed more comprehensive classification systems that apply to both anterior and posterior dislocations. These classification systems also have prognostic value but have not gained widespread use in clinical practice.

Mechanism of Injury

As stated previously, nearly all femoral head fractures are due to traumatic hip dislocations. As such, femoral head fractures are typically secondary to high-energy mechanisms such as motor vehicle accidents, pedestrians struck by automobiles, falls, and sports injuries.

The direction of hip dislocation and the position of the hip at the time of impact determine the presence and type of facture. Classically, femoral head fractures are caused by posterior hip dislocations. However, only approximately 15% of posterior dislocations have an associated fracture of the femoral head. Nevertheless, when these fractures occur, typically a portion of the head is sheared off by the acetabular rim as the head dislocates. This may leave a portion of the head within the acetabulum and block closed reduction attempts. In contrast, anterior dislocations commonly result in indentation-type fractures as the femoral head is levered out of the acetabulum.

Presentation

Patients with femoral head fractures usually have an accompanying hip dislocation. They will present with severe pain with inability to move the affected hip or bear weight. They may also complain of numbness in the sciatic or femoral nerve distributions. Often patients will have multiple injuries at presentation and may be obtunded or unconscious.

Physical Examination

The physical examination should initially be directed by the guidelines of the Advanced Trauma and Life Support System. Following a thorough trauma evaluation, examination of the injured extremity should begin with observation of the position of the limb as this will give clues to the direction of the hip dislocation and the potential type of femoral head fracture present. Posterior hip dislocations cause the limb to be fixed in flexion, adduction, and internal rotation. On the contrary, marked abduction and external rotation are evidence of an anterior dislocation. However, with a femoral head fracture or associated fracture of the femur or acetabulum, these signs may not be present. Inspection and palpation should include the entire extremity with emphasis on examination of the knee as these injuries are common with posterior hip dislocations. Additionally, a careful neurovascular examination should be performed and repeated after hip reduction.

Radiographic Examination

Evaluation begins with careful and systematic review of the AP pelvis radiograph (Fig. 16.21A). Dislocation is typically apparent with disruption of Shenton's line and incongruency between the femoral head and acetabulum. Often the fractured portion of the femoral head will remain in the acetabulum, held there by an intact ligamentum teres. Further inspection may reveal associated fractures of the acetabulum and femoral neck.

Following closed reduction or in the event of an irreducible dislocation, the five standard views of the pelvis (AP, inlet, outlet, obturator oblique, and iliac oblique) and a CT scan should be obtained. These studies will allow for the assessment of the congruency of reduction as well as identify intra-articular loose bodies and associated fractures (Fig. 16.21B). Additionally, the CT scan will accurately localize the fracture plane in the femoral head, which is useful in planning the surgical approach.

Special Tests

Bone scan or MRI may reveal vascular changes associated with AVN of the femoral head prior to evidence on plain

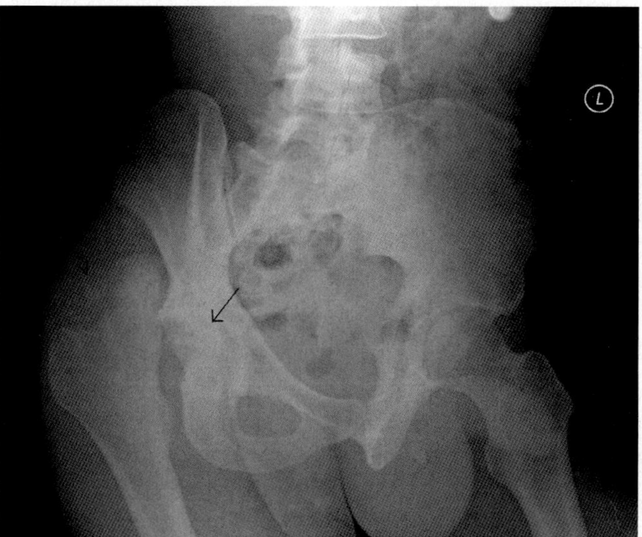

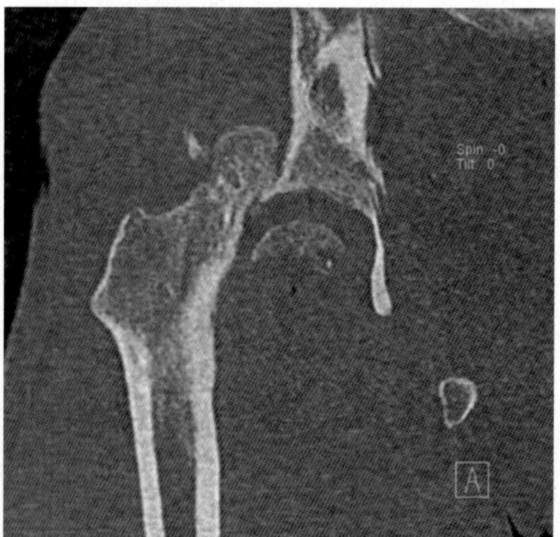

Figure 16.21 (**A**) Anteroposterior radiograph of the pelvis depicting a posterior hip dislocation with femoral head fracture. Note the portion of the femoral head remaining within the acetabulum (*arrow*) and the fracture of the posterior wall of the acetabulum (*arrow head*). (**B**) Coronal CT reconstruction in the same patient.

radiographs but have no current role in the acute management of femoral head fractures.

Differential Diagnosis

The differential diagnosis is limited and includes fractures of the pelvis, acetabulum, and proximal femur.

Treatment

Hip dislocation with femoral head fracture is an orthopedic emergency. The goal of initial treatment is to achieve reduction of the femoral head within 6 hours of the injury as this has been shown to decrease the rate of AVN.

Occasionally, a hip dislocation with femoral head fracture is irreducible. Often this is due to the blockage by femoral head fracture fragments. In this case, emergent open reduction is indicated. If a substantial delay is not anticipated, a CT scan should be obtained prior to open reduction to accurately identify the fracture fragments and aid in operative planning.

Once reduction of the femoral head is achieved, definitive management of the femoral head fracture depends on a number of variables including the stability of the hip reduction, size of the fragment, location of the fracture in relationship to the weight-bearing surface, and the quality of fracture reduction. Nonsurgical management should be considered for dislocations in which a congruent and stable reduction is achieved with associated fractures that have less than 2 mm of step off or do not involve the weight-bearing portion of the femoral head.

Surgical treatment is indicated for femoral head fractures in which the hip remains unstable or incongruent, intra-articular loose bodies are entrapped in the joint or fracture reduction that is nonanatomic. Simple excision is appropriate for loose bodies or fracture fragments that are comminuted or do not involve the weight-bearing portion of the femoral head. Large fracture fragments, especially those that involve the superior weight-bearing dome of the femoral head, should undergo open reduction with stable internal fixation.

For fractures managed nonoperatively or with open reduction and internal fixation, weight-bearing is typically protected for 8 weeks to ensure fracture healing. For those fractures in which fragments are simply excised, full weight-bearing may begin when tolerated. Regardless of treatment, early hip motion should be encouraged to minimize stiffness and adhesions. However, extremes in ROM should be avoided until the joint capsule has fully healed.

Outcomes and Complications

Historically, femoral head fractures have resulted in relatively poor functional outcomes. Modern surgical techniques and emergent hip reduction have led to somewhat improved results. However, as with hip dislocations, the overall outcome from a femoral head fracture is often dependent on the complications encountered such as post-traumatic arthritis, AVN of the femoral head, sciatic nerve injury, heterotopic ossification, and the treatment of associated fractures.

Femoral Neck Fractures

Femoral neck fractures are intracapsular fractures occurring between the articular surface of the femoral head and the intertrochanteric region of the proximal femur. These fractures occur in two distinct populations. In the elderly, these are common injuries typically due to low-energy falls and have associated 1-year mortality rates of 14% to 50%. Additionally, in elderly patients, it has been reported that only about half of the patients will regain their prefracture functional status. Much less commonly, these fractures occur in young patients and are generally secondary to high-energy trauma. In either case, a fracture of the femoral neck can be a devastating injury with an impact that reaches far beyond the fracture itself.

Classification

Femoral neck fractures are often classified according to the anatomic location of the fracture line. This includes basicervical fractures occurring at the base of the neck, transcervical fractures through the mid-portion of the neck, and subcapital fractures at the base of the head. However, it is often difficult to precisely define the exact location of the fracture line with plain radiography, and thus, this classification method has limited utility.

The most commonly used classification scheme is that proposed by Garden (Fig. 16.22). This classification system is based on the degree of displacement observed on plain radiographs. Garden I fractures are incomplete or impacted. Garden II fractures are complete fractures without displacement. Garden III fractures are complete fractures with partial displacement, while Garden IV fractures are completely displaced. However, distinction between Garden I and II or between Garden III and IV does not affect treatment. Thus, there has been a trend toward simply classifying these fractures as nondisplaced or displaced since this improves both interobserver and intraobserver reliability and has greater relevance to treatment and prognosis.

Femoral neck fractures have also been classified by Pauwel according to the angle at which the fracture line makes with the horizontal (Fig. 16.23). Type I fractures are 30 degrees from the horizontal; Type II, 50 degrees from the horizontal; and Type III, 70 degrees from the horizontal. This classification was based on the hypothesis that vertically oriented fracture lines are more unstable and lead to greater complications. However, further research has demonstrated that it is often difficult to accurately measure the angle of the fracture on prereduction radiographs and that the fracture angle does not correlate with nonunion or AVN. Thus, this classification is not commonly used today.

Additionally, the Orthopaedic Trauma Association has proposed a comprehensive classification system. This

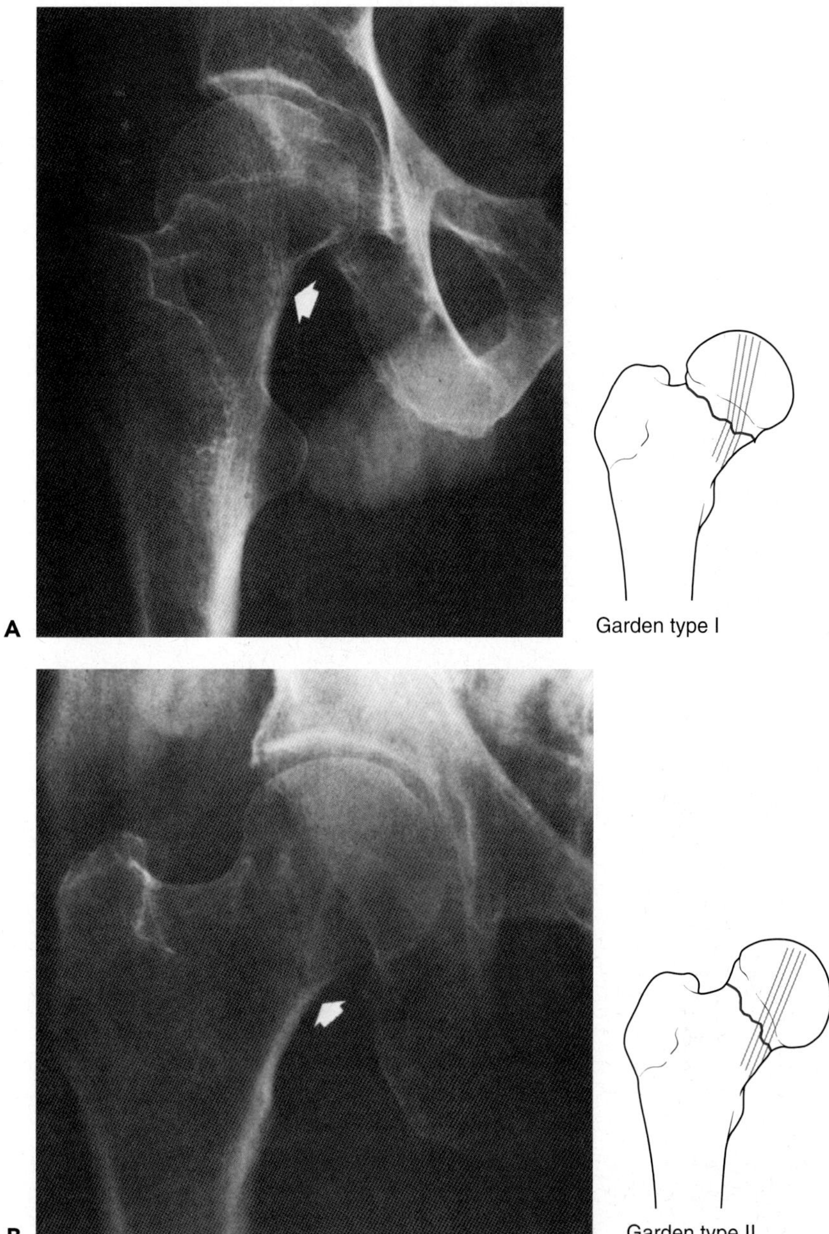

Figure 16.22 The Garden classification of femoral neck fractures. (*Reprinted with permission from* Bucholz RW, Heckman JD, Court-Brown CM, et al. *Rockwood and Green's Fractures in Adults.* 6th ed. Philadelphia, PA: Lippincott Williams & Wilkins, 2006.)

classification scheme is based on fracture location and displacement and is most useful for research purposes.

Mechanism of Injury

In the elderly, a fracture of the femoral neck is almost always an insufficiency fracture through osteoporotic bone. The mechanism may be a low-energy fall directly onto the greater trochanter causing in impaction fracture or an external rotation force that causes the femoral neck to lever and buckle off of the posterior acetabulum, leading to comminution of the posterior neck.

In younger patients, high-energy trauma, such as a motor vehicle accident or a fall from a height, is usually required to generate a fracture of the femoral neck. Typically, the mechanism is an axial force along the femoral shaft that may include a rotational component. This mechanism causes high Pauwel angle shear-type fractures and contributes to the association between fractures of the femoral shaft and concurrent fracture of the femoral neck in young patients.

Presentation

The clinical presentation of a patient with a femoral neck fracture can vary widely. Patients generally present with groin pain and an inability to bear weight; however, stress fractures and nondisplaced fractures may present with no obvious clinical deformity and only slight groin pain. Typically, there is noticeable shortening and external rotation of the involved extremity. Elderly patients who live alone may be discovered hours to days after a fall and present with

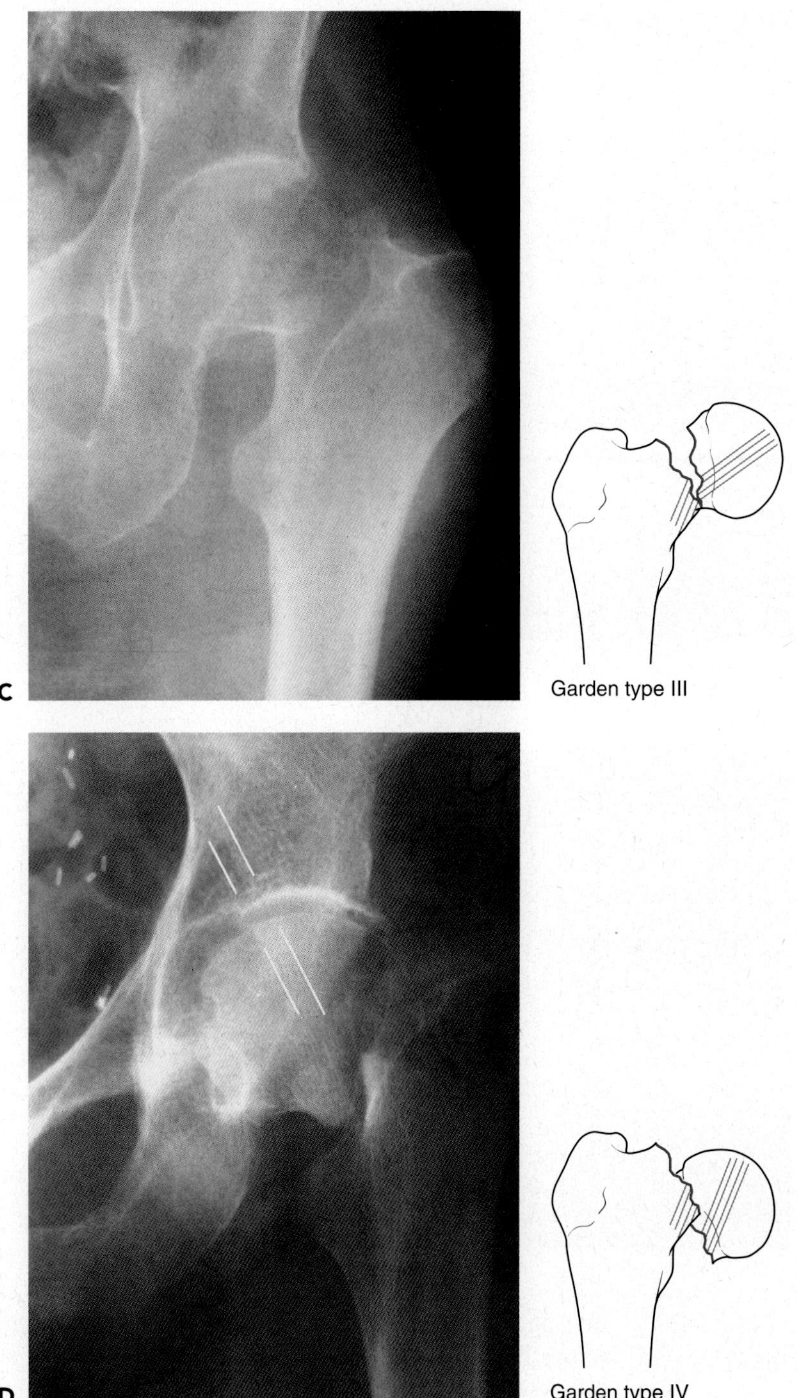

Figure 16.22 *(continued)*

dehydration, decubitus ulcers, or confusion. With elderly patients, it is important to inquire about the patient's prior functional level and the circumstances that lead to the fall. In younger patients, because of the high-energy nature of these injuries, there may be associated injuries as well as signs and symptoms of shock.

Physical Examination

For high-energy mechanisms and obtunded elderly patients, the initial examination should be directed by the guidelines of the Advanced Trauma and Life Support System. Following a thorough trauma evaluation, examination of the injured extremity should begin with close inspection of the skin for signs of an open fracture. Shortening and external rotation of the affected leg should be noted. ROM of the hip should be avoided as it may lead to further fracture displacement. In high-energy mechanisms, a detailed examination of the entire injured extremity is important with special attention to the examination of the knee. Elderly patients should be evaluated for concomitant fragility

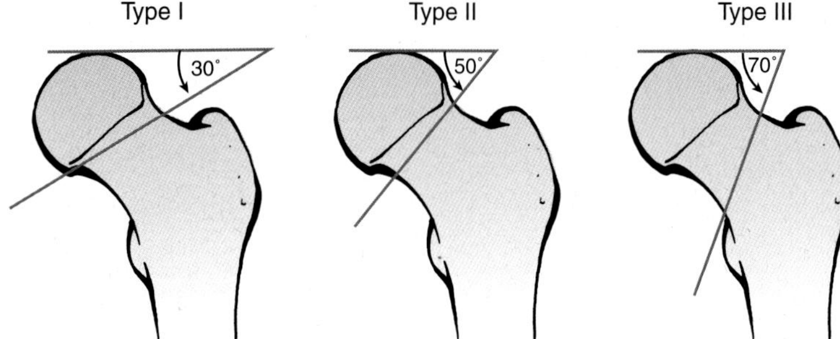

Figure 16.23 The Pauwels' classification of femoral neck fractures. (*Reprinted with permission from* Bucholz RW, Heckman JD, Court-Brown CM, et al. *Rockwood and Green's Fractures in Adults.* 6th ed. Philadelphia, PA: Lippincott Williams & Wilkins, 2006.)

fractures such as distal radius and proximal humerus fractures. While nerve or vessel injury is uncommon, a careful neurovascular examination should be performed in all patients.

Radiographic Examination

Radiographic evaluation begins with careful scrutiny of the AP pelvis radiograph as well as the AP and cross-table lateral views of the affected hip. An AP view of the hip in 10 to 15 degrees of internal rotation is often helpful as it offsets the femoral anteversion and provides a true AP of the femoral neck. Fracture displacement, the degree of osteoporosis, and presence of posterior comminution should be noted as these factors will affect the treatment.

Reduction can be assessed radiographically via two methods. Lowell described the radiographic appearance of the femoral head–neck junction (Fig. 16.24). Anatomic alignment should reveal the convex femoral head meeting the concave femoral neck, thus forming an S-curve on both of the visualized cortices. Malreduction will cause a C-shaped curve on one cortex and a sharp apex on the other.

A second method of assessing reduction is through the Garden Alignment Index (Fig. 16.25). This method measures the angle formed between the bony trabeculae of the femoral neck and the femoral head fragment on both the AP and lateral radiographs. In the AP plane, the normal alignment is 160 degrees. On the lateral radiograph, normally the trabeculae form a straight line (180 degrees). A Garden Alignment Index of 155 to 180 degrees on both AP and lateral radiographs indicates an acceptable reduction.

Special Tests

MRI and bone scan are helpful in diagnosing stress fractures or occult nondisplaced femoral neck fractures for those patients with groin pain and inconclusive radiographs. Bone scan should be delayed until 48 hours post injury to decrease the rate of false negatives; however, MRI will reveal fractures immediately. Additionally, MRI is appropriate for suspected pathologic fractures. While CT scans can be used to confirm a femoral neck fracture, they are not adequate to rule out a nondisplaced fracture and therefore have minimal utility in the assessment of these patients.

Differential Diagnosis

The differential diagnosis includes intertrochanteric femur fracture, fractures of the pubic rami, acetabular fracture,

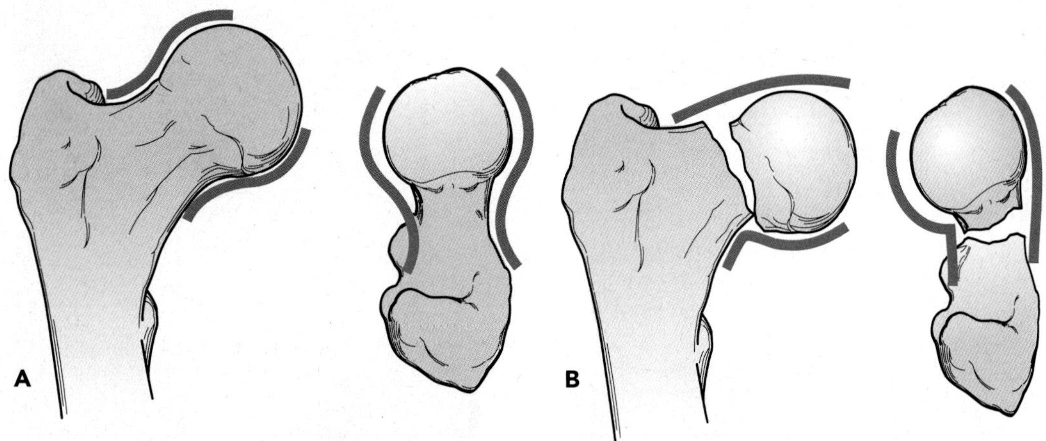

Figure 16.24 (**A**) The cortices of an anatomically reduced femoral neck fracture will from an S- or reverse S-shaped curve on both radiographic views. (**B**) Malreduction will cause a C-shaped curve on one side and a sharp apex on the opposite. (*Reprinted with permission from* Bucholz RW, Heckman JD, Court-Brown CM, et al. *Rockwood and Green's Fractures in Adults.* 6th ed. Philadelphia, PA: Lippincott Williams & Wilkins, 2006.)

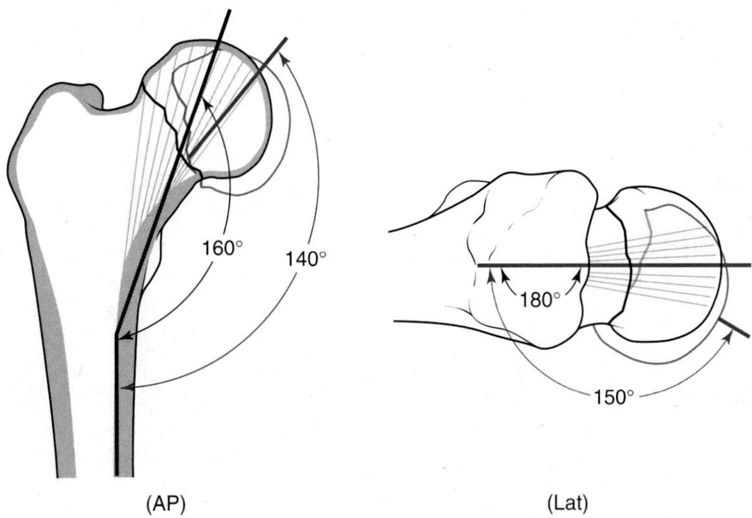

Figure 16.25 The Garden Alignment Index. Anatomic (*black*) and nonanatomic reductions (*blue*) are depicted. (*Reprinted with permission from* Bucholz RW, Heckman JD, Court-Brown CM, et al. *Rockwood and Green's Fractures in Adults.* 6th ed. Philadelphia, PA: Lippincott Williams & Wilkins, 2006.)

sacral insufficiency fracture, OA, AVN, tumor, or lumbar spine pathology.

Treatment

Fractures of the femoral neck are best treated with operative management that allows for early mobilization and full weight-bearing. Because of the significant morbidity and risks associated with prolonged recumbency, nonoperative treatment should only be considered in patients who are extremely poor surgical candidates or in nonambulatory patients who have minimal discomfort. In either case, early bed-to-chair mobilization should be instituted with knowledge that malunion will occur.

In elderly patients, the presence of fracture displacement, preexisting OA, and the functional demands of the patient are important factors in determining the appropriate method of surgical treatment. Fracture displacement has important implications regarding the viability of the femoral head. In nondisplaced fractures, rates of AVN have been reported to be 13% to 20%, compared with rates as high as 25% to 40% for displaced fractures. This discrepancy is believed to be due to differing degrees of damage to the ascending cervical vessels. These vessels travel within the joint capsule to supply a large portion of the femoral head and are thought to partially remain intact in nondisplaced fractures. Thus, nondisplaced fractures (Garden I and II) are generally treated with anatomic reduction and internal fixation utilizing parallel lag screws with the expectation of low rates of femoral head collapse from AVN (Fig. 16.26).

On the other hand, displaced fractures (Garden III and IV) are typically treated with prosthetic replacement due to the high probability of femoral head necrosis and subsequent collapse. Prosthetic replacement may consist of hemiarthroplasty in which a femoral stem with a metallic head is used to replace the femoral head and neck (Fig. 16.27). Alternatively, a total hip arthroplasty may be used, in which the acetabulum is resurfaced in addition to prosthetic replacement of the femoral head and neck. The decision to employ a hemiarthroplasty versus a total hip arthroplasty is dependent on the presence of preexisting hip pain, the degree of OA within the acetabulum, and the activity level of the patient. Preexisting hip pain, significant degenerative changes within the acetabulum, or a highly active patient would likely lead to progressive acetabular erosion and pain with hemiarthroplasty. In these cases, total hip arthroplasty is often the preferred option. However, the

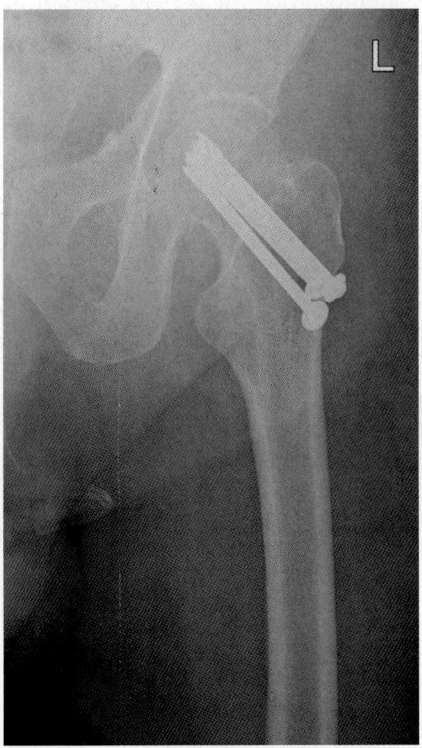

Figure 16.26 Anteroposterior radiograph of the hip demonstrating anatomic fixation of a femoral neck fracture with three parallel lag screws.

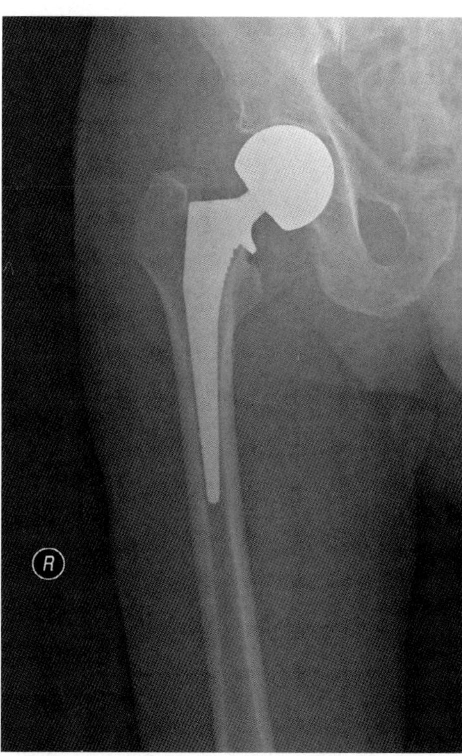

Figure 16.27 Anteroposterior radiograph of the hip, depicting a modular hemiarthroplasty in good position.

longer operative time, increased blood loss, and increased risk of postoperative dislocation must be considered on a case-by-case basis when choosing between total hip arthroplasty and hemiarthroplasty in the management of femoral neck fractures.

In contrast to elderly patients, femoral neck fractures in young patients are orthopedic emergencies. All attempts to save the patient's native femoral head and reduce the rate of AVN should be made through emergent reduction and stabilization within 6 hours of the injury. For displaced fractures, a single attempt at closed reduction should be made in the operating room, and if successful, percutaneous pinning should ensue. However, more commonly closed reduction is unsuccessful, and the surgeon should proceed with open reduction to achieve anatomic alignment. A detailed understanding of the vascular anatomy is required to minimize further damage to the femoral head blood supply during the surgical approach. Once reduction is obtained, the fracture should be rigidly stabilized with cancellous lag screws or a sliding screw and side-plate with a derotational screw.

Postoperatively, patients are mobilized immediately. It has been shown that the elderly will self-regulate weight-bearing and thus should be allowed to weight bear as tolerated in most instances, whether they undergo prosthetic replacement or internal fixation, as this promotes early mobilization. This is an important point to consider as partial and nonweight bearing are often not possible in elderly patients due to diminished functional capacity and upper extremity weakness. In younger patients, weight-bearing status will depend on the stability of the reduction but if often delayed for 6 weeks.

TABLE 16.5
COMPLICATIONS OF FEMORAL NECK FRACTURES

Nonunion
Malunion
Failure of internal fixation
Avascular necrosis of the femoral head
Pain
Deep venous thrombosis
Infection
Heterotopic ossification
Dislocation
Death

Complications

Treatment of femoral neck fractures may be complicated by loss of fixation, nonunion, malunion, pain, dislocation, deep vein thrombosis, infection, AVN, and death (Table 16.5). Early fixation failure is uncommon and is associated with fracture comminution and varus reduction. The rates of nonunion and AVN are related to fracture displacement with higher rates occurring for displaced fractures. Historically, nonunion rates for nondisplaced fractures have ranged from 0% to 5%, while nonunion rates as high as 35% have been reported for displaced fractures. However, rates of nonunion appear to be improving with modern treatment methods. More recently, nonunion rates in young patients are typically less than 10% and are likely related to improved fixation and timely surgical treatment. AVN with collapse complicates 11% of nondisplaced fractures and up to 27% of displaced fractures.

Intertrochanteric Hip Fractures

Intertrochanteric femur fractures are extracapsular fractures that occur in the transitional region between the base of the femoral neck and the lesser trochanter. This region is made up of dense trabecular bone and includes the calcar femorale, which is the strut of dense bone between the posteromedial femoral neck and shaft that acts to transfer stress from the femoral neck to the femoral shaft.

While different from femoral neck fractures anatomically and in the way in which they are managed, the epidemiology of intertrochanteric and femoral neck fractures is quite similar. Intertrochanteric fractures also occur in two distinct patient populations. The vast majority of these fractures occur in the elderly and are fragility fractures from low-energy mechanisms. In the elderly population, these

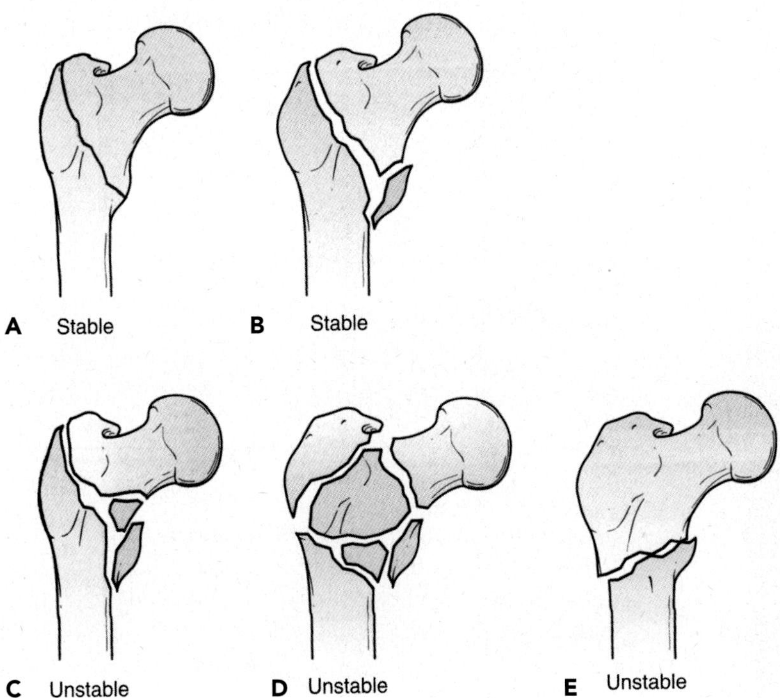

Figure 16.28 The Evans' classification of intertrochanteric hip fractures. (**A**) Stable with intact posteromedial cortex. (**B**) Stable with minimal comminution of posteromedial cortex. (**C**) Unstable with comminuted posteromedial cortex. (**D**) Unstable with global comminution. (**E**) Unstable with reverse obliquity fracture pattern. (*Reprinted with permission from* Bucholz RW, Heckman JD, Court-Brown CM, et al. *Rockwood and Green's Fractures in Adults.* 6th ed. Philadelphia, PA: Lippincott Williams & Wilkins, 2006.)

injuries can be devastating with an impact that reaches far beyond the fracture itself. It has been reported that only approximately half of the patients will regain their prefracture functional status, while 1-year mortality rates have ranged from 14% to 50%. Much less commonly, these fractures occur in young patients and are typically secondary to high-energy trauma.

Classification

Historically, intertrochanteric fractures have been classified according to the system introduced by Evans (Fig. 16.28). Evans recognized that the posteromedial cortex was the key to fracture stability. Subsequently, he divided intertrochanteric fractures into two groups (stable and unstable) on the basis of the integrity of the posteromedial cortex. In stable fractures, the posteromedial cortex is intact or has minimal comminution. Unstable fractures have a comminuted posteromedial cortex or have a reverse obliquity fracture pattern. Evans recognized that reverse obliquity fractures are inherently unstable with a tendency toward medial migration of the femoral shaft. He also noted that some unstable fractures can be converted to stable fractures through restoration of the posteromedial cortex. This fracture classification is important not only because it defines the stability of the fracture but because it also guides treatment through definition of a stable reduction. However, despite the important contributions of this classification, it has been plagued by poor interobserver reliability. Thus, today the underlying principles of the Evans' classification are utilized to facilitate communication and guide treatment by simply describing intertrochanteric fractures as stable or unstable.

Mechanism of Injury

The vast majority of intertrochanteric fractures are fragility fractures in the elderly secondary to low-energy mechanisms. Approximately 90% result from a simple fall, most often directly onto the lateral hip where there is little soft tissue to cushion the blow. In younger patients, high-energy trauma is required to fracture the intertrochanteric region of the femur. Motor vehicle accidents or a fall from a height causing a direct blow to the lateral hip or a rotational force to the leg are the most common mechanisms.

Presentation

The clinical presentation of an intertrochanteric fracture can vary widely. Patients with displaced fractures will complain of severe groin pain and will be unable to stand or bear weight. However, some nondisplaced fractures will cause slight groin pain and will lack the typical shortened and externally rotated posture present in displaced fractures. Thus, the diagnosis of a hip fracture should be considered for any patient complaining of groin pain. Elderly patients who live alone may be discovered hours to days after a fall and may present with dehydration, decubitus ulcers, or confusion. In younger patients, there may be associated injuries as well as signs and symptoms of shock.

Physical Examination

For high-energy mechanisms and obtunded elderly patients, the initial examination should be directed by the guidelines of the Advanced Trauma and Life Support System. Following a thorough trauma evaluation, examination of the injured extremity should begin with close inspection of the skin for signs of open fracture. Shortening and external rotation of the affected leg should be noted. ROM of the hip should be avoided as it may lead to further fracture displacement. In high-energy mechanisms, a detailed examination of the entire injured extremity is important with special attention given to the examination of the knee. As with femoral neck fractures, the elderly should be evaluated for concomitant fragility fractures such as distal radius and proximal humerus fractures. While neurovascular injury is uncommon, a careful neurovascular examination should be performed in all the patients.

Radiographic Findings

Radiographic evaluation begins with careful scrutiny of the AP pelvis radiograph as well as the AP and cross-table lateral views of the affected hip. An AP view of the hip in 10 to 15 degrees of internal rotation is often helpful as it offsets the femoral anteversion and provides a true AP of the proximal femur. Fracture displacement, the degree of osteoporosis, and presence of posteromedial comminution should be noted as these factors will affect the treatment. Radiographs of the contralateral hip may be helpful for preoperative planning.

Special Tests

In patients with groin pain and inconclusive radiographs, MRI and bone scan are helpful in diagnosing occult nondisplaced fractures of the proximal femur. Bone scan should be delayed until 48 hours post injury to decrease the rate of false negatives; however, MRI will reveal fractures immediately. Additionally, MRI is appropriate for suspected pathologic fractures.

Differential Diagnosis

The differential diagnosis includes femoral neck fracture, fractures of the pubic rami, acetabular fracture, sacral insufficiency fracture, OA, AVN, tumor, or lumbar spine pathology.

Treatment

Intertrochanteric femur fractures are best treated with operative management that provides for early mobilization and full weight-bearing. Because of the significant morbidity and risks associated with prolonged recumbency, nonoperative treatment should only be considered in patients who are extremely poor surgical candidates or in nonambulatory patients who have minimal discomfort. In either case, early bed-to-chair mobilization should be instituted with knowledge that malunion will occur.

Today, intertrochanteric femur fractures are typically treated with either a sliding screw plate device or a cephalomedullary device that incorporates a lag screw into the femoral head through an intramedullary nail. The appropriate choice of implant depends on the fracture pattern and stability. Cephalomedullary devices have generally been found to be most appropriate for very unstable fractures and reverse obliquity patterns. Regardless of the

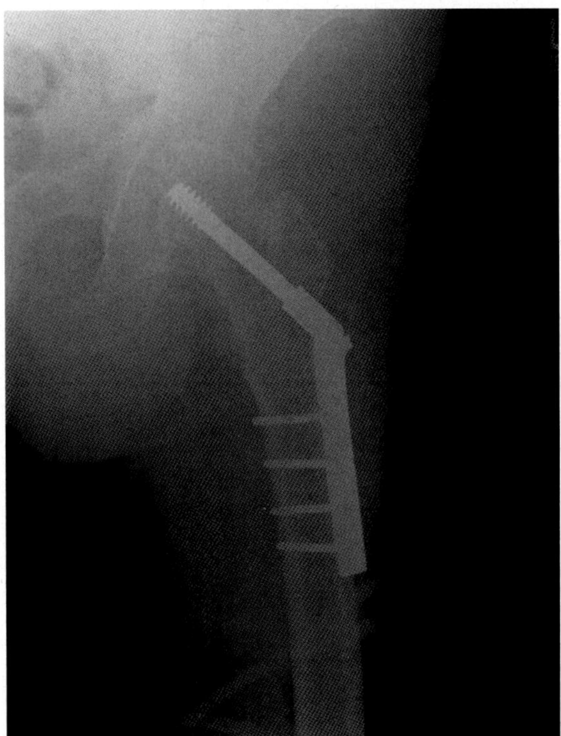

Figure 16.29 Anteroposterior radiograph of the hip, demonstrating the use of a sliding screw plate device.

device used, successful operative treatment begins with adequate reduction. Accurate reduction will restore the biomechanics of the hip and lessen the load on the implant. Reduction should restore the femoral neck-shaft angle and correct rotational deformity. Large posteromedial fragments should be reduced and secured with a cerclage wire or interfragmentary screw to improve the stability of the fracture.

The most common method of treating intertrochanteric fractures is with a sliding screw plate device (Fig. 16.29). This device allows for controlled fracture impaction through sliding of the lag screw within the barrel of the side-plate. The fracture impaction provided by this device promotes healing and decreases the stress on the implant through a reduction in the moment arm acting on the lag screw. An important factor in preventing superior cutout of the lag screw is placement of the screw within 1 cm of subchondral bone and in the center of the femoral head. Measurement of the tip–apex distance, defined as the sum of distances from the tip of the screw to the apex of the femoral head on both the AP and lateral radiographs, predicts the rate of screw cutout (Fig. 16.30). Increasing rates of cutout have been associated with tip–apex values greater than 25 mm. Overall, sliding screw plate devices have had the highest success rates; however, they should be avoided in reverse obliquity fracture patterns or very unstable fractures with subtrochanteric extension due to high failure rates.

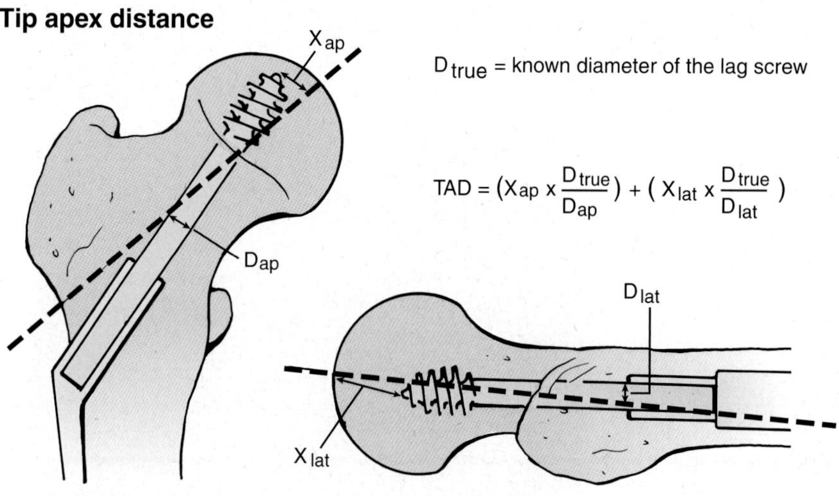

Figure 16.30 Illustration of the tip–apex distance. (*Reprinted with permission from* Bucholz RW, Heckman JD, Court-Brown CM, et al. *Rockwood and Green's Fractures in Adults.* 6th ed. Philadelphia, PA: Lippincott Williams & Wilkins, 2006.)

Recently, cephalomedullary devices with a sliding lag screw have risen in popularity (Fig. 16.31). These devices offer some theoretical advantages over the sliding screw plate devices. It is believed that cephalomedullary devices reduce the lever arm acting on the lag screw. Additionally, the intramedullary implant may buttress against excessive lateral translation of the proximal fragment during compression. Moreover, newer materials and designs have decreased the incidence of fracture at the tip of the nail, which plagued the first generation of these devices. Of note, the tip–apex measurement also applies to these devices when placing the lag screw. Despite these theoretical advantages, studies have shown that there is no difference in the outcome compared with the sliding screw plate devices for most intertrochanteric fractures; however, more frequent complications have been reported with the cephalomedullary nails.

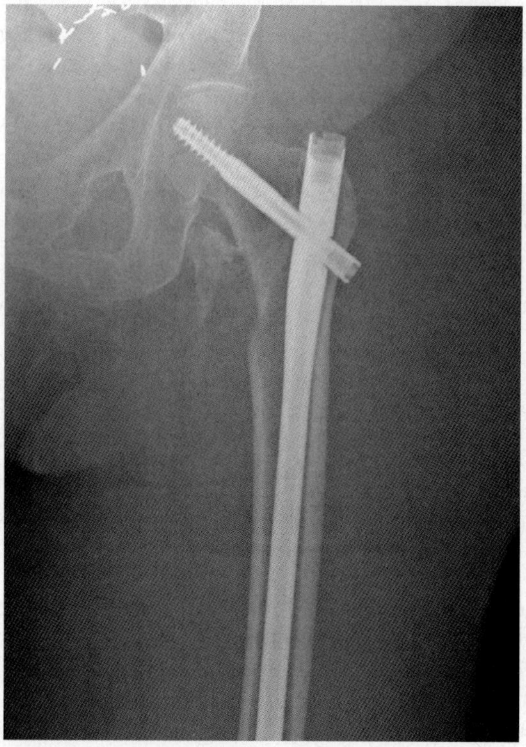

Figure 16.31 Anteroposterior radiograph of the hip, demonstrating the use of a long cephalomedullary device.

Treatment of highly unstable fracture patterns should be approached more cautiously and are worth special mention. These fracture patterns include highly comminuted fractures, fractures with subtrochanteric extension, and the reverse obliquity fracture. Often occurring in younger patients secondary to high-energy trauma, these fractures are notorious for excessive collapse, nonunion, and implant failure, especially when a sliding screw plate device is employed. Thus, highly unstable fractures are best treated with long cephalomedullary implants.

Postoperatively, patients should be mobilized immediately. It has been shown that the elderly will self-regulate weight-bearing and thus should be allowed to weight bear as tolerated in most instances to promote early mobilization. In younger patients, weight-bearing status will depend on the stability of the reduction.

Complications

Treatment of intertrochanteric fractures is most commonly complicated by loss of fixation and lag screw cutout, occurring in up to 20% of cases. Close attention to the tip–apex distance and avoiding the use of the sliding screw plate device for highly unstable fracture patterns should minimize these complications. Because of the extracapsular location of these fractures and the rich vascular supply, nonunion occurs in less than 2% of these fractures. Finally, careful scrutiny of the reduction is necessary to avoid rotational malunion.

Subtrochanteric Femur Fractures

Subtrochanteric fractures occur in a zone extending from the lesser trochanter to 5 cm distal to the lesser trochanter;

however, proximal involvement of the intertrochanteric region is not uncommon. The medial and posteromedial cortices of the subtrochanteric femur experience the highest compressive stresses in the body, while the lateral cortex is under a high degree of tensile stress. The action of the iliopsoas, the hip abductors (gluteus medius and gluteus minimus), and short external rotators cause the proximal fragment to flex, abduct, and externally rotate, respectively, while the pull of the adductors lead the distal fragment to adduct (Fig. 16.32). Because of these powerful muscle forces and the tremendous stresses on the bone, fracture reduction and maintenance of the reduction can be quite challenging.

Classification

Numerous classification schemes have been proposed for subtrochanteric fractures. The Fielding's classification is an anatomic classification based on the distance of the major fracture line from the lesser trochanter and is rarely used today. The Seinsheimer's classification factors in the integrity of the posteromedial cortex to predict fracture stability (Fig. 16.33). This classification guides treatment, predicts outcome, and is the most clinically useful.

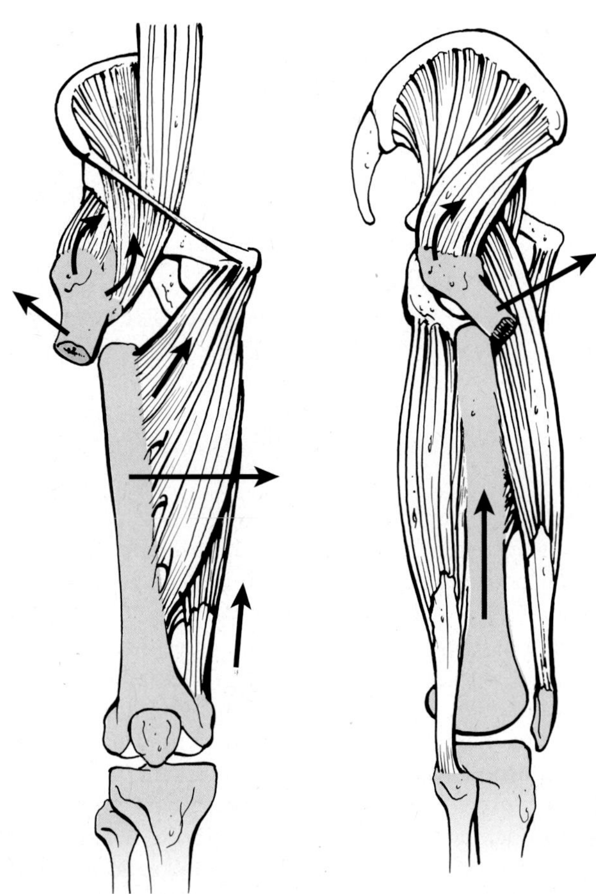

Figure 16.32 Drawing depicting the deforming forces acting on a subtrochanteric femur fracture. (*Reprinted with permission from* Bucholz RW, Heckman JD, Court-Brown CM, et al. *Rockwood and Green's Fractures in Adults*. 6th ed. Philadelphia, PA: Lippincott Williams & Wilkins, 2006.)

The Russell–Taylor's classification is based on the integrity of the piriformis fossa (Fig. 16.34). In this system, Type I fractures have an intact piriformis fossa, while Type II fractures have a fracture line extending into the piriformis fossa. These are subclassified as either A or B depending on the presence of posteromedial comminution. This classification was designed to guide the treatment of these fractures with a piriformis entry intramedullary nail. However, this classification is less important today due to the improvement in intramedullary techniques and the multitude of devices with extrapiriformis fossa entry points.

Additionally, the OTA and AO have offered descriptive classification systems on the basis of the fracture configuration. These classification schemes are quite comprehensive and thus, typically too cumbersome for routine clinical use.

Mechanism of Injury

In young patients, subtrochanteric fractures are typically the result of high-energy blunt trauma or gun shot wounds. A low-energy mechanism in a young patient should raise the suspicion of a pathologic fracture. In the elderly, these fractures typically occur through osteoporotic bone after a low-energy fall. Rarely, a subtrochanteric fracture may result from treatment of a femoral neck fracture with cannulated screws. If the starting point for the screws on the lateral femoral cortex is distal to the lesser trochanter, a stress riser is created and there is a risk of fracture.

Presentation

Patients typically present unable to ambulate due to significant pain. Typically, there is obvious shortening and external rotation of the leg with marked swelling of the proximal thigh. As these fractures are often secondary to high-energy trauma, the patient may present with associated injuries as well as signs and symptoms of shock.

Physical Examination

Initially, the physical examination should be directed by the guidelines of the Advanced Trauma and Life Support System as these are often high-energy fractures and may have associated injuries. Following a thorough trauma evaluation, examination of the injured extremity should begin with close inspection of the skin for signs of open fracture. The entire limb should then be inspected and palpated for evidence of ipsilateral extremity trauma. Careful attention should be given to the knee for signs of effusion, which may be indicative of ligamentous injury. Although neurovascular injuries are rare with subtrochanteric femur fractures, a detailed neurovascular examination should be performed.

Radiographic Examination

Radiographic evaluation involves detailed and systematic review of the AP radiograph of the pelvis as well as an

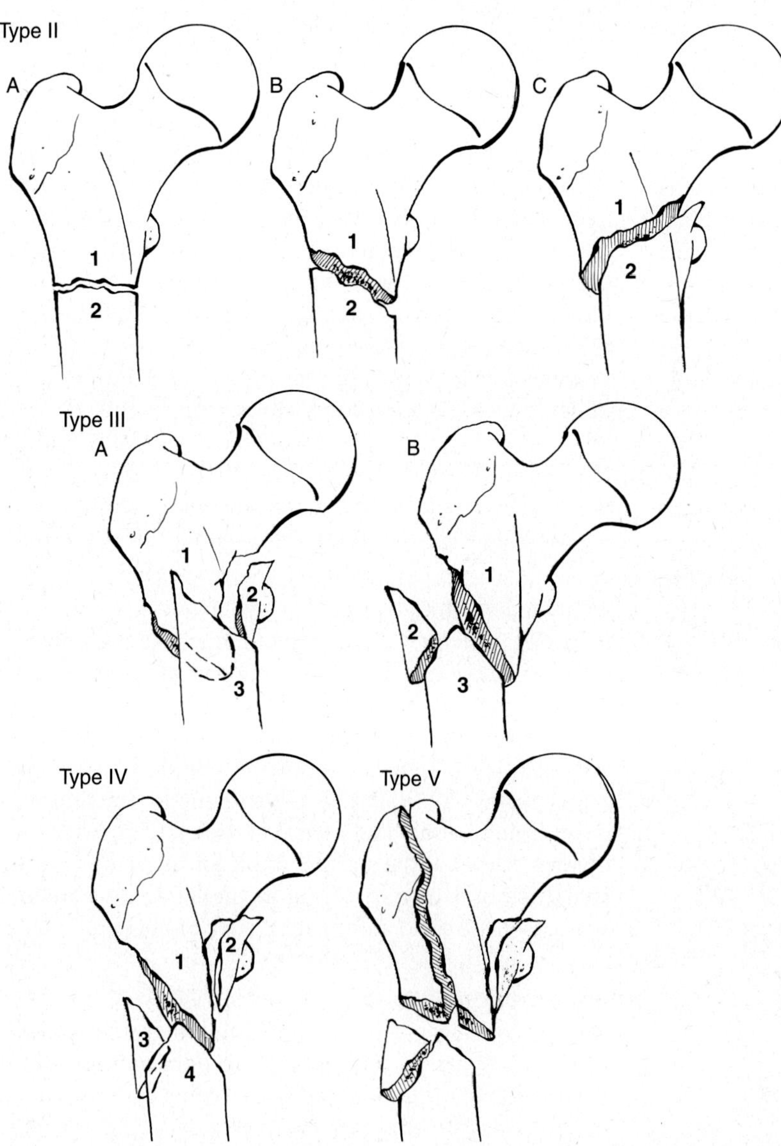

Figure 16.33 The Seinsheimer's classification of subtrochanteric femur fractures. Type I (not shown)—nondisplaced. Type II—two-part fracture. Type III—three-part fractures. Type IV—comminuted. Type V—subtrochanteric fracture with intertrochanteric extension. (*Reprinted with permission from* Bucholz RW, Heckman JD, Court-Brown CM, et al. *Rockwood and Green's Fractures in Adults.* 6th ed. Philadelphia, PA: Lippincott Williams & Wilkins, 2006.)

internal rotation AP view and cross-table lateral view of the affected hip and entire femur.

Special Tests

Plain radiographs are typically sufficient for diagnosis and preoperative planning; however, MRI is indicated if there is concern for pathologic fracture.

Differential Diagnosis

The differential diagnosis is limited and includes hip dislocation, femoral neck fracture, and peritrochanteric fracture.

Treatment

Subtrochanteric femur fractures are best treated with surgical fixation. Because of the significant morbidity and risks associated with prolonged recumbency, nonoperative treatment should only be considered for patients who are extremely poor surgical candidates. In the rare instance that nonoperative treatment is deemed appropriate, the patient should be placed in 90 to 90 skeletal traction for 8 to 12 weeks followed by hip spica casting. With 90 to 90 skeletal traction, the hip is held in a 90-degree flexed position and allowed to externally rotate in an attempt to bring the distal fragment in-line with the flexed and externally rotated proximal fragment, thus minimizing malunion.

While the surgical techniques and implants for the treatment of subtrochanteric femur fractures have evolved, the goals of achieving stability while restoring length, alignment, and rotation to allow rapid mobilization have remained the same. Historically, treatment of these fractures involved open reduction and the application of rigid internal fixation with plates, a sliding hip screw device, or blade plate. Because of size and strength of the implants required to control the powerful muscle forces inherent to these

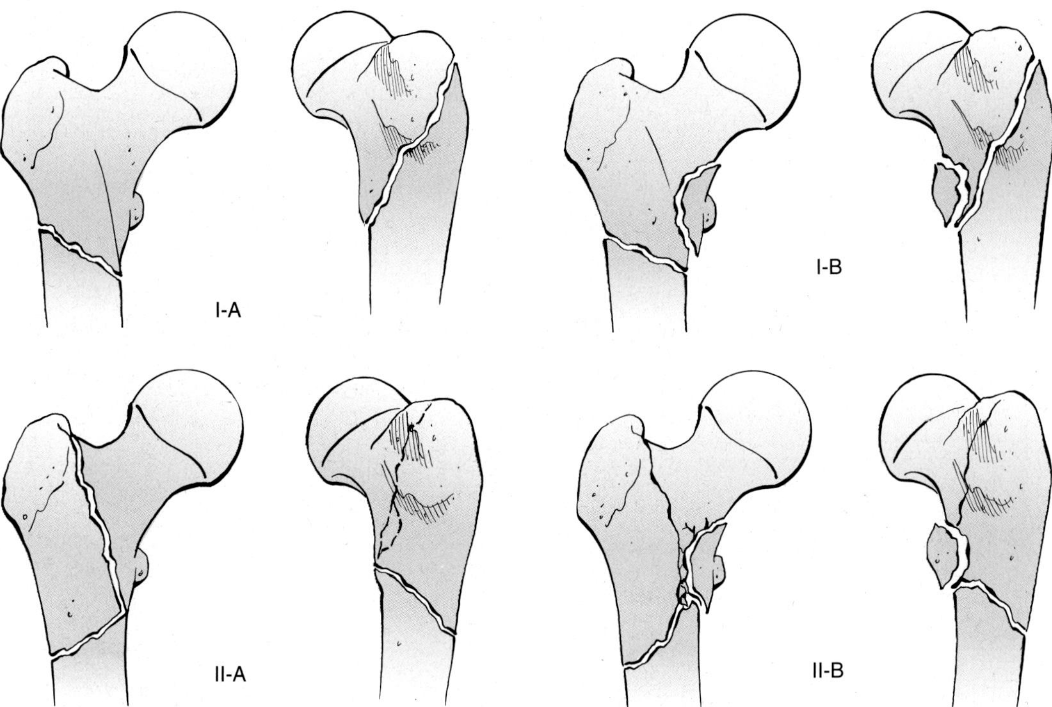

Figure 16.34 The Russell–Taylor's classification of subtrochanteric fractures. (*Reprinted with permission from* Bucholz RW, Heckman JD, Court-Brown CM, et al. *Rockwood and Green's Fractures in Adults.* 6th ed. Philadelphia, PA: Lippincott Williams & Wilkins, 2006.)

fractures, large dissections and soft-tissue stripping were typically necessary. This contributed to high rates of delayed union, nonunion, and ultimately to implant failure.

With advances in modern internal fixation principles and implants, closed reduction techniques have allowed for near anatomic reductions without disturbing the fracture hematoma or further damaging the local blood supply. However, closed reduction remains a demanding technique, and careful attention is required to avoid varus alignment, shortening, or rotational malunion. Following closed reduction, an interlocking antegrade intramedullary device is employed percutaneously to stabilize the fracture (Fig. 16.35). Use of an intramedullary device affords two additional advantages over traditional plating techniques by decreasing the moment arm on the implant through its intramedullary location and supplying local bone graft from the reaming required for canal preparation. Fractures with minimal comminution, an intact posteromedial cortex, and without proximal extension may be treated with a first generation intramedullary nail. For comminuted fractures or those with extension into the intertrochanteric region, a cephalomedullary nail offers superior fixation. Occasionally, closed reduction is unable to be achieved. In these cases, a limited open reduction with minimal soft-tissue dissection should be performed with consideration of bone grafting the posteromedial cortex.

Postoperatively, the patient's weight-bearing should be restricted until mature callus is noted on radiographs and the patient's pain has subsided. Often these fractures require 8 to 12 weeks for healing. Failure of the fracture to unite may be related to infection, the nutritional state of the patient, comorbid health conditions, extensive soft-tissue stripping, or inadequate fixation.

Femoral Shaft Fractures

Fractures of the femoral shaft occur in the portion of the diaphysis from 5 cm distal to the lesser trochanter to 5 cm proximal to the adductor tubercle. The femur is the strongest bone in the body and therefore typically requires a high-energy mechanism to fracture. Because of the high-energy nature of these fractures, associated injuries are common. Additionally, the excellent vascularity and sizable muscular compartments surrounding the femur can lead to significant blood loss requiring transfusion in nearly half of the patients. However, this significant soft-tissue coverage and vascularity also contributes to the low rate of nonunion. Advances in trauma resuscitation as well as surgical techniques have greatly improved the morbidity and mortality associated with these injuries.

Classification

Often for informal communication, these fractures are classified descriptively on the basis of the location (proximal, middle, or distal third) and fracture morphology (transverse, oblique, spiral, comminuted, or segmental).

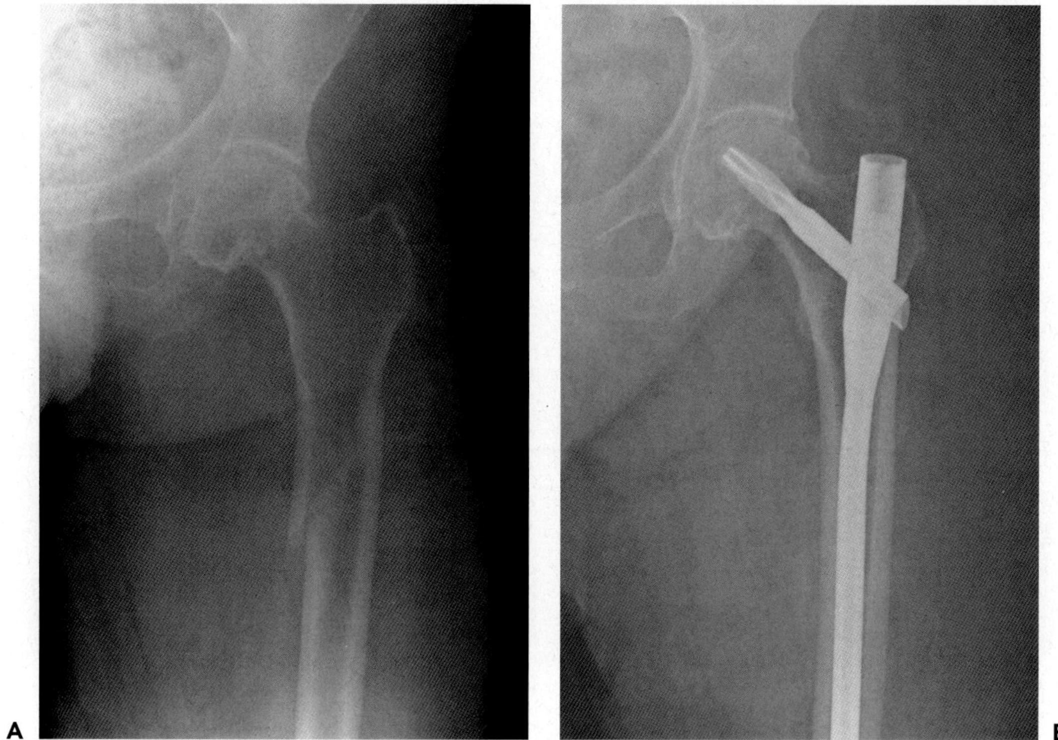

Figure 16.35 (**A**) Subtrochanteric femur fracture. (**B**) Anatomic stabilization with a cephalomedullary device.

Winquist and Hansen offered a more formal classification scheme that is also commonly employed (Fig. 16.36). It was designed to predict which fractures would be prone to shortening, and thus require treatment with an interlocked nail, o the basis of the amount of fracture comminution. Today, it is rare to consider the treatment with an intramedullary nail without employing interlocking screws. Nevertheless, this classification scheme remains useful, has prognostic significance, and aids in operative planning. Additionally, a comprehensive classification proposed by the

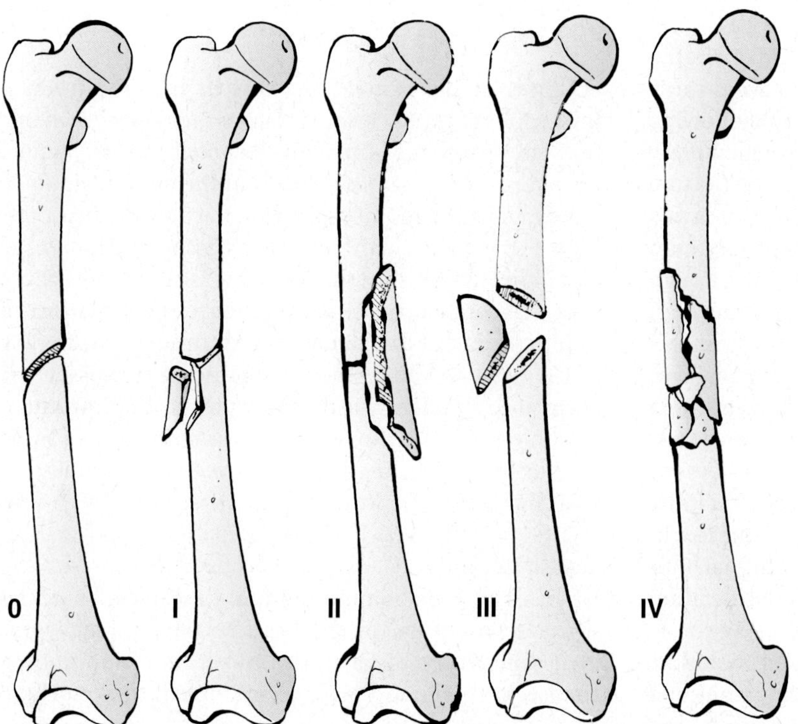

Figure 16.36 The Winquist–Hansen's classification for femoral shaft fractures. (**A**) No comminution. (**B**) Small butterfly fragment with minimal comminution. (**C**) Large butterfly fragment with at least 50% cortical contact remaining. (**D**) Large butterfly fragment with less than 50% cortical contact remaining. (**E**) Comminution with no cortical contact remaining. (*Reprinted with permission from* Bucholz RW, Heckman JD, Court-Brown CM, et al. *Rockwood and Green's Fractures in Adults.* 6th ed. Philadelphia, PA: Lippincott Williams & Wilkins, 2006.)

AO/Orthopaedic Trauma Association exists and is typically utilized for research purposes.

Mechanism of Injury

Femoral shaft fractures are almost always due to high-energy mechanisms such as motor vehicle accidents, falls, gunshots, or pedestrian injuries. Pathologic fracture should be suspected for any patient presenting with a femoral shaft fracture in the absence of high-energy trauma.

Since the femoral shaft is essentially a cylinder, the exact mechanism of injury can often be extrapolated from the fracture pattern. Transverse fractures are the result of a bending force. Torque applied to the femur causes a spiral fracture. An element of compression combined with a bending force creates an oblique fracture or a butterfly fragment. For comminuted fractures, it is the degree of energy and not the direction of force that determines this pattern.

Presentation

Typically, these patients present unable to ambulate, in a tremendous amount of pain and with obvious deformity of the thigh. In cases of associated trauma, patients may present obtunded, unconscious, or in shock.

Physical Examination

The initial physical examination should be directed by the guidelines of the Advanced Trauma and Life Support System as these are often high-energy fracture and may have associated injuries. Even in isolated fractures of the femoral shaft, blood loss of greater than 2.0 L into the thigh can be significant and results in hemodynamic instability.

Following a thorough trauma evaluation, examination of the injured extremity should begin with close inspection of the skin for signs of open fracture. Next, the entire limb should be inspected and palpated for evidence of ipsilateral extremity trauma. Careful attention should be paid to the knee for signs of effusion, which may be indicative of ligamentous injury or fracture. A detailed neurovascular examination must be performed in each patient who has sustained a femur fracture. Finally, the compartments of the thigh should be assessed for evidence of compartment syndrome, and if warranted, formal compartment pressure measurement should be undertaken.

Radiographic Examination

Radiographic assessment should begin with careful evaluation of full-length AP and lateral views of the femur for fracture pattern, bone quality, and length (Fig. 16.37). Full-length radiographs of the contralateral femur are useful in comminuted fractures for assessing the patient's normal length and anatomic bow. Alternatively, a CT scout view that includes both femurs may give useful information on femoral length. Measurement of the size of the femoral canal will guide preoperative planning for the intramedullary nail diameter. Additionally, it is imperative to carefully scrutinize high-quality internal rotation AP and lateral views of the ipsilateral hip for evidence of femoral neck fracture. Concomitant femoral neck fractures occur in up to 10% of femoral shaft fractures and are often subtle and nondisplaced. AP pelvis as well as AP and lateral radiographs of the knee should also be obtained and carefully reviewed for associated injuries.

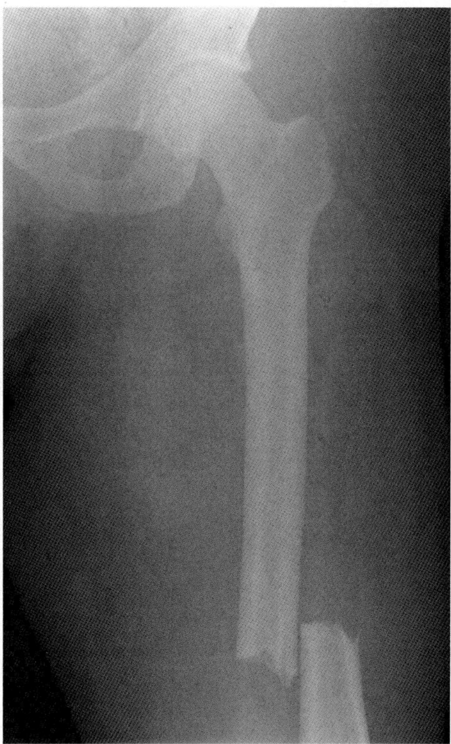

Figure 16.37 Anteroposterior radiograph of midshaft femur fracture.

Special Tests

MRI is indicated for evaluation of suspected pathologic fractures.

Differential Diagnosis

The differential diagnosis is limited and includes other fractures of the femur.

Treatment

The initial goal of the treatment for femoral shaft fractures is to expeditiously restore length, alignment, and rotation. Skeletal traction and external fixation are frequently used for this purpose in a temporary capacity. They serve to alleviate pain and minimize bleeding through a reduction in the volume of the thigh. Today, however, skeletal traction and external fixation have limited utility as definitive treatment of femoral shaft fractures due to frequent malunion, pin site infection, and knee stiffness. Additionally, skeletal traction requires prolonged recumbency leading to increased pulmonary complications and greater risk of decubitus ulcers. Thus, these methods should only be considered as definitive stabilization in patients who are extremely poor surgical candidates.

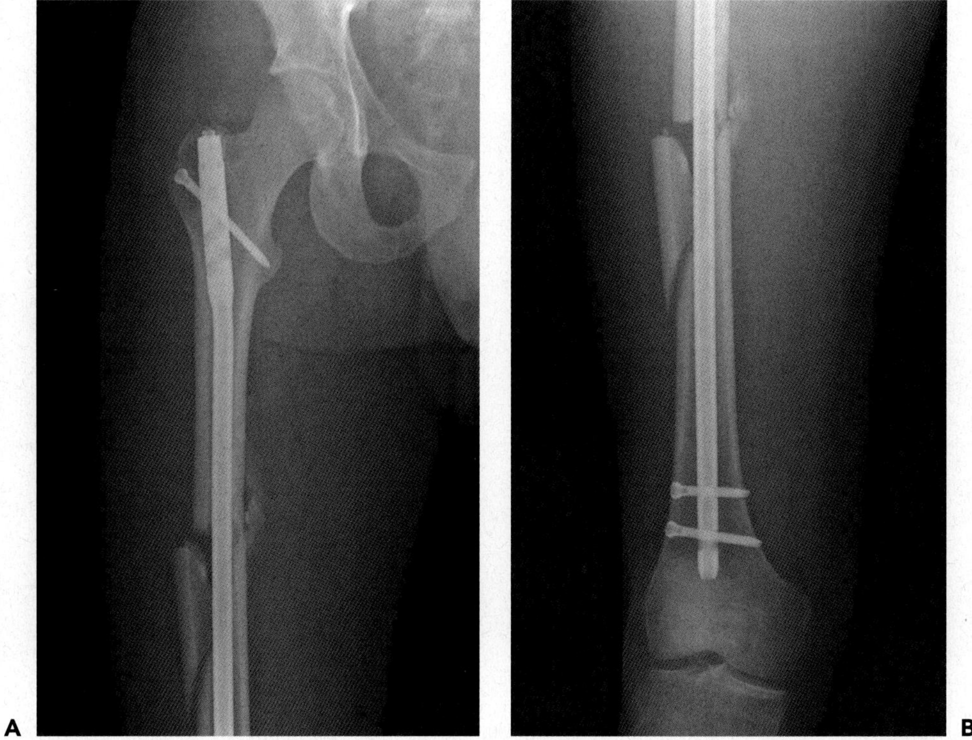

Figure 16.38 Anteroposterior radiographs of intramedullary nail fixation of midshaft femur fracture (**A & B**).

The goals of definitive treatment are to restore length, alignment, and rotation while providing stable fixation that allows early mobilization. Additionally, the timing of fixation is important. It has been demonstrated that early definitive fixation of femoral shaft fractures within 24 hours of the injury, in the absence of severe chest trauma or head injury, significantly decreases the incidence of pulmonary complications including acute respiratory distress syndrome.

Definitive fracture stabilization in the vast majority of femoral shaft fractures, including most open fractures, is best achieved with an intramedullary nail (Fig. 16.38). These devices provide for early mobilization and are inserted into the intramedullary canal at a site remote from the fracture. In closed injuries, this allows the fracture hematoma to remain undisturbed, which has beneficial effects on fracture healing.

Intramedullary nails are load sharing devices that act as internal splints. The load supported by the nail depends on the stability of the fracture, with gradual load transfer to the femur as the fracture heals. Interlocking screws should be used in nearly all cases and serve to maintain rotation and length. Typically, intramedullary nails are inserted in an antegrade fashion from the piriformis fossa or greater trochanter. However, the nail may be inserted in retrograde manner through a knee arthrotomy. This technique may be useful in floating knees, bilateral femoral fractures, extreme obesity, and pregnant patients.

Intramedullary nails may be inserted with or without reaming. Reaming allows for insertion of a larger diameter nail and provides bone graft at the fracture site; however, it disrupts the endosteal blood supply. Despite its effects on the endosteal blood supply, reaming has been shown to decrease the rate of delayed union and nonunion for femoral shaft fractures.

Although the majority of femoral shaft fractures are best treated with intramedullary nailing, fixation with a plate and screws remains a viable option. Plate fixation also provides for early mobilization; however, the extensive dissection necessary for insertion of the plate as well as the load-bearing nature of these devices are distinct disadvantages compared with intramedullary nailing. Plates remain a potential treatment alternative for femoral shaft fractures with an associated fracture of the femoral neck as well as for fractures occurring at the distal metaphyseal–diaphyseal junction. Percutaneous insertion techniques may broaden the indications for plate fixation in the future.

Postoperatively, patients should be mobilized immediately to diminish the risk of pulmonary complications and pressure sores. Unrestricted active and passive motion of the knee should be encouraged. Weight-bearing often depends on associated injuries. However, in an isolated fracture of the femoral shaft, regardless of comminution, modern large diameter-reamed intramedullary nails with two distal interlocking screws allow for immediate weight bearing as tolerated. Complications are relatively infrequent and include infection, nonunion, malunion, device failure, and thigh compartment syndrome.

ATRAUMATIC HIP CONDITIONS

Hip Arthritis

OA, also known as degenerative joint disease, is the most prevalent form of arthritis affecting the major joints of the lower extremity (e.g., hip and knee). Long-standing arthritis eventually results in end-stage joint deterioration and serves as a leading cause of physical disability worldwide. It is estimated that that approximately 16 million people in the United States suffer from OA and 1 in 3 people over the age of 60 are affected by the disease.

OA of the hip is characterized by focal degeneration of articular cartilage, typically located in the weight-bearing region of the femoral head and/or acetabulum. As the articular cartilage loss becomes more severe, the resulting altered joint reaction forces across these regions result in progressive cartilage loss. This self-perpetuating cycle results in bony remodeling and continued cartilage destruction. Patients suffering from hip OA typically present with an insidious onset of pain that accompanies activity and is relieved by rest in addition to gradual loss of ROM. Often, patients will complain of difficulty with ambulation, a decreased ability to ambulate long distances, and an increased struggle with rising from a seated position. Most symptoms will resolve with the first few steps of walking but will recur after sitting for any extended period of time. As the hip joint approaches end-stage degeneration, the patient may present with a limp or antalgic gait due to pain inhibition of the abductor complex.

Patients with symptoms suspicious of OA require at minimum an AP pelvis and an AP and lateral hip radiograph. Additional radiographic imaging modalities are not usually necessary to make the diagnosis of OA. The typical radiographic features of the diseased hip can assist in differentiating OA from inflammatory arthritis (Table 16.6).

TABLE 16.6
RADIOGRAPHIC CRITERIA FOR DIFFERENTIATING OSTEOARTHRITIS FROM INFLAMMATORY ARTHRITIS ABOUT THE HIP JOINT

Osteoarthritis	Inflammatory Arthritis
Eccentric joint space narrowing	Symmetric joint space narrowing
Bony	Periarticular osteopenia/osteoporosis
Subchondral cyst	Joint erosion
Osteophyte formation	Ankylosis

When determining the appropriate treatment regimen for a patient with hip OA, it is important to take into account patient's age, presence of significant comorbidities, symptom severity, limitation of function, extent of arthritic change, and expected activity level. As with most diagnoses in orthopedics, the initial treatment strategy should be focused on nonoperative management.

Nonpharmacologic therapy is the mainstay for the treatment of hip OA. There has been a clear association between obesity and the development and progression of hip OA. From the first office visit, patients should be counseled on the importance of diet and weight loss. Young, active patients should be encouraged to stay active through low-impact activities such as the elliptical machine or swimming. Patients who present with limited hip ROM may benefit from aquatic therapy to regain motion and minimize pain.

Pharmacologic therapy can also be a powerful adjunct to the nonoperative management of hip OA. Nonsteroidal anti-inflammatory drugs (NSAIDs) are often prescribed on a daily basis to provide pain relief. Patients should be advised that NSAIDs can affect renal and hepatic function and, as a result, long-term use may be detrimental. Cyclooxygenase-2 inhibitors are an alternative that offer a lower side-effect profile. Additionally, NSAIDs should be discontinued 5 to 7 days prior to any surgical intervention due to an inhibitory effect on platelet function and prolonged bleeding times.

For patients suffering from mild osteoarthritic symptoms, over the counter supplements such as Glucosamine Chondroitin Sulfate, a glycosaminoglycan derivative, have been shown to provide some benefit. Intra-articular administration of viscosupplementation agents is also an option, although it is much more readily accepted in the treatment of mild knee OA. This entails a series of three or five injections spaced 1 week apart. Typically, patients gain moderate relief lasting from 6 months to 1 year; however, the use of intra-articular viscosupplementation has not been FDA approved for hip arthritis.

The use of intra-articular glucocorticoid injections have also not been studied extensively for the treatment of hip OA. However, they can be used diagnostically in combination with an anesthetic agent in determining whether hip pain is referred (e.g., lumbosacral referred pain) or related to internal derangement of the hip joint itself. Often younger patients with suspected labral pathology will undergo intra-articular administration of corticosteroids along with a short-acting analgesic (e.g., Lidocaine) at the time of an MR arthrogram. Pain relief derived from the injection is diagnostic for hip pathology as the cause for hip symptoms. Given the substantial soft-tissue envelope surrounding the hip joint, intra-articular injections are generally performed under radiographic guidance to ensure accurate placement.

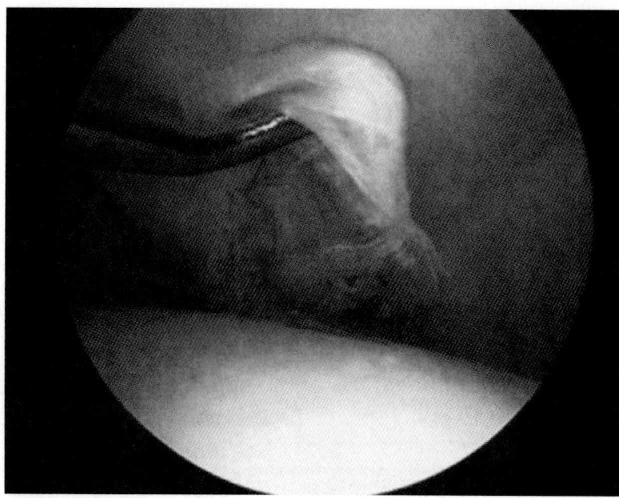

Figure 16.39 Arthroscopic photograph showing a labral tear with adjacent acetabular chondral lesion. The femoral head is shown at the bottom of the photograph. (*Reprinted with permission from* Barrack RL. *Master Techniques in Orthopaedic Surgery: The Hip.* 2nd ed. Philadelphia, PA: Lippincott Williams & Wilkins, 2005.)

Nonarthroplasty Alternatives for the Treatment of Hip Arthritis

Hip Arthroscopy

The use of hip arthroscopy has become increasingly popular in the treatment of the young adult arthritic hip. With the diagnosis of femoral–acetabular impingement as a leading cause for idiopathic hip OA, patients often present with mechanical hip symptoms due to labral tears (Fig. 16.39). This patient population typically will undergo hip arthroscopy for visualization of the joint and debridement versus possible repair of labral tears. Arthroscopic examination can aid in identifying the precise location and extent of chondral degeneration and additional pathology that may not have been clearly observed with plain radiographic or advanced imaging. Arthroscopic debridement of the hip facilitates the removal of inflammatory mediators, degenerative cartilage, and loose bodies. Debridement, chondroplasty, and removal of loose bodies is occasionally useful in the management of early-to-moderate arthritis, with associated mechanical symptoms, which may not be suitable for more extensive procedures such as total hip arthroplasty.

Hip Arthrodesis

The advent of technological advances in total hip arthroplasty (THA) over the past half century has made hip arthrodesis essentially obsolete for the treatment of OA of the hip. However, because of the concerns over the longevity of THA in younger patients, hip arthrodesis remains a possible treatment option. The main disadvantages of this procedure include progressive degeneration of the ipsilateral knee and lumbar spine and limitation of activities of daily living such as putting on socks. Young laborers and patients with a remote history of a septic arthritis are still considered good surgical candidates for hip arthrodesis with consideration given to conversion to THA in the future. The optimal hip fusion position is hip flexion of 20 to 25 degrees, adduction of 5 degrees, and neutral rotation.

Osteotomies

Osteotomies or bony procedures around the hip joint may be classified on the basis of location, pelvis, or proximal femur, or by purpose, reconstructive, or salvage. Reconstructive osteotomies are geared toward the treatment of a preexisting hip deformity such that the procedure will prevent degenerative changes from occurring prematurely. Salvage options rely upon operative correction of a preexisting degenerative hip pathology to reduce the patient's symptoms and delay the need for possible arthroplasty. The general goal of a hip osteotomy is to redirect forces across the hip joint from a degenerative area to a healthier region, preventing disease progression and preserving the remaining viable articular cartilage. A detailed discussion of the different hip osteotomies is beyond the scope of this textbook.

Total Hip Arthroplasty

Total hip replacement is one of the most successful surgical procedures performed today with nearly 95% good-to-excellent results at 15 years. Younger, more active patients are being considered surgical candidates for this procedure and nearly 250,000 THA procedures are performed annually in the United States. The overall goals of THA are to relieve pain and improve function through the restoration of joint mobility, joint stability, and anatomic alignment of the lower extremity.

Surgical Approaches to the Hip

There are several surgical approaches that may be employed to gain access to the hip joint, each with distinct advantages and disadvantages. The most common approaches include the anterior, anterolateral, the direct lateral, and the posterior approach.

The anterior or Smith–Peterson's approach uses the internervous plane between the Sartorius (innervated by the Femoral nerve) and the Tensor Fascia Lata (innervated by the Superior Gluteal nerve) (Fig. 16.40). The deeper dissection is carried out between the Rectus Femoris (innervated by the femoral nerve) and the Gluteus Medius (innervated by the Superior Gluteal nerve). This approach is typically used for irrigation and debridement of the pediatric septic hip. However, with the advent of minimally invasive techniques for THA, the two-incision approach uses the anterior approach for implantation of the acetabular cup.

The anterolateral or Watson–Jones' approach utilizes the intermuscular plane between the Tensor Fascia Lata (innervated by the Superior Gluteal nerve) and the Gluteus

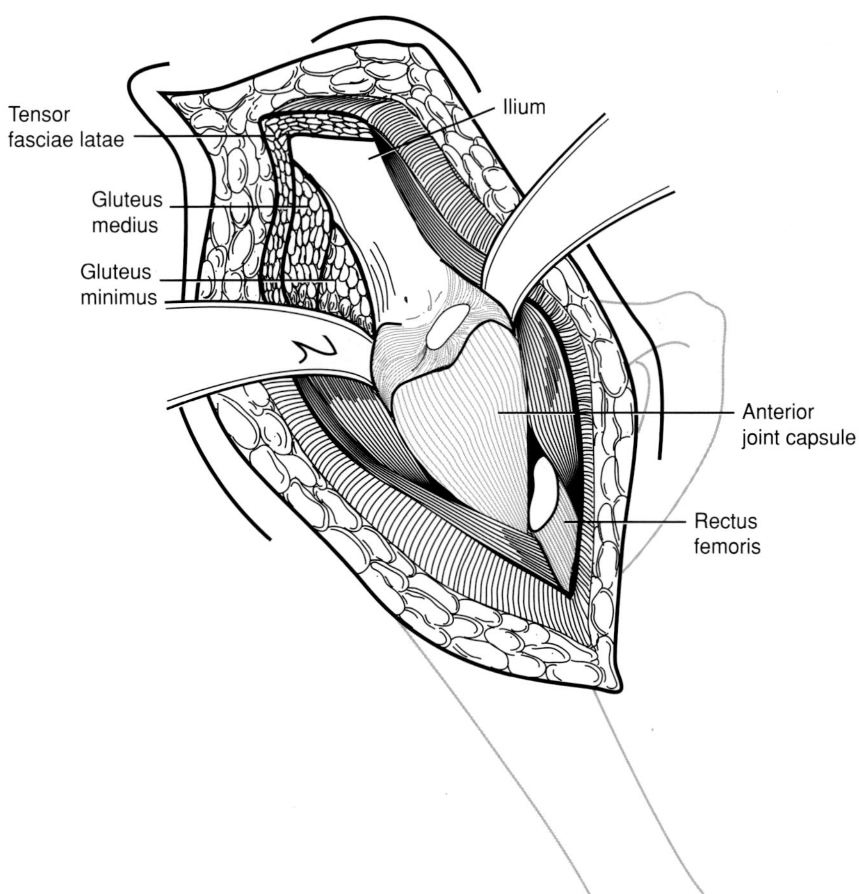

Figure 16.40 Smith–Peterson anterior approach to the hip. (*Adapted from* Hoppenfeld S, deBoer P. *Surgical Exposures in Orthopaedics: The Anatomic Approach.* 3rd ed. Philadelphia, PA: Lippincott Williams & Wilkins, 2003.)

Medius (innervated by the Superior Gluteal nerve). This is a true muscle sparing approach but is not considered an internervous approach since both muscles are innervated by the same nerve. This approach gives excellent visualization for acetabular preparation, but access to the femur is slightly more challenging than with the posterior approach.

The direct lateral or Modified Hardinge's approach is a Gluteus Medius splitting approach. The anterior one-third of the Gluteus Medius is divided to gain access to the hip capsule and joint. This approach also provides excellent visualization of the acetabulum but may result in an abductor lurch (Trendelenburg gait) in the postoperative period, while the abductor complex is healing. Access to the femur for femoral component preparation requires adduction and external rotation of the lower extremity.

The posterior or Moore's approach is the most common approach used for THA. This approach centers the incision over the greater trochanter. The incision extends distally along the femoral shaft, while it is curved proximally over the Gluteus Maximus. This is a true muscle splitting (Gluteus Maximus) approach and requires resection of the short external rotator (Piriformis, Superior and Inferior Gemellus, and Obturator Internus) muscles from their greater trochanteric insertion site (Fig. 16.41). Access to the hip joint is achieved by incising the posterior hip capsule. This approach also gives excellent visualization of the acetabulum and requires flexion, adduction, and internal rotation of the lower extremity for femoral component preparation. Upon closure of this approach, the posterior capsule and short external rotator muscles are reattached to the greater trochanter. The biggest disadvantage to this approach is the postoperative dislocation risk that has been reported to be as high as 2% to 7%. However, an adequate capsular repair has been shown to minimize the incidence of postoperative dislocation.

Hip Implant Design and Methods of Fixation

Total hip implants have evolved a great deal from the early 1970s, the time of the first modern THA performed in the United States. Initially, cemented fixation of both the acetabular and femoral component was advocated on the basis of the theory that cement interdigitated with cancellous bone resulted in superior immediate implant fixation. However, in the early 1980s, it was recognized that poor THA outcomes were associated microfracture and fatigue failure of the cement mantle. Cemented cups were found to fail at a higher rate than cemented stems because cement is less able to resist the shear and tension forces seen by the acetabulum compared with compression forces seen by the femur. The focus shifted toward using cementless fixation for the acetabulum, while cement technique was improved for the femur. Improvements in cement technique

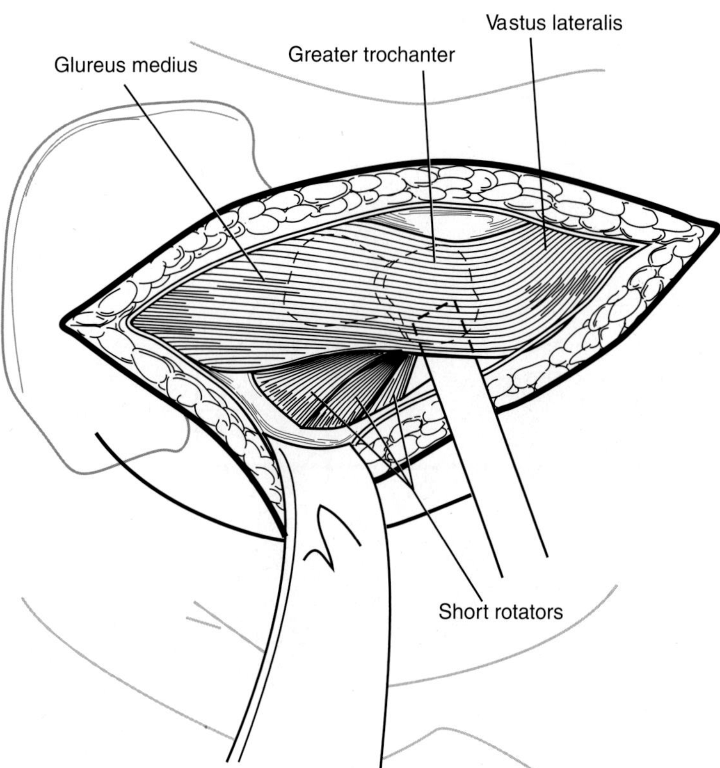

Figure 16.41 Posterior approach to the hip. (*Adapted from* Hoppenfeld S, deBoer P. *Surgical Exposures in Orthopaedics: The Anatomic Approach.* 3rd ed. Philadelphia, PA: Lippincott Williams & Wilkins, 2003.)

included the advent of vacuum mixing to decrease porosity, pressurization of the cement upon introduction into the femoral canal, and the use of a centralizer to ensure a uniform cement mantle. These improvements are referred to as third-generation cement technique and are currently used today.

Despite these technological and methodological advances in cement technique, cementless implantation of both components has gained popularity with widening surgical indications and younger, more active patients requiring THA. Today, most THA components are implanted using cementless fixation. The bone on-growth or ingrowth and remodeling potential associated with uncemented components is dynamic and life lasting. In the setting of revision THA, cementless fixation is preferred if there is adequate remaining bone stock.

There are two different techniques for cementless implant fixation: press fit and line-to-line. In *press fit,* the implant is slightly larger than the reamed size, creating compression hoop stresses for temporary fixation. In *line-to-line* fit, the same diameter implant as the reamer is used and extensive porous coating provides the initial interference fit between the prosthesis and the host bone. Screws provide initial fixation of the acetabular cup in the line-to-line fit but may also be required for adequate component stability when using the press fit technique. Safe acetabular screw placement is ensured by using quadrants on the basis of the ASIS and center of the acetabulum: posterior–superior is the safe zone; posterior–inferior is safe for screws less than 20 mm (sciatic nerve); anterior–inferior may injure the obturator nerve, artery, or vein; and anterior–superior is the "zone of death" (external iliac vessels) (Fig. 16.42).

Cementless acetabular shells typically have a coating of plasma spray, sintered beads, or mesh metal (e.g., fiber metal) that allows for bony on-growth and eventual biologic fixation of the implant. Newer porous metals such as porous tantalum are also being used as the acetabular shell backing that aids in obtaining better biologic fixation by bony in-growth. Initially, acetabular liners were implanted using cement, and cement may be used in salvage situations with a well-fixed acetabular shell. The current gold standard is to use an uncemented acetabular shell with placement of a modular acetabular liner within the shell.

Uncemented femoral components are classified as metaphyseal fitting or diaphyseal fitting stems. Metaphyseal stems are anchored in the trabecular bone of the intertrochanteric region of the proximal femur. Proximal loading of the femur decreases stress-shielding of the proximal femur. Diaphyseal stems bypass the trabecular bone of the proximal femur and rely upon cortical bone fixation within the femoral canal, typically requiring 4 to 5 cm of scratch fit (Fig. 16.43). Diaphyseal fixation results in greater proximal femoral stress-shielding and also may be associated with a higher incidence of anterior thigh pain. Older patients with osteoporotic bone may require distal fitting stems due to the inability to obtain adequate cancellous bone fixation in the proximal portion of the femur; however, these patients are at higher risk of thigh pain and stress-shielding. Both stem types are commonly used in the United States, and selection is based upon

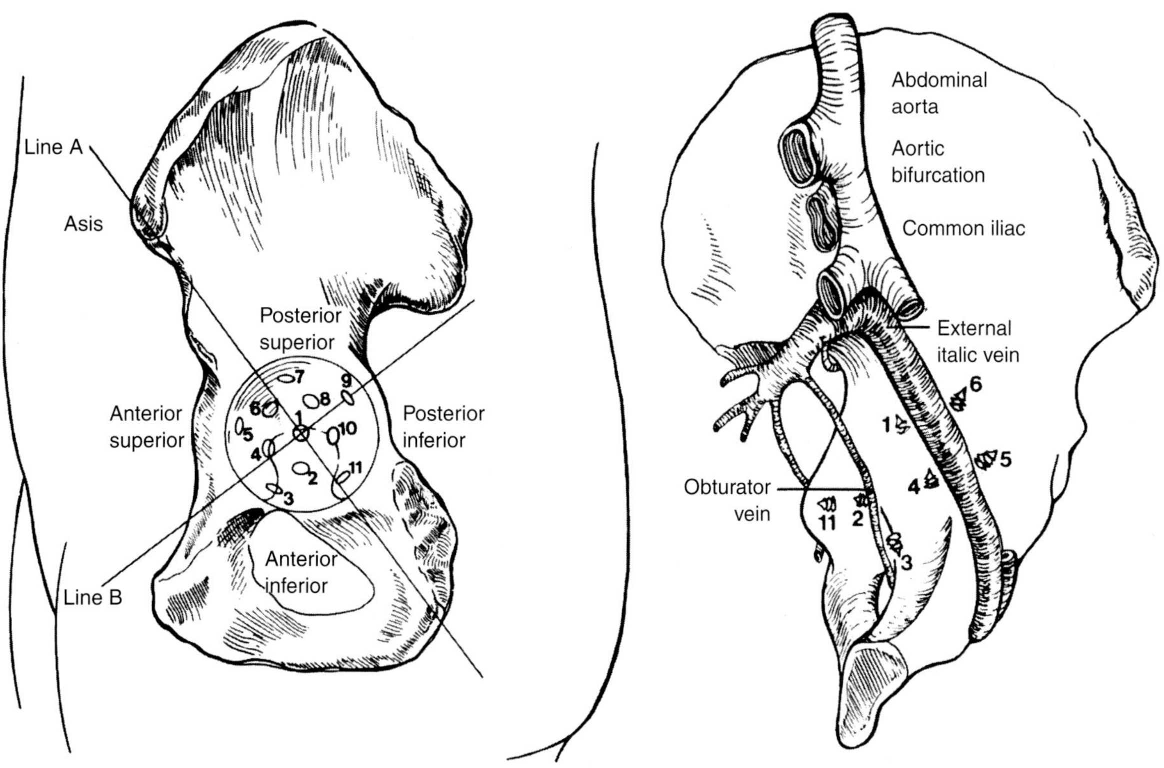

Figure 16.42 Acetabular quadrant system for screw placement (*Reprinted with permission from* Wasieleski RC, et al. Acetabular anatomy and the transacetabular fixation of screws in THA. *J Bone Joint Surg.* 1990;72A:501–508.)

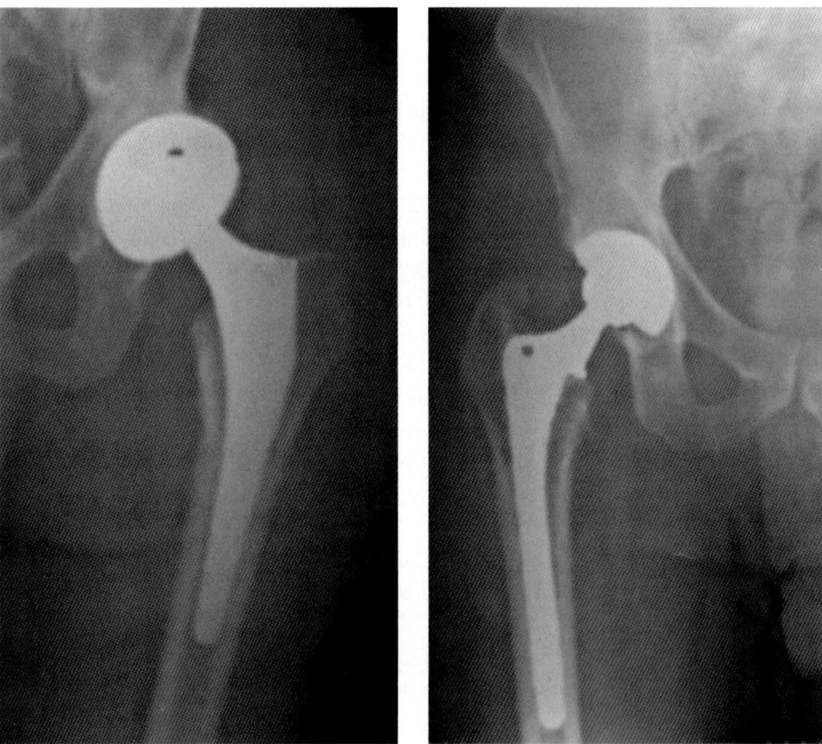

Figure 16.43 Radiographs of a cementless metaphyseal (**A**) and diaphyseal (**B**) fitting stems.

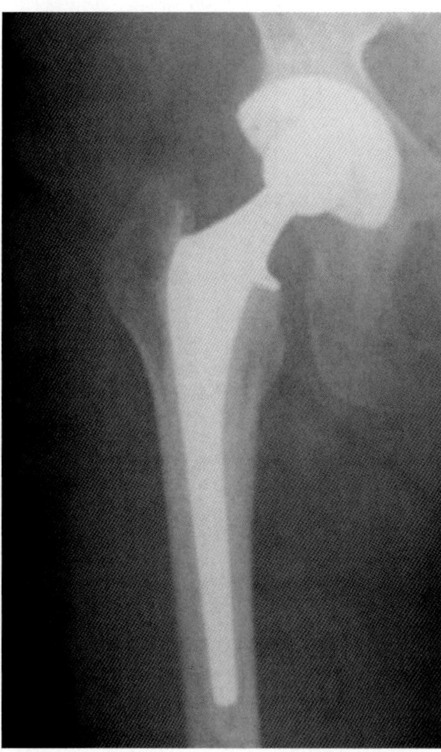

Figure 16.44 Cemented femoral stem with a 2-cm uniform cement mantle.

surgeon's preference as well as patient anatomy and bone quality.

In several institutions in the United States and worldwide, cemented femoral fixation is still considered the gold standard. Cemented femoral fixation has a long track record, and fixation is achieved via cement interdigitation with the interstices of cancellous bone. This technique can be utilized in patients with capacious canals where bony fixation is not possible with a cementless device; however, it is not ideal for young patients or femoral canals with thick cortices. When cement is used, it is important to obtain a uniform cement mantle and avoid mantle defects. A mantle defect is a region in a cement column where the prosthesis touches the bone and serves as an area of concentrated stress associated with a higher loosening rate. If the femoral stem is placed in a varus position (the distal aspect of the stem abuts the lateral femoral cortex), upon implantation, there is a higher likelihood of a stress riser and eventual fixation failure. A cement mantle of 2 mm around the entire prosthesis is generally recommended (Fig. 16.44).

Total hip Arthroplasty—General Principles and Hip Stability

Achieving a stable total hip arthroplasty is a function of component positioning, component sizing/fit, abductor complex/soft-tissue tension, and component fixation. Proper alignment of the acetabular and femoral components is typically 20 to 30 degrees of acetabular anteversion, 35 to 40 degrees of acetabular inclination (theta angle), and 10 to 15 degrees of femoral stem anteversion. Improper alignment can lead to anterior instability (increased acetabular anteversion), posterior instability (retroverted cup or stem), trochanteric impingement (decreased theta), or superior instability (increased theta angle) (Table 16.7). The end point of instability is dislocation and stability of the construct is typically confirmed on the operating room table prior to completion of the procedure.

One of the major contributors to hip stability and hip ROM is the ratio between the diameters of the implant head and implant neck, known as the head-to-neck ratio. The primary arc of motion of the hip depends on this ratio. The greater the head-to-neck ratio, the greater the ROM the femoral component can undergo prior to neck impingement on the acetabular shell.

Another determinant of hip stability is the excursion distance. Excursion distance is defined as the distance the head must travel to lever out of the acetabular liner once the neck impinges on the acetabular shell and is typically half the diameter of the head. A larger diameter head has a larger excursion distance and thus confers greater hip stability. In general, the largest head that can be implanted safely is recommended.

The soft tissues surrounding the hip are also of critical importance in attaining hip stability following THA. The hip abductor complex (gluteus medius and minimus) tension must be maintained for optimal hip stability. When there is significant abductor complex laxity (i.e., when the implanted components leave the limb short), the lack of tension results in instability of the implanted devices. The abductor tension is also affected by the degree of lateral offset of the components utilized (the more the lateral offset, the greater the abductor tension). Optimal soft-tissue balancing is determined intraoperatively with implant stability determining the degree of tension required. Any process that interferes with proper soft-tissue function (the distance between the center of the femoral head and the tip of the greater trochanter) or coordination, such as stroke, dementia, delirium, or cerebellar dysfunction, can increase the risk of postoperative hip instability.

One of the major problems facing THA today is osteolysis secondary to the generation of microscopic wear particles generated at the articulating surface. Traditional articular bearing surfaces were hard on soft (i.e., cobalt-chrome metal on polyethylene plastic). The high wear rates and particle generation associated with hard on soft bearings has led to the development of alternative bearing articulations that are hard on hard (metal on metal or ceramic on ceramic). These hard-on-hard bearings have greatly improved wear properties and have been developed to improve implant longevity for the increasing number of young, active patients requiring THA.

Complications

Complications associated with total hip arthroplasty can be classified as intraoperative, early, and late postoperative.

TABLE 16.7
TOTAL HIP INSTABILITY WITH REGARD TO ACETABULAR CUP POSITION

	Cup Position	Cup Angle (°)	Instability Pattern	Position of Compromise	Reduction Maneuver
VERSION	Anteverted	>25°	Anterior	■ Extension ■ External Rotation	Longitudinal traction ■ Hip extension ■ Abduction ■ Hip IR/ER
	Retroverted	<15°	Posterior	■ Flexion ■ Internal Rotation	■ Anterior traction ■ Hip flexion >90° ■ Adduction ■ Hip IR/ER
ABDUCTION	Vertical	>50°	Superior/Lateral	■ Adductin	Longitudinal traction ■ Adduction ■ Hip IR/ER
	Horizontal	<40°	Inferior	■ Abduction ■ Greater trochanter impingement	Longitudiral traction ■ Abduction ■ Hip IR/ER

Major intraoperative complications include fractures or nerve and vessel injury. Intraoperative fractures are more common on the femoral side than on the acetabular side. Implantation of an uncemented femoral component is more likely to result in a femoral fracture due to the tremendous forces generated to obtain rigid fixation of the device within the confines of the proximal femur. On the acetabular side, fractures typically occur when there is a large size discrepancy between the reamed acetabulum and the size of component chosen for implantation. Most fractures about the acetabulum are cortical defects, involve the posterior wall, and do not require formal open reduction and internal fixation.

While uncommon, injury to the sciatic, femoral, obturator, and superior gluteal, or lateral femoral cutaneous nerves can occur. The most common cause for nerve injury associated with THA is errant retractor placement. The most commonly injured nerve is the peroneal division of the sciatic nerve as it runs just posterior to the posterior wall of the acetabulum. Additionally, lengthening of the limb during THA by more than 3.5 to 4 cm has been associated with an increased risk for sciatic nerve neuropraxia or nerve stretch injury. Typically, nerve injuries that are neuropraxic in nature will recover spontaneously, but full recovery may take more than 6 months.

Vascular injury at the time of THA is typically associated with errant acetabular screw placement. As mentioned earlier, the acetabulum is divided into four quadrants on the basis of a line extending distally from the ASIS that bisects the acetabulum (Fig. 16.42). A second line is drawn to divide the acetabulum into four equal quarters. The safe zone is the posterior–superior quadrant, while screw placement in the anterior–superior quadrant is contraindicated due to the proximity of the iliac vessels. In the event of intraoperative injury to the iliac vessels, the THA procedure should be aborted, and the patient should be flipped into the supine position with immediate access of the abdomen by a general or vascular surgeon to obtain control of the bleeding source.

Early complications following THA include infection (deep joint), thromboembolic disease, and dislocation (Table 16.7). Infection following a primary joint replacement, although rare, is a potentially devastating complication. The incidence of primary deep joint infection is less than 1% at most large centers that perform a high volume of joint replacements annually. An important factor for preventing infection is the administration of intravenous antibiotics within 1 hour of making the surgical incision. The use of personal isolation suits and laminar flow have demonstrated only minor improvements in infection rates. However, the employment of all of these modalities may have a synergistic effect in minimizing infection following primary THA in the perioperative period (Fig. 16.45).

Any patient with new onset hip pain following primary THA must be considered to have an infected prosthesis until proven otherwise. The algorithm for diagnosing an infected prosthesis begins with plain radiographs, and laboratory work including a white blood cell count with differential, erythrocyte sedimentation rate and c-reactive protein. Nuclear imaging scans can be helpful in differentiating between aseptic and septic component loosening. Recently, the use of positron emission tomography scanning has gained popularity in the diagnosis of infection following total joint replacement. Acute infections, defined as an infection occurring within 2 weeks of symptom onset, may be effectively treated with irrigation, debridement, and liner exchange. Subacute and chronic infections diagnosed greater than 4 weeks after the onset of symptoms or implantation of the prosthesis are typically treated by a more

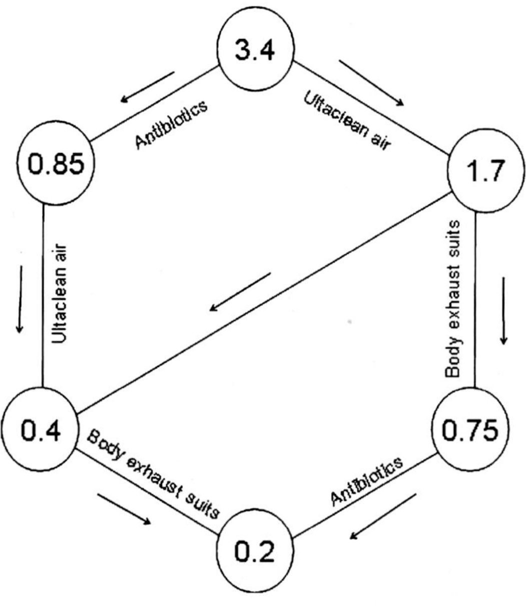

Figure 16.45 There is a synergistic effect seen with multiple modalities used to minimize the risk for infection in primary total hip arthroplasty. (*Reprinted with permission from* Callaghan JJ, Rosenberg AG, Rubash HE. *The Adult Hip*. 2nd ed. Philadelphia, PA: Lippincott Williams & Wilkins, 2007.)

TABLE 16.8

THE VANCOUVER'S CLASSIFICATION OF POSTOPERATIVE PERIPROSTHETIC FEMORAL FRACTURES

Type	Fracture Location	Subtype
A	Trochanteric region	A_G (greater trochanter) A_L (lesser trochanter)
B	Around or just distal to the stem	B1 (stable prosthesis) B2 (unstable prosthesis) B3 (inadequate bone stock)
C	Well distal to the stem tip	

Reprinted with permission from Callaghan JJ, Rosenberg AG, Rubash HE. *The Adult Hip*. 2nd ed. Philadelphia, PA: Lippincott Williams & Wilkins, 2007.

extensive protocol detailed below in the late complications section.

Thromboembolic disease refers to the formation of postoperative DVT, which may result in pulmonary emboli (PE). Thromboembolic disease is the most common complication following primary THA; however, most are subclinical and do not affect the clinical success of the procedure. Several regimens may be employed for prevention of DVT and PE and most utilize an anticoagulant agent, such

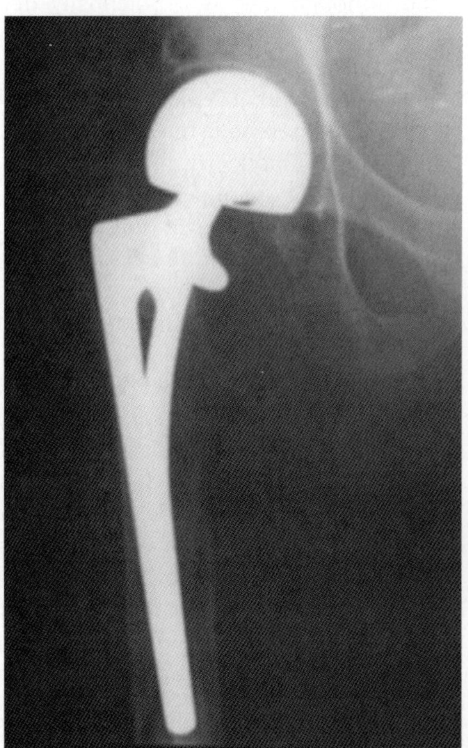

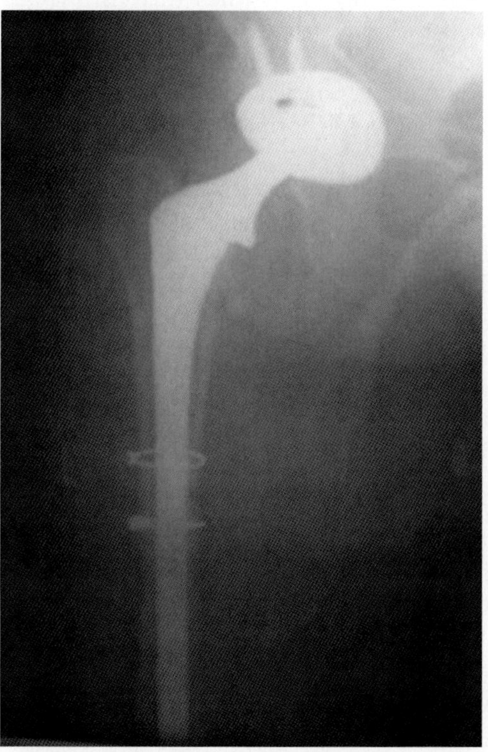

Figure 16.46 Periprosthetic fracture around a hip arthroplasty (**A**) preoperative x-ray, demonstrating a spiral fracture around a hemiarthroplasty and (**B**) postoperative radiograph. The fracture was treated with removal of the implant, cerclage of the fracture with two cables, and reimplantation of a total hip arthroplasty.

as warfarin, low molecular weight heparin, or aspirin for up to 6 weeks following surgery.

The major late complications following primary THA include delayed or chronic deep joint infection and periprosthetic fractures. When a subacute or chronic infection is diagnosed following THA, it is assumed that bacteria have formed a glycocalyx around the implant, and thus, simple irrigation and debridement would be inadequate to eradicate the infection. The typical treatment protocol for late infections requires removal of the implant, placement of an antibiotic cement spacer, a directed course of intravenous antibiotic therapy, and reimplantation of new THA components when laboratory and imaging studies demonstrate no signs of residual infection. Approximately 90% of patients will be able to clear the infection with the use of this two-stage reimplantation technique.

Periprosthetic fractures are fractures that occur around a well-fixed THA construct. Fractures about the femoral component are more common than fractures about the acetabulum; however, acetabular fractures may be seen in cases with significant acetabular bone loss and loss of medial wall integrity. Periprosthetic fractures of the femur are classified on the basis of (a) the level of the fracture about the femur and (b) the quality of fixation of the femoral stem. The Vancouver's classification is the most common periprosthetic fracture classification used to describe these fractures (Table 16.8).

Treatment is dictated on the basis of the stability of the prosthetic component, with loose or unstable components requiring revision THA. Fractures at the level of the intertrochanteric region often do not require surgical fixation. Fractures distal to the stem tip can be treated with a plate that overlaps the distal portion of the femoral stem. Fractures that extend through the region of the stem are treated with plates and cables or revision surgery on the basis of the stability of the femoral component. In general, a revision stem must extend two cortical diameters of the femur beyond the level of the fracture to get adequate fixation (Fig. 16.46).

Osteonecrosis

Osteonecrosis, also referred to as AVN, is defined as death of periarticular bone from an etiology other than infection, with the femoral head being the most commonly affected area in the body. The incidence is approximately 20,000 new cases in the Untied States annually, and osteonecrosis comprises the original diagnosis for nearly 10% of all total hip arthroplasties performed each year. Osteonecrosis typically results from a disruption of the blood supply either secondary to trauma or other causes such as systemic steroid use, alcohol abuse, blood dyscrasias such as sickle cell disease, coagulopathies (protein C or S deficiency or low lipoprotein level), caisson disease, excessive radiation therapy, and metabolic storage diseases such Gaucher's disease. Cases of idiopathic femoral head osteonecrosis is commonly seen in the pediatric population and is termed Legg–Calve–Perthes' disease.

Osteonecrosis typically involves the anterolateral portion of the femoral head and may result in head flattening and eventual head collapse. The pathogenesis of the disease leads to necrotic subchondral bone and subchondral collapse. The histopathologic changes are characterized as follows: (a) inflammation with invasion of primitive mesenchymal tissue and capillaries; (b) deposition of new lamellar bone on necrotic trabecular bone; and (c) remodeling of necrotic trabecular bone by a process known as creeping substitution. Bone is weakest during the remodeling phase, leading to potential subchondral collapse (crescent sign) and fragmentation.

On physical examination, patients typically present with decreased hip abduction and internal rotation and a slight limp during ambulation. Comparison to the contralateral hip is an important adjunct to the physical examination, although up to 80% of patients with steroid-induced AVN will have bilateral hip involvement.

Radiographic evaluation of AVN should start with plain radiographs of the pelvis and two views of the involved

TABLE 16.9
UNIVERSITY OF PENNSYLVANIA SYSTEM FOR STAGING AVASCULAR NECROSIS

Stage	Criteria
0	Normal or nondiagnostic radiography, bone scan, MRI
I	Normal radiographs, abnormal bone scan, and/or MRI
	A. Mild (<15% of femoral head affected)
	B. Moderate (15%–30%)
	C. Severe (>30%)
II	"Cystic" and sclerotic changes in femoral head
	A. Mild (<15% of femoral head affected)
	B. Moderate (15%–30%)
	C. Severe (>30%)
III	Subchondral collapse (crescent sign) without flattening
	A. Mild (<15% of articular surface)
	B. Moderate (15%–30%)
	C. Severe (>30%)
IV	Flattening of femoral head
	A. Mild (<15% of surface and <2-mm depression)
	B. Moderate (15%–30% of surface or 2- to 4-mm depression)
	C. Severe (>30% of surface or >4-mm depression)
V	Joint narrowing or acetabular changes
	A. Mild Average of femoral head involvement, as determined in stage IV, and estimated acetabular involvement
	B. Moderates
	C. Severe
VI	Advanced degenerative changes

Reproduced from Steinberg ME. Diagnostic imaging and the role of stage and lesion size in determining outcome in osteonecrosis of the femoral head. Tech Orthop. 2001;16:6–15.
Reprinted with permission from Steinberg ME, et al. *Tech Orthopaedics.* 2001;16:6–15.

hip. MRI can be utilized to detect early cases with very high sensitivity and specificity. Nuclear medicine bone scans can also be used for early diagnosis, demonstrating increased uptake in areas of bone remodeling.

Several classifications systems have been historically used to define the severity of involvement of the femoral head as well as patient prognosis. The University of Pennsylvania System for Staging Avascular Necrosis evaluates both the radiographic appearance of the lesion as well as the size of the lesion (Table 16.9). This classification determines the likelihood of success when using joint-preserving procedures such as core decompression.

Treatment for osteonecrosis of the hip range from conservative symptomatic therapy with a focus on maintaining hip ROM to joint-preserving alternatives for early AVN to hemiarthroplasty or THA for end-stage AVN. Joint-preserving alternatives include core decompression, vascularized fibular grafting, and proximal femoral osteotomy. Core decompression involves drilling a 6 to 10 mm whole up the femoral neck into the area of necrotic bone in an attempt to stimulate revascularization and healing. Some surgeons will augment the procedure by packing the area with bone graft. The results of this procedure decline rapidly if there is any collapse of the articular surface. In the end-stages of AVN with associated acetabular changes and hip joint degeneration, THA is the treatment of choice; however, there is an increased failure rate in this younger patient population compared with THA for OA.

RECOMMENDED READINGS

Lorich DG, Geller DS, Nielson JH. Osteoporotic pertrochanteric hip fractures: management and current controversies. *J Bone Joint Surg Am*. 2004;86:398–410.

Lieberman JR, Berry DJ, Montv MA, et al. Osteonecrosis of the hip: management in the twenty-first century. *J Bone Joint Surg Am*. 2002;84:834–853.

Sierra RJ, Trousdale RT, Ganz R, Leunig M. Hip disease in the young, active patient: evaluation and nonarthroplasty surgical options *J Am Acad Orthop Surg*. 2008;16:689–703.

Barrack RL. Dislocation after total hip arthroplasty: implant design and orientation. *J Am Acad Ortho Surg*. 2003;11:89–99.

Knee and Leg Injuries

17

Todd Rimington **John Klimkiewicz** **Freddie Fu**

INTRODUCTION

Pain or injury about the knee and leg is one the most frequent conditions prompting a patient to seek evaluation by an orthopaedist. The purpose of this chapter is to review the functional anatomy and evaluation of the knee and leg and to describe the presentation and treatment of the most common traumatic and atraumatic injuries to this area. Knee arthritis and arthroplasty, including periprosthetic fractures about the knee, will be discussed in Chapter 18.

FUNCTIONAL ANATOMY

The knee is composed of three separate articulations: the tibiofemoral, patellofemoral, and the proximal tibiofibular joints. The joint most commonly referred to when describing the "knee joint" is the tibiofemoral joint. The knee is also divided into three compartments: medial, lateral, and patellofemoral. The medial and lateral compartments comprise the tibiofemoral articulations (Fig. 17.1). The distal femur is composed of medial and lateral condyles with the slightly larger and distal medial condyle accounting for the valgus orientation of the normal knee joint. The patellofemoral compartment lies in the anterior knee and contains the patellofemoral articulation (Fig. 17.2). The sulcus between the femoral condyles is called the *trochlear groove*. The patella tracks within this groove as the knee is ranged through flexion and extension. At the distal end of the femur between the femoral condyles, there is an intercondylar notch. The cruciate ligaments of the knee are found within this intercondylar notch. On the medial aspect of the distal femur is the medial epicondyle, which serves as the insertion of the adductor magnus and the origin of the medial collateral ligament (MCL). The lateral epicondyle on the lateral aspect of the distal femur serves as the origin of the lateral collateral ligament (LCL).

The tibiofemoral joint is a modified hinge joint. The greatest range of motion occurs in the sagittal plane (flexion and extension). The knee can also move in the coronal plane (varus and valgus) and the axial plane (internal and external rotation). The chondral surfaces of the femoral condyles articulate with the chondral surfaces of the tibial plateaus. Both medial and lateral plateaus are relatively flat in shape when viewed in the coronal plane. However, in the sagittal plane, the contours of the plateaus are different. The medial plateau demonstrates a gentle concavity into which the medial condyle fits. On sagittal magnetic resonance imaging (MRI) scans, this is described as looking like a golf ball (medial femoral condyle) on a tee (medial tibial plateau) (Fig. 17.3). In contrast, the lateral plateau demonstrates a convexity and is slightly incongruous with the lateral femoral condyle. Therefore, the bony architecture of the tibiofemoral joint alone is relatively incongruent.

The menisci provide enhanced stability to the knee joint. They are medial and lateral fibrocartilaginous structures that provide an interface between the adjacent articular surfaces of the tibiofemoral joint. The medial meniscus is semicircular in shape, and the lateral meniscus is more circular (Fig. 17.4). They are firmly connected to the tibial plateaus through ligament fibers to the tibia called the *meniscotibial* or *coronary ligaments*. The menisci are also attached to the femur by the meniscofemoral ligaments. Although they are firmly attached, some movement is permitted. The lateral meniscus is more mobile than the medial meniscus, accounting for the decreased prevalence of lateral meniscus tears. The movement of the menisci allows them to conform to the moving joint surfaces and avoid positions of sheer. The lateral meniscus's greater mobility is approximately 1 cm in the anterior–posterior plane compared with the medial meniscus's 0.5 cm. This is the result of the lack of attachment of the lateral meniscus along the posterolateral aspect of the knee at the popliteal hiatus where the popliteal tendon passes intra-articularly through the popliteal hiatus.

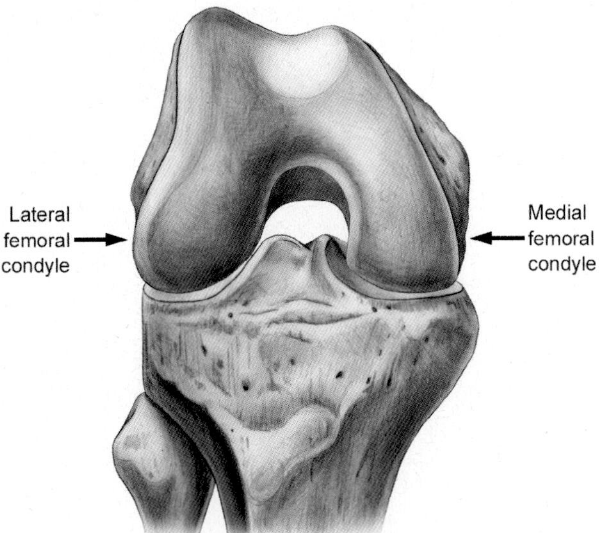

Figure 17.1 The medial and lateral condyles. (*Reproduced with permission from* Johnson DH and Pedowitz RA: *Practical Orthopaedic Sports Medicine and Arthroscopy.* Philadelphia: Lippincott Williams & Wilkins, 2006.)

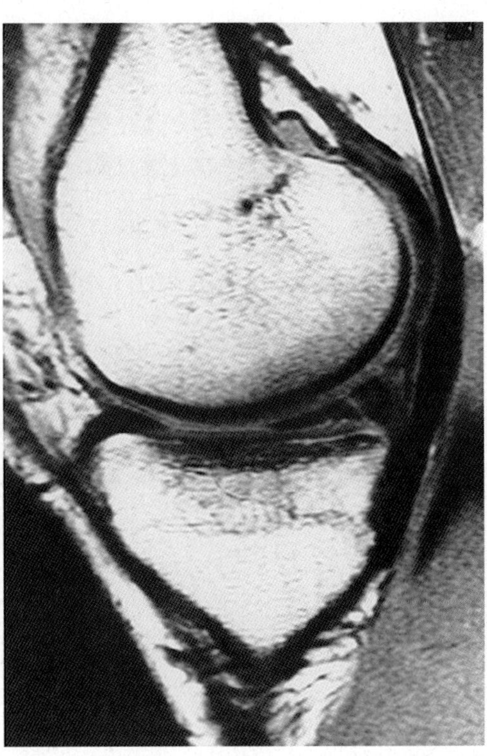

Figure 17.3 A sagittal magnetic resonance imaging of the medial compartment of the knee demonstration to conformity of the convex femoral condyle and the concave medial tibial plateau. A vertical tear of the posterior horn of the medial meniscus is also seen. (*Reproduced with permission from* Chapman MW, Szabo RM, Marder R, et al. *Chapman's Orthopaedic Surgery.* 3rd ed. Philadelphia, PA: Lippincott Williams & Wilkins, 2001.)

The menisci provide several important functions. First and most important is the transmission of joint stresses. As a result of their conforming anatomy, the menisci distribute the forces across the joint surfaces to a larger area and decrease the peak contact stresses. The presence of a meniscus helps to protect the articular surfaces of the knee from excessive peak contact stresses. Biomechanical studies have shown increases in contact pressures up to 300% following meniscus removal. The medial meniscus transmits 50% of the joint force and the lateral meniscus transmits up to 70% of the joint force across the knee. Additional functions of the meniscus include improved joint stability, impact absorption, and articular nourishment.

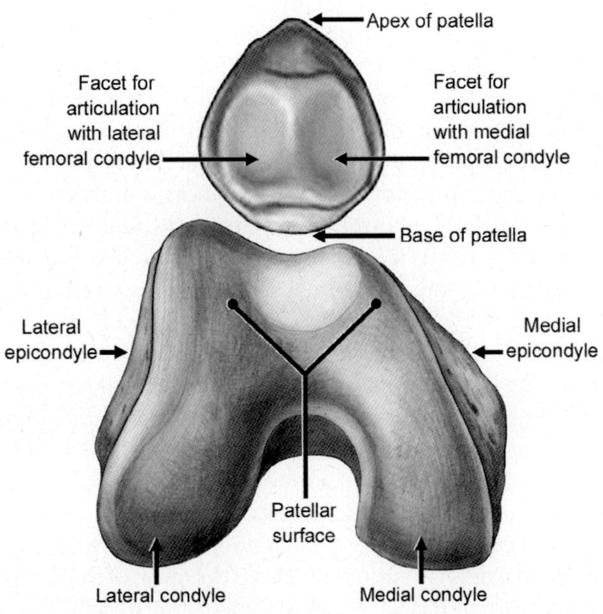

Figure 17.2 The patella articulation with the trochlea of the femur. (*Reproduced with permission from* Johnson DH and Pedowitz RA: *Practical Orthopaedic Sports Medicine and Arthroscopy.* Philadelphia: Lippincott Williams & Wilkins, 2006.)

The bone of the distal femur and proximal tibia is covered by a highly organized structure of hyaline cartilage. The articular cartilage thickness varies with location. The patella has the thickest articular cartilage in the human body, and it is 8 to 10 mm thick. The cartilage is composed of type II collagen, whose structure allows it to absorb impact and accommodate to the variable forces of compression, tension, and sheer seen in this joint.

Although joint congruence through the bone and meniscal anatomy provides some inherent stability, most joint security is conferred by the surrounding soft tissue structures, including the joint capsule and ligaments. The capsule of the knee is a variably thick structure lined by synovium. This layer is responsible for the synovial fluid production that accounts for the knee's low coefficient of friction. Perhaps the most important macromolecule synthesized by the synovium is hyaluronic acid, which serves to lubricate the joint surfaces. External to the synovium is the fibrous capsular envelope of the knee, which varies in

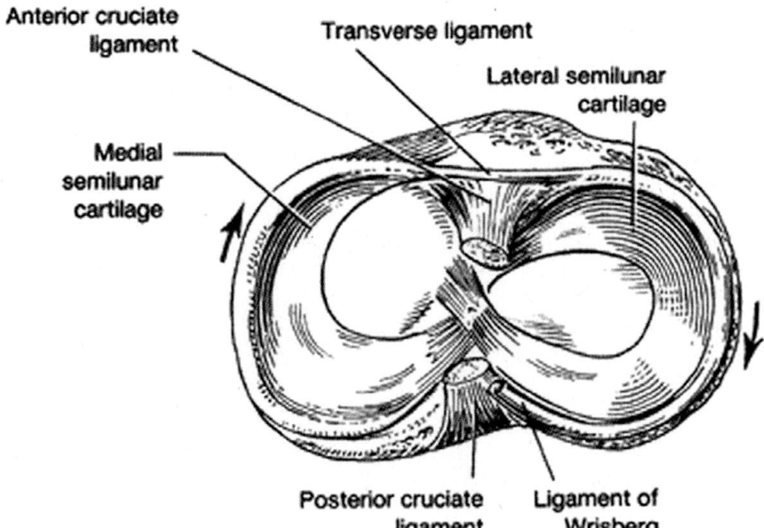

Figure 17.4 Superior surface of tibia with superimposed medial and lateral menisci. (After Helfet AJ. The Management of Internal Derangements of the Knee. Philadelphia: JB Lippincott, 1963. *Reproduced with permission from* Chapman MW, Szabo RM, Marder R, et al.: *Chapman's Orthopaedic Surgery*, 3rd ed. Philadelphia: Lippincott Williams & Wilkins, 2001.)

thickness according to the region. Somewhat thin in the anterior portion of the knee, it is thicker and reinforced by numerous discrete fibrous ligament complexes posteriorly. The posterolateral reinforcement is the arcuate ligament and posteromedially is the posteromedial oblique ligament.

The ligaments of the knee are responsible for most joint stability and include the collateral ligaments and the cruciate ligaments. These ligaments are discrete collagen bundles that connect one bone to another. The cruciate ligaments provide stability in the sagittal and axial planes. The cruciate ligaments work together to guide the articular surfaces during knee motion. They are critical in maintaining this normal relationship. The anterior cruciate ligament (ACL) originates from a broad footprint on the anteromedial tibia, passes through the intercondylar notch, and attaches to the posterolateral aspect of the intercondylar notch on the lateral femoral condyle. The average length of the ACL is 32 to 33 mm. The ACL is divided into two separate bundles, the posterolateral and anteromedial bundles. They are named by their tibial insertion. The anteromedial bundle is reconstructed in a traditional ACL reconstruction. The tension in the two bundles varies with the position of the knee; the anteromedial bundle is tight in flexion, and the posterolateral bundle is tight in extension (Fig. 17.5). The ACL is the primary restraint to anterior tibial translation. The middle geniculate artery is the blood supply of the cruciate ligaments.

The posterior cruciate ligament (PCL) crosses posterior to the ACL within the intercondylar notch. This cross formation with the notch is the reason they are called *cruciate ligaments*. The PCL arises on the posterior aspect of the tibial plateau, passes through the intercondylar notch posterior to the ACL, and inserts on the anteromedial aspect of the notch of the medial femoral condyle. The average length of the PCL is 38 mm. The two bundles of the PCL are the anterolateral and posteromedial bundles. The tension in the two bundles varies with the position of the knee; the anterolateral is tight in flexion, and the posteromedial is tight in extension (Fig. 17.6). The PCL is the primary restraint to posterior tibial translation.

The collateral ligaments provide stability in the coronal plane. The MCL is composed of two discrete bundles: a superficial bundle and a deep bundle (Fig. 17.7). The superficial MCL arises from the medial epicondyle of the femur and travels inferiorly to a broad proximal medial tibial

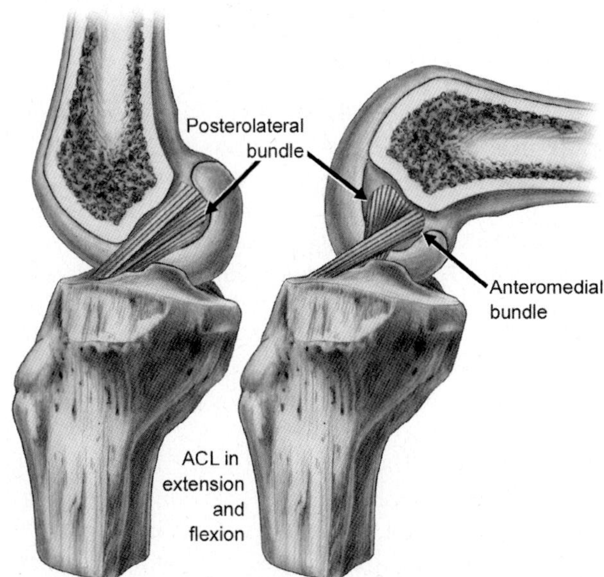

Figure 17.5 The two bundles of the anterior cruciate ligament (ACL). (*Reproduced with permission from* Johnson DH, Pedowitz RA. *Practical Orthopaedic Sports Medicine and Arthroscopy*. Philadelphia, PA: Lippincott Williams & Wilkins, 2006.)

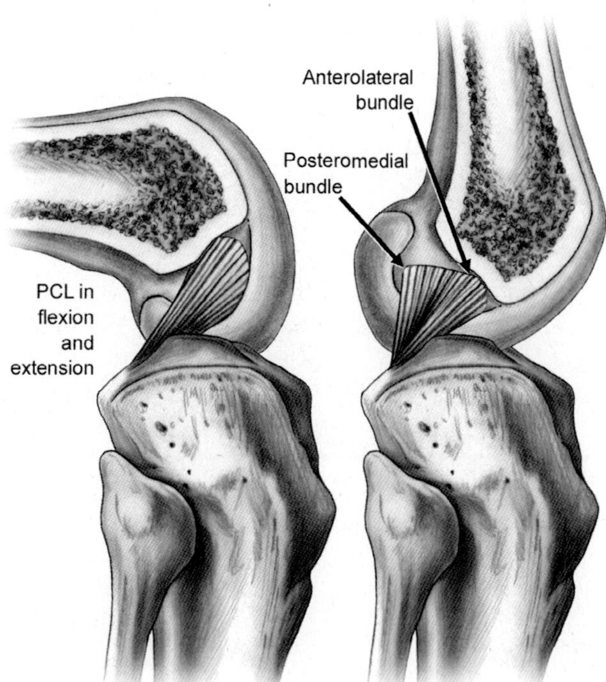

Figure 17.6 The two bundles of the posterior cruciate ligament (PCL). (*Reproduced with permission from* Johnson DH, Pedowitz RA. *Practical Orthopaedic Sports Medicine and Arthroscopy.* Philadelphia, PA: Lippincott Williams & Wilkins, 2006.)

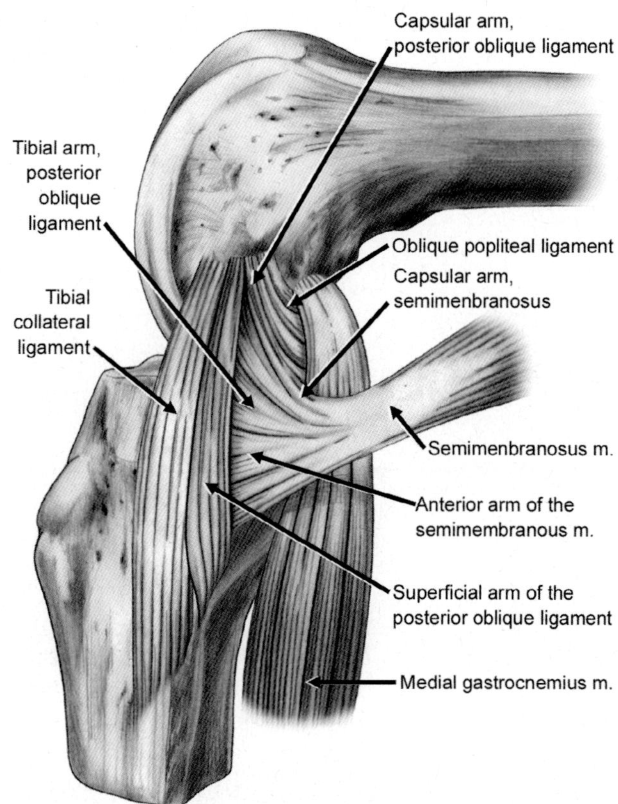

Figure 17.7 The structures of the medial side of the knee. (*Reproduced with permission from* Johnson DH, Pedowitz RA. *Practical Orthopaedic Sports Medicine and Arthroscopy.* Philadelphia, PA: Lippincott Williams & Wilkins, 2006.)

attachment approximately 8 cm inferior to the medial joint line. The deep MCL is composed of the capsule of the medial knee joint. The MCL is the primary restraint to valgus stress about the knee. The LCL travels from the lateral femoral epicondyle to the fibular head (Fig. 17.8). It can be palpated when the knee is in the "figure-of-four" position. The LCL is the primary restraint to varus force about the knee.

The patellofemoral joint consists of the intercondylar groove in the anterior distal femur and the patella. The patella is a sesamoid bone encased with the quadriceps mechanism. The patella increases the power of the quadriceps mechanism by moving the quadriceps mechanism anterior to the center of the knee joint. This increases the moment arm of the quadriceps and decreases the force necessary to actively extend the knee. Clinical data show that patients treated with removal of the patella (patellectomy) experience 30% weakness in their quadriceps mechanism.

The patella articulates with the distal femur in its trochlear groove. The posterior surface of the patella contains medial and lateral facets that congruently track within the trochlear groove in a very specific manner. The patella is loosely held in place by its anatomic convex–concave arrangement and by the medial and lateral retinacular ligaments. The patellofemoral joint carries large loads, particularly during activities in which the knee is flexed. During stair climbing the patellofemoral joint can experience loads 3 times the body weight, this increase to as much as 6 times the body weight with stair descent.

The final joint of the knee is the proximal tibiofibular joint. This joint is often overlooked and an occasionally unrecognized source of knee or leg pain. A diarthrodial joint, the articular surfaces are surrounded by a synovial-lined capsule with strong reinforcing anterior and posterior ligaments. This joint is at risk of developing the same pathology as that seen in other joints, including arthritis, trauma, and synovial disease.

The most important muscles around the knee include the quadriceps mechanism anteriorly, the hamstrings posteriorly, the pes tendons medially, and the iliotibial (IT) band laterally. The quadriceps mechanism is composed of four muscles: the rectus femoris, vastus lateralis, vastus intermedius, and the vastus medialis. The rectus femoris arises from the anterior inferior iliac spine and the hip capsule and inserts onto the tibia. The remaining quadriceps muscles originate on the femur and insert with the rectus femoris as the patella tendon at the tibial tubercle. All four muscles are innervated by the femoral nerve. The quadriceps mechanism is the primary extender of the knee.

Posteriorly, the hamstrings originate from the ischial tuberosity and travel distally to attach on the posterior tibia

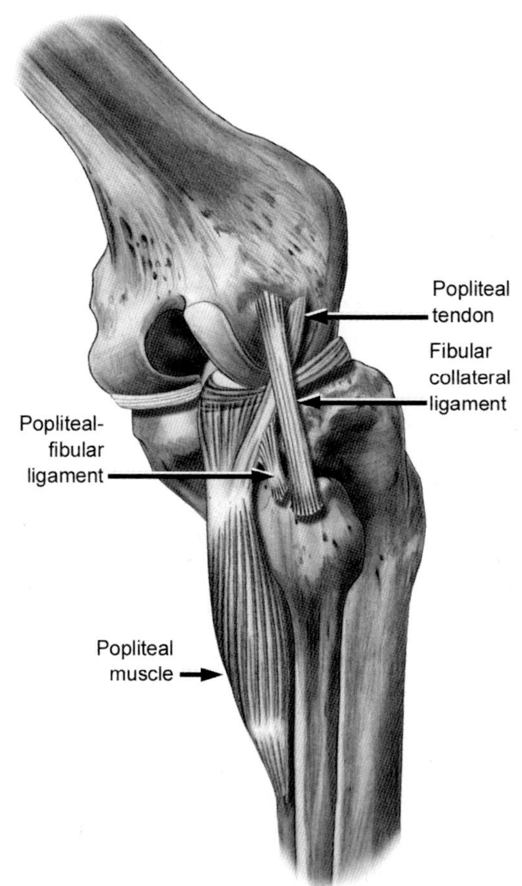

Figure 17.8 The structures of the lateral side of the knee. (*Reproduced with permission from* Johnson DH, Pedowitz RA. *Practical Orthopaedic Sports Medicine and Arthroscopy.* Philadelphia, PA: Lippincott Williams & Wilkins, 2006.)

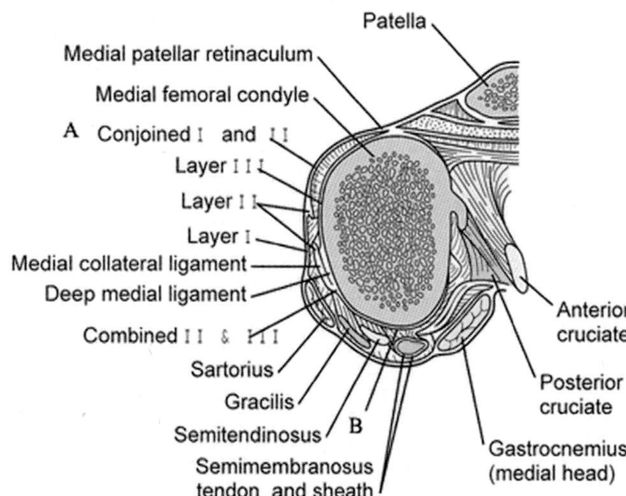

Figure 17.9 Transverse section through the distal femur. A: The retinacular fibers, which are the conjoined layers I and II. B: The conjoined layer-II and -III fibers posterior to the medial collateral ligament. (*Redrawn from* Warren LF, Marshall JL. The Supporting Structures of the Medial Side of the Knee. *J Bone Joint Surg* 1979; 61-A:56. *Reproduced with permission from Chapman MW, Szabo RM, Marder R, et al.: Chapman's Orthopaedic Surgery,* 3rd ed. Philadelphia: Lippincott Williams & Wilkins, 2001.)

and fibula. Medially, the semimembranosus and semitendinosus insert at the proximal tibia and posteromedial capsule. Laterally, the biceps femoris inserts along the fibular head. Branches of the sciatic nerve innervate the hamstring muscles. The hamstrings are the primary flexors of the knee.

The tendons of the gracilis, semitendinosus, and sartorius are found medially (Fig. 17.9). These tendons arise from the pubis, ischial tuberosity, and anterior superior iliac spine (ASIS), respectively, and insert over the anteromedial aspect of the proximal tibia superficial to the MCL. The appearance of these three structures led Greek observers to describe them structure as a *"pes anserine"* in its similarity to a duck's webbed foot. Clinically, this structure is responsible for symptoms when its underlying bursa become irritated (pes bursitis) and is a popular source of autograft tendons during reconstructive surgery.

Laterally, the IT band is a strong broad flat band that originates at the iliac crest, receives insertions of the gluteus maximus and tensor fascia lata, and travels inferiorly to insert at Gerdy's tubercle on the proximal anterolateral tibia (Fig. 17.10). From 0 to 30 degrees, the IT band contributes to knee extension. Beyond 30 degrees, the IT band contributes to knee flexion. The IT band is clinically relevant in causing a friction syndrome over the lateral aspect of the knee, known as *runner's* or *cyclist's* knee. The IT band is also thought to be mechanically responsible for the pivot shift maneuver seen in ACL deficiency.

Posteriorly, there are several other muscle groups of importance, including the medial and lateral gastrocnemii, which originate from their respective posterior femoral condyles along with an indirect slip from the joint capsule. The gastrocnemii combine with the soleus to from the triceps surae muscle, whose tendinous portion is known as the Achilles tendon. Deep to the gastrocnemii, originating from the midpoint of the posterior proximal tibia, is the popliteus muscle. The popliteus travels superolaterally and enters the knee joint capsule directly posterior to the lateral meniscus and exits again to attach just inferior to the lateral epicondyle. The insertion of the popliteus is anterior and distal to the LCL origin. This structure is important in contributing to normal knee function by unlocking the tibial plateau via internal rotation of the tibia at the beginning of knee flexion.

There are a number of bursae in the knee, including the prepatellar, pes, IT, and semimembranosus bursae. All of these bursae are synovial-lined potential sacs that serve as lubricated interfaces between adjacent moving surfaces. The prepatellar bursa is detected only when it becomes symptomatic and inflates in response to trauma or irritation, most commonly in patients with direct trauma to the anterior aspect of their knee. Repetitive or direct trauma leads to inflammation, occasional thickening, and

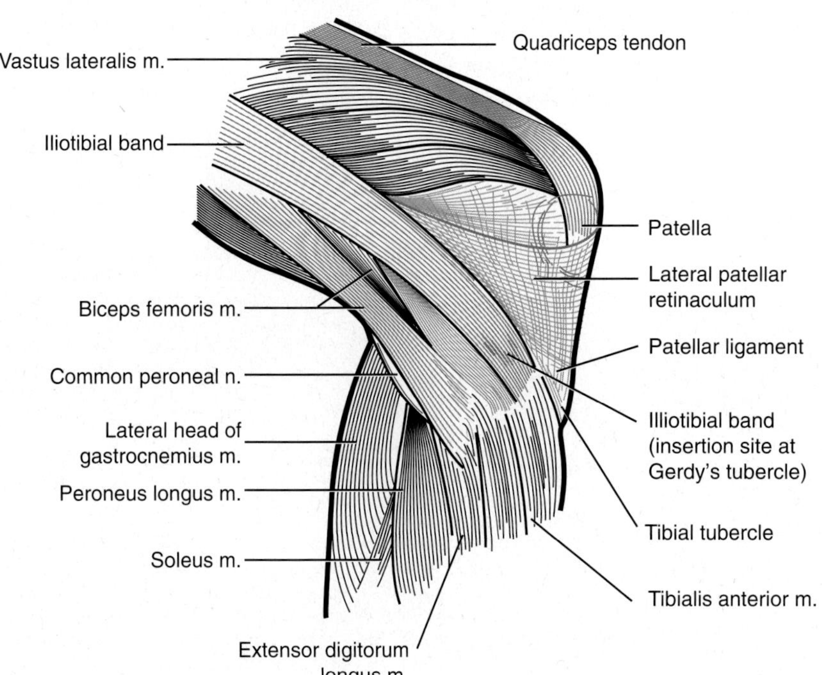

Figure 17.10 A slightly anterolateral view of the outer layer of the knee. The lateral patellar retinaculum, the biceps femoris, and the iliotibial band constitute the outer layer. (*Adapted from* Hoppenfeld S and deBoer P: *Surgical Exposures in Orthopaedics*, 3rd ed. Philadelphia: Lippincott Williams & Wilkins, 2004.)

swelling. The pes bursa lies between the pes tendons and the underlying anteromedial tibia. Inflammation here often leads to anteromedial knee pain. Laterally, inflammation and irritation of the IT band over the lateral epicondyle is a common problem in running athletes and cyclists, leading to IT band friction syndrome. Finally, a bursa in the posteromedial aspect of the knee between the posteromedial capsule and the semimembranosus can become swollen and historically has been called a Baker cyst. A Baker cyst is most commonly located between the semimembranosus and the medial head of the gastrocnemius. More recently, clinicians recognize that this structure is in fact a prominent semimembranosus bursa.

Important neurovascular structures about the knee include the posterior femoral artery, which becomes the popliteal artery at the adductor hiatus. Distal to the joint, the popliteal artery divides into three branches: an anterior branch, the anterior tibial artery, which travels anterior piercing the interosseous membrane; a posterior branch, the posterior tibial artery; and a lateral branch, the peroneal artery. This trifurcation is of clinical significance because it tethers the popliteal artery to the posterior tibia, making it vulnerable to injury during leg trauma. Important nerves include the sciatic nerve, which runs with the popliteal artery, and branches into the tibial nerve, which runs with the posterior tibial artery, and the common peroneal nerve, which travels laterally around the fibular neck. There are also several smaller nerves of clinical significance. The infrapatellar branch of the saphenous nerve travels along the medial aspect of the knee and provides sensation to the anteromedial and lateral sensory dermatomes. This nerve's proximity to the common anterior, midline surgical approach to the knee puts it at risk for damage with this approach. It is also at risk during harvesting of the medial hamstring tendons and medial exposures of the knee for open meniscal repair. Damage can result in a neuroma medially or a sensory deficit along the anterolateral aspect of the leg. The obturator nerve provides innervation to the distal medial thigh and is of little significance in the adult population, but in children, it may be a source of referred hip pain. The common peroneal nerve provides motor and sensory innervation to the anterior and lateral compartments of the leg and foot and is vulnerable as it courses anteriorly around the fibular neck. The nerve is vulnerable to both traumatic and iatrogenic injury from surgical exploration on the lateral side of the knee. The superficial peroneal nerve is at risk during surgery on the lateral compartment of the leg.

In the leg, there are four muscular compartments, including the anterior, lateral, superficial posterior, and deep posterior (Fig. 17.11). Each has specific muscle groups and neurovascular structures surrounded by a fascial envelope. The risk of increased pressure within this envelope due to trauma, disease, or overuse makes recognition and understanding of the anatomy of each of these compartments clinically important. The anterior compartment is composed of the tibialis anterior, extensor digitorum, and the extensor hallicus longus. The deep peroneal nerve and the anterior tibial artery supply the anterior compartment. The lateral compartment is composed of the peroneus longus and brevis. The superficial peroneal nerve contributes motor supply to this compartment, which is divided from the anterior compartment by the lateral intermuscular septum. Posteriorly, there are two separate compartments: the deep

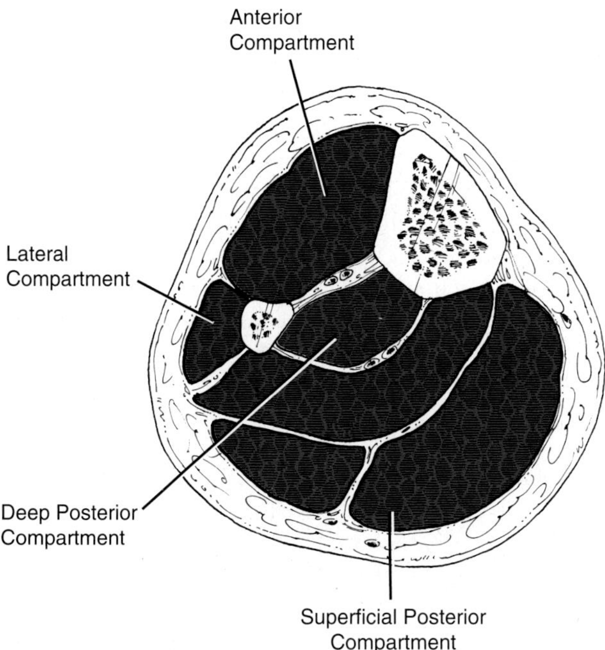

Figure 17.11 The four compartments of the leg. (*Reproduced with permission from* Bucholz RW, Heckman JD, Court-Brown C, Tornetta P. *Rockwood and Green's Fractures in Adults*, 6th Ed. Philadelphia: Lippincott Williams & Wilkins, 2005.)

and superficial compartments. The deep compartment is composed of the flexor digitorum, flexor hallucis longus, and posterior tibialis. The superficial compartment is composed of the soleus, the gastrocnemii, and the plantaris tendon. All posterior compartment muscles are supplied by the posterior tibial nerve.

EVALUATION OF THE KNEE AND LEG

The evaluation of the knee and leg depends on an understanding of normal knee anatomy, techniques of physical examination, and familiarity with common knee conditions. A history and physical examination, complemented as necessary by radiographs, can diagnose most problems. Special tests are not commonly required, although MRI is sometimes helpful.

Although familiarity with how to perform a systematic knee examination approach is important, a comprehensive examination is not usually required in every patient. Instead, the examination should be tailored to the patient's presentation. For example, examination of a 72-year-old with progressive knee pain should be different from the examination of an 18-year-old football player following a traumatic injury. Understanding how to perform a basic overall examination is an important skill, but knowing when to perform the various specific examination techniques is a learned art. A thorough history usually alerts the examiner to the most likely diagnostic conditions and facilitates a tailored examination in the context of the differential diagnosis.

The examiner should always take advantage of the body's symmetry. The opposite knee and leg serve as an excellent control that can help distinguish a normal from an abnormal examination with respect to atrophy, swelling, motion, strength, and stability. Because of normal variability within the population, the use of the patients opposite limb can make diagnostic evaluation more accurate.

Finally, it is important for the physician to remember that knee symptoms can be caused by pathology elsewhere. Common sources of referred pain in adults are the spine and hip, and in children, knee pain is considered hip pathology until proven otherwise.

History

Obtaining a careful history is as important as the actual physical examination. The most common presenting symptoms include pain, swelling, giving way, clicking, catching, and locking. First, determine the patient's chief complaint. The most common complaint is that of knee pain. Next, gather information about the chief complaint. The following 10 questions are important to any knee history.

1. When was the onset of the pain?

   Acute injuries are suggestive of ligament injuries, meniscus injuries, or fractures. It is important to determine the inciting event. The mechanism of a traumatic injury is important to determine the severity of the traumatic force applied to the joint. Chronic injuries are more likely degenerative in nature.

2. Where (point to it) does the pain hurt the most?

   Patients can generally localize their pain to a specific pain generator. The location of the pain can help limit the injury to a specific compartment of the knee. Anterior knee pain is typical of patella disorders. Medial or lateral joint line pain is generally a chondral injury or a meniscus injury.

3. What is the nature of the pain?

   Patella disorders are typically a dull ache. Meniscus injuries are typically a sharp, catching pain.

4. What makes the pain worse?

   Most knee injuries are worse with activity. Patella disorders are worse with ascending or descending stairs and sitting for prolonged periods in a chair. Meniscus injuries are worse with twisting, turning, or squatting movements. Cycling or rowing may exacerbate IT band syndrome.

5. When did the knee first swell, and does it continue to swell?

The onset of swelling after the injury is important. Intraarticular swelling or effusion within the first 2 hours after trauma suggests hemarthrosis. Hemarthrosis can be caused by ACL tear, peripheral meniscus tear, or chondral injury such as with a knee dislocation, whereas swelling that occurs overnight usually is an indication of acute traumatic synovitis. This can be a reaction to the traumatic injury and is less specific. The frequency of swelling should be determined. Causes of recurrent swelling include synovial disorders such as inflammatory arthritis, degenerative arthritis, gout, and pseudogout.

6. Does the knee "give way"?

This generally reflects a functional weakness in which the quadriceps suddenly stops contracting, allowing the knee to involuntarily bend or "give way." Giving way is a nonspecific symptom that can occur in patellofemoral pain syndrome, patellar instability, meniscus tears, ligament injuries, and chondral injuries. This process is often due to "reflex inhibition of pain," in which sudden impending joint overload or pain stimuli are transmitted through a reflex arc and cause the quadriceps to stop firing. A second reason for giving way is actual quadriceps weakness. Giving way can also occur with instability. The most common cause of instability is patellar instability with lateral patellar subluxation or dislocation. ACL-deficient knees can also sublux and give way with twisting, turning, or cutting movements.

7. Has the knee "locked"?

Locking is a very specific phenomenon and generally reflects meniscal pathology or a loose body, such as a displaced osteochondral fracture fragment. Locking implies a transient inability to flex or extend the knee, lasting from minutes to days. Generally the knee is fixed in 10 to 20 degrees of flexion and cannot be straightened. Episodes may occur spontaneously or follow a twist or squat. In locked knees with a torn meniscus, the meniscus is usually torn and subluxed within the joint in the configuration of a bucket handle. Some patients complain of locking episodes in which their knee seems to get stuck for a few seconds. This has been called "pseudolocking." This can occur for a variety of reasons such as chondral injury, loose bodies, patellofemoral pain syndrome, and synovial irritation. During knee range of motion, the typical smooth gliding and rotation does not occur and instead the knee joint surfaces jam together, creating a momentary pause in motion.

8. What improves the pain?

Rest and activity modification almost always improve knee pain. A red flag should be raised if the pain is constant and unrelated to activities. Constant pain should raise concern for more serious problems such as osteonecrosis, tumor, infection, thrombophlebitis, and neuropathic syndromes. It is also helpful to obtain a history about previous treatment with nonsteroidal anti-inflammatory drugs (NSAIDs), corticosteroid injections, and physical therapy to help formulate a treatment plan.

9. Does the pain radiate?

In children, hip pathology may present as knee pain. In adults, knee pain can radiate from the hip or low back. Asking about the hip and back as pain generators can sometimes reveal the true source of the pain. In addition, radiating pain can be the sign of a neurologic problem such as lumbar stenosis or a peripheral nerve compressive neuropathy.

10. How does the pain interfere with your activities?

This information will help you formulate a treatment plan. You must first understand patients' motivation and their goals before formulating a treatment plan. A sedentary elderly patient with knee pain should be treated differently than a young competitive runner. Once you understand how this injury affects their work and recreational lifestyle, you can formulate the best treatment plan for them.

These 10 questions should be combined with a detailed medical and surgical history to elucidate any medical problems that may affect treatment course. After a detailed but efficient history, orthopaedists should have a limited differential diagnosis in place that will allow them to use the physical examination to determine the correct diagnosis.

Physical Examination

The physical examination of the knee should include a basic knee examination combined with special tests based on the differential diagnosis established from the history. A basic knee examination should include inspection, palpation, range-of-motion, and stability testing. The basic examination is done first, followed by the appropriate special tests.

Inspection

Both lower extremities should be undressed completely for examination to allow comparison between the two extremities. Observe patients' gait as they walk down the hallway at their normal cadence. Note any evidence of pain that results in an antalgic gait. In this gait, more time is spent of the unaffected leg during the stance phase of gait. Also, note the presence of abnormal motion, either from stiffness or a varus, valgus, or hyperextension thrust. Observe the patient standing at rest to determine the overall alignment of the leg. Note the position of the patients' foot's medial arch while standing. If the arch collapses or the foot pronates, this can negatively affect patellofemoral disorders and medial tibial stress syndrome (shin splints); an orthotic can be effective form of treatment for these patients. Also note the alignment of the knee while standing. The normal alignment of the knee is 5 to 7 degrees of valgus. Last, evaluate the patients' skin for ecchymoses, erythema, abrasions, wounds, and swelling. Be certain to inspect the popliteal fossa to ensure that an occult laceration or abrasion does not escape detection.

Palpation

Knee palpation should be systematic so that you do not overlook areas of potential pain generators. First, the soft tissues and skin should be evaluated for swelling, turgor, integrity, tenderness, or crepitus. If swelling is detected, it must be determined whether the swelling is in the subcutaneous tissues or a knee joint effusion. A joint effusion can be detected by the ballottement test or the fluid wave test. The ballottement test is performed with the knee extended, first one hand milks fluid from the suprapatellar pouch inferiorly into the knee joint. Then the other hand applies a posterior force to the anterior aspect of the patella. This force compresses the patella into the fluid of the knee effusion, and when the pressure is released, the patella bounces back anteriorly. When swelling is present over the anterior patella and seems circumscribed but is not ballotable, a prepatellar effusion is present and not a joint effusion.

The fluid wave test can detect a smaller knee joint effusion. In the test, one hand milks fluid from the suprapatellar pouch while the other hand is positioned so that the index finger is placed on one side of the patella and the thumb is placed on the other side. Then the thumb is used to apply pressure while the index finger is used to detect the transmission of a fluid wave on the other side of the joint. The fluid wave test is subtle and requires practice.

Next, palpate the knee for soft tissue integrity and the presence of any soft tissue defect. This includes the presence of an extensor mechanism disruption. Palpate the quadriceps tendon superior to the superior pole of the patella for defects and then palpate the patellar tendon inferior to the inferior pole of the patella for defects.

Then palpate the knee for tenderness. This is the most familiar part of the knee examination and requires exact knowledge of the anatomy of the knee and attention to detail. The knee should be palpated from proximally to distally in a systematic manner to ensure completeness. Diagnostic accuracy and patient comfort can be improved by examining less symptomatic areas first for reassurance and demonstration of intended gentleness of the examination. Examination of the patient's countenance during the examination will often improve the examination reliability.

Anteriorly, palpate the extensor mechanism, including the rectus femoris, vastus lateralis, vastus medialis, the retinaculum, patella, patella tendon, and the tibial tubercle. Medially, palpate the medial epicondyle, medial joint line, course of the superficial MCL, MCL insertion, pes tendons, and pes insertion. Laterally, palpate the lateral epicondyle, lateral joint line, course of the LCL, LCL insertion, fibular head, and Gerdy tubercle. Palpate both joint lines from anterior to posterior. Palpate the medial and lateral patella facets by subluxing the patella to the medial or lateral side to facilitate palpation of its deep surface. Palpate posteriorly in the popliteal fossa for tenderness or a mass.

Last, palpate the knee for crepitus. Crepitus refers to a grating sensation that is felt by placing one's hand over the patellofemoral joint while the patient actively extends the knee. Although crepitus is not necessarily pathologic, the presence of crepitus should be compared with the opposite side. Crepitus can be suggestive of patellofemoral arthritis.

Range of Motion

The normal range of motion of the knee in flexion and extension is 0 to 140 degrees, but 5 to 10 degrees of hyperextension is often possible. When the knee is flexed at 90 degrees, passive rotation of the tibia on the femur can be demonstrated up to 25 or 30 degrees. The degree of passive rotation varies from patient to patient. However, the amount of internal rotation always exceeds that of external rotation. When the knee is fully extended, no rotation is possible. Sagittal displacement of the tibia on the fixed femur is detectable in both the anterior and posterior directions when the knee is flexed. The normal extent of sagittal displacement should not exceed 3 to 5 mm. When the knee is extended, lateral (abduction–adduction) motion at the knee joint occurs to a limited extent and should not exceed 6 to 8 degrees. With the knee hyperextended, no lateral motion should be present. With the knee flexed, lateral motion is possible but should not exceed 15 degrees.

The range of motion of the knee joint should be compared with that of the opposite, uninjured knee. Range of motion of the knee should be evaluated both actively and passively. Loss of flexion is nonspecific, and it is seen in nearly every situation where the knee is painful. It is important to pay careful attention to the loss of extension as it can help narrow the differential. The different degrees of active and passive motion can indicate possible pathology.

1. Decreased active and passive motion

   This motion is likely due to some type of mechanical block within the knee. Mechanical blocks within the knee can include a joint effusion, a displaced bucket handle meniscus tear, an ACL stump (cyclops lesion), and a loose body (chondral fragment). Pain can also limit both active and passive motion. In degenerative arthritis, a flexion contracture can form as the knee loses both active and passive extension. The loss of extension in the arthritic knee occurs from both pain and recurrent effusion that eventually results in tightening of the posterior capsule.

2. Decreased active but normal passive motion

This motion is likely due to pathology involving the extensor mechanism such as quadriceps tendon rupture, patella fracture, or patella tendon rupture. In addition, injury to the knee can cause reflex quadriceps inhibition, causing an inability of the quadriceps to actively contract with maintained passive motion. Quadriceps inhibition generally resolves with time or with resolution of the joint effusion. A femoral nerve lesion would also prevent quadriceps contraction and decrease active motion with normal passive motion.

One way to compare lack of extension is with heel height difference. The patient is placed prone, and the height difference of the affected heel is compared with the unaffected contralateral heel. Each centimeter of height difference is roughly equivalent to 1 degree of loss of extension. The degree of extension can also be measured with a goniometer and compared between the knees.

Ligament Evaluation

The examination of the knee ligaments can be one of the most difficult aspects of the knee physical examination. It is important to evaluate the uninvolved knee for comparison as this can be considered the normal degree of laxity for the patient in most cases. In general, ligament evaluation involves stressing the joint in the direction that is usually protected by the specific ligament in question. In addition, the ligament's origin, midsubstance, and insertion should be palpated if possible. The four major knee ligaments are the MCL, ACL, PCL, and LCL.

Ligament injuries are graded according to I-to-III (mild, moderate, severe) classification scale. A type I (mild) sprain involves ligament injury without detectable laxity and a solid endpoint. A type II (moderate) sprain involves minimal laxity with a soft endpoint and represents a partial disruption. A type III (severe) sprain involves complete disruption of the ligament without an endpoint. Injury is determined by the following:

1. The amount of "opening" compared with the opposite side, measured in either degrees or millimeters.
2. The abnormal quality of the endpoint with a soft feel upon application of stress rather than a firm or discrete endpoint.
3. The reproduction of symptoms, usually pain with stress testing.

The MCL is the most commonly injured ligament of the knee. The MCL prevents valgus movement of the knee. Although its course can be traced from the medial epicondyle of the femur to the proximal medial tibia, it cannot be palpated. However, tenderness to palpation along the course of the ligament does correspond to the site of the tear. Integrity of the MCL is tested by applying a valgus stress to the slightly flexed knee, 15 to 30 degrees. The patient is placed supine with the knee slightly flexed off the table. One hand applies a medial force to the distal femur and one hand grabs the distal tibia and applies a lateral force to it (Fig. 17.12). The degree of opening and the endpoint is evaluated. Injury to the MCL leads to both pain and opening of the knee when a valgus stress is applied.

The ACL is the next most common injured ligament of the knee. The ACL prevents anterior translation of the tibia on the femur. Physical examination of the ACL is more difficult than the MCL because it cannot be palpated. The main examinations for the ACL are the Lachman test, the anterior drawer test, and the pivot shift test. The Lachman test is the most sensitive test for an ACL tear. It is performed with the patient supine and the knee flexed 15 to 30 degrees off the edge of the table. The femur is held securely in one hand and the tibia is firmly grasped with the other hand, and an attempt is made to translate the tibia anteriorly (Fig. 17.13). The test is positive if the tibia translates anteriorly greater than the contralateral side or shows an abnormal endpoint. Generally the Lachman test is not painful. False negatives can occur if the patient's leg musculature is not relaxed, and it may help to put a pillow behind the patient's knee before performing the examination. The anterior drawer test is less sensitive than the Lachman test. In this test, the knee is flexed to 90 degrees with the patient supine. While the foot is fixed, usually with the examiner sitting on it, both hands grasp the proximal tibia and attempt to translate it anteriorly. As with the Lachman test, the test is positive if the tibia translates anteriorly greater than the contralateral side or shows an abnormal endpoint. The anterior drawer test is generally less reliable because of pain, swelling, and hamstring spasm. The pivot shift test is the most specific ACL test. This test evaluates the ACL's function on both anterior and rotational knee stability. The patient is placed supine and the foot is grabbed and internally rotated. Using the heel of the opposite hand, a valgus stress is applied to the proximal tibia as the knee is flexed from an extended position. Because the ACL-deficient knee is subluxed anterolaterally in the extended position, it reduces with a palpable and a visible clunk at 30 degrees of flexion. The clunk occurs as the IT band becomes a knee flexor at 30 degrees and reduces the tibia posteriorly. The pivot shift test demonstrates functional incompetence of the ACL. These patients are at risk for knee subluxation during cutting or twisting movements. This test is difficult to perform on awake, alert patients and often can be performed only once because it produces an uncomfortable instability sensation and pain. Therefore, the test is commonly used in the

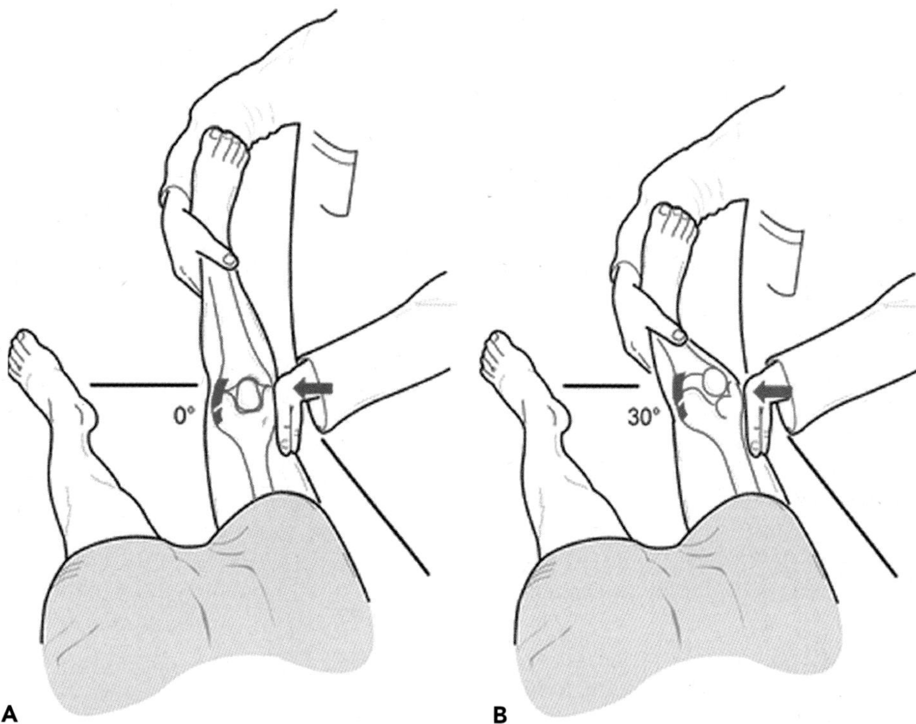

Figure 17.12 Test for varus and valgus laxity at 0° and 30° of knee flexion. (Redrawn from Tria AJ, Klein KS. *An Illustrated Guide to the Knee.* New York: Churchill Livingstone, 1992, with permission. *Reproduced with permission from* Chapman MW, Szabo RM, Marder R, et al.: *Chapman's Orthopaedic Surgery*, 3rd ed. Philadelphia: Lippincott Williams & Wilkins, 2001.)

operation room after the induction of general anesthesia to verify that the ACL is functionally incompetent prior to ACL reconstruction graft harvest/preparation.

The PCL is injured less frequently than the ACL. The PCL prevents posterior translation of the tibia on the femur. The PCL is examined with the sag sign, the posterior drawer test, and the quadriceps active test. The sag sign, "Godfrey test," is observed with the patient supine and the knee flexed to 90 degrees. The amount of posterior displacement of the tibia on the femur in this position is compared with the contralateral knee. The posterior drawer test is then performed. First, the tibia is reduced from its posteriorly subluxed position. Then both hands are used to force the proximal tibia posteriorly. The amount of translation and the end point are evaluated (Fig. 17.14). The quadriceps active test can also be performed in this position with the patient supine and the knee flexed to 90 degrees. The examiner sits on the patient's foot to prevent extension of the knee. Then the amount of posterior sag is noted, and the patient is asked to attempt to straighten out the leg. The contraction of the quadriceps reduces the posteriorly subluxed tibia.

The LCL is the least commonly injured knee ligament. The LCL prevents varus movement of the knee. The ligament can be palpated for tenderness along its course from the lateral epicondyle to the head of the fibula. The LCL

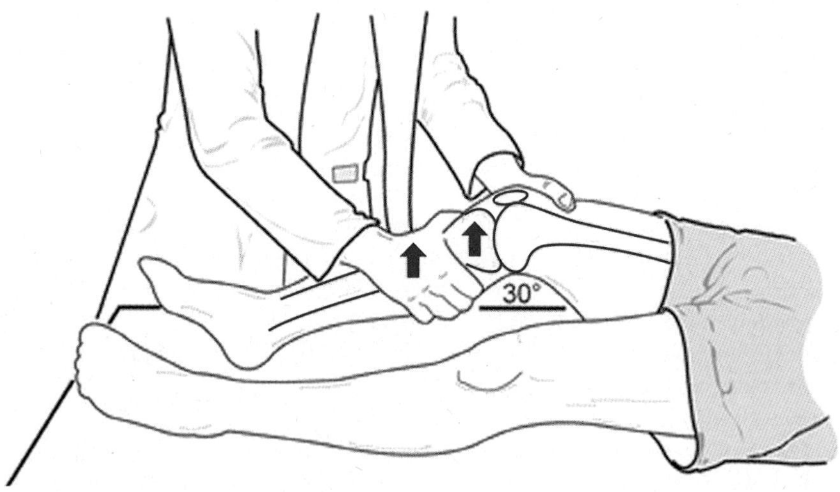

Figure 17.13 The Lachman test, performed at 30° of knee flexion, is the most sensitive test for integrity of the ACL. (Redrawn from Tria AJ, Klein KS. *An Illustrated Guide to the Knee.* New York: Churchill Livingstone, 1992, with permission. *Reproduced with permission from* Chapman MW, Szabo RM, Marder R, et al.: *Chapman's Orthopaedic Surgery*, 3rd ed. Philadelphia: Lippincott Williams & Wilkins, 2001.)

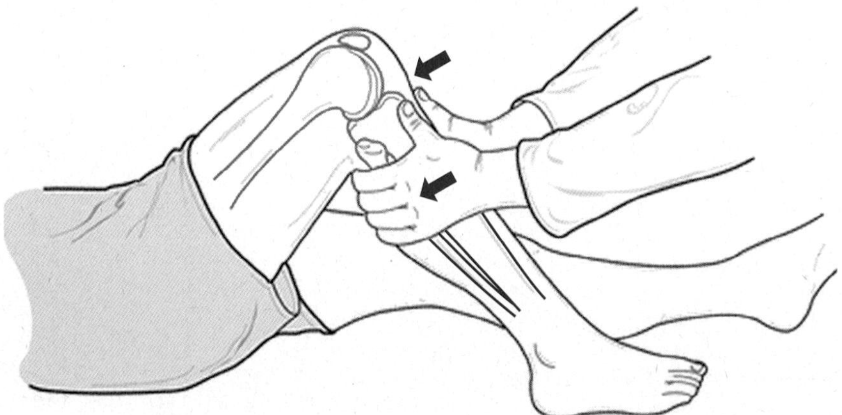

Figure 17.14 The posterior drawer test, performed at 90 degrees of knee flexion. (*Reproduced with permission from* Chapman MW, Szabo RM, Marder R, et al. *Chapman's Orthopaedic Surgery*. 3rd ed. Philadelphia, PA: Lippincott Williams & Wilkins, 2001.)

is best palpated in the figure-of-four position. Testing for ligament integrity is performed by placing a varus stress on the slightly flexed knee, 15 to 30 degrees. The degree of opening and the endpoint are evaluated.

Strength

Strength assessment should be conducted to determine muscle or nerve injury. Ask the patient to perform a straight leg raise, lifting the leg off of the examination table. He or she may not be able to do this owing to pain, swelling, and apprehension, but the ability to do so confirms function of the femoral nerve and the extensor mechanism. If additional abnormalities are suspected, then a thorough neuromuscular examination of the lower extremity should be performed.

Patellofemoral Joint Assessment

Examination of the patellofemoral joint begins with inspection, noting the dynamic gait, including the feet for pronation. The presence of pronation is a common accompaniment of patellofemoral pain syndrome. The examiner then inspects for atrophy with particular attention to quadriceps development. The vastus medialis obliquis (VMO) at the superomedial border of the patella strongly influences patellar tracking. Having the patient try to push the back of the knee into the examination table while lying supine allows for observation of VMO development. Next, malalignment is assessed. Patellofemoral pain due to malalignment and that due to patellar instability are two frequent clinical problems in which abnormal patella positioning or tracking plays a role. The quadriceps angle (Q angle) is measured; this angle is made by a line from the ASIS to the midpatella, intersecting a line from the midpatella to the patella tendon insertion at the tibial tubercle. The normal angle is approximately 15 degrees but is gender-dependent, with females having a greater angle than do males. Q angles greater that 15 degrees contribute to patella maltracking and malalignment (Fig. 17.15).

The extensor mechanism is palpated for tenderness, integrity, and crepitus. Palpation should include the medial and lateral patellar facets and retinaculum. Identifying the exact area of tenderness is important when formulating a proper treatment plan. The presence of medial facet tenderness is the most common location of pain in patients with patellofemoral pain syndrome. Patients with symptomatic

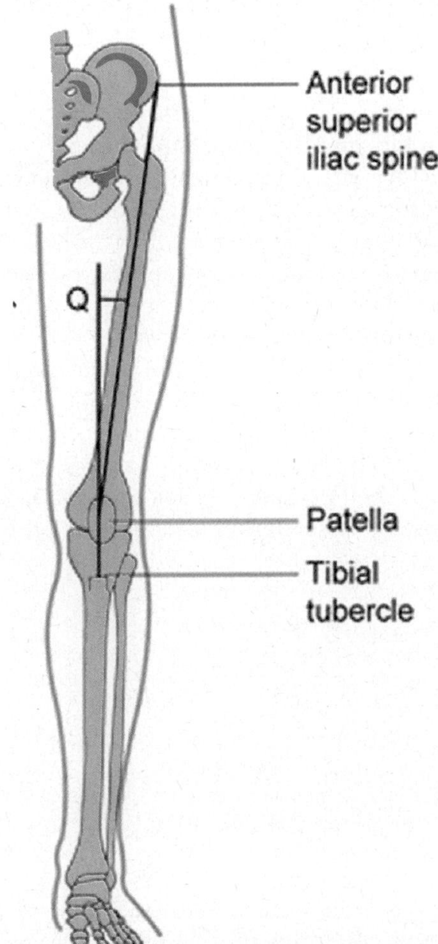

Figure 17.15 Q angle measured in full extension. In men, Q angles greater than 10 degrees and, in women, Q angles greater than 15 degrees are associated with patellofemoral disorders. (*Reproduced with permission from* Chapman MW, Szabo RM, Marder R, et al.: *Chapman's Orthopaedic Surgery*, 3rd ed. Philadelphia: Lippincott Williams & Wilkins, 2001.)

bipartite patella may have tenderness localized to the nonunited fragment. Alternatively, some patients with radiographically evident abnormal ossification centers will have no localized tenderness. Irregular ossification or scar tissue formation may lead to nodularity within the patellar tendon. Prominence of the tibial tubercle at the site of the patella tendon insertion, with or without tenderness, may be present due to Osgood Schlatter syndrome. Some examiners have described the patellofemoral compression test as a useful indicator of patellofemoral pathology. The test involves the gentle application of a compressive force to the patella into the trochlear groove, attempting to elicit pain that reproduces patients' symptoms. This test is nonspecific, as discomfort is frequently elicited as a result of painful impingement of the highly innervated synovial lining.

Next, the examiner inspects and palpates for patella alignment and tracking. The patella glide test is performed on a supine patient with the legs relaxed. The patella is translated both medially and laterally while noting the degree of translation and the amount of soft tissue restraint at the extremes of translation. Normally, the patella can be slightly translated both medially and laterally. Restriction may be normal for that patient, so it must be compared with the opposite side. Failure to translate the patella medially during the patellar glide test may suggest lateral patellar retinacular tightness. Translation of more than 50% of the patella's width laterally suggests medial retinacular laxity. Increased laxity in both medial and lateral translation suggests the possibility of generalized ligamentous laxity.

The patellar tilt test is also performed on a supine, relaxed patient. An attempt is made to evert the patella by lifting up its lateral side (Fig. 17.16). Normally the patella can evert at least to neutral. Failure to elevate the lateral side to approximately 15 degrees suggests a tight lateral retinaculum and is the most common physical finding in patients with patellofemoral pain syndrome.

Maltracking is evaluated by inspection of the patella. First, the examiner observes the resting position of the patella when the patient is seated. If the patella is oriented laterally from midline and looks like "grasshopper eyes," it is suggestive of patellar instability. Next, the seated patient should extend the knee. The course the patella as it tracks from flexion to terminal extension is followed. Normal excursion of the patella involves tracking in multiple planes, and its course is not simply direct superior translation. Slight medial to lateral movement and subtle rotational movement may accompany normal patella tracking. The asymptomatic knee is useful for comparison. The "J" or "jump" sign can sometimes be observed in patients with patellofemoral instability, in which the patella actually is seen to "jump" at approximately 20 degrees of flexion as it reduces into the trochlear groove from its laterally subluxed position. The course that the patella tracks takes on the shape of an inverted "J." Slight lateral excursion during terminal extension may be normal, especially if present bilaterally.

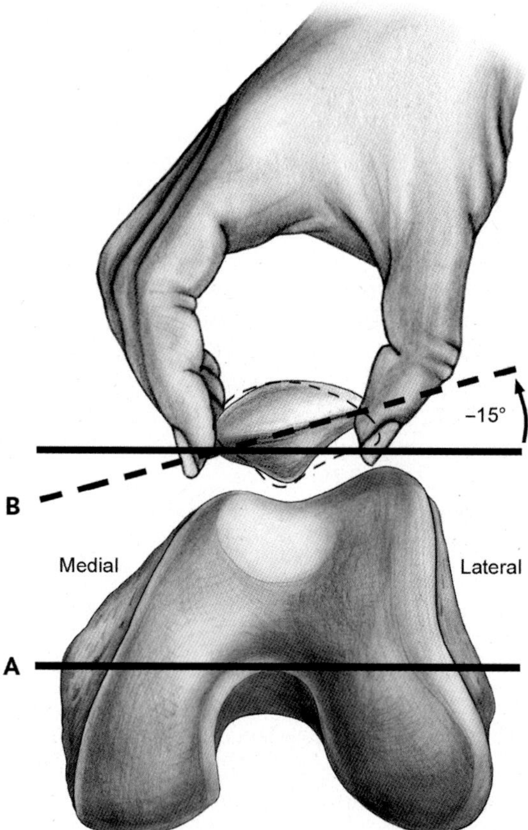

Figure 17.16 A positive patella tilt test is defined as inability to lift the lateral facet of the patella more than 15 degrees (or to neutral) and indicates a tight lateral retinaculum. (*Reproduced with permission from* Johnson DH and Pedowitz RA: *Practical Orthopaedic Sports Medicine and Arthroscopy*. Philadelphia: Lippincott Williams & Wilkins, 2006.)

Patellar instability assessment should also include an examination for apprehension. The patella apprehension test is performed with the patient supine and relaxed. Gentle pressure is applied to the patella to laterally translate the patella while observing the patient's countenance. The patient may become anxious and/or actually implore the examiner to discontinue the manipulation because of the feeling of impending instability.

Radiographic Analysis

Plain Radiography

Radiographs are helpful as an adjunct to a knee examination, particularly in the traumatized patient. In the absence of trauma, patients do not always require radiographic evaluation, particularly when the diagnosis is clinically apparent. Patients with persistent symptoms unresponsive to treatment, those with a history of acute or traumatic onset, and those with physical examination findings suggestive of mechanical or structural pathology (malalignment, crepitus, restricted motion, and loss of integrity) deserve radiographic evaluation.

The standard radiographs of the knee are a three-view series consisting of anteroposterior (AP), lateral, and a patellofemoral view. The AP view should be taken during weight-bearing to facilitate detection of malalignment or joint space narrowing. Both knees should be imaged for comparison. The AP should also be inspected for soft tissue abnormalities, bone density, and joint height. The lateral view can be taken while non–weight–bearing, with the knee flexed at 30 degrees. The patellofemoral joint can be evaluated on the lateral view along with the patellar height. The patellofemoral view (also know as the *sunrise, Merchant,* or *Laurin view* depending on the imaging technique used) demonstrates the relationship between the patella and the femur's trochlear groove. The patellofemoral view can demonstrate patellofemoral joint space narrowing, osteophytes, and maltracking.

Numerous other knee radiographs have been described, including the tunnel view, the posteroanterior (PA) flexion weight-bearing view, oblique joint views, and specific views to evaluate the tibial plateau. The tunnel view is obtained by directing the x-ray beam into the intercondylar notch or tunnel, with the knee flexed at 30 degrees. The knee flexion angle allows visualization of not only the intercondylar notch but also the posterior aspect of the femoral condyles. Lesions located more posteriorly on the femoral condyles, such as osteochondritis dissecans (OCD) lesions or osteonecrosis, may be seen only on this view. Likewise, osteochondral fragments within the knee may be more readily detected with the knee flexed. The weight-bearing PA view is taken in 30 degrees of flexion and demonstrates joint line narrowing earlier than the conventional weight-bearing AP view.

Computed Tomography

Computed tomography (CT) scans are routinely used to evaluate patients with distal femur or proximal tibia fractures as an adjunct to radiographs. Fine-cut (2 mm) CT scans with sagittal and coronal reconstructions provide excellent bony detail of the joint surfaces and allow demonstration of the degree of articular involvement and displacement. CT scans can also be of use in cases of patellofemoral malalignment to better visualize the bony articulation of the patellofemoral joint. CT scans are preferred over MRI for evaluation of bone. They are less helpful in the evaluation of knee soft tissue pathology.

Magnetic Resonance Imaging

MRI scans are unnecessary in the evaluation of most knee injuries. However, when indicated, they are highly sensitive and specific for the diagnosis of soft tissue injuries of the knee. Most commonly, they are used to diagnose or confirm the diagnosis of knee ligamentous and meniscus injuries. Knee MRI has been shown to be 90% to 100% sensitive and specific for these indications. MRI is also useful in detecting tibial stress fractures and neoplasms. MRI is highly sensitive and specific for knee pathology; however, it is expensive and requires a patient to be cooperative and remain motionless during the examination. Despite these limitations, it remains the "gold standard" for soft tissue injuries within and surrounding the knee.

Bone Scan

Some conditions are not visible using conventional plain radiographs. Three-phase technetium bone scans are used to detect areas of increased vascularization and bone turnover. However, bone scans are nonspecific. They are used to evaluate patients with shin splints. Increased focal uptake confirms the presence of a stress fracture, whereas diffuse uptake suggests medial tibial stress syndrome without fracture. Bone scan is cheaper than MRI; but it is less specific and requires contrast injection.

Arthroscopy

The gold standard for diagnosis of intraarticular pathology is knee joint arthroscopy. Introduced for clinical applications in the late 1970s, this modality has developed into a tool for diagnosis and immediate treatment for the majority knee pathology. Arthroscopy is a minimally invasive technique that is performed through two or three small, 1-cm, incisions. A fiber optic camera is placed within the knee, allowing visualization of the entire knee joint. Intraarticular pathology can be diagnosed, and then miniature instruments can be used to perform immediate treatment. Studies have shown decreased morbidity (pain, stiffness, infection, nerve injury) when compared with open arthrotomy. In addition, the magnification afforded by the fiber optic lens technology allows for superior visualization of the knee joint compared with conventional open techniques. Diagnostic arthroscopy is expensive and invasive and, therefore, should be utilized only when other more conservative measures of diagnosis and treatment have failed.

TRAUMATIC INJURIES OF THE KNEE

Distal Femur Fractures

Distal femur fractures account for approximately 7% of all femur fractures. There is a bimodal age distribution effecting young adults and osteoporotic elderly individuals. Fractures of the distal femur may occur in either the supracondylar or the intercondylar region and are often intraarticular. Their management is sometimes difficult, owing to fracture displacement and associated soft tissue injury.

Classification

Several classification systems exist, of which perhaps the most used is the AO/ASIF classification. It divides the fractures according to whether they are intraarticular or extraarticular. Type A is extraarticular, B is unicondylar, and C is intraarticular. In addition, there are several subtypes that are beyond the scope of this chapter.

Mechanism of Injury

Most fractures occur as a consequence of direct trauma. As mentioned previously, there is a bimodal age distribution based on the mechanism of injury. Younger patients have complex, intraarticular fractures as a result of high-energy trauma, often, a motor vehicle accident or a fall from height. Older, osteoporotic patients frequently have more simple extraarticular fractures that result from a minor fall from standing onto a flexed knee.

Presentation

Patients generally present with localized pain, deformity, and inability to bear weight. Approximately 5% to 10% of all distal femur fractures are open injuries.

Relevant Anatomy

The gastrocnemius muscle originates on the most distal portion of the femoral condyles. The pull of the gastrocnemius muscle on the distal piece causes the usual posterior displacement and angulation at the fracture site. The pull of the quadriceps and hamstrings muscles lead to shortening at the fracture site.

Physical Examination

Painful swelling and deformity present over the distal femur, often accompanied by false motion at the fracture site. The proximity of neurovascular structures to the fracture site mandates prompt assessment of the neurovascular status of the limb. Fullness in the popliteal space accompanied with weak distal pulses suggests vascular injury.

Radiographic Examination

Radiographs should include AP, lateral, and two oblique projections of the knee. In addition, two views of the hip should be obtained to evaluate the femoral neck.

Special Tests

CT scans are generally performed to evaluate the amount of intraarticular involvement and displacement.

Differential Diagnosis

The diagnosis is easily made if deformity is present and good radiographs are obtained. The differential includes femoral shaft fracture, tibial plateau fracture, and knee dislocation.

Treatment

Nonoperative treatment is possible in extraarticular and nondisplaced intraarticular fractures. Nonoperative treatment consists of fracture reduction and casting or functional bracing. For displaced fractures, traction is generally needed to obtain and maintain reduction. Nonoperative treatment of these fractures often requires traction for 6 to 12 weeks, so most displaced distal femur fractures are treated operatively with or without initial tibial pin traction. Articular components of the fracture are repaired with interfragmentary screws. The fractures are then fixed stabilized with a lateral plate and screws, intramedullary (IM) nail, or external fixator. Lateral plates can be inserted with conventional open methods or via newer, minimally invasive techniques (Fig. 17.17). The plates can be 95-degree condylar

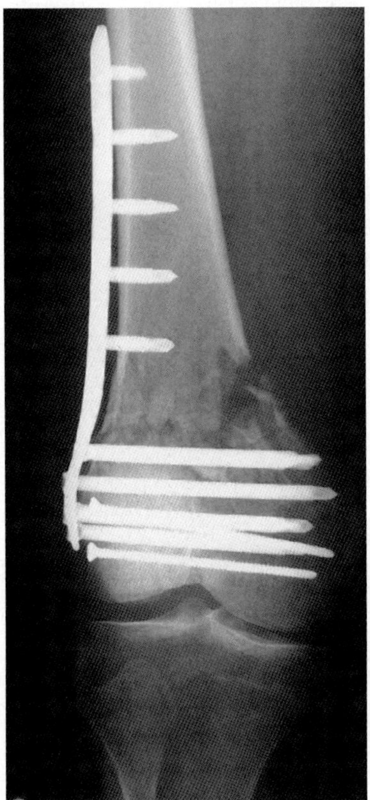

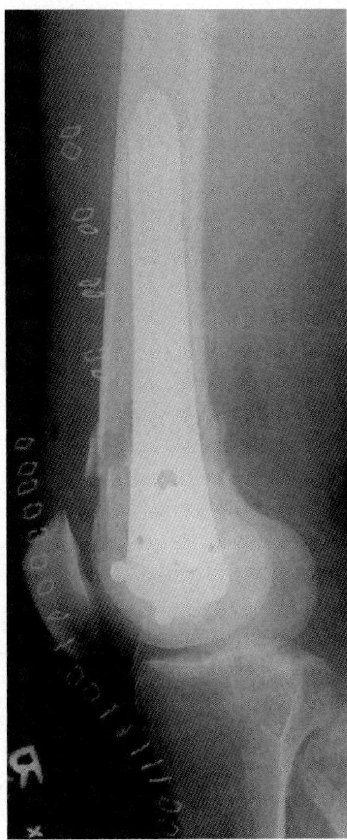

Figure 17.17 **(A)** AP and **(B)** lateral radiographs demonstrating locking plate fixation of a distal femur fracture. (*Reproduced with permission from* Bucholz RW, Heckman JD, Court-Brown C, et al. *Rockwood and Green's Fractures in Adults.* 6th ed. Philadelphia, PA: Lippincott Williams & Wilkins, 2005.)

plates, dynamic condylar screw plates, or contoured periarticular plates with locking or nonlocking screws. IM nails are limited to extraarticular distal femur fractures, with the fracture at least 5 cm superior to the joint line. The main limitation of IM nails is achieving adequate fixation of the distal fragment. IM nails can be inserted anterograde or retrograde. Retrograde IM nails have improved distal fixation with multiple distal interlocking screws at multiple angles. External fixation devices are generally used as a part of damage control orthopaedics with distal femur fractures; however, hybrid frames using fine-wire fixation distally and half-pin fixation proximally can be used for definitive treatment. Postoperatively, weight-bearing is initially delayed, but early range of motion of the knee is encouraged to decrease stiffness. Weight-bearing is advanced with radiographic evidence of healing at 6 to 12 weeks.

Complications

The most common complication of distal femur fractures is knee stiffness, and therefore, range-of-motion exercises are started early. Nonunion is rare, given the rich vascular supply of the cancellous bone of the distal femur. Varus malunion is the most common deformity. Posttraumatic osteoarthritis results from failure to restore articular congruity and altered knee biomechanics, as well as chondral damage at the time of the injury. Infection is greater with a high-energy mechanism and open injuries.

Tibial Plateau Fractures

Tibial plateau fractures constitute approximately 1% of all fractures.

Classification

There are several classification systems, the one that is most utilized is the Schatzker classification, which divides the plateau fractures according to their pattern, location, and level of trauma (Fig. 17.18). In type I, there is a split fracture of the lateral tibial plateau. Type II involves a split with associated depression of the lateral plateau. In type III, the lateral plateau is depressed. Type IV fractures involve a split, depression, or combination of both of the medial plateau. Type V fractures are bicondylar, involving both the medial and lateral plateaus. The type VI fractures extend proximal into the metaphysic of the tibia, causing dissociation between the metaphysis and diaphysis of the proximal tibia. Generally, types I to III are low-energy injuries, and types IV to VI are high-energy injuries.

Mechanism of Injury

The mechanism of injury is a varus or valgus load about the knee coupled with an axial load. Motor vehicle accidents account for the majority of injuries in younger patients; however, in older patients, this injury may occur with a simple fall. The quality of the patient's bone and the degree of force applied determine the type of fracture and the presence of associated ligamentous injuries. With a high-energy varus or valgus load to the knee, either the collateral ligament will tear or the plateau will fracture. The weaker structure will fail. In younger patients with strong, rigid bone, there is a high incidence of split-type fractures and a high rate of associated ligament injuries. In older patients, with bone that is weaker, there is a higher incidence of depression-type fractures and a lower incidence of ligament injuries. Type V bicondylar split fractures involve a high-energy axial load applied to an extended knee.

Presentation

Patients present with severe knee pain and swelling following major trauma to the knee due to a motor vehicle, industrial, or athletic accident. The patient typically cannot bear weight on the extremity. Traditionally, these injuries were called "bumper injuries" to describe the common mechanism of the fracture occurring to the knee of patients who stepped out into traffic and their knee was struck by a car's bumper.

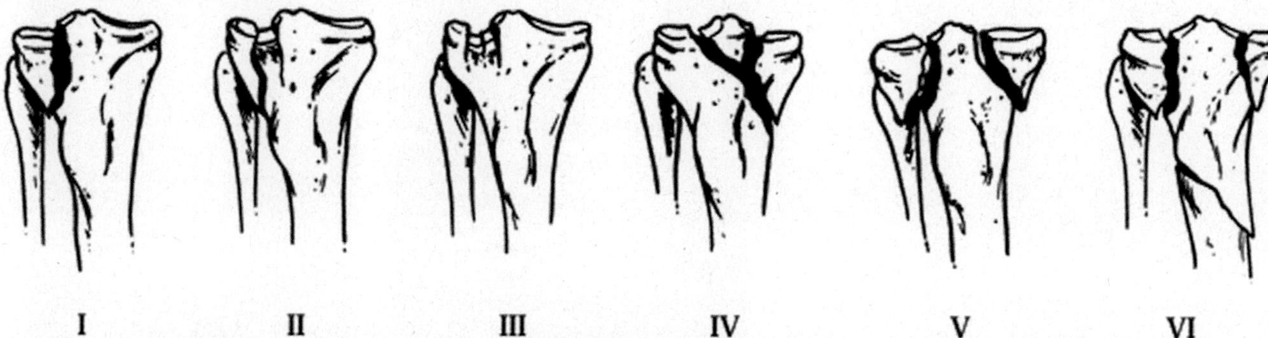

Figure 17.18 Schatzker's classification of tibial plateau fractures is shown. Types I to IV are defined as follows: I: A split fracture of the lateral tibial plateau. II: A pure depression fracture of the lateral tibial plateau. III: A split-depression fracture of the lateral tibial plateau. IV: A fracture of the medial tibial plateau. V: A bicondylar fracture of the tibial plateau. VI: A fracture of the tibial plateau with metaphyseal-diaphyseal dissociation. (*Reproduced with permission from* Chapman MW: *Chapman's Orthopaedic Surgery*, 3rd ed. Philadelphia: Lippincott Williams & Wilkins, 2001.)

Relevant Anatomy

The tibial plateau is composed of medial and lateral condyles. The medial condyle is larger and concave from anterior to posterior and medial to lateral. The lateral plateau is smaller in size and convex in shape. The plateaus are separated by an intercondylar eminence that serves as an attachment for the ACL. Because the medial articular surface and its associated condyle is stronger than the lateral plateau, and because of the normal valgus angle of the knee, fractures involving the lateral compartment are more common. Adjacent soft tissue and neurovascular structures are at risk in these injuries, particularly those that involve extensive comminution and a higher-energy injury. The popliteal vessel trifurcates just below the knee and is at risk with proximal tibial fractures. Laterally, the peroneal nerve is at risk as it winds around the neck of the fibula.

Physical Examination

Swelling and ecchymoses are frequently present and may be severe. Neurovascular assessment is critical, particularly in cases of high-energy trauma. Evaluation for stability is an important component in determining the treatment. This involves the application of gentle stresses to the knee to determine the degree of stability. With the knee in extension, a varus or valgus force is applied, depending on the compartment involved, and the tendency for the joint line to "open up" is determined. Similarly an anterior or posterior force may be gently applied to determine the presence of associated cruciate ligament injury. Pain often precludes a satisfactory evaluation, which requires intraarticular local anesthetic or general anesthesia.

Radiographic Examination

AP, lateral, and oblique radiographs of the knee are required.

Special Tests

Varus and valgus stress radiographs are sometimes helpful to establish the stability of an injury and assess for associated ligamentous damage. This sometimes requires anesthesia and can be performed under fluoroscopy. CT scans are helpful to determine the degree of intraarticular displacement. Because management often hinges on the amount of fracture displacement, CT scans are commonly indicated in the workup of tibial plateau fractures.

Differential Diagnosis

Because knee dislocations may be accompanied by a tibial plateau fracture, one must consider the possibility when evaluating any patient with distal femoral or proximal tibial trauma. The relatively high percentage of vascular injuries mandates the consideration in any knee trauma. There are a number of commonly associated injuries accompanying fractures of the tibial plateau. These include meniscus tears in up to 50% and associated ligament injury in up to 30%. Young patients with strong bone are at a higher risk for ligamentous injury.

Treatment

Nonoperative treatment may be sufficient for non- or minimally displaced fractures and those that are "stable." Treatment most commonly involves non–weight-bearing in a fracture brace for up to 3 months. Operative intervention is reserved for displaced (usually greater than 5 mm articular incongruity), unstable, or open fractures. Surgical treatment most commonly consists of open reduction and internal fixation (ORIF) with a contoured proximal tibia locking plate or an external fixator in patients with severe swelling and fracture blisters. Vascular injuries usually require repair. Nerve injuries are usually neuropraxias. When treating an open injury or performing an ORIF, nerve exploration may be warranted. A high index of suspicion for the development of compartment syndrome should be maintained.

Complications

Complications include stiffness, malunion, nonunion, posttraumatic osteoarthritis, infection, compartment syndrome, and nerve injury.

Patella Fractures

Fractures of the patella are relatively common, accounting for 1% of all skeletal injuries. They are more common in men than in women (2:1). They can occur in all age groups, but the most common age group is 20 to 50 years of age.

Classification

Patella fractures are divided into nondisplaced and displaced patterns. In addition, they can be described on the basis of fracture location and pattern: stellate, comminuted, transverse, vertical, polar (superior or inferior), or osteochondral (Fig. 17.19).

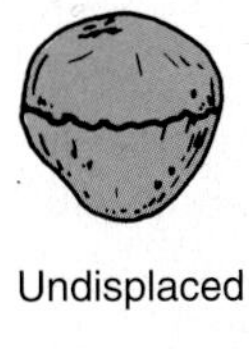
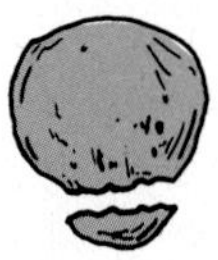
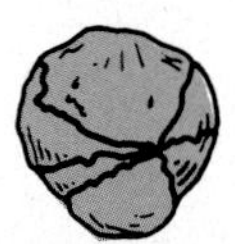

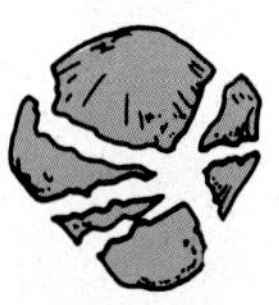
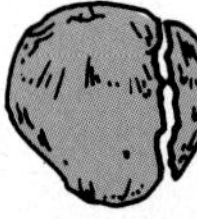
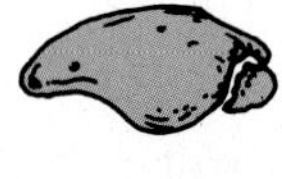

Figure 17.19 Classification of patella fractures. (*Reproduced with permission from* Bucholz RW, Heckman JD, Court-Brown C, Tornetta P. *Rockwood and Green's Fractures in Adults*, 6th Ed. Philadelphia: Lippincott Williams & Wilkins, 2005.)

Mechanism of Injury

The most common mechanism is indirect, from a forced eccentric contraction of the quadriceps as the knee is flexed. The intrinsic strength of the patella is exceeded by the pull of the extensor mechanism. The facture is generally transverse with variable inferior pole comminution. The degree of displacement is based on the degree of retinacular disruption. Patella fractures can also occur through direct trauma from a fall directly on the patella. Direct trauma results in a stellate or comminuted fracture pattern with preservation of the retinaculum.

Presentation

Patients present with acute anterior knee pain accompanied by localized tenderness and swelling.

Relevant Anatomy

The patella is the largest sesamoid bone in the body. The patella increases the mechanical moment arm of the quadriceps and protects the femoral condyles from direct trauma. The articular cartilage of the patella is the thickest in the body and can be up to 10 mm thick. The medial and lateral extensor retinacula are strong longitudinal expansions of the quadriceps and insert directly onto the tibia. If these remain intact, active extension may be preserved in the setting of a patella fracture.

Physical Examination

Patients have a tender, swollen, ecchymotic anterior knee. The physician must evaluate for active extension or the ability to do a straight leg raise to determine the integrity of retinacula.

Radiographic Examination

AP, lateral, and sunrise views of the knee are required.

Special Tests

Special tests are not necessary.

Differential Diagnosis

A bipartite patella, in which an ossification center persists, is occasionally mistaken for a fracture. A bipartite patella almost always has smooth superolateral margins, and 50% are bilateral. If a bipartite patella is suspected, consider imaging the contralateral patella. Quadriceps tendon rupture and patella tendon rupture should be ruled out by physical examination and radiographs.

Treatment

Nonoperative treatment with either a cylinder cast or a knee immobilizer is reserved for nondisplaced or minimally displaced fractures with an intact extensor mechanism. Operative treatment consists of ORIF or patellectomy. For the most common transverse fracture pattern, ORIF is performed with K-wires or screws placed longitudinally through the patella followed by an anterior or circumferential tension band wire (Fig. 17.20). Comminution is either excised or fixed with interfragmentary screws. Partial patellectomy is performed for comminuted polar fragments with reattachment of the patellar tendon. Total patellectomy is reserved for severe, unrepairable comminution and is rarely indicated. The retinaculum should be repaired with any type of treatment. Postoperatively, the patient is weight-bearing as tolerated in a knee immobilizer or cylinder cast for 6 weeks.

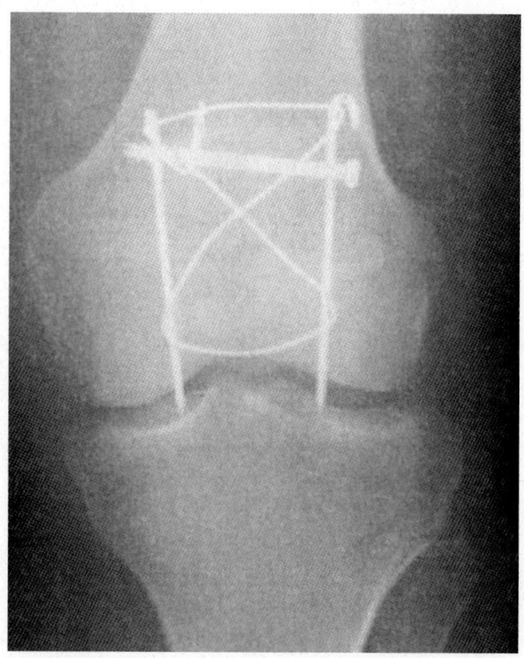

Figure 17.20 AP radiograph demonstrating ORIF of a patella fracture using tension band fixation and an interfragmentary screw. (*Reproduced with permission from* Bucholz RW, Heckman JD, Court-Brown C, et al. *Rockwood and Green's Fractures in Adults.* 6th ed. Philadelphia, PA: Lippincott Williams & Wilkins, 2005.)

Complications

Knee stiffness, extensor lag of approximately 5 degrees, and extensor weakness are the most common complications. Posttraumatic osteoarthritis has been shown to occur in up to 50% of patients in long-term studies. Symptomatic hardware is common and may necessitate removal after the healing has occurred. Nonunion and infection are rare. Osteonecrosis occurs with increasing comminution, but the majority of patients can be treated with observation with spontaneous revascularization in 2 years.

Quadriceps Tendon Rupture

Rupture of the quadriceps tendon is relatively common in middle-aged patients older than 40 years. The rupture generally occurs within 2 cm of the superior pole of the patella. Quadriceps tendonitis or tendinosis is a risk factor and can be caused by anabolic steroid use, local steroid injection, diabetes mellitus, inflammatory arthropathy, or chronic renal failure.

Classification

Quadriceps tendon injuries are known as *quadriceps strains*. They are classified from mild to severe or grade I to III. A grade III rupture is a complete tear. The most common classification is an incomplete or complete rupture based on the patient's ability to perform a straight leg raise or actively extend the knee.

Mechanism of Injury

The mechanism is the same as that for an indirect patella fracture, an eccentric load of the quadriceps. In the case of a quadriceps rupture, the quadriceps tendon is generally weakened through a degenerative process (tendinosis); and therefore, it is weaker than the patella and thus ruptures.

Presentation

Patients present after experiencing sharp, acute pain after a stumble or trip. Most are unable to walk because of pain and incompetence of their extensor mechanism. This injury commonly occurs in patients 40 to 70 years old, whereas patella tendon ruptures are more common in patients younger than 40 years.

Relevant Anatomy

As discussed in the knee anatomy section, the four quadriceps muscles become tendinous, and coalesce to form the quadriceps tendon. They then envelop the patella and attach distally at the tibial tubercle as the patella tendon. Longitudinal extensions, the retinacula, run medial and lateral to the extensor mechanism and attach directly onto the tibia. If retinacula are intact, a patient with a quadriceps rupture may still be able to perform active knee extension.

Physical Examination

The patient will have swollen, tender, anterior knee. The tenderness is greatest at the superior pole of the patella. A palpable defect is often present superior to the patella. The vast majority of patients are unable to actively extend the leg or perform a straight leg raise.

Radiographic Examination

AP and lateral radiographs of the knee demonstrate an intact patella with the presence of patella baja or a low-riding patella.

Special Tests

MRI can confirm the tear but is unnecessary with a positive physical examination. MRI or ultrasound can be utilized in inconclusive cases or cases where patient body habitus limits the physical examination.

Differential Diagnosis

The differential includes the two other injuries to the extensor mechanism: patella tendon rupture and patella fracture.

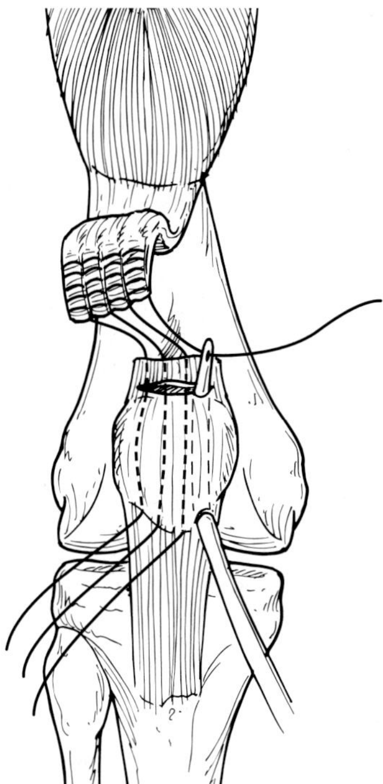

Figure 17.21 Quadriceps tendon repair technique. (*Reproduced with permission from* El Attrache NS, Harner CD, Mirzayan R, Sekiya JK: *Surgical Techniques in Sports Medicine*. Philadelphia: Lippincott Williams & Wilkins, 2006.)

Treatment

Nonoperative treatment is reserved for incomplete tears in which active, full-knee extension is preserved. Operative treatment consists of primary repair of the quadriceps tendon to the superior pole of the patella. Strong nonabsorbable suture is placed into the quadriceps tendon with a locked, running stitch. The tendon is then reapproximated to the patella through bone tunnels and secured (Fig. 17.21). For chronic ruptures, a quadriceps turndown, Scuderi technique, can be utilized for the repair. Postoperatively, the patient is weight-bearing as tolerated in a knee immobilizer or cylinder cast for 3 to 4 weeks. At that point, motion is started and slowly advanced over the next 6 to 8 weeks with a hinged knee brace.

Complications

Knee stiffness, extensor lag, and extensor weakness are the most common complications. Rerupture rates are low for acute, primary repair.

Patella Tendon Rupture

Patella tendon ruptures are less common than quadriceps tendon ruptures and occur in younger patients, generally those younger than 40 years. The rupture occurs at the inferior pole of the patella and is related to degenerative changes within the patella tendon. Risk factors include inflammatory arthritis, systemic lupus erythematous, diabetes mellitus, chronic renal failure, corticosteroid use, and chronic patella tendonitis.

Classification

Patella tendon ruptures can be classified by location of the rupture: proximal insertion, midsubstance, or distal insertion. The proximal insertion, at the inferior pole of the patella, is the most common location of rupture. In addition, patella tendon ruptures can be classified by the timing between the injury and surgery. Acute repair is performed within 2 weeks, and delayed repair is performed after 6 weeks. Repair during the acute period is the most important prognostic factor.

Mechanism of Injury

The injury occurs by the same mechanism as indirect patella fractures and quadriceps ruptures, an eccentric load of the extensor mechanism. In these younger patients, the quadriceps tendon has not undergone degeneration; and therefore, the patella tendon is the weakest component of the extensor mechanism.

Presentation

Patients present after experiencing sharp, acute pain after a stumble or a trip. Most are unable to walk because of pain and incompetence of their extensor mechanism.

Relevant Anatomy

The patella tendon runs from the inferior pole of the patella to the tibial tubercle. The greatest forces through the patella tendon occur at 60 degrees of knee flexion, and these forces can be as high as 3 to 4 times the body weight when climbing stairs.

Physical Examination

The patient has a swollen, tender, anterior knee. The tenderness is greatest at the inferior pole of the patella. A palpable defect is present inferior to the patella. The vast majority of patients are unable to actively extend or perform a straight leg raise.

Radiographic Examination

AP and lateral knee radiographs reveal an intact patella with patella alta, or a high-riding patella (Fig. 17.22).

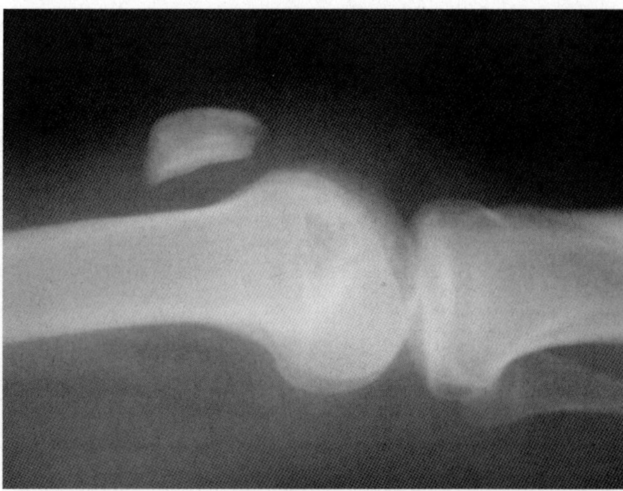

Figure 17.22 Lateral radiograph demonstrating patella alta after an acute patellar tendon rupture. (*Reproduced with permission from* El Attrache NS, Harner CD, Mirzayan R, Sekiya JK: *Surgical Techniques in Sports Medicine*. Philadelphia: Lippincott Williams & Wilkins, 2006.)

Special Tests

MRI or ultrasound can be used in cases where the physical examination is inconclusive.

Differential Diagnosis

The differential diagnosis includes quadriceps tendon rupture, patella fracture, or tibial tubercle avulsion.

Treatment

Nonoperative treatment is reserved for incomplete tears, in which active, full-knee extension is preserved. Operative treatment consists of primary repair of the patella tendon to the inferior pole of the patella. Acute repair, within 2 weeks, has better outcomes than delayed repair due to patella tendon scarring and quadriceps contraction. Strong nonabsorbable suture is placed into the patella tendon with a locked, running stitch, and the tendon is then reapproximated to the patella through bone tunnels. For delayed repairs, the primary repair may need to be augmented with hamstring or fascia lata autograft or Achilles tendon allograft. Postoperatively, the patient is weight-bearing as tolerated in a knee immobilizer or cylinder cast for 2 to 3 weeks. As with a quadriceps repair, motion is then started and slowly advanced over the next 6 to 8 weeks. Delayed repairs are managed more conservatively with delayed weight-bearing.

Complications

Knee stiffness, extensor lag, extensor weakness, and patella baja are the most common complications. Rerupture rates are low for acute, primary repair and higher for delayed repairs.

Patella Dislocation

Patella dislocation is relatively common and accounts for most patients complaining of a knee dislocation. The dislocation is always in the lateral direction. It is more common in women, owing to physiologic laxity, and patients with hypermobility and connective tissue diseases, such as Ehlers–Danlos and Marfan syndrome.

Classification

Patellar instability can occur in the form of frank dislocation or subluxation. In a subluxation, there remains a portion of articular contact between the patella and the femur. Patella dislocations can be classified as acute or chronic.

Mechanism of Injury

Patella dislocations usually occur during a maneuver in which the knee is slightly flexed and rotated. In such a position, the patella may be poorly engaged in its groove and vulnerable to lateral subluxation or dislocation. Predisposition to lateral dislocation of the patella falls into the main categories of hypoplasia or dysplasia, malalignment, and contracture or laxity. Hypoplasia of the lateral femoral condyle, patella alta, a shallow trochlea, dysplasia of the patella, and hypoplasia of the vastus medialis decrease the forces that keep the patella within the trochlea grove and increase the risk of dislocation. An increased Q angle, femoral anteversion, genu valgum, external tibial rotation, and lateralization of the tibial tubercle predispose to instability by increasing the laterally directed forces on the patella. Laxity of the medial retinaculum, tightness of the lateral retinaculum, and generalized ligamentous laxity also predispose the patient to patellar dislocations.

Presentation

Patients present with acute pain following an incident where the knee "went out of place." The patient may be unable to extend the knee if the patella is unreduced.

Relevant Anatomy

The *Q angle* is defined as the angle formed by a line from the ASIS to the midpatella and a line from the midpatella to the tibial tubercle. The normal range is 8 to 12 degrees, with a high Q angle being greater than 15 degrees. Patella tracking through the trochlear groove is balanced by the Q angle, the lateral retinaculum, the medial retinaculum, the medial patellofemoral ligament (MPFL, the major medial restraint to lateral displacement of the patella), and the VMO. Maltracking or lateral subluxation/dislocation can occur if any of the following three components are present: the Q angle is too great, the lateral retinaculum is too tight, or the VMO is too weak. When the patella dislocates, the medial retinaculum is torn and the MPFL is torn or stretched

Physical Examination

When the patella is dislocated, the contour of the knee is abnormal and displays a prominence laterally and a void anteriorly where the patella is usually located. Most patellar dislocations, however, are seen after either spontaneous or manipulated reduction, in which physical examination findings are nonspecific and include swelling, tenderness, and ecchymoses. Tenderness is often present over the lateral aspect of the knee, specifically over the lateral femoral condyle, and medially over the medial facet of the patella and the medial retinaculum.

Radiographic Examination

AP, lateral, and sunrise views of the knee are required. The lateral or sunrise views should be inspected for evidence of an osteochondral fragment.

Special Tests

Special tests are generally unnecessary. If the diagnosis is doubtful, MRI can be helpful to visualize retinacular and chondral injury as well as loose bodies.

Differential Diagnosis

Knee dislocation should be ruled out by physical examination. Additional differential diagnoses are patellofemoral pain syndrome, patella subluxation, MCL sprain, ACL tear, and meniscus tear. Each of these can typically be ruled out by physical examination, with the patient occasionally requiring an MRI.

Treatment

The treatment of patella dislocations should be based on the acuity of the injury and the patients symptoms. Patients with initial dislocations are treated differently than patients with chronic instability.

Initial Dislocation

The patient with an acute primary dislocation of the patella is managed with prompt reduction and evaluation to rule out associated displaced osteochondral fractures. Osteochondral fracture generally occurs as the patella is relocated and the medial facet of the patella impacts the lateral femoral condyle. Therefore, the medial patella facet and lateral femoral condyle are the typical locations of osteochondral fracture. Occasionally, aspiration of the hemarthrosis may be performed for comfort. If there is no osteochondral fracture, the patient's knee should be immobilized in either a knee immobilizer or a cylinder cast for 3 to 4 weeks. Operative treatment is reserved for the presence of displaced osteochondral fragments or recurrent instability. Once immobilization is discontinued, the patient is started on an aggressive quadriceps-strengthening physical therapy program focusing on VMO strengthening.

Chronic Instability

The patient with chronic patellar instability and patellofemoral pain has different surgical options depending on the exact etiology of the instability and pain. The major causes of patellofemoral pain are patella chondromalacia, malalignment, maltracking, and retinacular imbalance. These etiologies can present separately or together, and it is important that the surgical approach to the patient address all of the etiologies to be successful.

1. Arthroscopic debridement and a chondral procedure—Patients with patella chondromalacia can have partial- or full-thickness damage to the patella chondral surface. This chondral damage can be the source of their patellofemoral pain. The first step in treating these patients is to arthroscopically debride (chondroplasty) the unstable cartilage. A procedure to either stimulate cartilage growth or transplant cartilage tissue to the damaged area can then be performed. The purpose of this procedure is to replace the damaged cartilage with a new

cartilage surface to cover the underlying subchondral bone and prevent pain. Microfracture is the most commonly performed cartilage-stimulating procedure. It involves punching small holes into the underlying subchondral bone to cause a controlled fracture and subsequent bleeding. This causes fibrocartilage, which is essentially "scar cartilage" as it has inferior biomechanical properties when compared with hyaline cartilage, to grow into the defect. The cartilage transplant procedures are the osteochondral autograft transport system (OATS) and autologous chondrocyte implantation (ACI). OATS is difficult to perform on the patella but can be utilized for trochlear lesions. OATS involves taking plugs of cartilage and subchondral bone from a non–weight-bearing surface of the knee and transporting them to the damaged area. ACI is a two-step procedure in which cartilage is initially harvested from a non–weight-bearing area in the knee. This cartilage is sent to a laboratory where chondrocytes are isolated and proliferated. At a second procedure, these chondrocytes are implanted into the defect and covered with a periosteal patch. The exact procedure that is chosen depends on the size and the location of the lesion. Generally, microfracture is performed initially, followed by either OATS or ACI. Most of the times, these procedures are performed with a realignment procedure, especially in the setting of a large, full-thickness lesion, to off-load the damaged area.

2. Lateral retinacular release—A lateral release should be performed in patients who have significantly positive lateral tilt. This can be detected on physical examination and intra-articularly during arthroscopy. It involves incising the lateral retinaculum and letting it retract to create a gap in the retinaculum that results in a lengthening of the tight lateral structures.
3. Proximal realignment—This involves tightening up the medial retinaculum and MPFL. This procedure is performed if the etiology for the instability is a weak or "stretched out" medial patellar restraints. The surgery involved shortening the medial retinaculum and MPFL, thus tightening the medial patellar restraints. Generally, proximal realignment is performed in conjunction with a lateral release to weaken the lateral restraints.
4. MPFL reconstruction—This procedure is performed in patients with weak or torn medial restraints from patellar dislocation. The procedure does not realign or unload damaged chondral surfaces of the patella, instead it "tightens" the medial restraints by reconstructing the MPFL. This is accomplished with either an autograft hamstring tendon or an allograft soft tissue tendon. MPFL reconstructions are becoming popular for patients with instability without significant chondral damage.
5. Distal realignment (Fulkerson)—Distal realignment procedures are performed at the tibial tubercle. They accomplish two main goals. First, they elevate the tibial tubercle and, therefore, increase the moment arm of the quadriceps. This provides a mechanical advantage to the quadriceps, consequently unloading the total force seen by the patella. The specific areas that are loaded during knee flexion are also altered slightly to unload the damaged areas of the patella. Second, the distal realignment procedure moves the tibial tubercle medially to decrease the Q angle. This alters the direction of the patella tendon pull to increase the medial and decrease the lateral directed forces on the patella. Distal realignment procedures have developed into first-line treatments for patients with significant patellofemoral arthritis. However, for patients with instability, distal realignment procedures have become second-line treatments, after MPFL reconstruction.

Complications

Recurrent dislocation is more common in patients with a primary dislocation at an age younger than 20 years. Recurrent dislocation is an indication for surgical intervention. Knee stiffness may result from prolonged immobilization or postsurgical arthrofibrosis. Patellofemoral pain can result from chondral injury at the time of the dislocation or from retinacular injury that results in maltracking and subsequent chondral damage. Overall, 50% of patients with a primary patellar dislocation will improve with nonoperative treatment; however, the other 50% will have recurrent instability or patellofemoral pain.

Knee Dislocation

Dislocation of the knee is an uncommon but serious orthopaedic injury that may be limb-threatening and should be treated as an orthopaedic emergency. Tibiofemoral (knee) dislocation is much less common than patellar dislocation and is a much more serious injury. The true incidence is probably underestimated as 30% to 50% of dislocations spontaneously reduce before presentation.

Classification

Knee dislocations are classified according to the displacement of the tibia relative to the femur (Fig. 17.23). The most common dislocation is anterior due to knee hyperextension, accounting for 30% to 50% of knee dislocations. Posterior dislocations are the next most frequent ones due to a posteriorly directed force to the proximal tibia, most commonly from the dashboard of a car. Medial, lateral, and rotational dislocations are less common and result from a combination of mechanisms involving sagittal and coronal and rotational movements. Knee dislocations can also be described by the ligaments that are involved. Most commonly, the ACL and PCL are involved along with at least one of the collateral ligaments.

Mechanism of Injury

Knee dislocations occur after substantial trauma to the knee. High-energy injuries usually occur as the result of

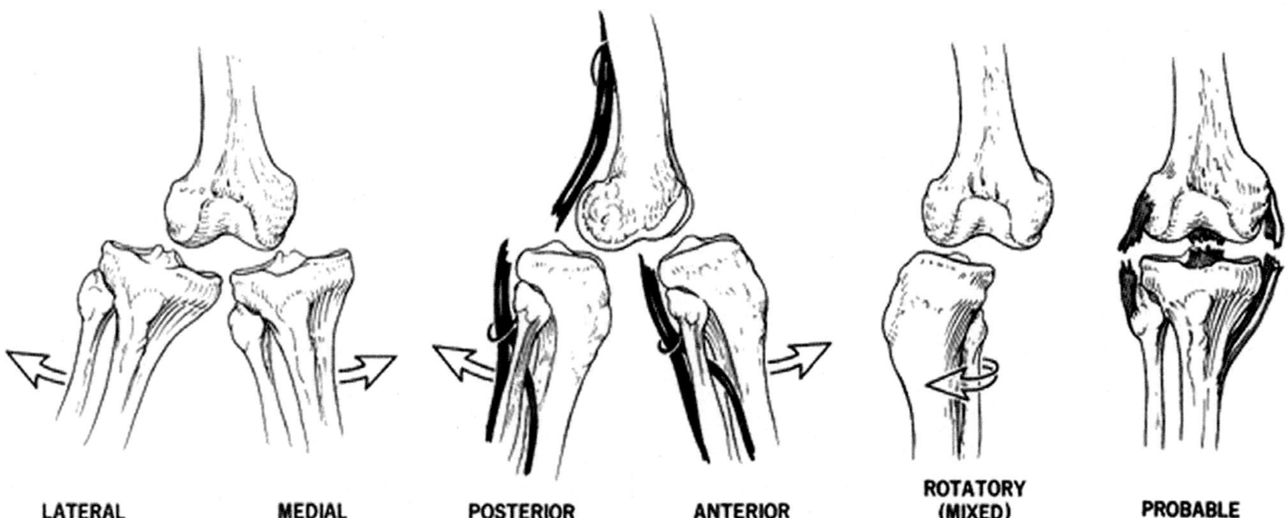

Figure 17.23 Classification of knee dislocations. (*Reproduced with permission from* Chapman MW, Szabo RM, Marder R, et al. *Chapman's Orthopaedic Surgery*. 3rd ed. Philadelphia, PA: Lippincott Williams & Wilkins, 2001.)

motor vehicle accidents. Lower-energy mechanisms occur during athletic events or falls.

Presentation

Patients with high-energy traumatic mechanisms can have multiple traumatic injuries. Lower-energy injuries are more commonly isolated. Patients will complain of severe pain and swelling and will be unable to bear weight. Patients or emergency personel may describe an awkward position of the knee that reduced while stabilizing the limb.

Relevant Anatomy

Tibiofemoral joint stability is provided predominantly by soft tissue restraints. For a knee dislocation to occur three of the four main constraining ligaments must be torn. Most commonly, the ACL and PCL are involved along with either the MCL or LCL. The posterior vascular structures of the knee, including the popliteal artery and vein, the tibial nerve, and the common peroneal nerve, can be damaged with a knee dislocation and cause a limb-threatening injury. The popliteal neurovascular bundle courses through a fibrous tunnel at the level of the adductor hiatus. Within the popliteal fossa, multiple branches arise from the popliteal artery, including the superior medial and lateral geniculate arteries, the middle geniculate artery, and the inferior medial and lateral geniculate arteries. The popliteal artery then runs through another fibrous tunnel deep to the soleus. These branches and the fibroosseous tunnels tether the popliteal artery to the popliteal space. Therefore, when a knee dislocation occurs, the popliteal artery is at great risk for kinking, tenting, or, rarely, tearing.

Physical Examination

The examination findings vary with the type of dislocation and the timing of the evaluation. The knee will be swollen and tender. Deformity may be present if the knee is still dislocated at the time of presentation. If the knee is still dislocated, it should be reduced immediately before continuing the examination. A thorough ligamentous examination should be performed to determine the extent of the ligamentous injury. Most importantly, a careful neurovascular examination should be performed, including ankle–brachial indices (ABIs). The neurovascular examination must be repeated serially over the next 24 to 48 hours as vasospasm or thrombosis from an intimal tear of the popliteal artery can cause delayed limb ischemia. Vascular injury with either initial damage or rupture occurs in 20% to 60% of knee dislocations. Collateral circulation is usually inadequate to perfuse the distal extremity. Capillary refill and distal pulses may be intact despite significant arterial injury. Neurologic injury, most commonly to the peroneal nerve, can occur in up to 35% of cases and requires careful neurologic evaluation.

Radiographic Examination

AP, lateral, and oblique radiographs of the knee before and after reduction are performed. Joint space widening may indicate incomplete reduction. Ligamentous or capsular avulsion fractures can often be visualized on radiographs.

Special Tests

The high incidence of vascular injury mandates a vascular surgery consultation and possible arteriography in every knee dislocation. Generally, if the initial ABI is normal, serial ABIs can be used in lieu of an arteriogram, although this decision should ultimately be made by the vascular surgeon. MRI is helpful to assess the extent of ligamentous injury and formulate a reconstructive approach (Fig. 17.24).

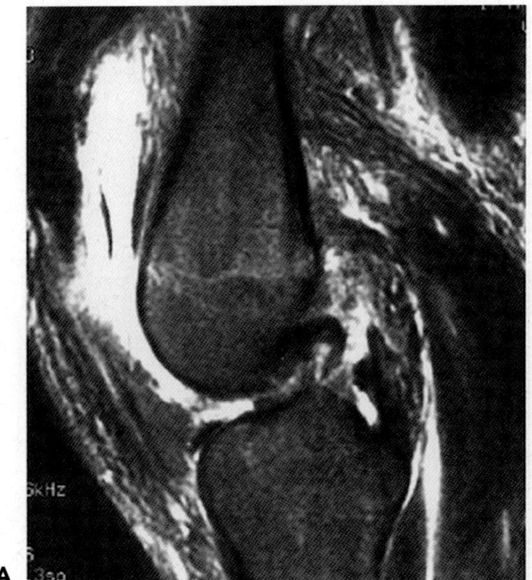
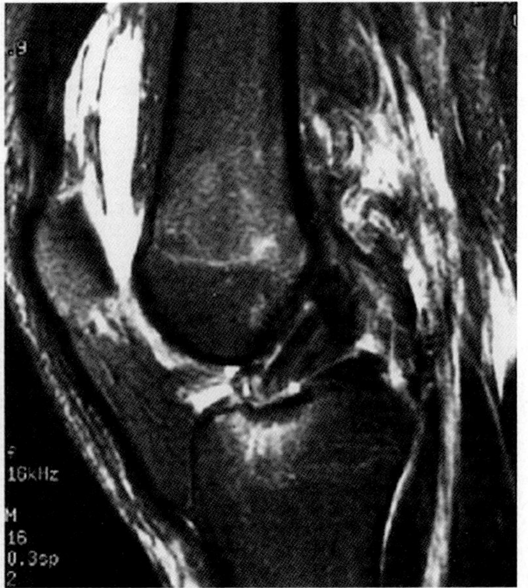

Figure 17.24 T2-weighted magnetic resonance images showing **(A)** PCL tear and **(B)** ACL avulsion following a knee dislocation. (*Reproduced with permission from* Chapman MW, Szabo RM, Marder R, et al. *Chapman's Orthopaedic Surgery*. 3rd ed. Philadelphia, PA: Lippincott Williams & Wilkins, 2001.)

Differential Diagnosis

The differential diagnosis includes distal femur, patella, and tibial plateau fractures. In addition, isolated ligamentous injury without dislocation should be included.

Treatment

Initially, a prompt reduction, after neurovascular assessment, should be performed, followed by a repeat neurovascular assessment and postreduction radiographs. Concern for limb ischemia mandates immediate vascular consult and likely intervention. Closed reduction is generally successful, although some dislocations are irreducible as a result of "button-holing" of the bone through the soft tissues. Indications for immediate open management include open injury, inability to achieve a closed reduction, associated residual soft tissue interposition, and vascular injury.

The definitive treatment is debated. The debate surrounds the timing of ligament repair and reconstruction. Some orthopaedists recommend immediate repair and reconstruction, whereas others recommend delayed repair or, more often, reconstruction. The cruciate ligaments generally require reconstruction, whereas the collateral ligaments may be amenable to repair when addressed acutely (within 2 to 3 weeks of injury) but require reconstruction in more chronic cases. Outcome studies have been mixed with outcomes of persistent pain, stiffness, and instability following both immediate and delayed treatment.

Complications

Initial complications include neurovascular injuries. Delayed complications include pain and stiffness.

MCL Sprain

MCL sprains are the most common knee ligament injuries. The MCL has superficial and deep layers. The MCL is the primary restraint to valgus stress about the knee.

Classification

MCL sprains are graded from I to III, with severity increasing from I to III. In grade I (mild) injuries, there is minor injury to the ligament without a full-thickness tear. There is no detectable laxity with grade I sprains. In grade II (moderate) sprains, there is more significant injury to the ligament, with stretching and partial tearing. There is minimal laxity present on examination. In grade III sprains, the MCL is completely disrupted. There is laxity on physical examination without a detectable endpoint.

Mechanism of Injury

MCL sprains occur when a valgus stress is applied to the knee. This frequently occurs when a player is tackled or tripped from the side during soccer or as a contact injury in football. If the injury involves more of a twisting mechanism, the MCL, the ACL, and the medial meniscus can also be torn; this is called the *unhappy triad of the knee*. MCL injuries may also occur in the setting of a knee dislocation.

Presentation

Patients with MCL sprains generally present with acute medial knee pain following a traumatic injury to the knee.

Relevant Anatomy

The MCL has both superficial and deep layers. The superficial MCL originates on the medial epicondyle of the femur and broadly inserts along the anterior medial proximal tibia. The deep MCL is a thickening within the medial capsule of the knee. The superficial MCL is the more important of the two structures in providing valgus stability to the knee. The MCL most commonly tears off its origin on the medial epicondyle of the femur.

Physical Examination

The specific physical examination elements of a knee with an MCL tear should include palpation of the medial knee and valgus stress testing. Palpation of the medial knee should include the entire length of the MCL: its origin on the medial epicondyle (the most common location of a tear), its midsubstance at the medial joint line, and its insertion on the anteromedial proximal tibia. Valgus stress testing should be tested at both 30 degrees of flexion and full extension. Valgus tress testing at 30 degrees of flexion is specific for the MCL, and at full extension, it tests the MCL, posteromedial corner, and cruciate ligaments. Valgus laxity at 30 degrees in a normal knee ranges from 0 to 10 degrees of opening with a solid endpoint and no tenderness. Physical examination findings differentiate between grades I to III injuries. In grade I injuries, there is minimal ecchymoses, swelling, and tenderness. Valgus stress testing in grade I sprains elicits tenderness without medial joint space opening and a solid endpoint. In grade II sprains, there is increased ecchymoses, swelling, and tenderness. Valgus stress testing at 30 degrees of flexion elicits tenderness and opening from 10 to 15 degrees with the presence of an endpoint. Valgus stress testing at full extension will be stable. In grade III injuries, there is complete tearing of the MCL with more severe ecchymoses, swelling, and tenderness. There is opening beyond 15 degrees without an endpoint with valgus stress testing at 30 degrees of flexion and instability can also be present at full extension depending on the severity of the injury.

Radiographic Examination

AP and lateral radiographs are generally negative. With chronic MCL tears, calcification can be seen at the origin of the MCL at the medial epicondyle, and this is called the *Pellegrini–Stieda sign.*

Special Tests

MRI is rarely necessary with an isolated MCL sprain; however, it is used commonly with multiligament knee injuries and/or knee dislocations. MRI is helpful in patients in whom an additional knee injury is suspected. It can confirm additional knee ligament injuries or meniscus injuries that may require surgical treatment. Stress radiographs can also be performed by placing valgus stress about the knee while an AP radiograph is taken. Stress radiographs are especially helpful in the pediatric population to differentiate physeal fractures from ligament sprains

Differential Diagnosis

The most important differential diagnosis is that of a distal femoral physeal fracture in skeletally immature patients. Other differential or concomitant injuries include ACL tears, meniscus tears, patella subluxation or dislocation, pes tendonitis, and chondral injuries. Medial meniscus tears can be differentiated on physical examination by the presence of instability with valgus stress testing in patients with MCL tears. In addition, patients with MCL tears are generally tender at the medial epicondyle, whereas patients with meniscus tears are tender at the medial joint line. The differential diagnosis for tenderness at the medial epicondyle is MCL tear and patellar dislocation or subluxation. In patellar dislocation, the MPFL tears off the medial epicondyle, resulting in tenderness.

Treatment

Treatment is nonoperative and involves immobilization for a duration that is dependent on the degree of injury and associated injuries. Grade I sprains are treated with early range of motion as tolerated and early return to activity without immobilization. Grade II sprains require a short period of immobilization with return to activity when the pain allows with a protective hinged knee brace at 3 to 4 weeks. Grade III injuries are immobilized with a cast or knee immobilizer at full extension for 2 to 4 weeks, followed by physical therapy to return-to-normal strength, with full return to activity by 6 to 8 weeks with a hinged knee brace. Associated injuries should be treated accordingly and at times warrant repair of grade III injuries. Protective, hinged knee braces are commonly used prophylactically to prevent MCL injuries in football lineman, with mixed results.

Complications

The main complication is recurrent valgus instability and pain that can result from early return to activity without brace protection.

ACL Sprain

ACL sprains or tears are the second most common knee ligament injury. They occur in an estimated 250,000 people annually.

Classification

ACL ligament injuries are graded from I to III, similar to other ligament injuries. It is difficult to distinguish between grade I and grade II injuries; however, the distinction between partial (I or II) and complete (III) is the most important for prognostic and therapeutic reasons.

Mechanism of Injury

ACL sprains are the result of a single traumatic event and are not due to overuse injuries. The exact mechanism varies according to the sport involved, but most injuries involve a twisting or pivoting mechanism of an extended knee on a planted foot. ACL injuries can also occur with hyperextension. ACL injuries commonly occur in contact sports, but they most commonly occur as a result of a noncontact mechanism. ACL injuries are common in soccer, football, basketball, and skiing.

Presentation

The classic presentation is the acute onset of pain and swelling after a traumatic event in which the patient landed awkwardly or twisted the knee and heard a "pop." The athlete is rarely able to continue activity.

Relevant Anatomy

The ACL is the most anterior of the two cruciate ligaments. The ACL arises from the anteromedial tibia, runs in the intercondylar notch, and inserts posteromedially on the lateral femoral condyle. The ACL is intraarticular and covered by a thin synovial membrane. The middle geniculate artery supplies the ACL and PCL. The ACL provides sagittal and rotary stability to the knee. It prevents rotation and anterior displacement of the tibia on the femur. The ACL most commonly tears off of its femoral insertion.

Physical Examination

Acute injuries of the ACL present with a tender hemarthrosis of the knee with difficulty bearing weight. The patient may not be able to fully extend the knee due to the effusion/hemarthrosis. The amount of swelling and tenderness may prevent an accurate examination of the ACL. Chronic injuries of the ACL present with a benign knee with no effusion and asymptomatic weight-bearing. The patient may not be able to fully extend the knee due to a cyclops lesion. A cyclops lesion results when the scarred down torn ACL remnant prevents full extension by obstructing the femoral notch The tests for ACL injuries include the Lachman test, the anterior drawer test, and the pivot shift test. These tests are described in the physical examination section of this chapter. The Lachman test is the most sensitive, and the pivot shift test is the most specific. It is important to perform a full-knee examination in a patient with a suspected ACL tear to evaluate for additional ligament or meniscus injury. All physical examination findings should be compared with the uninjured contralateral side.

Radiographic Examination

Radiographs are generally normal with an ACL tear. Occasionally, a small capsular avulsion fracture off of the lateral tibia can be present with an ACL tear; this is called a *Segund sign* (Fig. 17.25). Rarely, the ACL can avulse off of its origin at the tibial eminence, and the tibial eminence avulsion fracture fragment can be seen radiographically. ACL avulsion occurs most commonly in the adolescent population.

Special Tests

MRI is highly sensitive and specific for ACL tears and meniscus injuries. However, in a patient with obvious physical examination findings for an ACL tear, MRI adds little to the diagnosis and does not influence treatment. Another special test for ACL injuries is the KT-1000. The KT-1000 is a device that evaluates and quantifies anterior laxity of the tibia on the femur. It is not commonly used in clinical practice but is commonly used in research settings.

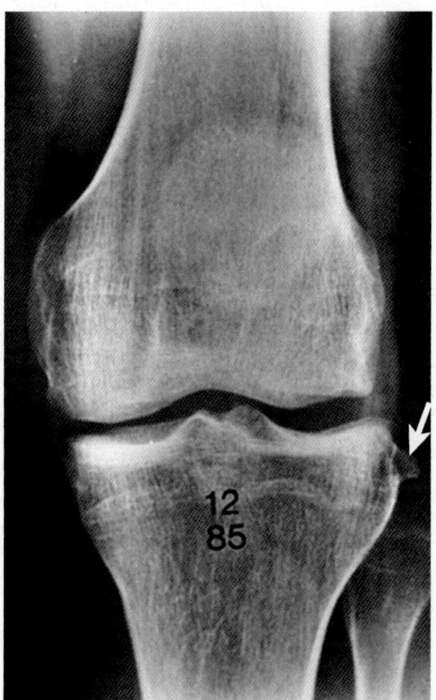

Figure 17.25 Anteroposterior radiograph of the knee showing a Segond fracture, which is pathognomonic of anterior cruciate ligament injury. (*Reproduced with permission from* Chapman MW, Szabo RM, Marder R, et al. *Chapman's Orthopaedic Surgery*. 3rd ed. Philadelphia, PA: Lippincott Williams & Wilkins, 2001.)

Differential Diagnosis

The differential diagnosis of an ACL tear involves the differential diagnosis for an acute knee hemarthrosis. This includes ACL tear, patellar dislocation, osteochondral injury, and a peripheral meniscus tear. If patients present acutely, the pain and effusion often prevent an appropriate examination of the knee. In these patients, an MRI is very helpful at differentiating between these diagnoses. Meniscus tears occur with approximately 50% of ACL tears. Lateral meniscus tears occur most commonly with acute ACL tears, and medial meniscus tears occur most commonly with chronic ACL tears.

Treatment

The options for an ACL tear involve nonoperative treatment with physical therapy or operative ACL reconstruction. The ACL has poor healing potential due to its intraarticular location and limited blood supply. The natural history of the ACL-deficient knee involves recurrent instability, progressive meniscus injury, progressive chondral damage, and eventual sports disability and arthritis. Interestingly, current long-term outcome studies suggest that the risk of osteoarthritis after ACL injury is not dependent on treatment, suggesting that the arthritis may be caused by damage sustained by the articular cartilage at the time of the original injury.

Patients best suited for nonoperative treatment are lower level recreational athletes or athletes involved in less-demanding straight-line activities (cycling, swimming, running, cross-country skiing, and rollerblading) with limited residual laxity after appropriate physical therapy. Age can be a relative indication for conservative treatment, as older patients are less active. Nonoperative treatment emphasizes physical therapy to restore motion and improve strength in the hamstring muscles, which act as a dynamic anterior stabilizer of the knee. Activity modification includes limiting and more aggressive sports (football, rugby, soccer, volleyball, basketball, and singles tennis). Protective bracing is also used as an element of nonoperative treatment.

Operative treatment involves surgical reconstruction with either autograft (tissue from the patient) or allograft (tissue from a cadaver) that is arthroscopically implanted as a substitute for the deficient ACL. The most common grafts are central third patella tendon and hamstring tendon autograft. Allografts are less commonly used. Current long-term outcome studies show no difference between the different types of grafts. ACL reconstruction is highly effective with approximately 90% to 95% of patients returning to full brace-free activity following a postoperative rehabilitation program. Concurrent meniscus injuries should be treated appropriately. Meniscus tears that can be repaired (peripheral, horizontal tears) have better outcomes when repaired at the time of ACL reconstruction than when performed in isolation.

Complications

The most common technical error in ACL reconstruction surgery is inappropriate tunnel placement that can result in recurrent laxity and limited flexion. The goal of ACL reconstruction is an anatomic reconstruction. Some studies have shown that arthrofibrosis (knee stiffness) can occur more commonly with acute ACL reconstruction (<2 weeks after injury).

PCL Sprain

Injury to the PCL is much less common than the ACL. The relative infrequency has led to a poorer understanding of the natural history of the injury. PCL injuries are most commonly associated with knee dislocations.

Classification

PCL injuries are graded from I to III, similar to other ligaments. Grade III injuries represent complete tears. Associated ligament injury to the posterolateral corner (PLC) may cause a greater degree of laxity than isolated PCL injuries.

Mechanism of Injury

The mechanism varies, but the most common mechanism involves a direct blow to the anterior aspect of a flexed knee with the ankle plantar flexed. In this position, the majority of the posterior force is absorbed by the PCL instead of the patella. The PCL is usually torn in its midportion. PCL injuries can also occur with hyperextension.

Presentation

The patient presents with a painful swollen knee. The degree of symptoms depends on the degree of trauma and the associated injuries. PCL injuries can be missed in a patient with distracting injuries, the most common is a posterior hip dislocation or posterior wall acetabular fracture in a patient presenting after a motor vehicle accident. In this patient the same force that dislocated the hip also caused the PCL injury. Associated injuries with a PCL include ACL, MCL, LCL, PLC, and meniscus injuries.

Relevant Anatomy

The PCL provides approximately 95% of the primary restraint to posterior tibial translation on the femur. The PCL originates from the center of the posterior tibia just distal to the articular surface, travels through the intercondylar notch, and inserts on the lateral aspect of the medial femoral condyle. Its fibers are stout and stronger than the ACL. Directly anterior and posterior to the femoral insertion of the PCL lie the meniscofemoral ligaments of Humphrey and Wrisberg, respectively, which serve as attachments of the PCL to the posterior horn of the lateral meniscus.

Physical Examination

The primary test for the PCL is the posterior drawer test. The posterior drawer test is performed on a supine patient with the knee flexed 90 degrees. The examiner sits on the patient's foot and pushes posteriorly on the tibia to detect the amount of posterior displacement. Before performing the test, it is important to take note of the position of the proximal tibia to the distal femur in relationship to the uninjured side to detect any degree of posterior subluxation before performing the examination. The posterior sag sign is the test to determine the degree of posterior subluxation at rest, if the tibia is less than 1 cm anterior to the femur and also less than the unaffected side it is a positive. The quadriceps active test is performed in the same position as the sag sign, by asking the patient to contract quadriceps, taking note of the reduction of the sag sign when the quadriceps are contracted. The degree of knee tenderness, swelling, and ecchymoses on physical examination increases with increasing grade of PCL injury from grade I to III. A grade I injury has mild swelling and tenderness with no detectable posterior laxity. Grade II injuries have some posterior laxity with an endpoint and may have a positive sag sign. Grade III injuries have increased subluxation without an endpoint and a positive sag sign.

Radiographic Examination

Radiographs are usually normal in PCL injuries. Chronic PCL injuries may exhibit degenerative changes in the patellofemoral and medial compartments.

Special Tests

MRI is highly sensitive and specific for PCL injuries. MRI is performed when multiligamentous injury and/or knee dislocation is suspected. Stress radiographs can be performed with a posterior force applied to the anterior tibia while a lateral radiograph is taken.

Differential Diagnosis

The differential diagnosis includes all of the knee ligamentous injuries and knee dislocation. The PCL must be considered injured until proven otherwise with a knee dislocation. The most important differential is to determine an isolated PCL injury from that associated with injury to the PLC. The anatomic description of the postero-PLC has been inconsistent and includes the LCL, popliteus, and the popliteofibular ligament. With injury to the PLC in addition to the PCL the knee will be increasingly unstable. In addition, PLC injuries have been met with poorer results if they are not repaired acutely primarily. The primary physical examination maneuvers for PLC injuries are the posterolateral drawer and the dial test. The posterolateral drawer test involves applying a posterolaterally directed force while the patient is in the same position as the posterior drawer test. The dial test is performed on a relaxed, prone patient. The patient's knees are flexed to 30 and 90 degrees and the amount of external rotation of the feet is determined. A difference of greater than 10 degrees from the uninjured side is a positive test. Increased external rotation at 30 degrees of flexion but not 90 degrees suggests an isolated PLC injury, whereas increases at both 30 and 90 degrees suggest a combined PLC and PCL injury.

Treatment

Treatment is generally nonoperative for isolated PCL injuries. This includes hinged bracing and physical therapy to regain the range of motion and strength. The natural history of the PCL-deficient knee is variable with some patients functioning well and other developing progressive instability. Surgical reconstruction is reserved for patients who fail nonoperative treatment, patients with knee dislocations, or patients with grade III injuries with excessive posterior instability. Reconstruction involves open or arthroscopic autograft or allograft ligament reconstruction. Long-term results have not approached the success seen following ACL reconstruction.

Complications

Complications include knee stiffness and recurrent or chronic instability. PCL deficient knees are at increased risk for patellofemoral and medial compartment degeneration.

LCL Sprain

LCL injuries are very uncommon, and when they do occur, they are usually in association with other ligament injuries such as knee dislocations or PLC injuries.

Classification

LCL injuries are graded from I to III, similar to those of other ligaments. Grade III injuries represent complete tears. Associated ligament injuries to the PLC may cause a greater degree of laxity than isolated LCL injuries.

Mechanism of Injury

An acute varus stress is responsible for the injury as the LCL is the primary restraint of varus motion about the knee. With multiligamentous knee injuries, injury to the LCL can result from a twisting mechanism of the knee.

Presentation

The presentation is that of a significantly traumatized knee with pain, swelling, and an inability to bear weight.

Relevant Anatomy

The LCL is a distinct collagenous structure traveling from the lateral epicondyle of the femur to attach to the fibular head. Other structures of importance on the lateral side include the arcuate ligament complex composed of the thickening of the posterolateral capsule, the biceps tendon, the IT band, and the popliteus tendon. The peroneal nerve courses around the fibular neck and dives into the anterior compartment as the deep peroneal nerve while sending a branch into the lateral compartment as the superficial peroneal nerve. The nerve is vulnerable during injury to the lateral side of the knee. Tears of the LCL are variable but are typically midsubstance or off its distal insertion on the fibular head.

Physical Examination

Pain, swelling, ecchymoses, and tenderness over the lateral side of the knee are common. Examination for associated nerve injury is important due to the peroneal nerve's proximity of the LCL. Ligament integrity can be palpated with the knee in the figure-of-four position and tested by applying a varus stress with the knee in slight flexion. Associated injury to the PLC is suggested if there is increased external rotation or posterior translation of the tibia at 30 degrees of knee flexion. Lateral opening with varus stress in full extension suggests additional injury to the ACL and/or PCL.

Radiographic Examination

AP and lateral radiographs of the knee should be performed to evaluate for avulsion fractures and to rule out additional fractures or injuries.

Special Tests

MRI can confirm the injury and exclude or include additional ligamentous, meniscus, or chondral injuries.

Differential Diagnosis

Associated ligamentous injuries should be included in the differential diagnosis, especially the PLC, ACL, PCL, and the possibility of knee dislocation.

Treatment

Treatment of isolated LCL injuries is usually nonoperative, with immobilization with a cast or knee immobilizer for 6 weeks followed by a rehabilitation program. For patients with associated PLC injuries, early primary repair is recommended, as outcomes with primary repair are better than with secondary reconstruction. In patients with varus malalignment, corrective valgus osteotomy should be considered prior to LCL repair to decrease the varus stress on the LCL and decrease the risk of recurrent instability.

Complications

Complications include knee stiffness and recurrent or chronic instability.

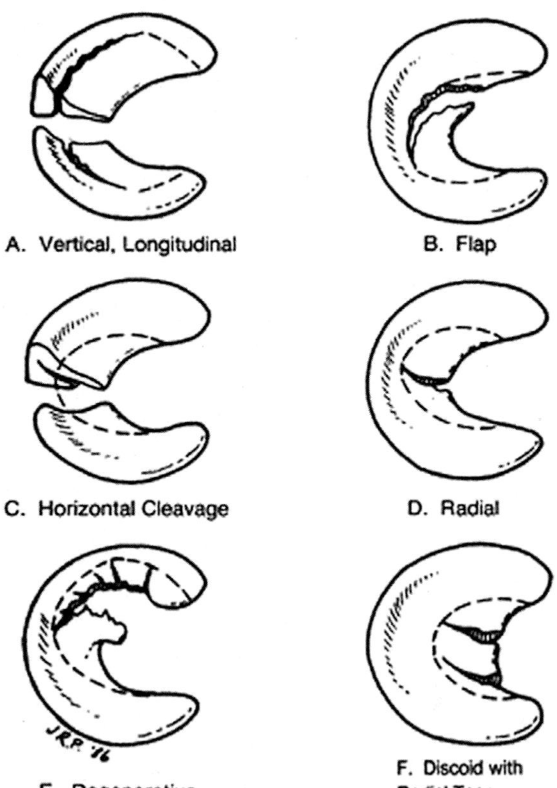

Figure 17.26 Types of meniscus tears, shown with the typical lines of resection. (*Reproduced with permission from* Chapman MW, Szabo RM, Marder R, et al.: *Chapman's Orthopaedic Surgery*, 3rd ed. Philadelphia: Lippincott Williams & Wilkins, 2001.)

NONTRAUMATIC INJURIES OF THE KNEE

Meniscus Tears

Meniscus tears are one of the most common problems seen in the knee and account for the most common indication for knee arthroscopy. In younger patients, they are generally traumatic in origin, whereas they are more commonly degenerative in patients older than 40 or 50 years.

Classification

Meniscus tears are classified by their configuration and location (Fig. 17.26).

The main tear configurations are as follows:

1. Longitudinal or horizontal—Tears that are parallel to the circumference of the meniscus.
2. Radial—Tears that are perpendicular to the circumference of the meniscus.
3. Cleavage—Tears that are in the plane of the meniscus, parallel to its superior and inferior surfaces.
4. Complex—Tears that are a combination of more than one specific pattern.

The meniscus is divided into thirds based on its relative blood supply and capacity to heal (Fig. 17.27):

1. Peripheral third—The peripheral third has the best blood supply and capacity to heal and is called the *red–red zone*.
2. Middle third—The middle third has an intermediate blood supply and is called the *red–white zone*.
3. Central third—The central third is avascular and lacks the capacity to heal. It is called the *white–white zone*.

Mechanism of Injury

Trauma can be responsible for meniscus tearing, although with age, the fibrocartilaginous menisci stiffen, degenerate, and tear with little trauma. Simple sheer or rotational stress can be sufficient to cause a tear.

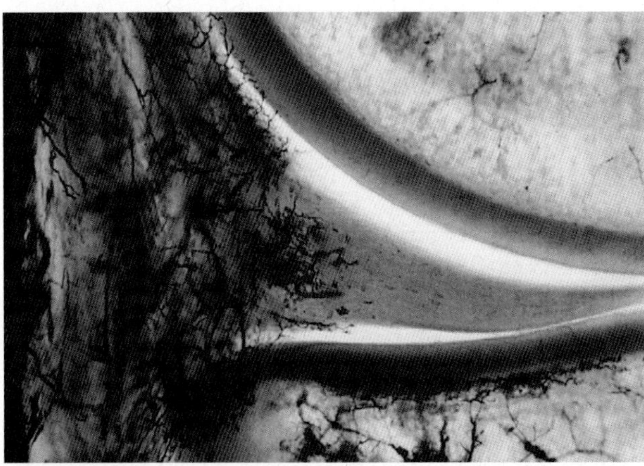

Figure 17.27 The blood supply of the meniscus. (*Reproduced with permission from* Johnson DH and Pedowitz RA: *Practical Orthopaedic Sports Medicine and Arthroscopy*. Philadelphia: Lippincott Williams & Wilkins, 2006.)

Presentation

Acute or insidious onset of pain or aching may herald a tear of the medial or lateral meniscus. Occasionally, in addition to pain, there may be a history of having heard a pop at the time of injury, usually when the patient twisted, squatted, or came down on the leg in an awkward manner. In older patients, symptom onset is usually related to a low-energy activity, such as stepping off a curb or getting out of a car. There may or may not be a history of swelling associated with the pain. Occasionally, there may be a history of mechanical locking in which the knee is temporarily stuck in a flexed position.

Relevant Anatomy

The menisci are the fibrocartilaginous semilunar-shaped disks that occupy the medial and lateral compartments of the knee. They provide congruency between the convex femoral condyles and the flat tibial plateau. Their predominant function is that of load distribution with a secondary contribution to stability, shock absorption, and cartilage nutrition. The medial meniscus is circumferentially attached to the capsule and has little mobility. In contrast, the lateral meniscus has no capsular attachment posterolaterally at the popliteal hiatus, accounting for its significantly greater mobility. The differential in mobility contributes to the fact that symptomatic medial meniscus tears outnumber lateral meniscus tears by an average of 4 to 1. The blood supply to the menisci come from the inferior medial and lateral geniculate arteries. As described earlier, the peripheral portion of the meniscus is relatively vascular and the central portion is avascular.

Physical Examination

The knee examination includes an examination for quadriceps atrophy, knee effusion, and restricted range of motion. The most sensitive finding is joint line tenderness that reproduces the patient's pain. The McMurray test, in which internal and external rotation of the knee from full flexion to 90 degrees of flexion causes a palpable click, is specific for a meniscus tear. The palpable click reflects an intermittently entrapped and freed meniscus fragment in the joint line.

Radiographic Examination

Standard views of the knee (weight-bearing AP, lateral, and sunrise views) should be taken to evaluated for osteoarthritis. They are generally negative in the younger population. In patients who have undergone complete meniscectomy (surgical resection of the meniscus), early arthritis with Fairbanks classic radiographic changes will often be present. Fairbanks changes are joint space narrowing, osteophyte formation, subchondral sclerosis, and subchondral cysts.

Special Tests

MRI is highly sensitive (90%–95%) and specific (90%–95%) for meniscus tears. However, as patients age, the likelihood of finding an asymptomatic meniscus tear on MRI is relatively high. Therefore, MRI should be utilized in cases when the diagnosis is uncertain to maximize the utility of the MRI.

Differential Diagnosis

The differential diagnosis includes articular cartilage injury (osteoarthritis, chondral, or osteochondral fracture), synovial disorders, or ligamentous injury.

Treatment

Meniscus tears are often successfully treated with nonoperative treatment including NSAIDs, activity modification, and a quadriceps-strengthening physical therapy program. A large portion of proven meniscus tears, especially in older, more sedentary patients, will improve with a significant duration of nonoperative treatment (1–2 months). Indications for surgical treatment include failed conservative treatment, a locked knee in which the meniscus is mechanically blocking knee extension, and meniscus pathology diagnosed during ligament surgery.

Historically, surgical treatment involved opening the knee joint (arthrotomy) and removing the entire meniscus (meniscectomy), which predictably led to arthritis in the involved compartment. Currently, with the development of knee arthroscopy, meniscus tears are treated with either meniscus repair or partial meniscectomy. Efforts are made to preserve as much of the meniscus as possible to prevent the development of degenerative arthritis. Unfortunately, despite such efforts, many studies show that even partial meniscectomy can lead to degenerative changes with time. Certain meniscus tears can be repaired. The gold standard is an "inside-out" meniscus repair, during which sutures are threaded through the meniscus from inside the knee and a knot is tied outside of the capsule to secure the repair. "Outside-in" and "all-inside" meniscal repairs can also be performed. Repairable meniscus tears are longitudinal in configuration and in the peripheral aspect of the meniscus. The peripheral tears exist in the vascular portion of the meniscus and are therefore capable of healing. Only approximately 5% of meniscus tears are repairable. Meniscus tears that are repaired at the same time as ACL reconstruction have the highest success rate of healing. Greater success has been attributed to returning stability to the knee and the fact that a hemarthrosis occurs secondary to the ACL reconstruction in the knee. Lateral meniscus tears occur more commonly with acute ACL tears, whereas medial meniscus tears occur more commonly in chronically ACL deficient knees.

The final surgical treatment for meniscus tears in patients who remain symptomatic after meniscal removal without arthritic involvement is meniscus replacement.

Allograft (from cadaver tissue) meniscus replacement is indicated in a small percentage of patients with meniscal-deficient knees. These are patients who are meniscus deficient without arthritis, have normal alignment, and have a stable knee. Surgical correction of knee malalignment with a high tibial osteotomy or surgical corrected knee instability with an ACL reconstruction may need to be performed prior to or with a meniscus allograft. Moderate long-term success can be expected with meniscus allograft replacement. Currently, research is ongoing regarding synthetic total and partial meniscus replacement.

Complications

The main complication of meniscus tears is degenerative arthritis as previously described.

Patellofemoral Pain Syndrome

Patellofemoral pain syndrome is one of the most common causes of knee pain. Historically termed *chondromalacia* (literally, softening of the articular cartilage), the pain is usually due to patellar malalignment rather than chondral breakdown.

Classification

There is no specific classification system for patellofemoral pain syndrome. Patellofemoral pain syndrome is a broad classification that includes multiple etiologies including trauma, overuse, instability, and idiopathic causes.

Mechanism of Injury

Most patients with patellofemoral symptoms have underlying patellar malalignment. Abnormal patella tracking leads to abnormal pressure on the articular cartilage. Although the articular cartilage is without sensory nerve endings, the underlying subchondral bone is not, and the abnormal forces from asymmetrical loading are perceived as pain. Rarely is there actual structural injury to the patella articular surface, whose thickness of 8 to 10 mm is the thickest hyaline cartilage in the body. When such softening does occur, it is known as *chondromalacia*. The terms *chondromalacia* and *patellofemoral pain syndrome* are not synonyms. Chondromalacia specifically refers to the condition in which there is pathologic softening of the cartilage surface.

Presentation

Patients present with vague pain in the front of the knee, often bilaterally, and usually with no history of specific injury. Pain is exacerbated by activities in which the knee is flexed, such as rising from a chair, stair climbing, and squatting. Descending stairs may be the most painful activity because the stress felt at the patellofemoral joint with descending stairs is 6 times the body weight, versus 3 times the body weight with ascending stairs. Unlike other mechanical knee problems, activity such as walking usually makes the symptoms better rather than worse.

Relevant Anatomy

The patella functions to effectively lengthen the lever arm of the quadriceps muscle. In full extension, standing or supine, the patella lies superior to the trochlear groove. As the knee is flexed, the patella begins articulating with the trochlear groove, with progressively increasing contact with knee flexion.

Physical Examination

First, the patient's overall alignment is evaluated. Passive malalignment is evaluated by noting the Q angle. The Q angle is the angle formed from a line drawn from the ASIS to the patella and a line drawn from the patella to the tibial tubercle (Fig. 17.28). The normal Q angle is approximately 10 degrees and is slightly greater in women. The Q angle should not exceed 15 degrees. As the patient stands

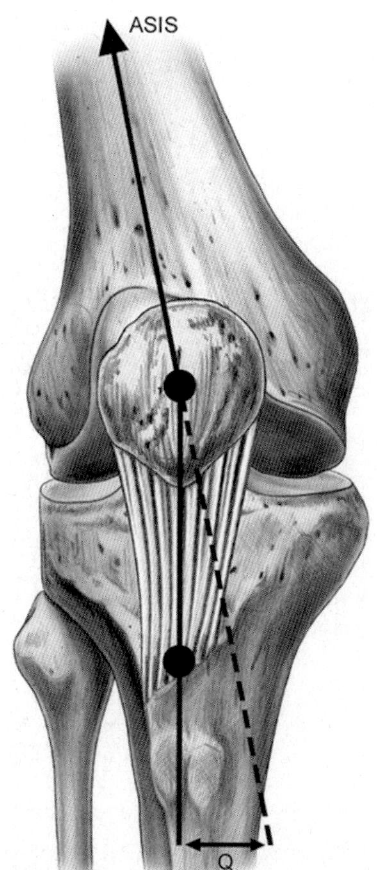

Figure 17.28 The Q angle is a helpful measure of patella tracking. There are differing opinions as to whether the Q angle is best measured in extension, 30 degrees, or 90 degrees of flexion. (*Reproduced with permission from* Johnson DH, Pedowitz RA. *Practical Orthopaedic Sports Medicine and Arthroscopy.* Philadelphia, PA: Lippincott Williams & Wilkins, 2006.)

and walks, careful attention is paid to the position of the foot to identify any pronation that will increase the Q angle. With the patient seated, observe the position of patellae. In patients with excessive lateral tilt, the patellae appear as "grasshopper eyes" tilting laterally away from each other. Inspect for active malalignment by having the patient actively extend the knee while seated. The "J" sign occurs when the patella reduces medially into the trochlear groove as the knee moves from full extension to flexion.

The quadriceps is inspected for overall development, specifically the VMO. Quadriceps atrophy or hypoplasia contributes to maltracking. With the patient supine, the physician should evaluate the mobility of the patella. Inability to elevate the lateral aspect of the patella to a neutral position indicates tightness of the lateral retinaculum, which is also known as a positive "patellar tilt" sign. Ability to laterally displace the patella more than 50% of its width suggests lax medial retinacular restraints, a finding in both malalignment and instability. If the patient displays apprehension when attempting lateral patellar displacement, there may be actual instability contributing to or responsible for the patient's symptoms.

In the seated position, the examiner palpates over the patellofemoral joint while the patient actively extends the knee, noting any crepitus. The opposite knee must be palpated as well, since crepitus may be a normal finding. Crepitus may reflect articular pathology or may be due to intermittently entrapped and bowstringed synovial bands within the patellofemoral joint. Palpation of the medial and lateral patellar facets is often tender.

Radiographic Examination

Radiographs should include AP and lateral views of the knee and a view tangential to the patellofemoral joint. A tangential view (sunrise, Merchant, Laurin) helps evaluate patellofemoral congruency, tracking, and arthritis (Fig. 17.29).

Special Tests

There are no special tests necessary to confirm the diagnosis of patellofemoral pain syndrome. Some clinicians have found tangential radiographs at different angles of knee flexion helpful to better evaluate the relationship of the patella to the trochlear groove. However, such tests are static and do not take into account dynamic forces of muscle pull during activity. This limits the usefulness not only of radiographs but also of CT and MRI.

Differential Diagnosis

In children, anterior knee pain is presumed hip pathology until proven otherwise. When tenderness is localized to the tibial tubercle, the condition may be Osgood–Schlatter syndrome, a consequence of repetitive traction stresses to the vulnerable tibial tubercle apophysis. Local tenderness and radiographic changes with fragmentation and enlargement of the tibial tubercle apophysis confirm the diagnosis. In older adolescents and adults, anterior knee pain may occur more over the patellar tendon rather than the patella itself and is known as *patellar tendonitis* (*jumper's knee*). Another cause of anterior knee pain is bipartite patella, in which a separate ossification center persists, most commonly at the superolateral aspect of the patella. This is usually incidental and rarely accounts for patient symptoms. However, if tenderness is present directly over the fragment, the fragment may need to be excised to improve symptoms.

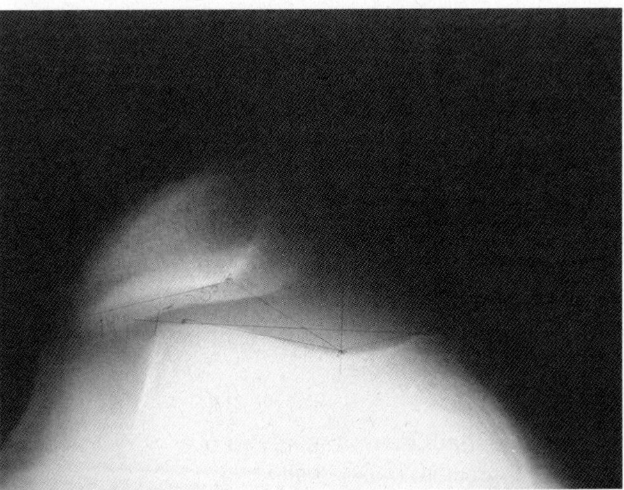

Figure 17.29 Merchant view of the patella, showing severe lateral patella tilt. (*Reproduced with permission from* Johnson DH, Pedowitz RA. *Practical Orthopaedic Sports Medicine and Arthroscopy.* Philadelphia, PA: Lippincott Williams & Wilkins, 2006.)

Treatment

It is important to remember that most patients with patellofemoral pain syndrome have no actual articular cartilage damage. The mainstay of treatment is to identify and correct malalignment or maltracking. Physical therapy emphasizes quadriceps-strengthening, specifically the VMO, through short-arc quadriceps exercises. Some patients benefit from McConnell taping of the patella into a corrected tracking position.

Surgical treatment is reserved for patients who are unresponsive to conservative treatment, have a suspected articular cartilage lesion, or have significant malalignment. Surgical treatment involves appropriate treatment of the articular cartilage lesion and treatment of the malalignment as detailed in the patella instability section of this chapter. An arthroscopy is performed to evaluate the articular surface. If an articular lesion is present, the patient is treated with chondroplasty, microfracture, or possibly ACI. Then the malalignment is addressed. If the patient has a positive patella tilt test and arthroscopically the patella is tilted in the trochlear groove, a lateral release of the lateral retinaculum can be performed. The lateral release weakens the lateral constraints of the patella to decrease the amount of lateral maltracking. If the patient has a large Q angle, a distal realignment procedure can be performed. The most commonly performed distal realignment procedure is the Fulkerson procedure. During this procedure, the tibial tubercle is cut and shifted anteriorly and medially. The medial shift decreases the Q angle. The anterior shift off-loads the damaged articular cartilage of the patella and increases the moment arm of the quadriceps muscle.

Complications

Complications include recurrent pain, patellar instability, nonunion, and patellofemoral arthritis.

IT Band Syndrome

IT band syndrome is an overuse injury of the lateral knee. It is also called *cyclist's* or *runner's knee.*

Presentation

The patient will present with pain along the lateral knee that usually relates to running or cycling. Symptoms are often preceded by a change in training regimen, such as an increase in mileage, intensity, terrain surface, or changed shoe wear.

Mechanism of Injury

IT band syndrome is a friction syndrome over the lateral part of the leg. Repetitive motion of the tense IT band over the lateral epicondyle is thought to cause a bursitis between the tendon and the lateral epicondyle.

Relevant Anatomy

The IT band originates on the gluteus maximus as the tensor fascia lata and inserts at Gerdy tubercle on the anterolateral aspect of the tibia. As it travels to the knee, it runs over the greater trochanter of the hip and the lateral epicondyle of the femur. A friction syndrome involving the IT band can develop at the greater trochanter as trochanteric bursitis, the femoral epicondyle, or Gerdy tubercle. Female patients have a wider pelvis and greater valgus alignment of their knees, which predispose them to IT band syndrome.

Physical Examination

The patient will have focal tenderness over the lateral epicondyle. Occasionally, the Ober test will be positive. The Ober test is performed by lying the patient laterally on the uninvolved side. Then the hip is adducted and the knee is flexed 90 degrees; the hip is then gently extended, abducted, and the knee is extended. Tightness and irritation over the IT band will result in pain, which is a positive Ober test.

Radiographic Examination

Standard radiographic views of the knee are negative.

Special Tests

Rarely, an MRI is obtained and can show increased signal at Gerdy tubercle or the lateral epicondyle.

Differential Diagnosis

The differential diagnosis for lateral knee pain includes lateral meniscus tear, LCL sprain, lateral compartment arthritis, proximal tibiofibular joint pathology, peroneal nerve pathology, or IT band syndrome.

Treatment

Treatment is nonoperative for the vast majority of patients and includes activity modification, NSAIDs, and physical therapy to include a thorough stretching program of the IT band, hamstrings, and glutei. A compression strap worn above the lateral epicondyle during activity may improve symptoms. Most patients are able to return to their previous level of activity. Rarely, corticosteroid injections or surgical release are needed.

Osteochondritis Dissecans

Although chondral or osteochondral injuries can be caused by acute trauma, a more common cause is OCD. In this condition, a portion of the normal articular cartilage is dissected away from its underlying subchondral bed. The most common location in the knee is the lateral aspect of the medial femoral condyle, in more than 80% of cases.

Classification

Osteochondral injuries have been classified on the basis of the fragment's relationship to the bone from which it arises. A grade I lesion is incomplete without actual complete fracture line extending from the underlying subchondral bone into the joint. In a grade II lesion, there is a complete fracture line extending from the subchondral bone to the joint, but the fragment is still within the bed and minimally displaced. In a grade III lesion, the fragment is loose with a fracture plane around the lesion, which loosely lies in its bed. In a grade IV lesion, the fragment has become detached and is free within the joint.

Mechanism of Injury

This condition has been attributed to a vascular insult of the growing epiphysis of skeletally immature patients. The condition is most frequently seen in the lateral aspect of the medial femoral condyle of the knee; however, it has been described in the elbow on the capitellum and the ankle on the talus.

Presentation

The most common presentation is that of an adolescent or young adult with knee joint symptoms of intermittent pain, swelling, or catching related to knee activities.

Physical Examination

Physical findings are usually nonspecific, and the diagnosis is afforded by imaging studies.

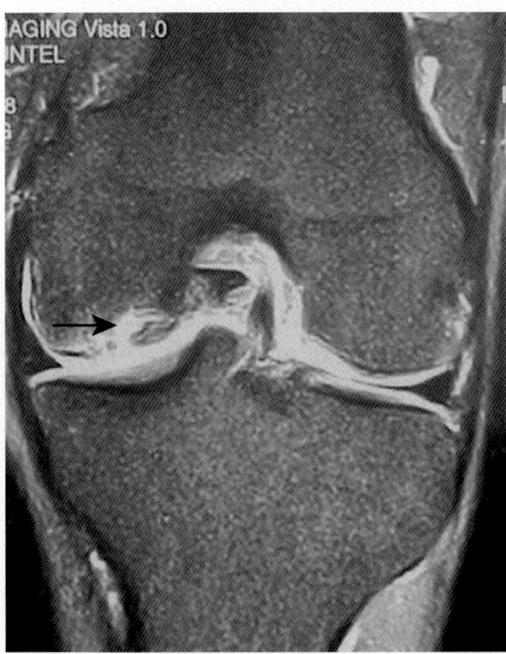

Figure 17.30 T2 weighted MRI of the knee demonstrating high signal behind osteochondral fragment, indicating an unstable fragment. (*Reproduced with permission from* El Attrache NS, Harner CD, Mirzayan R, Sekiya JK: *Surgical Techniques in Sports Medicine.* Philadelphia: Lippincott Williams & Wilkins, 2006.)

Radiographic Examination

Standard radiographs of the knee show a localized area of radiolucency (decreased density) in the area of the OCD. Often, the osteochondral fragment is sclerotic (increasingly dense) and may be partially or completely detached from its underlying bed.

Special Tests

MRI is useful to localize the lesion and determine its size and stability. Unstable lesions have fluid behind the lesion that can be seen on T2-weighted MRI images (Fig. 17.30).

Treatment

Treatment varies according to the lesion's size, location, stage, and the patient's age. In skeletally immature patients, nondisplaced osteochondral fragments are thought to have healing potential with immobilization. Conversely, in older adolescents or young adults, particularly when there is evidence of fragment displacement, definitive treatment involves debridement and, if possible, fixation of the fragment with headless screws. A number of strategies have been devised for treating the defect left behind following debridement of an OCD. These include microfracture, OATS, and ACI, as discussed previously in the patellar instability section of this chapter.

Complications

The major complication is the development of degenerative arthritis in the involved compartment.

Baker cyst

Described by Baker in the late 1800s, this condition is a well-known accompaniment of several knee disorders. Rather than a discrete entity, it is actually a normal anatomic structure that becomes prominent in response to knee pathology.

Presentation

Most Baker cysts come to the physician's attention when discovered by MRI. Occasionally, the patient will note a prominence in the popliteal area. Less commonly, patients may present with acute pain and swelling in their proximal calf as a consequence of cyst rupture, with spilling of the synovial contents into the posterior compartments of the leg.

Relevant Anatomy

This structure is a normal bursa of the semimembranosus and is present in an estimated 35% to 50% of patients. Synovial fluid generated within the knee in response to meniscal, chondral, or synovial pathology can lead to bursa distention due to direct communication with the joint.

Physical Examination

Baker cysts are almost always located posteromedially in the knee. Usually, there is an indistinct area of tenderness in the popliteal fossa.

Radiographic Examination

Radiographs are usually negative, although occasionally osteochondral fragments can be seen posteromedially.

Special Tests

Special test are unnecessary in patients with a typical history. Imaging by MRI demonstrates the cyst and other intraarticular pathology and is the diagnostic test of choice. Aspiration of the mass yields golden-yellow viscous synovial fluid. Its viscosity mandates the use of a large-bore needle, such as an 18-gauge, to ensure successful aspiration.

Differential Diagnosis

The presence of a neoplasm must be considered in the patient presenting with fullness or a palpable mass in the popliteal fossa. Imaging is almost always conducted to rule out this possibility. In the patient with acute pain and swelling of the proximal calf, consideration must be given to a deep vein thrombosis. Meniscal cysts are differentiated in their size and location. They are very discrete grape-like structures that occur directly along the joint line and are most commonly associated with meniscus tears.

Treatment

Baker cysts are often diagnosed as an incidental finding on MRI performed for knee symptoms. Most cysts will resolve on definitive treatment of the intraarticular pathology, such as partial meniscectomy. Occasionally, the cyst itself produces symptoms due to its size. Aspiration, followed by corticosteroid injection, is an alternative but, if unsuccessful, surgical excision is often curative

TRAUMATIC INJURIES OF THE LEG

Midshaft Tibia and Fibula Fractures

Fractures of the tibia and fibula shafts are the most common long bone fractures. Men are more affected than women, with the average age being 37 years.

Classification

Fractures are described by fracture pattern type: transverse, spiral, oblique, and comminuted; the location: proximal, middle, and distal; and the type and degree of displacement. The presence of associated soft tissue injuries are also characterized according to the Gustilo and Anderson classification of open fractures. Grade I fractures are clean, with a wound less than 1 cm. Grade II fractures have more extensive soft tissue damage and a wound generally greater than 1 cm and less than 10 cm. Grade IIIA fractures are complex fracture patterns or crush injuries with extensive soft tissue damage. Grade IIIB are extensive injuries with periosteal stripping requiring soft tissue flap coverage. Grade IIIC are fractures with associated vascular injuries requiring repair.

Mechanism of Injury

There are three common mechanisms of injury. Direct trauma can be from high-energy injury, such as a motor vehicle accident, or a low-energy direct blow, such as during a sporting event. Indirect trauma can occur when the foot is fixed and the leg is torqued, as can occur in sporting events or a fall from a short height. Finally, fractures can occur as a result of penetrating injury such as gunshot wounds.

Presentation

Patients present with acute leg pain accompanied with deformity and swelling following a traumatic injury.

Relevant Anatomy

The tibia and fibula are long bones, with the tibia demonstrating a triangular shape when viewed in axial cross section. Its anterior border is rather sharp, subcutaneous, and quite vulnerable to trauma. The fibula is joined proximally to the posterolateral proximal tibia at the proximal tibiofibular joint. Distally, the fibula articulates with the distal tibia laterally at the ankle mortise. Four distinct compartments contain the soft tissue and neurovascular components of the leg and include the anterior, lateral, superficial posterior, and deep posterior compartments (Fig. 17.11). The blood supply is almost entirely from the popliteal artery, which in the proximal third of the leg sends branches anteriorly through the interosseous membrane to provide blood supply to the anterior and lateral compartments. The origin of this vasculature, at the trifurcation in the proximal leg, is a site of vulnerability with potential vascular compromise, ischemia, and limb loss following trauma to this area. Nerve supply is via the common peroneal nerve and the posterior tibial nerve.

Physical Examination

Physical examination should focus on close inspection to rule out open fracture. In addition, a thorough secondary survey should be performed to rule out associated injury. Compartment syndrome is a consideration with all tibia fractures with pain severe with passive dorsiflexion or the foot or toes one of the earliest physical findings.

Radiographic Examination

Radiographs should include AP and lateral views of the full length of the tibia and fibula; AP and lateral views of the knee; and AP, lateral, and mortise views of the ankle.

Special Tests

Further radiographs are obtained depending on the clinical suspicion of associated injuries. If the fracture line extends into the knee or ankle joints, CT scans of these joints should be considered. Doppler evaluation and ankle–brachial indices should be used to evaluate vascular status in the setting of a possible injury. An arteriogram is the definitive test for suspected vascular injury.

Differential Diagnosis

There is little in the differential diagnosis; however, correct and prompt diagnosis of associated neurovascular injury including compartment syndrome should be made. A high index of suspicion for the development of compartment syndrome should be maintained before and after definitive treatment of these fractures.

Compartment syndrome is a clinical diagnosis based on tenderness with passive stretch of the involved compartment, pain out of proportion to examination, and a tense compartment. If the diagnosis is questioned, the compartment pressure can be directly measured. This is obtained with a hand-held monometer or arterial line that is placed directly into the compartment. Compartment syndrome is a cyclic process started when the compartment pressure exceeds the venous outflow pressure of the compartment. This results in venous stasis, resultant increased pressure and eventual ischemia. Intervention needs to occur before the process starts so the cutoff of the compartment pressure above which a fasciotomy should be preformed is 30 mm Hg or within 30 mm Hg of venous pressure. The treatment for compartment syndrome is fasciotomy.

Treatment

Treatment depends on the type of fracture. For closed fractures, nonoperative treatment is often acceptable, with closed reduction and long leg cast application. General guidelines for acceptable reduction include less than 5 degrees of varus and valgus angulation, less than 10 degrees of rotational deformity, less than 1 cm of shortening, less than 5 mm of distraction, and more than 50% cortical contact. When treated nonoperatively, a long leg cast is placed with initial non–weight-bearing transitioning to progressive weight-bearing as the fracture begins to heal. Healing averages 16 weeks and the risk of displacement warrants frequent follow-up evaluation to ensure maintenance of reduction. Closed treatment is most effective for low-energy fractures with little displacement, with healing rates as high as 97%.

Unstable fractures, those in which reduction cannot be achieved or maintained, are usually candidates for IM nail fixation. Plates and screws can be utilized for proximal or distal fractures and intraarticular fractures. The IM nail has become the standard of care for extraarticular midshaft tibia fractures. The IM nail allows for immediate weight-bearing, low nonunion rates, and low infection rates.

Open fractures must be treated with attention to wound management and fracture stability. Antibiotics should be instituted immediately in the emergency department along with tetanus prophylaxis. Open wounds should be sterilely covered, splinted, and treated as a surgical emergency with prompt surgical irrigation and debridement and fracture fixation. Repeat debridement and flap coverage or vascular repair may be required. The options for fracture fixation include IM nails or external fixation devices. For grade I and some grade II fractures, an IM nail can often be placed at the time of the initial debridement. For higher grade injuries, an external fixator is applied until the wound is stable and then the external fixation device is often removed and an IM nail is placed for definitive fracture treatment. Conversion from an external fixator to a nail is performed only within the first 3 weeks to decrease the risk of spreading osteomyelitis to the tibial canal from infection around the external fixator pins.

Complications

Complications are numerous, the most common complications are soft tissue related, including infection. Other complications include delayed union, nonunion, malunion, knee or ankle stiffness, thromboembolic disease, compartment syndrome, and limb loss.

NONTRAUMATIC INJURIES OF THE LEG

Tibial Stress Fractures

Tibial stress fractures are most often encountered in athletes and military recruits. The majority of stress fractures occur in the lower extremity, with 50% of cases in the tibia or fibula. Stress factures are seen most commonly in women and are can be related to malnutrition.

Mechanism of Injury

A stress fracture occurs when repetitive loads exceeding the remodeling capability of the involved bone are applied. Cyclic loading above the level of normal bone remodeling causes osteoclastic to exceed osteoblastic activity. This results in weakening of the bone and fracture.

Presentation

Tibial stress fractures are considered overuse injuries. They are most commonly seen with rapid increases in frequency, duration, or intensity of athletic activity. Pain is the most common symptom associated with tibia stress fractures. It is generally located in the anterior leg at the midaspect of the tibia. Pain is worse with activity such as jumping.

Relevant Anatomy

The tibia has a normal bow that has its aspect along the anterior midshaft. The most common location for tibia shaft fractures is the anterior midshaft of the tibia. As a result of the anterior tibia bow the anterior aspect of the tibia is under tensile load and the posterior aspect of the tibia is under compressive load.

Physical Examination

Physical examination reveals a point tender area along the anterior midshaft of the tibia. There may be an irregular thickening palpable at the tender aspect of the anterior tibia. In addition, axial compression to the tibia exacerbates the pain.

Radiographic Examination

AP and lateral radiographs of the tibia may reveal signs of a stress fracture. Cortical hypertrophy may be present at the stress fracture. In addition a "dreaded black line" can occur in the cortex. This is an infraction line that is considered the sign of an impending fracture (Fig. 17.31).

Special Tests

Radiographs can be negative for as long as 3 weeks after the onset of symptoms. If radiographs are negative, MRI or bone scan can be performed. Increased T2 intensity on MRI or increased uptake on bone scan are the signs of stress fracture.

Differential Diagnosis

The differential diagnosis is medial tibial stress syndrome and exertional compartment syndrome. This can generally be distinguished from tibial stress fracture by history and physical examination.

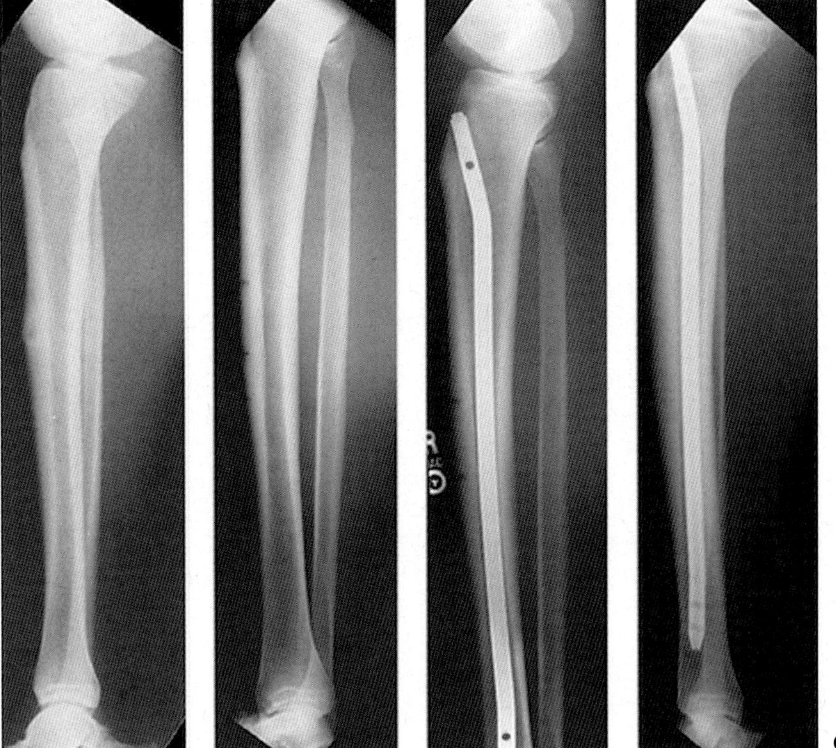

Figure 17.31 Stress fracture of the anterior middiaphysis of the tibia. Notice the extensive cortical hypertrophy in addition to the transverse infraction **(A)** and the multiple horizontal translucencies **(B)**. **C:** Immediately after IM nailing. **D:** Healed fractures with extensive anterior cortical thickening. (*Reproduced with permission from* Chapman MW, Szabo RM, Marder R, et al.: *Chapman's Orthopaedic Surgery*, 3rd ed. Philadelphia: Lippincott Williams & Wilkins, 2001.)

Treatment

Most tibial stress fractures improve with activity modification by avoiding impact loading activities for 4 to 8 weeks. This is achieved with crutches and with or without casting. Tibial stress fractures can result in nonunion because of their location on the tensile aspect of the tibia, which results in fracture distraction and the relative hypovascularity of the tibia. A difficult tibial stress fracture can be treated with an external bone stimulator and a patella tendon bearing cast. If the patient continues to be symptomatic after 4 to 6 months of nonoperative treatment, then surgical treatment with an IM rod is indicated.

Complications

Complications of tibial stress fractures include nonunion and overt fracture of the midshaft of the tibia.

Medial Tibial Stress Syndrome (Shin Splints)

One of the most common problems seen among runners is "shin splints," also known as *medial tibial stress syndrome.*

Mechanism of Injury

The pathophysiology of this condition is not well understood. Historically, this condition was thought to be a consequence of one of several entities, including periostitis, posterior tibial tendonitis, soleus tendonitis, or early stress reaction in the bone. There is no absolute consensus on the etiology of this condition, although there is wide agreement that it is an overuse injury. Periostitis of the soft tissue muscular attachments along the posteromedial tibia is thought to be the most likely cause of this syndrome.

Presentation

The presentation is indicative of its name. Pain over the shin and posteromedial tibia occurs, usually as a consequence of running, often on hard, flat terrain. Discomfort is usually during activity, but with continued running, it can lead to pain even with walking.

Relevant Anatomy

Medial tibial stress syndrome occurs over the posterior mid to distal third of the tibia.

Physical Examination

Diffuse tenderness to palpation is usually present over the posteromedial mid to distal third of the tibia.

Radiographic Examination

Radiographs are negative.

Special Tests

A number of special tests have been described, including injection into adjacent soft tissue with local anesthetic. However, relief does not completely confirm the diagnosis or definitively exclude the possibility of a stress fracture. Bone scans demonstrate diffuse uptake of the tracer along the distal third of the tibia.

Differential Diagnosis

The main differential to consider is that of a tibial stress fracture, which is well demonstrated on the bone scan as a focal hot spot in comparison with the more diffuse dye take-up in tibial stress syndrome.

Treatment

Definitive treatment is rest. Usually, activity modification results in near-immediate improvement. When athletes can return to their running depends upon the severity, intensity, duration, and goals of individual patients. Ice massage several times a day over the painful area combined with the use of NSAIDs can improve symptoms. Some studies have suggested that the use of arch supports may help those with marked pronation. Heel cord stretching may also be useful in some patients. Cross-training to maintain conditioning through swimming, cycling, and even running with a weighted vest in a pool are encouraged until the condition resolves. Importantly, prevention of this condition is possible through correcting any identified training errors such as excessive mileage, hard surfaces, and inadequate shoe wear.

Exertional Compartment Syndrome

Compartment syndrome, in which the elevated compartment pressure can lead to muscle ischemia, pain, and potential necrosis, most commonly occurs in the traumatized extremity. However, this condition can also occur in the absence of discrete trauma and is seen among athletes as exertional compartment syndrome. This most commonly affects the anterior and deep posterior compartments of the leg.

Mechanism of Injury

Exertional compartment syndrome occurs as a consequence of progressive increased compartmental pressure due to activity, most commonly occurring in the leg while running. Progressive muscle hypertrophy and swelling during activity compromises the normal blood supply, leading to potential ischemia and pain.

Presentation

Unlike stress reactions or shin splints, where pain is bearable and the patient can continue running with the pain, pain with exertional compartment syndrome is severe enough to force the athlete to stop running. Unlike stress reactions or fractures, the symptoms promptly vanish after cessation of activity.

Physical Examination

Physical examination is unremarkable. There is no particular focal tenderness or neurologic abnormality.

Radiographic Examination

Radiographs are negative.

Special Tests

The diagnosis of exertional compartment syndrome is established by compartment pressure measurements at rest and following activity. Using a small needle attached to a pressure manometer setup, each of the four compartments are measured in both the legs and recorded. The athlete runs on a treadmill until symptomatic and then compartment pressures are measured again and compared to preexercise levels. The exact criteria necessary for diagnosing compartment syndrome are somewhat variable, but in general, pressure measurements in excess of 15 mm Hg at rest or more than 20 mm Hg 5 to 15 minutes postexercise are suggestive of exertional compartment syndrome.

Differential Diagnosis

In the patient with equivocal intracompartmental pressure readings and the presence of bone tenderness, medial tibial stress syndrome is a more likely diagnosis.

Treatment

Athletes can either modify their activity (i.e., give up running) or have the affected compartment(s) surgically decompressed. This surgical procedure involves a small incision over the affected compartment, followed by an incision of the surrounding fascial envelope. The outcome is predictably good.

Complications

The major risks with compartment release are superficial peroneal nerve injury and inadequate release.

RECOMMENDED READINGS

Albert MJ. Supracondylar fractures of the femur. *J Am Acad Orthop Surg.* 1997;5:163–171.

Berkson EM, Virkus WW. High-energy tibial plateau fractures. *J Am Acad Orthop Surg.* 2006;14:20–31.

Browne JE, Branch TP. Surgical alternatives for treatment of articular cartilage lesions. *J Am Acad Orthop Surg.* 2000;8:180–189.

Greis PE, Bardana DD, Holmstrom MC, et al. Meniscus injury, I: basic science and evaluation. *J Am Acad Orthop Surg.* 2002;10:168–176.

Greis PE, Holmstrom MC, Bardana DD, et al. Meniscus injury, II: management. *J Am Acad Orthop Surg.* 2002;10:177–187.

Pell RF IV, Khanuja HS, Cooley GR. Leg pain in the running athlete. *J Am Acad Orthop Surg.* 2004;12:396–404.

Post WR. Anterior knee pain: diagnosis and treatment. *J Am Acad Orthop Surg.* 2005;13:534–543.

Rihn JA, Cha PS, Groff YJ, et al. The acutely dislocated knee: evaluation and management. *J Am Acad Orthop Surg.* 2004;12:334–346.

Knee Arthroplasty

18

John A. Johansen *Brian G. Evans*

INTRODUCTION

Osteoarthritis (OA) of the knee is a degenerative condition that affects a large number of people during the aging process and is by far the most common cause of knee pain in those older than 50 years. Pain tends to be progressive and is often debilitating, thus leading to a significant decline in the quality of life in these individuals. While there are many nonoperative treatment options and joint-sparing procedures available for the management of early OA, the gold standard for treatment of end-stage OA is total knee arthroplasty (TKA). Currently, there are approximately 200,000 total knee replacements done in the United States annually, and this number can be expected to increase substantially as the population ages. This chapter will serve as a comprehensive review of the diagnosis and treatment of OA of the knee and the expected outcomes and complications of TKA.

ANATOMY

The osseous anatomy of the knee consists of the proximal tibia, distal femur, and the patella, which combine to form three compartments in the knee: medial, lateral, and patellofemoral. (Fig. 18.1)

The medial compartment of the knee is formed by the articulation between the medial femoral condyle and the medial tibial plateau, whereas the lateral compartment is formed by the lateral femoral condyle and the lateral tibial plateau. The medial and lateral menisci are attached to the proximal tibia in the respective compartments and function mainly to increase the surface area for weight-bearing (Fig. 18.2). By decreasing the stress transmitted to the articular surface on both the distal femur and proximal tibia, these menisci help preserve the joint surface. Biomechanical studies have indicated that there is approximately a 300% increase in contact pressures on the articular cartilage following meniscal removal.

The patellofemoral compartment is formed by the articulation between the trochlea, which is located on the anterior aspect of the distal femur, and the patella. The patella is a sesamoid bone located within the tendon of the quadriceps mechanism and is composed of medial and lateral facets. The lateral facet is typically broader, whereas the medial facet is more acutely oriented in relation to the trochlea (Fig. 18.3). The undersurface of the patella contains the thickest layer of articular cartilage in the human body. The trochlear groove is located between the condyles anteriorly on the distal femur and has both a medial and a lateral rim. The lateral rim is frequently more prominent, allowing for proper patellar tracking with flexion and extension of the knee.

BIOMECHANICS

The mechanical axis of the lower extremity extends from the center of rotation of the hip to the center of the ankle joint and normally crosses the knee joint in the lateral third of the medial tibial plateau. However, the anatomic axis is in 5 to 7 degrees of valgus, as the femoral shaft extends more laterally than the center of the femoral head (Fig. 18.4). When the knee is loaded, the medial compartment experiences 60% of the weight-bearing stress, whereas the lateral compartment experiences 40%. This difference in the applied load in the normal knee is the reason the medial tibial plateau and the medial femoral condyle are larger than the lateral side. Patients with significant angular deformity in the knee have altered weight-bearing, which results in increased stress in the medial (with varus or bowlegged deformity) or lateral (with valgus or knock-knee deformity) compartment. The increased stress frequently results in early arthritis in the affected compartment.

The highest joint forces, however, are found in the patellofemoral articulation, as forces up to 5 to 8 times body weight can be noted for activities such as stair climbing and jumping. The function of the patella is predominantly to

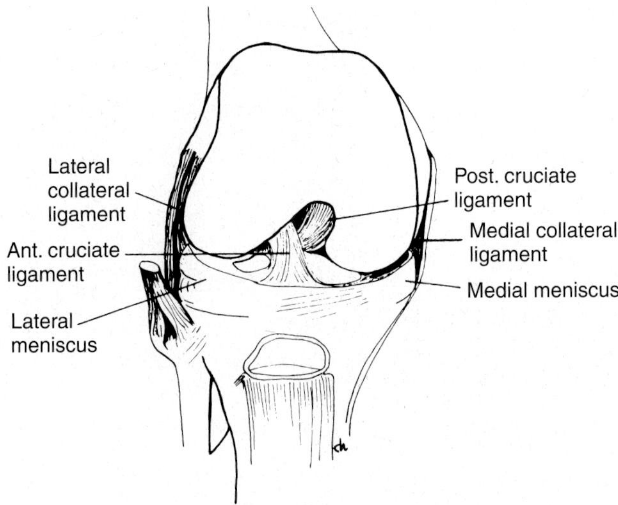

Figure 18.1 Diagram of the knee joint with the patella and capsule removed. The medial compartment contains the medial meniscus, the lateral compartment contains the lateral meniscus, and the patellofemoral compartment is anterior to the distal femur. (*Reproduced with permission from* Koopman WJ, Moreland LW. *Arthritis and Allied Conditions: A Textbook of Rheumatology.* 15th ed. Philadelphia, PA: Lippincott Williams & Wilkins, 2005.)

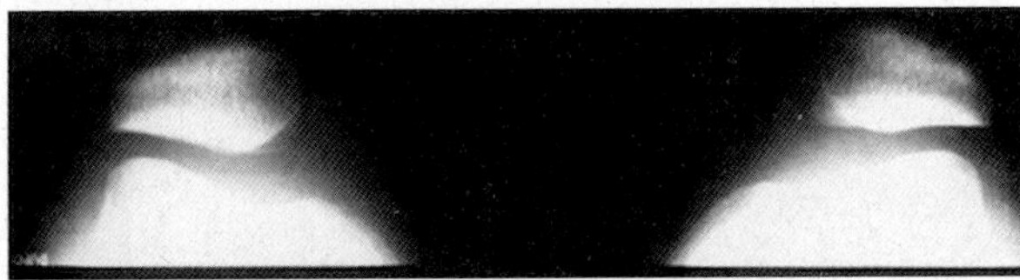

Figure 18.3 Bilateral axial views of the patella. Note the broad lateral facet in relation to the relatively acutely angled medial facet. Also note the relative prominence of the lateral rim of the trochlea. (*Reproduced with permission from* Chapman MW, Szabo RM, Marder R, et al. *Chapman's Orthopaedic Surgery.* 3rd ed. Philadelphia, PA: Lippincott Williams & Wilkins, 2001.)

provide a mechanical advantage to the quadriceps muscle during knee extension. The patella moves in the line of pull of the quadriceps further away from the center of rotation of the knee, thereby acting as a lever and reducing the force required to extend the knee. Patients who have had a patellectomy due to arthritis, trauma, and other causes are noted to have approximately a 30% reduction in knee extension strength.

OA OF THE KNEE

OA, or degenerative joint disease, of the knee is an extremely common condition that affects approximately 10% to 15% of people older than 60 years. This translates to approximately 26 million people in the United States alone, with more than 200,000 total knee replacements being performed annually in this country and more than 500,000 worldwide. OA causes a substantial physical burden on the population as approximately 80% of these patients have some degree of movement limitation, with up to 25% having difficulty performing routine daily activities. It also leads to significant reduction in job productivity with reports indicating that patients with knee arthritis missed up to 2 weeks per year of work because of their condition. The economic burden of the disease is also quite remarkable. When including OA of all joints, it is estimated that the cost in the United States is $60 billion per year, whereas job productivity lost costs anywhere from $3 billion to $10 billion. In fact, OA is second only to ischemic heart disease as a cause of work disability.

Risk Factors

OA is characterized by disruption of the highly organized articular cartilage overlying the subchondral bone and can be caused by different factors. The first and the most common type is primary, or idiopathic, degenerative arthritis,

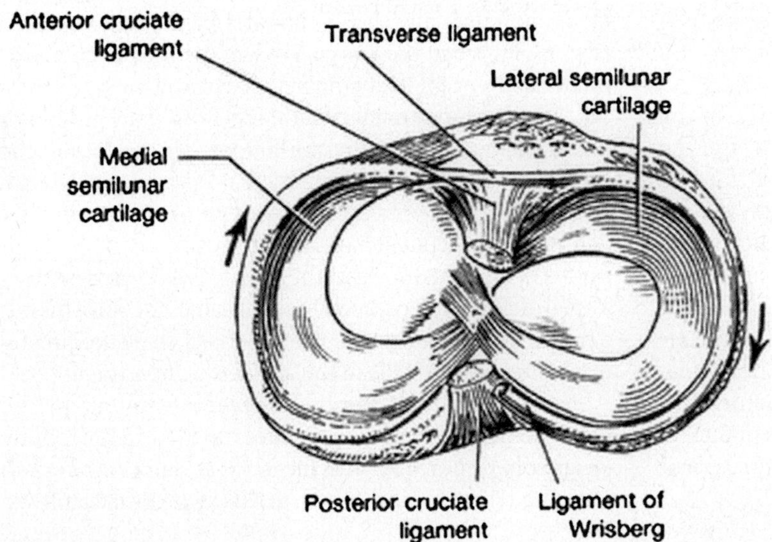

Figure 18.2 Superior surface of the tibia with superimposed medial and lateral menisci. (*Reproduced with permission from* Chapman MW, Szabo RM, Marder R, et al. *Chapman's Orthopaedic Surgery.* 3rd ed. Philadelphia, PA: Lippincott Williams & Wilkins, 2001.)

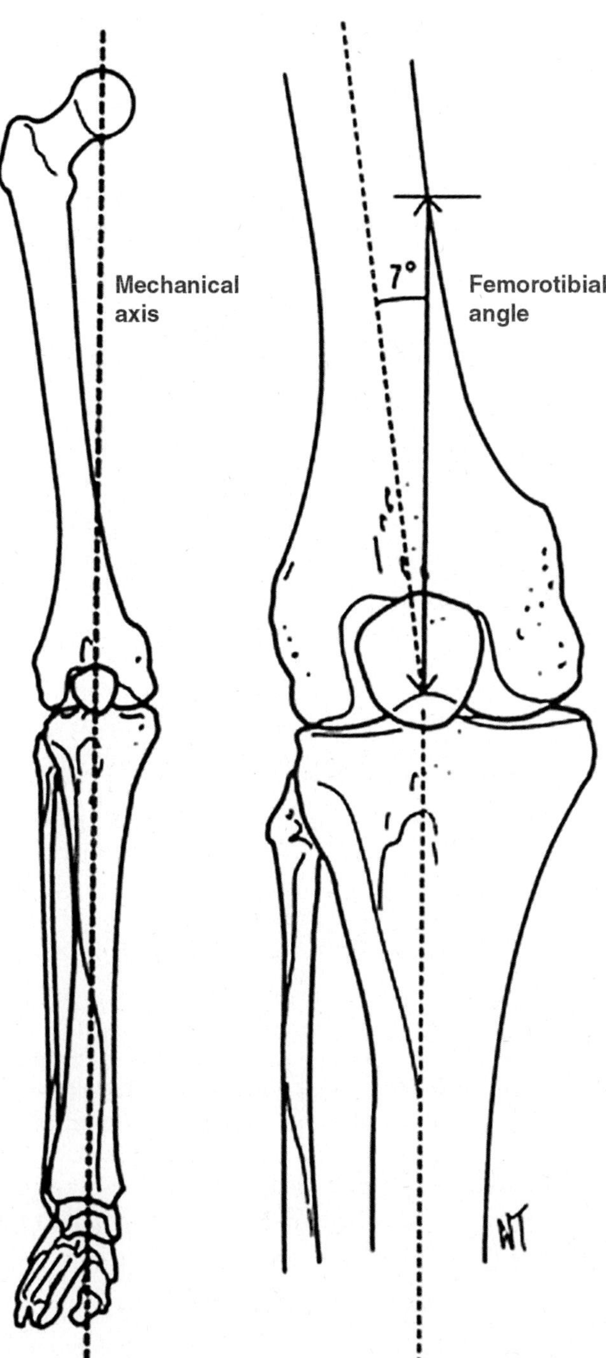

Figure 18.4 Mechanical and anatomic axes of the knee. The mechanical axis goes from the center of the femoral head to the center of the ankle. The anatomic axis is along the femoral and tibial shafts and forms approximately a 7-degree angle to the mechanical axis. (*Reproduced with permission from* Chapman MW, Szabo RM, Marder R, et al. *Chapman's Orthopaedic Surgery*. 3rd ed. Philadelphia, PA: Lippincott Williams & Wilkins, 2001.)

and in this group, the most important risk factor is age. This is a condition caused by repetitive "wear and tear" on the joint, so as time progresses, it tends to worsen. Primary OA is rare in those younger than 40 years, but after the age of 60 years, it becomes quite common, with approximately 60% of people demonstrating radiographic signs of arthritis. There can also be a genetic predisposition, as there is a much higher rate of occurrence in first-degree relatives. Obesity is also commonly associated with OA, as patients who are overweight put a greater load on the weight-bearing joints of the lower extremities, which tends to accelerate wear. Women tend to be affected more often than men.

There are several secondary causes of OA. Posttraumatic OA occurs from prior injury to the articular surface and can potentially affect a much younger patient population. Previous intraarticular fracture to the distal femur, proximal tibia, or patella will often lead to degenerative disease if anatomic alignment of the extremity and articular surface is not maintained. At the time of these injuries, the articular cartilage is damaged and often left with irregularities that can lead to asymmetric loading and accelerated articular cartilage injury. Therefore, one of the mainstays in the operative treatment of articular fractures is anatomic restoration of the joint surface.

Ligamentous injuries can also lead to accelerated joint degeneration, although the mechanism is somewhat unclear. Anterior cruciate ligament (ACL) injuries have been observed to lead to early knee degeneration, but it is not known whether this is caused by the chondral injury sustained at the time of the traumatic event or whether it is from the subsequent instability of the knee. It is most likely a combination of the two, but although the injury cannot be reversed, it is possible to limit future instability. Therefore, one major reason to reconstruct the ACL is to limit the further injury to the chondral surfaces by stabilizing the knee. Meniscal tears are another important injury to consider, as the menisci function to provide a broader weight-bearing surface between the proximal tibia and distal femur. Treatment of meniscal tears is often by arthroscopic meniscectomy, which drastically alters the force experienced by the articular cartilage. Therefore, prior meniscectomy is a well-known risk factor for the development of OA.

Deformities, some of which start in childhood, can also place a patient at risk for OA at a young age. Osteochondritis dissecans causes chondral damage mainly in teenagers and can be very difficult to manage. Blount's disease or any other condition that leads to malalignment of the lower extremities places one at risk. A knee that develops significant varus alignment will lead to wear on the medial side of the joint, whereas valgus alignment will cause wear on the lateral side.

Pathophysiology

Knee OA is felt to occur because of repetitive stresses placed on the joint over time, which gradually leads to a breakdown of the articular cartilage. This process begins as a simple softening of the chondral surface and is followed by fraying, which will eventually lead to enough articular cartilage destruction to expose the subchondral bone. Once the subchondral bone is directly experiencing the weight-bearing stresses, microfractures begin to appear in its surface, which in turn lead to the development of subchondral cysts. Thinning of the cartilage also manifests itself as a narrowing of the joint space, which in turn leads to a subtle degree of instability in the knee. The bone's response to this phenomenon is to form osteophytes, which are simply areas of reactive bone formation that act to stabilize the joint. The clinical effect of chondral wear is the development of pain in addition to possible malalignment and loss of motion. Malalignment is the result of asymmetric wear, most commonly in the medial compartment, thus causing a varus deformity, whereas motion loss results from capsular contracture, which typically occurs posterior and appears clinically as a loss of terminal extension.

PATIENT EVALUATION

Clinical Presentation/History

Patients with OA can present in a variety of ways, but most commonly, they complain of knee pain that has been insidious in onset, often over the course of many years. Frequently, this is associated with stiffness and intermittent swelling of the knee that is typically worse with activity and relieved with rest. Patients will also commonly state that they have been getting progressively more "bowlegged" over the course of time.

When a younger patient presents with complaints that seem consistent with degenerative knee pain, it is also important to take a thorough history to determine the probable cause. First, the physician should consider potential sources of referred pain, which can include either the lumbar spine or the hip. Lumbar disc disease can frequently cause radicular symptoms that manifest as knee pain, while hip pathology can also be referred to the knee along the course of the obturator nerve. A history of injuries or surgeries on the knee, such as intraarticular fractures, ligamentous or meniscal tears, or prior knee surgery, is important as these are potential risk factors. As previously mentioned, genetics also plays a prominent role in the development of OA, so family history of early-onset arthritis should be determined. One should also take a complete medical history as other conditions such as gout, rheumatic diseases, recent infection, and hemophilia can cause knee pain and lead to arthritic changes.

Physical Examination

The physical examination should always begin with inspection, and there are several important things to look for in the degenerative knee. First, the static longitudinal alignment of the lower extremity should be observed in the standing patient. The normal alignment of the lower extremity is approximately 5 to 7 degrees of valgus, and degenerative changes can cause either varus or valgus malalignment, with varus malalignment being more common

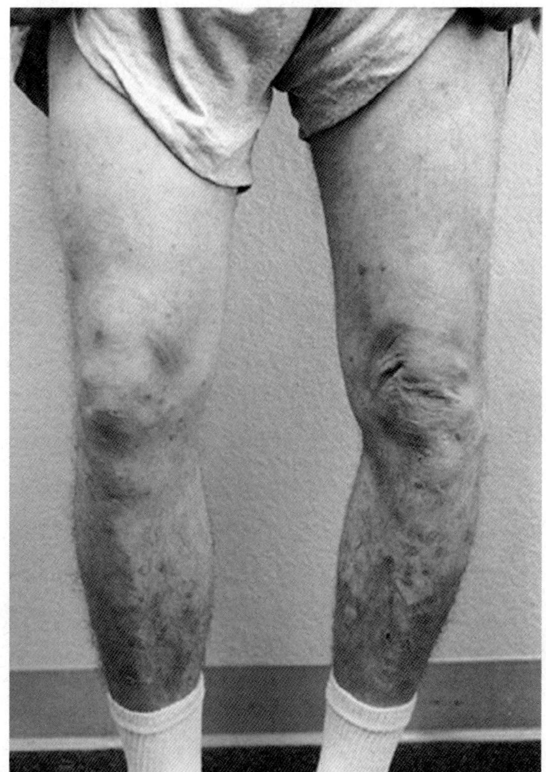

Figure 18.5 This patient is seen to have significant varus alignment of the left lower extremity when observed in the standing position. (*Reproduced with permission from* Chapman MW, Szabo RM, Marder R, et al. *Chapman's Orthopaedic Surgery*. 3rd ed. Philadelphia, PA: Lippincott Williams & Wilkins, 2001.)

(Fig 18.5). The examiner should also observe the patients gait, which is frequently seen to be antalgic, meaning that there is a shortened stance phase on the affected extremity. A lateral thrust is also commonly seen due to the attenuation of the lateral collateral ligament (LCL). This typically occurs in patients with a long-standing varus deformity of the knee (Fig. 18.6). Medial thrusts can also be seen with valgus deformity but are much less common in the osteoarthritic patient.

Palpation will often reveal the presence of an effusion, which is present during an exacerbation, or an "arthritic flare." Medial and lateral joint line tenderness is commonly present, with medial tenderness being more often associated with varus deformity. Range of motion should also be assessed and is frequently limited. A flexion contracture (loss of passive extension) is seen early, and as the condition progresses, a loss of flexion is also appreciated. During the range of motion, patellofemoral crepitus is commonly observed.

Imaging

Plain radiographs are the only imaging study necessary for the diagnosis of OA, with the classic findings being joint space narrowing, osteophyte formation, subchondral cysts, and subchondral sclerosis (Fig. 18.7). The

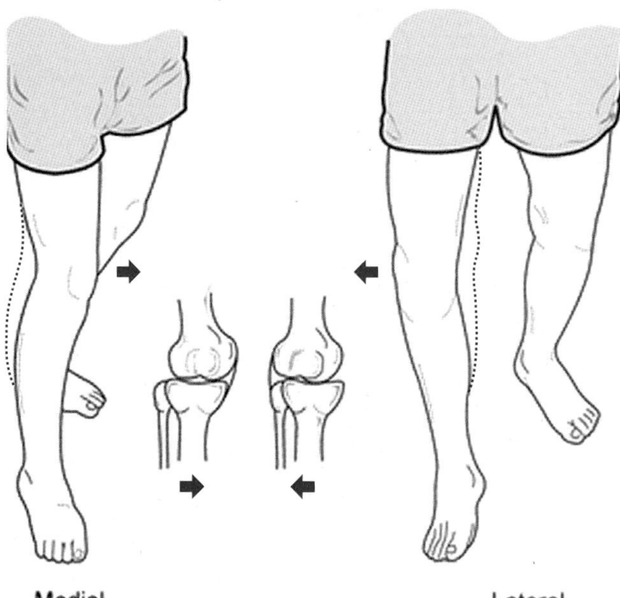

Figure 18.6 A lateral thrust is seen in the stance phase of gait in a patient with a long-standing varus deformity, whereas a medial thrust can be seen with a valgus deformity. (*Reproduced with permission from* Chapman MW, Szabo RM, Marder R, et al. *Chapman's Orthopaedic Surgery*. 3rd ed. Philadelphia, PA: Lippincott Williams & Wilkins, 2001.)

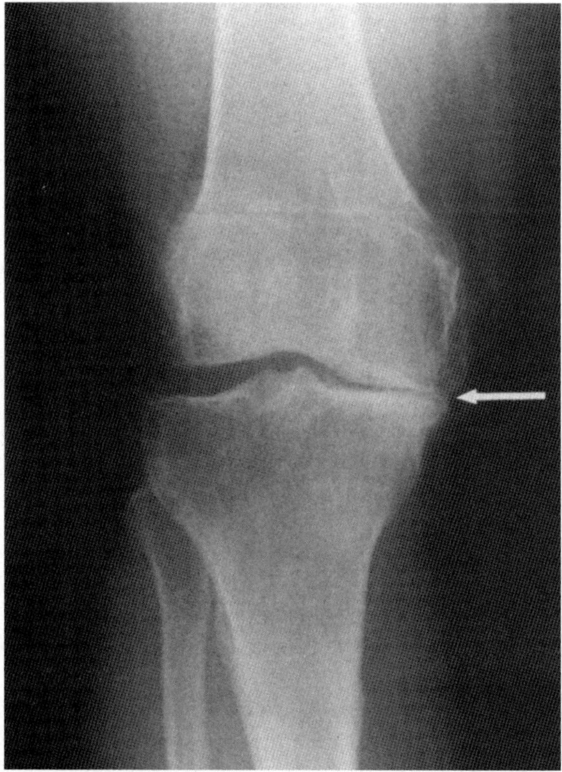

Figure 18.7 Osteoarthritis of the knee. Note the asymmetric joint space narrowing, osteophyte formation, and the subchondral sclerosis on the medial side of the joint. (*Reproduced with permission from* Weinstein SL, Buckwalter JA. *Turek's Orthopaedics: Principles and Their Application*. 6th ed. Philadelphia, PA: Lippincott Williams & Wilkins, 2005.)

evaluation should start with a weight-bearing anteroposterior (AP), lateral, and sunrise view of the knee. The need for weight-bearing radiographs cannot be overemphasized, as they more accurately show the condition of the joint when placed under a load. It is not uncommon for significant varus alignment and medial joint space narrowing to be missed on non–weight-bearing radiographs (Fig. 18.8). Lateral views show both the tibiofemoral and patellofemoral joints, whereas the sunrise view more thoroughly images the patellofemoral joint. Often with early arthritis the weight-bearing AP view will fail to show any significant changes as this loads only the anterior and middle weight-bearing portions of the tibial femoral joint. A 30- to 45-degree weight-bearing posteroanterior flexion view can be used to more accurately assess the middle and posterior aspects of the femoral condyles. This study will frequently show a more significant arthritis than what was visualized on the standard AP view (Fig. 18.9).

Differential Diagnosis

The differential diagnosis for OA includes other conditions that can lead to knee pain and swelling. These include inflammatory arthritis, crystalline arthropathy, septic arthritis, and osteonecrosis.

The main conditions to consider are the inflammatory arthritides, the most common of which is rheumatoid arthritis. However, other conditions include lupus, ankylosing spondylitis, Reiter's syndrome, psoriatic arthritis, and arthritis associated with inflammatory bowel disease. These conditions can all present similarly with an insidious onset and long duration of knee pain. However, there are several important differences. First, many of these patients will have involvement of multiple joints, and they classically have pain that is worse with rest and relieved by activity. Bilateral knee involvement can certainly be seen with OA, but it is normal in those with rheumatoid disease. One must also be cognizant of the review of systems, as inflammatory arthritis can be associated with conditions involving the eyes, skin, and gastrointestinal tract and may also be associated with a family history. Physical examination is important for distinguish inflammatory arthritis, as again, multiple joints are frequently involved. In addition, soft tissue bogginess and swelling is more common than a true effusion. Valgus alignment of the knee is also associated with inflammatory arthritis, although it can be seen in the osteoarthritic patient. Radiographic changes are also different, as the classic changes in rheumatic disease include symmetric joint space narrowing, osteopenia, and periarticular erosions, along with the absence of osteophyte formation (Fig. 18.10). The conservative treatment options between these two conditions are significantly different, although the gold standard for end-stage disease is total knee replacement in both instances.

Crystalline arthropathies, such as gout and pseudogout, must also be considered, particularly in those who

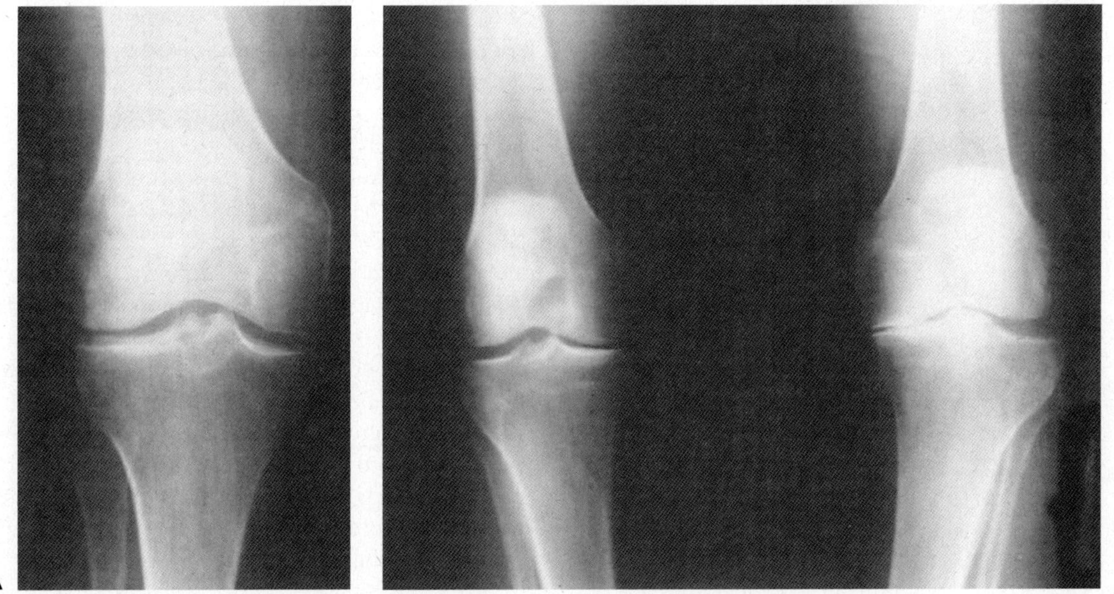

Figure 18.8 **(A)** Supine anteroposterior in a patient presenting with knee pain. **(B)** Weight-bearing radiograph of the same patient taken a short time later. Note the medial joint space narrowing and the obvious varus alignment, thus confirming the diagnosis of osteoarthritis. (*Reproduced with permission from* Koopman WJ, Moreland LW. *Arthritis and Allied Conditions: A Textbook of Rheumatology.* 15th ed. Philadelphia, PA: Lippincott Williams & Wilkins, 2005.)

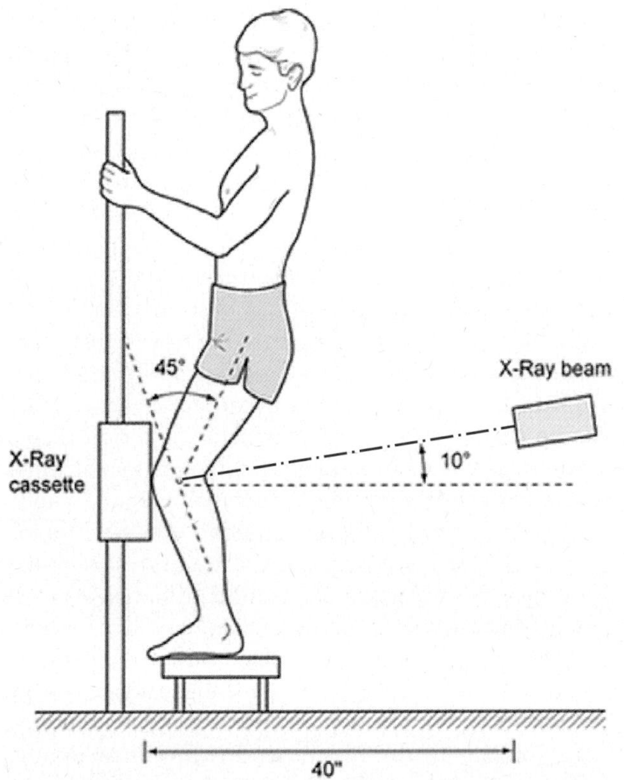

Figure 18.9 Technique for the 45-degree posteroanterior flexion weight-bearing radiograph of the knee. (*Reproduced with permission from* Chapman MW, Szabo RM, Marder R, et al. *Chapman's Orthopaedic Surgery*. 3rd ed. Philadelphia, PA: Lippincott Williams & Wilkins, 2001.)

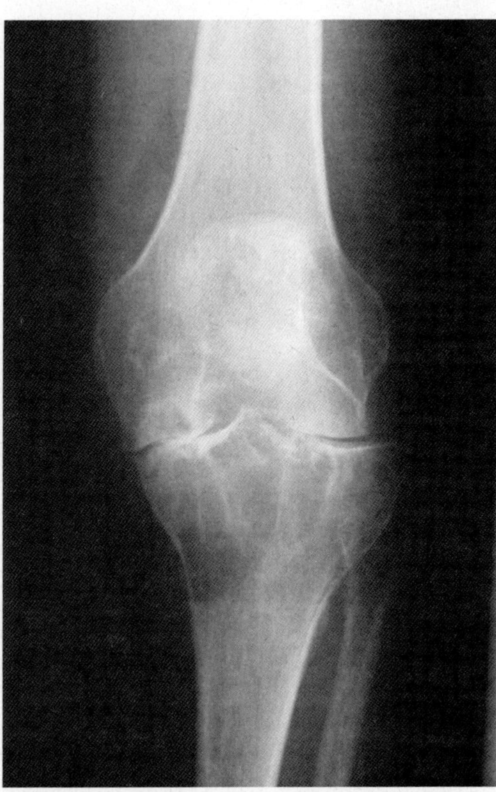

Figure 18.10 Rheumatoid arthritis of the knee. Note the large subchondral cysts, symmetric joint space narrowing, and the generalized osteopenia. There is also a complete absence of osteophytes. (*Reproduced with permission from* Koopman WJ, Moreland LW. *Arthritis and Allied Conditions: A Textbook of Rheumatology*. 15th ed. Philadelphia, PA: Lippincott Williams & Wilkins, 2005.)

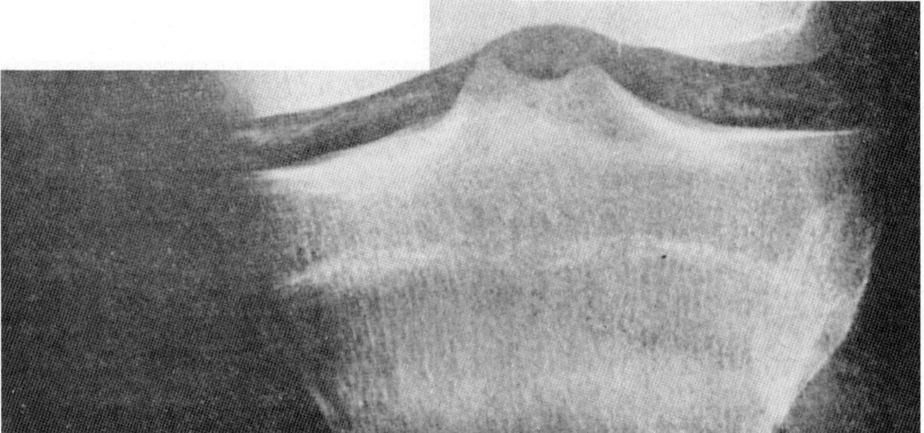

Figure 18.11 Pseudogout. Note the typical punctate and linear deposits of calcium in both the medial and lateral menisci. (*Reproduced with permission from* Koopman WJ, Moreland LW. *Arthritis and Allied Conditions: A Textbook of Rheumatology*. 15th ed. Philadelphia, PA: Lippincott Williams & Wilkins, 2005.)

have a history of gout in other joints. Gout is caused by the buildup of sodium urate crystals in the joint, which leads to significant pain. However, the pain often presents more acutely than degenerative joint disease. An effusion is often present, and diagnosis is definitively made by arthrocentesis with the presence of negatively birefringent crystals in the aspirate. Pseudogout is caused by a buildup of calcium pyrophosphate crystals, which are often seen as calcifications in the menisci on radiographs (Fig. 18.11). Diagnosis is by presence of rhomboid-shaped crystals on aspiration.

Septic arthritis is possible, although this should be seen and diagnosed on a much more acute basis. These patients will have an acute onset of pain and swelling with an inability to move the knee. Diagnosis is by the presence of more than 75,000 white blood cells in the synovial fluid. Osteonecrosis can also be considered, although it too is seen much more acutely. Known as the "heart attack of the knee", osteonecrosis typically occurs in the medial femoral condyle and will cause persistent pain.

NONOPERATIVE TREATMENT

Treatment of OA of the knee is similar to the management of OA in other joints, so there are multiple nonsurgical options available. The first-line therapy is typically nonsteroidal anti-inflammatory drugs (NSAIDs), which function by reducing pain and swelling associated with the knee. Although all NSAIDs function in a similar fashion, there is a wide variation to patient response to each individual medication. Therefore, at minimum, two to three different NSAIDs should be attempted before abandoning this treatment option. One must also be cognizant of the gastrointestinal side effects, as patients with a history of ulcers and gastroesophageal reflux should not be given these medications without consultation from the their primary caregivers. Other oral medications that have been tried include the recently popularized over-the-counter supplements glucosamine and chondroitin sulfate. These substances are part of the building blocks of articular cartilage and work theoretically by intestinal absorption of the substances, followed by their incorporation into the articular cartilage of the damaged joint. A recent large clinical trial conducted at the National Institutes of Health indicated that there was no clinical benefit to using these products, but there is certainly anecdotal evidence that they lead to symptomatic improvement in some patients. With that said, there does not appear to be any harm, other than cost, to using these products, so they are certainly worth trying in those who have been unable to get symptomatic relief via other methods.

The second-line treatment is the use of intra-articular corticosteroid injections, which are mainly used for controlling the acute exacerbations of pain. These medications function as strong anti-inflammatory agents and are used to "quiet down" patients' pain in an effort to restore them to their baseline level of discomfort. However, when overutilized, cortisone has actually been shown to accelerate degeneration of the articular cartilage. Therefore, steroid injections should not be used to control baseline pain and typically should not be given more than three times over the course of a year. If a patient is requiring more than this, other treatment options should be explored. A second form of injections that are used include the hyaluronic acid derivatives. Hyaluronic acid is the substance that provides the lubricating function in normal synovial fluid and is often deficient in the arthritic knee. These injections are theoretically used to decrease the coefficient of friction between the opposing chondral surfaces, thus leading to less degeneration of the cartilage. This has shown some clinical efficacy in certain trials, although basic science proof of its mechanism is lacking. However, these injections have also been shown to cause minimal harm, other than the small risk of infection, so they are a reasonable option in the patient who is attempting to delay surgery.

Physical therapy can be very helpful in the treatment of arthritis of the knee. The soft tissue sleeve is important to knee function, so its optimization can diminish the symptoms of osteoarthritis. Therapy should be directed at maintaining the range of motion of the knee and strengthening the quadriceps and hamstring muscles. However, in the late stages of degenerative disease, therapy can worsen the symptoms and should be limited only to the patient's tolerance.

Assistive devices such as a cane, crutch, or walker may also be helpful in the management of OA. These aids can limit the stress across the painful knee and improve the patient's walking tolerance. Last, if all else fail, patients may modify their activities. This includes eliminating activities that overload the joint, some of which include running or playing tennis, and changing to less demanding activities such as swimming. Patients with degenerative joint disease are also frequently overweight, so weight loss can be an effective method to reduce symptoms by reducing the stress experienced by the joint.

SURGICAL TREATMENT

Nonoperative management can include some or all of the therapies previously mentioned; however, as pain continues to progress, limitation of activities will increase. When the patient is unable to obtain acceptable symptomatic relief with nonoperative care, surgical treatments should be discussed. These can be broken down into procedures that spare the patient's native articular cartilage and those that remove or replace it. The timing of the surgery depends on the patient's situation. In the younger patient with unicompartmental disease, an early intervention may be necessary to prevent rapid progression of the disease. However, in the patient older than 60 years with tricompartmental disease, there is little change in the complexity or the outcome of a total knee replacement with advanced disease, so timing should be based on the patient's symptoms.

Arthroscopy

Arthroscopy of the knee is by far the simplest operative treatment that can be chosen for management of the arthritic knee. This is an outpatient procedure that can generally be completed in less than 30 minutes, and the complete recovery time is often less than 2 weeks. However, its effectiveness is controversial. The procedure is done simply to "clean out" the knee by removing any loose chondral flaps, debris in the joint, or torn or frayed meniscus. Arthroscopy cannot be used to off-load or replace any of the diseased cartilage and exists only to delay the need for more invasive intervention. Several well designed studies have indicated that there is no benefit to arthroscopy in the degenerative knee, indicating that some patients may even get worse, whereas others have shown that it is an effective way to postpone a knee replacement by up to several years. The actual results are likely somewhere in between these extremes. There is good evidence that doing an arthroscopic debridement on patients with advanced OA is unlikely to provide any substantial relief; however, if done on patients with earlier-stage disease, it will often make them symptomatically better for variable periods.

Osteotomy

Angular deformities of the knee commonly occur in patients with OA. This malalignment causes an asymmetrical loading between the medial and lateral compartments, thus leading to accelerated degenerative changes on the overloaded side. Varus deformity is the most common in OA, and it can lead to increased stress on the medial compartment. When this occurs there are benefits to addressing just the diseased compartment with surgical intervention. However, it is important to recognize that the vast majority of patients presenting with a varus deformity in an arthritic knee have disease that also involves the other compartments. With that said, chondral-sparing procedures are frequently indicated in younger patients as they can be used to delay the need for total knee replacement. The best option for treating unicompartmental medial disease in the younger patient (<60 years) is by high tibial osteotomy (HTO). HTO is done to off-load the diseased medial compartment by correcting, and in fact overcorrecting, the malalignment of the lower extremity by placing it back into valgus (Figs. 18.12 and 18.13).

The primary benefit of doing an HTO as opposed to a TKA is that it preserves patients' native articular cartilage, thus eliminating the concern about material wear seen with TKA. This leaves patients with no activity restrictions following union of the osteotomy site, which is particularly important in younger active patients who are likely to quickly wear out a prosthetic joint. The two principal drawbacks to HTO are that it should be used only in those with unicompartmental disease and that the results of the procedure progressively deteriorate with time. HTO functions by transferring the weight-bearing load over to the lateral compartment, so it is important to determine the condition of the lateral side preoperatively. If there are already degenerative changes there, it is likely that the procedure will fail because of increased lateral-sided pain. Regarding longevity, new instrumentation has increased the average survival rates of this procedure to approximately 10 years, but this is nowhere near the proven long-term results that are seen with TKA. For this reason, HTO is generally discouraged in older patients with a more sedentary lifestyle in which TKA is more likely to give them more complete and enduring success.

Valgus producing osteotomies (for varus deformity) are performed as either medial opening wedge or lateral closing wedge procedures. Lateral closing wedge osteotomies were described first and are done by taking a wedge of bone out of the lateral border of the proximal tibia. The gap is then closed and typically held with internal fixation (Fig. 18.12). However, medial opening wedge osteotomies are currently used more frequently as they allow for easier

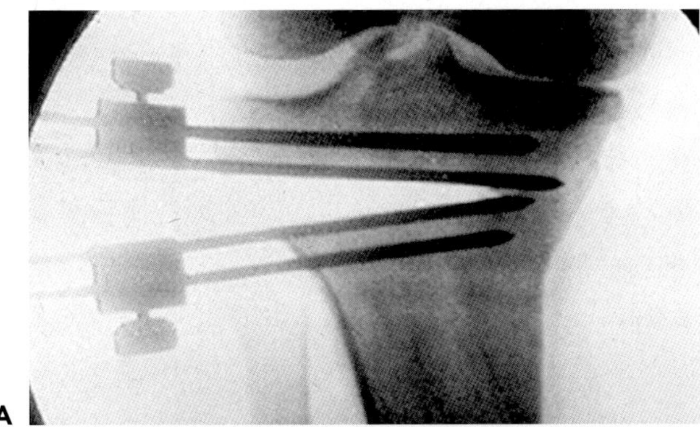

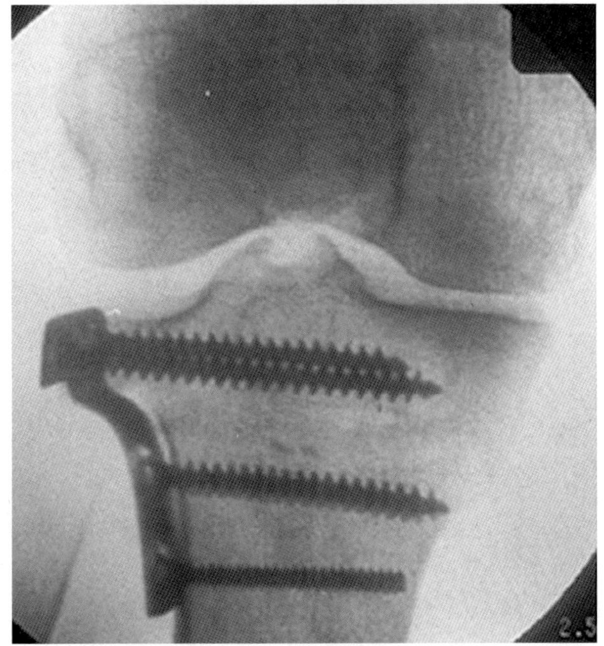

Figure 18.12 High tibial lateral closing wedge valgus osteotomy: **(A)** after the bone wedge is removed and **(B)** following closing of the wedge and internal fixation to correct a varus deformity. (*Reproduced with permission from* Chapman MW, Szabo RM, Marder R, et al. *Chapman's Orthopaedic Surgery*. 3rd ed. Philadelphia, PA: Lippincott Williams & Wilkins, 2001.)

adjustment at the osteotomy site (Fig. 18.13). With opening wedge procedures, only one saw cut is made, and the bone is levered open while keeping the lateral cortex intact. This osteotomy is also typically held in place with internal fixation devices.

Valgus deformities can also be corrected with a varus-producing osteotomy, although this is much less common. The technique of choice is typically a distal femoral osteotomy and can be either a lateral opening wedge or a medial closing wedge procedure.

Unicompartmental Knee Arthroplasty

Unicompartmental knee arthroplasty (UKA) is another treatment option for those with single compartment disease. Just as with the HTO, it is used most commonly

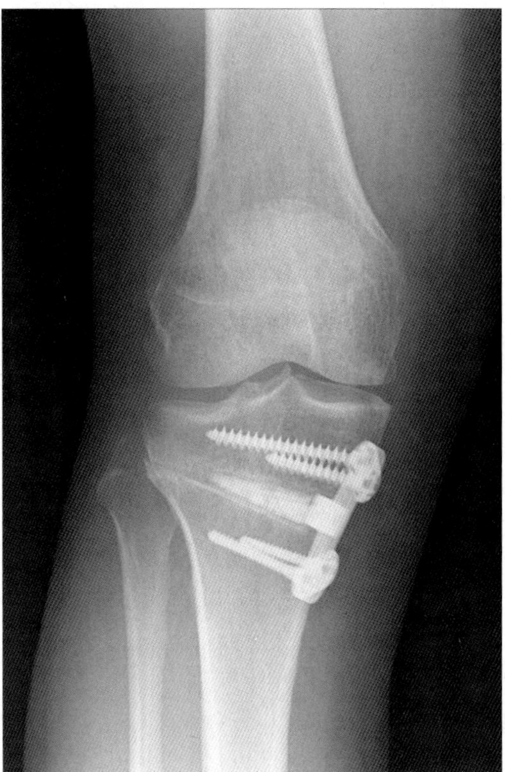

Figure 18.13 Medial opening wedge high tibial osteotomy following correction with placement of internal fixation. Bone graft substitute has been used to fill in the osteotomy site.

in those with a varus deformity that has led to isolated degeneration of the medial compartment. This procedure entails a resurfacing, or replacement, of the degenerative compartment by removing the native articular cartilage from the medial femoral condyle and medial tibial plateau and replacing it with prosthetic components (Fig. 18.14). The primary advantage of UKA over HTO is that it allows for a much faster recovery and permits immediate weight-bearing in the postoperative period. However, it does replace a portion of the patient's native joint with prosthetic components, which are in turn susceptible to wear, particularly in those who are more active. When comparing UKA with TKA, the primary advantage is that the entire joint is not replaced. Patients' native cruciate ligaments are maintained, leading to more natural kinematics than that following TKA. Furthermore, it is less invasive with a smaller incision, there are fewer short-term complications, and the early recovery and rehabilitation is felt to be faster. However, the major disadvantage is that the long-term survivorship has been unable to approach the well-documented track record of total knee replacement.

UKA is a procedure that certainly has a role in the management of OA, but it is important to adhere to strict surgical indications to achieve success. First, and most important, patients must have isolated one compartment disease, as failure to address other diseased compartments with surgery will lead to continued pain. Also, patients younger

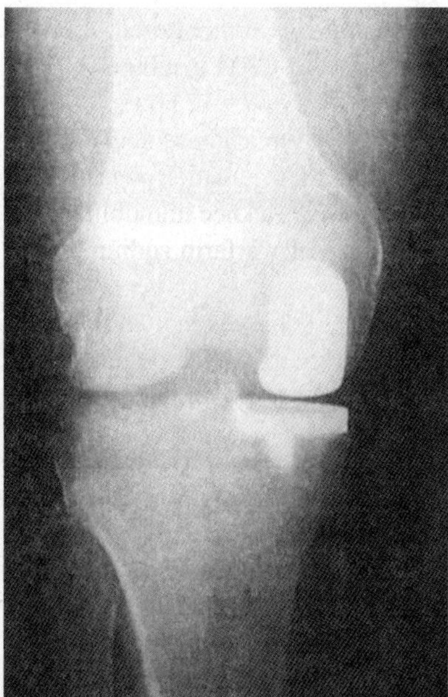

Figure 18.14 Unicompartmental knee arthroplasty of the medial compartment. (*Reproduced with permission from* Lotke PA, Lonner JH. *Master Techniques in Orthopaedic Surgery: Knee Arthroplasty*. 2nd ed. Philadelphia, PA: Lippincott Williams & Wilkins, 2003.)

than 60 years, or active patients older than 60 years, should be considered for HTO in the setting of unicompartmental disease, as the prosthetic components used in UKA are likely to fail early in this cohort. Other contraindications to UKA include ACL deficiency, fixed varus deformity of the knee, knee flexion contractures, and inflammatory arthritis. Again, UKA does have a role in a small group of patients, but in most cases, it is difficult to argue with the proven success rate of TKA in the degenerative knee.

While UKA of the medial compartment is the most common partial joint replacement, there are various others that can be done. Isolated lateral disease is less common, but when present, one can consider either a distal femoral osteotomy or a lateral UKA. Patellofemoral arthritis is also seen, and in rare circumstances, an isolated patellofemoral replacement can be used. In addition, there have been bicompartmental replacements designed to replace the medial and patellofemoral compartments, but at this time, long-term data are lacking.

Knee Arthrodesis

Arthrodesis, or fusion, of the knee is another seldom-used option for the osteoarthritic knee (Fig. 18.15). This procedure is very effective for pain relief, but because it does so by completely eliminating all knee motion, it is an unappealing option. It does allow for full weight-bearing and ambulation, although the resultant gait pattern is significantly abnormal. At this time, fusion is considered only in young active patients, particularly in physical laborers, or in those with failed and nonsalvageable prior joint replacement.

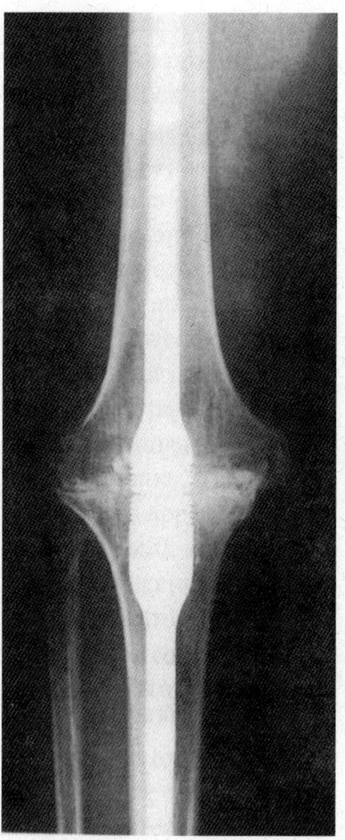

Figure 18.15 Right knee arthrodesis done with a modular intramedullary nail. (*Reproduced with permission from* Lotke PA, Lonner JH. *Master Techniques in Orthopaedic Surgery: Knee Arthroplasty*. 2nd ed. Philadelphia, PA: Lippincott Williams & Wilkins, 2003.)

TOTAL KNEE ARTHROPLASTY

The gold standard for the treatment of end-stage OA of the knee is total knee replacement (Fig. 18.16). This is an extremely common operation, and it has a proven track record for both survival and pain relief. The average age of patients undergoing knee replacement in the United States is approximately 65–70 years, but it is often used in those who are much younger and older. As mentioned earlier, there are several surgical alternatives, but none has been able to approach the long-term results of TKA.

Indications

The major indication for TKA is the presence of persistent mechanical knee pain that can no longer be controlled by other nonsurgical or surgical means. The pain is most typically caused by OA, either primary or posttraumatic, but it can also be from rheumatoid arthritis or other inflammatory disorders. Patients will benefit from a course of conservative management, but the progressive nature of the disease eventually results in many patients requiring a surgical treatment.

Total knee replacement is an elective procedure, so the decision for when to proceed with the operation is left up to

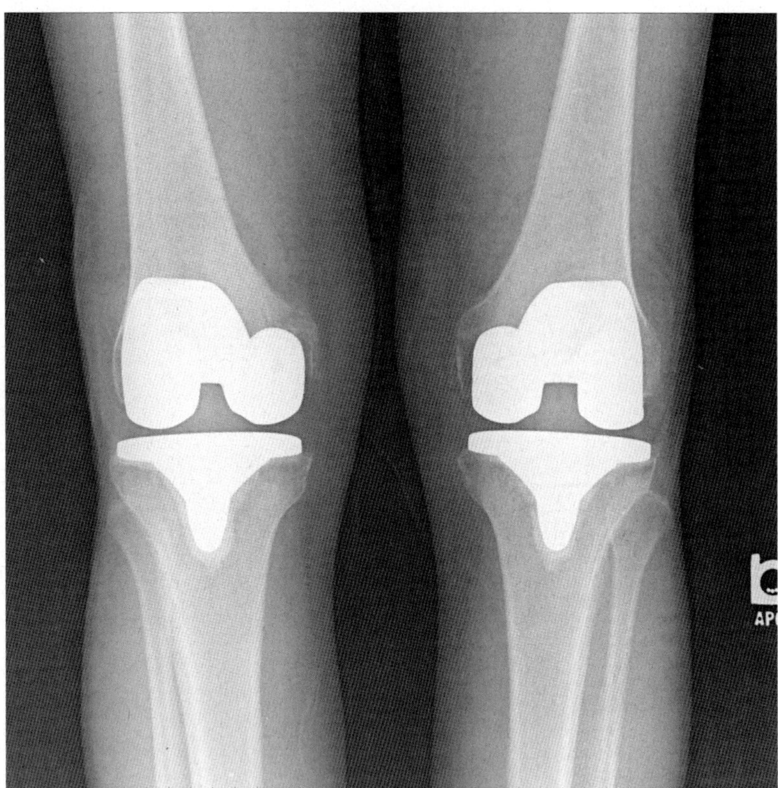

Figure 18.16 Postoperative radiograph of a patient who had bilateral total knee arthroplasties.

patients. When patients are experiencing enough pain and functional limitation that they feel it is worthwhile to undergo a major operation with a prolonged recovery, then it is time for the surgery. Radiographs can also be somewhat misleading, as some patients with rather mild-appearing radiographs will have severe pain, whereas others with severe changes on radiograph will be functioning quite well. With that said, patients should be informed that the purpose of the surgery is to relieve pain, and it is able to do this effectively in the vast majority of cases.

Surgical Procedure

The knee joint is approached through an anterior midline incision, followed by a medial parapatellar arthrotomy. The patella can then be everted, which in turn exposes the entirety of the knee joint. At that point, the proximal tibia is cut perpendicular to the long axis of the shaft of the tibia and the femoral articular surface is cut by using specific guides to remove the femoral trochlea and the distal and posterior femoral condyles. The patella is normally resurfaced as well by resecting the articular surface with a cut parallel with its anterior surface. The ACL is removed, whereas the medial collateral ligament (MCL) and the LCL are retained and carefully balanced. The posterior cruciate ligament (PCL) can be either resected or retained, depending on the design of the implant chosen. This allows for a classification of knee designs into two types: posterior cruciate retaining and posterior cruciate substituting designs. Use of the two designs is approximately equal in the United States. Those who prefer the retaining designs argue that keeping the PCL allows for a more biomechanically normal knee motion, particularly in late flexion, whereas those who are against it claim that in the osteoarthritic knee, the PCL is already diseased and should be resected. Substituting designs replace the PCL with a mechanical block that prevents posterior translation of the tibia (Fig. 18.17).

The components used in TKA are a combination of metal alloys and polyethylene (Fig. 18.18). The femoral and tibial sides of the joint are typically resurfaced with metal alloys shaped to fit the surfaces, while there is an intervening polyethylene component between them. Therefore, the bearing surfaces used for TKA at this time are metal on polyethylene. In addition, when the decision is made to resurface the patella, it too is typically done with an all-polyethylene component. Metal backing has been used for this component, but this led to substantial stress shielding of the remaining patellar bone and later risk for fracture.

There has been a trend toward noncemented components in hip replacement surgery, but knee replacement is typically done with all of the components cemented. Polymethylmethacrylate is the substance that is used as bone cement, and it holds the components in place by interdigitating with the adjacent metaphyseal bone. Noncemented components, which have a porous surface for bone ingrowth, have been associated with a higher incidence of component loosening in long-term studies, so their use is discouraged. This is particularly true on the tibial side,

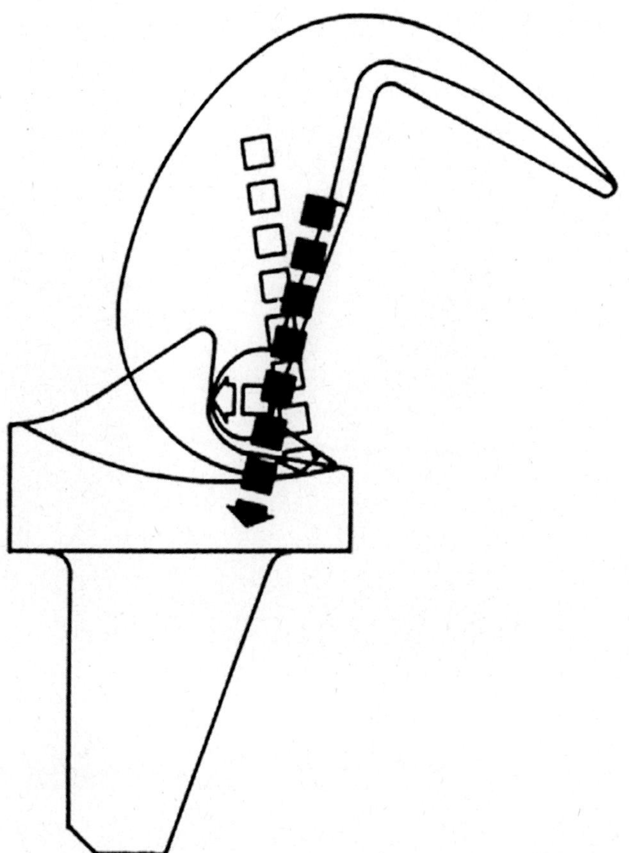

Figure 18.17 Posterior substituting total knee arthroplasty. When the knee goes into flexion, posterior translation of the tibia is blocked by the polyethylene post abutting the distal femur. (*Reproduced with permission from* Chapman MW, Szabo RM, Marder R, et al. *Chapman's Orthopaedic Surgery*. 3rd ed. Philadelphia, PA: Lippincott Williams & Wilkins, 2001.)

where the highest force on the components fixation is experienced due to the shear stress that felt during knee flexion. Therefore, if noncemented components are chosen, they should be limited to the femoral side of the arthroplasty.

Postoperative Recovery

The patient is mobilized into a chair on the first postoperative day, and full weight-bearing may be allowed immediately. However, a knee immobilizer should be used to protect the knee from acute flexion while walking, and this is continued until the quadriceps function returns. The critical element of the postoperative therapy is the restoration of motion. If the motion is not restored within the first 3 to 6 weeks, maturation of the scar tissue will prevent major gains in motion. Many surgeons elect to use a continuous passive motion (CPM) machine in the immediate postoperative period to encourage motion, although it has not been shown to have any substantial impact in the long term. Total hospital time postoperatively in most centers averages between 3 and 4 days, and most patients require home physical therapy to continue work on range of motion and ambulation in the first few weeks after surgery. The total rehabilitation period after TKA is between 3 and 6 months, although patients are functionally mobile after 2 to 3 weeks.

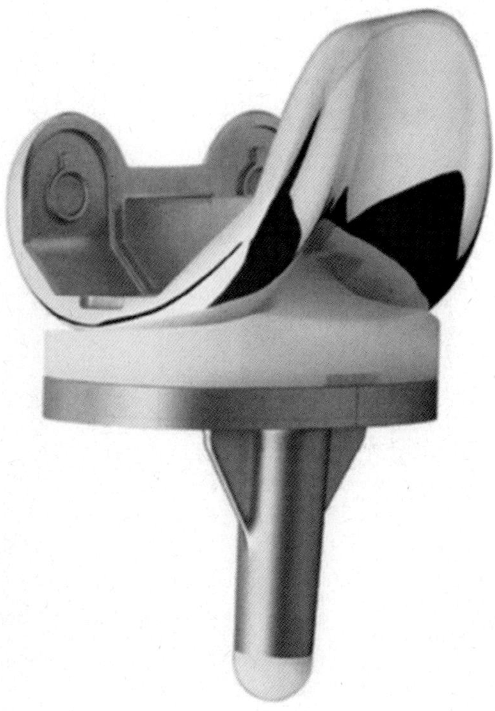

Figure 18.18 The Depuy PFC sigma total knee arthroplasty. (*Reproduced with permission from* Courtesy of DePuy Orthopaedics, Inc.)

Outcomes

The ultimate goal of all total knee replacement surgeries is pain relief, and in most cases, it is successful. The long-term outcomes of the procedure have been well documented in the literature and have repeatedly shown excellent results. Survivorship numbers for modern prostheses are cited as being as high as 95% at 10 years, 90% at 15 years, and up to 80% at 20 years. Longevity is improved in those older than 70 years, women, and those with an underlying diagnosis of inflammatory arthropathy. Younger male patients, however, tend to put more stress on the prosthesis, which leads to earlier and higher rates of component wear and loosening. In addition to impressive longevity of these implants, it must also be noted that in the majority of cases, these patients will have near-complete pain relief in addition to significant functional benefits from the procedure.

Complications

The majority of total knee replacements are successful operations, but there are several common and significant complications that need to be discussed. Particularly when considering the large volume of knee replacements done, it is important to be familiar with the causes of continued pain and the medical complications that can be encountered following arthroplasty.

Postoperative Pain

Continued pain after TKA is seen in less than 10% of patients, and the majority of these complaints are from the patellofemoral joint. This can be the result of poor soft tissue alignment at the time of arthroplasty and may lead to painful subluxation or dislocation of the patellar component. If inadequate bone is resected from the patella at the time of resurfacing, a marked increase in the patellofemoral stress can be noted, and this may lead to pain. Several authors have advocated not resurfacing the patella for this reason, but studies now demonstrate a higher rate of patellofemoral complaints after TKA without patellar resurfacing. If significant patellofemoral arthritis exists at the time of arthroplasty, patients with weight more than 60 kg and height more than 160 cm will have more pain postoperatively if the patella is not resurfaced.

When evaluating the patient with pain following TKA, it is important to do a thorough investigation of the possible causes, and infection must always be ruled out. If infection is not present, then one must search for other sources of pain, and in many cases, there is not one that is identifiable. In these instances, the surgeon should be hesitant to return to the operating room for revision surgery, as the success rates are much higher in the setting of a problem that has been clearly identified preoperatively and is correctable.

Thromboembolic Disease

The most common complication after TKA is thromboembolic disease, which can range from deep venous thrombosis (DVT) to fatal pulmonary embolism (PE). At the present time, the rate of DVT identified by ultrasound in the postoperative setting is approximately 5% in patients who complain of calf pain. However, studies using venography in all postoperative patients have reported rates of DVT ranging from 25% to 50%. PE is reported to occur in approximately 1% of patients, and this can potentially be fatal, although the mortality risk is only approximately 0.01%.

In an effort to prevent these occurrences, all patients should be given lower extremity compressive devices for mechanical prophylaxis and be mobilized on postoperative day 1. Both these interventions have been shown to significantly reduce the number of thromboembolic events. The standard of care is for chemical prophylaxis to be given as well. At present, there are a variety of medications from which to choose and there is conflicting evidence regarding their risks and effectiveness. Warfarin (Coumadin) given for 6 weeks postoperatively has the greatest volume of literature to support its use, although the international normalized ratio (INR) needs to be closely monitored. While Coumadin is undoubtedly effective when the INR is kept at a safe range, it can be difficult to control in the outpatient setting, and dangerous elevations of the INR are a distinct possibility. This can lead to bleeding and hematoma not only at the operative site but also at other locations, including the brain. Low-molecular-weight heparin formulations can also be used, with the prime advantage being that they do not require outpatient monitoring. In addition to this, recent literature has shown that they provide effective prophylaxis with only a 10-day course postoperatively. Disadvantages of low-molecular-weight heparin are that it is contraindicated in patients with renal failure; it comes only as an injection, which many patients do not like; and it has a tendency to cause prolonged drainage from the incision site postoperatively. Aspirin has also been used for DVT prophylaxis due to its ease of administration, although there is minimal data to directly support it for this indication.

Thromboembolic disease is a significant complication of TKA, and a high index of suspicion must always be maintained in the postoperative period. Any patient complaining of calf pain or shortness of breath following joint replacement surgery warrants further workup, and appropriate treatment should be started immediately after the diagnosis is made.

Infection

The most devastating complication after TKA is deep sepsis, which is estimated to occur in approximately 1% of patients. The most common organisms are skin flora, primarily *Staphylococcus aureus* and *S. epidermidis*. These organisms often gain entrance via the relatively thin soft tissue envelope at the inferior aspect of the wound, which must be monitored in the early postoperative period. Any area of skin breakdown after TKA should be treated aggressively to prevent deep infection, particularly in patients with prior incisions and in those with diabetes or significant vascular disease. Diagnosis is made by history and physical examination combined with laboratory and imaging studies. Patients who present with pain in a previously well-functioning arthroplasty should always be worked up for infection, which includes erythrocyte sedimentation rate, C-reactive protein level, and joint aspiration. Radiographs should be evaluated for the presence of component loosening.

Early postoperative infection is less common than late infection, but recognition is critical for optimal treatment. If detected within the first 3 weeks postoperatively, aggressive open debridement, synovectomy, and polyethylene exchange combined with intravenous antibiotics can be successful. However, if the infection recurs after debridement or if it is detected beyond 3 weeks, treatment must include removal of the prosthetic components and all cement. An antibiotic-impregnated cement spacer should be placed at the time of debridement, which serves as a local depot of antibiotic at the site of the infection and also provides stability to soft tissues during treatment. After completion of a minimum of 6 weeks of intravenous antibiotic therapy, repeat laboratory studies and repeat aspiration should be

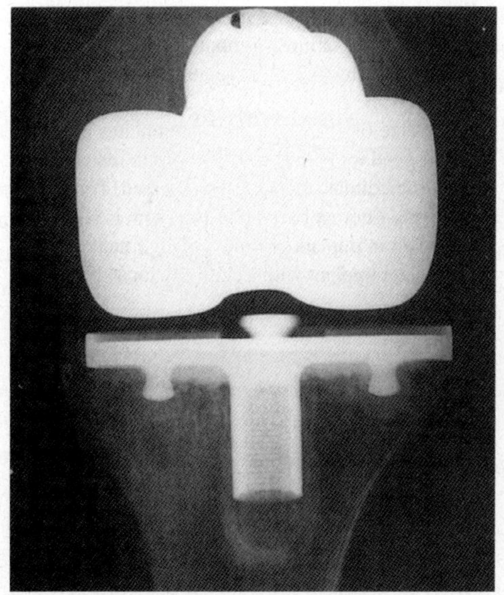
A

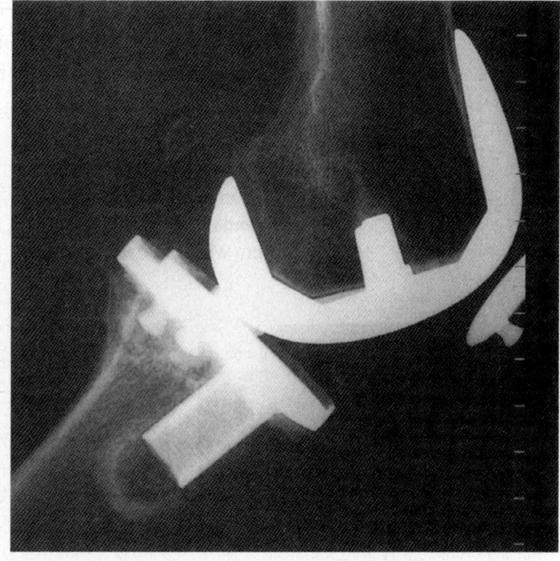
B

Figure 18.19 **(A)** Anteroposterior and **(B)** lateral radiographs showing radiolucent lines around both the tibial and femoral components indicative of loosening of this total knee arthroplasty. (*Reproduced with permission from* Lotke PA, Lonner JH. *Master Techniques in Orthopaedic Surgery: Knee Arthroplasty*. 2nd ed. Philadelphia, PA: Lippincott Williams & Wilkins, 2003.)

completed, and if these studies are negative, one may proceed with revision total knee replacement. However, as a result of the inevitable scarring and probable bone loss, the clinical result is compromised to some degree, and the infection rate following revision surgery is significantly higher than that seen following primary arthroplasty.

Loosening/Wear

While current implants have significantly improved durability, the long-term effect of placing prosthetic components into the knee joint is the generation of wear particles from the implants. This is more pronounced in patients who place more stress on the implant, particularly those who are younger, more active, or obese. In TKA, aseptic loosening of the components occurs at a low rate, but over the expected survivorship of an implant, it eventually becomes significant. Loosening of components will lead to knee pain, so the most common presentation is that of a patient with a well-functioning implant for many years who then develops the gradual onset of pain, especially with activity. Of note, any component loosening prior to 5 years postoperatively should be considered infected until proven otherwise. The diagnosis of loosening is made radiographically, as areas of implant loosening will appear as radiolucent lines around the components (Fig. 18.19). Serial radiographs will show progression of the radiolucent areas and possibly migration of the component. Once the symptoms are severe enough, revision surgery is generally required to provide a stable implant.

Wear in TKA has other significant effects, particularly in regard to the polyethylene component (Fig. 18.20). The bearing surface in TKA is metal on polyethylene, and the result of repeated loading of the joint is particulate debris originating from the polyethylene. The microscopic polyethylene particles are released into the local tissues where they are ingested by macrophages, which attempt to digest the particles with catabolic enzymes and superoxides. The debris accumulates in the cell, which eventually breaks down and releases the polyethylene and the enzymes back into the local environment. The release of the catabolic enzymes into the tissue causes osteolysis of the bone, which can have severe consequences (Fig. 18.21). Loss of bone support can lead not only to prosthetic loosening and clinical failure but also to significant weakness of

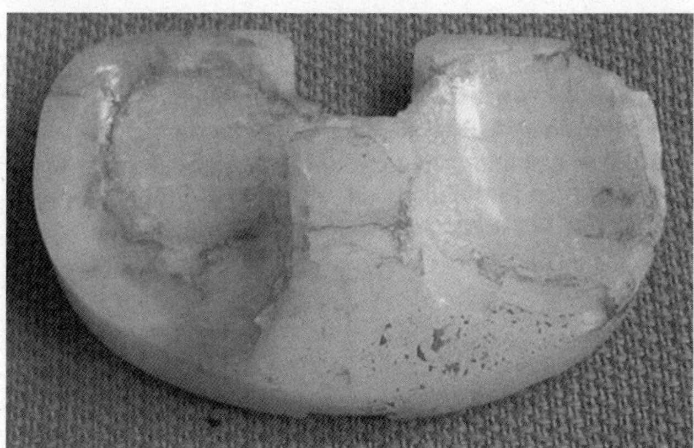

Figure 18.20 Polyethylene just removed from a knee that had been in place for 6 years. Note the delamination of the polyethylene both medially and laterally. (*Reproduced with permission from* Lotke PA, Lonner JH. *Master Techniques in Orthopaedic Surgery: Knee Arthroplasty*. 2nd ed. Philadelphia, PA: Lippincott Williams & Wilkins, 2003.)

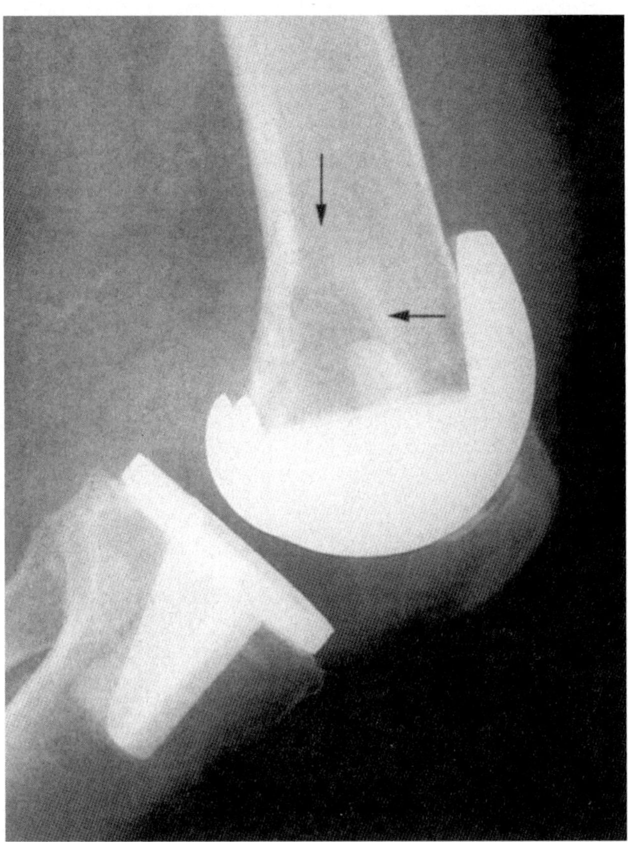

Figure 18.21 Lateral radiograph of a total knee arthroplasty that has been in place for 6 years. Note the extensive osteolysis of the distal femur shown by the *arrows*. (*Reproduced with permission from* Lotke PA, Lonner JH. *Master Techniques in Orthopaedic Surgery: Knee Arthroplasty.* 2nd ed. Philadelphia, PA: Lippincott Williams & Wilkins, 2003.)

the bone, which predisposes one to periprosthetic fracture. The timing of surgical intervention in these patients is actually somewhat controversial, as many surgeons favor early intervention in asymptomatic individuals with significant, progressive osteolysis to avoid future complications.

Stiffness/Arthrofibrosis

Patients' pre-operative range of motion is the best indicator of postoperative range of motion of the knee, meaning that those with good motion before surgery will have the best motion after surgery. However, in some cases, range of motion following TKA does not reach optimal levels. Approximately 100 degrees of knee flexion is needed for activities of daily living, and failure to reach this can have many possible causes, including poor patient compliance with rehabilitation, excessive postoperative swelling and pain, or poorly implanted components. CPM is used in the postoperative period to encourage motion, but in some cases, patients do not reach their goals. If patients are less than 2 to 6 weeks from the time of surgery, manipulation of the knee under a general anesthesia can be done in an attempt to restore motion by "breaking up" the scar tissue. If the motion cannot be restored, particularly if patients are beyond 6 weeks from surgery, additional surgery with an open lysis of adhesions may be indicated.

Instability

The most common type of instability following TKA is in the varus–valgus plane. This can occur from several different mechanisms, some of which include incompetence of the collateral ligaments, poorly made bone cuts, failure to correct preoperative deformity, or an inadequately sized polyethylene component. In general, the majority of these problems can be identified and corrected intraoperatively. One must be careful to protect the collateral ligaments while making the bone cuts to avoid injury, and the surgeon must also carefully balance the knee prior to implanting the components. This is particularly problematic in the valgus knee, which can be quite difficult to correct and balance with surgery, and when done incompletely will lead to laxity on the medial side of the knee. Patients with varus–valgus instability will often present with a stiff-legged gait, which is done to avoid flexion of the knee. When the knee is flexed at heel strike, instability will cause a painful medial or lateral thrust depending on the direction of the instability.

Instability in the anterior–posterior plane is less common but can occur with both cruciate-retaining and cruciate-substituting devices. This can result from excess resection of bone from the posterior femoral condyles, from using too small a femoral component, or from placing excess slope on the proximal tibial cut. If this is done with a cruciate-retaining prosthesis, the PCL will gradually attenuate and will rupture in some cases. This will lead to significant instability of the knee, with the tibia sliding posteriorly relative to the femur. In a cruciate-substituting prosthesis, the stability is provided by the polyethylene post, but when the flexion space is too loose, the femur can actually jump the post and dislocate with the knee in deep flexion (Fig. 18.22).

Periprosthetic Fracture

Periprosthetic fracture following TKA is seen in approximately 2% of patients, and of these, supracondylar femur fractures are the most common (Fig. 18.23). They are generally secondary to minor trauma, and risk factors include osteoporotic bone, limited range of motion in flexion, and notching of the distal femur. Limited range of motion is important because when one falls onto the leg with a flexed knee, the force is typically absorbed by increasing the flexion of the knee. However, if flexion is limited, the force is dissipated elsewhere, which in most cases is to the distal femur. Notching occurs when the anterior femoral shaft is cut while preparing the femur and is a risk factor for fracture (Fig. 18.24).

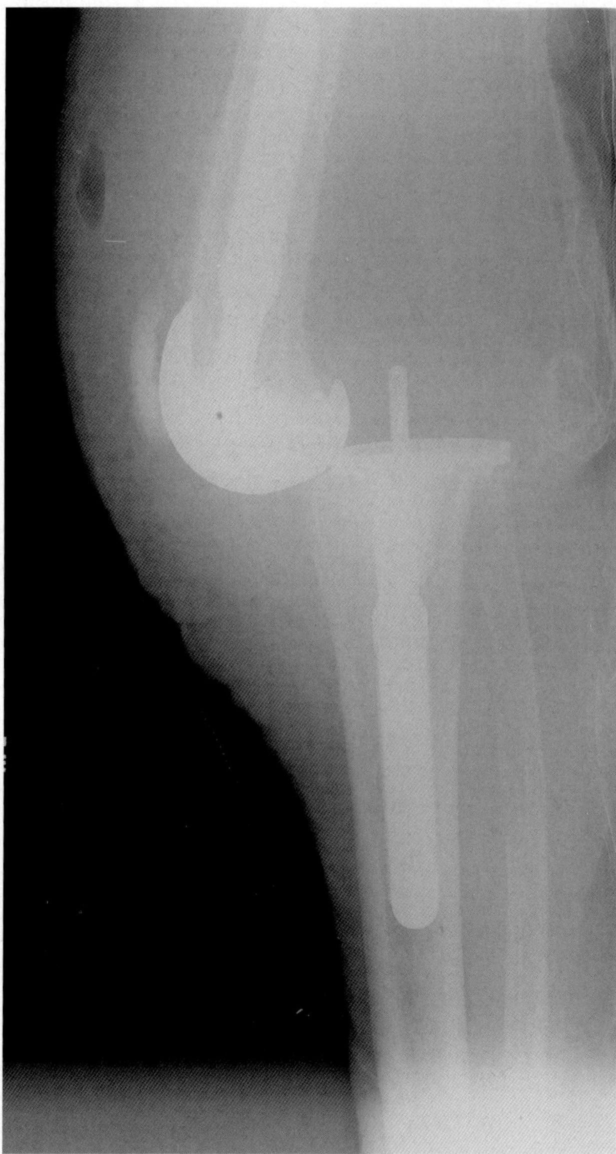

Figure 18.22 Postoperative radiograph following revision total knee arthroplasty where the femoral component has jumped the polyethylene post, leading to a knee dislocation.

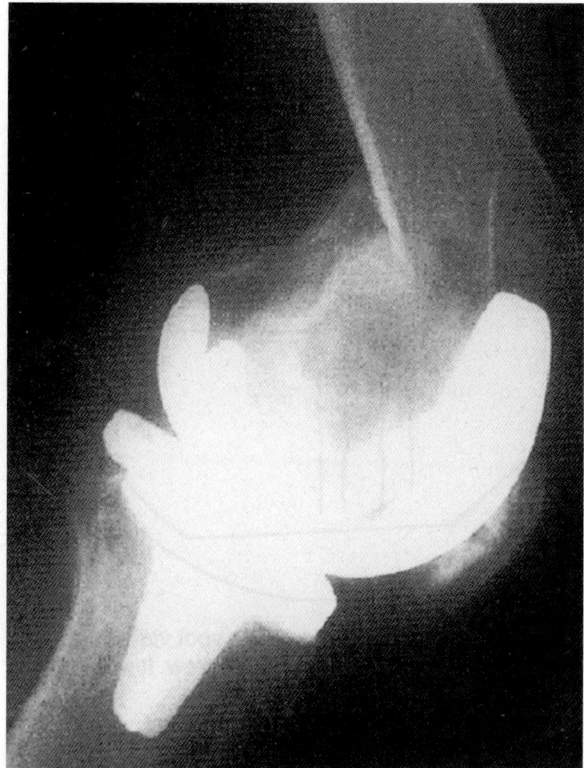

Figure 18.23 Periprosthetic fracture of the distal femur after a fall. (*Reproduced with permission from* Lotke PA, Lonner JH. *Master Techniques in Orthopaedic Surgery: Knee Arthroplasty.* 2nd ed. Philadelphia, PA: Lippincott Williams & Wilkins, 2003.)

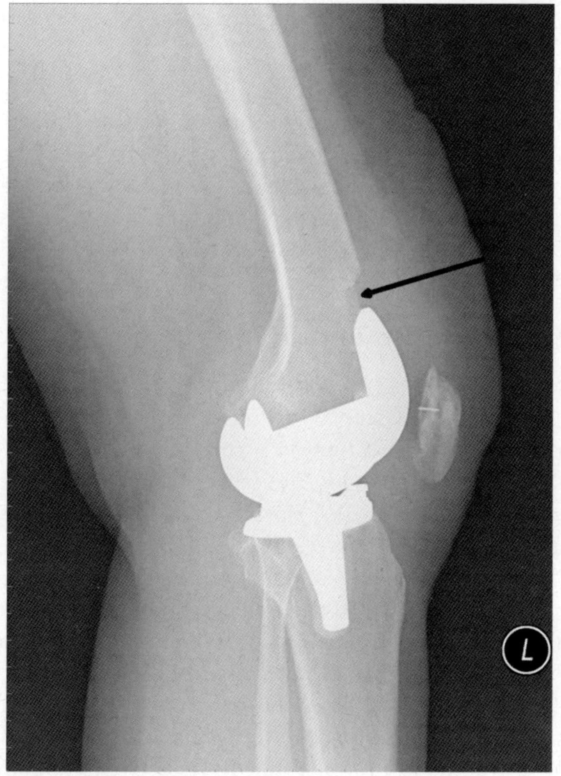

Figure 18.24 Notching (*arrow*) of the anterior cortex of the distal femur after a total knee arthroplasty.

Treatment of periprosthetic distal femur fractures depends on the degree of displacement and the status of the arthroplasty. If the femoral component is already loose, then revision should be undertaken in addition to treatment of the fracture. When the femoral component is well fixed, the fracture can be treated either operatively or nonoperatively. Nondisplaced and minimally displaced fractures are generally treated nonoperatively, which consists of non–weight-bearing in either a long leg cast or a brace for 6 to 8 weeks. Displaced fractures should be treated operatively, the options for which most commonly include open reduction internal fixation (ORIF) or retrograde intramedullary nailing. ORIF is typically accomplished with a plate-and-screw construct placed on the lateral femur and is frequently done with a locking plate, which adds stability

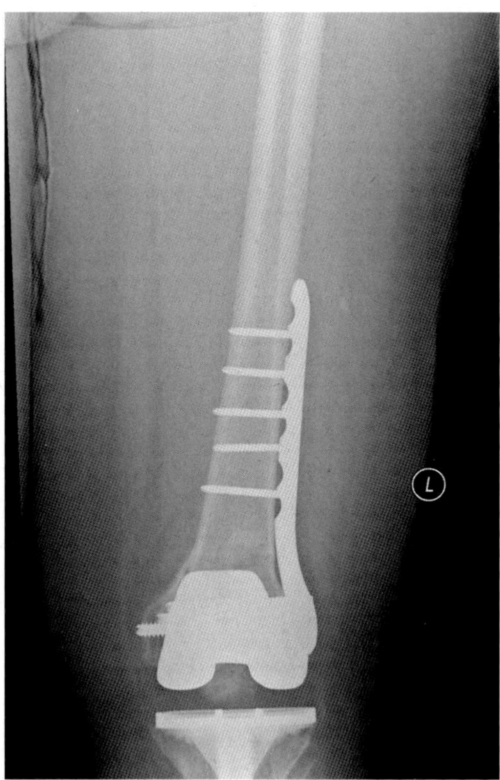

Figure 18.25 Open reduction internal fixation of a distal femoral periprosthetic fracture with a locking plate.

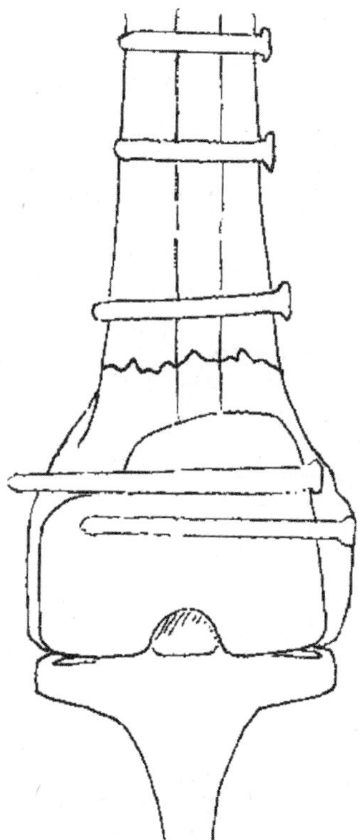

Figure 18.26 Retrograde intramedullary nailing of a periprosthetic distal femur fracture. (*Reproduced with permission from* Lotke PA, Lonner JH. *Master Techniques in Orthopaedic Surgery: Knee Arthroplasty*. 2nd ed. Philadelphia, PA: Lippincott Williams & Wilkins, 2003.)

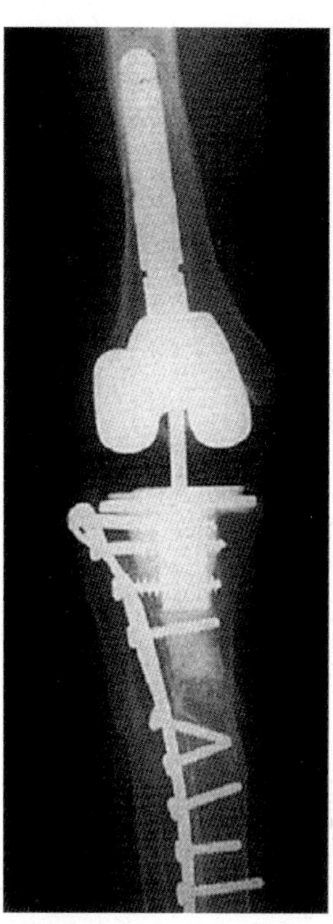

Figure 18.27 Open reduction internal fixation following a periprosthetic proximal tibia fracture. (*Reproduced with permission from* Lotke PA, Lonner JH. *Master Techniques in Orthopaedic Surgery: Knee Arthroplasty*. 2nd ed. Philadelphia, PA: Lippincott Williams & Wilkins, 2003.)

in patients with osteoporotic bone (Fig. 18.25). Nailing is also an option (Fig. 18.26), but this requires placing the device through an opening in the femoral component, which is not present on all prosthetic designs. Therefore, one must first identify the implant that was used and then determine whether or not it is conducive to retrograde nailing.

Periprosthetic tibial fractures also occur, although they are much less common. In many cases, these are tibial shaft fractures resulting from significant trauma (Fig. 18.27). The standard treatment for tibial shaft fractures is intramedullary nailing, which cannot be done with a TKA in place. Therefore, treatment is altered and limited to either casting or ORIF. Tibial fractures also occur in the setting of tibial component malalignment, which place excess stress on the underlying bone. In most cases, these are minimally displaced, and nonoperative treatment can be utilized. However, in many cases, tibial component revision is needed.

SUMMARY

OA of the knee is a significant problem that is experienced by a large proportion of the aging population. There are many options for conservative treatment of OA, but there is no way to reverse the progression of the disease. Therefore, surgical intervention becomes necessary in a large number of individuals. Joint-sparing operations include arthroscopy, HTO, and UKA, all of which have a role in certain patient populations, but the gold standard of surgical treatment continues to be TKA. TKA has a well-established track record of providing symptomatic relief to patients with OA, and survivorship continues to improve as better prostheses are developed. While results are generally excellent, it is important to be aware that significant complications can occur from what is a very invasive surgery. These range from minor functional deficits to fatal PE, so the surgeon must always be aware of their possible development, particularly in the early postoperative period.

RECOMMENDED READINGS

Buckwalter JA, Saltzman C, Brown T. The impact of osteoarthritis: implications for research. *Clin Orthop Relat Res*. 2004;427(suppl): S6–S15.

Dixon MC, Brown RR, Parsch D, Scott RD. Modular fixed-bearing total knee arthroplasty with retention of the posterior cruciate ligament: a study of patients followed for a minimum of fifteen years. *J Bone Joint Surg Am*. 2005;87(3):598–603.

Gonzalez MH, Mekhail AO. The failed total knee arthroplasty: evaluation and etiology. *J Am Acad Orthop Surg*. 2004;12(6):436–446.

Naudie, DD, Ammeen DJ, Engh GA, Rorabeck CH. Wear and osteolysis around total knee arthroplasty. *J Am Acad Orthop Surg*. 2007;15(1):53–64.

Rand JA, Trousdale RT, Ilstrup DM, Harmsen WS. Factors affecting the durability of primary total knee prostheses. *J Bone Joint Surg Am*. 2003;85A(2):259–265.

Windsor RE, Bono JV. Infected total knee replacements. *J Am Acad Orthop Surg*. 1994;2(1):44–53.

Foot and Ankle

19

Benjamin D. Martin **Francis X. McGuigan**

The tibia, fibula, and the 26 major bones of the foot work in concert as essential components of the locomotion system. Congenital, acquired, and traumatic conditions are common in this region and cause significant morbidity and disability.

FUNCTIONAL ANATOMY

Osteology

The tibia is a triangular long bone that expands proximally to form the plateau at the knee and distally to form the plafond and medial malleolus. The fibula is also triangular and is oriented slightly posterior and lateral to the tibia. The distal flare forms the lateral malleolus. These two bones articulate both proximally and distally in arthrodial joints, allowing for slight translational and rotational movements.

Distally, the tibia and fibula form the ankle joint. The joint is secured through multiple ligamentous connections—the interosseous membrane, the anterior inferior tibiofibular ligament, and the posterior inferior tibiofibular ligament. Together, the tibia and fibula create the mortise of the ankle, which articulates with the dome of the talus, allowing for dorsiflexion and plantarflexion.

The foot is divided into three separate regions—the hindfoot, midfoot and forefoot, and three groups of bones: the tarsus, metatarsus, and phalanges. The hindfoot includes the talus and calcaneus. The midfoot is composed of the navicular, cuboid, and the three cuneiforms. The forefoot region incorporates the metatarsals and the phalanges.

The anatomy of the talus is critical to understanding the hindfoot. More than 60% of the talus is covered with hyaline cartilage. It consists of a head, neck, and body and has no muscle or tendon attachments. Stability is dependent on bone articulations, joint capsules, and ligaments. The body of the talus has a unique trapezoidal shape, being wider anteriorly. This provides extra stability to the ankle mortise in dorsiflexion. The medial and lateral concave aspects of the body articulate with the respective malleoli. Posteriorly, a sulcus is formed between two tubercles to accommodate the flexor hallucis longus (FHL). The os trigonum is an accessory bone seen in 50% of people that is attached to the posterolateral process of the talus and is usually bilateral. The inferior aspect of the talus has the anterior, middle, and posterior facets that articulate with the calcaneus to form the subtalar joint. The talar neck is oriented medially and in a plantar direction and creates the roof of the sinus tarsi. The neck is the most at risk for fracture. The talar head articulates with the navicular and anterior process of the calcaneus. The calcaneonavicular ligament, or spring ligament, acts as a sling to support the talar head.

Because most of the talus is covered with cartilage, there is limited area for the blood supply to enter. Three main arteries—the posterior tibial, the anterior tibial, and the perforating peroneal arteries—and their branches provide the blood supply. The artery of the tarsal canal, a branch of the posterior tibial artery, and the artery of the tarsal sinus, a branch of the perforating peroneal artery, create an anastomotic sling under the talar neck (Fig. 19.1). The artery of the tarsal canal supplies the medial half to two-thirds of the talar body, whereas the sinus tarsi artery supplies the lateral 25%. A fracture of the talar neck can result in disruption of blood flow and avascular necrosis of the body.

The calcaneus, or os calcis, transmits body weight to the ground and serves as a lever arm for the Achilles tendon. The anterior, middle, and posterior facets articulate with the corresponding facets of the talus, with the posterior facet being the largest and most important. The middle facet overlies the sustentaculum tali, under which the FHL tendon runs and is often confluent with the anterior facet. The sustentaculum tali also serves as the insertion site of the spring ligament and the tibiocalcaneal part of the deltoid ligament. The lateral wall of the calcaneus contains the trochlear process, which forms a groove for the peroneus longus tendon. Distally, the calcaneus articulates with the

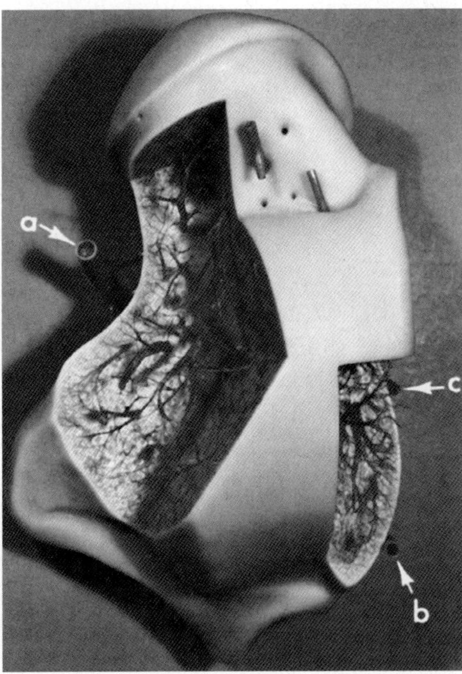

Figure 19.1 The blood supply to the talus is primarily from an anastomotic sling that originates from the artery of the tarsal sinus **(A)** laterally and the artery of the tarsal canal **(B)** medially. Additional blood vessels enter dorsally through the neck and medial body **(C)**. (*Reproduced with permission from* Rockwood CA, Green DP, Bucholz RW. *Rockwood and Green's Fractures in Adults*. 6th ed. Philadelphia, PA: Lippincott Williams & Wilkins, 2006.)

cuboid via a saddle joint. The cortical bone of the calcaneus is weak in the central body and is susceptible to compression fracture.

The midfoot consists of the navicular, cuboid, and three cuneiform bones. The navicular serves as the keystone for the medial longitudinal arch of the foot, articulating with the talus proximally and the cuneiforms distally. The posterior tibial tendon inserts on the medial side of the navicular. An accessory navicular, or os tibiale externum, is present in 10% of people. The cuboid forms the lateral column through an articulation with the calcaneus proximally and the fourth and fifth metatarsals distally. A groove on the undersurface of the cuboid accommodates the peroneus longus tendon. The cuneiforms are trapezoidal in shape, tapering plantarly, contributing to the formation of the transverse arch of the foot (Fig. 19.2). Distally, the cuneiforms articulate with the first, second, and third metatarsals. The second cuneiform is shorter than the others, allowing for the second metatarsal to be recessed proximally (Fig. 19.3), providing added stability to the second tarsometatarsal joint.

The forefoot is composed of the five metatarsals and phalanges, which articulate to form the metatarsophalangeal (MTP) joints. Normally, the first metatarsal is the shortest and widest and bears one-third of the body weight. The plantar surface of the head of the first metatarsal articu-

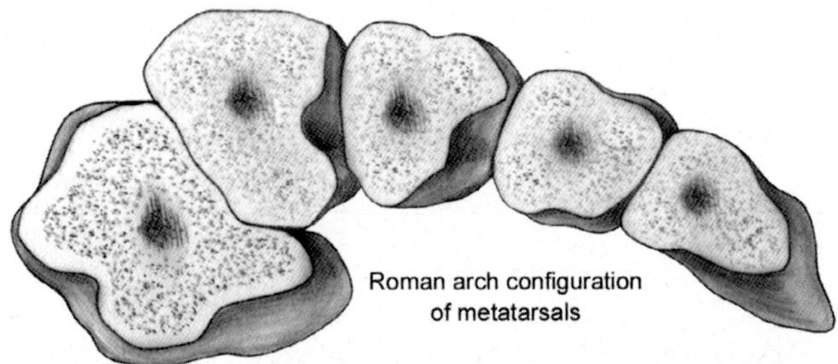

Figure 19.2 The wedge shape of the three cuneiforms creates the transverse arch of the foot, often compared to a Roman arch. (*Reproduced with permission from* Johnson D, Pedowitz RA. *Practical Orthopaedic Sports Medicine and Arthroscopy*. Philadelphia, PA: Lippincott Williams & Wilkins, 2007.)

lates with two sesamoid bones that are encased by the flexor hallucis brevis (FHB) tendon. These sesamoids provide a mechanical advantage by increasing the level arm for flexion, much like the patella for knee extension. The second metatarsal is usually the longest and is recessed proximally between the cuneiforms. Mobility of the second metatarsal is sacrificed for this extra stability. The third, fourth, and fifth metatarsals are successively shorter, creating a curved appearance of the foot. The fifth metatarsal has a prominence at its base for insertion of the peroneus brevis tendon. The lesser four metatarsals bear two-thirds of the body weight equally.

The phalanges of the foot are similar to those in the hand. The proximal aspect of the proximal phalanges is concave to allow articulation with the convex head of the metatarsals. The distal ends have more of a trochlear shape that articulates with the corresponding middle phalanx. Each distal phalanx terminates in a tuft of bone to serve as an anchor for the toe pad.

Ankle Joint

The mortise formed by the tibia and fibula is dynamic but stable due the bone anatomy, thick posterior capsule, and ligamentous structures. As the foot dorsiflexes, the fibula moves proximally, posteriorly, and externally and rotates to provide room for the trapezoid-shaped talus, which is wider anteriorly. The axis of the ankle joint is not perpendicular to the malleoli, such that the foot externally rotates 15 degrees with dorsiflexion and internally rotates 15 degrees with plantarflexion.

The medial deltoid complex and the lateral ligaments provide added stability. The deltoid is fan-shaped ligament with deep and superficial components (Fig. 19.4). The superficial components include the posterior tibiotalar, tibiocalcaneal, and the tibionavicular ligaments. The anterior tibiotalar ligament forms the deep component and is important to maintaining the medial joint space. The lateral complex consists of the posterior talofibular ligament (PTFL), the calcaneofibular ligament (CFL), and the

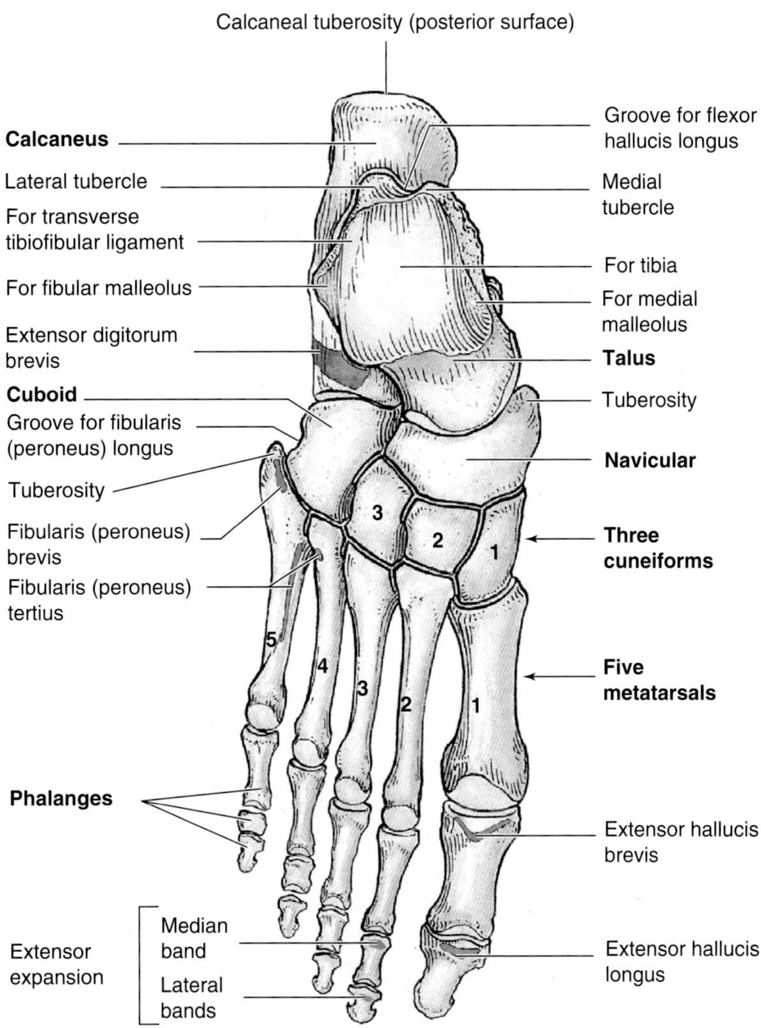

Figure 19.3 The second metatarsal is recessed between the medial and lateral cuneiform, adding to the stability of the foot. (*Adapted from* Hoppenfeld S, DeBoer P. *Surgical Exposures in Orthopaedics: The Anatomic Approach*. 3rd ed. Philadelphia, PA: Lippincott Williams & Wilkins, 2003.)

anterior talofibular ligament (ATFL) (Fig. 19.5). The ATFL, running from the anteroinferior aspect of the fibula to the neck of the talus, is the primary restraint against anteriorly directed forces when the ankle is in the neutral position and also resists inversion in the plantarflexed foot. The CFL, which extends from the tip of the fibula to the lateral tubercle of the calcaneus, prevents varus talar tilt when the ankle is in neutral or dorsiflexed position. The PTFL runs from the posterior aspect of the distal fibula to the lateral tubercle of the talus. A tear in one or more of these lateral ligaments results in an ankle sprain, which is common after an inversion or plantarflexion injury. The ATFL is the most vulnerable and commonly injured. The normal angle between the CFL and ATFL averages 105 degrees in

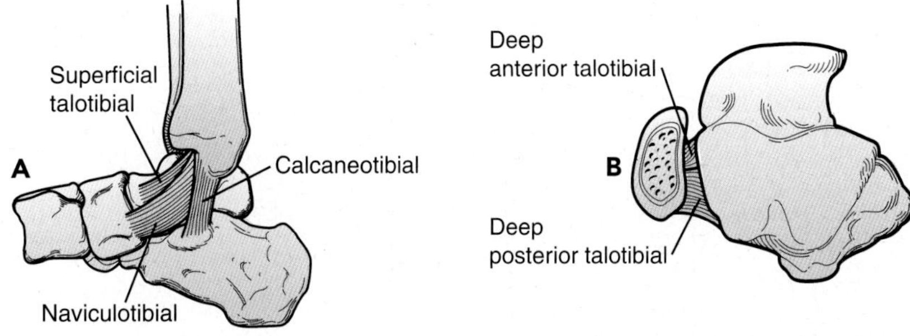

Figure 19.4 The medial deltoid ligament complex is comprised of superficial **(A)** and deep **(B)** components. (*Reproduced with permission from* Rockwood CA, Green DP, Bucholz RW. *Rockwood and Green's Fractures in Adults*. 6th ed. Philadelphia, PA: Lippincott Williams & Wilkins, 2006.)

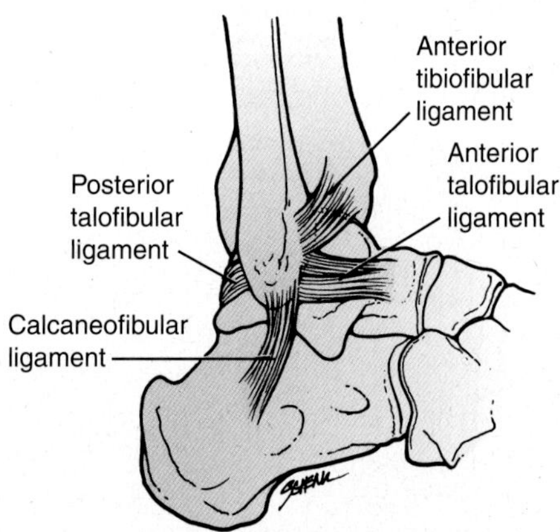

Figure 19.5 The posterior talofibular ligament (PTFL), the calcaneofibular ligament (CFL), and the anterior talofibular ligament (ATFL) together form the lateral collateral structures of the ankle. The anterior tibiofibular ligament is part of the syndesmosis. (*Reproduced with permission from* Rockwood CA, Green DP, Bucholz RW. *Rockwood and Green's Fractures in Adults.* 6th ed. Philadelphia, PA: Lippincott Williams & Wilkins, 2006.)

the sagittal plane. It is thought that individuals with greater angles may be more susceptible to injury.

The syndesmosis provides stability to the distal tibiofibular articulation and thus the mortise (Fig. 19.6). The anterior tibiofibular, the posterior tibiofibular, inferior transverse ligament, and the interosseous membrane form the syndesmosis. Injury to these structures can result from hyperdorsiflexion and external rotation. These are often referred to as "high" ankle sprains and are associated with a slower functional recovery than injury to the lateral ligaments.

Subtalar Joint

The subtalar joint is essentially a hinge joint between the talus and calcaneus, creating an axis for inversion and eversion. Functionally, this translates into the ability to ambulate on uneven ground. The axis of the joint averages 23 degrees medially from the longitudinal axis of the foot and 42 degrees from the horizontal plane and usually has approximately 10 degrees to 60 degrees of motion. The range of motion varies depending on anatomy. For example, a cavus (high-arched) foot has much less motion than a planovalgus (flat) foot. Ligamentous resistance to inversion is provided by the inferior extensor retinaculum when the foot is in neutral and dorsiflexion. The CFL, joint capsule, interosseous talocalcaneal ligament, and the ligament of the tarsal canal also contribute to stability.

Transverse Tarsal Joint

The transverse tarsal joint, or Chopart joint, is the sum of the saddle-shaped calcaneocuboid and concave talonavicular joints. The orientation of these joints changes with the position of the calcaneus such that when the calcaneus is in valgus, the joints are parallel and mobile. During heel strike, this allows the dissipation of forces. When the calcaneus is in varus, the joints diverge, resulting in a rigid midfoot, which is essential to effective push-off.

Midfoot Joints

The midfoot joints are stabilized by multiple ligaments and by the intrinsic bony architecture of the wedge-shaped cuneiform bones. This section of the foot is primarily a

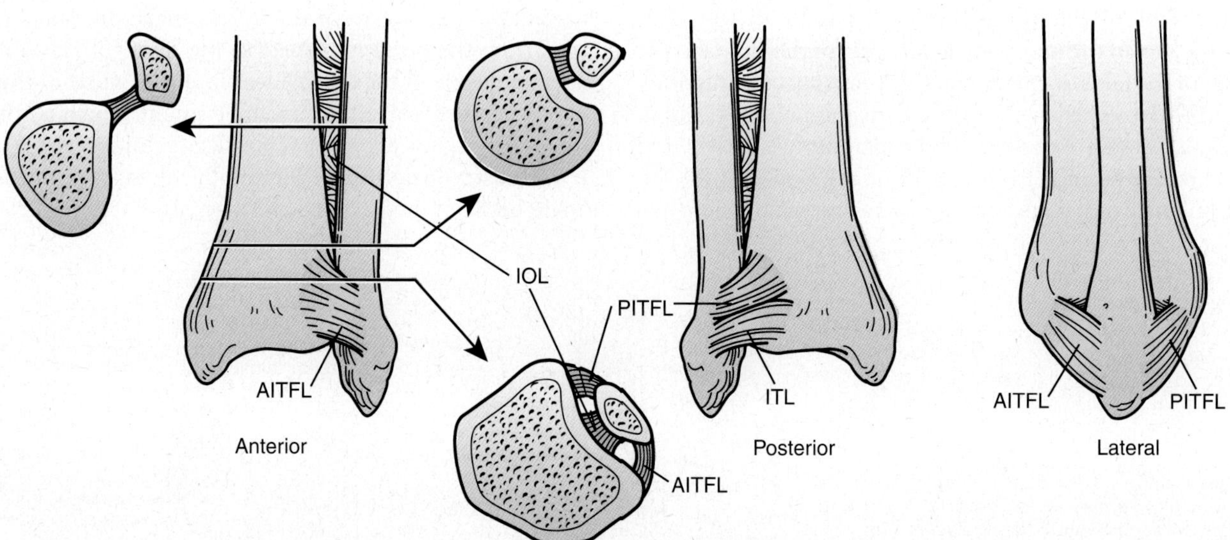

Figure 19.6 The syndesmosis is composed of the anterior inferior tibiofibular (AITFL), the posterior inferior tibiofibular (PITFL), inferior transverse ligament (ITL), and the interosseous membrane (IOM). (*Reproduced with permission from* Rockwood CA, Green DP, Bucholz RW. *Rockwood and Green's Fractures in Adults.* 6th ed. Philadelphia, PA: Lippincott Williams & Wilkins, 2006.)

stable segment designed to handle the stresses of the stance phase of gait. Little motion actually occurs through these articulations. The Chopart ligament, long plantar ligament, and short plantar ligament provide stability to the joints and to the longitudinal arch of the foot.

Tarsometatarsal Joints

Dorsal, plantar, and interosseous ligaments stabilize the tarsometatarsal joints, or the joint of Lisfranc. The interosseous ligaments are transverse connections between the adjacent metatarsal bases, except between the first and second metatarsals. Joint stability for that articulation is instead conferred via the oblique ligament, or Lisfranc ligament, that spans from the medial cuneiform bone to the second metatarsal. The first tarsometatarsal joint is the only one with significant motion because of the lack of connection to the neighboring metatarsal. Significant dorsiflexion, plantarflexion, and rotation all occur during the gait cycle.

Metatarsophalangeal Joints

The MTP joints of the lesser toes are stabilized by the bony shape, the fibrocartilaginous plantar plates originating from the metatarsal heads and inserting on the bases of the proximal phalanges, the deep transverse metatarsal ligament, and the collateral ligaments. Attenuation of these structures can result in dorsal subluxation and dislocation. The MTP joint of the hallux has a range of motion of 70 degrees allowing for the toe-off phase of the gait cycle.

Interphalangeal Joints

The interphalangeal joints are ginglymus joints with cam-shaped condyles analogous to those in the hand, with similar anatomy and ligamentous support. More flexion occurs through the proximal interphalangeal (PIP) joints, whereas both the proximal and distal interphalangeal (DIP) joints have little extension.

Extrinsic Muscles of the Foot

The extrinsic muscles of the foot are separated into four fascial compartments in the leg—the superficial and deep posterior compartments, the lateral compartment, and the anterior compartment. The superficial posterior compartment includes the gastrocnemius, plantaris, and the soleus muscles. The gastrocnemius originates from the medial and lateral femoral condyles and joins the soleus muscle, which originates from the posterior tibia and fibula, to form the Achilles tendon. The Achilles tendon, also referred to as the *tendo calcaneus*, rotates 90 degrees as it inserts onto the posterosuperior tuberosity of the calcaneus. This is the largest and strongest tendon in the body. The plantaris originates from the lateral femoral condyle and is mostly tendinous along its length as it courses between the soleus and the gastrocnemius to insert just medial to the Achilles tendon on the calcaneus. The plantaris can be used as a tendon graft but is absent in approximately 7% of people. These three muscles, often referred to as the *triceps surae*, are innervated by the tibial nerve and function as the primary plantarflexors of the ankle. They also assist in inversion of the hindfoot.

The tibialis posterior, the flexor digitorum longus (FDL), and the FHL are the three muscles of the deep posterior compartment and serve as inverters of the foot and secondary plantarflexors. These muscles originate from the posterior tibia and interosseous membrane and pass together as tendons behind the medial malleolus in the tarsal canal under the flexor retinaculum along with the posterior tibial artery and nerve (Fig. 19.7). The tibialis posterior inserts on the navicular, medial and middle cuneiforms, and the bases of the second, third, and fourth metatarsals. Its

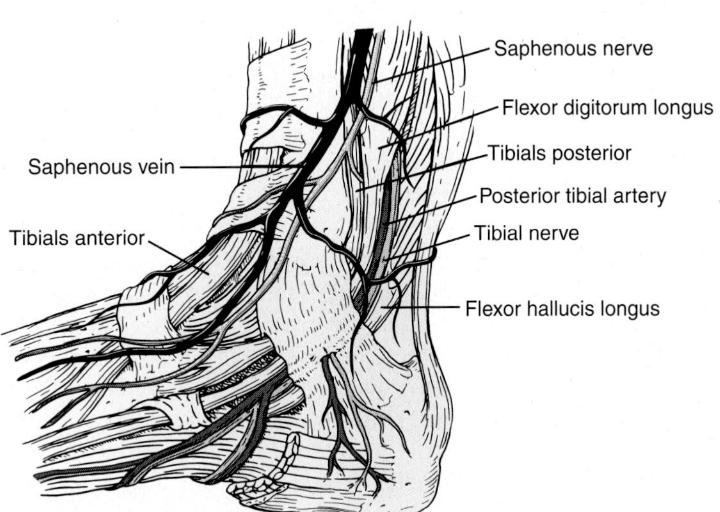

Figure 19.7 Anatomy of the medial neurovascular structures as they course behind the medial malleolus. (*Reproduced with permission from* Rockwood CA, Green DP, Bucholz RW. *Rockwood and Green's Fractures in Adults.* 6th ed. Philadelphia, PA: Lippincott Williams & Wilkins, 2006.)

primary function is inversion of the foot, but it also contributes to the support of the longitudinal arch. The FDL travels behind the medial malleolus with the tibialis posterior superficial to the deltoid ligament and into the plantar aspect of the foot just plantar to the FHL. After joining with the quadratus plantae, it divides into four slips and inserts onto the base of the distal phalanx of the lesser toes. The FDL flexes the MTP, PIP, and DIP joints of the lesser toes and serves as a weak ankle plantarflexor. The FHL is the most lateral muscle of the deep posterior compartment and courses between the posterior talar processes, under the sustentaculum tali, and through the second layer of plantar aspect of the foot to insert on the distal phalanx of the great toe. It is the primary flexor of the hallux and a weak ankle plantarflexor. The tibial nerve innervates these three muscles.

The lateral compartment contains the peroneus longus and peroneus brevis muscles, which are innervated by the superficial peroneal nerve. The peroneus longus is more superficial and is posterolateral to the peroneus brevis behind the lateral malleolus. The peroneus longus originates from the upper two-thirds of the lateral fibula and intermuscular septum and inserts on the plantar base of the first metatarsal and medial cuneiform after traveling beneath the cuboid. The muscle plantarflexes the first ray and contributes some ankle plantarflexion and foot abduction. The peroneus brevis originates from the distal two-thirds of the intermuscular septum and inserts onto the base of the fifth metatarsal and serves as the primary evertor of the foot. In some individuals, a third muscle, the peroneus tertius, parallels the peroneus brevis and inserts on the dorsal base of the metatarsal. The tendons are held within the peroneal groove as they pass posteriorly and around the lateral malleolus by the superior and inferior peroneal retinaculum. The CFL lies deep to both tendons at the tip of the lateral malleolus.

The tibialis anterior, the extensor hallucis longus (EHL), and the extensor digitorum longus (EDL) form the anterior compartment of the leg and are innervated by the deep peroneal nerve. As a group, these muscles dorsiflex the foot and ankle. The tibialis anterior originates from the lateral tibial condyle and the interosseous membrane and inserts on to the medial border of the medial cuneiform and base of the first metatarsal. In addition to dorsiflexion of the ankle, it inverts the subtalar joint and supports the longitudinal arch of the foot. The tibialis anterior muscle is the antagonist of the peroneus longus muscle. The EHL, the primary extensor of the hallux, arises from the middle two-thirds of the anterior fibula and interosseous membrane and inserts onto the distal phalanx of the hallux. The EHL weakly dorsiflexes the ankle and inverts the foot. The EHL crosses from lateral to medial over the dorsalis pedis artery and deep peroneal nerve just proximal to the ankle joint. The dorsalis pedis artery and deep peroneal nerve are bordered by the EHL medially and the EDL laterally at the level of the ankle joint. The EDL originates from the lateral tibial condyle, interosseous membrane, and the intermuscular septum. Combined with fibers from the lumbricals and interossei muscles, it forms a broad aponeurosis at the proximal phalanx of each lesser toe. The aponeurosis splits at the distal end of the proximal phalanx to form a central and two lateral slips. The central slip inserts onto the middle phalanx, and the lateral slips form the extensor hood over the DIP joint. Thus the EDL can extend the MTP joints as well as the PIP and DIP joints. However, PIP and DIP extensions can occur only when the MTP joint is in neutral or slight flexion.

Intrinsic Muscles of the Foot

While there are four layers of plantar muscles in the foot, there is only one dorsal muscle. The extensor digitorum brevis (EDB), innervated by the lateral branch of the deep peroneal nerve, originates from the sinus tarsi and superolateral calcaneus and forms four tendons. The three lateral tendons join the lateral aspect of the tendons of the EDL. The most medial part of the EDB is often distinct and referred to as the *extensor hallucis brevis*. This tendon inserts on the base of the proximal phalanx of the hallux.

The medial and lateral plantar nerves innervate all the plantar muscles. The superficial layer of the plantar muscles consists of three muscles that are deep to the plantar fascia, originate from the calcaneal tuberosity, and insert into the toes. The abductor hallucis is the most medial. Its tendon merges with the medial slip of the FHB tendon to insert on the base of the proximal phalanx of the hallux. The flexor digitorum brevis (FDB) forms four tendons, one for each of the lesser toes. Prior to insertion on the middle phalanx of the respective toe, each divides into a medial and lateral slip through which pass the FDL tendon. This is analogous to the anatomy of the flexor tendons of the upper extremity. The abductor digiti minimi (ADM), the most lateral muscle, crosses under the fifth metatarsal to insert on the lateral side of the proximal phalanx of the small toe.

The second layer contains the quadratus plantae, lumbrical muscles, and the tendons of the FHL and FDL. The quadratus plantae originates from the calcaneal tuberosity as a medial and lateral head and ultimately forms tendons that join the FDL tendons to the lesser toes. It assists in toe flexion and is also referred to as the *flexor digitorum accessorius*. The anatomy of the quadratus varies. The muscle may be congenitally absent. There are four lumbricals, each originating from the medial side of a FDL tendon and inserting on the dorsal extensor aponeurosis of the proximal phalanges. The lumbricals flex the MTP joints and extend the PIP joints.

The third layer contains the FHB, the adductor hallucis, and the flexor digiti minimi. The FHB originates from the posterior tibial tendon and divides into two heads. Each head contains a sesamoid under the first metatarsal head and inserts on the base of the first metatarsal. The medial head joins the abductor hallucis tendon and the lateral joins the adductor hallucis tendon. The adductor hallucis is formed from oblique and transverse heads. The oblique head originates from the base of the cuboid and second, third, and forth metatarsals. The transverse head originates from the plantar plates and transverse metatarsal ligaments of the third, fourth, and fifth metatarsals. The adductor hallucis provides reinforcement to the transverse metatarsal ligaments. In a bunion (hallux valgus), contracture of the adductor muscle is part of the deformity. The flexor digiti minimi originates from the fifth metatarsal, and its tendon combines with the ADM to insert on the lateral side of the proximal phalanx of the fifth toe. Together, they flex and abduct the fifth digit.

The fourth and deepest layer contains the interossei muscles and the tendons of the peroneus longus, posterior tibialis, and anterior tibialis. There are four bipennate dorsal and three unipennate plantar interossei muscles. The dorsal group abducts the second, third, and fourth toes relative to the second metatarsal, whereas the plantar group adducts the third, fourth, and fifth toes. Along with the lumbricals, the interossei assist in flexion of the MTP joints and extension of the PIP and DIP joints via the extensor aponeurosis.

Neurovascular Structures

Five major nerve branches and three arteries supply the foot and ankle. Most of the sensory and motor innervation to the foot and ankle come from the two portions of the sciatic nerve, the common peroneal (L4–S2) and tibial nerves (L4–S3). The common peroneal nerve divides in the anterior compartment into the deep and superficial peroneal nerves after crossing around the neck of the fibula. At this point, the nerve is most susceptible to injury, especially compression neuropathy. The deep peroneal nerve innervates the anterior compartment muscles and travels with the anterior tibial artery across the ankle under the extensor retinaculum. Ultimately, it innervates some of the intrinsic muscles of the foot and provides sensation in the first dorsal webspace. The superficial peroneal nerve innervates the lateral compartment muscles and provides sensation to the dorsum of the foot and toes. This nerve is at risk during exposure of the fibula approximately 10 to 15 cm above the lateral malleolus. It becomes subcutaneous at that level passing from the lateral into the anterior compartment of the leg. Care should be taken when exposing fractures of the fibula above the lateral malleolus. The sural nerve is another branch of the common peroneal nerve that provides sensation to the lateral side of the foot. It travels separately from the superficial and deep peroneal nerves running posteriorly over the gastrocsoleus complex and eventually passing midway between the lateral malleolus and Achilles tendon at the level of the ankle.

The tibial nerve lies deep in the posterior compartment of the leg with the posterior tibial artery and continues underneath the flexor retinaculum behind the medial malleolus. Under the flexor retinaculum, the medial calcaneal nerves branch from the tibial nerve, perforate the retinaculum, and provide sensation to the heel and medial sole of the foot. After exiting the tarsal tunnel, the tibial nerve divides into the medial and lateral plantar nerves that innervate the intrinsic muscles and the skin of the bottom of the foot.

The saphenous nerve, a terminal branch of the femoral nerve (L2–L4), which provides sensation to the medial aspect of the leg and foot, is the only innervation of the foot that is not derived from the sciatic nerve. The nerve travels posterior to the greater saphenous vein.

The anterior tibial, posterior tibial, and peroneal arteries supply the lower leg. The anterior and posterior tibial arteries are the terminal branches of the popliteal artery. The anterior tibial artery enters the anterior compartment through the interosseous membrane below the proximal tibiofibular joint. It travels along the interosseous membrane medial to the deep peroneal nerve. Before passing under the superior and inferior extensor retinaculum, it gives off the anterior medial and lateral malleolar branches to supply the malleoli. Below the retinaculum, it becomes known as the *dorsalis pedis artery* and is superficial enough to be palpable as an arterial pulse. The dorsalis pedis artery sends a lateral branch to the sinus tarsi, a deep branch known as the *arcuate artery* that contributes to the deep arterial arch, and a terminal branch that forms the first dorsal metatarsal artery. The posterior tibial artery gives off a lateral branch high in the calf, called the *peroneal artery*. The peroneal artery travels posterior to the interosseous membrane deep to the FHL. It terminates at the distal tibiofibular joint, forming an anastomosis with the lateral malleolar artery of the anterior tibial artery. The posterior tibial artery runs deep to the gastrocnemius and soleus muscles, providing a blood supply to the posterior compartment. After passing under the flexor retinaculum with the tibial nerve, the posterior tibial artery terminates as the medial and lateral plantar arteries.

Gait Analysis

The gait cycle consists of events occurring from heel strike to the next heel strike of the same foot. It is divided into the stance and swing phases. The stance phase makes up 62% of the cycle and the swing phase makes up the remaining 38%. The stance phase is further separated into three segments: the initial double-limb support (loading response), the single-limb stance, and the terminal double-limb support (preswing). Similarly, the swing phase is separated into initial swing, midswing, and terminal swing phases.

Although most limb motion takes place in the sagittal plane, coronal and transverse motions do occur. With foot strike, the transverse tarsal joint is unlocked to allow axial forces to dissipate. Toward the end of the stance phase, the subtalar joint inverts, locking the transverse tarsal joint and allowing effective push-off from the forefoot. The five prerequisites of normal gait are appropriate foot prepositioning for initial contact, stance phase stability, swing phase clearance, adequate step length, and maximization of energy conservation.

EVALUATION OF FOOT AND ANKLE PROBLEMS

History

A pertinent history guides the physical examination and is the basis of a preliminary differential diagnosis. A well-directed questionnaire provides an accurate and complete documentation of patient's complaint, medical history, and review of systems. The mechanism of injury; the location, duration, and character of the pain; the relationship of the pain to activities and the effectiveness of alleviating factors such as over-the-counter medications and ice help to narrow the likely cause of the patient's pathology. Other symptoms to note include timing and duration of swelling, instability, and changes in ankle and foot alignment. Existing systemic disorders—including inflammatory, infectious, neoplastic, metabolic, and congenital conditions – should be elicited, with a specific emphasis on gout and diabetes mellitus. A medical and surgical history, with emphasis on the appendicular and extremity musculoskeletal systems is helpful in creating a diagnostic and therapeutic plan of treatment. Activity level, occupation, level of education, and socioeconomic status assist in determining the impairment imposed by the patient's condition and any obstacles to patient compliance with treatment. Family history is helpful because many of the foot and ankle disorders arise from a hereditary predisposition, including congenital abnormalities and inflammatory metabolic disorders.

Physical Examination

A sound foot and ankle examination should follow the principles of any orthopaedic examination: inspection, palpation, range of motion, manipulation, and neurovascular examination. A fundamental understanding of the anatomy discussed earlier is critical in performing a complete focused physical. The examination begins as the patient walks into the examination room, providing an opportunity to evaluate gait patterns. It is important to remove shoes and socks for complete evaluation. Extremity alignment should be assessed from the front and back with the subject standing and sitting. Gait should again be observed without shoes and supports. The sole of the patient's shoes are inspected, and abnormal shoe wear is noted. Lateral sole wear is associated with a cavovarus foot and medial wear with a planovalgus foot. Special attention is given to the hindfoot alignment and its relation to the forefoot. The longitudinal arch is noted both with and without weight-bearing. Callous formation over bony prominences that indicate areas of excessive pressure should be evaluated. The condition of the soft tissues is critical, especially in the setting of trauma and in patients with diabetes. Palpation will depend on where the patient is having symptoms and the underlying pathology. More details will be discussed in the following sections; however, a brief discussion on the examination of the major joints of the foot and ankle follows.

The ankle joint should be checked for the presence of an effusion versus local tissue swelling. Palpating the ankle joint either medial to the tibialis anterior tendon or lateral to the EDL tendon best assesses this. The normal range of motion for the ankle is 20 degrees of dorsiflexion and 50 degrees of plantarflexion. Loss of ankle dorsiflexion, an equinus contracture, can be associated with heel cord tightness, posterior capsule contracture, or anterior bony impingement. Contracture of the heel cord occurs from shortening of either one or both of the gastrocnemius and soleus musculotendinous units. To distinguish the cause of the contracture, ankle dorsiflexion is tested with the knee extended and again with the knee flexed to 90 degrees. By flexing the knee to 90 degrees, the gastrocnemius muscle, which crosses the knee, is relaxed. The gastrocnemius is contracted only when there is no restriction to dorsiflexion in this position. If restriction is present in both positions, both musculotendinous units are contracted. The lateral side of the ankle is a common site of pathology because ankle sprains are so common. Tenderness over the ATFL, with or without pain along the CFL, is characteristic of a lateral ankle sprain. Stability is tested with the anterior drawer and inversion stress tests. The anterior drawer test examines the competency of the ATFL. With the tibia stabilized with one hand, the examiner applies an anteriorly directed force by pulling anteriorly, with the second hand grasping the posterior heel (Fig 19.8). Inversion stress tests of the ankle should be applied in both dorsiflexion and plantarflexion to assess the laxity of the CFL and ATFL, respectively.

The subtalar joint typically allows for more inversion than eversion by a factor of three to one. Typically, inversion is approximately 20 degrees and eversion is 7 degrees; however, this depends on the patient's anatomy. For example, a cavovarus foot will have a decreased range of motion, whereas a planovalgus foot will have an increased range of motion.

Imaging

Plain radiographs of the foot and ankle are the best initial forms of imaging; however, arthrography, computed

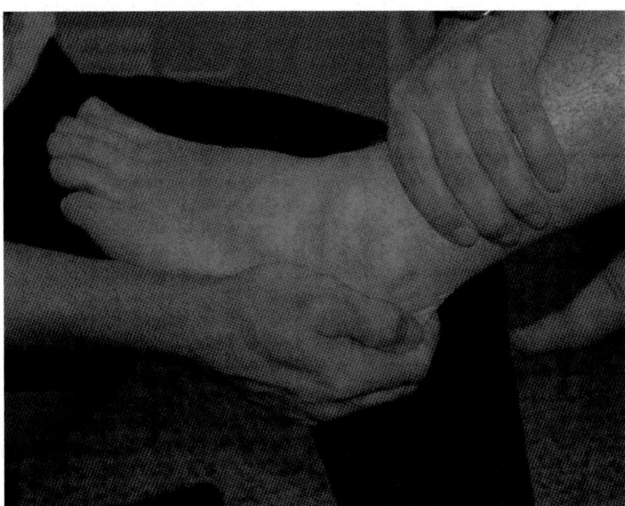

Figure 19.8 The anterior draw test is used to examine the competency of the ATFL. An anterior force is applied to the posterior heel with the ankle in 10 degrees of plantarflexion while the tibia is stabilized. (*Reproduced with permission from* Johnson D, Pedowitz RA. *Practical Orthopaedic Sports Medicine and Arthroscopy*. Philadelphia, PA: Lippincott Williams & Wilkins, 2007.)

tomography (CT) scans, and magnetic resonance imaging (MRI) scan can be useful in certain situations. When possible, radiographs should be taken while weight-bearing and include an anteroposterior (AP), lateral and oblique views for the foot and AP, lateral, and mortise views for the ankle. For the AP view of the foot, the beam is directed 15 degrees from the vertical toward the hindfoot, with the beam centered at the level of the talonavicular and calcaneocuboid joints. The AP view allows for assessment of the forefoot and midfoot. The oblique view is used to evaluate the relationship of the lateral tarsometatarsal joints. It is obtained with the knee flexed and the side of the foot angled at 30 degrees to the surface of the cassette with the beam directed vertically. Additional images such as sesamoid views, the Harris axial heel view, and Broden view are available to evaluate specific pathology. These variations will be discussed later in sections dealing with specific foot and ankle conditions.

As mentioned, a standard ankle series includes an AP, lateral, and mortise views. The AP radiograph allows evaluation of the distal tibia and fibula, the talar dome, and the integrity of the syndesmosis. The mortise view aids in assessing the ankle joint spaces. It is obtained with the ankle internally rotated 20 degrees to orient the joint axis parallel to the radiographic beam. Ankle stress views are helpful in diagnosing instability patterns.

CT scans are helpful to detect occult bone lesions, evaluate intraarticular pathology like bony coalitions, and assess fracture patterns in calcaneus injuries. Images of the subtalar joint are taken perpendicular to the posterior facet of the calcaneus. MRI is used to evaluate soft tissue pathology including tumors, ligament and tendon abnormalities, and articular cartilage injuries. It is also useful to evaluate avascular necrosis and osteomyelitis.

TRAUMATIC INJURIES TO THE FOOT AND ANKLE

Pilon Fractures

Pilon fractures are injuries of the distal tibial articular surface or plafond. They are typically high-energy injuries and are associated with significant soft tissue injury. The extent of the soft tissue involvement varies, but it affects the manner in which these fractures are treated. Most often these fractures require open reduction and internal fixation (ORIF) to restore the joint surface and provide the best possible outcome. These injuries account for 10% of all lower extremity fractures.

Classification

Pilon fractures have historically been classified according to Rüedi and Allgöwer (Fig. 19.9). Type I fractures are nondisplaced. Type II fractures are displaced with minimal comminution, whereas type III fractures are displaced with significant comminution. The AO/OTA classification is more descriptive and has three main types. Type A fractures are nonarticular. Type B fractures involve part of the articular surface, and type C fractures involve the entire articular surface. These three types are further subclassified based on the amount of comminution.

The soft tissue envelope can be classified on the basis of a scale of 0 to 3, according to Tschern and Goetzen. Increasing grades are associated with more damage to the surrounding soft tissue.

Mechanism of Injury

Pilon injuries result from axial loads, with or without a rotational component, most commonly as a result of falls from a height or the impact of motor vehicle crashes. The position of the foot at the time of impact affects the fracture location (Fig. 19.10). If the foot is in dorsiflexion, the anterior portion of the tibia is fractured, whereas in plantarflexion, the posterior tibia is fractured because of the impact of the talar dome. With the ankle in neutral at the time of impact, the middle portion of the distal tibia is maximally involved. Pilon fractures are distinguished from ankle fractures with intraarticular extension by their mechanism and degree of injury. Ankle fractures are typically rotational injuries with the main fracture lines involving the lateral, medial, and posterior malleoli (Table 19.1).

Presentation

Patients commonly present with significant pain and swelling about the ankle and varying degrees of soft tissue damage. Because of the high-energy mechanisms associated with these injuries, many patients may have sustained additional orthopaedic or organ system injuries.

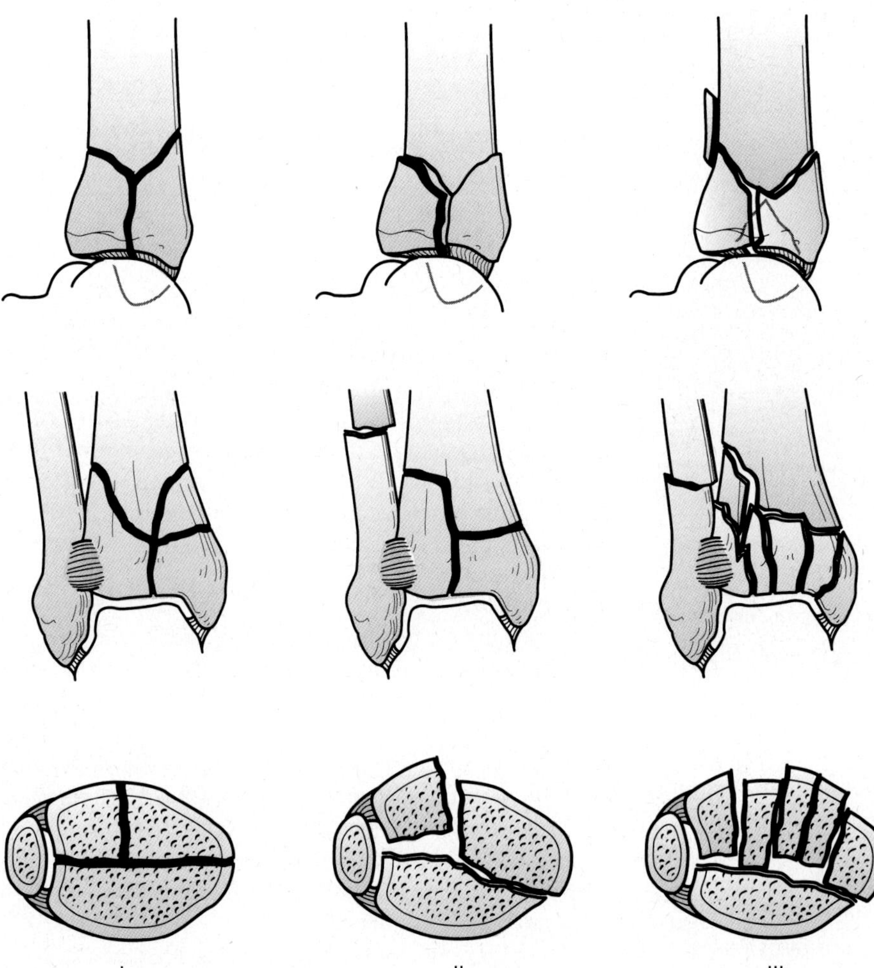

Figure 19.9 The classification of distal tibia fractures according to Rüedi and Allgöwer. The type corresponds to the degree of articular comminution. (*Reproduced with permission from* Rockwood CA, Green DP, Bucholz RW. *Rockwood and Green's Fractures in Adults.* 6th ed. Philadelphia, PA: Lippincott Williams & Wilkins, 2006.)

Physical Examination

The extent of soft tissue injury is important as it directs treatment. An open injury or an injury that results in vascular compromise, such as a fracture dislocation, is a surgical emergency. If the injury is several hours old, fracture blisters about the lower extremity are often present. The full extent of soft tissue injury may not declare itself immediately, and so serial examination is warranted. In addition to evaluating the soft tissue status and documenting a thorough neurovascular examination, it is essential to perform a complete secondary survey on patients involved in any high-energy trauma, to avoid missing additional life- or limb-threatening injuries.

Imaging

Standard ankle radiographs are the primary imaging study. CT scan is helpful to delineate fracture patterns and determine the amount of comminution for surgical planning.

TABLE 19.1

CHARACTERISTICS OF ROTATIONAL COMPARED WITH AXIALLY LOADING FRACTURES

Rotation	Axial Load
Slow rate of load application	Rapid rate of load application
Little energy released at failure (yield point)	Large amount of energy released
Predominant translational displacement of talus	A component of proximal displacement of talus
Little comminution	Comminuted articular surface and metaphysis
Minimal soft tissue injury	Severe soft tissue injury

Reproduced with permission from Rockwood CA, Green DP, Bucholz RW. *Rockwood and Green's Fractures in Adults.* 6th ed. Philadelphia, PA: Lippincott Williams & Wilkins, 2006.

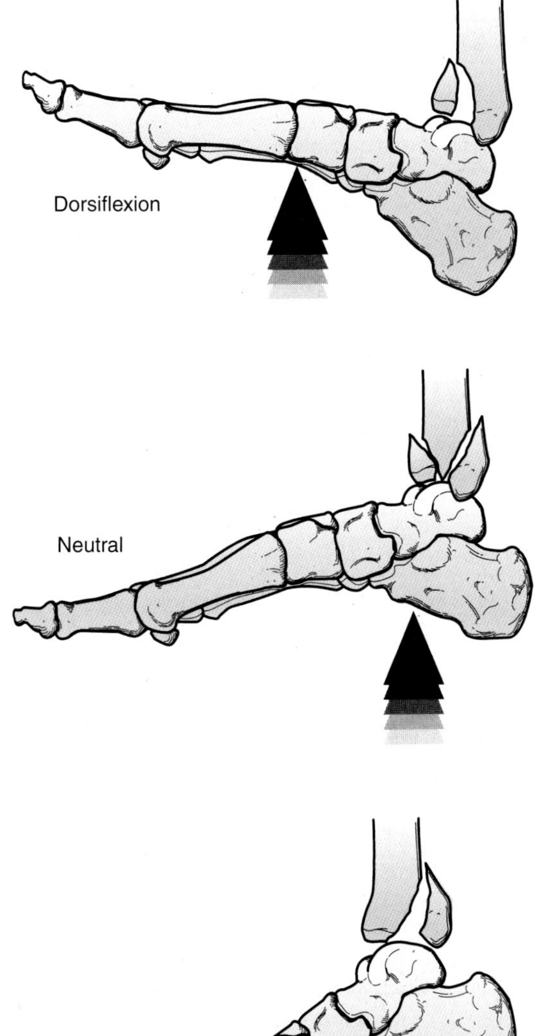

Figure 19.10 The area of the tibial plafond fracture depends on the position of the foot at the moment of axial load. (*Reproduced with permission from* Rockwood CA, Green DP, Bucholz RW. *Rockwood and Green's Fractures in Adults.* 6th ed. Philadelphia, PA: Lippincott Williams & Wilkins, 2006.)

If a temporizing external fixator is planned because of the degree soft tissue injury, it is best to wait to obtain the CT scan until after it has been placed.

Treatment

Gross malalignment and associated dislocations should be reduced immediately and the limb immobilized. This reduces the patient pain and minimizes additional soft tissue trauma. Frequently, soft tissue swelling and injury prevent immediate surgical fixation of the fracture; in these situations, an external fixator spanning the joint provides temporary immobilization and definitive fixation is often delayed for 10 days to 2 weeks. Once the soft tissue injury has subsided enough to allow surgery, an ORIF using plates and screws is performed. Most principles of intraarticular fracture treatment apply to pilon fractures. The surgical goals are anatomic reduction of the joint surface and rigid fixation to allow early range of motion. Immediate weight-bearing is often delayed for up to 3 months following surgical reduction. External fixation with fine wires and limited internal fixation can also serve as definitive fixation.

Ankle Fractures

Ankle fractures are among the most common injuries treated by orthopaedic surgeons. These are often low-energy rotational injuries that occur in people of all ages, with the highest incidence in elderly women.

Classification

There are a number of classifications systems used, but the Weber and Lauge–Hansen systems receive the most recognition. The Weber system is based on the level of the fibula fracture: type A are below the level of the syndesmosis, type B fractures are at the level of the syndesmosis, and type C fractures are above the level of the syndesmosis (Fig. 19.11). Type C fractures are most likely to be associated with a significant syndesmotic injury. The Lauge–Hansen classification system is based on the mechanism of ankle fractures. Injuries to bones and soft tissues structures are taken into account. The terminology describes the position of the foot at the moment of injury and then the direction of the deforming force (Fig. 19.12). For instance, in a supination-external rotation (SER) injury, the foot is in

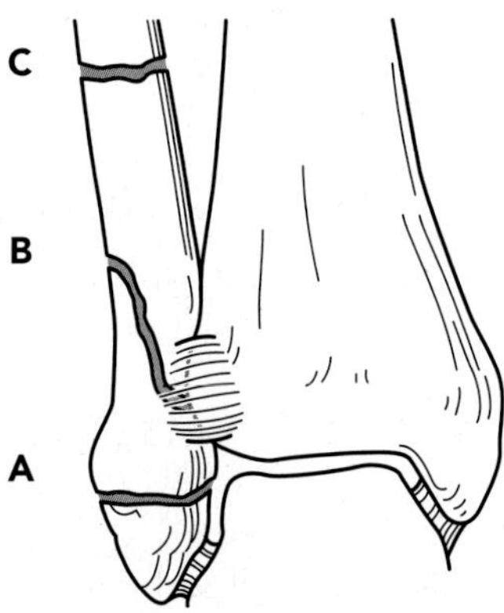

Figure 19.11 The Weber classification of ankle fractures depends on the level of the fibula fracture in relation to the syndesmosis. (*Reproduced with permission from* Rockwood CA, Green DP, Bucholz RW. *Rockwood and Green's Fractures in Adults.* 6th ed. Philadelphia, PA: Lippincott Williams & Wilkins, 2006.)

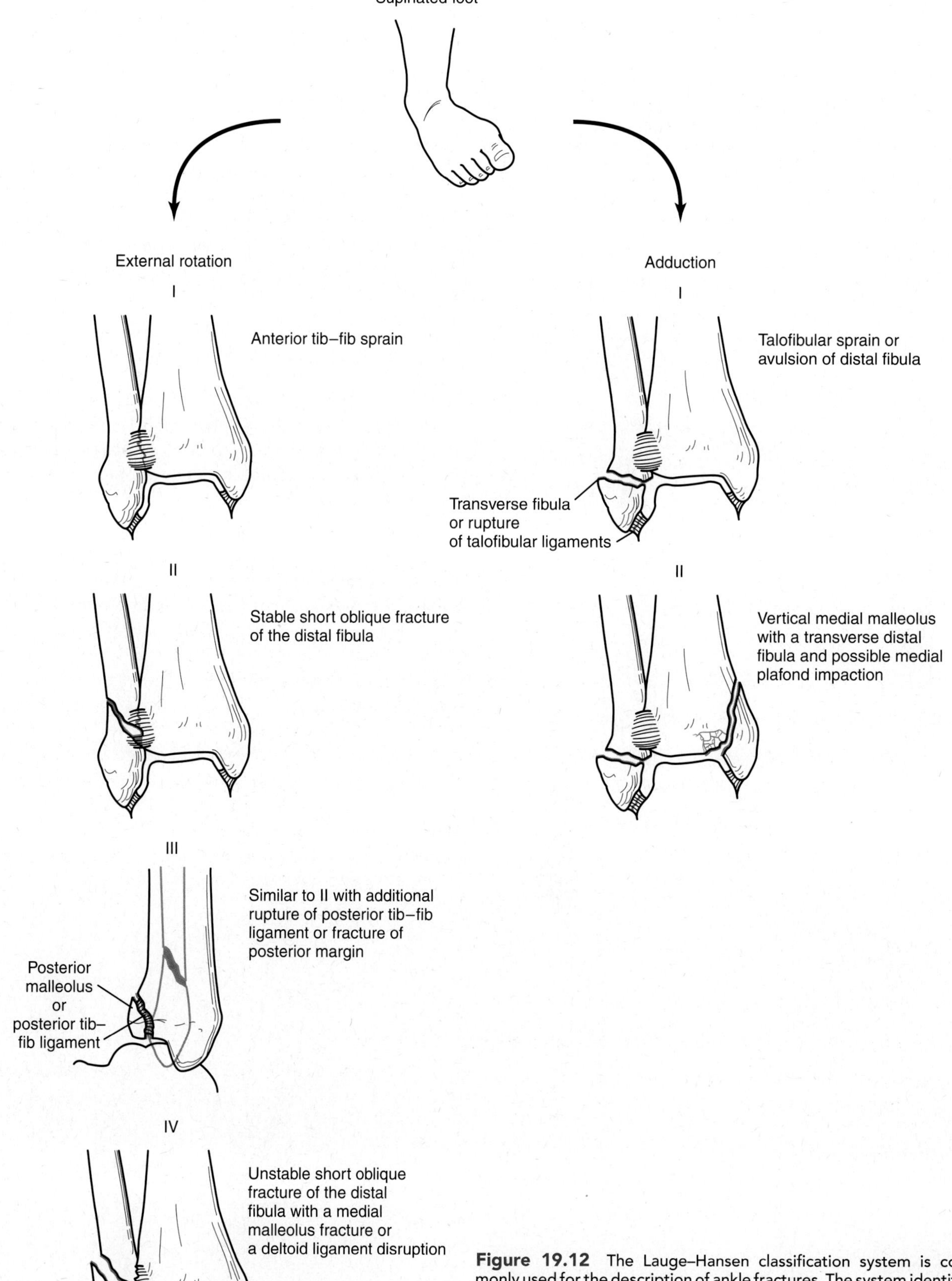

Figure 19.12 The Lauge–Hansen classification system is commonly used for the description of ankle fractures. The system identifies the position of the foot at the time of injury as either supinated **(A)** or pronated **(B)** followed by the direction of forces acting on the ankle. (*Reproduced with permission from* Rockwood CA, Green DP, Bucholz RW. *Rockwood and Green's Fractures in Adults*. 6th ed. Philadelphia, PA: Lippincott Williams & Wilkins, 2006.)

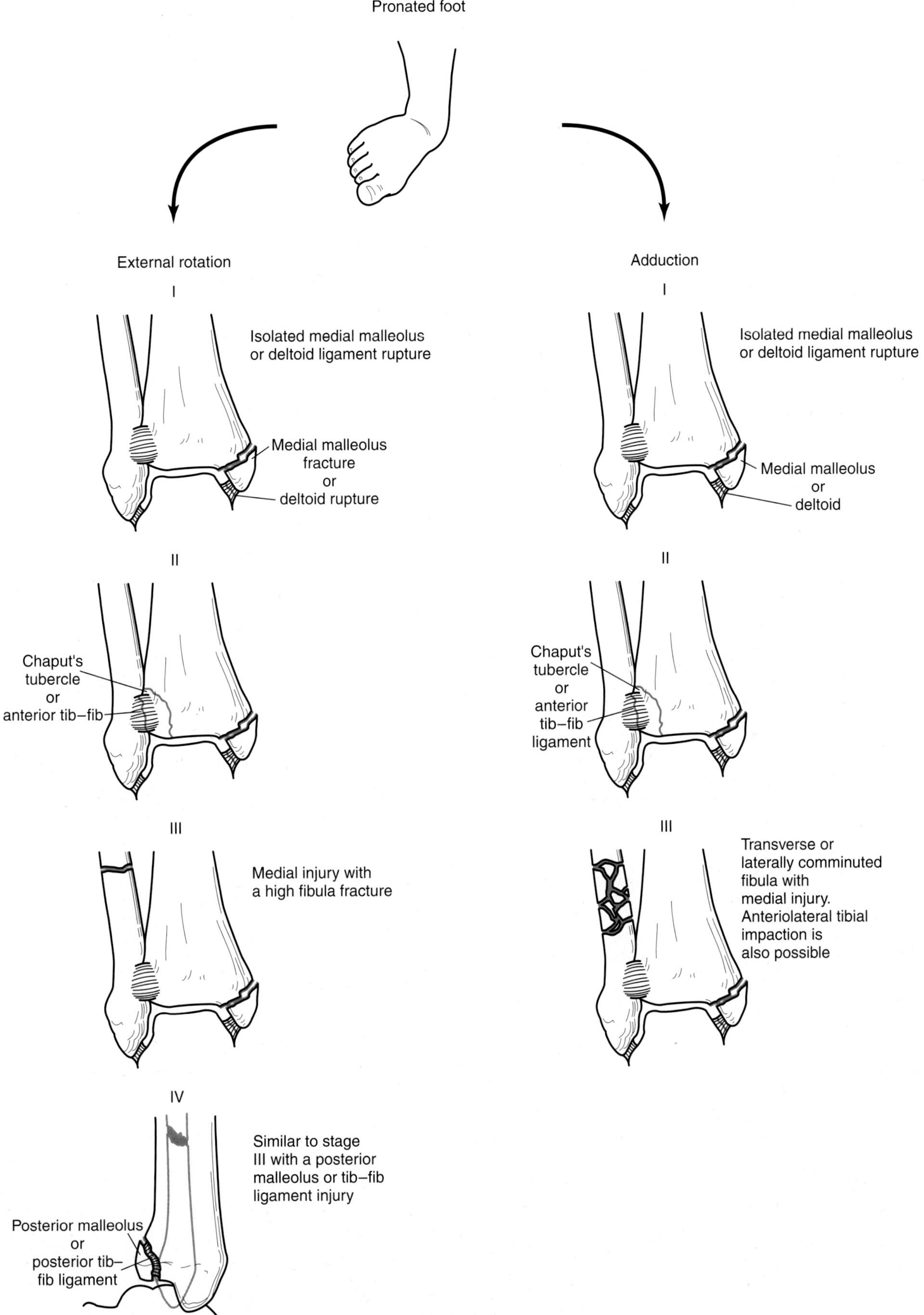

Figure 19.12 *(Continued)*

a supinated position and an external rotation force is applied. Four types are described: supination-adduction, SER, pronation-abduction, and pronation-external rotation. Each type is further subclassified on the basis of the degree of involvement of different soft tissue and bone structures. Supination injuries are the most common and account for approximately 75% of all ankle fractures. In supination injuries, the lateral side of the ankle is affected first, whereas in pronation injuries, the medial sided structures fail first. The mechanism of injury is often reflected by the fracture pattern of the fibula. For supination injuries, the fibula fracture follows a predictable anteroinferior to posterosuperior pattern, whereas in pronation injuries, the opposite pattern is commonplace with the fracture line running from anterosuperior to posteroinferior. A transverse fibula fracture with lateral comminution, often represented as a butterfly fragment, typifies pronation-abduction injuries. Supination-adduction injuries are typically transverse avulsion fractures of the distal fibula fractures at or below the joint line. Unfortunately, the Lauge–Hansen classification has low interobserver reliability, does not direct treatment, and does not predict prognosis. Nevertheless, it is commonly used and is useful for conceptually understanding this injury.

Beyond describing the gross morphology of fractures, it is often more helpful to classify ankle fractures as stable and unstable. Stable fractures have the ability to resist displacement under physiological loads, whereas unstable patterns do not. In general, stable fractures carry a better prognosis and can be treated nonoperatively. Unstable fractures most often need surgical reduction and internal fixation.

A Maisonneuve variant is a particular type of ankle fracture associated with a high fibular fracture. The external rotation force exerted on the ankle propagates from the deltoid ligament through the interosseus membrane and exits through the proximal fibula creating the characteristic fracture pattern and instability of the ankle.

Mechanism of Injury

Ankle fractures usually result from low-energy forces that have a rotational component as seen in athletic activities or slight falls.

Presentation

Patients present with acute ankle pain and swelling and, often, the inability to bear weight.

Physical Examination

Ecchymosis and swelling are usually present. Obvious deformity is a sign of an associated dislocation. Impending open and open injuries are uncommon, but a thorough examination of the skin is imperative. A neurovascular examination is required before and after any manipulation of the extremity. The entire length of the tibia and fibula should be palpated, especially the proximal fibula, to evaluate for a Maisonneuve fracture.

Imaging

Standard radiographs are sufficient for most ankle injuries. Stress radiographs help rule out a syndesmosis injury. The Ottawa Ankle Rules provide direction as to when radiographs are indicated. These four rules drastically decreased the number of radiographs performed in emergency departments while maintaining 100% sensitivity. If a patient is 55 years or older, unable to bear weight, or has bone tenderness along the posterior edge or tip of either malleoli, a radiograph is indicated. In a normal ankle, the talus should sit under the tibia with a tibiotalar space that is equal to the distance from lateral border of the medial malleolus to the medial border of the talus on the mortise view, or approximately 4 mm (Fig. 19.13A–D). Any translation of the talus indicates an unstable fracture pattern. The talocrural angle helps to judge fibular length and is usually 83 degrees (Fig. 19.13B). The tibiofibular clear space is the best way to evaluate an unstable syndesmosis injury on radiograph. It is the distance between the medial fibula and the incisura of the tibia measured 1 cm above the joint; it should be less than 6 mm (Fig. 19.13D). This measurement is minimally affected by rotation. The entire length of the tibia and fibula should be imaged if there is any concern for a proximal fracture line.

Differential Diagnosis

A pilon fracture, simple ankle dislocation, subtalar dislocation, and even severe ankle sprain can also present with either a deformity or an ankle swelling. In addition, patients may describe ankle pain, when in reality the foot is the site of pathology, for example, in a fracture of the base of the fifth metatarsal. Appropriate imaging studies aid in determining the correct diagnosis.

Treatment

If the injury is a fracture-dislocation, the ankle should be reduced immediately. Definitive treatment is dependent on stability of the fracture pattern. Stable fibula fractures, displaced less than 5 mm, without a medial ankle injury can be treated with a walking cast or a fracture boot for 6 weeks. A fracture boot is necessary only for ambulation and thus can be removed for range-of-motion exercises to prevent stiffness. It is important to repeat radiographs at 1 week to ensure there is no late displacement. For unstable fractures, operative intervention is recommended. The fibula is usually approached first. When possible, an interfragmentary screw should be placed from the proximal fragment into the distal fragment and perpendicular to the fracture line. A neutralization plate provides rotational stability to the construct. Recently, there have been a number

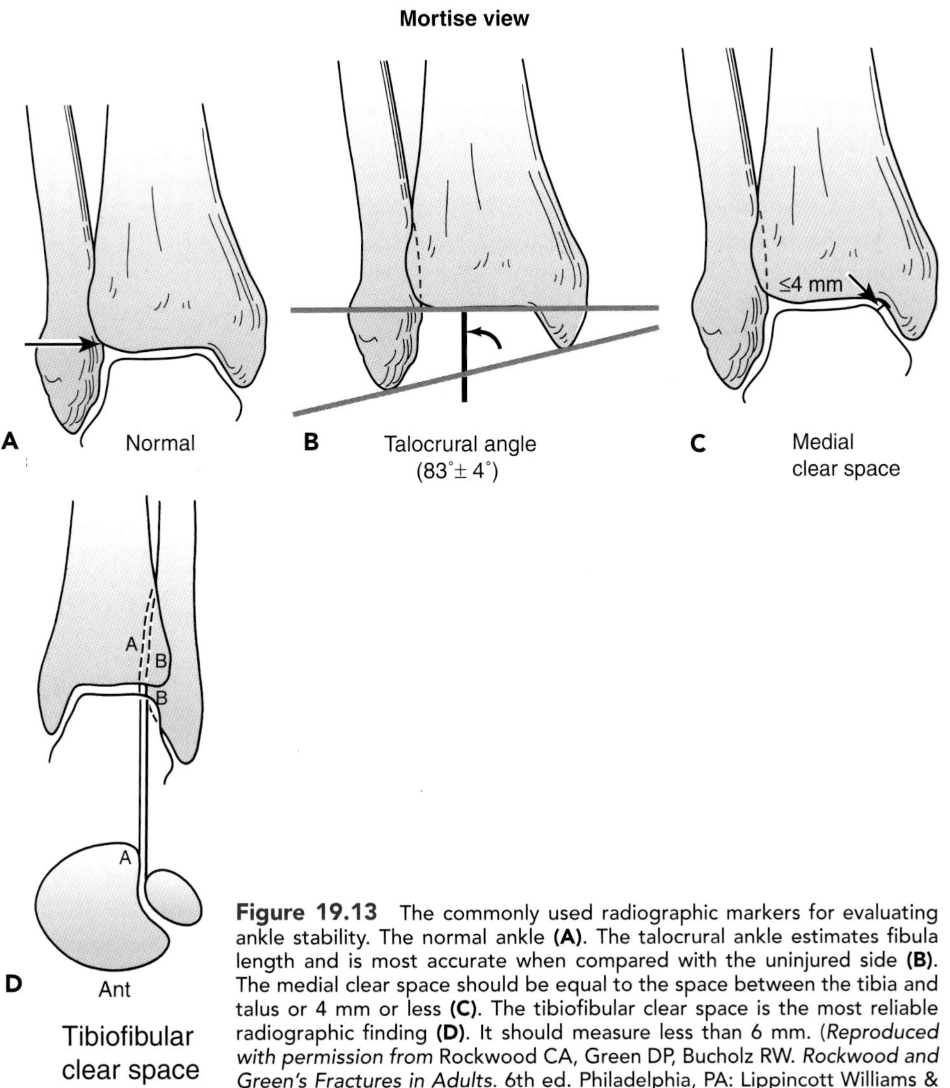

Figure 19.13 The commonly used radiographic markers for evaluating ankle stability. The normal ankle **(A)**. The talocrural ankle estimates fibula length and is most accurate when compared with the uninjured side **(B)**. The medial clear space should be equal to the space between the tibia and talus or 4 mm or less **(C)**. The tibiofibular clear space is the most reliable radiographic finding **(D)**. It should measure less than 6 mm. (*Reproduced with permission from* Rockwood CA, Green DP, Bucholz RW. *Rockwood and Green's Fractures in Adults*. 6th ed. Philadelphia, PA: Lippincott Williams & Wilkins, 2006.)

of precontoured plates introduced, which can simplify plate application. The medial malleolus should then be reduced and fixed with two cancellous screws or with a tension band technique if the fragment is small. On rare occasions, a torn deltoid may flip into the joint and impede reduction. When this is the case, an arthrotomy is performed to remove the interposed ligament, otherwise a deltoid tear does not usually require repair. The stability of the syndesmosis must be checked on all ankle fractures before leaving the operating room. If there are signs of instability, one 4.5 mm or two 3.5 mm screws should be placed from the lateral fibula across the syndesmosis and into the tibia. The screws can engage one or both of the tibia cortices depending on surgeon preference. To avoid overcompression of the syndesmosis, the screw should be a fully threaded cortical screw placed parallel to the joint, and inserted without using a lag technique. Most surgeons remove the syndesmosis screw(s) 12 weeks following surgery. A separate posterior malleolus fragment requires repair only when it is greater than 25% of the articular surface. Postoperatively, patients are usually made touchdown weight-bearing for 6 weeks. Starting range of motion early in the postoperative course decreases swelling and stiffness.

Ankle Sprains and Syndesmosis Injuries

Ankle sprains are the most common sports-related injuries and can result in chronic pain and/or instability if not treated appropriately. Injury to the lateral side of the ankle occurs in most of the cases, with the ATFL being the most commonly injured structure. The CFL is involved in approximately 50% of cases, whereas PTFL injury occurs in less than 10%. Syndesmotic injuries are often referred to as "high ankle" sprains.

Classification

It is easiest to divide ankle sprains into acute injuries and chronic instability. Chronic instability results from repeated sprains and manifests as persistent pain and a feeling of giving way. Acute sprains are graded on the basis of severity. In grade I injuries, the ATFL is stretched or partially torn, without complete disruption. Pain, swelling, and tenderness over the ATFL are characteristic of this injury. There is, however, no laxity appreciable on physical examination. Grade II injuries involve a complete tear of the ATFL and may include injury to the CFL. Laxity may be evident. In grade III injuries, the ATFL and CFL are torn, and the PTFL or anterolateral capsule of the ankle joint may also be affected. There is a complete loss of the normal hindfoot contours due to swelling.

Mechanism of Injury

The normal mechanism for lateral sided injuries is plantarflexion-inversion. Inversion injuries occurring with the ankle positioned in neutral or in dorsiflexion create isolated CFL disruption or subtalar dislocation. An external rotation-eversion injury may cause a sprain of the deltoid and syndesmotic ligaments. Isolated syndesmosis injuries result from dorsiflexion-eversion injuries.

Presentation

The patients typically present with pain, swelling, and ecchymosis over the lateral side of the ankle depending of the severity of injury. With higher grades of injury, patients tend to have significant difficulty bearing weight.

Physical Examination

The origins and insertions of the ankle ligaments should be palpated, but this can be difficult in the presence of significant swelling. As pain allows, the ankle is tested for evidence of instability. The anterior drawer test, a test of the ATFL, is performed with the ankle in 10 degrees of plantarflexion. While stabilizing the tibia, an anteriorly directed force is applied to the hindfoot. Translation of the talus is an indication of incompetence of the ATFL and is measured in millimeters. Grade I injuries have minimal translation with a firm endpoint. Grade II injuries have laxity but a firm endpoint, whereas grade III injures have a soft endpoint. For the talar tilt test, which stresses the CFL, the hindfoot is inverted with the ankle held in maximal dorsiflexion. Translation and tilt of the talus with varus stressing is compared with the uninjured side.

The fibular squeeze test, performed by squeezing the fibula and tibia together at the midpoint of the calf, elicits pain with syndesmosis injury. The external rotation test, in which the foot is externally rotated with the ankle in neutral flexion and the knee flexed to 90 degrees, produces pain over the interosseous membrane and distal tibiofibular joint when a syndesmosis injury is present.

Imaging

Standard three ankle views are obtained to rule out fracture or frank translation of the talus. Stress views can be helpful to diagnose ligament tears of the lateral side of the ankle. Anterior translation of greater than 5 mm is considered abnormal. There is no consensus on the degree of talar tilt that is abnormal, but if there is doubt, a stress radiograph of the uninjured ankle can be taken for comparison. To assess syndesmotic injury, weight-bearing radiographs and external rotation stress views can be obtained to evaluate mortise widening.

Differential Diagnosis

The differential diagnosis of lateral hindfoot injuries associated with a plantarflexion-inversion mechanism includes peroneal tendon tears, peroneal tendon subluxation or dislocation, and fractures of the anterior process of the calcaneus, base of the fifth metatarsal, lateral process of the talus, and os trigonum.

Treatment

Grade I and II ankle sprains are uniformly treated with rest, ice, compression, elevation, (RICE) and protected weight-bearing for 5 to 7 days, followed by physical therapy emphasizing proprioception using trampolines or wobble boards, strengthening, and stretching. The rehabilitation protocol then focuses on agility and sport-specific exercises to return the patient to the previous level of athletic activity and prevent recurrent sprains. Grade III sprains are treated with a brief period of immobilization followed by rehabilitation, functional rehabilitation alone, or surgical repair. Immobilization for 3 weeks with either a walking cast or a removable walker boot with the ankle in neutral or 10 degrees of dorsiflexion to approximate the torn ends of the ATFL should be reserved for low-demand patients. After the period of immobilization, rehabilitation is the same as that for grade I and II injuries. For athletes, it is best to avoid immobilization and associated stiffness, by initiating early mobilization with the protection of an external support, such as a lace-up brace or Aircast. Taping is less effective as it loosens rather rapidly during athletic activity. Patients treated with early mobilization have higher satisfaction rates than those treated with cast immobilization and return to sports earlier. While there is no good evidence to support it, anatomic repair is an option for high-performance athletes.

Chronic ankle instability requires surgery when functional rehabilitation fails to relieve pain and symptoms of giving way. Surgical reconstruction can be either anatomic or nonanatomic. Anatomic reconstructions recreate normal ankle and subtalar motion and mechanics, whereas nonanatomic reconstructions do not. The Brostrum procedure is the most popular anatomic procedure, in which the ruptured ligament ends are imbricated and retensioned. Variations include shortening the ligaments due to attenuation and reinforcement with the extensor retinaculum (Gould modification) or fibular periosteum. There are a number of non-anatomic reconstructions that use a portion of the peroneus brevis tendon, free gracilis autograft tendon, or an allograft tendon to stabilize the lateral ankle. These more robust reconstructions have a greater complication rate with motion loss, wound healing, and sural nerve injury as the most common. At the time of surgical intervention, all patients should undergo an ankle arthroscopy, as the rate of intraarticular pathology associated with chronic instability is as high as 90%. Injuries include osteochondral lesions of the talus, chondromalacia, meniscoid lesions, and anterior impingement from osteophytes. Appropriate treatment of these associated injuries increases the chance of successful resolution of symptoms.

Achilles Tendon Ruptures

The Achilles tendon is the largest and strongest tendon in the body. Acute ruptures commonly do not have antecedent symptoms and occur in middle-aged men who are in moderately poor physical condition, at a rate of 18 per 100,000. Treatment strategies have changed over the last 20 years, but there is no consensus on the ideal treatment.

Pathophysiology and Classification

Ruptures most commonly occur 2 to 6 cm proximal to the insertion site of the tendon in the hypovascular zone (Fig. 19.14). Most commonly, the injury is the result of a forceful eccentric contraction; however, uncontrolled dorsiflexion of the ankle and rarely direct trauma may also be responsible. When rupture occurs from a trivial event, one must rule out metabolic abnormalities, inflammatory arthroses, and steroid and fluoroquinolone use.

Presentation

Patients present after a severe, sudden pain in the back of the calf that is described as being struck from behind and is often associated with swelling. Unfortunately, the pain resolves rather quickly and some may still be able to participate in sporting activities, which contributes to the 25% rate of missed and delayed diagnoses.

Physical Examination

Diagnosis is made by palpating a defect 2 to 6 cm above the insertion of the Achilles tendon. It is often accentuated by holding the foot in maximal dorsiflexion, which places the Achilles on stretch. In obese patients and individuals with severe swelling, a gap may not be evident. Strength of the gastrocsoleus complex can be tested by having the patient perform a single-leg heel rise or by testing plantarflexion against resistance. Because of the participation of the posterior tibialis muscle and toe flexors, patients can have rather significant plantarflexion strength even with an Achilles rupture.

Having the patient lie prone on the examination table is helpful. The passive resting tension of the tendon and position of the foot should be noted. With a defect in the Achilles tendon, the foot rests at 90 degrees to the body compared with the unaffected extremity, which rests in relative plantarflexion. A similar observation can be made with the knee flexed to 90 degrees according to the Matles test. The torn side will fall into relative dorsiflexion with gravity and the loss of tension from the Achilles tendon. The Thompson, or calf squeeze, test is performed by squeezing the mid portion of the gastrocnemius, which should result in passive plantarflexion of the foot if the Achilles tendon is in continuity (Fig. 19.15).

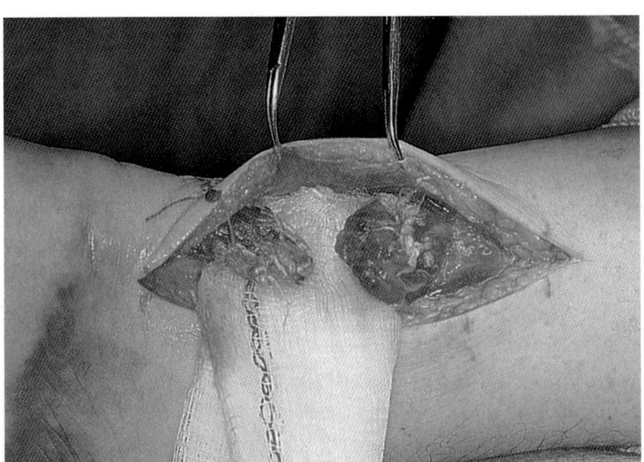

Figure 19.14 Ruptures of the Achilles tendon occur 4 to 6 cm proximal to the insertion on the calcaneus, which is a relative hypovascular zone. (*Reproduced with permission from* Kitaoka HB. *The Foot and Ankle*. 2nd ed. Philadelphia, PA: Lippincott Williams & Wilkins, 2002.)

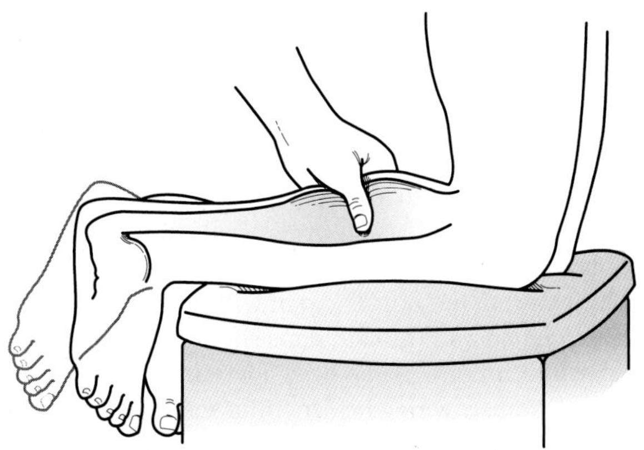

Figure 19.15 The Thompson test evaluates the continuity of the gastrocsoleus complex. When intact the complex is intact, squeezing the midcalf results in plantarflexion of foot. (*Reproduced with permission from* Rockwood CA, Green DP, Bucholz RW. *Rockwood and Green's Fractures in Adults*. 6th ed. Philadelphia, PA: Lippincott Williams & Wilkins, 2006.)

Radiographic Findings

Radiographs may reveal blunting of the retrocalcaneal space or rarely a bony avulsion fracture of the posterior calcaneus.

Special Tests

If there is any confusion in the diagnosis, ultrasound and MRI are useful in evaluating the continuity of the tendon. MRI also provides the added benefit of revealing any degenerative changes of the tendon that may have played a role in the rupture. In up to 25% of cases, patients report previous symptoms in the Achilles. Pathological studies have indicated all ruptured tendons have some degree of degeneration prior to rupture.

Treatment

Historically, Achilles tendon injuries were treated nonoperatively because of wound complication rates approaching 30%. However, more recently, the relatively high rerupture rates have lead surgeons to surgical intervention. Nonoperative treatment typically involves 6 to 8 weeks in a non–weight-bearing cast with the foot in gravity equinus followed by an additional 4 weeks in a walking cast. After this period of immobilization, a supportive lace-up shoe with a heel lift is worn for an additional 1 to 2 months. Some authors support weight-bearing from the outset of treatment and the use of functional bracing rather than casting. The advantage of nonoperative methods is the avoidance of surgical complications, most notably wound breakdown and infection. The major disadvantage of nonoperative treatment is the rerupture rate of approximately 13%. Other disadvantages include a longer time before returning to work and activity.

The high rates of wound complications have often deterred surgeons from pursuing surgery for the treatment of Achilles tendon ruptures. However, with advances in techniques, these rates have dropped. These injuries can be approached in an open fashion or percutaneously and should be repaired within 7 to 14 days. When performing the surgery open, it is imperative to respect the soft tissue envelope. The tendon is repaired end-to-end, using a Krackow stitch with nonabsorbable heavy suture. Obtaining appropriate tension of repair is difficult but using the plantaris tendon and observing the resting posture of the foot can be helpful. The paratenon should be closed over the repair, and the skin flaps should be closed with a no-touch technique. Some have advocated for augmentation of the repair with gastrocnemius fascia, the plantaris, or artificial materials; however, these have yet to have a proven benefit. While percutaneous techniques may have less wound complications, the suture placement may not be optimal and there is a greater chance of sural nerve injury. Operative intervention also allows for early functional rehabilitation (weight-bearing and range of motion), which is thought to hasten the healing of the tendon.

There is no consensus on optimal treatment for acute tendon ruptures. Nonoperative treatment is effective; however, there is a significant rerupture rate. Operative treatment with early functional rehabilitation results in a quicker return to full function and a lower rerupture rate at the sacrifice of wound complications. Percutaneous treatment is an attempt to minimize the major complications of each group; however, there is the risk of sural nerve injury.

Chronic ruptures are Achilles tendons that go untreated for 4 to 6 weeks due to a delayed diagnosis. Patients often complain of weakness without significant pain. The pain and swelling associated with the initial injury subsides fairly quickly. Fibrous scar tissue does form between tendon ends; however, it does not restore correct tension or strength. Patients are able to plantarflex the foot by recruiting the FHL, FDL, posterior tibialis and peroneal muscles but with relative weakness. One should also observe for calf wasting, claw toes, and a high arch deformity as a result of the FDL activity. Management is typically operative unless the patient has low demands or is not healthy enough to undergo surgery. For nonoperative treatment, an ankle foot orthosis (AFO) should be prescribed. There are numerous options for surgical reconstruction, most of which involve augmentation with a graft. The peroneus brevis, FDL, FHL, fascia lata, gracilis, and allografts have all been described. Unfortunately, functional results are not as predictable as those after repair of acute Achilles tendon ruptures.

Talus Fractures

Fractures of the talus are typically high-energy injuries that are difficult to treat and can be debilitating even when treated appropriately. Fractures can involve the head, neck, body, lateral process, and posterior process. Displaced body and neck fractures require extra diligence and are treated as emergencies due to the associated complications.

Classification

Talus fractures are most easily divided by the anatomic location, that is, head, neck, body, lateral process, and posterior process. Talar neck fractures are further classified on the basis of a description by Hawkins, which was subsequently modified by Canale (Fig. 19.16). Type I fractures are nondisplaced fractures without an associated joint dislocation. Type II fractures are displaced with subluxation or dislocation of the subtalar joint. Type III fractures have dislocations of the subtalar joint and the ankle. Type IV fractures have dislocations of the subtalar, ankle, and talonavicular joints. The risk of osteonecrosis increases with the injury grade such that nearly all type IV fractures develop osteonecrosis.

Mechanism of Injury

Talar neck fractures, historically referred to as *aviator astragalus*, result from hyperdorsiflexion with an axial load usually from a fall from height or a motor vehicle crash. As the

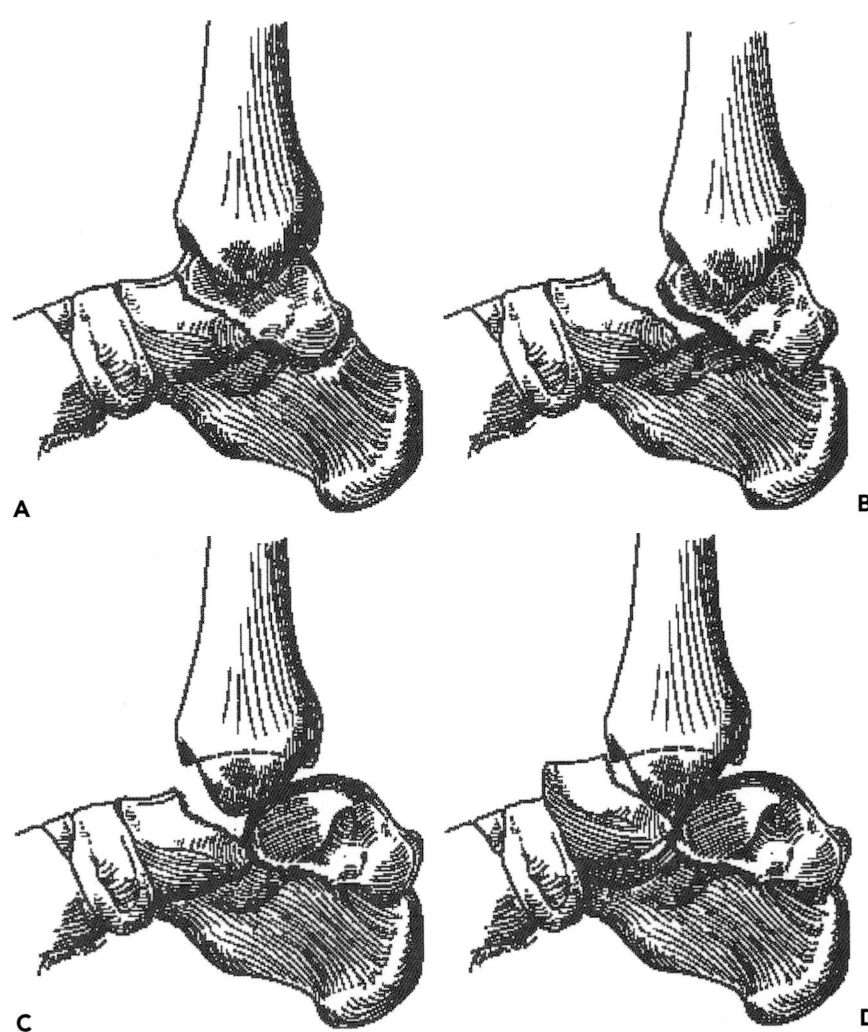

Figure 19.16 The Hawkins classification of talus fractures. (*Reproduced with permission from* Kitaoka HB. *The Foot and Ankle*. 2nd ed. Philadelphia, PA: Lippincott Williams & Wilkins, 2002.)

foot dorsiflexes, the neck of the talus impacts the anterior distal tibia. When there is sufficient force, the body of the talus can displace posteromedially to lie behind the medial malleolus, rotating on the deltoid ligament. Fractures of the talar body result from high-impact axial loading, most commonly motor vehicle crashes, and are associated with talar neck fractures in about 40% of cases. Axial loading is also responsible for head fractures, but the forces are transmitted through the navicular. Lateral process fractures commonly occur while snowboarding and result from ankle inversion and dorsiflexion with axial loading. Posterior process fractures occur from avulsion or direction compression. With inversion of the ankle, the PTFL can avulse the process; however, direct compression of the process between the calcaneus and tibia is the more common mechanism.

Presentation

When resulting from high-energy trauma, patients will have swelling and deformity if a dislocation is present. Low-energy mechanisms may present similar to ankle fractures or sprains.

Physical Examination

A thorough neurovascular and skin examination is imperative. It is important to rule out other injuries that require emergent treatment.

Imaging

AP, lateral, and mortise views of the ankle provide good visualization of the talar body, neck, and processes. Additional information concerning the medial talar neck can be obtained by positioning the ankle in plantarflexion, the foot in 15 degrees of pronation, and directing the beam 75 degrees to the perpendicular (Fig. 19.17). This view is especially helpful in the operating room to confirm adequate reduction. CT can help to further define the fracture pattern and plan surgical reduction. MRI is less useful acutely but is a sensitive test for avascular necrosis.

Differential Diagnosis

Low-energy injuries such as lateral process fractures can resemble ankle sprains and fractures due to their similar mechanism of injury. The swelling and ecchymosis of

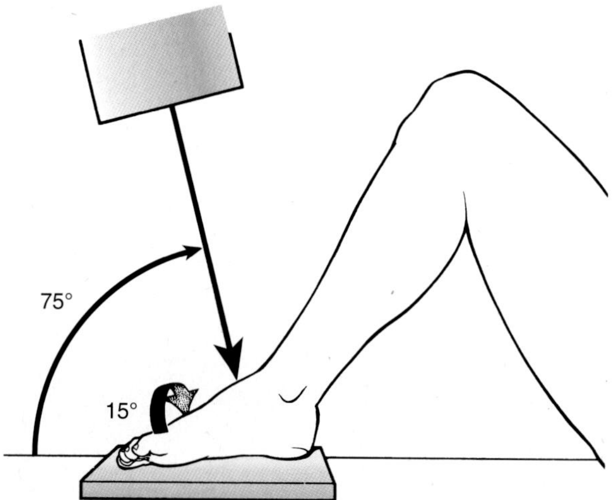

Figure 19.17 The Canale and Kelly view for evaluation of the talar neck. (*Reproduced with permission from* Rockwood CA, Green DP, Bucholz RW. *Rockwood and Green's Fractures in Adults.* 6th ed. Philadelphia, PA: Lippincott Williams & Wilkins, 2006.)

high-energy mechanisms can resemble calcaneus and pilon fractures.

Treatment

Talar neck and body fractures are true orthopaedic emergencies. Displaced fractures and joint dislocations require immediate reduction to decrease the risk of osteonecrosis and protect the overlying soft tissue. The goal of definitive treatment is to maintain anatomic reduction while minimizing posttraumatic arthrosis, osteonecrosis, and varus malalignment. Varus malalignment greater than 5 degrees and displacement more than 5 mm have adverse effects on the kinematics of the hindfoot.

All displaced talar neck fractures require reduction and surgical fixation. Nondisplaced fractures can be treated successfully closed but must be monitored closely with serial imaging. Non–weight-bearing is maintained for at least 6 weeks or until there is evidence of revascularization. Surgical fixation can be performed either percutaneously through a posterolateral approach or open via an anteromedial approach. In the anteromedial approach, the interval of dissection is between the tibialis anterior tendon and the tibialis posterior tendon. This allows for adequate visualization of the medial aspect of the neck and can be extended by a medial malleolar osteotomy. Fixation constructs are usually screws supplemented with small plates if comminution is present. Postoperatively, the patient is immobilized and made non–weight-bearing for at least 6 weeks. To avoid stiffness early range of motion can be initiated.

Signs of osteonecrosis typically manifest by 8 to 10 weeks. The Hawkins, or crescent, sign seen on AP and mortise radiographs is an indication of a viable talar body. With sufficient vascularity the talar body will be relatively osteoporotic compared with the surrounding bone because of disuse and revascularization. This is differentiated from dense, sclerotic bone seen with osteonecrosis. MRI is useful to evaluate for osteonecrosis. Other major complications include skin necrosis, infection, malunion, nonunion, and posttraumatic arthritis. Varus malunion has a locking effect on the midfoot and may occur in up to 50% of type II, III, and IV fractures. Posttraumatic arthritis of the ankle and subtalar joints can result from avascular necrosis, articular damage, malunion, and prolonged immobilization.

Similar to talar neck fractures, talar body fractures with associated joint dislocation require emergent reduction. Surgical fixation is recommended for nearly all body fractures and is usually accomplished with cortical screws. Nondisplaced head fractures are treated conservatively in a short-leg, non–weight-bearing cast. Small, displaced fractures can be excised or rigidly fixed with headless screws countersunk below the articular surface. Head fractures often result in talonavicular arthritis.

The treatment of lateral process fractures mainly depends on the size of the fragment and degree of comminution. Nondisplaced or fractures with small fragments are treated with cast immobilization and progressive weight-bearing. Larger fragments that are displaced are treated with ORIF. Posterior process fractures are treated with a non–weight-bearing cast for 4 weeks followed by a walking cast for 2 weeks. Excision of symptomatic fragments is recommended for persistent pain in the retromalleolar area especially with forced plantarflexion.

Osteochondral Lesions of the Talus

Osteochondral lesions of the talus are a relatively common cause of ankle pain and are most often related to ankle trauma and chronic ankle instability. Although commonly used for all lesions of the talus, the term *osteochondritis dissecans* (OCD) refers specifically to the nontraumatic spontaneous necrosis of bone. *Osteochondral lesion* is probably more encompassing and appropriate term for the majority of talus articular injuries. The workup and treatment of these lesions have changed with the advent of ankle arthroscopy and the advances made in the treatment of cartilage lesions in the knee.

Pathophysiology and Classification

Osteochondral lesions of the talus are best broken down into traumatic and atraumatic causes. Injury to the talus can occur with an ankle injury or with chronic ankle instability. Nontraumatic causes include ossification defects, abnormal vasculature, emboli, and endocrine disorders.

Lesions are typically seen posteromedially and anterolaterally. Lateral lesions are almost universally related to trauma resulting from inversion and dorsiflexion. Trauma is also the cause of most medial lesions; however, there is a significant incidence of nontraumatic lesions of the medial side. Traumatic lesions on the medial aspect of the talus occur with inversion, plantarflexion, and external rotation forces.

Berndt and Harty described the classification referenced most frequently on the basis of radiographs. Stage I denotes a lesion with a small area of subchondral compression. In stage II lesions, there is an osteochondral fracture that is only partially displaced. If the osteochondral fragment is completely detached but remains in the bed, it is considered stage III. Stage IV lesions are completely displaced from the bed. Numerous classifications have since been described on the basis of CT and MRI accounting for the presence of sclerosis and subchondral cyst formation. However, intraoperative findings during arthroscopy are probably the most reproducible and prognostic.

Presentation

The highest incidence occurs in the third decade of life. Complaints of chronic ankle pain with or without intermittent swelling and instability after an episode of minor trauma such as an inversion ankle sprain is common. Locking can occur if the lesion becomes displaced.

Physical Examination

The ankle should be examined for signs of joint laxity. Anterolateral lesions can be tender to palpation with the ankle in maximum plantarflexion. Tenderness behind the medial malleolus with the foot in maximum dorsiflexion can be a sign of a posteromedial lesion.

Radiographic Findings

Standard ankle radiographs are sufficient to diagnose lesions with evidence of a subchondral fracture (Fig. 19.18), subchondral cysts, or localized sclerosis.

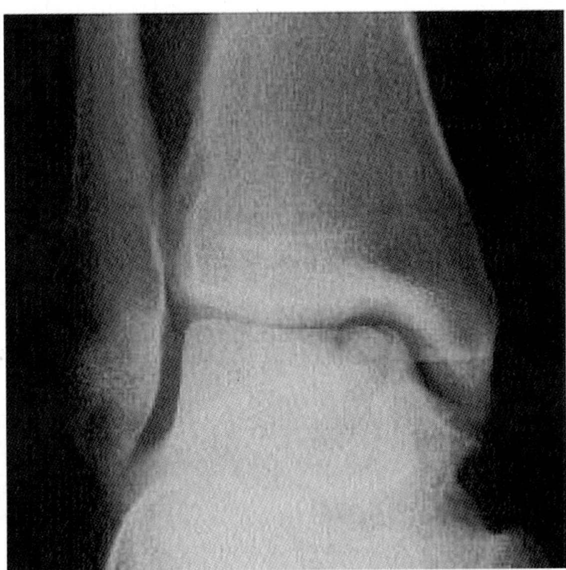

Figure 19.18 A posteromedial osteochondral lesion is seen on a standard radiograph. (*Reproduced with permission from* Kitaoka HB. *The Foot and Ankle*. 2nd ed. Philadelphia, PA: Lippincott Williams & Wilkins, 2002.)

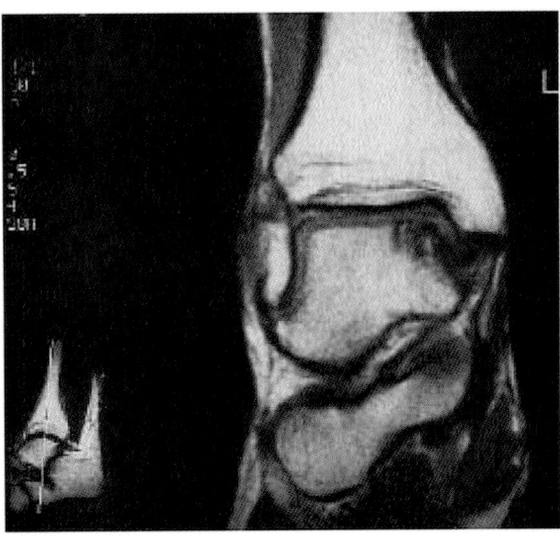

Figure 19.19 A coronal magnetic resonance image showing a posteromedial lesion of the talar dome. (*Reproduced with permission from* Kitaoka HB. *The Foot and Ankle*. 2nd ed. Philadelphia, PA: Lippincott Williams & Wilkins, 2002.)

Special Tests

MRI is highly sensitive for identifying lesions before changes are apparent on radiographs (Fig. 19.19). MRI has the added benefit of providing insight into the stability and viability of the fragment. A CT scan can be useful for surgical planning and accurately identifying the location and extent of the bone lesion.

Treatment

Stage I and II lesions are treated with immobilization in a non–weight-bearing short-leg cast for 6 to 12 weeks. Nonoperative treatment is effective in less than 50% of cases overall. Stage III and IV lesions and stage I and II lesions that do not respond to nonoperative treatment should be treated operatively either arthroscopically or through an open approach. Treatment options include chondroplasty, debridement and internal fixation, anterograde or retrograde drilling, excision with marrow stimulation, excision with osteochondral transplantation, or excision alone. The stability of the lesion, size of the lesion, and condition of the cartilage determine outcome.

Chondroplasty is the simplest intervention. The goal is to restore a stable edge to the lesion. Drilling of the subchondral lesion to stimulate healing can be performed using either an anterograde or retrograde technique. Retrograde drilling techniques avoid injury to the cartilage. If the fragment is not salvageable, it should be excised and the lesion debrided. The resulting defect is treated with a microfracture technique to stimulate fibrocartilage formation. Alternative options include the transplant of osteochondral autograft plugs taken from the non–weight-bearing portion of the knee into the defect or the use of autologous chondrocyte transplantation.

There have been no good studies comparing the outcomes of the various treatment methods; however, there does appear to good short-term results regardless of the treatment technique.

Calcaneus Fractures

The calcaneus is the most commonly fractured tarsal bone usually resulting from axial loading during falls or motor vehicle crashes. Seventy-five percent of these fractures are intraarticular and comminuted, making them challenging to treat. The severity of these injuries is highlighted by the fact that 25% of patients will have an associated lower extremity fracture and 10% a spine fracture. Unfortunately, even appropriate treatment can result in long-term disability.

Classification

Fractures were historically classified according to radiographs but are now more commonly classified by information obtained with a CT scan. Fractures are divided into extraarticular or intraarticular types. Extraarticular fractures involve the anterior process, the tuberosity, the body, the medial process, and the lateral process. Intraarticular fractures based on radiographs are divided into tongue-type and joint-depression-type fractures. With the tongue-type fractures, the posterior facet remains attached to the tuberosity fragment, whereas in the joint-depression-type, the fragments are separate. The most commonly used classification for intraarticular fractures is the Sanders classification based on coronal CT images taken through the widest aspect of the posterior facet (Fig. 19.20). The location and number of fragments determines the type. The posterior facet is divided into three columns—the lateral, central and medial—or A, B, and C, respectively. Nondisplaced fractures regardless of the number of fracture lines are type I. Type II, III, and IV fractures have two, three, and four fracture lines, respectively. Each type is then amended on the basis of where the individual fracture lines enter the joint with the letters A, B, and C.

Mechanism of Injury

High-energy injures including falls from heights and motor vehicle crashes are the usual cause of calcaneal fractures. Because of the force involved, they are often associated with spine fractures. The position of the foot determines the exact fracture pattern. As the lateral talar process is driven into the superior calcaneal surface, a primary fracture line runs from the posterior facet in a lateral to posteromedial direction, creating anteromedial and posterolateral fragments. The anteromedial fragment usually contains the sustentaculum tali, which is nondisplaced because of its attachments to the talus via the interosseous ligament, and is often called the "constant" fragment. Secondary fracture lines may occur and extend through the calcaneocuboid joint and lateral calcaneal wall.

Extraarticular fractures of the calcaneus are typically lower-energy and occur by different mechanisms. Forced dorsiflexion from a fall can result in avulsion of the tuberosity via the pull of the Achilles tendon. Inversion and plantarflexion injuries can result in injury to the anterior process of the calcaneus. Body fractures of the calcaneus without extension into the subtalar joint are also possible.

Presentation

Pain and swelling may be the only presenting complaints for low-energy injuries such as those of the anterior process and tuberosity. Patients with high-energy, intraarticular fractures are often in significant pain and have obvious deformities. In addition, these patients often have other injuries.

Physical Examination

Determining the appropriate timing and treatment for calcaneus fractures requires adequate assessment of the soft tissues. Fracture blisters, open wounds, and compartment syndrome effect how these injuries are approached. It is essential to respect the soft tissue envelope, as failure to do so has devastating consequences. Patients should be evaluated for lower extremity fractures. The entire spine, especially the lumbar spine, should be inspected and palpated.

Imaging

AP, lateral, the Harris heel, and Broden views should be initially taken for diagnosis. In addition, radiographs of the pelvis and thoracolumbar spine may be indicated to rule out associated fractures. Helpful radiographic angles, the tuber angle of Böhler, and the crucial angle of Gissane are measured on the lateral view (Fig. 19.21). The tuber angle of Böhler is formed by the most posterosuperior aspect of the calcaneal tuberosity, the posterior facet, and the anterior process and is normally 20 to 40 degrees. With fracture and collapse of the posterior facet, this angle decreases. The crucial angle of Gissane is formed by lateral margin of the posterior facet and a strut of bone leading to the beak of the calcaneus and usually measures about 100 degrees. With fracture of the posterior facet and collapse the angle increases. The Harris heel view assesses the loss of height, increase in width, and malalignment of the calcaneal tuberosity, usually into varus (Fig. 19.22). The Broden view helps to assess the status of the posterior facet. The view is similar to a mortise view of the ankle with the foot in internal rotation, and by changing the angle x-ray beam, different aspects of the posterior facet are visualized (Fig. 19.23). With the wide availability of CT scans, they are now becoming a standard radiographic study. These scans provide fast and accurate views of the fracture pattern and amount of displacement of the posterior facet that is critical in directing surgical intervention.

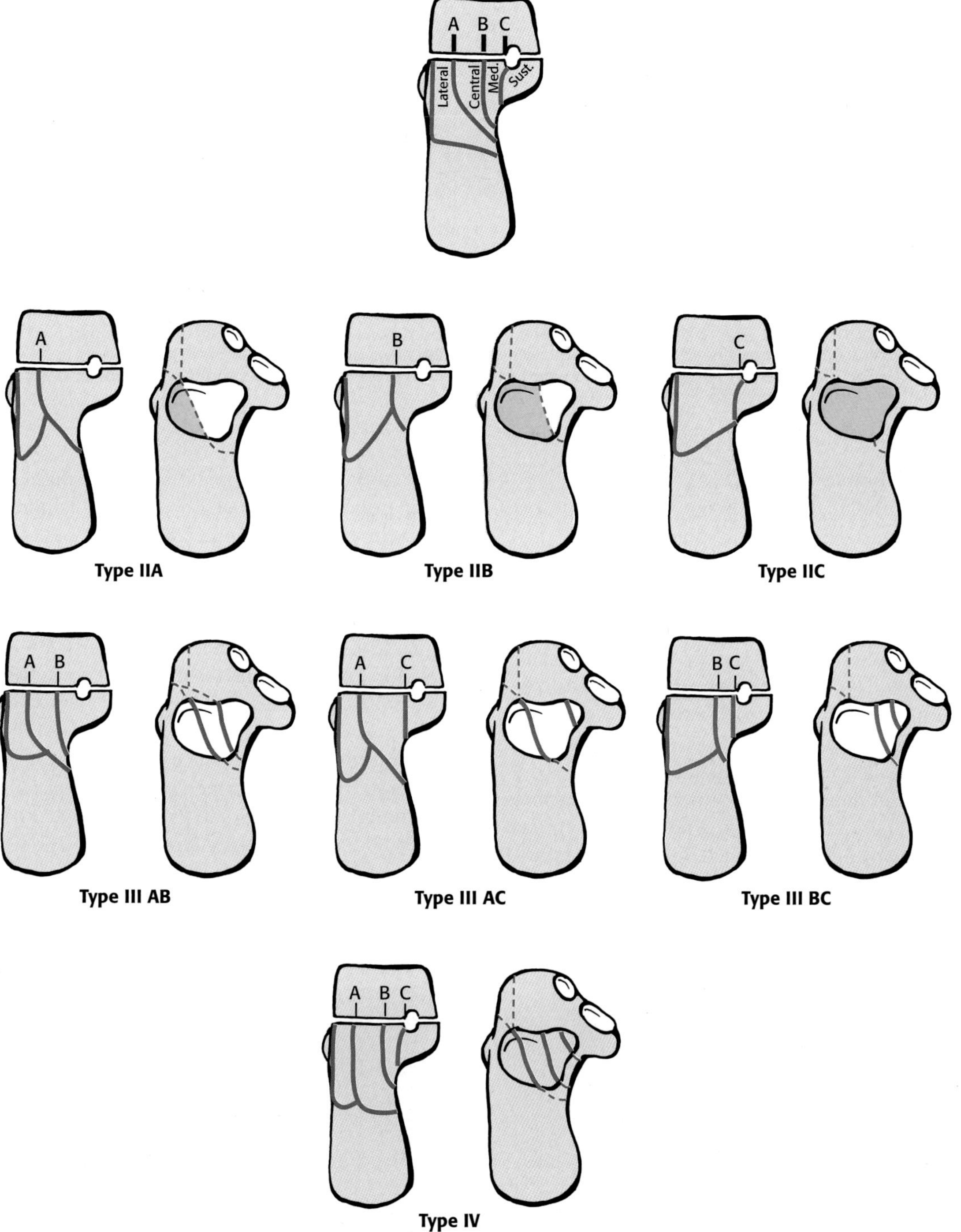

Figure 19.20 The Sanders classification of calcaneus fractures. This is based on coronal computed tomography images taken through the widest aspect of the posterior facet, which is divided into three columns **(A–C)**. The number of displaced fractures determines the subtype. (*Reproduced with permission from* Rockwood CA, Green DP, Bucholz RW. *Rockwood and Green's Fractures in Adults.* 6th ed. Philadelphia, PA: Lippincott Williams & Wilkins, 2006.)

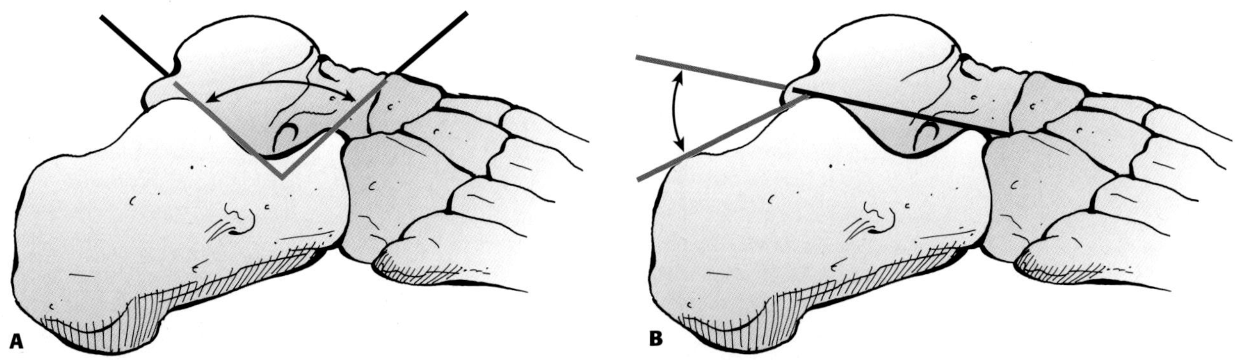

Figure 19.21 The crucial angle of Gissane **(A)** and the tuber angle of Böhler **(B)** help to identify calcaneus fractures and to evaluate adequacy of reduction. (*Reproduced with permission from* Rockwood CA, Green DP, Bucholz RW. *Rockwood and Green's Fractures in Adults*. 6th ed. Philadelphia, PA: Lippincott Williams & Wilkins, 2006.)

Differential Diagnosis

High-energy injuries are usually obvious. Anterior process fractures can be mistaken for ankle sprains.

Treatment

Calcaneus fractures are challenging to treat, and this is made more complicated by a lack of consensus on acceptable treatment. Nonoperative treatment is typically reserved for nondisplaced fractures. However, recent studies have shown better functional outcomes with nonoperative treatment for smokers, laborers, patients involved in workers' compensation suits, bilateral injuries, and fractures with significant comminution of the posterior facet. Cast immobilization for approximately 3 months is required before weight-bearing is initiated. Displaced fractures treated nonoperatively usually result in malunions, which can lead to tibiotalar impingement with loss of ankle dorsiflexion and calcaneofibular abutment with peroneal tendon entrapment or dislocation. Varus malunion alters the ankle and hindfoot kinematics, resulting in a locked forefoot and ambulating on the outer border of the foot. Plantarflexion strength is also lost because of the altered mechanics of the Achilles tendon.

The goal of operative intervention is to restore the articular congruity and avoid the complications of malunion. Surgery should be performed within 3 weeks but delayed long enough to allow the soft tissue envelope to calm down, usually about 7 to 10 days. Until surgery, the leg is maintained in a Jones dressing and elevated. When wrinkling of the skin over the lateral hindfoot returns, it is usually safe

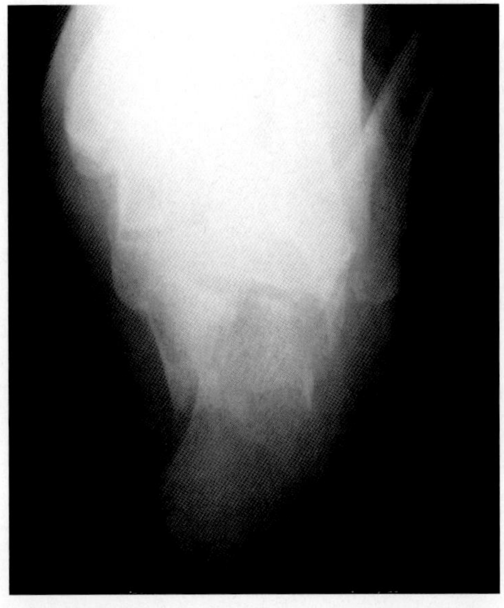

Figure 19.22 A Harris heel view showing a loss of height, increase in width, and varus alignment of the calcaneus. (*Reproduced with permission from* Rockwood CA, Green DP, Bucholz RW. *Rockwood and Green's Fractures in Adults*. 6th ed. Philadelphia, PA: Lippincott Williams & Wilkins, 2006.)

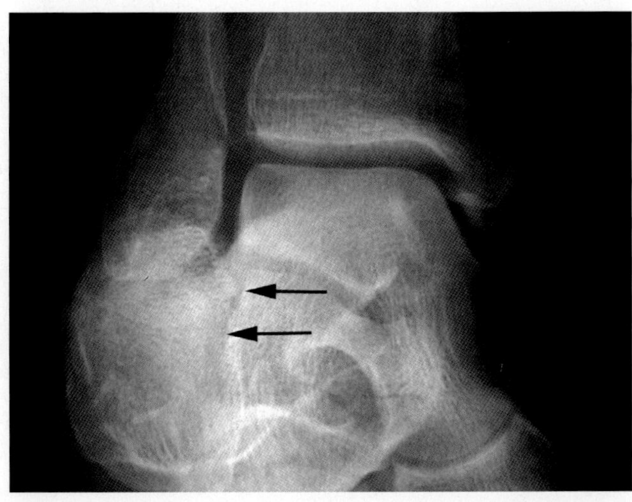

Figure 19.23 Broden view is similar to the mortise view of the ankle and helps in assessment of the posterior facet. An intraarticular fracture is denoted with arrows. (*Reproduced with permission from* Rockwood CA, Green DP, Bucholz RW. *Rockwood and Green's Fractures in Adults*. 6th ed. Philadelphia, PA: Lippincott Williams & Wilkins, 2006.)

to proceed. Surgical dissection is carried laterally using an L-shaped incision with a full-thickness subperiosteal flap including the peroneal tendons, sural nerve, and CFL. Fixation involves initially reducing and stabilizing the posterior facet and then attaching the laminate portion of the calcaneus to the main tuberosity and anterior process. Intraoperative imaging is useful to ensure restoration of radiographic landmarks and angles. Fixation is typically achieved with a low-profile locking plate designed for the lateral wall of the calcaneus. The use of bone graft is controversial.

Non–weight-bearing is maintained for 10 to 12 weeks until fracture union, and early range of motion is initiated once the wound has safely healed. Complications include soft tissue breakdown, infection, subtalar and calcaneocuboid arthritis, malunion, chronic regional pain syndrome, and sural nerve injury. Given the minimal amount of soft tissue available, rotational or free flaps may be necessary for coverage if wound breakdown occurs. This should be performed quickly to avoid deep infection and osteomyelitis. Arthritis can develop rapidly especially if adequate reduction is not achieved.

Patients with significant comminution of the posterior facet or delamination of the articular cartilage are candidates for ORIF with primary subtalar fusion. This avoids the potential complications of arthritis and may allow for earlier return to work.

For anterior process fractures involving more than 25% of the calcaneocuboid joint, ORIF is recommended. Nondisplaced tuberosity avulsion fractures can be treated closed with immobilization in plantarflexion for 3 weeks followed by an additional 3 to 6 weeks in neutral. Displaced patterns require ORIF. Close monitoring of the soft tissues is necessary.

Navicular Fractures

The tarsal navicular bone is an important structure of the medial column involved in both hindfoot motion through its articulation with the talus and maintenance of the longitudinal arch via the cuneiforms. Navicular fractures are classified as dorsal lip, tuberosity, body, and stress fractures. AP, lateral, and medial oblique radiographs of the foot are usually adequate for diagnosis.

Dorsal lip fractures are the most common, occurring from an eversion mechanism, resulting in talonavicular joint capsule and deltoid ligament avulsing a fragment of bone. The fracture fragment is best identified with a lateral radiograph. The differential diagnosis includes an accessory ossicle of the navicular and talus. The majority of cases are treated with a short-leg walking cast for 4 to 6 weeks. With significant articular surface involvement, ORIF should be performed. Persistent displacement can generate a painful prominence and is treated with excision.

Tuberosity fractures result from an eversion mechanism and eccentric contraction of the posterior tibial tendon. Local tenderness is elicited, and there is pain on resisted inversion. Displacement is often minimal because of the broad attachment of the posterior tibial tendon. AP and medial oblique radiographs best demonstrate the fracture. If an accessory navicular is suspected, which is present in 12% of the population and bilateral in 64% of cases, radiographs of the contralateral foot can be obtained. Treatment for nondisplaced or minimally displaced fractures is immobilization for 4 to 6 weeks in a short-leg cast. Fractures displaced 1 cm or more should be opened and reduced to preclude dysfunction of the posterior tibial tendon. Symptomatic nonunions may be treated by excision of the fragment, advancement of the tendon to the remaining tuberosity, and immobilization for 4 to 6 weeks. Proper function of the posterior tibial tendon is the most important factor in determining appropriate treatment.

Navicular body fractures can occur in isolation but frequently occur with other foot injuries. Typically, they involve both the talonavicular and navicular cuneiform joints. Body fractures are classified on the basis of the location and orientation of the fracture line. Type I fractures are transverse in the coronal plane without associated angulation of the forefoot. Type II fractures are oblique, running dorsolateral to plantar medial. The forefoot is displaced medially with a large dorsomedial fragment. Type III fractures have central or lateral comminution with lateral displacement of the forefoot. Attention should be paid to associated fractures and dislocations of the midfoot and metatarsals on the radiographs. A CT is useful for defining the fracture pattern and determining the amount of comminution of the articular surface. The goal of surgery is to anatomically reduce the articular surface of all joints and restore length to the medial column. Options for fixation include screws and mini-fragment plates for reducible patterns, whereas transarticular fixation or temporary bridge plating may be necessary for highly comminution patterns. weight-bearing should be delayed for 3 months.

Stress fractures occur in the avascular central third of the navicular bone and are typically seen in young male athletes performing repetitive high-intensity activities. Clinically, the pain is localized to the dorsolateral aspect and is worse with activity. Frequently, the fracture is not visible on plain radiographs. Bone scan, CT, and MRI are useful to confirm diagnosis when radiographs are negative. Treatment of incomplete stress fractures requires 6 to 8 weeks of cast immobilization. Displaced fractures and nonunions exhibiting sclerosis require ORIF with bone grafting. Chronic untreated conditions may result in debilitating pain caused by talonavicular arthrosis, which may ultimately require arthrodesis.

Cuboid Fractures

Cuboid fractures are typically associated with other injuries of the midfoot and rarely occur in isolation. The two common patterns are the avulsion type and compression injuries to the cuboid. The avulsion-type injury results from an inversion mechanism. A "fleck" sign may be visible on radiographs. These are treated with short-term immobilization.

Compression, or nutcracker, fractures of the cuboid occur as the forefoot displaces laterally with a Lisfranc injury. This results in loss of axial length of the lateral column and creates an asymmetrical flatfoot pattern. The goal of treatment is to restore the articular surfaces, length of the lateral column, and kinematics of the foot. Length is restored by external fixation or plating. Bone graft may be necessary to fill defects of the cuboid. The foot is immobilized in a short-leg, non–weight-bearing cast for up to 12 weeks. Late arthrodesis may be necessary if arthrosis of the calcaneocuboid joint develops.

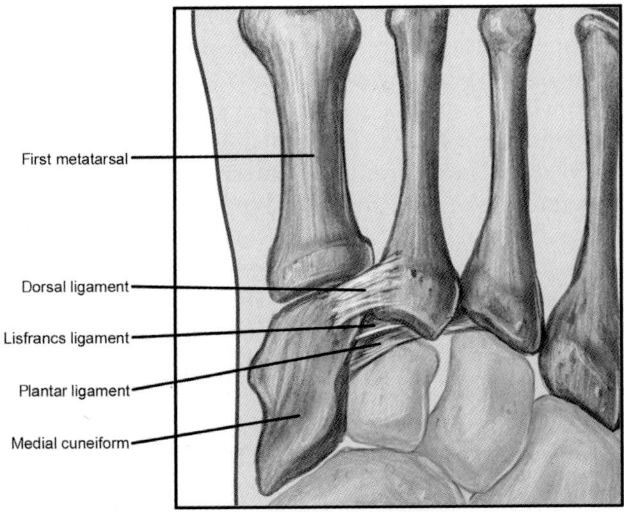

Figure 19.24 The Lisfranc ligament spans from the medial cuneiform to the base of the second metatarsal. (*Reproduced with permission from* Johnson D, Pedowitz RA. *Practical Orthopaedic Sports Medicine and Arthroscopy.* Philadelphia, PA: Lippincott Williams & Wilkins, 2007.)

Lisfranc Injuries

Injuries to the tarsometatarsal joint, or Lisfranc joint, include a spectrum from subtle sprains to frank dislocations. Unfortunately, even when appropriately diagnosed and treated with anatomic reduction of the joint, functional outcomes can be poor, especially with high-energy injuries. The tarsometatarsal joint complex is composed of the three cuneiforms, the cuboid, and the five metatarsal bases. The bony architecture is similar to that of a Roman arch in design and stability. The keystone of the arch is the second metatarsal, which has a wedge-shaped base recessed between the medial and lateral cuneiforms. The strong plantar interosseous ligaments and transverse intermetatarsal ligaments further support the stable bone configuration. The intermetatarsal ligaments connect the four lesser metatarsal; however, there is no such ligament between the first and second metatarsal. The Lisfranc ligament spans the plantar–lateral aspect of the medial cuneiform to the medial base of the second metatarsal and functions to resist lateral translation of the lesser metatarsals (Fig. 19.24). The first metatarsal–medial cuneiform joint is stabilized by the joint capsule and by the insertions of the anterior tibialis and peroneus longus tendons. The lack of ligamentous support between the first and second metatarsal renders it susceptible to injury and is the weak link of the tarsometatarsal joint complex. Successful treatment is most dependent on restoring and maintaining this anatomy.

Classification

A number of classification systems have been proposed; however, not a single classification system provides an algorithm for treatment or prognostic value. Quenu and Kuss described three types based on the pattern of displacement of the metatarsals—isolated, homolateral, and divergent (Fig. 19.25). In isolated type, one or two of the metatarsals displaces relative to the others. Homolateral refers to all of the metatarsals displacing either medially or laterally. In the divergent type, the first ray is displaced medially while the lesser ones laterally. It is probably most helpful to divide these injuries into purely ligamentous and those involving a fracture as these two patterns heal differently and should potentially be approached differently for treatment.

Mechanism of Injury

Both direct and indirect mechanisms have been described (Fig. 19.26). The direct mechanism is a crush injury to the dorsum of the foot, resulting in plantar displacement of the metatarsals. High-energy trauma and heavy crush injuries produce significant injury to the soft tissue, vascular injuries, compartment syndromes and open wounds. Axial and rotational loading on a plantarflexed foot can injury the Lisfranc joint indirectly. This pattern is seen in motor vehicle crashes, equestrian injuries, falls, and during sports participation. The metatarsals are usually displaced laterally and dorsally. With abduction of the forefoot, the cuboid can be fractured.

Presentation

Patients with low-energy injuries usually complain of pain in the midfoot and inability to bear weight after a twisting injury to the foot. Crush mechanisms are more obvious, and these patients may also have other injuries.

Physical Examination

Up to 20% of these injuries are missed on initial evaluation because of their broad spectrum of presentation. Gross deformity of the midfoot may not be apparent if there was spontaneous reduction. Tenderness, ecchymosis, and swelling over the tarsometatarsal joints are typical. Pronation-abduction stress may recreate the pain and deformity. Incongruity and crepitus of the midfoot is noted on severely unstable injuries. Careful inspection of the soft tissues and a thorough neurovascular examination is

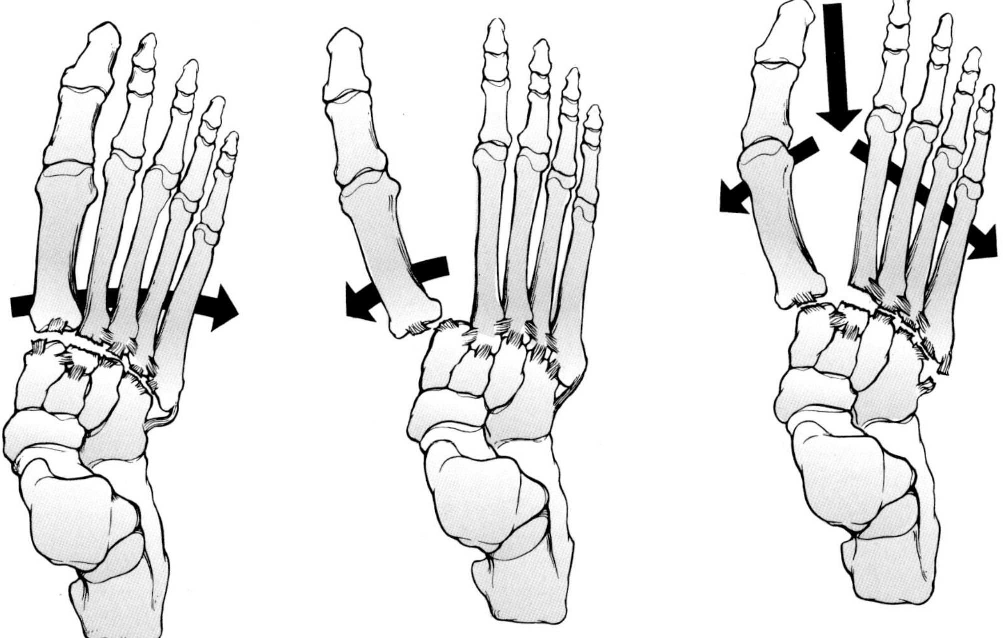

Figure 19.25 Quenu and Kuss classified Lisfranc injuries as homolateral, isolated, or divergent. (*Reproduced with permission from* Rockwood CA, Green DP, Bucholz RW. *Rockwood and Green's Fractures in Adults.* 6th ed. Philadelphia, PA: Lippincott Williams & Wilkins, 2006.)

necessary. Signs and symptoms of compartment syndrome should be investigated.

Imaging

AP, lateral, and 30-degree medial oblique radiographs are obtained to evaluate the injury. On the AP, the first metatarsal should line up with the medial cuneiform and the medial border of the second metatarsal base should line up with the medial aspect of the middle cuneiform. An avulsion fracture from the base of the second metatarsal, from the pull of the Lisfranc ligament, is diagnostic for the injury occurring in more than 90% of cases. On the oblique view, the lateral border of the third metatarsal should line up with the lateral edge of the lateral cuneiform and the medial aspect of the fourth metatarsal should align with the medial aspect of the cuboid. On the lateral view, the dorsal borders of the first and second metatarsals should line up with their respective cuneiforms without evidence of step-off. Because these injuries may spontaneously reduce, it is best to obtain weight-bearing, simulated weight-bearing, or stress views to identify instability of the tarsometatarsal joint complex if non–weight-bearing radiographs are normal (Fig. 19.27). Comparison views or CT scans are helpful when the injury is subtle.

Differential Diagnosis

The differential diagnosis includes navicular fracture, cuboid fracture, second metatarsal base fracture, stress fracture, and rupture of the posterior tibialis tendon.

Treatment

The management of tarsometatarsal joint injuries involves obtaining a stable, painless plantigrade foot by means of anatomic restoration of articular congruency. Treatment options range from closed reduction and cast immobilization for nondisplaced injuries to ORIF for displaced injuries. Given that K-wire fixation frequently fails, these are best stabilized with screw fixation. All fracture-dislocations should be reduced and immobilized urgently to minimize the risk of vascular and soft tissue compromise. Incisions are made over the first and third intermetatarsal spaces on the dorsum of the foot. Care should be taken to maintain the soft tissue bridge between. Reduction and preliminary fixation starts medially and proceeds laterally. After confirming anatomic reduction with appropriate imaging, definitive screw fixation follows. If there is instability of the fourth and fifth tarsometatarsal joints, these should be reduced and held with K-wires (Fig. 19.28). The lateral side of the foot is rather mobile; therefore, screw fixation is too rigid. If a nutcracker injury to the cuboid is present, restoration of the lateral column length is necessary. An external fixator may be needed to maintain length of the lateral column. Postoperatively, the patient is placed in a non–weight-bearing cast for 6 to 8 weeks, followed by progressive weight-bearing in a cast for an additional 4 to 6 weeks. If K-wires are used for the fourth and fifth tarsometatarsal joints, they should be removed at 8 weeks. Screws are removed 6 to 9 months after treatment. Complications include posttraumatic arthrosis, chronic pain, malunion, and deformity. Secondary arthrosis develops in

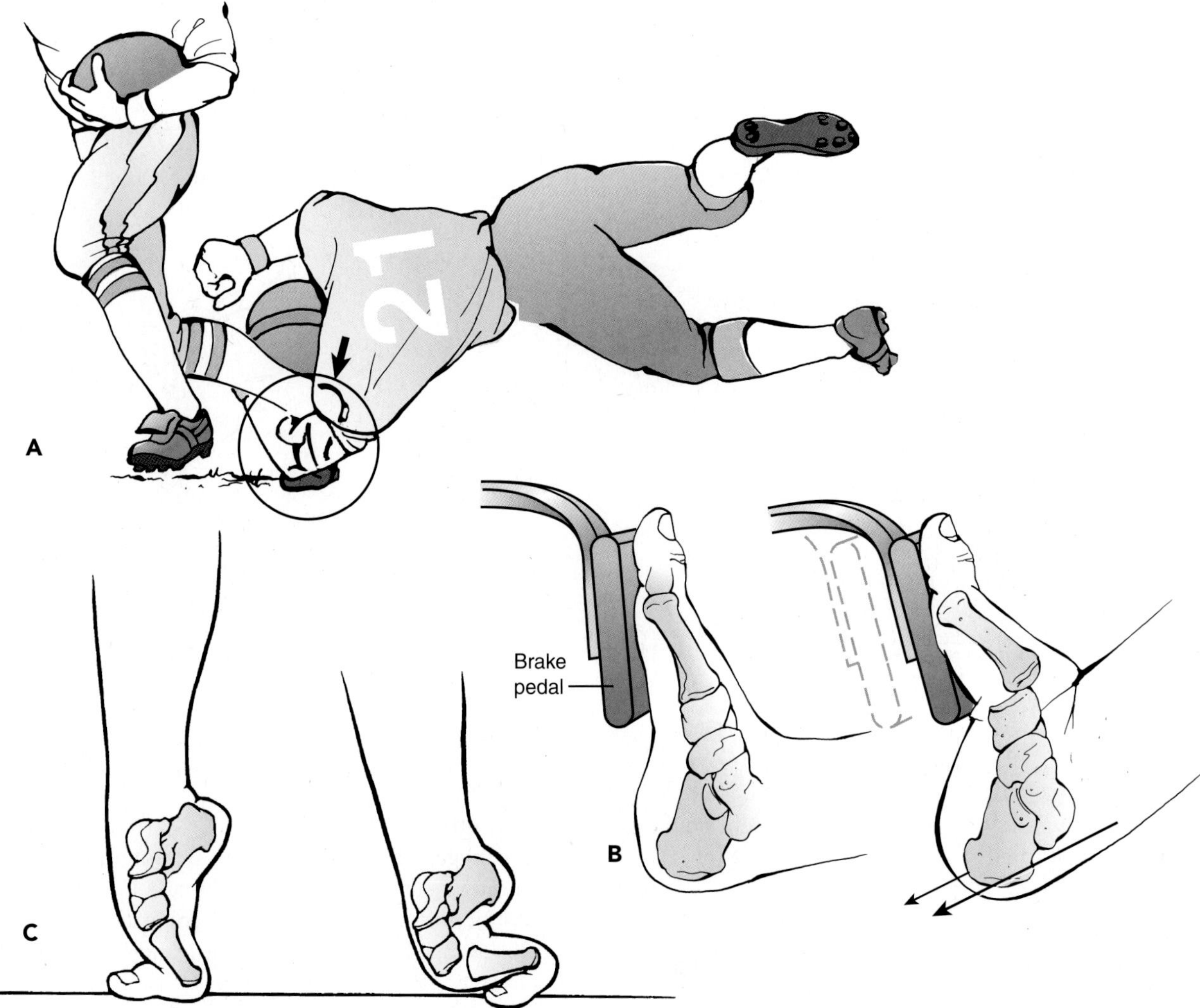

Figure 19.26 Lisfranc injuries occur from axial loads to the foot during athletics **(A)**, direct forces related to motor vehicle crashes **(B)**, and axial loads due to a fall from height **(C)**. (*Reproduced with permission from* Rockwood CA, Green DP, Bucholz RW. *Rockwood and Green's Fractures in Adults.* 6th ed. Philadelphia, PA: Lippincott Williams & Wilkins, 2006.)

up to 70% of cases and can be treated with medial column arthrodesis.

There is increasing evidence that patients with purely ligamentous injuries may benefit from primary arthrodesis of the medial column, because of the poor healing potential of the joint capsules and ligaments. Given the potential for improved outcomes, fusion should be considered for patients with these injuries.

Metatarsal Fractures

Metatarsal fractures are the most common fracture of the foot and usually occur from a direct blow. For high-energy injuries such as those sustained in motor vehicle crashes or by heavy objects, injury to the soft tissue can be significant. AP, lateral, and oblique radiographs are usually adequate for diagnosis and treatment. Low-energy injuries with minimal displacement are treated conservatively with non–weight-bearing immobilization for 3 to 4 weeks. Fractures with significant deformity are best treated surgically with anatomic reduction. Residual deformity can result in chronic pain and transfer metatarsalgia. Distal fractures are more likely to displace due to lack of soft tissue attachments providing stability to the metatarsal neck and head. ORIF with plate and screw constructs are generally used for the first metatarsal, whereas K-wire fixation may be adequate for the lesser metatarsals. For intraarticular fractures, the articular congruity should be restored. The goals of surgery are to restore the length, rotation, and angulation to ensure proper weight distribution among the metatarsals.

Fractures of the base of the fifth metatarsal are divided into three zones (Fig. 19.29). Zone 1 fractures, the most common type, are avulsion fractures of the peroneal brevis or lateral plantar fascia caused by a plantarflexion and inversion force. The fracture line travels into the tarsometatarsal joint through cancellous bone, giving these

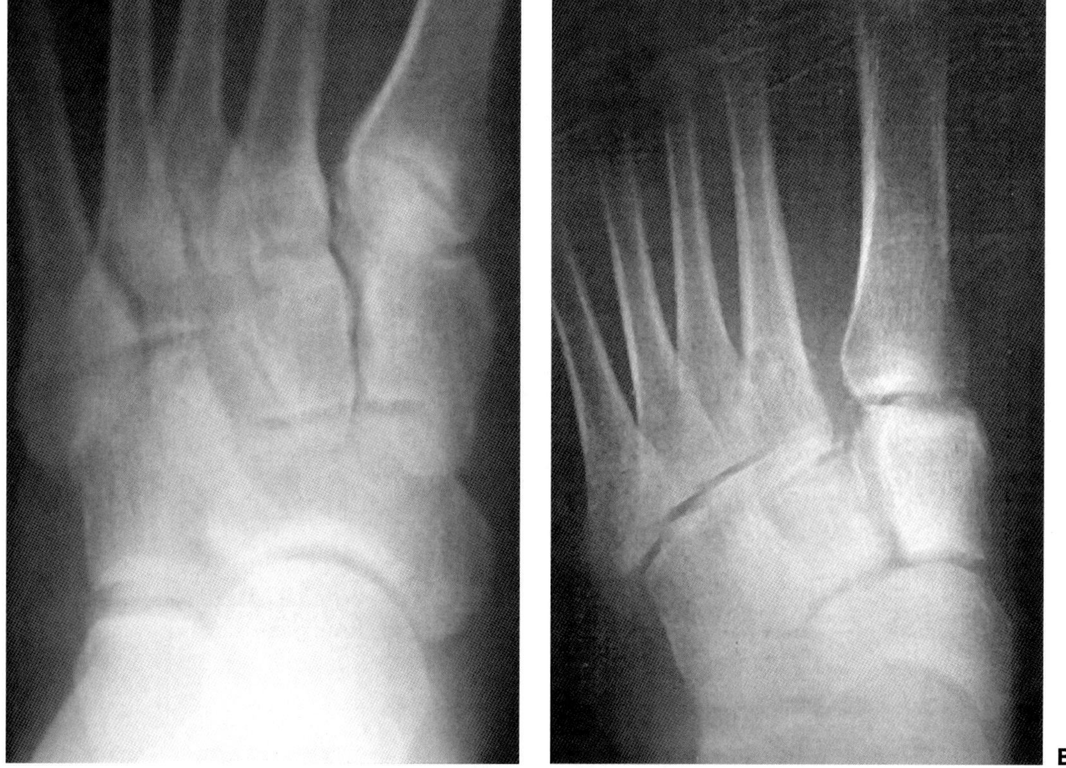

Figure 19.27 Stress views are important in the evaluation of Lisfranc injuries. A normal-appearing radiograph **(A)** taken without stress. A weight-bearing view of the same foot indicates gross instability **(B)**. (*Reproduced with permission from* Rockwood CA, Green DP, Bucholz RW. *Rockwood and Green's Fractures in Adults*. 6th ed. Philadelphia, PA: Lippincott Williams & Wilkins, 2006.)

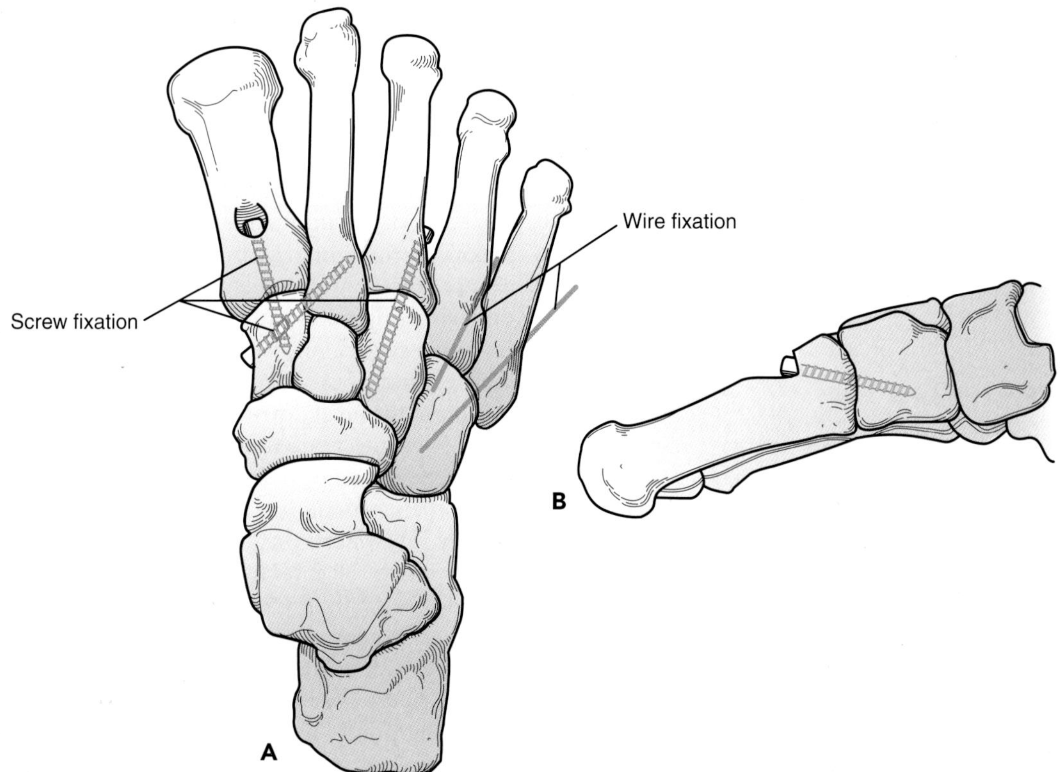

Figure 19.28 A typical construct for fixation of tarsometatarsal injuries. (*Reproduced with permission from* Rockwood CA, Green DP, Bucholz RW. *Rockwood and Green's Fractures in Adults*. 6th ed. Philadelphia, PA: Lippincott Williams & Wilkins, 2006.)

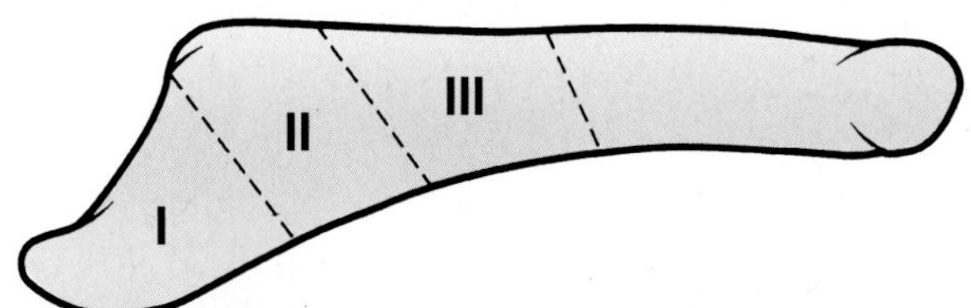

Figure 19.29 Fractures of the base of the fifth metatarsal are divided into three zones. Zone 1 fractures enter the tarsometatarsal articulation. Zone 2, or Jones, fractures enter the intermetatarsal joint. Zone 3 fractures occur distal to the diaphyseal–metaphyseal junction (*Reproduced with permission from* Rockwood CA, Green DP, Bucholz RW. *Rockwood and Green's Fractures in Adults.* 6th ed. Philadelphia, PA: Lippincott Williams & Wilkins, 2006.)

an excellent chance of healing. Zone 1 injuries are treated with a hard sole shoe. Patients are allowed to bear weight as tolerated. Zone 2 injuries, or Jones fractures, occur through the intermetatarsal articulation. These fractures occur as a result of a nutcracker effect, in which the fifth metatarsal is levered against the stable base of the fourth metatarsal. An avascular watershed zone between the nonoverlapping intramedullary and extraosseous blood supply contributes to the high rate of nonunion. Zone 2 fractures are treated with a non–weight-bearing cast for 6 weeks followed by progressive weight-bearing for an additional 4 to 6 weeks until union. Closed reduction and percutaneous screw fixation using an intramedullary screw is an option for high-performance athletes and those who need an early return to work. Delayed unions and nonunions are treated with open bone grafting and intramedullary screw fixation. The postoperative regimen is similar to acutely treated fractures. Zone 3 fractures occur in the distal metaphyseal–diaphyseal junction and are most commonly stress fractures. Acute fractures can be managed with a short-leg non–weight-bearing cast for 6 weeks. Intramedullary screw fixation is reserved for chronic fractures with medullary sclerosis.

Sesamoid Fractures

Fractures of the sesamoid bones occur as a result of direct trauma, frank overuse, or avulsion injuries associated with hyperdorsiflexion ("turf toe"). Disruption of the soft tissue surrounding the sesamoid complex and dislocation causing diastasis of the intersesamoid ligament can occur. Radiographic evaluation includes AP, lateral, and axial views. It is important to distinguish fractures from a bipartite sesamoid, which occur in approximately 25% of individuals. While fractures have irregular edges, a bipartite sesamoid has smooth, sclerotic edges. Contralateral radiographs or bone scan can assist in diagnosis. Acute fractures are treated with a cast or hard-soled shoe for 3 to 6 weeks. Pain associated with a nonunion may require partial or total excision. Complications include hallux valgus and hallux varus with excision of the tibial and fibular sesamoid bone, respectively. Transfer sesamoiditis of the remaining sesamoid is common. As an alternative, bone grafting has been successfully performed for symptomatic nonunions.

Phalangeal Fractures

Injury to the toes caused by stubbing, axial loads, or a dropped object may result in joint dislocation or phalangeal fracture. The proximal phalanx of the fifth toe is the most commonly involved. Phalangeal fractures may either be displaced or nondisplaced, but there is frequently angulation. The fracture should be reduced and "buddy-taped" to the adjacent toe, and the patient should wear a stiff-soled shoe or sandal. A fracture that extends into the joint should be reduced and stabilized with either K-wires or screw fixation. Sequela of these injuries includes joint instability, incongruence, and arthrosis.

ATRAUMATIC CONDITIONS OF THE FOOT AND ANKLE

The Rheumatoid Foot

Rheumatoid arthritis is a systemic autoimmune disease that commonly afflicts the foot, and its extent is related to the duration of systemic illness. The disease affects both the synovial lining of the joints and the tendons of the foot and ankle. The forefoot and hindfoot are most commonly affected.

Pathophysiology and Classification

The underlying cause of rheumatoid arthritis is not entirely understood. Environmental, genetic, and even infectious factors are thought to be involved. The synovium becomes a target of the immune system, resulting in the infiltration with inflammatory cells and synovial hyperplasia. The inflamed synovium, referred to as *pannus,* ultimately covers the articular cartilage and releases proteolytic enzymes, leading to the breakdown of cartilage and bone. The disease also affects the vascular system, which complicates surgical interventions of the foot and ankle. Neuropathy from entrapment, vasculitis, and drug toxicity is common but is usually subclinical.

Clinically, the forefoot is the most commonly affected area, followed by the hindfoot. Chronic synovitis of the lesser MTP joints leads to destruction of the articular cartilage, collateral ligaments, and joint capsule. With disease progression, the MTP joints sublux dorsally as a result of ground reaction forces. The destabilization of the MTP joints pulls the plantar weight-bearing pad and plantar plate distally, uncovering the metatarsal head and creating severe metatarsalgia. The PIP and DIP joints typically develop fixed flexion contractures due to imbalance between

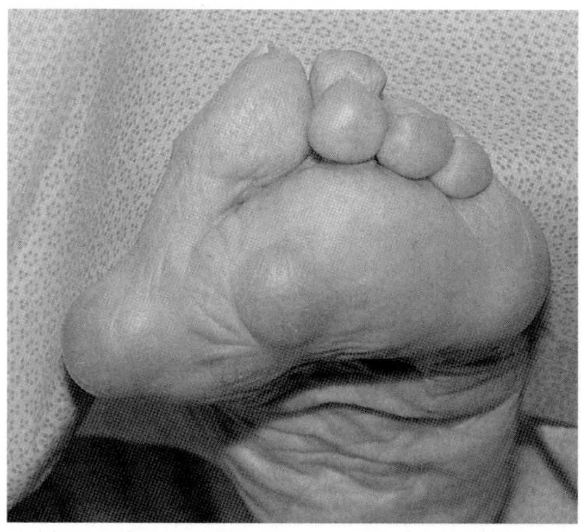

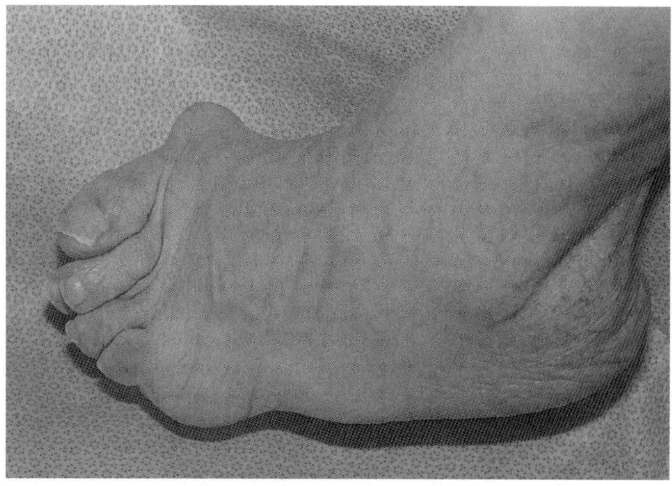

Figure 19.30 A typical appearance of the rheumatoid forefoot. (*Reproduced with permission from* Kitaoka HB. *The Foot and Ankle.* 2nd ed. Philadelphia, PA: Lippincott Williams & Wilkins, 2002.)

the intrinsic and extrinsic musculature. Painful callosities can develop over the dorsal aspects of these prominent and rigid joints. Hallux valgus, an angular deformity of the great toe at the MTP joint, develops secondary to abduction forces with ambulation and the loss of the second toe buttress from the claw toe deformity (Fig. 19.30).

The hindfoot falls into valgus as destruction of the articular cartilage, the ligaments, the posterior tibial tendon, and joint capsules of the subtalar and ankle joints progresses. Depending on the severity, the deformity can be flexible or fixed. An increasing valgus deformity can result in calcaneofibular abutment and sinus tarsi impingement.

Midfoot degeneration is not as common as forefoot and hindfoot degeneration in rheumatoid arthritis. Synovitis results in capsular attenuation and joint subluxation with collapse of the longitudinal arch, and eventually a painful flatfoot. When a planovalgus foot deformity develops with progressive failure of the posterior tibial tendon, the highly mobile fourth and fifth metatarsal cuboid joints are often spared. This results in forefoot abduction relative to the hindfoot, shortening of the peroneal tendons, and contracture of the gastrocnemius–soleus complex.

Presentation

Nearly 95% of patients with rheumatoid arthritis develop foot and ankle pain. It is the initial manifestation of the disease in 15% of cases. Pain, swelling, and stiffness in the affected joints are early complaints. Pain in the ball of the foot, metatarsalgia, is due to the prominence of the plantar metatarsal heads. Shoe wear leads to callosities and pain over the PIP joints of the lesser toes. When the hindfoot is involved, patients most often complain of vague ankle pain or lateral pain secondary to peroneal tendon or fibular impingement. With progression of the disease, the characteristic deformities described earlier develop.

Physical Examination

The physical examination should be systematic while focusing on the most commonly involved areas of the ankle and foot. The relative flexibility or rigidity of the deformity should be determined. The forefoot will typically show claw toe deformities of the lesser toes, with calluses under the metatarsal heads and over the PIP joints. Evidence of a symptomatic hallux valgus deformity is noted. The ankle and subtalar joints are inspected to determine the joint responsible for a hindfoot valgus deformity. Laxity of the deltoid ligament and resultant ankle instability will often masquerade as hindfoot valgus. An AP weight-bearing radiograph of the ankle assists in making the distinction. In the midfoot, manual stress may reveal hypermobility of the midtarsal joints in both the sagittal and transverse planes and detect the presence of mild warmth and edema. Discomfort is elicited with range of motion of the central three tarsometatarsal joints. Patients tend to walk with a prolonged stance phase, short strides, and a slow velocity to decrease stresses through a painful forefoot.

Radiographic Findings

weight-bearing radiographs are helpful to document the progression of disease and for surgical planning. Juxtaarticular osteopenia, subchondral cyst formation, narrowing of the joint space, bone destruction, and soft tissue swelling are common findings on plain radiographs. Radiographic changes usually precede clinical symptoms and the development of gross deformity.

The severity of lesser digit MTP subluxation and hallux valgus is noted. The cause of hindfoot valgus is assessed and attributed to either the ankle or subtalar joint. The midfoot is inspected for subluxation of the first tarsometatarsal joint. An increased talar-first metatarsal angle is consistent with an acquired flatfoot and forefoot abduction deformity.

Treatment

Pharmacological treatments for rheumatoid arthritis include nonsteroidal anti-inflammatory drugs (NSAIDs), corticosteroids, and disease-modifying antirheumatic drugs (DMARDs). A rheumatologist typically manages these medications; however, it is important for the orthopaedic surgeon to verify that patients receive appropriate treatment.

In the forefoot, nonoperative management seeks to decrease peak pressures on the metatarsal heads and dorsal aspects of the PIP joints. Soft trilaminate full-length orthotics and stiff-soled rocker shoes offload the MTP joints and minimize deforming stresses. These measures relieve symptoms but do not restore normal gait. Toe spacers, toe sleeves, and toe crests pad painful callosities, and paring of calluses provide short-term pain relief. Physical therapy aimed at increasing mobility may also improve function. When nonoperative management fails to provide relief, surgery is indicated. Operative intervention aims to reduce pain, improve ambulatory status, simplify shoe-wear alterations, and enhance cosmesis. Surgery involves the stabilization of the first ray, the reduction of the lesser MTP joints, and the relocation of the fat pads so as to provide a suitable weight-bearing structure. It includes arthrodesis of the first MTP joint to provide permanent stability to the medial column along with PIP and metatarsal head resectional arthroplasty to align the lesser toes. Complications include problems with wound healing, infection, nonunion, malunion, recurrence of deformities of the lesser toes, and recurrent metatarsalgia.

Nonoperative treatment of hindfoot arthrosis includes the use of a soft University of California Biomechanics Laboratory (UCBL) orthosis with a rocker sole, a small heel lift, and medial or lateral flaring on the outer sole to add stability. With early hindfoot collapse (increased valgus), an off-the-shelf athletic ankle brace is helpful for stabilization but an ankle–foot orthosis is necessary for advanced deformities. Operative treatment of rheumatic disorders of the hindfoot includes arthrodesis of the subtalar joint, the talonavicular joint, and the calcaneocuboid joint (triple arthrodesis). A tendoachilles lengthening is normally a part of this procedure. Hindfoot surgery, in the presence of other major involvement of the lower extremity, requires that the hip or knee be aligned initially so as to determine overall alignment and thus position the hindfoot properly. The goal of hindfoot arthrodesis in a rheumatoid patient is to provide pain relief, improve function and alignment, and provide a stable platform for ambulation.

Management of a rheumatoid ankle arthrosis includes activity modification, intermittent corticosteroid injections, the use of an ankle–foot orthosis and shoe modifications. Surgical options include synovectomy, ankle arthrodesis, and total ankle arthroplasty. Synovitis in the ankle can be treated with an open or arthroscopic synovectomy. Irrigation procedures may decrease the synovitic load on the ankle joint but are temporizing measures at best. Arthrodesis remains the only reliable and durable procedure to treat a painful rheumatoid ankle. Indications include intractable pain, significant deformity, loss of range of motion, and failed total arthroplasty. Techniques are similar to those described for osteoarthritis of the ankle, but there is the need for additional fixation due to the poor bone quality. In the presence of subtalar joint involvement, as seen in cases of global talar avascular necrosis resulting from steroid use, a tibiotalar calcaneal arthrodesis may be required. It can be performed by internal fixation using cannulated screws, specialized plates, or a retrograde intramedullary rod.

Total ankle arthroplasty has historically been plagued by dismal long-term results; however, newer systems appear to yield better results. Its advantage over arthrodesis in the rheumatoid patient is the minimization of stress transference to adjacent joints as occurs following an isolated ankle fusion. In addition, maintaining a mobile segment between the MTP and knee joints avoids a severely stiff gait if there is bilateral involvement. Total ankle arthroplasty is contraindicated with severe coronal plane deformity.

Management of midfoot arthritis consists of arresting painful synovitis by means of a short-leg, weight-bearing cast for 4 weeks followed by an orthosis with a medial heel wedge or, in advanced cases, an ankle–foot orthosis. Stretching the Achilles tendon helps relieve midfoot stresses. Cortisone injections are normally limited to the first tarsometatarsal joint in conjunction with a short period of immobilization. Surgery is reserved for patients with greater functional demands who cannot tolerate bracing. The technique involves stabilizing the medial arch with arthrodesis. Typically, the first, second, and third tarsometatarsal joints are fused; rarely, the fourth and fifth metatarsal cuboid joints are included.

The Diabetic Foot

Diabetes mellitus is a devastating disease causing multiple problems in various organ systems throughout the body. Manifestation in the foot is common and can lead to serious consequences. It is estimated that 20% of diabetic patients have at least one serious foot infection during their lifetime. Prevention of ulceration and infection is important. However, once these occur, treatment must be aggressive.

Pathophysiology and Classification

Diabetes mellitus affects the peripheral nerves and the vascular system, placing patients at risk for ulcers, infections, and potentially amputation. Diabetic neuropathy is the most common foot and ankle manifestation of the disease affecting sensory, motor, and autonomic nerves. Light-touch and proprioceptive sensory neuropathy typically occur first, progressing from distal to proximal in a stocking and glove distribution, and placing patients at risk for ulceration. While diabetic patients tend to have a loss of sensation, they can also suffer from neuropathic paresthesias, which present as contact hypersensitivity, burning pain, and aching. This may be treated with gabapentin. Motor changes can lead to an imbalance between the intrinsic and extrinsic muscles of the foot and the development of claw toes. In addition equinus contracture is common. Together these deformities produce areas of high stress under the metatarsal heads and the dorsal aspect of the PIP joints with shoe wear. With the loss of autonomic control of blood vessels, sweat glands, and lubricating glands, the skin becomes dry and less pliable. With repetitive trauma the skin can fissure providing access for infection.

Arthrosclerosis affects both large and small vessels, resulting in poor circulation, especially in the feet. Most commonly the anterior tibialis, posterior tibialis, and peroneal arteries are affected just below the trifurcation of the popliteal artery. Lack of appropriate blood flow limits healing potential of ulcers and infection.

Foot ulcers are classified according to the system described by Wagner. Grade 0 lesions still have intact skin. Grade 1 lesions are superficial ulcers. Grade 2 lesions are deep with full-thickness ulcerations. Grade 3 signifies the development of an abscess or osteomyelitis. Forefoot gangrene is considered grade 4. Extensive gangrene is considered grade 5.

Presentation

Diabetic patients are often unaware of the sensory and vascular changes occurring in their feet placing them at risk for areas of breakdown and infection. Patients can experience neuropathic symptoms such as burning, deep aches, and hypersensitivity. However, even with these symptoms, they often lack protective sensation. Patients may also present for evaluation of a worsening foot deformity.

Physical Examination

Routine foot examinations are essential for diabetic patients. While a yearly comprehensive examination by a physician is recommended, patients should be proactive in their own care, inspecting their feet on a regular basis for callosities and areas of skin breakdown. Light touch, pin-prick, two-point discrimination, and proprioception should be evaluated. Most typically, the sensation loss follows a stocking and glove distribution. Semmes–Weinstein monofilament testing is helpful to determine a patient's threshold of sensation, and the ability to feel a 5.07 monofilament indicates protective sensation. Chronic vascular insufficiency can manifest as hair loss and thin, shiny skin. The presence or absence of the dorsalis pedis and posterior tibial pulses should be noted.

Diabetic patients often present for the evaluation of a red, swollen foot, and it is imperative to distinguish infection from Charcot arthropathy of the foot. On physical examination, the limb should be elevated above the level of the heart. Any erythema and swelling related to Charcot arthropathy will resolve, whereas it often does not when caused by infection.

All deformities of the foot and associated areas of plantar prominence (rocker-bottom deformity) should be evaluated and noted, as these may require preventative treatment to avoid future skin breakdown.

Radiographic Findings

Standard radiographs of the foot and ankle should be obtained if there is suspicion of trauma, Charcot arthropathy, or osteomyelitis.

Special Tests

If the diagnosis of infection is in question, MRI is helpful for establishing the diagnosis, determining the extent of disease, and distinguishing it from Charcot arthropathy. Technetium-99m and indium-111–labeled leukocyte scans are alternatives but are used less frequently with the widespread availability and speed of MRI.

Vascular evaluations are important to determine the healing potential of chronic ulcers and infections. The arterial pressure at different levels in the leg can be measured with Doppler ultrasound. Toe pressures greater than 45 mm Hg are thought to be necessary for healing. Transcutaneous oxygen measurement is the most accurate measure of healing potential. A level greater than 30 mm Hg indicates adequate circulation for healing.

Treatment

Ideally the treatment of the diabetic foot should focus on prevention of ulcers and infection. Tight glycemic control is an essential. The orthopaedist should always inquire how well patients are managing their glucose levels and ensure physicians are overseeing their medications. Patients should inspect their feet daily and keep their skin well moisturized. Areas of pressure should be relieved with shoe modifications and the use of inserts. Extradepth shoes with a wide toe box are recommended. Rigid insoles should be avoided as these can hasten skin breakdown. Orthotics and bracing may help unload areas of high pressure, especially when deformity is present. Surgery may be necessary to address bone deformities causing areas of high pressure.

Once ulceration occurs, early and aggressive treatment must be initiated to prevent a deep infection. Necrotic tissue and areas of hyperkeratosis should be debrided, and local wound care is essential. If there is no evidence of infection, patients are treated with total contact casting to unload the area of breakdown to allow healing. Casts are placed with little padding to allow appropriate molding and, therefore, must be placed by an individual experienced in their application. Unfortunately, it is necessary to change them frequently to monitor healing and ensure the correct fit of the cast.

Infections require a combination of surgery and antibiotic treatment. The vascular workup is critical to operative planning to assess healing potential. Serial debridements are performed until the infection is controlled. Diabetic foot infections are most often polymicrobial and involve gram-negative organisms. *Staphylococcus aureus* is the most commonly found organism, followed by *Streptococcus, Enterococcus, Proteus mirabilis, Staphylococcus epidermidis, Peptostreptococcus,* diphtheroids, and *Pseudomonas aeruginosa.* Unfortunately, many patients ultimately require amputation to control the infection, especially in the setting of inadequate tissue perfusion. There are a number of amputation options depending on the extent of infection, healing potential, and quality of the soft tissue. The same principles apply to all amputations—resections through viable bone outside the zone of soft tissue infection and with a tension-free wound closure. The most common amputations are digital, ray, transmetatarsal, and below-knee amputations. Patients must often decide between limb salvage requiring multiple surgeries and amputation, which often provides a faster recovery and a superior functional result.

Charcot Arthropathy

Charcot, or neuropathic, arthropathy is a progressive destruction of joints, resulting in deformity, ulceration, and potentially amputation. While underlying causes include syringomyelia, myelomeningocele, alcoholism, syphilis, heavy metal intoxication, congenital insensitivity to pain, and leprosy, the most common cause in the United States is diabetes mellitus.

Pathophysiology and Classification

While multiple theories exist to explain Charcot arthropathy, the common clinical findings are loss of proprioception and vasomotor instability. Minor repetitive trauma is not perceived by patients and therefore not treated, resulting in joint instability, dislocations, osteophyte formation and subchondral fracture. In addition, there is a loss of autonomic control, leading to a local hyperemia of bone and relative osteopenia. The exact incidence of arthropathy among diabetic patients is unknown, but the incidence is approximately 3%, with 6% to 40% of patients being affected bilaterally.

Eichenholtz developed the classic classification system of Charcot arthropathy. Stage I, or the fragmentation stage, is the acute phase of the disease process characterized by subchondral fragmentation, periarticular fracture, subluxation, and dislocation. Stage II, or the coalescence stage, is the beginning of the reparative process. This is best identified with serial imaging—the resorption of bone debris, the formation of new bone, and sclerosis of bones. Stage III, or the consolidation phase, is a period of remodeling and healing. Deformity and the ankylosis of joints may be the end result of the Charcot process. Authors subsequently added a Stage 0, or inflammatory stage. Radiographs are normal; however, MRI and bone scan studies show changes. This stage may last up to 1 year before stage I changes occur.

The midfoot is affected in approximately 60% to 70% of cases, with the most severe deformity occurring at the tarsometatarsal articulations. The ankle and subtalar joints account for approximately 30% of cases.

Presentation

Patients with stage 0 and I disease present with erythema, swelling, hyperemia, and warmth. These stages are commonly confused with infection. Fevers are not typical with Charcot and support the diagnosis of infection when present. The swelling may be severe enough that ordinary shoe wear is difficult. In stage II, the symptoms of erythema, swelling, and warmth diminish, and by stage III, these usually resolve. Even though many patients have significant neuropathy, up to 75% have discomfort in the foot and ankle associated with this pathology. Only approximately 20% recall a traumatic event before developing the symptoms related to Charcot.

Physical Examination

As noted earlier, patients in the early stage have erythema, swelling, and warmth of the foot and ankle. The swelling and erythema related to Charcot often respond to elevation above the level of the heart as opposed to infection, which does not. Patients typically exhibit a dense neuropathy. Good vascular perfusion may be present. The limb should be thoroughly inspected for ulceration and areas of skin breakdown.

Radiographic Findings

Radiographs of the foot and ankle should be obtained on all diabetic patients presenting with a red, swollen foot. First, radiographs may aid in ruling out osteomyelitis. Second, the radiographs help to determine the stage of the disease process and the appropriate treatment. The radiographic findings for each stage have been discussed earlier. Third, characterizing the deformity is necessary to plan surgical intervention. Ideally these radiographs should be weight-bearing to identify subtle instability patterns.

Special Tests

MRI is becoming more popular, especially in diagnosing early stages of disease. Stress reactions and bone marrow edema are evident in the periarticular and subchondral regions of multiple bones. These findings differ from osteomyelitis, which most often is diffuse within one bone. Bone scans can also be used, but they have low specificity. They are more useful to rule out osteomyelitis when negative.

Differential Diagnosis

Clearly, it is most important to distinguish Charcot arthropathy from osteomyelitis in its early stages. Patients with infection often have fevers, open wounds, hyperglycemia above their normal blood sugar levels, nondependant rubor, and associated MRI findings. Charcot can also be misdiagnosed as gout, rheumatoid arthritis, ankle sprain, and deep venous thrombosis. A thorough history and physical examination in conjunction with appropriate imaging usually resolves any question in diagnosis.

Treatment

The treatment goal is to establish a stable, plantigrade foot without deformity. Treatments vary depending on the stage of disease, the presence of open wounds, and the joints affected. For patients who present early in the disease course, nonoperative management should be attempted. Total contact casting is initiated after a few days of elevation to decrease the swelling. Total contact casting allows for the even distribution of the forces across the plantar aspect of the foot. Every 2 to 4 weeks, the cast is changed until the process has entered the coalescence phase when the foot is no longer warm, erythematous, and swollen and radiographs show signs of stability. Approximately 4 months of casting is expected; afterwards, patients are transitioned to custom-made shoes with orthotics. Historically, patients were told to remain non–weight-bearing; however, some specialists now allow modified weight-bearing. There is no definitive evidence that non–weight-bearing increases the risk of developing Charcot in the other limb due to the increases in forces. Deep ulcers complicate the nonoperative management of Charcot arthropathy because of the risk of osteomyelitis. When associated with infection, ulcers require debridement and evidence of local control prior to initiation of total contact casting. Alternatives to total contact casting include removable casts and Charcot restraint orthotic walker (CROW) devices. These function in a manner similar to total contact casts by distributing forces on the plantar aspect of the foot. Their advantages over total contact castings is that soft tissue can be more closely monitored and they do not require specialized training in their application.

With significant deformity, recurrent ulceration, and joint instability surgical intervention may be necessary for the treatment of Charcot arthropathy and its residual deformity. Traditionally, surgery was not performed during the fragmentation phase of the disease because of the risk of nonunion, malunion, and infection. It was typically delayed until the consolidation phase. More recently, this has been questioned, especially with techniques using external fixation. There is no consensus on the optimal timing of surgical intervention. Surgical interventions range from exostectomy to complex reconstructions and arthrodesis. Immobilization is continued until the erythema, swelling, and warmth resolve. Patients are then placed into custom-molded orthotics.

Achilles Tendon Pathology

The terms referring to tendon conditions can be confusing and are often used inaccurately. Even though one may be able to distinguish tendinosis versus tendonitis based on history and physical examination, it is best to use tendinopathy when making a clinical diagnosis. Tendinopathy is a broad term that encompasses both tendinitis and tendinosis, which are confirmed with pathological evaluation. Tendinitis has an acute inflammatory component, whereas tendinosis is more of a chronic degenerative noninflammatory condition.

Pathology of the Achilles tendon must be divided into insertional and noninsertional as well as acute and chronic. Noninsertional pathology occurs approximately 4 to 6 cm proximal to the insertion site in an area of relative poor vascularity. Symptoms can result from acute inflammation of the paratenon (paratenonitis) or from a more chronic degeneration of the tendon itself (tendinosis). Insertional pathology causes posterior heel pain and is commonly associated with retrocalcaneal bursitis and a Haglund deformity.

Pathophysiology and Classification

Tendinosis is the result of the repetitive stress of lengthening and shortening of the Achilles tendon during ambulation. Without appropriate rest to allow for normal tendon repair, continued overuse can result in the degeneration of the collagen structure of the tendon 4 to 6 cm proximal to the insertion. This form of noninsertional Achilles tendinopathy is typically seen in long-distance runners. Collagen is not produced normally, neovascularization occurs, fibroblasts proliferate, and mucoid material is deposited, which manifests as a palpable nodule and thickening of the tendon. The pathological tendon has less tensile strength and elasticity. Tendinosis typically lacks an inflammatory component.

Inflammatory conditions of the paratenon and tendon can occur at the insertion and proximally. Insertional pathology is most commonly related to retrocalcaneal bursitis and irritation of the Achilles tendon itself. The retrocalcaneal bursa is located between the posterior angle of the os calcis and the Achilles tendon. This can become inflamed and thickened, often due to shoe wear. An enlarged posterosuperior calcaneal process, commonly referred to as a *Haglund deformity*, predisposes a person to retrocalcaneal bursitis. Calcification of the insertion site can also develop with chronic inflammation.

Presentation

Noninsertional Achilles tendinosis occurs most commonly in runners with a history of altered training or shoe wear. Pain is present along the Achilles tendon approximately 4 to 6 cm proximal to its insertion. The pain is aggravated by activity and relieved with rest. Uphill running or walking is especially painful.

Insertional tendinitis and retrocalcaneal bursitis commonly presents in middle-aged to elderly women with posterior heel pain.

Examination

A tender fusiform nodule is present within the substance of the Achilles with tendinosis. With peritendinitis, the mass is typically mobile and is associated with common signs of inflammation, including pain, stiffness, swelling, and diffuse tenderness. Tenderness medial and lateral to the Achilles tendon at the insertion site is typical of retrocalcaneal bursitis. With insertional inflammation of the Achilles, there is tenderness directly at the point of posterior insertion. In both insertional and noninsertional pathology, there is no loss in continuity of the Achilles tendon, so patients can perform a heel rise test, and the Thompson test is negative. Contracture of the Achilles is usually a constant finding in both forms of tendinopathy.

Imaging Studies

Standard radiographs are not usually necessary for noninsertional pathology but may show calcifications related to the tendinosis. More distally, radiographs can show a Haglund deformity or calcification of the tendon. MRI is more useful to evaluate the underlying pathology both proximally and at the insertion site. This can easily distinguish between peritendinitis, thickening of the outer sheath, tendinosis, and intratendinous degeneration.

Differential Diagnosis

Systemic disorders such as gout and spondyloarthropathies should be ruled out. Posterior insertional heel pain must also be distinguished from plantar fasciitis and calcaneal stress fractures. Reiter syndrome may present with insertional Achilles tendon pain and retrocalcaneal bursitis. There is also a known association of Achilles tendon pathology and fluoroquinolone use.

Treatment

The goal of treatment for noninsertional Achilles tendinosis is to reverse the degenerative process and allow normal healing of the tendon. Nonoperative management is recommended initially; however, it tends to be less effective when the condition is more chronic. Treatment typically includes NSAIDs, rest, shoe modification, and physical therapy. Incorrect therapy regimens such as concentric strengthening can often worsen symptoms. Eccentric strengthening is recommended. A heel lift and the use of open-backed shoes may be helpful in reducing symptoms during daily activities. Alternative modalities including ultrasound and extracorporeal shock wave therapy have shown good results. Use of local steroid injections is not recommended because of the potential for tendon rupture and subcutaneous atrophy.

If nonoperative management has failed to provide relief of symptoms after 4 to 6 months, surgery may be indicated. The tendon is split longitudinally and all pathological tissue is excised. The remaining tendon is repaired side-to-side. In cases of severe, extensive tendinosis, augmentation with the adjacent FHL tendon is recommended.

The treatment of isolated retrocalcaneal bursitis is nonoperative. Heel lifts help to move the bursal prominence forward and away for the Achilles tendon. NSAIDs and occasional immobilization can be beneficial. When a Haglund deformity is present, surgical intervention may be required to remove the posterosuperior process of the calcaneus. Attention is also directed toward debridement and repair of the Achilles tendon insertion and resection of any calcific deposition or osteophytes.

Tarsal Tunnel Syndrome

Entrapment of the posterior tibial nerve within the fibro-osseus tunnel posterior and distal to the medial malleolus is referred to as *tarsal tunnel syndrome*. The tarsal tunnel is the distal extension of the deep fascia of the posterior compartment, formed by medially by the talus, sustentaculum tali, and calcaneus, and laterally by the flexor retinaculum (laciniate ligament). The posterior tibialis, FDL, and the FHL tendons traverse the canal within individual sheaths, with the posterior tibial nerve and artery lying between sheaths.

Pathophysiology and Classification

Compression the posterior tibial nerve can occur from within or outside the tunnel. Space occupying lesions such as varicosities, lipomas, ganglia, perineural fibrosis, bony exostoses, flexor retinaculum hypertrophy, rheumatoid synovitis, and anomalous muscles may create compression. Foot deformities such as hindfoot varus with forefoot pronation and hindfoot valgus with forefoot abduction are associated with this condition. Trauma including displaced fractures of the distal tibial and hindfoot as well as ankle sprains have led to tarsal tunnel symptoms. In reality, an etiology is identifiable in only approximately 50% of cases.

Presentation

Patients characteristically complain of burning pain in the arch, vague numbness in the toes, night pain, and pain that is accentuated by ambulation. Extremes of dorsiflexion place the nerve under tension and may exacerbate symptoms. Pain may radiate proximally into the midcalf. Motor deficits and intrinsic paralysis are late findings. Some patients report a minor trauma preceding the symptoms.

Physical Examination

Physical findings in approximately half of patients include a positive percussion test (Tinel sign) over the posterior tibial nerve reproducing the symptoms. Two-point discrimination on the plantar aspect of the foot should be tested, since this is the first sensory abnormality seen in the condition. Motor weakness is uncommon but can affect the intrinsic toe flexors, the abductor hallucis, and the abductor digiti mini. If the condition is caused by an accessory muscle or hypertrophy of the abductor hallucis longus, fullness in the area may be appreciable.

Given the association with certain deformities, the position of the hindfoot should be noted.

Radiographic Findings

While the overall yield of radiographs may be low, these help to evaluate the anatomy of the foot and rule out certain space-occupying lesions such as exostoses, accessory ossicles, and fractures.

Special Tests

Electromyographic nerve conduction studies are helpful in ruling out lumbar disk disease as the source of symptoms. Diagnostic findings for medial plantar nerve involvement include terminal latency in the abductor hallucis of more than 6.32 milliseconds. Similarly, a prolonged latency of more than 7 milliseconds in the abductor digiti mini is consistent with lateral plantar nerve involvement. Sensory latencies are the most sensitive tests because these are the first fibers affected. MRI is useful to delineate space-occupying lesions.

Differential Diagnosis

Radicular lumbar pathology, plantar fasciitis, peripheral neuropathy, stress fractures, and inflammatory arthropathies can present with similar symptoms.

Treatment

Treatment includes NSAIDs to control pain and orthotics to control hindfoot valgus and decrease the tension across the tunnel. Cortisone injections to decrease inflammation and bracing to rest the nerve may be helpful. Surgery involves decompressing from the proximal aspect of the flexor retinaculum to the bifurcation of the tibial nerve. This should be extended to release the superficial calcaneal branch of the tibial nerve and trace the plantar branches distally through the abductor hallucis muscle. Resection of any space-occupying lesion should be performed, including anomalous muscles. Internal neurolysis is indicated if there is evidence of nerve fibrosis. Good results are expected in up to 95% of patients when a space-occupying lesion is identified. When there is not, approximately 75% of patients improve after tarsal tunnel release.

Peroneal Tendon Pathology

The peroneal tendon complex consists of the peroneus brevis and longus, which course behind the lateral malleolus. Above the level of the ankle joint, the two tendons travel in a common synovial sheath. The peroneus longus lays posterolateral to the peroneus brevis as they pass behind the lateral malleolus in the retromalleolar groove. The superior retinacular ligament, the primary lateral restraint to dislocation of the tendons, forms the roof of the groove. More distally, the sheath diverges such that each tendon travels in its own sheath separated by the peroneal tubercle as they pass under the inferior peroneal retinaculum 2 cm distal to the tip of the fibula. The peroneus brevis then inserts on the base of the fifth metatarsal while the peroneus longus travels under the cuboid to insert onto the base of the first metatarsal. A small pisiform bone is contained within the peroneus longus as it passes around the cuboid. This flat disc can appear as an avulsion fracture on oblique foot radiographs.

Conditions affecting the peroneal tendon complex fall into three categories—tendonitis/tenosynovitis, tendon tears/ruptures, and subluxation/dislocation. These tendon pathologies are uncommon and unfortunately often missed.

Pathophysiology and Classification

Tendinitis/tenosynovitis is commonly related to an increase in repetitive activity such as running after a period of inactivity and is caused by a mechanical irritation. Varus hindfoot alignment is a risk factor for developing tendinitis. Inversion injuries, chronic tenosynovitis, ankle sprains, ankle fractures, chronic ankle instability, and stenosis of the retrofibular groove can all cause ruptures and tears of the peroneal tendons. Peroneal tendon subluxation or dislocation is usually a sports-related injury. An inversion injury to a dorsiflexed foot with eccentric loading is the most common mechanism for peroneal tendon subluxation.

Presentation

Lateral ankle pain and swelling are the most common presenting complaints. When patients present acutely, an isolated injury is often identifiable. In chronic injuries with a history of multiple ankle sprains, there are often associated pathologies present. Peroneal tendon pathology commonly accompanies lateral ankle instability.

Examination

The anatomy and alignment of the foot should be inspected given the association between a cavovarus foot and peroneal tendon pathology. Swelling and tenderness may be appreciable along the peroneal tendons. Passive inversion of the hindfoot and resisted eversion with dorsiflexion can reproduce peroneal tendon pain. Eversion strength is not usually affected. Snapping of the tendons behind the fibula can be associated with tendon subluxation or frank instability. It is important to test the stability of the ankle ligaments and rule out other causes of lateral ankle pain, such as an osteochondral defect.

Radiographs

AP and lateral radiographs of the foot and ankle should be obtained to evaluate for os peroneum, fibular impingement, and arthrosis. Avulsion fractures of the calcaneus and base of the fifth metatarsal can be ruled out. A fleck sign may be visible on an AP image, which is a small piece of bone avulsed off the fibula by the superior peroneal retinaculum. MRI is the standard for evaluating pathology of the tendons. Ultrasound is potentially a relatively inexpensive but highly sensitive and specific alternative if performed by appropriately trained technicians.

Treatment

First-line treatment of peroneal complex pathology is nonoperative and includes activity modification, brief immobilization, and NSAIDs. After the acute phase, physical therapy can be initiated. When this fails and surgery is planned, it is essential to address the underlying condition and anatomic variation responsible. The most important and probably most common is lateral ankle instability. This must be addressed to improve the chances of successful treatment.

Tendinitis and tenosynovitis are treated with synovectomy and debridement. Tendon tears less than 50% of the cross-sectional area are treated with debridement and tubularization. If the tear is complete, a tenodesis is performed between the peroneus longus and peroneus brevis. For a tear or rupture of both tendons, a tendon transfer or tendon graft may be necessary. Transfer options include FDL to peroneus brevis and plantaris to peroneus longus. Surgical treatment options for peroneal tendon subluxation or dislocation include anatomic repair of the superior retinaculum, tissue transfers for reconstruction, groove-deepening procedures, and tendon rerouting under the CFL.

Acquired Adult Flatfoot Deformity

Dysfunction of the posterior tibial tendon can range from mild tendinitis to complete rupture and an asymmetrical flatfoot deformity. Underlying causes include trauma, inflammatory arthropathies, and attritional degenerative conditions.

Pathophysiology and Classification

The posterior tibial tendon is involved with maintenance of the longitudinal arch and bringing the hindfoot into varus for push-off. When the posterior tibial muscle contracts, it provides a varus force to the hindfoot, causing transverse tarsal joint to lock and creating a rigid foot to transmit the force of the gastrocsoleus complex. With attenuation and degeneration, the hindfoot falls into valgus, the forefoot into more abduction, and effective push-off is not possible. While posterior tibial tendon dysfunction in acquired adult flatfoot deformity is usually the cause of pain and swelling, it is not the only pathological structure in the disease process. With hindfoot valgus and abduction of the forefoot, the Achilles tendon and deltoid ligament also become dysfunctional over time.

The classification system proposed by Johnson and modified by Meyerson focuses on the flexibility of the flatfoot deformity. Stage I describes pain and swelling with minor weakness of the posterior tibialis muscle and the absence of deformity. Stage II involves posterior tibial tendon disruption with medial column collapse and a flexible flatfoot deformity. Stage III is reserved for a rigid flatfoot and potentially arthrosis. Asymmetry of the tibiotalar joint associated with a rigid flatfoot is considered stage IV.

Presentation

Patients present with pain, swelling, and fullness localized to the posterior medial hindfoot and note difficulty with ambulation. Only approximately 50% of patients report a traumatic event. With progressive deterioration of the tendon and incompetent function, a progressive asymmetrical flatfoot deformity develops. Late symptoms include progression of deformity, difficulty with shoe wear, and lateral calcaneal-fibular impingement.

Examination

Clinical examination in the early stages reveals tender, boggy edema at the level of the medial malleolus, a secondary Achilles contracture, and weakness of isolated posterior tibial tendon strength testing (resisted inversion with the foot in a plantarflexed and abducted in a non–weight-bearing position). Patients are unable to perform a single-leg heel rise and often there is no inversion of the hindfoot on double-stance toe rise (Fig. 19.31). Flexibility of the subtalar and transverse tarsal joint is evaluated, as this alters treatment. The Jack test consists of passively dorsiflexing the hallux, which results in restoration of the medial longitudinal arch in flexible conditions. With advanced forefoot abduction and collapse, the "too many toes" sign occurs when observing a patient from behind in resting stance (Fig. 19.32). With advanced collapse, there is evidence of loss of medial longitudinal arch, and there are varying degrees of rigidity. Because of the association with Achilles tendon contracture, the range of the motion of the ankle should be noted. When doing so, the talonavicular joint should be reduced to avoid misinterpreting motion through the midfoot as dorsiflexion.

The lateral side of the ankle should be examined as significant valgus deformity can result in impingement of the fibula onto the calcaneus. Tenderness in this area may be appreciated.

Radiographs

Diagnostic studies consist of weight-bearing AP and lateral radiographs of the foot, as the deformity may not be appreciated on non–weight-bearing films (Fig. 19.33). On the AP view, the coverage of the talus is evaluated for talonavicular subluxation. This is estimated by calculating the angle between the medial articular edge of the talus and the navicular. A coverage angle greater than 10 degrees is considered an abnormal amount of forefoot abduction. On the lateral radiograph, Meary angle is formed between the axis of the talus and the first metatarsal ray. Normally, these two axes are parallel; however, they become divergent with collapse of the midfoot. weight-bearing radiographs of the ankle should be evaluated for asymmetry and arthrosis.

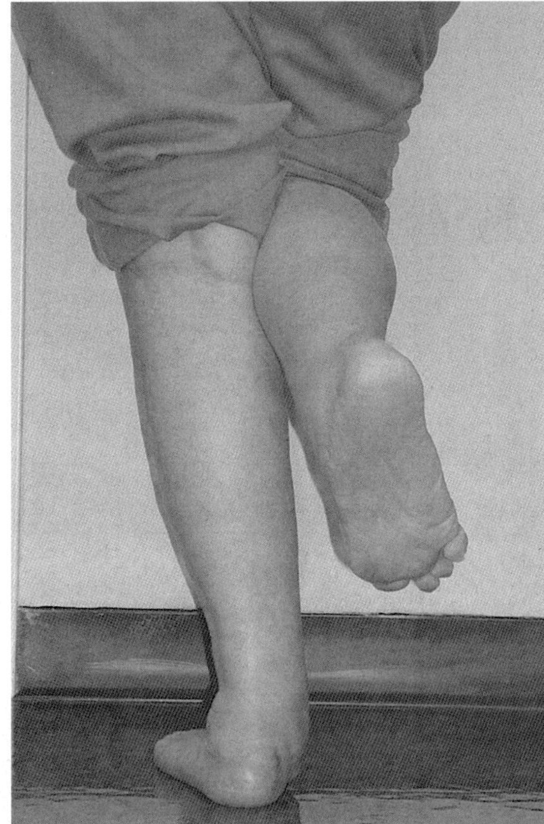

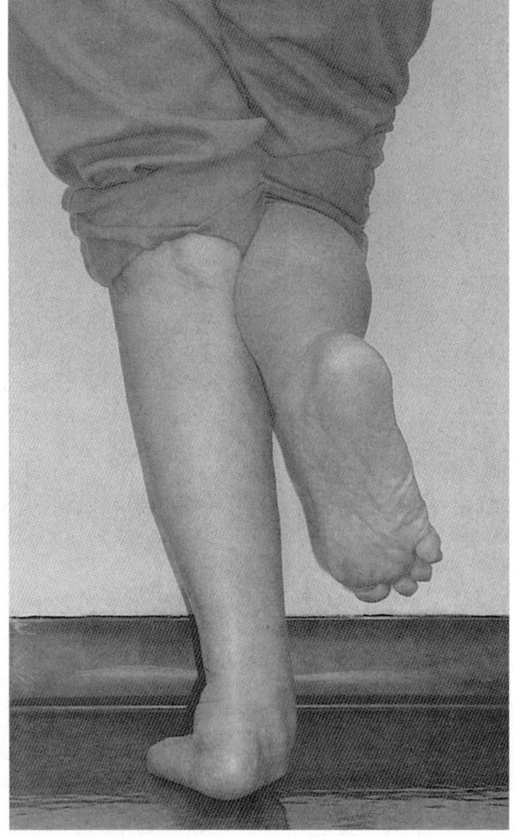

Figure 19.31 **(A)** Posterior photograph demonstrating the flatfoot deformity associated with posterior tibial tendon dysfunction. **(B)** When the patient attempts to perform a single heel rise the heel does not leave the ground. (*Reproduced with permission from* Kitaoka HB. *The Foot and Ankle*. 2nd ed. Philadelphia, PA: Lippincott Williams & Wilkins, 2002.)

Treatment

The stage of the disease dictates the treatment. Stage I disease with minimal deformity is treated with NSAIDs, orthotics, and physical therapy. In fulminate tenosynovitis, cast immobilization or a modified ankle–foot orthosis is used to decrease tendon strain. An orthosis such as the UCBL semi-rigid orthosis supports the medial arch while maintaining the hindfoot in neutral position. If refractory to nonoperative measures, a tenosynovectomy may relieve pain and halt the formation of tendinosis.

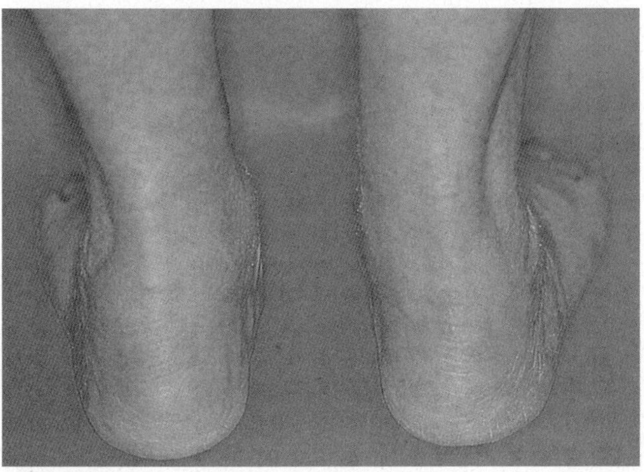

Figure 19.32 The "too many toes" sign due to advanced forefoot abduction. (*Reproduced with permission from* Kitaoka HB. *The Foot and Ankle*. 2nd ed. Philadelphia, PA: Lippincott Williams & Wilkins, 2002.)

The treatment of stage II disease is controversial. Historically, it has been treated similarly to stage I, with nonoperative management and triple arthrodesis if that failed. Currently, stage II disease is treated with a combination of soft tissue reconstruction and various osteotomies to maintain motion. FDL and FHL transfers for augmentation of the posterior tibial tendon are options for surgical reconstruction. Lengthening of the Achilles tendon or gastrocnemius is often necessary. Bony procedures include calcaneal medial displacement osteotomy, lateral column lengthening, and medial cuneiform osteotomy.

For severe stage II and stage III deformities, arthrodesis is the mainstay of treatment. Isolated arthrodesis that include the subtalar joint, talonavicular joint, or calcaneocuboid joint have been proposed. In severe rigid deformities, and those associated with forefoot varus, a triple arthrodesis is recommended.

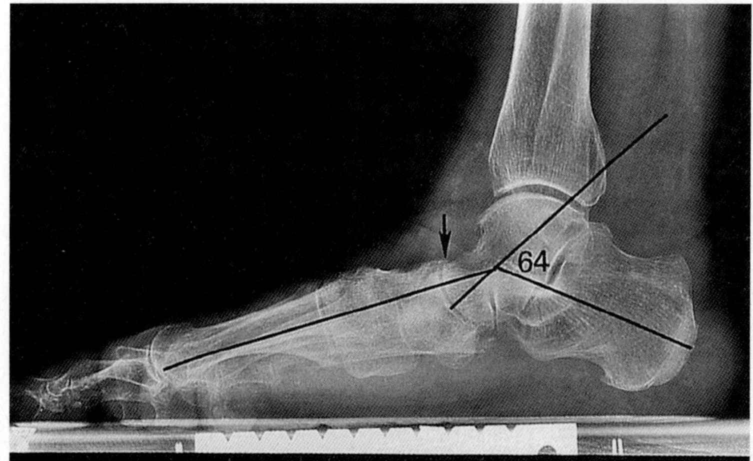

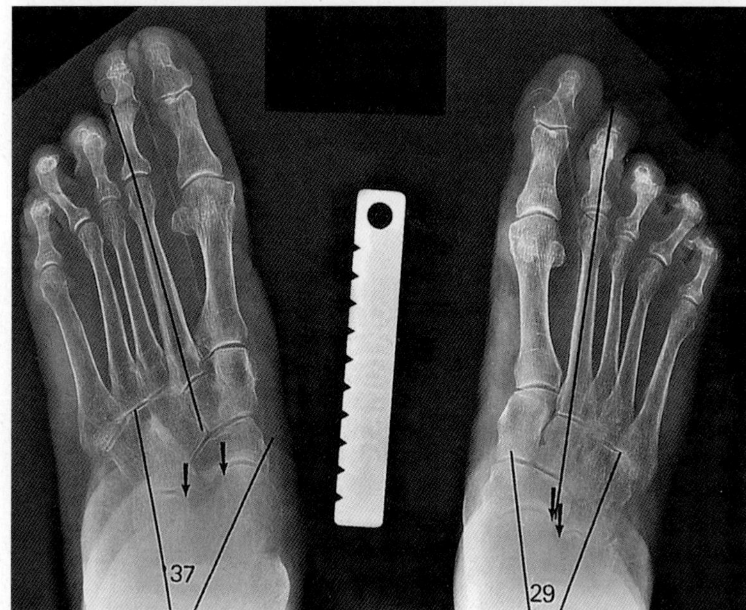

Figure 19.33 weight-bearing radiographs taken in a patient with posterior tibial tendon dysfunction and flatfoot. On the lateral, there is collapse of the midfoot with loss of parallelism between the talus and the axis of the first metatarsal (Meary angle) and a decrease in calcaneal pitch **(A)**. Anteroposterior radiographs of both feet clearly show the typical deformities in the left foot when compared with the normal right foot **(B)**. The peritalar subluxation is evident by the increase in the talocalcaneal angle, seen as a separation between the lateral margin of the talar head and medial margin of the anterior calcaneus (*arrows*). Abduction of the forefoot, represented by the second metatarsal axis, is seen. The talar head is uncovered medially. (*Reproduced with permission from* Kitaoka HB. *The Foot and Ankle*. 2nd ed. Philadelphia, PA: Lippincott Williams & Wilkins, 2002.)

Plantar Fasciitis

Heel pain is one of the most common and potentially disabling conditions to affect the foot. There are a multitude of potential causes for heel pain, including tumors, infection, stress fractures, inflammatory arthropathies, and compressive or metabolic neuropathies. The most common plantar heel pain is associated with a chronic injury-reparative process that leads to microtears, necrosis, and chondroid metaplasia at the origin of the plantar fascia on the medial calcaneal tuberosity. The condition is more of a chronic degenerative one than a true inflammatory process and is more appropriately referred to as *plantar fasciosis*.

Pathophysiology

The plantar fascia originates on the medial aspect of the calcaneal tuberosity and inserts on the base of the proximal phalanx of each toe after dividing into five bands. With dorsiflexion of the MTP joints during toe-off, significant tensile forces act through the plantar fascia to elevate the arch and lock the transverse tarsal joints creating what has been described as the "windlass mechanism." Repetitive microtrauma to the fascia results in necrosis and degeneration at the origin of the plantar fascia.

Presentation

The onset is insidious and is often preceded by overuse in women aged 40 to 65 years old. Symptoms include morning stiffness and pain that resolves during the day with walking. Classically, pain is most severe when arising in the morning or getting up after sitting and taking the first step. Jumping and running can exacerbate the pain. Night pain is not common, and its presence should warn the physician to rule out more serious conditions. High-heeled shoes typically alleviate symptoms, whereas going barefoot and wearing flat shoes worsens symptoms.

Examination

Physical examination reveals a point of tenderness at the plantar medial origin of the plantar fascia on the os calcis. There is often a moderate to severely tight Achilles tendon complex and restricted ankle dorsiflexion. There may be some fullness and warmth in the area of the plantar medial heel and, occasionally, heel pad atrophy. The central band in the midfoot is typically not tender, but passive dorsiflexion of the toes resulting in tension on the plantar fascia may elicit pain.

Radiographs

Diagnosis of plantar fasciitis is based on history and physical examination. While radiographs may reveal specific findings, they are reserved for patients who do not respond to treatment to rule out other causes of heel pain. Lateral weight-bearing views may demonstrate a plantar spur at the origin of the FDB in approximately 50% of patients, which signifies chronicity of the condition. It is thought that the spur is a result of the disease process and not a cause of it. A spur does not usually develop at the origin of the plantar fascia. A bone scan is positive in almost all cases, but this finding is not specific and is of little value. MRI and ultrasound can also help to confirm diagnosis when needed.

Differential Diagnosis

The differential diagnosis for heel pain is a long procedure but can be easily separated into neurological, bony, and soft tissue causes. Neurological causes include tarsal tunnel syndrome, entrapment of the first branch of the lateral plantar (Baxter) or medial calcaneal nerves, peripheral neuropathy, or S1 radiculopathy. Atrophy of the heel pad, tendinitis of the Achilles, FHL, or posterior tibial tendons, and plantar fibromatosis can all cause heel pain. Bone sources include stress fractures, infections, contusions, tumor, and arthritis.

Treatment

In almost all cases of heel pain, management is primarily nonoperative. Treatment usually consists of rest, cold therapy, NSAIDs, Achilles stretching, and orthotic devices; however, there is little evidence to support these modalities individually. Studies have shown that an inexpensive, over-the-counter heel cushion is as effective as a custom-made orthosis when combined with a stretching regimen. Various stretching programs have been described and usually are plantar fascia–specific or focus on the Achilles tendon. Night splinting helps to keep the posterior calf muscles and plantar fascia on stretch while sleeping. For patients who have failed to show progress within 2 months, a cortisone injection at the medial calcaneal tuberosity can be given. Regardless of the regimen chosen, it is important to stress to patients that patience and dedication to stretching is required. Relief from pain may take 6 months to 1 year.

An alternative therapy receiving more attention is extracorporeal shock wave therapy for refractory cases of plantar fasciitis treated with at least three other nonoperative modalities for 6 months. The exact mechanism is not known, but it is thought to stimulate revascularization of the tissue to promote appropriate healing.

Surgery is relegated to chronic conditions that do not respond to nonoperative measures and is necessary in less than 10% of cases. Interventions include partial and complete plantar fasciotomy performed either open or endoscopically. Care should be taken, as releasing the plantar fascia does have consequences on the biomechanics of the foot. The longitudinal arch can collapse, and increased stresses are transferred to the ligaments and bones of the midfoot and metatarsals. For patients with heel cord contracture, a partial release of the Achilles or gastrocnemius may alleviate the pain.

Hallux Valgus

Hallux valgus is a disorder of the first ray that involves metatarsus primus varus, lateral deviation of the great toe, and a medial prominence of the first MTP joint. This prominence is the most visible aspect of the condition and is commonly referred to as a *bunion* (Fig. 19.34). While genetics and certain anatomic factors such as a planovalgus foot deformity, heel cord contracture, and ligamentous laxity predispose patients to developing the condition, it is almost exclusively related to shoe wear.

Pathophysiology and Classification

The pathophysiology of hallux valgus involves a derangement of the intrinsic musculature of the foot, resulting in

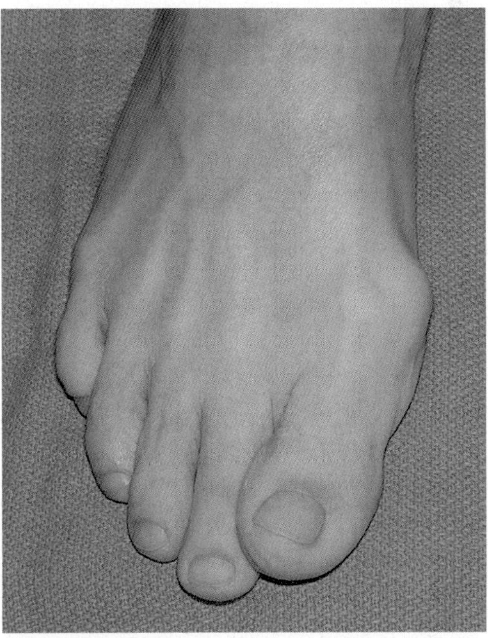

Figure 19.34 A clinical picture of a typical bunion showing the prominent medial eminence. (*Reproduced with permission from* Kitaoka HB. *The Foot and Ankle.* 2nd ed. Philadelphia, PA: Lippincott Williams & Wilkins, 2002.)

lateral deviation of the great toe and medial displacement of the first ray. The abductor hallucis usually balances the adductor hallucis; however, with the development of hallux valgus, the abductor hallucis displaces plantarward. With the loss of balance, the adductor hallucis becomes a deforming force pulling the toe further into valgus and pronation due to its insertion on the plantar aspect of the lateral base of the proximal phalanx. As the deformity worsens, the abductor hallucis, adductor hallucis, FHB, FHL, and even the EHL become deforming forces, leaving the thin dorsal capsule as the only medial restraint. Ultimately, the sesamoids can displace laterally from under the metatarsal head. Hallux valgus is usually classified as mild, moderate, and severe on the basis of the radiographic parameters discussed later.

Presentation

Symptoms associated with hallux valgus deformity include pain, swelling, and inflammation over the medial eminence caused by shoe wear as well as secondary hypertrophy of the overlying bursa. Patients often complain that they are unable to find comfortable shoes, while being able to ambulate barefoot without difficulty. By contrast pain in the hallux MTP joint while ambulating barefoot is a sign of first MTP joint arthritis.

Physical Examination

Evaluation of the foot should be performed while sitting and weight-bearing, as this may make the deformity more obvious. The foot should be assessed for a pes planovalgus deformity, Achilles tendon contracture, ligamentous laxity, and signs of a neuromuscular disorder. Associated lesser toe deformities, including subluxation or dislocation of the lesser MTP joints (especially the second digit commonly referred to as a *crossover toe*), transfer callosities under the metatarsal heads, bunionette deformity, corns, and hammertoes are noted. The degree of pronation and the correctibility of the deformity should be judged. Range of motion of the MTP joint should be measured, keeping in mind that 70 degrees of dorsiflexion is necessary for normal gait. The presence of crepitus is a sign of osteoarthritic change within the joint. Finally, the first metatarsocuneiform joint should be assessed for hypermobility by comparing motion of this articulation to that of the fifth metatarsal with the cuboid.

Radiographic Findings

weight-bearing AP and lateral radiographs are essential for proper diagnosis of the deformity and surgical planning, as not all bunions are treated the same. The degree of hallux valgus and metatarsus primus varus deformity, first MTP joint congruity, degenerative changes of the MTP joint, and evidence of sesamoid subluxation determine the optimal treatment approach and are assessed on radiographs (Fig. 19.35).

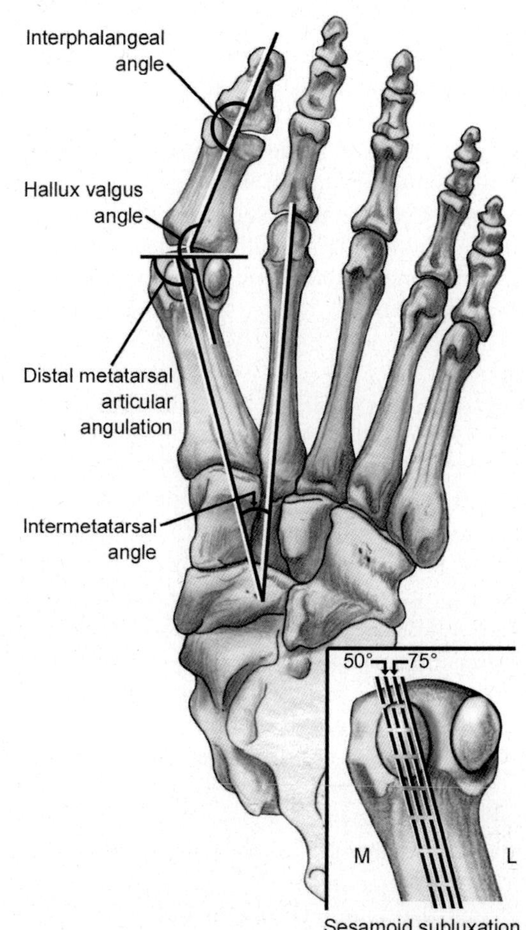

Figure 19.35 The angles and degree of sesamoid subluxation used to assess severity of hallux valgus. (*Reproduced with permission from* Johnson D, Pedowitz RA. *Practical Orthopaedic Sports Medicine and Arthroscopy*. Philadelphia, PA: Lippincott Williams & Wilkins, 2007.)

The hallux valgus angle, subtended by a line bisecting the first metatarsal and the proximal phalanx, is normally less than 15 degrees. The intermetatarsal angle of the first and second metatarsals is determined by bisecting the longitudinal axis of each, and an angle of 9 degrees or less is normal. A hallux valgus angle of less than 20 degrees with an intermetatarsal angle less than 11 degrees and sesamoid subluxation of less than 50% are considered a mild deformity. A hallux valgus angle of 20 to 40 degrees, an intermetatarsal angle less than 16 degrees, and sesamoid subluxation 50% to 75% are considered moderate. Hallux valgus angles greater than 40 degrees, intermetatarsal angles greater than 16 degrees, and sesamoid subluxation more than 75% are considered severe. Severe hallux valgus is usually associated with first MTP joint incongruity.

The distal metatarsal articular angle describes the orientation of the articular surface in relation to the longitudinal axis of the ray. A line connecting the medial and lateral articular margins of the hallux metatarsal head and a line bisecting the longitudinal axis of the first metatarsal form the angle. This angle can impact the surgical treatment plan.

Differential Diagnosis

Hallux valgus interphalangeus is a deformity of the interphalangeal joint of the great toe. The angle between the proximal and distal phalanx on an AP radiograph normally measures 10 degrees. This deformity can resemble hallux valgus.

Treatment

Treatment of hallux valgus in the early stage is nonoperative and includes selection of appropriate shoes with a high, wide toe box. If an associated planovalgus deformity exists, orthotic devices may be helpful. Surgical intervention is indicated when conservative measures fail, and there is progression of the deformity, increasing difficulty with shoe wear, and involvement of the second MTP joint manifested as a crossover deformity. Contraindications include spasticity, ligamentous laxity from Marfan or Ehlers–Danlos syndrome, and vascular or skin insufficiency.

The principle of surgical treatment is to correct all deformities while maintaining a functional foot. A number of surgical options exist, ranging from soft tissue procedures to multiple osteotomies and fusions. There is no clear-cut consensus on optimal treatment (Fig. 19.36). Decisions are

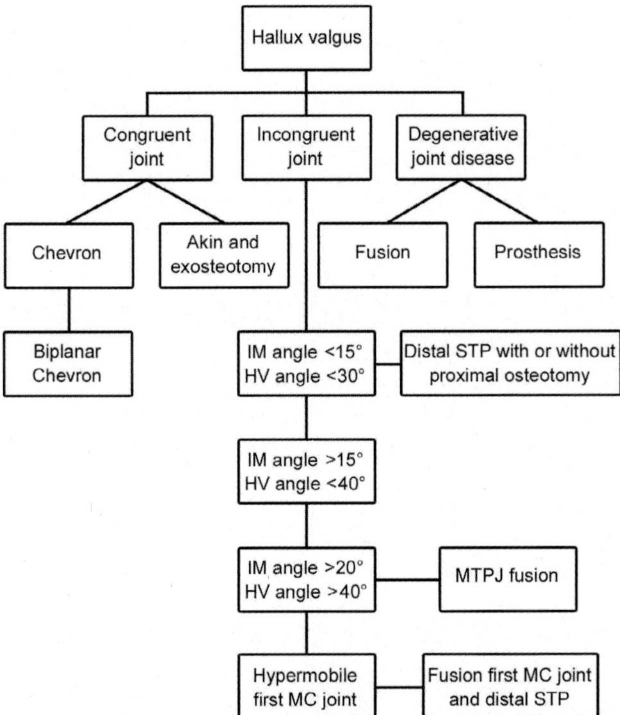

Figure 19.36 An algorithm for the treatment of hallux valgus (HV). IM, intermetatarsal; MC, metatarsal cuneiform; MTPJ, metatarsophalangeal joint; STP, soft tissue procedure. (*Reproduced with permission from* Johnson D, Pedowitz RA. *Practical Orthopaedic Sports Medicine and Arthroscopy*. Philadelphia, PA: Lippincott Williams & Wilkins, 2007.)

based on the age and activity level of the patient, the presence of arthrosis, hypermobility of the first ray, congruency of the MTP joint, physical shape of the metatarsal head, and the hallux valgus and intermetatarsal angles.

A distal metatarsal osteotomy is the preferred treatment for a mild hallux valgus deformity, with the Mitchell and chevron osteotomies being most common. In most bunionectomies, a distal soft tissue procedure to realign the MTP joint is performed. The modified McBride procedure achieves this by correcting all soft tissue components of the MTP joint deformity. A moderate hallux valgus is treated in a similar fashion but may require a proximal osteotomy, rather than a distal osteotomy.

For severe hallux valgus, a proximal metatarsal osteotomy is commonly performed in conjunction with a distal soft tissue procedure. Proximal metatarsal osteotomy provides powerful correction of metatarsus primus varus greater than 15 degrees. Techniques include crescentic, opening and closing wedge osteotomies, as well as a proximal chevron osteotomy. When hypermobility of the first ray is present, a metatarsocuneiform fusion may be required with a distal soft tissue procedure.

Arthrosis of the first MTP joint associated with hallux valgus can be aggravated by surgery. In this situation, a resection arthroplasty or arthrodesis of the first MTP joint is indicated. A resection arthroplasty, or Keller procedure, involves excising a segment of the proximal phalanx and the medial eminence. This decompresses the MTP joint, resulting in relaxation of the contracted lateral structures. Although it was a popular procedure in the past, current primary indications for its use include impending medial skin breakdown and patients who walk only minimally. Occasionally, it is used as a salvage procedure in failed bunion surgery. Arthrodesis of the first MTP joint has been a reliable and durable procedure that is indicated for management of severe deformities associated with degenerative joint disease, neuromuscular conditions, and salvage procedures. The toe should be fused in 10 to 15 degrees of dorsiflexion and 15 to 20 degrees of valgus.

Hallux Rigidus

Hallux rigidus is a painful loss of motion of the first MTP joint due to arthrosis. Degenerative changes result in a dorsal metatarsal osteophyte and loss of dorsiflexion. Although it may occur bilaterally, often one side is usually more advanced. It generally occurs in middle-aged and older persons but may also occur in active young people.

Pathophysiology and Classification

Hallux rigidus is a manifestation of arthrosis of the first MTP joint and is caused by trauma, OCD of the metatarsal head, congenital deformity, and systemic arthritides. Mechanical blocks from osteophytes on the dorsal aspect of the proximal phalanx and the metatarsal head reduce the available range of motion, especially dorsiflexion (Fig. 19.37).

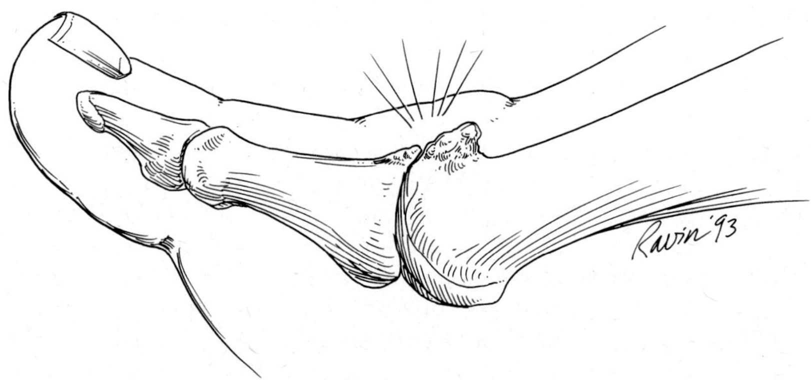

Figure 19.37 Dorsal osteophytes result in loss of range of motion and pain with dorsiflexion. (*Reproduced with permission from* Kitaoka HB. *The Foot and Ankle*. 2nd ed. Philadelphia, PA: Lippincott Williams & Wilkins, 2002.)

Presentation

Patients commonly complain of pain, swelling, and loss of motion in the great toe. Symptoms are worse in the morning and are aggravated by prolonged walking or standing. Shoes with elevated heel lifts exacerbate pain by further limiting the amount of dorsiflexion.

Examination

The first MTP joint tends to be enlarged, warm, and swollen with decreased dorsiflexion. If the pain is severe, patients may limp into the office. A dorsal prominence is most often palpable at the dorsomedial metatarsal head, and significant joint line tenderness may be present. With time and severity, a mediolateral exostosis may develop.

Radiographs

Radiographs show a decrease in the joint space, sclerotic joint margins, flattening of the first metatarsal head, and subchondral cyst formation consistent with progressive arthrosis.

Treatment

Initial treatment is nonoperative management with NSAIDs and shoe and activity modification. NSAIDS help to reduce the inflammation and pain related to synovitis about the first MTP joint. High-impact activities can be substituted with low-impact activities such as swimming and biking. Modifications to shoe wear include a stiff sole with a steel shank or carbon fiber footplate, or a rocker-bottom attachment to minimize stress and motion across the MTP joint during the toe-off phase of gait. Intraarticular steroid injections should be used sparingly.

When nonoperative management fails, surgical options include cheilectomy, interpositional arthroplasty, joint replacement, MTP joint fusion, and resectional arthroplasty. A cheilectomy is indicated for patients with mild to moderate disease, whose symptoms are related to the dorsal impingement during toe-off. Approximately 20% to 30% of the dorsal aspect of the metatarsal head is removed along with the dorsal exostosis and osteophytes on the proximal phalanx to achieve 60 degrees to 80 degrees of dorsiflexion (Fig. 19.38). If arthrosis of the joint is severe and more diffuse, a first MTP fusion is a reliable operation to relieve

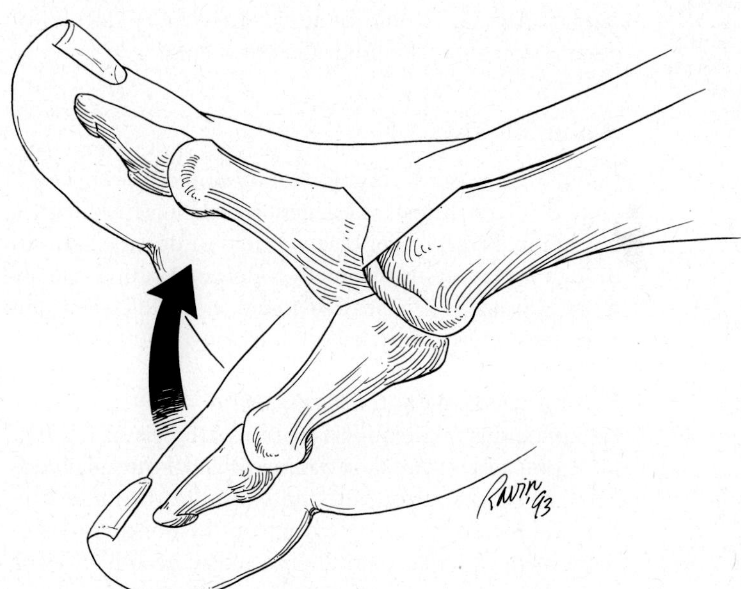

Figure 19.38 A cheilectomy removes approximately 20% to 30% of the dorsal metatarsal head and the dorsal osteophyte to regain motion at the first metatarsophalangeal joint. (*Reproduced with permission from* Kitaoka HB. *The Foot and Ankle*. 2nd ed. Philadelphia, PA: Lippincott Williams & Wilkins, 2002.)

pain. This provides a stable joint for patients who wish to remain active. Some authors have advocated resurfacing the joint with either biologic materials or implants. For lower-demand patients with severe arthrosis of the joint, a Keller resectional arthroplasty can also provide pain relief. This should not be performed if there is significant transfer metatarsalgia. A downside to the procedure is a loss of push-off strength at the MTP joint.

Morton Neuroma

Morton neuroma is a compression neuropathy of the plantar interdigital nerves that is a common cause of forefoot pain.

Pathophysiology and Classification

The plantar digital nerves, which are the terminal branches of the medial and lateral plantar nerves, are compressed by the distal edge of the transverse intermetatarsal ligament at the level of the metatarsal heads as they pass inferiorly (Fig. 19.39). The repetitive trauma with toe flexion and extension results in perineural fibrosis, demyelinization, degeneration of the nerve, and endoneural edema. Because there is no axonal proliferation and overgrowth, this condition is not truly a neuroma but rather an interdigital neuritis. Tight and high-heeled shoes are thought to contribute to the development. Activities that result in excessive extension of toes, such as running, lifting, and ballet dancing may increase the risk of Morton neuroma.

The second and third interdigital nerves are most commonly affected—with approximately 85% of cases involving the third web space and 15% involving the second. The third interdigital nerve is at higher risk because of its unique anatomy receiving contributions from both the lateral and medial plantar nerves. Neuromas of the first and fourth web spaces are rare.

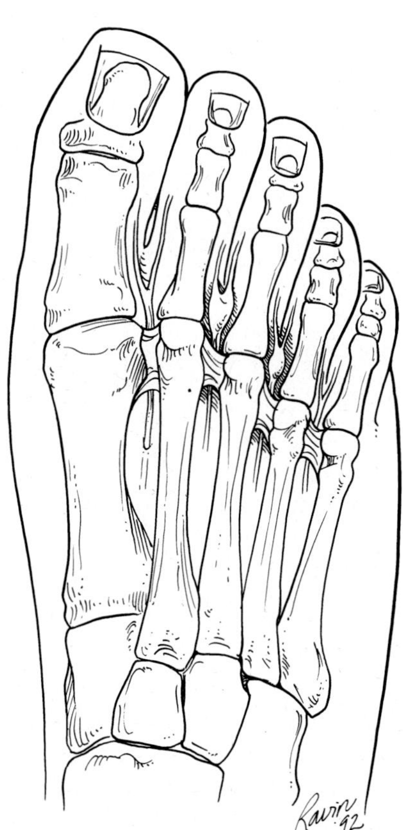

Figure 19.39 In Morton neuroma, the digital nerves are compressed by the intermetatarsal ligament. (*Reproduced with permission from* Kitaoka HB. *The Foot and Ankle.* 2nd ed. Philadelphia, PA: Lippincott Williams & Wilkins, 2002.)

Presentation

Patients present with vague, intermittent, burning pain in the area of the metatarsal heads that increases in intensity and duration during weight-bearing. The adjacent toes may have numbness. Wearing wide shoes and rubbing the feet typically helps.

Physical Examination

Deep palpation between the metatarsal heads or passive extension of the toes may reproduce the pain. Sensation may be diminished in the third and fourth toes. Compression of the metatarsal heads may result in a palpable Mulder click as the neuroma pops out between the metatarsal heads. Diagnosis is confirmed by injecting a local anesthetic into the webspace with relief of symptoms.

Special Tests

CT, MRI, and ultrasound have all been used to diagnose Morton neuroma; however, these are seldom necessary and should not be obtained routinely.

Differential Diagnosis

Other causes of forefoot pain include metatarsalgia, osteonecrosis of the metatarsal head, stress fractures, inflammatory arthropathy, and ganglion cysts.

Treatment

Treatment consists of modifying shoes and placing metatarsal pads proximal to the third and fourth metatarsal heads to help spread the transverse metatarsal ligament and unload the impingement on the nerve. External shoe modifications, including a metatarsal bar, may also help to unload the forefoot. Physical therapy, cryotherapy, and ultrasound are alternatives. Steroid and/or alcohol injections have also been advocated.

Operative intervention is reserved for refractory cases. Options include neurectomy with or without nerve burial into muscle, transverse intermetatarsal ligament release, and endoscopic decompression. Morton neuroma is most commonly approached dorsally but can exposed via a plantar incision. Surgical intervention has excellent results in up to 85% of cases. Complications include symptomatic end-stump neuroma and recurrence. With recurrence, a plantar approach should be used because it is extensile, allowing a more proximal excision of the nerve.

RECOMMEND READINGS

Herscovici D Jr, Anglen JO, Archdeacon M, Cannada L, Scaduto JM. Avoiding complications in the treatment of pronation-external rotation ankle fractures, syndesmotic injuries, and talar neck fractures. *J Bone Joint Surg Am*. 2008;90:898–908.

Mann RA. Disorders of the first metatarsophalangeal joint. *J Am Acad Orthop Surg*. 1995;3:34–43.

Recht MP, Donley BG. Magnetic resonance imaging of the foot and ankle. *J Am Acad Orthop Surg*. 2001;9:187–199.

Robinson HN, Pasapula C, Brodsky JW. Surgical aspects of the diabetic foot. *J Bone Joint Surg Br*. 2009;91:1–7.

Index

Note: Page numbers followed by f and t indicates figure and table respectively.

B

C

I

N

P

Q

LIBRARY
ACCESSION No.
CLASS
MONKLANDS HOSPITAL
AIRDRIE ML6 0JS

U

V

W

Z

CCS1110